For Ch.

with best wishes

Eelco Wijdicks

THE PRACTICE OF EMERGENCY
AND CRITICAL CARE NEUROLOGY

SECOND EDITION

THE PRACTICE
OF EMERGENCY
AND CRITICAL CARE
NEUROLOGY

EELCO F. M. WIJDICKS, MD, PhD, FACP, FNCS, FANA

Professor of Neurology, Mayo Clinic College of Medicine
Chair, Division of Critical Care Neurology
Consultant, Neurosciences Intensive Care Unit
Mayo Clinic Hospital, Saint Marys Campus
Mayo Clinic Rochester, Minnesota

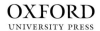

OXFORD
UNIVERSITY PRESS

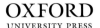

Oxford University Press is a department of the University of Oxford. It furthers
the University's objective of excellence in research, scholarship, and education
by publishing worldwide.Oxford is a registered trade mark of Oxford University
Press in the UK and certain other countries.

Published in the United States of America by Oxford University Press
198 Madison Avenue, New York, NY 10016, United States of America.

First Edition published in 2010
Second Edition published in 2016

Library of Congress Cataloging-in-Publication Data
Wijdicks, Eelco F. M., 1954- , author.
The practice of emergency and critical care neurology / Eelco F.M Wijdicks. — Second edition.
p. ; cm.
Includes bibliographical references and index.
ISBN 978–0–19–025955–6 (alk. paper)
I. Title.
[DNLM: 1. Critical Care—methods. 2. Neurologic Manifestations. 3. Central Nervous System Diseases—diagnosis.
4. Central Nervous System Diseases—therapy. 5. Emergency Treatment—methods. WL 340]
RC350.N49
616.8′0428—dc23
2015033653

9 8 7 6 5 4 3 2 1
Printed by Walsworth, USA

CONTENTS

LIST OF CAPSULES

PREFACE TO THE SECOND EDITION

A legitimate subspecialty allows neurointensivists to manage patients with acute and critical neurologic disease. Here is what I think—the neurointensivist is now a more recognized specialist and provides better care of patients with large scale clinical problems associated with acute neurologic disease. The disorders that shape this field are better defined, and all of us in the trenches, so to speak, have now a good idea of how to approach these problems. Revisions of textbooks—and also this one—are required to assimilate and critique new information and to put more modern approaches into practice. Single authored textbooks will remain useful not only because it forces the author to discipline approaches to patient management, but also to bring a consistent practical perspective to the whole of it's care. I hope this book not only provides an adequate grounding for newcomers, but also appeals to a broad audience of experienced practitioners.

This new edition of *The Practice of Emergency and Critical Care Neurology* continues the same organizational principles. My approach has been to pose the significant questions differently: How does the patient with an acute neurologic condition present to us? What are the distinguishing characteristics of the clinical picture, and how do we best anticipate clinical worsening? What do we do to stabilize the patient neurologically and medically? This book is much less about theorizing and more about management—progressing from an initial relatively straightforward approach to more complex decisions in a rapidly deteriorating situation. What practitioners need is an operational definition of the degree of deterioration and what can lead to bad outcomes.

The chapters have been revised to incorporate new information and new ideas. The management of the patient changes when information changes. Because there is a considerable proportion of patients with a new medical critical illness after a neurocritical illness, I have added a new section on critical care support adapted to the critically ill neurologic patient. Such an addition is needed to update neurointensivists on practice changes in critical care medicine. Other new sections are on multimodal monitoring, cooling techniques, and on the quality improvement in the NICU—topics that have been heavily written about in the years since the previous edition. Although a companion monograph on the neurological complications of critical illness has been published, (*Neurologic Complications of Critical Illness (Contemporary Neurology Series) third edition Oxford University Press, 2009*) I felt it necessary to summarize common requests for consults in other ICUs in four new chapters.

In total this new edition has 12 new chapters, over 50 new original illustrations and neuroimaging figures and I have added numerous new sections, subsections and capsules, which further complete the work. As with prior editions, this book has a pocketbook with a selection of the most relevant tables and figures. This pocket book can physically accompany practitioners, but it is also easily downloaded on portable devices.

This book before you is as recent and updated as possible, and we will be planning future editions every 5 years to keep the information fresh.

All that said, I hope this textbook—a work which originally started as a 3 volume work and now is condensed in a nearly 1000 page volume—will continue its lineage. So what follows I hope is a book which provides practical and data-driven advice to any physician caring for seriously ill neurologic patients.

E. F. M. Wijdicks

PREFACE TO THE FIRST EDITION

The specialty of critical care neurology considers its province acute neurologic disease presenting in the emergency department or the neurosciences intensive care unit and neurologic complications of medical or surgical critical illness.

The Practice of Emergency and Critical Care Neurology combines two monographs previously published with Oxford University Press, amalgamating the unique structure of each book, but in a more condensed form after eliminating overlap. I believe that with these changes, it is now a many-sided textbook on the management of a patient with an acute, definitely serious, and primarily critical neurologic disorder. (The neurologic complications of medical or surgical critical illness have been published last year in a companion monograph, also with Oxford University Press and now in a third edition.)

The Practice of Emergency and Critical Care Neurology follows patients from the very moment they enter the emergency department (ED)—where the neurologist makes on-the-spot decisions—to their admission to the neurologic intensive care unit (NICU)—where mostly specialists in the neurosciences assume full responsibility for patient care. This book differs from conventional textbooks by specifically following the time course of clinical complexities as they emerge and change.

Part I introduces the presenting neurologic emergency and the responsibilities of specialists interacting in the ED. Triage of acute neurologic disease has been defined arbitrarily, but many neurologists opt for brief observation in an intensive care setting rather than admission to the ward. Guidance for more appropriate triage is provided.

Part II encompasses the evaluation of presenting symptoms that indicate urgency, and their conversational titles echo the patient's main concerns or common requests for urgent consultation. As one would expect, the differential diagnosis of these symptoms is very broad. However, the intentionally brief chapters emphasize the red flags. They are intended only to orient readers, and to set the priorities and direction of the clinical approach.

Part III discusses the four most common presenting symptoms that indicate a critical neurologic emergency and, above all, require prompt action. These conditions often need immediate care even before the patient is triaged out of the ED.

Part IV discusses the organization of intensive care units (ICUs), including options for different types and models that can be used in ICUs all over the world. In some hospitals, the closed unit form fits nicely; in others, logistics, manpower, and economics may not allow such a model. In two chapters, the main attributes of a physician practicing critical care neurology and the organization of NICUs are explained. These chapters are included for readers who want to pursue a career in this field or set up a NICU.

Part V is devoted to the basic treatment of patients with critical neurologic illness and, next to the section on complex nursing care, includes the basic principles of pain and agitation management, mechanical ventilation, nutritional requirements, and fluid management. The use of anticoagulation, or its reversal in some instances, and the current practice of thrombolytic therapy in acute ischemic stroke are presented in detail. All these measures may have an impact on existing brain injury, and therefore this section concludes with the management of increased intracranial pressure.

Part VI encompasses the technology used in the NICU and the current monitoring capabilities—of which some are standard, whereas others are experimental and still being tested for usefulness and cost-effectiveness. It has been a truism that clinical examination trumps any monitoring device; however, the neurologic assessment of ongoing brain injury continues to be an approximation, and much better technology is needed.

Part VII is the core of the book and is devoted to specific disorders in critical care neurology. Each chapter is structured in a unique way, in that it focuses on diagnosis, interpretation of neuroimaging, first steps in management, problem solving for deteriorating patients, and an estimation of outcome.

Part VIII contains three chapters on the management of common postoperative neurosurgical and neurointerventional complications, but I have abbreviated these sections to match their scope to the needs of neurologists.

Part IX comprises chapters on medical complications that can be expected for any patient with an acute serious neurologic illness. These complications involve a consuming part of day-to-day care and may endanger the patient in many ways. Practical advice is provided to manage them effectively.

Part X concentrates on the diagnosis of brain death and the assessment of irrevocable damage to the brain. These situations lead to withdrawal of support, and may lead to organ donation. This section also highlights some of the current ethical controversies and legal risks.

Part XI closes the book with dosing tables and equations.

Finally, in order to show commitment to evidence-based medicine, useful references to academy and society guidelines pertaining to critical care neurology have been included.

In an attempt to present the field in its entirety and to fill some of the gaps, seven new chapters have been written for this new edition. They include a chapter on the role of the neurologist in the ED and how to collaborate effectively with colleagues of other disciplines. New chapters on specific neurologic conditions, management of complications in the NICU, and end-of-life care (the DCD protocols) have been added.

My main focus has been not only to inform the reader about the presentation of acute neurologic illness but also to assist directly in its management. I have expanded the information on the pathophysiology of brain injury and used a special format (capsules) to set it apart from the text. These capsules will be helpful for quickly understanding certain topics without cluttering the text with impractical information. Some can be used for teaching pearls during rounds.

Buyers of the book can expect even more changes. First, more than 1,000 references and over 100 new figures—many in full color—have been added. This book again comes with a pocketbook of selected tables and figures. The contents of this pocketbook also can be uploaded to any mobile device for quicker searching capability.

I hope that its text, without being too unwieldy to carry or too dense to read, has wide appeal and is a source of answers to clinical questions. This book not only amasses and interprets the available literature but is also based on our published clinical research at Mayo Clinic for nearly 2 decades.

As promised, it is tailored toward neurologists and neurosurgeons, neurointensivists, medical and surgical intensivists, emergency physicians, residents in neurology and neurosurgery and fellows in critical care. Any newly arrived neurointensivist may use this information to study for a certification exam. I hope the information in this book is also a useful resource for neuroscience nursing staff, respiratory therapists, physical therapists, ICU pharmacists, and other allied health providers.

This book serves as a reference on care of the patient with a critical neurologic disorder, at risk of deterioration, and in need of immediate attention. But there is more than that. I wish for this book to contribute to the best possible care of patients with a critical neurologic disorder. That remains my main motivation.

E. F. M. Wijdicks

ACKNOWLEDGMENTS

I am indebted to many persons over the years, but I have to single out those who made considerable contributions in the research and compilation of this book. I have enjoyed the advantage of access to Mayo Library, Media Support Services and Section of Presentation and Design. These are incredible resources. I have worked together on many projects with David Factor, whose wonderful color drawings are again interspersed throughout the book. I very much value his creativity, and it is difficult to thank him adequately. Paul Honermann (scientific illustrator) expertly formatted the neuroimaging and other photographs. Kevin Youel (presentation designer) was very helpful in modernizing the algorithms and other drawings. The cover created by Jim Rownd is inspired by the "untitled" paintings of Willem de Kooning. It is a great privilege to work with him through multiple ideas and he has been responsible for many of my book covers over the years.

I thoroughly thank Lori Reinstrom who was kind enough to type parts of the text, format, and reference. She lived with my books for many years. Writing is one thing, proofing is another (the writer's bane). In the final stages of the book production Newgen Knowledge Works diligently worked through several proofs until we felt it was right. I would like to express my gratitude to all involved.

I benefit greatly from the insights of my Mayo neurointensivist's colleagues (Alejandro Rabinstein, Sara Hocker, and Jennifer Fugate), but also the neurosurgery and neuroradiology staff admitting to the NICU (mostly notably Giuseppe Lanzino, Harry Cloft, and David Kallmes). Their friendship means much to me.

My deepest gratitude is to the neurosciences nursing staff. For all the time here at Mayo Clinic they have stood with me, and I have never seen such compassion and determination to patient care.

I am honored to be connected with Oxford University Press and greatly thank my editor Craig Panner, I appreciate their continuing interest in publishing my books.

This book is dedicated to my dearly loved wife Barbara and admirable children Coen and Marilou. They have been continually and crucially supportive.

E. F. M. Wijdicks

PART I

General Principles of Recognition of Critically Ill Neurologic Patients in the Emergency Department

1

The Presenting Neurologic Emergency

Acute neurologic disease is bound to get worse. In some it is critical and unquestionably life-threatening. Acute neurologic conditions can be seen everywhere in the hospital, but this chapter introduces the emergency department (ED), with all its complexities, as seen from a neurologist's perspective.[28]

Acute neurologic manifestations are a consequence of major trauma, acute stroke, emerging infection, or intoxication. Patients may also come to the hospital as an urgent referral or even as a walk-in. In these circumstances, acutely unfolding neurologic signs are obvious, yet difficult to interpret, and physicians feeling "uncomfortable" with such a progressive neurologic picture have a low threshold for sending patients to the ED. A major reason for the ED admission of patients with a critical neurologic manifestation lies in the fact that the ED may provide immediate advanced care and triage. But in other situations, patients with a not yet known neurologic emergency may present with nonspecific symptoms, such as weakness, twitching, agitation, dizziness, or headaches, or they may be simply not reacting and staring into space. All these symptoms carry a broad differential diagnosis and therefore are a serious test to any physician in any field.

Generally, emergency physicians are often faced with diagnostic scruples, but their uncertainty is most apparent with acute neurologic conditions. Emergency physicians are trained to recognize acute neurologic disease, but often they consult a neurologist for such cases. The American Board of Emergency Medicine has identified core competencies for critical neurologic disorders that include demyelinating disorders, acute headaches, acute hydrocephalus, central nervous system infection, dystonic reactions, Guillain-Barré syndrome and myasthenia gravis, seizures, spinal cord compression, stroke, and traumatic brain injury.[20] However, this list leaves out a gamut of other disorders that, if unrecognized and unmanaged, may lead to neurologic morbidity.[28] This chapter promotes close communication between neurologists and emergency physicians to achieve maximal effectiveness.

THE EMERGENCY DEPARTMENT

The ED is a separate place in the hospital, staffed by emergency physicians, and functions under unique characteristics. Emergency physicians are routinely required to make a string of decisions in rapid succession. The department is characterized by high activity levels, frequent interruptions and distractions, shift work, and a need to work in teams. The ED may handle both critical conditions and less-emergent presentations. In the United States and many other countries, the ED is also where the uninsured, needy, and poverty stricken go for medical help.

The physical structure of the ED is highly dependent on location, and EDs in inner-city locales have a different patient mix when compared with rural areas. Many EDs are packed: This crowding is a multifaceted problem and includes such causes as nonurgent visits, patients who frequent the ED for trivial reasons ("frequent flyers"), viral epidemics (e.g., influenza season), inadequate staffing, inpatient boarding, and hospital bed shortages. These conditions have led to the notion of compromised care and poor patient satisfaction.[2,10,12,26,29]

The ED has a designated critical care area where a patient's condition is stabilized and the patient is resuscitated and readied for triage (Figure 1.1). In each emergency center, levels of trauma activation have been defined and customized.

Trauma activation provides a strictly circumscribed number of skilled personnel who are available for different categories of medical severity. A level 1 trauma activation may suddenly deplete the nursing staff, and thus nurses may not be immediately available to assist other patients in unstable physical condition (Table 1.1).

Severity scales and scores for certain neurologic disorders have been proven to facilitate

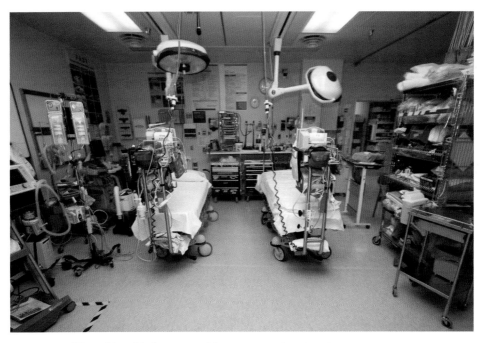

FIGURE 1.1: View of the critical care area of the emergency department.

TABLE 1.1. LEVEL 1 TRAUMA
ACTIVATION: RESPONSE OF STAFF
FOR INITIAL RESUSCITATION OF THE
ACUTELY INJURED ADULT PATIENT
AT MAYO CLINIC

Trauma consultant
Emergency physician
Trauma critical care and general surgery resident
or trauma physician assistant or nurse practitioner
Radiology technician
Phlebotomist
Respiratory therapist
Transfusion medicine registered nurse
Urology technician
Emergency medicine registered nurse

understanding, treatment, and triage.[6] Most recognizable for first responders are the Glasgow
Coma Scale and the National Institutes of Health
Stroke Scale (NIHSS).[19] A commonly used scale
is the Injury Severity Score (Capsule 1.1), but
this scoring system undervalues the impact of
trauma to the brain.[18] Severity scales may be helpful because they assist the physician in testing the
most important elements of a neurologic examination. Unfortunately, guidelines for other many
acute neurologic conditions are inadequate in

assisting emergency physicians, and some guidelines have not yet been developed because solid
data are not available.[9,21,22]

THE NEUROLOGIC EMERGENCY AND ITS ASSESSMENT

A neurologic consultation is often triggered by
the presence of any obvious localizing sign or
abnormal responsiveness. A neurologic emergency is defined by certain clinical manifestations, abnormality on neuroimaging, and, most
important, by a progression of symptoms. In
most instances, the presentation is dramatic,
attracts attention, and requires specialty care.
The condition of some patients worsens rapidly, and in these cases an acute neurosurgical
intervention is necessary. Typical examples are
an acute hemispheric lesion with mass effect,
resulting in brainstem displacement or acute
spinal cord compression.

Neurologic symptoms often fluctuate, and an
improvement in symptoms may not necessarily mean that the patient is improving. A classic
example is a patient with a basilar artery occlusion who presents with a transient hemiparesis,
only to have the symptoms re-emerge with acute
unresponsiveness and abnormalities of brainstem
reflexes. Fluctuating consciousness may indicate
ongoing seizures rather than a postictal state.

CAPSULE 1.1   INJURY SEVERITY SCORE

Injury severity scoring systems have included neurologic findings but with little detail. Scoring systems may include the Glasgow Coma Scale, Acute Physiology and Chronic Health Evaluation (APACHE), or may simply note the presence of cerebral contusion (Injury Severity Score [ISS]). The ISS has continued to be the most useful test for trauma severity and has been summarized by a calculation that takes the three highest scores and adds the squares of these three scores to an injury severity score. It defaults to the highest score of 75 if injury is assigned 6 (unsurvivable). An example is shown below. The major weaknesses of ISS are that different injury patterns yield a same score, and substantial errors in scoring may exist. Any patient with an ISS of more than 16 should be treated in a tertiary level 1 trauma center; Other scoring systems have been used, such as TRISS (a combination of revised trauma score, ISS, and age) and a severity characterization of trauma (ASCOT), without gaining sufficient acceptance. The APACHE scoring system includes comorbid conditions and an acute physiology score; however, it underestimates the probability of death when patients are transferred to the ICU and is less certain in predicting death for injured patients.[18]

Region	Injury Description	AIS
Head and neck	Cerebral contusion	4
Face	No injury	0
Chest	Flail chest	4
Abdomen	Minor contusion of liver	2
	Complex ruptured spleen	5
Extremity	Fractured femur	3
External	No injury	0

Rating for the Abbreviated Injury Scale (AIS)

AIS Score	Injury
1	Minor
2	Moderate
3	Serious
4	Severe
5	Critical
6	Unsurvivable

To obtain an injury severity score, square the 3 highest scores and add them. In this example $25 + 16 + 16 = 57$

A neurologic emergency can be deconstructed according to the acute presentation of certain signs, but it also can be defined by a need for immediate diagnostic or therapeutic action (Table 1.2).

Four neurologic tests—computed tomography (CT) scanning, magnetic resonance imaging (MRI), cerebrospinal fluid (CSF) examination, and electroencephalography (EEG)—should be immediately available and may narrow the diagnostic evaluation substantially. CT and CT angiogram (or MRI and MR angiogram) of the brain are mandatory in the timely evaluation of a stroke. CSF examination and EEG are needed when

TABLE 1.2. SIGNS AND SYMPTOMS THAT MAY CONSTITUTE A NEUROLOGIC EMERGENCY

Worsening and changing neurologic signs
Acutely dilated pupil or anisocoria
Acute eye movement abnormality
Abnormal level of consciousness
Seizure
Severe, unexpected, split-second headache
Acute vertigo
Acute cranial nerve deficit
Inability to stand or walk

certain clinical suspicions (e.g., central nervous system infection or inflammation, nonconvulsive status epilepticus) are strong. None of these studies can replace a neurologic examination, however, and emergency physicians would benefit from some guidance in the proper procedure for this type of evaluation.

Few studies have addressed the effectiveness of the neurologist in the ED. Prior studies have suggested that neurologists are rarely involved in the management of ischemic stroke[4,11] and that this lack of involvement potentially could lead to a delay in and a lack of treatment with thrombolytic agents. However, over the last few years the involvement of neurologists has increased due to Telestroke programs, which have increased the number of patients treated with IV thrombolytics and guided ED physicians to triage the patient to endovascular neurointervention.[8] Few institutions have a neurology resident in the emergency room, and even less often is a neurologist physically present in the ED to assess the urgency of a case. Far more often, physicians send patients to the ED to be seen by emergency physicians, only to have a neurologist called in because of conspicuous neurologic manifestations.

Ideally, a neurologist with expertise in acute critical neurologic illness would visit patients who are going to be triaged to an intensive care unit (ICU). This situation applies not only to patients admitted to specialized neurologic ICUs (NICUs), but also to patients with an acute neurologic illness who are transferred to a surgical, medical, or more general ICU. Neurointensivists are in a good position to expand their role in the ED and to become more directly involved in the management of acute neurologic conditions. Having such specialized neurologists ready to see patients during the so-called golden hour following initial presentation of symptoms may lead to improved assessment and, ultimately, to improved care and outcome. Their presence when decisions are made may also reduce second-guessing. The reality, however, is different, and we suspect that neurologists are rarely called in except when part of a designated management protocol (e.g., a rapid-response stroke protocol).[3]

Cross-training is equally important for resident emergency physicians rotating in the NICU and for neurology residents and fellows spending time in the critical care section of the ED. Additional training of emergency physicians in critical care neurology may be helpful,

but may be resisted in a currently cramped curriculum.[20,23,24]

The relationship between a neurologist and an emergency physician has been a subject of discussion, but much of it is hyperbole.[11] Some experts have argued that neurologists are rarely available on an urgent basis. In a large urban tertiary teaching hospital and trauma center, consultation with a neurologist increased the length of stay in the ED by an average of 3.5 hours.[10] Others have argued that emergency physicians are out of their depth on acute neurologic issues[15] and that failure of the timely presence of a neurologist may increase errors in the recognition and management of a neurologic emergency.[5,15]

CLINICAL JUDGMENT IN THE EMERGENCY DEPARTMENT

There are plenty of potential errors to consider (Table 1.3), and emergency physicians are often subject to blame and critique.[27] Some have categorically and unfairly characterized the ED as a "natural laboratory for the study of error."[7] Studies of diagnostic errors and management failures have been retrospective, biased, and confrontational (i.e., usually resulting in finger-pointing at ED physicians). Diagnostic errors are difficult to gauge, particularly when the diagnosis has been deferred to the accepting physician in charge of further workup.[16] There continues to be a broad-brush characterization of the ED as insufficient neurology of any kind, but it serves no purpose.

A frequently reported misjudgment is the diagnosis of subarachnoid hemorrhage (SAH). This finding is curious because many EDs may see on average two SAHs a month. A recent study in

---

TABLE 1.3. ERRORS THAT MAY OCCUR IN THE EMERGENCY DEPARTMENT

Failure to recognize acute brain injury on computed tomographic scanning
Failure to perform a cerebrospinal fluid examination
Failure to recognize acute hydrocephalus
Failure to recognize locked-in syndrome
Failure to recognize brainstem involvement
Failure to recognize status epilepticus
Failure to recognize spinal cord compression
Failure to recognize neurointerventional options
Failure to recognize brain death and potential for organ donation

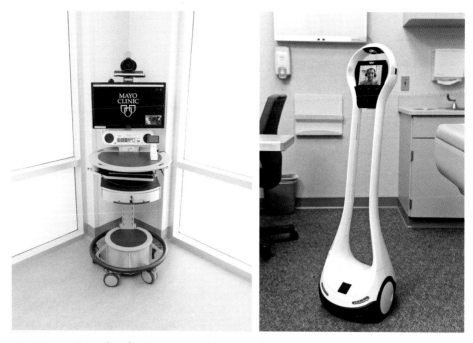

FIGURE 1.2: Examples of stationary or mobile robotic devices used in emergency departments..

Canada found that 1 in 20 cases of SAH were not recognized, but most of these involved a missed diagnosis in a nonteaching institution, followed by its recognition in another ED visit (often on the same day). The mortality rate was higher in the missed cases.[25]

Recognition of TIA or ischemic stroke in the ED has been an area of concern, and some experts have noticed a failure to recognize cerebellar ischemic stroke in patients presenting with "dizziness."[5,13,14]

Medication errors in the ED largely involve dosage miscalculation; an inappropriate dosage, drug, or route; and, rarely, failure to identify a drug interaction. Having a pharmacist assigned to the ED resulted in a 60%–75% decrease in medication errors.[4]

At issue is whether ED physicians have a sufficient comfort level in the management of critically ill neurologic patients. The worst-case scenario is that of an ED physician who handles an acute neurologic emergency, orders neuroimaging tests and interprets them without neurologic expertise, then intubates, sedates, or even paralyzes the patient (and thus making a neurologic examination pointless). The best-case scenario is that of a specialist in the neurosciences seeing any acute neurologic or neurosurgical emergency and handling it competently together with the attending ED physician, and in fact, our experience is just like that. Tertiary centers should have (or should develop) this expertise.

In rural areas, telemedicine may become a solution, once the logistics and technology can be put in place. Telemedicine involves a hub-and-spoke model. The hub is in an urban hospital with an expert neurologist on staff, and the spokes are hospitals without a readily available neurologist (may be up to 30 hospitals). Spoke hospitals are selected on the basis of volume of patients with acute neurologic disease. Communication is through interactive audiovisual teleconferencing equipment. Multiple hospitals from remote areas can communicate with one single hub. Robots are available and reliable (Figure 1.2). There is growing experience with stroke and ICU telemedicine in Europe and the United States, and some preliminary studies suggest reliable assessment of the NIHSS via high-quality videoconferencing and reliable neuroimaging interpretation over teleradiology systems, and thus eventual benefit to the patient. However, in the United States the costs of telemedicine implementation and support personnel, cross-state licensing barriers, and malpractice threats remain real.[1,8,17]

CONCLUSIONS

- Neurologic symptoms often fluctuate, and an improvement in symptoms may not necessarily mean that the patient is improving.

- Signs and symptoms indicating a neurologic emergency are worsening or changing neurologic signs, any abnormal level of consciousness, acute split-second onset headache, acute vertigo, acute cranial nerve deficit, and an inability to stand or walk.

REFERENCES

1. Audebert HJ, Schultes K, Tietz V, et al. Long-term effects of specialized stroke care with telemedicine support in community hospitals on behalf of the Telemedical Project for Integrative Stroke Care (TEMPiS). *Stroke* 2009;40:902–908.
2. Bogner MS. *Human Error in Medicine*. Hillsdale, NJ: Lawrence Erlbaum Associates; 1994.
3. Brown DL, Lisabeth LD, Garcia NM, Smith MA, Morgenstern LB. Emergency department evaluation of ischemic stroke and TIA: the BASIC Project. *Neurology* 2004;63:2250–2254.
4. Brown JN, Barnes CL, Beasley B, et al. Effect of pharmacists on medication errors in an emergency department. *Am J Health Syst Pharm* 2008;65:330–333.
5. Caplan LR. Dizziness: how do patients describe dizziness and how do emergency physicians use these descriptions for diagnosis? *Mayo Clin Proc* 2007;82:1313–1315.
6. Chawda MN, Hildebrand F, Pape HC, Giannoudis PV. Predicting outcome after multiple trauma: which scoring system? *Injury* 2004;35:347–358.
7. Croskerry P, Sinclair D. Emergency medicine: a practice prone to error? *CJEM* 2001;3:271–276.
8. Demaerschalk BM, Miley ML, Kiernan TE, et al. Stroke telemedicine. *Mayo Clin Proc* 2009;84:53–64.
9. Fuller G, Lawrence T, Woodford M, Lecky F. The accuracy of alternative triage rules for identification of significant traumatic brain injury: a diagnostic cohort study. *Emerg Med J* 2014;31:914–919.
10. Han JH, France DJ, Levin SR, et al. The effect of physician triage on emergency department length of stay. *J Emerg Med* 2010;39:227–233.
11. Hemphill JC, 3rd, White DB. Clinical nihilism in neuroemergencies. *Emerg Med Clin North Am* 2009;27:27–37, vii–viii.
12. Hoot NR, Aronsky D. Systematic review of emergency department crowding: causes, effects, and solutions. *Ann Emerg Med* 2008;52:126–136.
13. Kothari RU, Brott T, Broderick JP, Hamilton CA. Emergency physicians: accuracy in the diagnosis of stroke. *Stroke* 1995;26:2238–2241.

14. Kowalski RG, Claassen J, Kreiter KT, et al. Initial misdiagnosis and outcome after subarachnoid hemorrhage. *JAMA* 2004;291:866–869.
15. Manno EM. Safety issues and concerns for the neurological patient in the emergency department. *Neurocrit Care* 2008;9:259–264.
16. Moulin T, Sablot D, Vidry E, et al. Impact of emergency room neurologists on patient management and outcome. *Eur Neurol* 2003;50:207–214.
17. Schwamm LH, Holloway RG, Amarenco P, et al. A review of the evidence for the use of telemedicine within stroke systems of care: a scientific statement from the American Heart Association/American Stroke Association. *Stroke* 2009;40:2616–2634.
18. Senkowski CK, McKenney MG. Trauma scoring systems: a review. *J Am Coll Surg* 1999;189:491–503.
19. Stead LG, Bellolio MF, Suravaram S, et al. Evaluation of transient ischemic attack in an emergency department observation unit. *Neurocrit Care* 2009;10:204–208.
20. Stettler BA, Jauch EC, Kissela B, Lindsell CJ. Neurologic education in emergency medicine training programs. *Acad Emerg Med* 2005;12:909–911.
21. Stuke LE, Duchesne JC, Greiffenstein P, et al. Not all mechanisms are created equal: a single-center experience with the national guidelines for field triage of injured patients. *J Trauma Acute Care Surg* 2013;75:140–145.
22. Tang N, Stein J, Hsia RY, Maselli JH, Gonzales R. Trends and characteristics of US emergency department visits, 1997–2007. *JAMA* 2010;304:664–670.
23. Teixeira PG, Inaba K, Hadjizacharia P, et al. Preventable or potentially preventable mortality at a mature trauma center. *J Trauma* 2007;63:1338–1346.
24. Thomas HA, Beeson MS, Binder LS, et al. The 2005 Model of the Clinical Practice of Emergency Medicine: the 2007 update. *Ann Emerg Med* 2008;52:e1–17.
25. Vermeulen MJ, Schull MJ. Missed diagnosis of subarachnoid hemorrhage in the emergency department. *Stroke* 2007;38:1216–1221.
26. Vieth TL, Rhodes KV. The effect of crowding on access and quality in an academic ED. *Am J Emerg Med* 2006;24:787–794.
27. Wears RL. The error of counting "errors." *Ann Emerg Med* 2008;52:502–503.
28. Wijdicks EFM, Menon DK, Smith M. Ten things you need to know to practice neurological critical care. *Intensive Care Med* 2015;41:318–321.
29. Yoon P, Steiner I, Reinhardt G. Analysis of factors influencing length of stay in the emergency department. *CJEM* 2003;5:155–161.

2

Criteria of Triage

Ideally, the main priority for physicians with a patient with acute neurologic disease is to quickly triage to the neurosciences intensive care unit (NICU). In many medical institutions without a specialized ICU, patients are admitted to a general ICU or, depending on the cause of injury and neurosurgical involvement, to a trauma or surgical ICU. By its nature, the NICU is used for the medical and neurosurgical management of critical neurologic disorders and for the postoperative care of neurosurgical patients. As befits any major emergency, an active neurologic problem belongs in the NICU, but admission may also be strongly considered with severe physiologic derangements or any other progression of a prior medical illness.[3] The ICU case mix may differ among locations and may involve differences in utilization according to patient age and do-not-resuscitate status.[2,4]

Uniform criteria for admission to the NICU are difficult to establish, and some ambiguity will always remain. As may be expected, decisions to triage are physician specific and personal, and there is some leeway. Decisions could well be guided by bed availability. This all may seem easy in times of plenty, but it becomes definitively more complicated when (barely) recovered patients in the NICU may have to give way to new admissions. The economic pressure on physicians to reduce the length of hospital stay is always a factor, and this may also have an impact on ICU admission[7] (Capsule 2.1). In some ICUs, fast-track programs are in place. These postoperative programs involve early extubation, reduced use of postoperative sedation, and pre-authorized implementation of ICU transfer orders.[6,7]

Admission to the NICU must be free of bias and requires excellent rapport among the physician, nurse manager, and charge nurse. Criteria for NICU admission should be flexible.[8] For instance, sedation for marked agitation or monitoring of airway patency alone may justify admission for some patients. Also, although the suitability of NICU admission may be questioned for patients with an unsalvageable acute brain injury, transition to comfort care is rarely performed in the emergency department, and these patients may be admitted to the NICU to await the arrival of patients' families and to allow time for the families to come to grips with the situation. Palliation may also involve the activation of an organ procurement protocol, and these complex logistics are better handled in the NICU.

Criteria can be developed to assist in the initial assessment of NICU eligibility. These criteria can involve signs and symptoms (Figure 2.1) or specifically refer to major neurologic or neurosurgical disorders. The admission criteria for each of these neurologic disorders (discussed in Part VII of this book) are summarized in Table 2.1 for easy reference. Admission to the NICU after elective neuroendovascular procedures seems undisputed, but others found that step-down units may suffice in patients with coiling of unruptured cerebral aneurysms. Recognition of sudden new complications that may require intervention would need to be guaranteed, and thus many opt for safety in the NICU setting.[10,15]

While little disagreement exists regarding triage to an ICU, how much care—beyond appropriate support and initial management—should be provided in the emergency department before transfer is debatable. Most physicians would want to see the patient in an NICU promptly after initially resuscitated and stabilized. Transfer documentation between the emergency department and the NICU (known in hospital jargon as "sign-outs" or "hand-offs") best includes certain essential elements about the patient's condition (Table 2.2) and is best communicated between the attending emergency physicians and the attending neurointensivists and charge nurse. Information about the patient's neurologic condition should include level of consciousness, focal findings, seizure control (if any), and a summary of computed tomographic (CT) or magnetic resonance

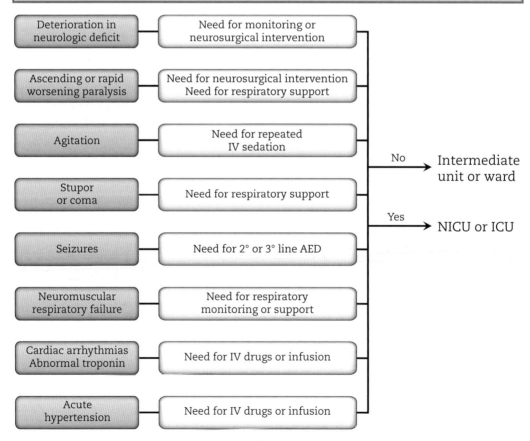

FIGURE 2.1: Common signs and symptoms associated with acute neurologic illness when triaging patients to an intensive care unit or other wards.

AED, antiepileptic drug; ICU, intensive care unit; IV, intravenous; NICU, neurosciences intensive care unit.

TABLE 2.1. COMMON REASONS FOR ADMISSION TO THE NEUROSCIENCES INTENSIVE CARE UNIT

Aneurysmal subarachnoid hemorrhage
Drowsiness, stupor, or coma
Mechanical ventilation
Any neurologic deterioration
Seizures
Neurogenic pulmonary edema
Aspiration pneumonia
Cardiac arrhythmias
Abnormal electrocardiogram
S/P coil placement
S/P clipping of aneurysm

Ganglionic or lobar hemorrhage
Drowsiness, stupor, or coma
Mechanical ventilation
CT scan evidence of brain shift
Hypertensive surges
Recurrent seizures
Coagulopathy or warfarin use
S/P ventriculostomy
S/P craniotomy

Cerebellum or brainstem hemorrhage
Drowsiness, stupor, or coma
Mechanical ventilation
CT or clinical signs of brainstem compression
Cardiac arrhythmia
S/P ventriculostomy
S/P craniotomy

Major hemispheric ischemic stroke syndromes
Drowsiness, stupor, or coma
Mechanical ventilation
CT scan evidence of early swelling
    or hemorrhagic conversion
Seizures
Cardiac failure or arrhythmias
S/P craniotomy
S/P endovascular intervention

Basilar artery occlusion
Drowsiness, stupor, or coma
Mechanical ventilation
S/P thrombolysis
S/P endovascular intervention

Cerebellar infarct
Drowsiness, stupor, or coma
Mechanical ventilation
CT scan or clinical evidence
    of brainstem compression
Cardiac arrhythmias
S/P ventriculostomy
S/P craniotomy

Acute bacterial meningitis
Drowsiness, stupor, or coma
Mechanical ventilation
CT scan evidence of edema
Any neurologic deterioration despite antibiotic
    therapy
Seizures
Shock
Pulmonary infiltrates

Brain abscess
Drowsiness, stupor, or coma
Mechanical ventilation
CT scan evidence of mass effect
Seizures
S/P drainage
S/P stereotactic puncture

Acute encephalitis
Drowsiness, stupor, or coma
Mechanical ventilation
CT scan evidence of swelling
Seizures
S/P brain biopsy

Acute spinal cord disorders
Mechanical ventilation
Cervical lesion
Ascending paralysis
Associated traumatic brain injury
Pulmonary infiltrates
Dysautonomia or acute bladder distension
Anticipated surgical intervention

Acute white matter disorders
Drowsiness, stupor, or coma
Mechanical ventilation
Seizures
Need to monitor plasma exchange

Acute obstructive hydrocephalus
Drowsiness, stupor, or coma
Mechanical ventilation
Ventriculostomy

Malignant brain tumors
Drowsiness, stupor, or coma
Mechanical ventilation
CT scan evidence of cerebral edema
Recurrent seizures

Status epilepticus
Drowsiness, stupor, or coma
Mechanical ventilation
Need for more intravenous antiepileptic drugs
Need for video/EEG monitoring

(*continued*)

TABLE 2.1 (CONTINUED)

Cerebral venous thrombosis	**Traumatic brain injury**
Drowsiness, stupor, or coma	Drowsiness, stupor, or coma
Mechanical ventilation	Mechanical ventilation
CT scan evidence of hemorrhagic infarct	CT scan evidence of contusions or early brain swelling
Seizures	Seizures
Suspected pulmonary embolus	Evidence of multitrauma
S/P endovascular intervention	S/P craniotomy
Guillain-Barré syndrome	**Myasthenia gravis**
VC < 20 mL/kg, PI_{max} < −30 cm H_2O, PE_{max} < 40 cm H_2O or 30% decrease in any of these values	Myasthenic crisis with neuromuscular respiratory failure (VC< 20 mL/kg or 30% decrease)
Mechanical ventilation	Bulbar weakness
Pulmonary infiltrates	Mechanical ventilation
Rapid clinical progression	
Dysautonomia	
Pneumonia or sepsis	

CT, computed tomography; EEG, electroencephalography; ICH, intracranial hemorrhage; PE_{max}, maximal expiratory pressure; PI_{max}, maximal inspiratory pressure; S/P, status post; VC, vital capacity.

imaging (MRI) findings. Information about medical conditions should include vital signs, airway control (and mechanical ventilator settings), pharmaceutical support, procedures and interventions used in the emergency department, and pending laboratory test results. Triage out of the NICU is not an exact reversal of the original indication and is more complex to regulate.[5] Inability to clear secretions, continuous agitation, lability of blood pressure measurements, and occasional need for IV hypertensive drugs are all reasons for return to

the ICU ("bounce-back").[9] Medication reconciliation is of utmost importance before transfer. Bounce-backs within 24 hours seem less common but more often are scrutinized for errors. It is unclear if mortality or morbidity is significantly higher with patients who have returned. Bounce-backs and unplanned transfers can be substantial when closely surveyed.[11] The frequency of these incidents can be targeted by administrators as a quality measure (see Chapter 14).

CONCLUSIONS

- Triage to the NICU could be based on certain criteria. Any patient with a neurologic disorder and unstable vital signs (pulse rate, blood pressure, respiratory rate, core temperature) or a progressive neurologic presentation should be admitted.
- Communication between the physician in the emergency department and the NICU attending physician requires special effort.
- Triage out the NICU requires assessment of neurologic and respiratory stability and no recent use of IV antihypertensives or IV cardiac drugs.

TABLE 2.2. CONSIDERATIONS FOR TRANSFER OF THE NEUROLOGIC PATIENT (ESSENTIALS OF PATIENT HANDOFFS)

Detailed neurologic examination and clinical course
FOUR score (EMBR 0–16)*
Mechanical ventilator settings
Review of dose of vasopressors
Review of recent use of neuromusculzar blocking agents and sedatives
Review of antiepileptic drugs
Review of neuroimaging
Consult with interventional neuroradiologist
Meeting with family members for their understanding of patient's condition and assessment of level of care.

*For FOUR score description, see Chapter 12.

REFERENCES

1. The Society of Critical Care Medicine Ethics Committee. Attitudes of critical care medicine professionals concerning distribution of intensive care resources. *Crit Care Med* 1994;22:358–362.

2. Bagshaw SM, Webb SA, Delaney A, et al. Very old patients admitted to intensive care in Australia and New Zealand: a multi-centre cohort analysis. *Crit Care* 2009;13:R45.

3. Cohen RI, Eichorn A, Motschwiller C, et al. Medical intensive care unit consults occurring within 48 hours of admission: a prospective study. *J Crit Care* 2015;30:363–368.

4. Cohen RI, Lisker GN, Eichorn A, Multz AS, Silver A. The impact of do-not-resuscitate order on triage decisions to a medical intensive care unit. *J Crit Care* 2009;24:311–315.

5. Coon EA, Kramer NM, Fabris RR, et al. Structured handoff checklists improve clinical measures in patients discharged from the neurointensive care unit. *Neurol Clin Prac* 2015;5:42–49.

6. Daly K, Beale R, Chang RW. Reduction in mortality after inappropriate early discharge from intensive care unit: logistic regression triage model. *BMJ* 2001;322:1274–1276.

7. Einav S, Soudry E, Levin PD, Grunfeld GB, Sprung CL. Intensive care physicians' attitudes concerning distribution of intensive care resources: a comparison of Israeli, North American and European cohorts. *Intens Care Med* 2004;30:1140–1143.

8. Escher M, Perneger TV, Chevrolet JC. National questionnaire survey on what influences doctors' decisions about admission to intensive care. *BMJ* 2004;329:425.

9. Fakhry SM, Leon S, Derderian C, Al-Harakeh H, Ferguson PL. Intensive care unit bounce back in trauma patients: an analysis of unplanned returns to the intensive care unit. *J Trauma Acute Care Surg* 2013;74:1528–1533.

10. Gaughen J, Jr, Hawk H, Evans A, Dumont A, Jensen M. The necessity of intensive care unit monitoring following elective endovascular treatment of unruptured intracranial aneurysms *J Neurointerv Surg* 2009;1:75–76.

11. Gold CA, Mayer SA, Lennihan L, Claassen J, Willey JZ. Unplanned transfers from hospital wards to the neurological intensive care unit. *Neurocrit Care* 2015;23:159–165.

12. Hurst SA, Hull SC, DuVal G, Danis M. Physicians' responses to resource constraints. *Arch Intern Med* 2005;165:639–644.

13. Manara AR, Pittman JA, Braddon FE. Reasons for withdrawing treatment in patients receiving intensive care. *Anaesthesia* 1998;53:523–528.

14. Nuckton TJ, List ND. Age as a factor in critical care unit admissions. *Arch Intern Med* 1995; 155:1087–1092.

15. Richards BF, Fleming JB, Shannon CN, Walters BC, Harrigan MR. Safety and cost effectiveness of step-down unit admission following elective neurointerventional procedures. *J Neurointerv Surg* 2012;4:390–392.

16. Rosenberg AL, Hofer TP, Strachan C, Watts CM, Hayward RA. Accepting critically ill transfer patients: adverse effect on a referral center's outcome and benchmark measures. *Ann Intern Med* 2003;138:882–890.

17. Ward NS, Teno JM, Curtis JR, Rubenfeld GD, Levy MM. Perceptions of cost constraints, resource limitations, and rationing in United States intensive care units: results of a national survey. *Crit Care Med* 2008;36:471–476.

PART II

Evaluation of Presenting Symptoms Indicating Urgency

3

Confused and Febrile

Confusion is a common presenting problem in the emergency department, and one should pity the physician (mostly the neurologist) who must make sense of an irritable, impulsive, desultory, and markedly uncooperative patient.[7,15] This chapter not only considers the evaluation of a patient presenting with an acute confusional state, but also closely examines the more commonly encountered confused patient with fever. The additional common presence of fever in patients with altered consciousness is often tied to an acute neurologic illness. Infection of the central nervous system (CNS) should be typically suspected, and decisions may have to be made quickly, based on few clinical clues.[9]

The causes of febrile confusion cover a broad spectrum. For example, neurologic examination could indicate that confusion means aphasia or nonconvulsive status epilepticus. Other unusual signs may point to a noninfectious explanation. These are muscle rigidity and trismus (strychnine in illicit drugs, tetanus), or myoclonus (serotonin syndrome).[4] Fever and confusion can be associated with marked rigidity and tremors in the face and arms, and these should suggest an acute autonomic storm (neuroleptic malignant syndrome or lethal catatonia). Hyperthermia could worsen signs of neurologic disease but fever alone may deteriorate many patients with Parkinson's disease.[24]

A too-narrow focus linking it only to meningoencephalitis can be a disadvantage when interpreting the clinical signs in patients with such a generalized presentation. Evidence of an infection outside the CNS may not be immediately obvious, and this situation presents a great number of diagnostic possibilities. Fever resulting in confusion can be caused by bacteremia, focal bacterial infection (upper respiratory tract, skin, and soft tissue infection), and nonbacterial illness such as viremia, malignancy, connective tissue disease, and thromboembolism.

This chapter provides diagnostic steps for organizing the evaluation of these patients.

Details on CNS infections and management are provided in Chapters 33–35.

CLINICAL ASSESSMENT

The diagnostic possibilities for the confused and febrile patient can be narrowed by the presence of additional distinctive symptoms. The most useful inquiries in the patient's history are shown in Table 3.1.[6,19,22]

The neurologic examination of a confused and febrile patient should include a serious attempt to assess demeanor and orientation, followed by thought content, attention, language, memory, and visuospatial skills. Delirium remains difficult to define (Capsule 3.1).[1,15] Emergency departments have developed a two-step approach to diagnose delirium (with 82% sensitivity and 95% specificity)[12] (Figure 3.1). Unfortunately, each of these cognitive spheres may be judged in only a cursory manner when agitation or delirium is prominent.

First, it is important to observe the patient's poise. Uneasiness and restlessness may also indicate a medical disorder (e.g., hyperthyroidism, hypoglycemia, severe hypoxemia) or drug intoxication (e.g., theophylline, lidocaine). Impulsivity and emotional outburst and their opposite manifestation, abulia, are largely due to acute frontal lesions. Second, orientation is addressed; this requires simple questions such as "How did you get here?" or "Where are you?" or "What is the month and year?" or "Why are you here?" However, the content of the answers may be abnormal with perseveration (continuation of thoughts) and intrusions (words from prior context, often due to aphasia). Attention, language, memory, orientation, and visuospatial tests are only possible in a patient with a willingness to respond. Attention can be tested by spelling words backward, reciting the days of the week in reverse order, or other spelling tests. Language should at least include the assessment of fluency, inflection and melody, rate, volume, articulation, and comprehension. Memory testing is challenging in confused febrile patients,

TABLE 3.1. OBSERVATIONS AND CLUES IN THE CONFUSED FEBRILE PATIENT

Debilitated, wasted, underfed (drug abuse, alcoholism, cancer)

Exposure to ticks, mosquitoes and beginning of endemic encephalitis (arboviruses)

Exposure to wilderness, tropics, animal bite (rabies)

Exposure to excessive heat (heat stroke)

Recent travel or immigration from developing country (neurocysticercosis, fungal meningitis)

Recent vaccination (ADEM)

Prior transplantation or AIDS (*Toxoplasma* encephalitis or *Aspergillus*)

ADEM, acute disseminated encephalomyelitis; AIDS, acquired immunodeficiency syndrome.

but remote memory (significant life events in the family) or recent breaking news can be assessed. Visuospatial orientation may be briefly assessed by having the patient localize body parts or interlock two circles formed by closed index finger and thumb of each hand.

Confusional behavior may be due to mass lesions, which often produce language disorders. Masses in the right frontal lobe (in right-handed persons) may enlarge to impressive tumors that may not be detected by even the most meticulous neurologic examination. A left frontal lobe mass, particularly if the lesion extends posteriorly and inferiorly, is manifested by Broca aphasia. Its characteristics are distinct; the patient is constantly unable to repeat an exact sentence, speaks in short phrases and with revisions, and makes major grammatical errors, together with loss of cohesion, in lengthier narratives. Frontal lobe syndrome has been well recognized and appears in many guises, such as loss of vitality and notable slow thinking. It may be manifested by strange behavior, sexual harassment, cynically inappropriate remarks in an attempt to be humorous, or intense irritability. Any executive function requiring planning is disturbed, but this may be covered up by euphoria, platitudes in speech, or "robot-like" behavior—in many with a preservation of social graces.

Masses in the temporal lobe may also generate changes in behavior and therefore may remain unnoticed or may be delayed in recognition. Dominant (left in right-handed persons) temporal masses may change a normal personality into one of depression and apathy. More posterior localization in the dominant temporal lobe may produce Wernicke aphasia. This classic type of aphasia is recognized by continuously "empty" speech, often with syllables, words, or phrases at the end of sentences and characteristically with incomprehensible content (e.g., one of our patients, when asked to define *island*, responded "place where petos . . . no trees . . . united presip thing" and to define *motor*, responded "thing that makes the drive thing"). Involvement of the nondominant temporal lobe may be manifested only by an upper quadrant hemianopia and nonverbal *auditory agnosia* (inability to recognize familiar sounds, such as a loud clap or tearing of paper).

CAPSULE 3.1   DSM-5 DIAGNOSTIC CRITERIA FOR DELIRIUM

A. A disturbance in attention (i.e., reduced ability to direct, focus, sustain, and shift attention) and awareness (reduced orientation to the environment).

B. The disturbance develops over a short period of time (usually hours to a few days), represents a change from baseline attention and awareness and tends to fluctuate in severity during the course of a day.

C. An additional disturbance in cognition (e.g., memory deficit, disorientation, language, visuospacial ability, or perception).

D. The disturbances in criteria A and C are not better explained by a preexisting, established or evolving neurocognitive disorder and do not occur in the context of a severely reduced level of arousal, such as coma.

E. There is evidence from the history, physical examination, or laboratory findings that the disturbance is a direct physiologic consequence of another medical condition, substance intoxication or withdrawal, or exposure to a toxin, or is due to multiple etiologies.

With permission from American Psychiatric Association, Diagnostic and Statistical Manual of Mental Disorders, 5th ed. Washington, DC: American Psychiatric Association, 2013.

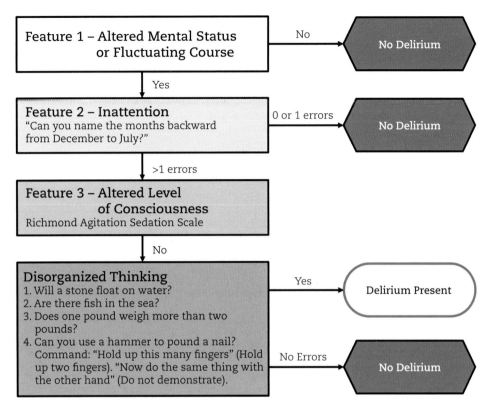

FIGURE 3.1: Two-step delirium triage screen used in emergency departments.

From Han et al. (2103) with permission.

Parietal lobe masses also produce effects that depend on localization. Nondominant right parietal lesions usually cause neglect of the paralyzed left limb (up to entire unawareness of the limb), but can also cause marked inertia and aloofness. A dominant parietal lobe lesion impairs normal arithmetical skills, recognition of fingers, and right–left orientation. A nonfluent aphasia may occur as well.

Occipital lobe masses produce hemianopia. When only the inferior occipital cortex is involved, *achromatopsia* (loss of color vision in a hemianopic field) or abnormal color naming ("What is the color of the sky, an apple, a tomato?") may result. Extension into the subcortical area from edema might produce alexia without agraphia, but the symptoms occur in a dominant left occipital lesion.

Many systemic illnesses may produce a confusional state and agitation, and the major considerations are shown in Table 3.2.[3,8,9,14,17,18,26] Many drugs have been implicated but we do not know how often (benzodiazepine infusions)[27] have been implicated but other drug associations are less clear and in susceptable patients (corticosteroids, histamine receptor antagonists). Systemic

signs can provide a clue to the infectious agent. Obviously, an illness beginning with a cough suggests a primary respiratory infection, but a broad differential diagnosis exists. Community-acquired respiratory infections with a proclivity for systemic manifestations include influenza A and B,

TABLE 3.2. SYSTEMIC ILLNESSES WITH FEVER AND CONFUSION

Septic shock
Lobar pneumonia
Acute osteomyelitis
Abdominal suppuration
Endocarditis
Erysipelas
Measles
Psittacosis
Influenza
Yellow fever
Typhoid fever
Cholera
Heat stroke
Thyrotoxicosis

adenoviral infection, *Mycoplasma pneumoniae,* *Legionella pneumophila,* and reactivation of tuberculosis. All of these disorders may have neurologic manifestations. An illness with a prominent rash, fever, and confusion could be due to viral, bacterial, or fungal agents, with a possibility of seeding in the CNS (Table 3.3). The patient should be questioned about recent travel.[22] Whether the patient presents in the summer (West Nile encephalitis[14] or equine encephalitis[16]) or the fall, and whether he or she is immunocompromised, must also be taken into consideration.[5,9]

The multisystem involvement (myocarditis, pneumonia, lymphadenopathy, or hepatorenal dysfunction) associated with encephalopathy could indicate a certain infectious agent. Diagnostic considerations should include Q fever[3] (periventricular or focal edema on magnetic resonance imaging [MRI]), pneumonia, lymphocytic pleocytosis caused by the zoonotic agent *Coxiella burnetii*), leptospirosis (meningitis, hepatic dysfunction, muscle pain, conjunctivitis), tularemia (ulceroglandular disease, conjunctivitis, and lymphadenopathy), *Mycoplasma pneumoniae* (pneumonia, transverse myelitis, conjunctivitis), and cat-scratch disease (lymphadenopathy, vasculitis caused by *Bartonella henselae*).[25] In any patient, it is important to consider an immunocompromised state, which raises an entirely different set of possibilities.[5,11] Acute human immunodeficiency virus (HIV) infections can be present in a young adult with fever, confusion, lymphadenopathy, pharyngitis, and rash. One may consider questioning patients about sexual practices or intravenous drug abuse.

Febrile neutropenia is a common finding in patients with recently treated malignancies, particularly when recently treated with aggressive myelosuppressive drugs. Infections become frequent and severe with neutrophil counts of less than 100 cells/mm³. Remission induction therapy for acute leukemia is commonly followed by a prolonged period of virtually absent neutrophils. The most common pathogens in patients with neutropenia are *Staphylococcus epidermidis, Streptococcus* spp., *Staphylococcus aureus, Escherichia coli,* and *Pseudomonas aeruginosa.* Many yeasts or fungi can be implicated.

In hematologic malignancies, *Listeria monocytogenes, Cryptococcus neoformans, Toxoplasma gondii,* and *Nocardia* are common CNS infections when patients present with febrile neutropenia. When an Ommaya reservoir is in situ for chemotherapeutic delivery in leptomeningeal disease, coagulase-negative staphylococci and other skin microorganisms may be implicated. Patients seen in the emergency department with neutropenia, prior induction therapy or bone marrow transplant, pneumonia, or other documented infection, as well as a major comorbid condition, should be admitted starting empirical broad-spectrum antibiotics followed by aggressive evaluation of the infection's source.

TABLE 3.3. GENERAL CLINICAL SIGNS INDICATING CAUSES IN CONFUSED FEBRILE PATIENTS

Signs	Disorder
Skin rash	Rickettsial diseases
	Vasculitis
	Aspergillosis
Petechiae	Thrombocytopenic purpura
	Meningococcemia
	Endocarditis
	Drug eruption from intoxication
	Leukemia
Splenomegaly	Toxoplasmosis
	Tuberculosis
	Sepsis
	Human immunodeficiency virus infection
	Lymphoma
Pulmonary infiltrates	*Legionella* species
	Fungi
	Tuberculosis
	Mycoplasma
	Pneumonia
	Q fever
	Tick-borne diseases

LINE OF ACTION

Any high fever impairs consciousness, and therefore the physician can expect difficulty with the assessment of newly presenting febrile patients. It is virtually impossible to approach these patients from every conceivable angle. Clearly, primary disorders of the CNS need rapid assessment because therapeutic options are limited and time-locked. The mortality and morbidity from the ravages of infection of the brain as a result of delayed treatment are very high.

To narrow the diagnosis in patients who present with multiple converging problems, the most reasonable sequence of evaluation is first to obtain laboratory data that could suggest a possible systemic infection. The chance of a bacterial infection increases with age (> 50 years), erythrocyte sedimentation rate (> 30 mm/hr), white blood cell

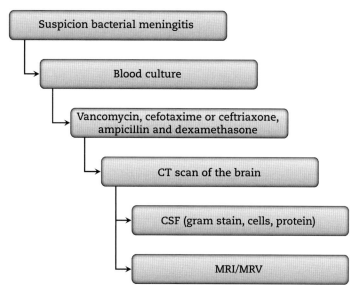

FIGURE 3.2: Critical steps in the evaluation of the febrile confused patient suspicious of acute bacterial meningitis.

CSF, cerebrospinal fluid; CT, computed tomography; MRI, magnetic resonance imaging; MRV, magnetic resonance venography.

count (> 15,000 mm³), bands (> 5%), and comorbid illness.[11,17,20] Laboratory tests should include a toxicology screen and drug levels, if needed, in addition to routine chemistry and hematology markers.

The recommended line of action for a patient with acute bacterial meningitis is shown in Figure 3.2. Blood cultures are followed by immediate administration of antibiotics and corticosteroids, followed by a computed tomography (CT) scan of the brain to exclude an empyema or abscess. Both disorders rarely produce focal signs or papilledema and may be very difficult to detect clinically, and urgent neurosurgical intervention is needed.[11] If the CT is abnormal, an MRI and magnetic resonance venography (MRV) follow. If the CT is normal, a cerebrospinal fluid (CSF) specimen is obtained.

In patients suspected of encephalitis, studies with the highest yield and that can be completed in the shortest period of time are needed. These can be prioritized according to the steps shown in Figure 3.3. When the suspicion of intracranial disease is high and suspicion of a systemic illness is

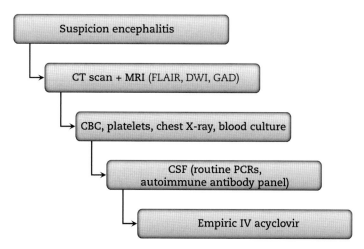

FIGURE 3.3: Critical steps in the evaluation of the febrile confused patient suspicious of encephalitis.

CBC, complete blood count; CSF, cerebrospinal fluid; CT, computed tomography; DWI, diffusion-weighted imaging; FLAIR, fluid-attenuated inversion recovery; GAD, gadolinium enhancement; PCR, polymerase chain reaction.

Class of Microorganism	General Diagnostic Evaluation
Viruses	Culture of respiratory secretions and nasopharynx, throat, and stool specimens[a]
	DFA of sputum for respiratory viruses
	PCR of respiratory specimens
	Culture and/or DFA of skin lesions (if present) for herpes simplex virus and varicella-zoster virus
	Serologic testing for HIV[b]
	Serologic testing for Epstein-Barr virus
	Serologic testing (acute and convalescent phase) for St. Louis encephalitis virus,[c] Eastern equine encephalitis virus,[c]
	Venezuelan equine encephalitis virus,[c] La Crosse virus,[c]
	West Nile virus[c]
	CSF IgM for West Nile virus,[c] St. Louis encephalitis virus,[c] varicella-zoster virus
	CSF PCR for herpes simplex virus 1, herpes simplex virus 2, varicella-zoster virus, Epstein-Barr virus,[d] enteroviruses
Bacteria	Blood cultures
	CSF cultures
	Serologic testing (acute and convalescent phase) for *Mycoplasma pneumoniae*
	PCR of respiratory secretions for *Mycoplasma pneumoniae*
Rickettsiae and ehrlichiae[c]	Serologic testing (acute and convalescent phase) for *Rickettsia rickettsi, Ehrlichia chaffeensis,* and *Anaplasma phagocytophilum*
	DFA and PCR of skin biopsy specimen (if rash present) for *Rickettsia rickettsiae*
	Blood smears for morulae
	PCR of whole blood and CSF specimens for *Ehrlichia* and *Anaplasma* species[e]
Spirochetes	Serum RPR and FTA-ABS
	Serologic testing for *Borrelia burgdorferi* (ELISA and Western blot)
	CSF VDRL
	CSF *Borrelia burgdorferi* serologic testing (ELISA and Western blot); IgG antibody index
	CSF FTA-ABS[f]
Mycobacteria	Chest radiograph
	PCR and culture of respiratory secretions
	CSF AFB smear and culture
	CSF PCR (Gen-Probe Amplified *Mycobacterium tuberculosis* Direct Test)
Fungi	Blood cultures
	CSF cultures
	Serum and CSF cryptococcal antigen
	Urine and CSF *Histoplasma* antigen[g]
	Serum and CSF complement fixing or immunodiffusion antibodies for *Coccidioides* species
Protozoa	Serum IgG for *Toxoplasma gondii*[h]

Note: These tests may not be required in all patients with encephalitis; certain tests should not be performed unless a consistent epidemiology is present. Additional tests should be considered on the basis of epidemiology, risk factors, clinical features, general diagnostic studies, neuroimaging features, and CSF analysis. Recommended tests should not supplant clinical judgment; not all tests are recommended in all age groups. AFB, acid-fast bacilli; CSF, cerebrospinal fluid; DFA, direct fluorescent antibody; ELISA, enzyme-linked immunosorbent assay; FTA-ABS, fluorescent treponemal antibody, absorbed; PCR, polymerase chain reaction; RPR, rapid plasma reagin; VDRL, Venereal Disease Research Laboratory.

[a] Additional diagnostic studies for immunocompromised patients are CSF PCR for cytomegalovirus JC virus, human herpesvirus 6, and West Nile virus.

[b] In patients who are HIV seronegative but in whom there is a high index of suspicion for HIV infection, plasma HIV RNA testing should be performed.

[c] Depending on time of year or geographic locale.

[d] Results should be interpreted in conjunction with Epstein-Barr virus serologic testing; quantitative PCR should be done, because a low CSF copy number may be an incidental finding.

[e] Low yield of CSF PCR.

[f] CSF FTA-ABS is sensitive but not specific for the diagnosis of neurosyphilis; a nonreactive CSF test result may exclude the diagnosis, but a reactive test result does not establish the diagnosis.

[g] Depends on a history of residence in or travel to an area of endemicity.

[h] Positive results may suggest the possibility of reactivation disease in an immunocompromised host.

Adapted from Tunkel et al. The management of encephalitis: clinical practice guidelines by the Infectious Diseases Society of America. *Clin Infect Dis* 2008;47:303–327, with permission of publisher.

low, it is quite justifiable to temporarily sedate the patient (e.g., propofol), intubate, administer antibiotic agents and acyclovir, and obtain CT or MRI and CSF. Initially, an electroencephalogram (EEG) should have some priority but may be artifactually abnormal or show a medication effect when sedative drugs are needed to control agitation. Early in the disease course, MRI may document characteristic findings in herpes simplex encephalitis (temporal lobe and in subinsular region), mosquito-borne encephalitis (cortical spotted lesions and basal ganglia) or fungal encephalitis (hyperintensities and nodular enhancing meninges).[10] Almost simultaneously, CSF analysis should be sent for multiple polymerase chain reaction (PCR); failure to do so is a lost opportunity to diagnose the underlying organism.[13,16] Polymerase chain reaction studies are specific in documenting the presence of herpes simplex, Epstein-Barr virus, and varicella-zoster DNA, and may detect organisms that do not grow in culture.[13]

The CSF in herpes simplex encephalitis will show a characteristic formula of normal or raised pressure, 10–200 cells/mm^3 (mostly lymphocytes), normal glucose, and increased protein, but all can be normal in 5% of presenting cases.[2,23] Cerebrospinal fluid and serum antibodies (immunoglobulins M and G) should be obtained specific to any mosquito-borne viral encephalitis and should be repeated after 1 week. Indirect immunofluorescent assays are useful if Rocky Mountain spotted fever or ehrlichiosis is considered.[21] Fungal meningoencephalitis is very uncommon, but cryptococcosis, coccidioidomycosis, *Histoplasma capsulatum*, and *Blastomyces dermatitidis* are more endemic.[10] Detection by growth in CSF or of specific antibody is possible, but multiple CSF specimens are needed to detect a positive culture. A diagnostic evaluation in patients with suspected encephalitis has been proposed by an expert panel of the Infectious Diseases Society of America and is shown in Table 3.4 (Part XIV, Guidelines). Not all encephalitis is infectious and in fact in younger adults many are autoimmune. A full panel of serum and CSF antibodies is needed (Chapter 35).

When CSF is suggestive of an infection, it is prudent to start with a multipronged approach directed against possibly resistant bacteria (fourth-generation cephalosporin and vancomycin), herpes simplex (acyclovir), and rickettsial and ehrlichial infections (doxycycline), while awaiting test results.

CONCLUSIONS

- Most confused and febrile patients have an underlying systemic infection.
- Confusion may indicate a more specific language disorder.
- Multisystem involvement and confusion point to certain infectious agents.
- Abnormal immune status should be investigated because its presence has a different set of diagnostic possibilities.

REFERENCES

1. American Psychiatric Association: *Diagnostic and Statistical Manual of Mental Disorders,* 5th ed. Washington, DC: American Psychiatric Association; 2013.
2. Baringer JR. Herpes simplex virus encephalitis. In: Davis LE, Kennedy PGE, eds. *Infectious Diseases of the Nervous System.* Woburn, MA: Butterworth-Heinemann; 2000:139–164.
3. Bernit E, Pouget J, Janbon F, et al. Neurological involvement in acute Q fever: a report of 29 cases and review of the literature. *Arch Intern Med* 2002;162:693–700.
4. Brendel DH, Bodkin JA, Yang JM. Massive sertraline overdose. *Ann Emerg Med* 2000;36:524–526.
5. Cunha BA. Central nervous system infections in the compromised host: a diagnostic approach. *Infect Dis Clin North Am* 2001;15:567–590.
6. Deresiewicz RL, Thaler SJ, Hsu L, Zamani AA. Clinical and neuroradiographic manifestations of eastern equine encephalitis. *N Engl J Med* 1997;336:1867–1874.
7. Ferrando SJ, Freyberg Z. Neuropsychiatric aspects of infectious diseases. *Crit Care Clin* 2008;24:889–919.
8. Fong TG, Tulebaev SR, Inouye SK. Delirium in elderly adults: diagnosis, prevention and treatment. *Nat Rev Neurol* 2009;5:210–220.
9. Frank LR, Jobe KA. *Admission and Discharge Decisions in Emergency Medicine.* Philadelphia: Hanley & Belfus; 2001.
10. Gottfredsson M, Perfect JR. Fungal meningitis. *Semin Neurol* 2000;20:307–322.
11. Hall WA, Truwit CL. The surgical management of infections involving the cerebrum. *Neurosurgery* 2008;62 Suppl 2:519–530.
12. Han JH, Wilson A, Vasilevskis EE, et al. Diagnosing delirium in older emergency department patients: validity and reliability of the delirium triage screen and the brief confusion assessment method. *Ann Emerg Med* 2013;62:457–465.
13. Johnston RT. *Viral Infections of the Nervous System.* 2nd ed. Philadelphia: Lippincott-Raven; 1998.

14. Kramer LD, Li J, Shi PY. West Nile virus. *Lancet Neurol* 2007;6:171–181.

15. Kyomen HH, Whitfield TH. Psychosis in the elderly. *Am J Psychiatry* 2009;166:146–150.

16. Lambert AJ, Martin DA, Lanciotti RS. Detection of North American eastern and western equine encephalitis viruses by nucleic acid amplification assays. *J Clin Microbiol* 2003;41:379–385.

17. Leibovici L, Cohen O, Wysenbeek AJ. Occult bacterial infection in adults with unexplained fever: validation of a diagnostic index. *Arch Intern Med* 1990;150:1270–1272.

18. Lorenzo M, Aldecoa C, Rico J. Delirium in the critically ill patient. *Trends in Anaesthesia & Critical Care* 2013;3:257–264.

19. McJunkin JE, de los Reyes EC, Irazuzta JE, et al. La Crosse encephalitis in children. *N Engl J Med* 2001;344:801–807.

20. Mellors JW, Horwitz RI, Harvey MR, Horwitz SM. A simple index to identify occult bacterial infection in adults with acute unexplained fever. *Arch Intern Med* 1987;147:666–671.

21. Ratnasamy N, Everett ED, Roland WE, McDonald G, Caldwell CW. Central nervous system manifestations of human ehrlichiosis. *Clin Infect Dis* 1996; 23:314–319.

22. Shlim DR, Solomon T. Japanese encephalitis vaccine for travelers: exploring the limits of risk. *Clin Infect Dis* 2002;35:183–188.

23. Steiner I, Kennedy PG, Pachner AR. The neurotropic herpes viruses: herpes simplex and varicella-zoster. *Lancet Neurol* 2007;6:1015–1028.

24. Umemura A, Oeda T, Tomita S, et al. Delirium and high fever are associated with subacute motor deterioration in Parkinson disease: a nested case-control study. *PLoS One* 2014;9:e94944.

25. Wormser GP. Discovery of new infectious diseases: bartonella species. *N Engl J Med* 2007;356:2346–2347.

26. Zaal IJ, Slooter AJ. Delirium in critically ill patients: epidemiology, pathophysiology, diagnosis and management. *Drugs* 2012;72:1457–1471.

27. Zaal IJ, Devlin JW, Hazelbag M, et al. Benzodiazepine-associated delirium in critically ill adults. *Intensive Care Med* 2015;41:2130–2137.

4

A Terrible Headache

Emergency departments (EDs) are frequently visited by patients with acute or treatment-refractory headaches.[27] Within this undifferentiated melee of patients presenting suddenly in the ED are some patients with potentially life-threatening conditions, and the outcome can have serious consequences if not recognized in time. The ED physician and neurologist are both commonly involved with the triage of these patients.[17,18,21] When faced with a patient presenting with severe headache, the physician must tread a narrow line between "playing it safe" by ordering a series of tests that may produce negative or false positive results, and running the risk of litigation due to incomplete investigations.[52] Not all patients with a "severe sudden headache" have a neurologic or medical illness; in fact, most do not. Many patients presenting with a new severe headache require CT scan or cerebrospinal fluid (CSF) examination, but the overwhelming proportion of patients will have a normal result. However, a split-second onset of persistent severe ("terrible") and completely unexpected and sustained headache bad enough to go to the ED may indicate aneurysmal subarachnoid hemorrhage (SAH) or another potentially acute neurovascular disorder (Capsule 4.1). Other patients frequently visit the ED to treat debilitating migraine or other headache syndromes. Many can be helped with urgent pharmacologic intervention.

A description of the scope of problems with diagnosing causes of acute headache is necessary for neurologists consulted in the ED. This chapter also briefly considers other non-neurologic disorders responsible for acute headache syndromes. First-line therapies for most of these acute headache syndromes are provided.

CLINICAL ASSESSMENT

The exact analysis of the onset and character of a presenting headache requires considerable skill, and most of the time the diagnosis is reached after discovering certain characteristic features. Most disorders presenting with serious warning signs are acute neurologic conditions (Table 4.1.) Acute severe headache may indicate equally serious non-neurologic disorders, such as acute sphenoid sinusitis, a first manifestation of malignant hypertension, or acute-angle glaucoma (Table 4.2).[22] All of these disorders require different therapeutic approaches, but should be considered by the neurologist and may prompt evaluation by other specialists. Severe unilateral headache may be without any physical signs until zoster rash appears[62] (Figure 4.1).

One should look out for a so called "thunderclap" headache. This unusual headache refers to a split-second, extremely intense ("10 out of 10"), totally unexpected headache. The patient feels as if struck by lightning, partly explaining the term *thunderclap* (although there is no sound). The sudden onset can often be recognized by the patient if the examiner demonstrates a handclap or finger snap. Headache of this character may be short in maximal intensity but typically persists for hours and remains severe.[12,14,21] Many patients describe a brief sense of panic because they are very worried by the unexpected presentation. The often-quoted "worst headache of my life" in textbooks may not necessarily indicate acute onset or precisely define the severity of the headache (e.g., patients with chronic headaches or migraine have episodes that they commonly first classify as "the worst headache ever").

Unfortunately, clinical signs, such as nuchal rigidity (rarely in the first hours), retinal or sub-hyaloid hemorrhage (predominantly in patients in a very poor condition from SAH), or cranial nerve deficits (third- or sixth-nerve palsy), are all uncommon leads. If SAH remains the main diagnostic consideration, the diagnosis is established by computed tomography (CT), in most cases when seen within 12 hours of onset. In the vast majority of patients with SAH on CT scan—and no history of trauma to the head—the symptom will be due to aneurysmal rupture. Other infrequent conditions have been associated with thunderclap-like headaches, all very serious (Table 4.3).[13,15,53]

CAPSULE 4.1   ACUTE SERIOUS HEADACHE IN THE EMERGENCY DEPARTMENT

Because so many headaches look the same, are physicians able to pick out a patient with a ruptured aneurysm (or any other serious disease)? (see accompanying Figure 4.1). There are five warnings. First, physicians in the ED have to avoid "anchoring" (The emergency physician or consulted neurologist fixates on certain features of a presentation too early and makes a premature assessment). Second, a careful detailed history of the characteristics of the headache is required. Third, examination of a patient with thunderclap headache should at least include carotid artery auscultation (bruits in dissection), testing of eye movements (for VI and III cranial nerve deficits), neck movement (stiffness), and ophthalmoscopy (for hypertensive retinopathy in posterior reversible encephalopathy syndrome, retinal hemorrhage, or Terson's syndrome). Fourth, carefully scrutinize the CT scan for areas where subarachnoid hemorrhage can be hidden and to have it reviewed by others if doubt remains. Fifth, is to perform a lumbar puncture and evaluate for xanthochromia even if the CTA is negative (CTA may miss a ruptured aneurysm more often than we think.)

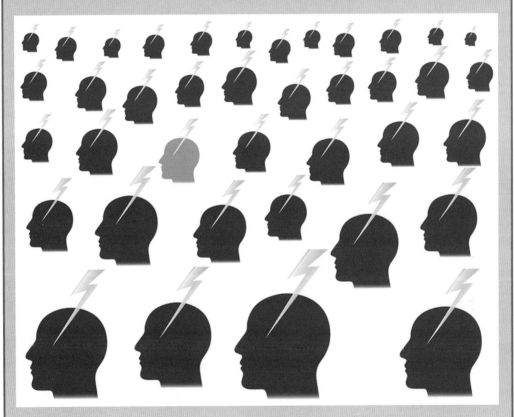

All acute headaches may sound identical but one is different.

TABLE 4.1. WARNING SIGNS IN ACUTE HEADACHE

Signs and Symptoms	Diagnosis to Consider
Split-second onset, unexpected, and excruciating	Aneurysmal subarachnoid hemorrhage
Loss of consciousness, vertigo, or vomiting	Cerebellar hematoma
Acute cranial nerve deficit (particularly oculomotor palsy)	Carotid artery aneurysm
Carotid bruit (in young individuals)	Carotid artery dissection
Fever and skin rash	Meningitis
Shock, Addison's disease	Pituitary apoplexy
Fall and coagulopathy or anticoagulation	Subdural, epidural, or intracerebral hematoma
Facial edema and vesicular rash	Herpes zoster ophthalmicus

TABLE 4.2. ACUTE SEVERE HEADACHE SYNDROMES
FROM NON-NEUROLOGIC CAUSES

Disorder	Location	Time Profile	Characteristic Features
Acute-angle glaucoma	Eye, frontal	Acute	Red eye, midrange pupil, decreased vision
Temporal arteritis	Temporal, frontal	Rapidly built up	Temporal artery painful, sedimentation rate > 55 mm/hr
Acute sinusitis	Frontal and maxilla	Hours	Fever, pressure pain on maxillary or frontal sinus
Pheochromocytoma	Entire head	Rapidly increasing intensity	Sweating, pallor, systolic blood pressure > 200 mm Hg

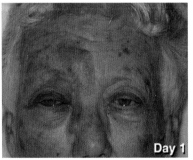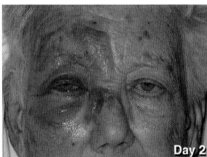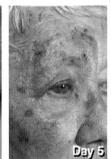

FIGURE 4.1: Serial photos of a patient with extreme headache and acute zoster trigeminal neuralgia. The first photograph shows early rash evolving into more characteristic skin crusting in subsequent photographs.
From Wijdicks EFM, Win PH. Excruciating headache but nothing obvious, look at the skin! *Pract Neurol* 2004;4:302–303. With permission of the publisher.

Thunderclap headache may be unaccompanied by any objective abnormalities on neuroimaging (CT and all other magnetic resonance [MR] modalities) and CSF examination, but this benign form is rather uncommon.[61] The term for this clinical entity was coined by Day and Raskin,[12] and is also known as *crash* or *blitz migraine*.[23] Some patients may go on to develop common migraine but not invariably so, and the link with established types of migraine is uncertain. Onset associated with exertion or orgasm is relatively common in thunderclap headaches.[29]

In a few patients with a thunderclap headache, diffuse segmental vasospasm is found by MR angiography (MRA) or cerebral angiogram.[15] Recurrences do occur in 10%–15% of cases, mostly within the first 6 months. Calcium channel blockers

TABLE 4.3. SYMPTOMATIC THUNDERCLAP HEADACHE OTHER THAN ANEURYSMAL SUBARACHNOID HEMORRHAGE

Diagnosis	Clues in History	Clues in Examination	MR Features
PRES	Poorly controlled hypertension	Systolic blood pressure > 200 mm Hg	Abnormalities predominantly in parieto-occipital lobes
Cerebral vasoconstriction syndrome	Recurrence	Use of vasoactive agents, migraine	Convexity subarachnoid hemorrhage, cerebral hematoma or infarct
Cerebral venous thrombosis	None	Increased CSF opening pressure	Transverse or sagittal sinus obstruction on MRV
Retroclival hematoma	None	CSF xanthochromia	Clot posteriorly and at level of clivus
Pituitary apoplexy	Cranial nerve deficit	Hypotension, hyponatremia	Pituitary tumor with hemorrhage
CSF hypotension	Marfan characteristics	Headache posture-related	Meningeal enhancement; subdural hematomas "sagging brain"
Carotid or vertebral artery dissection	Trauma, chiropractic therapy	Horner's syndrome, carotid bruit, dysarthria	Recent cerebral infarcts; double lumen sign on MRI

CSF, cerebrospinal fluid; MRI, magnetic resonance imaging; MRV, magnetic resonance venography; PRES, posterior reversible encephalopathy syndrome.

(i.e., nifedipine) may be helpful in some cases.[14,32] This syndrome is now recognized and is named reversible cerebral vasoconstriction syndrome.[42,43] Its ED presentation may be even more confusing, and patients may develop—next to a thunderclap headache—small lobar hematomas and sulcal hemorrhages and initially the cerebral angiogram is normal. A subsequent cerebral angiogram (2 weeks later) may show marked vasoconstriction resembling vasculitis. Most patients have a benign course, but poor outcome has been reported.[50]

Status migrainous, refractory trigeminal neuralgia, and cluster headache are other causes for acute severe headache,[1,4,5] usually accompanied by severe intensity, pulsating, unilateral headache that is aggravated by normal physical activity and is

TABLE 4.4. "BENIGN" ACUTE HEADACHE SYNDROMES

Disorder	Location	Time Profile	Quality	Characteristic Features
Cluster headache	Oculofrontal, temporal	30–90 minutes	Severe, stabbing	Rocking, restless, Horner syndrome, rhinorrhea
Chronic paroxysmal hemicrania	Unilateral	2–30 minutes	Severe	Conjunctival injection, not restless, lacrimation on symptomatic side (common in females)
Acute migraine	Mostly unilateral	6–30 hours	Moderately severe	Nausea and photophobia in 80%
Trigeminal neuralgia	Face	Seconds	Severe, electrical	Provoked by chewing, cold wind against face, shaving, tooth brushing

associated with nausea and vomiting. Photophobia and sonophobia are common features in all of these disorders, but differences between these more or less benign headaches are apparent (Table 4.4).

Refractory trigeminal neuralgia is characterized by episodic electrical sharp jabs of facial pain triggered by facial touch, chewing, talking, or tooth brushing, and is commonly refractory to medication. In some patients, medication doses are so high that intolerance has become a limiting factor.

Refractory cluster headache is fairly certain when patients present with excruciating retro-orbital forehead, jaw, or cheek pain following the first division of the trigeminal nerve, with lacrimation, nasal congestion, ptosis, and eyelid swelling. Attacks last approximately 1 hour and are commonly accompanied by restlessness and rocking motions.[23,45]

LINE OF ACTION
The critical treatment steps in patients with a new thunderclap headache are shown in Figure 4.2.[33] If the suspicion is very high, a CT can be supplemented with CTA or CTV, which may show a possible ruptured aneurysm, carotid or vertebral dissection dural AVM, and cerebral venous thrombosis when the suspicion is high as a result of prior pregnancy or prior manifestations of a coagulopathy.

Subtle SAH can be very difficult to detect on CT scan (Figure 4.3), and certain areas should be carefully inspected for traces of blood (Table 4.5). If the CT scan is negative, CSF examination is still able to document xanthochromia for up to 2 weeks following onset. CSF examination should be deferred until 4 hours have passed from

TABLE 4.5. REASONS FOR FAILURE TO RECOGNIZE SUBARACHNOID HEMORRHAGE ON COMPUTED TOMOGRAPHY SCANS

Blood in prepontine cistern is not visualized but is present on repeat CT scan

Blood in a part of the pentagon is not visualized from tilting of the gantry but is present on repeat CT scan

Absent unilateral sylvian fissure from isodense SAH

Sedimentation of blood in dependent part of the posterior ventricular horns

Blood in basal cisterns misinterpreted as contrast enhancement

Blood on tentorium misinterpreted as calcification

CT, computed tomography; SAH, subarachnoid hemorrhage.

onset, to allow the detection of xanthochromia from hemolyzed erythrocytes freeing up oxyhemoglobin. Cerebrospinal fluid examination should include cell count and morphology, protein, and CSF pressure before sampling, as well as assessment of xanthochromia.[16] In a recent study of 4,662 patients presenting with headache, 14% had their headache characterized as "the worst of their lives," but only 3% had a thunderclap-like headache. About one in four patients refused a lumbar puncture after a normal CT scan, but none had rebleeding at 2-year follow-up. In 15% of patients with a normal CT, xanthochromia was detected, and 72% had a ruptured cerebral aneurysm (sensitivity 93%, specificity 95%).[16] Cerebrospinal fluid in patients with a ruptured aneurysm more

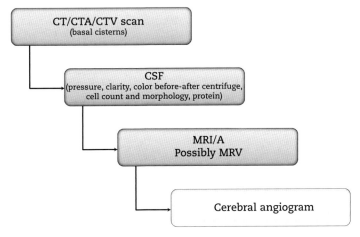

FIGURE 4.2: Critical steps in the evaluation of severe new acute headache.

CSF, cerebrospinal fluid; CT, computed tomography; MRI/A, magnetic resonance imaging/angiography; MRV, magnetic resonance venography.

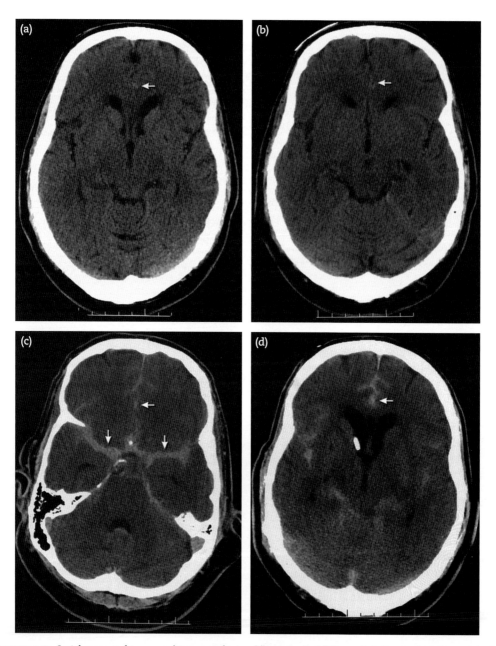

FIGURE 4.3: Serial computed tomographic scans of missed "warning leak." Very subtle hemorrhage (arrow) in the interhemispheric fissure in a patient with thunderclap headache initially interpreted as normal (a and b). Follow-up 2 months later (c and d) documents more dramatic presentation of ruptured anterior communicating artery aneurysm after recurrent severe headache. Ventriculostomy for acute hydrocephalus.

commonly shows high red blood cell counts, increased protein, and an increased total nucleated cell count. Spectrophotometry is a valuable method to prove xanthochromia that is due to bilirubin or oxyhemoglobin, but the technique is not used in the United States. Visual inspection of the CSF—with its obvious flaws—is currently most used (Capsule 4.2).[2,10,38,46]

A new rule—the Ottawa subarachnoid hemorrhage rule—received some attention, and it claimed high sensitivity and specificity. This rule includes the following items: First, it is assumed that there is no prior neurologic disorder that could have caused the headache. High-risk variables include age more than 40 years old, neck

CAPSULE 4.2   BLOOD IN CEREBROSPINAL FLUID

When blood enters the cerebrospinal fluid, the usually clear and colorless fluid changes to red or yellow. This color change is the result of the degradation of erythrocytes releasing oxyhemoglobin. In a time- and pH-dependent process, hemoglobin dissociates into heme and globin, and heme is converted to bilirubin. Bilirubin absorbs the blue part of the spectrum and transmits in the yellow. Substantial amounts of bilirubin must be present to be detected by the human eye (see accompanying figure), and spectrophotometry is more sensitive.[10,37] Oxyhemoglobin and bilirubin have overlapping spectra but can be distinguished reasonably well.[48] In some patients, the spectrophotometry calculations may fall in the equivocal zone and might produce imprecise bilirubin absorption measurements in analyzers. Hemolysis may occur when atmospheric air in the capped vial releases CO_2 and increases the pH, thus increasing the oxyhemoglobin content and falsely suggesting subarachnoid hemorrhage.[35]

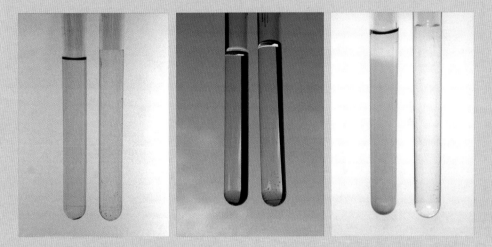

Left image: Tube (bloody cerebrospinal fluid) in a patient with subarachnoid hemorrhage compared with water. Note subtle xanthochromia after spinning in the laboratory, obscured by viewing in daylight (middle image), most evident against a strong light source (right image).

pain or stiffness, witnessed loss of consciousness, onset during exertion or sexual activity, instantly peaking pain in a thunderclap fashion, and limited neck flexion on examination. If one or more of these symptoms are present, there is an overall sensitivity of 99.2% (95% confidence interval 97.3%–99.8%) and a specificity of 99.6% (95% confidence limit 97.9%–99.9%) for subarachnoid hemorrhage.[44,47]

However, no emergency physician would defer a CT scan in any new headache, even if the pretest probability is low, but the real unresolved question is if these factors could determine the need for a lumbar puncture when CT scan is normal. Only about 4 patients among 3,000 patients with a normal CT scan (performed within 6 hours of onset) were eventually diagnosed with subarachnoid hemorrhage by lumbar puncture.[6,11]

MRI may detect subarachnoid hemorrhage where CT fails to show it (Figure 4.4). It remains a possible alternative in patients refusing lumbar puncture, but the negative and positive predictive value of MRI for detecting SAH is not known. Conditions other than aneurysmal SAH can be recognized by MRI and thus undermine the generally held tenet that CSF and CT should be sufficient to exclude underlying causes. No series of MRIs have been published on patients with thunderclap headaches; thus, recommendations to proceed with MRI or MRA in all cases are not solidly based on data. MRI has documented thunderclap headache associated with PRES

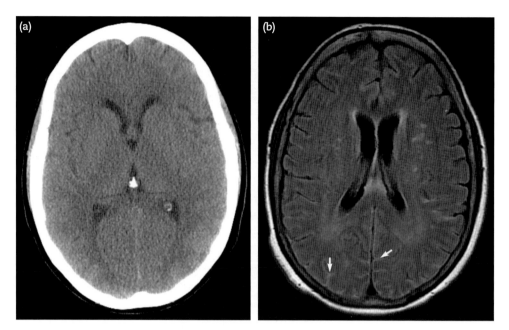

FIGURE 4.4: Negative CT (a) and FLAIR positive MRI (b) in patient with thunderclap headache and aneurysmal subarachnoid hemorrhage, imaged within 24 hours of each other.

pituitary apoplexia, signs of intracranial hypotension and meningeal enhancement, and retroclival hematoma.[13,15,53] Magnetic resonance angiography has documented carotid or vertebral artery dissection but should include the entire region from the origin of the arch to the circle of Willis to scrutinize for arterial dissection. Magnetic resonance venography (MRV) may discover cerebral venous thrombosis. However, upon retrospective analysis, each of these disorders had other clinical or laboratory clues suggesting the diagnosis.

In uncertain cases or in patients with ambiguous results, it is appropriate to proceed with a four-vessel cerebral angiogram. A CT angiogram may detect an aneurysm but it is just not good enough to confidently exclude an aneurysm. (One study found that DSA did have a 13% yield in patients with negative CTA).[29]

A cerebral angiogram may also seem appropriate in patients with a personal or family history of SAH and disorders associated with cerebral aneurysms (e.g., polycystic kidney disease). In all other patients, a cerebral angiogram is probably not recommended if neurologic examination, CT, and CSF are normal.[36,38,39,61]

Some patients with a migraine attack respond well to 900 mg of aspirin, 1,000 mg of acetaminophen, or high doses of nonsteroidal anti-inflammatory agents (NSAIDs). However, triptans and droperidol have been used,

including in the ED.[3,4,27,34,56,60] Contraindications include familial hemiplegic migraine, basilar migraine, ischemic stroke, ischemic heart disease, Prinzmetal angina, uncontrolled hypertension, combination with monoamine oxidase inhibitors or ergot compounds, and pregnancy. Abortive treatments for patients with therapy-resistant, persistent headaches lasting for hours are shown in Table 4.6.[7–9,23,26,30,59] and new agents have emerged.[20,31,49]

The designation of severity is very difficult to define, and the boundaries of rebound headache and analgesic-induced headache are not always that clear. The success of each of these pharmaceutical approaches in refractory migraine comes more from anecdotal clinical experience than clinical trials, and the mechanisms remain incompletely understood.[25]

Several other therapeutic options deserve mention. Dexamethasone has been commonly used in acute migraine treatment. However, a recent randomized trial of 10 mg IV dexamethasone found no effect in controlling acute migraine in the ED in patients with migraine lasting less than 72 hours (a positive effect may still prevail in patients with prolonged migraine and possibly at a higher dose).[24] There is interest in the use of valproate infusion. The lack of sedation makes it a good alternative; however, a nonrandomized trial found it no better than

TABLE 4.6. ABORTIVE THERAPIES IN UNRELENTING HEAD PAIN

Disorder	Therapy Options
Migraine	Sumatriptan (6 mg SC) or nasal spray 5 mg; repeat after 1 hour, if needed
	Droperidol (2.75–8.25 mg IM)
	Meperidine (100 mg IM) and hydroxyzine (50 mg IM)
	Valproate sodium (1,000 mg IV in 50 mL normal saline over 60 min)
	Dihydroergotamine (1–3 mg IV at hourly intervals) and metoclopramide (10 mg IM)
	Butorphanol nasal spray 1mg
	Ketorolac 30–60 mg IM
	Prochlorperazine 10 mg (in 10 mL saline infused in 2 min)
Cluster headache	Oxygen therapy (7 L/min face mask)
	Metoclopramide (10 mg IM)
	Sumatriptan (6 mg SC)
	Nasal butorphanol (1 mg/1 puff)
	Intranasal lidocaine 4% (4 sprays)
Trigeminal neuralgia	Fosphenytoin IV loading (15–20 mg/kg IV)
	Carbamazepine (1,200 mg/day)
	Lamotrigine (50–100 mg/day)
	Topiramate (50–100 mg/day)
Acute herpetic neuralgia	Tramadol (50–400 mg/day)
	Pregabalin (75–600 mg/day)
	Gabapentin (300–3600 mg/day)

IM, intramuscular; IV, intravenous; SC, subcutaneous.
References[39,54]

prochlorperazine.[58] A randomized trial of intravenous magnesium sulfate and metoclopramide in migraine showed a less favorable response than did metoclopramide alone.[9]

The treatment of evolving herpes zoster neuralgia is a major challenge. Apart from a likely benefit effect of valacyclovir or famciclovir (and possibly a corticosteroid course), the treatment is focused on (relatively rapid) escalating doses of opioids, gabapentin, or pregabalin until tolerated.[8]

In the treatment of refractory trigeminal neuralgia, antiepileptic drugs, antispasticity drugs, and tricyclic antidepressants, often in combination, may not be effective. In these patients, a preliminary study has shown that fosphenytoin loading (15–20 mg/kg) was rapidly successful. Lamotrigine or topiramate may take weeks to exert a maximal effect.[63,64] Other options are surgical, including ganglionic opioid analgesia, stereotactic radiosurgery, microvascular decompression, or percutaneous balloon compression.[19,54,57]

The response of cluster headache to subcutaneous sumatriptan or oxygen by nasal cannula is excellent, and refractory cases are quite uncommon.[40,41] Intranasal lidocaine or zolmitriptan is a good abortive therapy in cluster headache.[51] The options for severe cluster headache are shown in Table 4.6.

CONCLUSIONS

- The evaluation of severe headaches in the ED is common, and they often are not due to a major neurologic illness. The challenge is to identify that single patient with an emergency.
- The distinctive nature of a "thunderclap headache" needs to be recognized.
- Acute headache syndromes may be refractory migraine or cluster headache, and good treatment options exist in the ED.
- Acute severe headache may have a non-neurologic cause.

REFERENCES

1. Bahra A, May A, Goadsby PJ. Cluster headache: a prospective clinical study with diagnostic implications. *Neurology* 2002;58:354–361.
2. Beetham R, Fahie-Wilson MN, Park D. What is the role of CSF spectrophotometry in the

diagnosis of subarachnoid haemorrhage? *Ann Clin Biochem* 1998;35:1–4.

3. Brandes JL, Kudrow D, Stark SR, et al. Sumatriptan-naproxen for acute treatment of migraine: a randomized trial. *JAMA* 2007;297:1443 1454.

4. Cady R, Dodick DW. Diagnosis and treatment of migraine. *Mayo Clinic Proc* 2002;77:255–261.

5. Cheshire WP. Trigeminal neuralgia: for one nerve a multitude of treatments. *Expert Rev Neurother* 2007;7:1565–1579.

6. Chu K, Hann A, Greenslade J, Williams J, Brown A. Spectrophotometry or visual inspection to most reliably detect xanthochromia in subarachnoid hemorrhage: systematic review. *Ann Emerg Med* 2014;64:256–264.

7. Colman I, Friedman BW, Brown MD, et al. Parenteral dexamethasone for acute severe migraine headache: meta-analysis of randomised controlled trials for preventing recurrence. *BMJ* 2008;336:1359–1361.

8. Colman I, Rothney A, Wright SC, Zilkalns B, Rowe BH. Use of narcotic analgesics in the emergency department treatment of migraine headache. *Neurology* 2004;62:1695–1700.

9. Corbo J, Esses D, Bijur PE, Iannaccone R, Gallagher EJ. Randomized clinical trial of intravenous magnesium sulfate as an adjunctive medication for emergency department treatment of migraine headache. *Ann Emerg Med* 2001;38:621–627.

10. Cruickshank A, Auld P, Beetham R, et al. Revised national guidelines for analysis of cerebrospinal fluid for bilirubin in suspected subarachnoid haemorrhage. *Ann Clin Biochem* 2008; 45:238–244.

11. Czuczman AD, Thomas LE, Boulanger AB, et al. Interpreting red blood cells in lumbar puncture: distinguishing true subarachnoid hemorrhage from traumatic tap. *Acad Emerg Med* 2013;20:247–256.

12. Day JW, Raskin NH. Thunderclap headache: symptom of unruptured cerebral aneurysm. *Lancet* 1986;2:1247–1248.

13. de Bruijn SF, Stam J, Kappelle LJ. Thunderclap headache as first symptom of cerebral venous sinus thrombosis. CVST Study Group. *Lancet* 1996;348:1623–1625.

14. Dodick DW. Thunderclap headache. *J Neurol Neurosurg Psychiatry* 2002;72:6–11.

15. Dodick DW, Brown RD, Jr., Britton JW, Huston J, 3rd. Nonaneurysmal thunderclap headache with diffuse, multifocal, segmental, and reversible vasospasm. *Cephalalgia* 1999;19:118–123.

16. Dupont SA, Wijdicks EFM, Manno EM, Rabinstein AA. Thunderclap headache and normal computed tomographic results: value of cerebrospinal fluid analysis. *Mayo Clinic Proc* 2008;83:1326–1331.

17. Edlow JA. Diagnosis of subarachnoid hemorrhage. *Neurocrit Care* 2005;2:99–109.

18. Edlow JA, Malek AM, Ogilvy CS. Aneurysmal subarachnoid hemorrhage: update for emergency physicians. *J Emerg Med* 2008;34:237–251.

19. Elias WJ, Burchiel KJ. Microvascular decompression. *Clin J Pain* 2002;18:35–41.

20. Evans RW. Treating migraine in the emergency department. *BMJ* 2008;336:1320.

21. Evans RW, Dilli E, Dodick DW. Sentinel headache. *Headache* 2009;49:599–603.

22. Field AG, Wang E. Evaluation of the patient with nontraumatic headache: an evidence based approach. *Emerg Med Clin N Am* 1999;17: 127–152, ix.

23. Fisher CM. Honored guest presentation: painful states: a neurological commentary. *Clin Neurosurg* 1983;31:32–53.

24. Friedman BW, Greenwald P, Bania TC, et al. Randomized trial of IV dexamethasone for acute migraine in the emergency department. *Neurology* 2007;69:2038–2044.

25. Goadsby PJ. The vascular theory of migraine: a great story wrecked by the facts. *Brain* 2009;132:6–7.

26. Goadsby PJ, Lipton RB, Ferrari MD. Migraine: current understanding and treatment. *N Engl J Med* 2002;346:257–270.

27. Green MW. The emergency management of headaches. *Neurologist* 2003;9:93–98.

28. Green MW. A spectrum of exertional headaches. *Med Clin N Am* 2001;85:1085–1092.

29. Heit JJ, Pastena GT, Nogueira RG, et al. Cerebral Angiography for Evaluation of Patients with CT Angiogram-Negative Subarachnoid Hemorrhage: An 11-Year Experience. *AJNR* 2016;37:297–304.

30. Hill CH, Miner JR, Martel ML. Olanzapine versus droperidol for the treatment of primary headache in the emergency department. *Acad Emerg Med* 2008;15:806–811.

31. Ho TW, Ferrari MD, Dodick DW, et al. Efficacy and tolerability of MK-0974 (telcagepant), a new oral antagonist of calcitonin gene-related peptide receptor, compared with zolmitriptan for acute migraine: a randomised, placebo-controlled, parallel-treatment trial. *Lancet* 2008;372:2115–2123.

32. Jacome DE. Exploding head syndrome and idiopathic stabbing headache relieved by nifedipine. *Cephalalgia* 2001;21:617–618.

33. Jagoda AS, Dalsey WC, Fairweather PG, et al. Clinical policy: critical issues in the evaluation and management of patients presenting to the emergency department with acute headache. *Ann Emerg Med* 2002;39:108–122.

34. Jamieson DG. The safety of triptans in the treatment of patients with migraine. *Am J Med* 2002;112:135–140.

35. Kristensen SR, Salling AM, Kristensen ST, Hansen AB. Unrecognized preanalytical problem with the spectrophotometric analysis of

cerebrospinal fluid for xanthochromia. *Clin Chem* 2008;54:1924–1925.

36. Linn FH, Rinkel GJ, Algra A, van Gijn J. Follow-up of idiopathic thunderclap headache in general practice. *J Neurol* 1999;246:946–948.

37. Linn FH, Voorbij HA, Rinkel GJ, Algra A, van Gijn J. Visual inspection versus spectrophotometry in detecting bilirubin in cerebrospinal fluid. *J Neurol Neurosurg Psychiatry* 2005;76:1452–1454.

38. Linn FH, Wijdicks EFM, van der Graaf Y, et al. Prospective study of sentinel headache in aneurysmal subarachnoid haemorrhage. *Lancet* 1994;344:590–593.

39. Markus HS. A prospective follow up of thunderclap headache mimicking subarachnoid haemorrhage. *J Neurol Neurosurg Psychiatry* 1991;54:1117–1118.

40. Marmura MJ, Silberstein SD, Schwedt TJ. The acute treatment of migraine in adults: the American Headache Society evidence assessment of migraine pharmacotherapies. *Headache* 2015;55:3–20.

41. Matharu MS, Goadsby PJ. Persistence of attacks of cluster headache after trigeminal nerve root section. *Brain* 2002;125:976–984.

42. Miller TR, Shivashankar R, Mossa-Basha M, Gandhi D. Reversible cerebral vasoconstriction syndrome, part 1: epidemiology, pathogenesis, and clinical course. *AJNR Am J Neuroradiol* 2015;36:1392–1399.

43. Miller TR, Shivashankar R, Mossa-Basha M, Gandhi D. Reversible cerebral vasoconstriction syndrome, part 2: diagnostic work-up, imaging evaluation, and differential diagnosis. *AJNR Am J Neuroradiol* 2015;36:1580–1588.

44. Newman-Toker DE, Edlow JA. High-stakes diagnostic decision rules for serious disorders: the Ottawa subarachnoid hemorrhage rule. *JAMA* 2013;310:1237–1239.

45. Olesen J, Goadsby PJ. *Cluster Headache and Related Conditions*. Oxford: Oxford University Press; 1999.

46. Perry JJ, Spacek A, Forbes M, et al. Is the combination of negative computed tomography result and negative lumbar puncture result sufficient to rule out subarachnoid hemorrhage? *Ann Emerg Med* 2008;51:707–713.

47. Perry JJ, Stiell IG, Sivilotti ML, et al. Clinical decision rules to rule out subarachnoid hemorrhage for acute headache. *JAMA* 2013;310:1248–1255.

48. Petzold A, Sharpe LT, Keir G. Spectrophotometry for cerebrospinal fluid pigment analysis. *Neurocrit Care* 2006;4:153–162.

49. Potrebic S, Raskin NH. New abortive agents for the treatment of migraine. *Adv Intern Med* 2001;46:1–29.

50. Purdy RA, Ward TN. Dangerous and thunderclap headaches. *Headache* 2012;52 Suppl 2:56–59.

51. Rapoport AM, Mathew NT, Silberstein SD, et al. Zolmitriptan nasal spray in the acute treatment of cluster headache: a double-blind study. *Neurology* 2007;69:821–826.

52. Saper JR. Medicolegal issues: headache. *Neurol Clin* 1999;17:197–214.

53. Schievink WI, Thompson RC, Loh CT, Maya MM. Spontaneous retroclival hematoma presenting as a thunderclap headache: case report. *J Neurosurg* 2001;95:522–524.

54. Silberstein SD. Migraine. *Lancet* 2004;363:381–391.

55. Silberstein SD. Practice parameter: evidence-based guidelines for migraine headache (an evidence-based review): report of the Quality Standards Subcommittee of the American Academy of Neurology. *Neurology* 2000;55:754–762.

56. Silberstein SD, Young WB, Mendizabal JE, Rothrock JF, Alam AS. Acute migraine treatment with droperidol: a randomized, double-blind, placebo-controlled trial. *Neurology* 2003;60:315–321.

57. Skirving DJ, Dan NG. A 20-year review of percutaneous balloon compression of the trigeminal ganglion. *J Neurosurg* 2001;94:913–917.

58. Spacek A, Bohm D, Kress HG. Ganglionic local opioid analgesia for refractory trigeminal neuralgia. *Lancet* 1997;349:1521.

59. Trainor A, Miner J. Pain treatment and relief among patients with primary headache subtypes in the ED. *Am J Emerg Med* 2008;26:1029–1034.

60. Vinson DR. Emergency department treatment of migraine headaches. *Arch Intern Med* 2002;162:845; author reply 846.

61. Wijdicks EFM, Kerkhoff H, van Gijn J. Long-term follow-up of 71 patients with thunderclap headache mimicking subarachnoid haemorrhage. *Lancet* 1988;2:68–70.

62. Wijdicks EFM, Win PH. Excruciating headache but nothing obvious, look at the skin! *Practical Neurology* 2004;4:302–303.

63. Zakrzewska JM, Chaudhry Z, Nurmikko TJ, Patton DW, Mullens EL. Lamotrigine (lamictal) in refractory trigeminal neuralgia: results from a double-blind placebo controlled crossover trial. *Pain* 1997;73:223–230.

64. Zvartau-Hind M, Din MU, Gilani A, Lisak RP, Khan OA. Topiramate relieves refractory trigeminal neuralgia in MS patients. *Neurology* 2000;55:1587–1588.

5

Blacked Out and Slumped Down

Transient loss of consciousness, or syncope, may account for approximately 5% of emergency department (ED) admissions. The recurrence rate is high, with about a third of the patients having multiple events. The incidence of syncope is increased in the elderly, but in many instances the presentation is presyncope and falls. Finding the causes of syncope is never easy, and clinicians often find themselves considering several diagnostic possibilities. Very frequent episodes of syncope, delayed recovery of consciousness, the absence of prodromes, atypical triggers, eye closure, and syncope less than 1 minute may suggest psychogenic pseudosyncope but this diagnosis is very difficult to reliably assess in the ED.[2] The cause of a single syncopal episode continues to be unknown in about a third of the patients and is mostly due to neurally mediated syncope, such as a vasovagal attack, situational syncope, or carotid sinus syncope. In fewer than 1 in 10 patients, syncope is symptomatic of neurologic disease.[22,25] Substance abuse remains a common associated and possible contributing finding in certain ED surveys.[29] Syncope in elderly persons can often be attributed to the use of antihypertensives, neuroleptics, tricyclic antidepressants, or dopaminergic agents, or to some other trigger, such as dehydration. What is more challenging is that in the ED, the decision to admit a patient with syncope must be made on the basis of few clinical cues.

The evaluation of syncope is facilitated by the use of numerous algorithms that, when followed, may eventually lead to a diagnosis, but unexplained syncope nonetheless often leads to admission.[23,24] Generally, admission for diagnostic evaluation is mandatory for a patient with structural heart disease, with symptoms suggestive of arrhythmia or ischemia, or with electrocardiographic (EKG) abnormalities. Frequently, patients are admitted for treatment of orthostatic hypotension or for evaluation of whether to discontinue or modify the use of a likely offending drug. Syncope as a sign of acute occlusive vertebrobasilar disease

is rare, but this potential cause has remained a reason for consultation with a neurologist. A more common quandary is the distinction between syncope and seizure, and neurologists and cardiologists often courteously spar over this one.

CLINICAL ASSESSMENT

Syncope is typically defined as a transient, self-limiting loss of consciousness. Most patients fall as a result of syncope, but the recovery of consciousness is rapid. Although most studies have identified syncope duration as approximately 10 seconds, syncope may be clinically noticeable for a full minute. Studies have found that sudden cessation of cerebral blood flow for 6–8 seconds may cause a complete loss of consciousness, but tilt-table testing also found that a decrease in systolic blood pressure to 60 mm Hg could cause syncope. Most remarkable is that the return of orientation after syncope is immediate.

The diagnosis of syncope might seem straightforward, but history taking should include questions about the circumstances before the syncope attack, about body position and whether (a) the patient was supine, sitting, or standing; (b) the patient was active, at rest, or changed posture; (c) the syncope occurred during urination, defecation, cough, or swallowing; and (d) predisposing factors were present (for example, a crowded or warm environment, prolonged standing, or the immediate postprandial period, or sudden excruciating pain.[4,12,28] Some syncope attacks are preceded by nausea, vomiting, abdominal discomfort, blurred vision, dizziness, and a feeling of cold sweat. The history of the event is even more complete if it includes details such as the way in which the patient fell (slumped or keeled over); skin color; duration of loss of consciousness; breathing pattern, particularly loud breathing and snoring; movements and their duration; incontinence; and tongue biting. Medication use should be carefully reviewed for the presence of antihypertensives, antianginal medications, antidepressants,

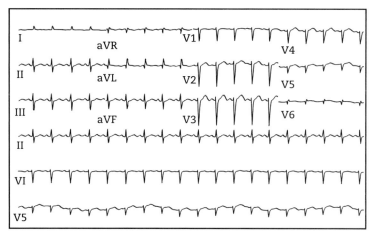

FIGURE 5.1: Prolonged QT syndrome in a patient with a history of multiple syncope attacks and marked hypotension. A normal QT is less than half the preceding RR interval and increases with slower heart rates.

antiarrhythmics, diuretics, and QT-prolonging agents (Figure 5.1 and Table 5.1).[15,16]

For the neurologist—evaluating a patient and knowing a priori that neurologic disease is not likely—specific questions about a prior neurologic history, such as Parkinson's disease, progressive neurodegenerative disorder, epilepsy, or perhaps most important, the possibility of narcolepsy, should be asked. The distinction between a seizure and syncope may be difficult to make and is certainly difficult to resolve in the ED. Any physician who has witnessed syncope appreciates the difficulty of differentiating it from acute stroke symptoms or a seizure. During syncope, a standing person rarely falls down suddenly but often gradually slumps sideways; the person may develop slurred speech, followed by head nodding, eye closure, and loss of postural tone.[18] Twitching and jerking, and particularly myoclonus, are often seen, and these signs are misinterpreted as seizures. Patients may be incontinent, which may simply reflect a full bladder at the time of the event. Pallor, a bitten tip of the tongue, and marked fatigue after the event may all be seen in syncope, and none indicates an epileptic seizure. Confusion that lasts more than 2 minutes, a lateral bite of the tongue, movement that is tonic and then clonic, and cyanosis are more typical features of a seizure that may be helpful in differentiating syncope from a true seizure. Most seizures occur with no warning. (By comparison, many patients with syncope recall that the "world was closing in" before they passed out.) Seizures are most likely to be suspected when the patient had tonic-clonic movements that were witnessed. Inquiries about automatisms such as chewing, lip smacking, or frothing at the mouth; tongue biting; a blue instead of pale face; the patient noting a funny or strange smell; prolonged confusion; or even combativeness after the event may be useful and may point to a seizure rather than syncope.

The most common type of syncope is termed neurally mediated syncope (Capsule 5.1). This syncope is caused by inhibition of vasomotor centers in the medulla (e.g., compression of the carotid baroreceptors, emptying of a distended bladder or bowel, overwhelming emotional shock or pain), which causes bradycardia. Vasodilatation plays a major role in this type of syncope. Several categories of neurally mediated syncope have been identified: central (emotionally generated), postural (due to suddenly becoming upright), and situational (caused by sneezing or coughing). Often, patients with this situational of syncope have a prior history of vasodilatory events prompted by an unexpected and unpleasant sight, sound, smell, or pain; by presence in a crowded, hot place; or by nausea and vomiting during a meal or postprandially. These features all suggest syncope. In addition, swallowing may cause syncope.[4] When swallowing is extremely painful (glossopharyngeal neuralgia), repeated bradycardia and asystole spells may occur. Cough syncope is seldom neurologic in origin and is mostly seen in patients with chronic pulmonary disease who may also have severe asymptomatic occlusive carotid and vertebral disease.

TABLE 5.1. CAUSES OF SYNCOPE

Neurally Mediated (Reflex) Syncope

Vasovagal syncope (common faint)
Carotid sinus syncope
Situational syncope
– Cough, sneeze, swallow, defecation, visceral pain
– Micturition
– After exercise
– After a meal
– Other causes
Glossopharyngeal neuralgia

Orthostatic Hypotension

Autonomic failure
– Primary autonomic failure syndromes (e.g., pure
  autonomic failure, multiple-system atrophy,
  Parkinson's disease with autonomic failure)
– Secondary autonomic failure syndromes (e.g.,
  diabetic neuropathy, amyloid neuropathy)
– Drugs and alcohol
– After exercise
– After a meal
Volume depletion
– Hemorrhage, diarrhea, Addison disease

Cardiac Arrhythmias

Sinus node dysfunction (including bradycardia-
  tachycardia syndrome)
Atrioventricular conduction system disease
Paroxysmal supraventricular and ventricular
  tachycardias
Congenital syndromes (e.g., long QT syndrome)
Malfunction of an implanted device (e.g., pacemaker,
  implantable cardioverter-defibrillator)
Drug-induced arrhythmias

Structural Cardiac or Cardiopulmonary Disease

Obstructive cardiac valvular disease
Acute myocardial infarction
Obstructive cardiomyopathy
Atrial myxoma
Acute aortic dissection
Pericardial disease
Pulmonary embolus and pulmonary hypertension

Data from Soteriades ES, Evans JC, Larson MG, et al. Incidence
and prognosis of syncope. *N Engl J Med* 2002,347.878–885; and
Strickberger SA, Benson W, Biaggioni I, et al. American Heart
Association Councils on Clinical Cardiology, Cardiovascular
Nursing, Cardiovascular Disease in the young, and, Stroke; Quality
of Care and Outcomes Research Interdisciplinary Working Group;
American College of Cardiology Foundation in collaboration with
the Heart Rhythm Society; American Autonomic Society. AHA/
ACCF scientific statement on the evaluation of syncope. *Circulation*
2006; 113:316–327. With permission of the publishers.

Orthostatic hypotension is suggested when syncope occurs after standing up, recent to the introduction of a medication that may lead to hypotension, in the presence of a neurodegenerative disease, or in the period after exertion. Cardiac syncope is often preceded by palpitation and may occur during exertion or when in a supine position. Often, a patient with cardiac syncope has evidence of structural heart disease.

In the initial assessment, it is necessary to identify whether the patient fits into a higher-risk group. Patients in this group have chest pain compatible with an acute coronary syndrome, have signs of congestive heart failure and moderate to severe valvular disease, or have a history of ventricular arrhythmia, prior abnormal EKG findings, persistent sinus bradycardia, and atrial fibrillation. During the diagnostic assessment, the EKG provides an important initial evaluation.[5,7,8,21] The most crucial and concerning EKG abnormalities suggestive of arrhythmic syncope are shown in Table 5.2. Some patients have bradycardia during an epileptic seizure, which complicates the diagnostic evaluation.[19,27] Several cases of ictal bradycardia have been described in which the patients had a partial seizure followed by marked bradycardia (Figure 5.2). For most of these patients, the seizure originated in the temporal lobe. Bradycardia may occur in approximately 5% of cases and may be particularly severe, even causing a true syncope after the initial seizure. Its treatment is similar to that of any other type of syncope, and usually involves pacemaker placement. However, ictal tachycardia is far more common, occurring in about two-thirds of patients, and is less of a concern.

Finally, *narcolepsy* is an unusual cause of blackouts. Usually, onset of symptoms is between 15 and 25 years of age, but it may occur at a much younger age or, in women, in the postmenopausal stage. Sudden loss of muscle tone (cataplexy) with laughing, anger, or an emotional response to a major surprise may cause these symptoms and is a common manifestation. Sleep paralysis (the inability to move limbs or to speak upon awakening or at sleep onset) may often occur, sometimes accompanied by vivid visual hallucination.[30]

LINE OF ACTION

Risk stratification in the ED may be helpful for patients with syncope. A low-risk group (in which the syncope is likely benign) are patients younger than 50 years who have no previous history of

> **CAPSULE 5.1 AUTONOMIC CONTROL IN NEURALLY MEDIATED SYNCOPE**
>
> Several theories have been proposed to explain the pathophysiology in neurally mediated syncope. The ventricular theory is complex and disputed, but it postulates that baroreceptors detect a decrease in blood pressure followed by an increase in sympathetic activity. This heightened sympathetic tone increases vascular resistance and cardiac inotropy, resulting in increased contraction and, eventually, an "empty chamber." This empty chamber stimulates the left ventricular efferents, resulting in an inhibitory response that causes hypotension, increased vagal tone, and bradycardia, resulting in syncope. The baroreflex dysfunction theory postulates that the baroreceptor responses may have been reset or suppressed by a depressor reflex from the heart. The reduced blood volume theory has been discarded because most changes are in blood volume redistribution and not in a reduced total blood volume. The neurohumoral theory proposes increased plasma epinephrine concentration or serotonin surges but is not supported by experimental studies. The active vasodilatation theory postulates that hypotension is a result of cholinergic stimulation. Finally, and most interesting, is the cerebrovascular blood flow dysregulation theory, which implies an abnormal response to orthostatic stress and is supported by the documentation of cerebral vasoconstriction and reduced cerebral blood flow in patients with recurrent syncope. The possible mechanisms of syncope are shown in the accompanying figure.
>
>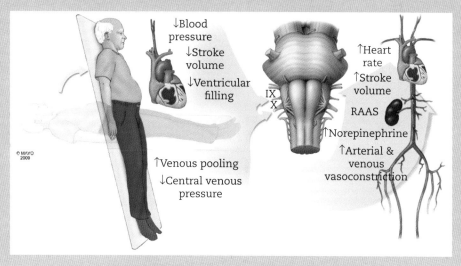
>
> Neurohumoral responses to an induced orthostatic challenge.
> IX, glossopharyngeal nerve; RAAS, renin angiotensin system; X, vagal nerve.

cardiovascular disease, have normal cardiovascular examination results, and have symptoms suggestive of a reflex-mediated or vasovagal syncope.[6,9,10,26] Simple measures may be possible in the treatment of vasovagal syncope in an elderly person and include physical counter-maneuvers, salt supplementation, and use of fludrocortisone acetate and midodrine hydrochloride.[14] Other patients may be admitted to a coronary care unit for further evaluation of a possible cardiac arrhythmia.

During evaluation in the ED, specific attention is directed toward recognition of a long QT syndrome that mimics seizures, and interpretation errors are comparatively common.[20] Holter monitoring is typically used for patients with syncope, but 24 hours may not be enough time for identifying potentially important arrhythmias.[3,17]

TABLE 5.2. ELECTROCARDIOGRAM ABNORMALITIES SUGGESTIVE OF ARRHYTHMIC SYNCOPE

Bifascicular block (defined as either a left bundle-branch block or a right bundle-branch block combined with a left anterior or left posterior fascicular block)

Other intraventricular conduction abnormalities (e.g., a QRS duration ≥ 0.12 seconds)

Mobitz I second-degree atrioventricular block

Asymptomatic sinus bradycardia (< 50 beats/min), sinoatrial block, or sinus pause (≥ 3 seconds) in the absence of negatively chronotropic medications

Pre-excited QRS complexes

Prolonged QT interval

Right bundle-branch block pattern with ST elevation in leads V1–V3 (Brugada syndrome)

Negative T waves in right precordial leads, epsilon waves and ventricular late potentials suggestive of arrhythmogenic right ventricular dysplasia

Q waves suggestive of myocardial infarction

Data from Soteriades ES, Evans JC, Larson MG, et al. Incidence and prognosis of syncope. *N Engl J Med* 2002;347:878–885; and Strickberger SA, Benson W, Biaggioni I, et al. American Heart Association Councils on Clinical Cardiology, Cardiovascular Nursing, Cardiovascular Disease in the young, and, Stroke; Quality of Care and Outcomes Research Interdisciplinary Working Group; American College of Cardiology Foundation in collaboration with the Heart Rhythm Society; American Autonomic Society. AHA/ACCF scientific statement on the evaluation of syncope. *Circulation* 2006; 113:316–327. With permission of the publishers.

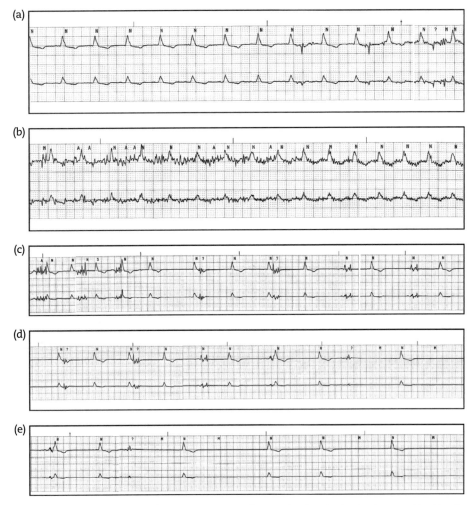

FIGURE 5.2: Electrocardiogram (EKG) strip in a patient with generalized tonic-clonic seizure and ictal bradycardia.

The beginning of the EKG strip (a and b) shows constant muscle artifact as a result of a clonic phase followed by intermittent periods of muscle artifact indicative of clonic activity (b and c) gradually diminishing (d) and followed by bradycardia (e).

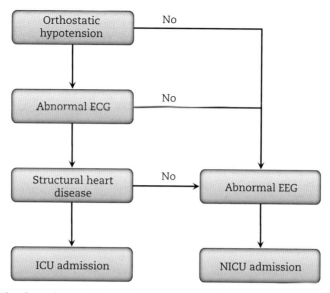

FIGURE 5.3: Algorithm for evaluation of syncope in the emergency department.

ECG, electrocardiogram; EEG, electroencephalogram; ICU, intensive care unit; NICU, neurosciences intensive care unit.

One study found that the diagnostic value of monitoring for evaluation of syncope was approximately 9%.[1] Continuous-loop event monitoring may increase yield, but its role has not been completely defined. An implantable continuous-loop recorder inserted subcutaneously has the capability of monitoring for about 18 months; however, the incidence of an event is low. Bradycardia in the setting of seizures requires not only treatment of seizures but in most instances a pacemaker to prevent life-threatening events.

Admission to the NICU is justified for a patient with seizures, and associated cardiac arrhythmias, glossopharyngeal neuralgia, and multiple episodes of bradycardia, clinical signs suggestive of occlusive basilar artery disease, or neurodegenerative disease, with autonomic failure. The yield of computed tomographic (CT) scan abnormalities is extremely low (one infarction in the posterior circulation in 128 patients with syncope) but may identify lesions that may point to seizures to some degree.[13] The yield of EKG in syncope is equally low.[11] The evaluation of syncope is summarized in Figure 5.3.

CONCLUSIONS

- Syncope rarely heralds an acute neurologic disease but may be part of an undiagnosed chronic neurologic illness.
- Narcolepsy may look like syncope.
- Syncope may be provoked by valsalva, cough, and swallowing.
- Cardiac arrhythmias can mimic seizures or may be caused by seizures.
- Patients with ictal bradycardia likely need a pacemaker.

REFERENCES

1. Bass EB, Curtiss EI, Arena VC, et al. The duration of Holter monitoring in patients with syncope. Is 24 hours enough? *Arch Intern Med* 1990;150:1073–1078.
2. Blad H, Lamberts RJ, Gert van Dijk J et al. Tilt-induced vasovagal syncope and psychogenic pseudosyncope: Overlapping clinical entities. *Neurology* 2015;85:2006–2010.
3. Blanc JJ, L'Her C, Touiza A, et al. Prospective evaluation and outcome of patients admitted for syncope over a 1 year period. *Eur Heart J* 2002;23:815–820.
4. Boos CJ, Martin U, Cherry RC, Marshall HJ. Dangerous sandwiches. *Lancet* 2008;372:2164.
5. Brignole M. Different electrocardiographic manifestations of the cardioinhibitory vasovagal reflex. *Europace* 2009;11:144–146.
6. Brignole M, Alboni P, Benditt DG, et al. Guidelines on management (diagnosis and treatment) of syncope: update 2004. *Europace* 2004;6:467–537.
7. Brignole M, Disertori M, Menozzi C, et al. Management of syncope referred urgently to general hospitals with and without syncope units. *Europace* 2003;5:293–298.
8. Brignole M, Menozzi C, Bartoletti A, et al. A new management of syncope: prospective

systematic guideline-based evaluation of patients referred urgently to general hospitals. *Eur Heart J* 2006;27:76–82.

9. Chen LY, Benditt DG, Shen WK. Management of syncope in adults: an update. *Mayo Clinic Proc* 2008;83:1280–1293.

10. Chen LY, Shen WK, Mahoney DW, Jacobsen SJ, Rodeheffer RJ. Prevalence of syncope in a population aged more than 45 years. *Am J Med* 2006;119:1088 e1-7.

11. Davis TL, Freemon FR. Electroencephalography should not be routine in the evaluation of syncope in adults. *Arch Intern Med* 1990;150:2027–2029.

12. Freeman R. Clinical practice. Neurogenic orthostatic hypotension. *N Engl J Med* 2008;358: 615–624.

13. Giglio P, Bednarczyk EM, Weiss K, Bakshi R. Syncope and head CT scans in the emergency department. *Emerg Radiol* 2005;12:44–46.

14. Guzman JC, Armaganijan LV, Morillo CA. Treatment of neurally mediated reflex syncope. *Cardiol Clin* 2013;31:123–129.

15. Jhanjee R, van Dijk JG, Sakaguchi S, Benditt DG. Syncope in adults: terminology, classification, and diagnostic strategy. *Pacing Clin Electrophysiol* 2006;29:1160–1169.

16. Kapoor WN. Syncope. *N Engl J Med* 2000;343: 1856–1862.

17. Kuhne M, Schaer B, Moulay N, Sticherling C, Osswald S. Holter monitoring for syncope: diagnostic yield in different patient groups and impact on device implantation. *QJM* 2007;100:771–777.

18. Lempert T, Bauer M, Schmidt D. Syncope: a videometric analysis of 56 episodes of transient cerebral hypoxia. *Ann Neurol* 1994;36:233–237.

19. Leutmezer F, Schernthaner C, Lurger S, Potzelberger K, Baumgartner C. Electrocardiographic changes at the onset of epileptic seizures. *Epilepsia* 2003;44:348–354.

20. MacCormick JM, McAlister H, Crawford J, et al. Misdiagnosis of long QT syndrome as epilepsy at first presentation. *Ann Emerg Med* 2009;54:26–32.

21. Ruwald MH, Zareba W. ECG monitoring in syncope. *Prog Cardiovasc Dis* 2013;56:203–210.

22. Saklani P, Krahn A, Klein G. Syncope. *Circulation* 2013;127:1330–1339.

23. Silverstein MD, Singer DE, Mulley AG, Thibault GE, Barnett GO. Patients with syncope admitted to medical intensive care units. *JAMA* 1982;248:1185–1189.

24. Smars PA, Decker WW, Shen WK. Syncope evaluation in the emergency department. *Curr Opin Cardiol* 2007;22:44–48.

25. Soteriades ES, Evans JC, Larson MG, et al. Incidence and prognosis of syncope. *N Engl J Med* 2002;347:878–885.

26. Strickberger SA, Benson DW, Biaggioni I, et al. AHA/ACCF Scientific Statement on the evaluation of syncope: from the American Heart Association Councils on Clinical Cardiology, Cardiovascular Nursing, Cardiovascular Disease in the Young, and Stroke, and the Quality of Care and Outcomes Research Interdisciplinary Working Group; and the American College of Cardiology Foundation: in collaboration with the Heart Rhythm Society: endorsed by the American Autonomic Society. *Circulation* 2006;113:316–327.

27. Tinuper P, Bisulli F, Cerullo A, et al. Ictal bradycardia in partial epileptic seizures: autonomic investigation in three cases and literature review. *Brain* 2001;124:2361–2371.

28. Wieling W, Thijs RD, van Dijk N, et al. Symptoms and signs of syncope: a review of the link between physiology and clinical clues. *Brain* 2009;132:2630–2642.

29. Wiener Z, Chiu DT, Shapiro NI, Grossman SA. Substance abuse in emergency department patients with unexplained syncope. *Intern Emerg Med* 2014;9:331–334.

30. Wise MS, Arand DL, Auger RR, Brooks SN, Watson NF. Treatment of narcolepsy and other hypersomnias of central origin. *Sleep* 2007;30:1712–1727.

6

See Nothing, See Double, See Shapes

Much like acute "often more recognizable" focal signs, sudden loss of visual acuity or clarity, or the appearance of newly formed images, may actually indicate a major neurologic condition, and additional investigations are required to diagnose acute neuro-ophthalmologic conditions. A certain presentation is obvious to the patient and examining neurologist—such as ptosis in third nerve palsy- and requires immediate magnetic resonance imaging (MRI) or cerebral angiography. Acute (transient) monocular vision loss may suggest a blockage involving the anterior cerebral circulation,[8] and acute binocular vision loss may point to occlusion in the territory of the posterior cerebral circulation—all requiring cerebrovascular neurology expertise.

If it can be obtained in the emergency setting additional consultation by an ophthalmologist is very helpful because many enigmatic presentations of monocular blindness are due to acute retinal or optic nerve disorders.

The emergency department (ED) may not be the place to commit one to definitively resolving the differential diagnosis of any of these conditions, and these patients may need admission. This chapter is included for the purpose of describing common urgent neuro-ophthalmologic disorders associated with decreased vision and positive visual phenomena.

CLINICAL ASSESSMENT

Poor vision due to a refractive error is easily discovered by having the patient look through a pinhole punched in a piece of paper. (Vision will improve if an error of refraction is the cause.) Other testing methods in the ED are limited, but certain tests should be performed on every patient presenting with major symptoms of a defective visual system. The first test in a patient with marked reduction in vision is to assess "blink to threat." This is a test preferably performed in patients with reduced level of consciousness or those who claim to have no vision. The best technique is to approach both eyes from the lateral visual field with a closed fist and then open up the fist to a hand with spread-out fingers several inches before the eyes. Absence of blinking to threat is often is noticed in hemianopic fields. Confrontation field testing is useful to delineate hemianopic and altitudinal defects, but it requires quiet cooperation from the patient and is not very accurate (a small red pin is much better).[10] The good technique is to present two fingers in each visual field quadrant of both eyes, typically midway between the patient and the examiner. Movement or finger counting can be used to indicate vision. Testing is followed by examination of the pupillary size and pupillary reaction to light.

Pupillary abnormalities are important telltale signs, but the interpretation is much more difficult than is appreciated. A common mnemonic, *PERRLA*, reminds the investigator of the different components of pupil assessment (*p*upils *e*qual, *r*ound, *r*eactive, *l*ight response, *a*ccommodation response).

Anisocoria without any change in dim or bright light is physiologic. In a Horner syndrome, anisocoria increases in dim light. It also increases in structural pupillary abnormalities, such as prior synechia or uveitis. In Horner syndrome, interruption of the oculosympathetic pathway also produces ptosis or reduced upper lid folding. A recognized cause for an acute Horner syndrome is carotid artery dissection (distention of the injured arterial wall damages the sympathetic fibers). In Horner's syndrome the face may be warm and the skin dry but *anhidrosis* is typically absent in Horner's syndrome due to lesions above the bifurcation (the fibers supplying the face accompany the external carotid artery below the carotid artery bifurcation).

Anisocoria increasing in bright light is virtually always caused by mydriasis due to pharmacologic effects but could be due to a third-nerve palsy if the reaction to diluted pilocarpine (0.1%) is negative and constriction occurs with 1.0% pilocarpine. Dilating the pupils with phenylephrine, which stimulates the iris dilator, generally should

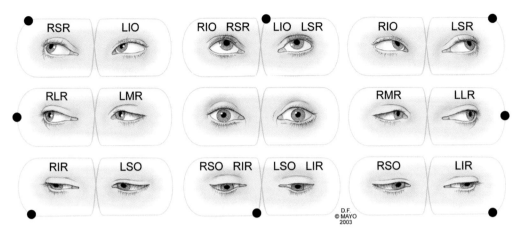

FIGURE 6.1: Baseline examination of eye movements and responsible muscles using standard figure-of-eight tracking (patient follows black dot).

LIO, left inferior oblique; LIR, left inferior rectus; LLR, left lateral rectus; LMR, left medial rectus; LSO, left superior oblique; LSR, left superior rectus; RIO, right inferior oblique; RIR, right inferior rectus; RLR, right lateral rectus; RMR, right medial rectus; RSO, right superior oblique; RSR, right superior rectus.

be discouraged in acutely progressive neuro-ophthalmologic disorders because it may take several hours for the pupil to regain its response to light.

Funduscopy is necessarily limited to the optic disk and retinal vasculature, and specific note should be made of the caliber of the arteries, flame-like hemorrhages, edema, or change in color of the retinal pigment. Examination is followed by testing of ocular eye movements in the horizontal and vertical directions with the intent of detecting misalignment. Voluntary gaze in all fields includes up, down, left, and right, but it is also useful to test figure-of-eight tracking (Figure 6.1).

Blindness

Blindness is usually defined as vision of less than 20/200 with correction or a field not subtending an angle greater than 20 degrees (legal blindness; see Capsule 6.1). *Functional blindness* is not further considered here but is easily diagnosed when a large mirror or a newspaper page with multiple images is moved in front of the patient and results in brief saccades.

Acute blindness may involve both eyes and, excluding ophthalmologic disorders, points to bilateral involvement of the occipital lobes. Differential diagnosis involves acute basilar artery occlusive disease, cerebral venous thrombosis, posterior reversible encephalopathy syndrome (PRES), and many drug-induced encephalopathies with PRES like pictures that include vincristine, methotrexate, cyclosporine, and tacrolimus.

Monocular blindness is more common than acute loss of entire vision. In addition, transient monocular visual loss is more commonly encountered in the ED than is persistent monocular defect. Transient monocular visual loss often includes embolization due to lesions of the aortic arch, heart valves, or carotid artery but may also include abnormalities associated with increased viscosity or hypercoagulability. Many patients would need admission to further evaluate its mechanism.

Visual loss (uni- or bilateral) may result from lesions at any topographic location of the afferent visual system ending in the occipital poles. Monocular vision loss often indicates an ophthalmologic disorder, and these are shown in Table 6.1.[17,35] A neurologic cause for monocular visual loss is most likely optic neuropathy. It typically manifests with markedly reduced visual acuity (20/200), inability to recognize color or its

CAPSULE 6.1	DEGREE OF VISUAL LOSS
20/200	Legal blindness
20/800	Finger counting
2/1000	Arm movements
20/∞	Light perception
0	No light perception

TABLE 6.1. OPHTHALMOLOGIC DISORDERS

Diagnosis	Findings
Central retinal artery occlusion	Afferent pupil defect Retinal edema Optic disk pallor and cherry- red spots
Retinal vein occlusion	"Blood-and-thunder" fundus (extensive intraretinal hemorrhages)
Retinal detachment	Translucent gray wrinkled retina
Ischemic optic neuropathy	Pale optic nerve Milky, swelling Scalp tenderness and absent temporal artery pulsation (giant cell arteritis)
Optic neuritis	Normal findings ("patient sees nothing, doctor sees nothing") Early pallor
Vitreous hemorrhage	Diabetes, hypertension

brightness (particularly red), and often no obvious findings on neurologic examination except an afferent pupil defect.[3] The optic disk may take time to become abnormal but may show pallor or elevation. Such an afferent pupillary defect (*Marcus-Gunn pupil*) is traditionally examined using the swinging flashlight test. The patient is asked to fixate on a distant target to eliminate the miotic effect of accommodation. A bright light is moved from one eye to the other. The response may vary from minimal asymmetry to pupils failing to constrict or dilate when the penlight moves to the affected eye. In its most pronounced form, pupils dilate immediately when the light shines into the diseased eye. Afferent pupillary defect is linked to optic neuropathy, but a retinal lesion or massive intravitreous hemorrhage (Terson syndrome) may produce similar findings.

Optic neuritis is associated with periocular pain and pain with eye movement in 90% of cases.[16] The causes of optic neuritis are manyfold and can typically be divided into inflammatory causes and the first manifestations of multiple sclerosis (5-year probability of later MS is 30%).[31] Inflammatory causes may include common bacterial infections, as by *Streptococcus* and *Staphylococcus*, but also extremely serious infections, such as toxoplasmosis, cryptococcosis, aspergillosis, and mucormycosis in susceptible immunosuppressed patients. In other patients, optic neuritis may occur after a vaccination or viral illness, or in the setting of connective tissue disease or sarcoidosis. Hereditary optic neuropathy may also present with acute monocular visual loss; and in approximately 50% of patients, family history can be elicited. Certain toxic optic neuropathies have been described; these include methanol, ethambutol, isoniazid, thiamine (B1), and folate deficiency.

Diplopia

Acute diplopia is complex to analyze, and the underlying deficit may remain ambiguous. Monocular diplopia, almost always due to abnormalities in the refractive media, precludes further neurologic workup. Binocular diplopia is difficult to assess because in some patients multiple cranial nerve involvement is present. Questions that could clarify the chief complaint in acute diplopia should include mode of onset, diplopia disappearing after one eye is closed, whether vertically or horizontally oriented, whether always present or fluctuating, and whether more pronounced in a certain gaze. A survey in the emergency department found, unsurprisingly, that additional neurologic symptoms in a patient presenting with diplopia pointed to a "secondary cause." Stroke was found in nearly half of 200 patients, multiple sclerosis in nearly 20%.[25]

Figure 6.2 shows nine cardinal positions of gaze in oculomotor palsies, each providing fairly characteristic deviations of the globe. In addition, Table 6.2 provides a simplified practical guide for sorting out the different cranial nerve palsies associated with diplopia.[7,23,33,37] Table 6.3 lists disorders that indicate the need for urgent evaluation.[23] *Skew deviation* may be associated with diplopia and indicates an internuclear lesion. It is a result of abnormalities in fibers ascending vertically from vestibular nuclei within the medial longitudinal fasciculus. Not infrequently, it is due to a pontine stroke in elderly patients and multiple sclerosis in younger patients (Figure 6.3). It is important to

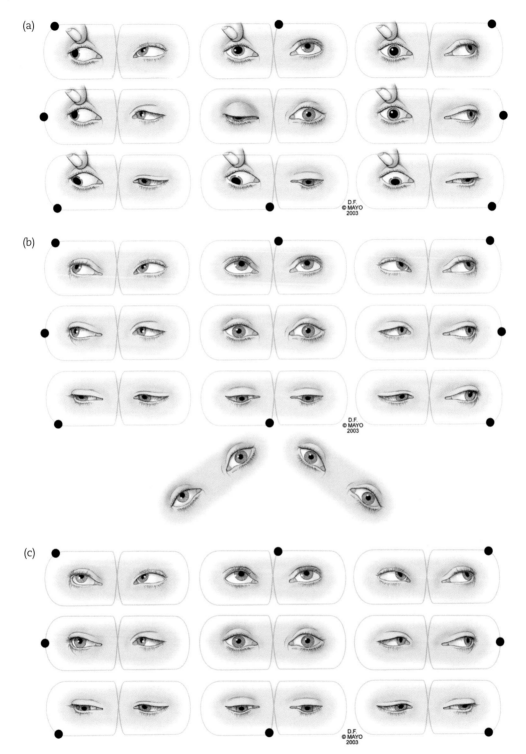

FIGURE 6.2: Nine gaze positions in (a) third-nerve palsy, (b) fourth-nerve palsy, and (c) sixth-nerve palsy (patient follows black dot).

TABLE 6.2. DIPLOPIA DUE TO CRANIAL NERVE PALSY

Cranial Nerve	Position of Eye	Diplopia	Additional Features
III	Down and out	Crossed	Ptosis, dilated fixed pupil
IV	Higher	Vertical	Head tilted away from affected side, chin down
VI	Inward	Uncrossed*	Head turned to affected side

* The image appears on the same side as the eye that sees it.

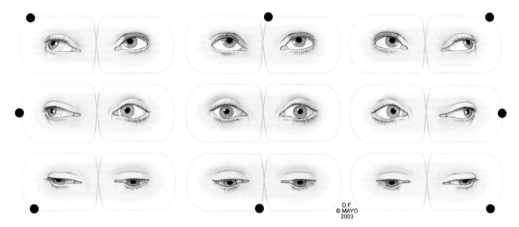

FIGURE 6.3: Internuclear ophthalmoplegia (patient follows black dot).

TABLE 6.3. URGENT DISORDERS IN ACUTE DIPLOPIA

Acute third-nerve palsy	Basilar artery aneurysm, posterior communicating artery aneurysm*
	Pituitary apoplexy
	Acute midbrain infarct or hemorrhage
	Mucormycosis*
	Carotid cavernous fistula
	Granulomatous inflammation (Tolosa-Hunt)
	Diabetic microvascular disease†
Acute fourth-nerve palsy	Trauma
	Meningitis, infectious or neoplastic*
	Herpes zoster ophthalmicus*
Acute sixth-nerve palsy	Carotid aneurysm
	Cavernous sinus thrombosis*
	Nasopharyngeal carcinoma
	Increased intracranial pressure

*Also known as the painful ophthalmoplegias.[11]
†More often pupil-sparing.

additionally recognize a painful ophthalmoplegia, which has a different differential diagnosis (Table 6.3).[16] The cause of acute diplopia, however, may also include other factors, such as difficulty with movement of the globe due to mass effect in the orbit[5] (thyrotoxicosis), diplopia caused by an acute manifestation of myasthenia gravis, and chronic progressive external ophthalmoplegia, particularly if ptosis is bilateral. A cavernous sinus lesion should be considered when an abducens lesion is associated with Horner's syndrome. Acute oculomotor palsy with preceding retro-orbital pain may be a sign of unruptured posterior communicating aneurysm,[9] and two-thirds may be smaller than 6 mm; it may herald rupture and indicate rapid aneurysm growth.[38] Development of pupil involvement, albeit uncommon, may be particularly worrisome for pending rupture

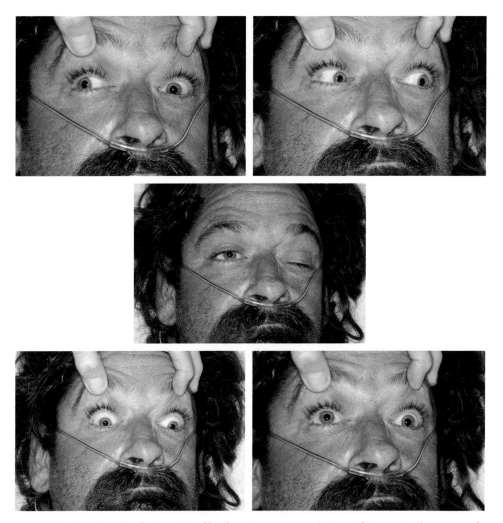

FIGURE 6.4: Third-nerve palsy due to ruptured basilar artery aneurysm. Note pupil asymmetry (compare with gaze positions in Figure 6.2a).

(Figure 6.4).[21] Pupil-sparing may indicate a recent ischemic stroke in the mesencephalon (Figure 6.5).[34] The differential diagnosis also includes multiple sclerosis.[29]

A very urgent condition is *carotid cavernous fistula*,[13,18,22,26] in which trauma to the orbit may be remote (e.g., hit against windshield) or early, such as after transsphenoidal pituitary surgery, carotid endarterectomy, or ethmoidal surgery.[22,26] Associations with Ehlers-Danlos syndrome and pregnancy have been noted in carotid cavernous fistula, or it may occur spontaneously. Lid swelling and orbital pain with characteristic pulsating exophthalmos and tortuous conjunctival vessels point to its diagnosis (Figure 6.6). Funduscopy may demonstrate pulsating venous dilation and, in more extreme forms, disk edema and ophthalmoplegia. Ophthalmoplegia may be due to restricted excursions or cranial nerve injury in the segments traversing the cavernous or petrosal sinus. Visual loss is a consequence of increased intraocular pressure and reversal of flow or thrombus in the superior ophthalmic vein. There is a need for full angiographic documentation. Immediate opacification of the cavernous sinus is seen after carotid injection.

Complete Ptosis

A curious phenomenon is apraxia of eyelid opening (the patient is unable to open the eyes).[6,36] The orbicularis oculi does not contract, and the frontalis muscles are used to try

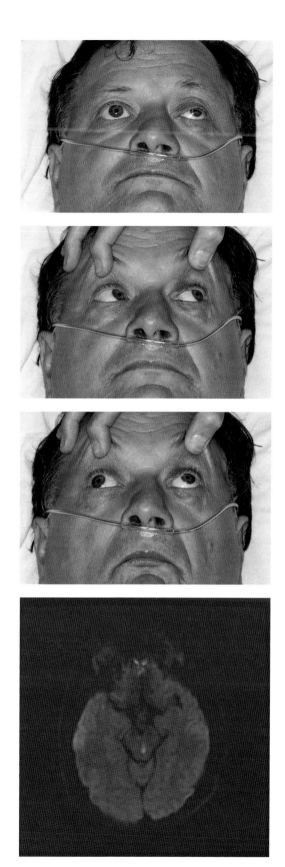

FIGURE 6.5: Third-nerve palsy due to mesencephalon infarct on MRI DWI (pupil-sparing).

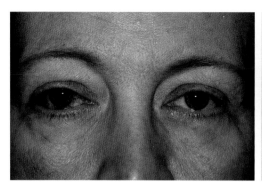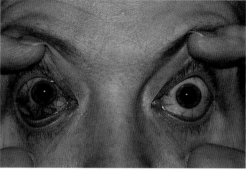

FIGURE 6.6: Exophthalmos, chemosis, and red eye (right) in traumatic carotid cavernous fistula. The abnormality is barely seen but becomes clear with further retraction of the eyelids.

to perform this act, but the eyes may remain completely closed. This disorder has been linked to acute nondominant hemispheric lesions[6,12] (e.g., putaminal hemorrhage and large hemispheric infarcts) but also to paraneoplastic encephalitis.[36] The pathways are unknown but involve supranuclear connections in the nondominant hemisphere. Lesions may be at brainstem level, and this condition is more common when brainstem displacement occurs[2,6,12] (Chapter 29).

Visual Illusions

Positive visual phenomena may need careful attention and evaluation. Images perceived as false may indicate an acute hemispheric lesion or significant neurotoxicity. Visual hallucinations may take many forms, from dots, geometric shapes, and lines to dream-like descriptions of figures, animals (often frightening), and detailed movie-like scenes (midbrain peduncular hallucinations). First, neurotoxicity should be excluded by history. Drugs to treat Parkinson's disease (e.g., levodopa, lisuride, mesulergine, pergolide) or depression (e.g., amitriptyline, imipramine, lithium carbonate), stimulants (amphetamine, cocaine), and immunosuppressive agents (cyclosporine, tacrolimus) should be considered as causes of visual hallucinations. Hallucinations with migrainous components, such as fortifications (zigzag lines in parallel) that are constantly in the same visual field, could point to an arteriovenous malformation.[20] Visual hallucinations may be due to seizures, albeit rarely, when isolated, not accompanied by head or eye deviation or rapid blinking, or associated with a transient hemianopic field defect. However, it is not always appreciated that colored comma shapes

or white streaks flashing in a vertical direction may be due to vitreous detachment.

Palinopsia involves an image that persists after looking at a subject, rapidly fades or returns hours later, and is superimposed on certain objects.[4,14,28,30] It has been noted with encephalitis, fulminant multiple sclerosis, and brain tumors, but seizures,[24] illicit drugs (lysergic acid diethylamide),[19] and major psychiatric pathology are equally common causes.[15]

Micropsia (objects appear smaller) is rarely caused by cerebral lesions and is more typically seen with retinal lesions. Unilateral *metamorphopsia* (illusion that objects are distorted; also common in macular degeneration) may indicate a parietal lobe lesion and may be limited to facial images. It probably only occurs as an ictal phenomenon.[39]

LINE OF ACTION

Many conditions are associated with diplopia or visual loss. Some acute neuro-ophthalmologic conditions may point to an acute neurologic condition that needs immediate evaluation. The critical steps in gathering key features of the presentation of a patient with the most urgent concerns are shown in Figure 6.7. This most likely involves immediate MRI or cerebral angiography. A neurosurgical consult is mandated in any patient with a painful ophthalmoplegia, due to its correlation with lesions that may require skull base surgery or endovascular procedures. A compressive or infiltrative lesion that affects the optic nerve should be excluded by an MRI scan. An MR angiogram to exclude an intracranial aneurysm should be considered when appropriate because an anterior cerebral aneurysm can leak into the

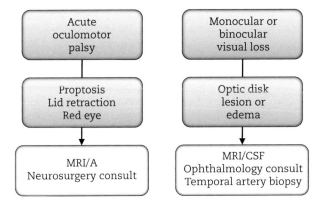

FIGURE 6.7. Critical steps in acute neuro-ophthalmology.

CSF, cerebrospinal fluid; MRI/A, magnetic resonance imaging/angiography.

optic sheath and can be responsible for acute monocular blindness.[8] Balloon or coil occlusion in carotid cavernous fistula has been successful, including reversibility of blindness.[1,16,22,27]

Unexpected loss of vision may have many causes and can be further delineated by an emergent ophthalmology examination. Giant cell arteritis usually presents with severe headache, jaw claudication, and scalp tenderness; but visual loss may be a presenting feature (estimated 20%). Color duplex sonography of the superficial temporal artery is the first imaging modality, and when positive a hypoechoic halo around the lumen of the temporal artery is found. Temporal artery biopsy should follow, but not necessarily before administration of corticosteroids, usually prednisone 60 mg daily for 4 weeks. However, immediate administration of methylprednisolone 1 g IV for 3 days is needed when there is visual loss due to anterior ischemic optic neuropathy. The erythrocyte sedimentation rate is elevated (normal age plus 12 in males; normal age plus 10 to 12 in females). There is an urgency in the administration of methylprednisolone because it may prevent involvement of the opposite eye.

In patients with optic neuritis, abnormal cerebrospinal fluid findings (oligoclonal bands) or typical magnetic resonance abnormalities in spinal cord or elsewhere will predict later disability from multiple sclerosis.[31,32]

CONCLUSIONS

- Neurologic causes of acute monocular (optic neuropathy) or binocular (occipital lobes) vision loss are less common than ophthalmologic causes.

- Painful ophthalmoplegia has a broad spectrum of causes and needs urgent evaluation.
- Positive visual phenomena rarely indicate acute neurologic disease and more often are associated with neurotoxicity.

REFERENCES

1. Albuquerque FC, Heinz GW, McDougall CG. Reversal of blindness after transvenous embolization of a carotid-cavernous fistula: case report. *Neurosurgery* 2003;52:233–236.
2. Averbuch-Heller L, Leigh RJ, Mermelstein V, Zagalsky L, Streifler JY. Ptosis in patients with hemispheric strokes. *Neurology* 2002;58:620–624.
3. Balcer LJ. Clinical practice. Optic neuritis. *N Engl J Med* 2006;354:1273–1280.
4. Bender MB, Feldman M, Sobin AJ. Palinopsia. *Brain* 1968;91:321–338.
5. Bhatti MT. Orbital syndromes. *Semin Neurol* 2007;27:269–287.
6. Blacker DJ, Wijdicks EFM. Delayed complete bilateral ptosis associated with massive infarction of the right hemisphere. *Mayo Clinic Proc* 2003;78:836–839.
7. Bruce BB, Biousse V, Newman NJ. Third nerve palsies. *Semin Neurol* 2007;27:257–268.
8. Chan JW, Hoyt WF, Ellis WG, Gress D. Pathogenesis of acute monocular blindness from leaking anterior communicating artery aneurysms: report of six cases. *Neurology* 1997;48:680–683.
9. Chen PR, Amin-Hanjani S, Albuquerque FC, et al. Outcome of oculomotor nerve palsy from posterior communicating artery aneurysms: comparison of clipping and coiling. *Neurosurgery* 2006;58:1040–1046.

10. Cooper SA, Metcalfe RA. Assess and interpret the visual fields at the bedside. *Practical Neurology* 2009;9:324–334.

11. Dargin JM, Lowenstein RA. The painful eye. *Emerg Med Clin N Am* 2008;26:199–216.

12. Defazio G, Livrea P, Lamberti P, et al. Isolated so-called apraxia of eyelid opening: report of 10 cases and a review of the literature. *Eur Neurol* 1998;39:204–210.

13. Fattahi TT, Brandt MT, Jenkins WS, Steinberg B. Traumatic carotid-cavernous fistula: pathophysiology and treatment. *J Craniofac Surg* 2003;14:240–246.

14. Fournier AV, Zackon DH. Palinopsia: a case report and review of the literature. *Can J Ophthalmol* 2000;35:154–157.

15. Gersztenkorn D, Lee AG. Palinopsia revamped: a systematic review of the literature. *Surv Ophthalmol* 2015; 60:1–35.

16. Gladstone JP, Dodick DW. Painful ophthalmoplegia: overview with a focus on Tolosa-Hunt syndrome. *Curr Pain Headache Rep* 2004;8:321–329.

17. Hickman SJ, Dalton CM, Miller DH, Plant GT. Management of acute optic neuritis. *Lancet* 2002;360:1953–1962.

18. Karaman E, Isildak H, Haciyev Y, Kaytaz A, Enver O. Carotid-cavernous fistula after functional endoscopic sinus surgery. *J Craniofac Surg* 2009;20:556–558.

19. Kawasaki A, Purvin V. Persistent palinopsia following ingestion of lysergic acid diethylamide (LSD). *Arch Ophthalmol* 1996;114:47–50.

20. Kupersmith MJ, Vargas ME, Yashar A, et al. Occipital arteriovenous malformations: visual disturbances and presentation. *Neurology* 1996;46: 953–957.

21. Lee AG, Hayman LA, Brazis PW. The evaluation of isolated third nerve palsy revisited: an update on the evolving role of magnetic resonance, computed tomography, and catheter angiography. *Surv Ophthalmol* 2002;47:137–157.

22. Miller NR. Diagnosis and management of dural carotid-cavernous sinus fistulas. *Neurosurg Focus* 2007;23:E13.

23. Miller NR, Newman NJ, Biousse V, Kerrison JB, eds. *Walsh & Hoyt's Clinical Neuro-Ophthalmology: The Essentials.* 2nd ed. Philadelphia: Lippincott Williams & Wilkins; 2007.

24. Muller T, Buttner T, Kuhn W, Heinz A, Przuntek H. Palinopsia as sensory epileptic phenomenon. *Acta Neurol Scand* 1995;91:433–436.

25. Nazerian P, Vanni S, Tarocchi C, et al. Causes of diplopia in the emergency department: diagnostic accuracy of clinical assessment and of head computed tomography. *Eur J Emerg Med* 2014;21:118–124.

26. Ou RJ, Lee AG. Direct carotid-cavernous fistula following carotid endarterectomy. *Can J Ophthalmol* 1999;34:401–406.

27. Paullus WS, Norwood CW, Morgan HW. False aneurysm of the cavernous carotid artery and progressive external ophthalmoplegia after transsphenoidal hypophysectomy: case report. *J Neurosurg* 1979;51:707–709.

28. Ritsema ME, Murphy MA. Palinopsia from posterior visual pathway lesions without visual field defects. *J Neuroophthalmol* 2007;27:115–117.

29. Seery LS, Hurliman E, Erie JC, Leavitt JA. Bilateral pupil-sparing third nerve palsies as the presenting sign of multiple sclerosis. *J Neuroophthalmol* 2011;31:241–243.

30. Smith PE, Shah P, Sharpe J, Todd A, Goringe AP. Palinopsia. *Lancet* 2003;361:1098.

31. Soderstrom M, Ya-Ping J, Hillert J, Link H. Optic neuritis: prognosis for multiple sclerosis from MRI, CSF, and HLA findings. *Neurology* 1998; 50:708–714.

32. Swanton JK, Fernando KT, Dalton CM, et al. Early MRI in optic neuritis: the risk for disability. *Neurology* 2009;72:542–550.

33. Thurtell MJ, Halmagyi GM. Complete ophthalmoplegia: an unusual sign of bilateral paramedian midbrain-thalamic infarction. *Stroke* 2008;39:1355–1357.

34. Tokunaga M, Fukunaga K, Nakanishi R, Watanabe S, Yamanaga H. Midbrain infarction causing oculomotor nerve palsy and ipsilateral cerebellar ataxia. *Intern Med* 2014;53:2143–2147.

35. Vortmann M, Schneider JI. Acute monocular visual loss. *Emerg Med Clin N Am* 2008;26:73–96.

36. Wagner J, Schankin C, Birnbaum T, Popperl G, Straube A. Ocular motor and lid apraxia as initial symptom of anti-Ma1/Ma2-associated encephalitis. *Neurology* 2009;72:466–467.

37. Woodruff MM, Edlow JA. Evaluation of third nerve palsy in the emergency department. *J Emerg Med* 2008;35:239–246.

38. Yanaka K, Matsumaru Y, Mashiko R, et al. Small unruptured cerebral aneurysms presenting with oculomotor nerve palsy. *Neurosurgery* 2003;52: 553–557.

39. Young WB, Heros DO, Ehrenberg BL, Hedges TR, 3rd. Metamorphopsia and palinopsia. Association with periodic lateralized epileptiform discharges in a patient with malignant astrocytoma. *Arch Neurol* 1989;46:820–822.

7

Spinning

Emergency physicians are painfully aware of the potentially imminent danger of dizziness in some patients and have listed it as one of the top priorities of clinical teaching.[7,26] Akin to other equally less precise descriptions, "spinning" (or the perception of movement) may have different meanings. Naturally, it is essential to recognize potentially urgent disorders in patients reporting signs such as acute floating, wooziness, drunkenness, tilting, and imbalance.

"Spinning" as a predominant symptom is frequently outside the purview of acute neurology. The sensation of spinning in a patient acutely admitted to the ED can be due to near fainting, acute peripheral vestibular disease,[3,4,6,8,19,23] or other causes such as the ubiquitous anxiety and hyperventilation or medication side effects[26] (see Capsule 7.1). Moreover, acute dizziness is not a common reason to visit emergency departments (EDs), and accounts for not more than one or two of each 100 ED presentations.[7,12]

For the ED physician faced with a dizzy patient, the main task is to find convincing arguments for a lesion in the central nervous system (CNS) as the cause. Certain elements in the history may point to a lesion of the central vestibular system (brainstem or cerebellum); when present, these justify an urgent magnetic resonance imaging (MRI) study for which the patient may be transferred to a tertiary center. Some of these disorders are discussed in more detail in Part VII and include vertigo as a presenting sign of cerebellar hematoma, acute embolus to the basilar artery, and dissection of the vertebral artery; in these cases, other key neurologic signs and neuroimaging features usually point to the diagnosis.

Both otologic and neurologic emergencies must be considered. Otologic emergencies should be considered early in the diagnosis, because emergent antibiotic or antiviral therapy may minimize long-standing sequelae. These disorders are summarized in Table 7.1.[6]

CLINICAL ASSESSMENT

When acute spinning represents vertigo, the history may provide additional clues. Autonomic symptoms such as vomiting, nausea, pallor, and sweating are less pronounced in central lesions, but these symptoms are so common and come in so many degrees of severity that they cannot be used as major discriminating factors. Vertigo due to positional change, coughing, sneezing, fluctuating hearing loss, nonpulsatile tinnitus, and hearing loss may be more typical of peripheral (vestibular) disease but all that is certain is that nothing is certain.[4,17,18]

Oscillopsia is another important symptom, in which patients feel images are moving or bouncing. When combined with spontaneous nystagmus and transient vertigo, a peripheral source is likely. Central causes may be strongly considered when oscillopsia is induced by head movement. Lesions in the cerebellum produce a spinning sensation, but more often scanning speech, and impaired finger-to-nose and heel-knee-shin testing predominate in the clinical picture. Ipsilateral hearing loss points to an occlusion of the anterior inferior cerebellar artery.[14,22] When oscillopsia is associated with Ipsifacial numbness, hypophonia, and Horner's syndrome the lesion localizes in the lateral medulla oblongata.

It goes without saying that attention to the presence of a nystagmus is a number one priority. The characterization of nystagmus into central (brainstem—cerebellum) or peripheral (vestibular) causes is an important determinant.[2,25]

Central nystagmus has a characteristic direction dependence. Common central types of nystagmus are shown in Table 7.2.[16] When present, gaze turned to where the fast component of nystagmus beats increases the frequency and amplitude in any type of nystagmus. In central causes of nystagmus, gaze turned away from the direction of the fast component will achieve the opposite effect and may abolish it or, in extremes of gaze, reverse the direction of nystagmus. A vertical

---

CAPSULE 7.1   SYSTEMIC ILLNESS AND DRUG-INDUCED DIZZINESS

Medical illness could produce a profound (and sometimes permanent) effect on the vestibular system. Long-standing juvenile diabetes mellitus, fat emboli, and hyperviscosity syndromes may acutely occlude the common cochlear artery. Less clear mechanisms known to cause acute vertigo are dialysis, acute anemia, and hypothyroidism; and many of the vasculitic syndromes such as polyarteritis nodosa, granulomatosis with polyangiitis, Behçet disease, and connective tissue disorders may be implicated. Vertigo can be a paraneoplastic manifestation. Drugs known to damage the auditory system are aminoglycosides, antiepileptic drugs, loop diuretics, and cisplatin. Exposure to these drugs may be only brief, and toxic levels are not always required to produce permanent impairment of auditory and vestibular systems.[4]

TABLE 7.1. VERTIGO AND OTOLOGIC EMERGENCIES

Diagnosis	Clues	Therapy
Herpes zoster oticus	Ear lobe vesicles, hearing loss, facial palsy	Acyclovir 10–12 mg/kg IV every 8 hours for 10 days
Bacterial labyrinthitis	Acute deafness, prior cholesteatoma, meningitis	Surgical management or specific antibiotics
Malignant external otitis	Extreme ear pain, facial palsy (*Pseudomonas aeruginosa*)	Ciprofloxacin 750 mg orally twice daily or gentamicin 1.7 mg/kg/dose every 8 hours
Perilymph fistula	Tinnitus, hearing loss, position vertigo, prior strain or valsalva or barotrauma	Conservative first, then surgery
Labyrinth hemorrhage	Nausea, vomiting, hearing loss, trauma	Correct coagulopathy

Data from Cummings CW, Fredrickson JM, Harker LA, et al. *Otolaryngology*, 3rd ed. St. Louis: Mosby, 1998. With permission of the publisher.

TABLE 7.2. NYSTAGMUS IN ACUTE LESIONS OF THE CENTRAL VESTIBULAR SYSTEM

Type	Features	Lesion
Downbeat	Increasing amplitude with downgaze	Cervicomedullary junction
Upbeat	Increasing amplitude with upgaze	Paramedian medulla oblongata or brainstem
Rebound	With continuous lateral position, reversal or disappearance	Cerebellum
Dissociated	Disconjugate	Brainstem
Bobbing	Downward jerk with slow return to midposition	Pons

---

nystagmus (up- or downbeat) is almost always central but can be drug-induced (particularly opioids).[11] Gaze-evoked nystagmus with similar amplitudes in both directions is due to medication, but has been reported in myasthenia gravis, multiple sclerosis, and cerebellar atrophy. Periodic alternating nystagmus (nystagmus changing in direction) has typically been considered in disease of the craniocervical junction but can be due to phenytoin or lithium overdose.[15]

Examination should focus on three components, which are summarized as follows. First, the type of nystagmus is noted and is a good indication of the source of the lesion (horizontal, rotational, or vertical). Second, the direction of the nystagmus is considered. In vestibular lesions, the unidirectional nystagmus with fast-phase beating does not change in either direction. In central lesions, the nystagmus becomes more intense in the fast-beating direction and less intense in the slow-beating direction. Third, the vestibular ocular reflex is tested. This reflex is abnormal in a peripheral vestibular lesion. To test this reflex, the patient is asked to fix his or her gaze on the examiner's nose (this requires the patient's cooperation and attention, which may be impaired in brainstem lesions). A fast 15–20-degree head tilt to one side should maintain this gaze fixation with a central lesion, but fixation is temporarily lost with a peripheral lesion.[25] The salient differences between "central" and "peripheral" signs are summarized in Table 7.3.[4]

Peripheral vestibular and *congenital nystagmus* can be markedly muted when the patient fixes his or her gaze.[16,25] Nystagmus can be observed with eye closure, but it is easier to examine the eye with an ophthalmoscope covering the opposite eye. This maneuver eliminates fixation and brings on the alternating drift and correcting jerks of the retina that are a manifestation of nystagmus. Frenzel glasses (30-plus lenses) also eliminate fixation, and both eyes can be observed due to the great magnification (Frenzel glasses are rarely available in emergency rooms and require ear, nose, and throat consultation).

Positional nystagmus can be documented by performing the Dix-Hallpike maneuver, in which the physician changes the patient's position rapidly, from sitting on the examination table, to hanging the head over the edge of the table, with the head turned sideways. In most cases, a torsional and vertical nystagmus appears after delay of several seconds and produces a vertiginous sensation that fades away with repeated testing. Both delay and fatiguability are characteristic of positional nystagmus, and are helpful in localizing a vestibular lesion, mostly due to canalithiasis. The absence of delay and fatiguability may suggest a central cause.[21,27]

Disorders of the vestibulospinal reflexes (i.e., neuronal connections from labyrinths and vestibular neurons to anterior horn cells) are tested by past-pointing, the Romberg test, and tandem walking. Past-pointing is tested by having the patient touch the hand of the examiner with an extended arm, close his or her eyes, point up, and try to touch the examiner's hand again in a repeated to and fro movement but with eyes closed. Past-pointing occurs toward the damaged side. Abnormalities of the past-pointing test may not be replicated by the more traditional finger-to-nose test because joint and muscle proprioception during this coordinated movement may compensate. Another technique is vertical writing with eyes closed. This test identifies unilateral vestibular dysfunction, but this may occur in both peripheral and central causes.[9]

Static posture is tested by the Romberg test. A standing position with feet close together and eyes closed can be maintained for 30 seconds in normal individuals younger than 70 years. Crossing the arms against the chest adds complexity to the test and may bring on more subtle swaying. Tandem gait walking (10 steps) evaluates vestibular function when done with eyes closed and cerebellar function with eyes opened. Imbalance due to an acute vermian or cerebellar hemisphere lesion can be dramatic because patients are unable to sit steadily upright or to stand unassisted.

LINE OF ACTION

A few patients presenting with spinning will have an emergent neurologic disorder. In many, an acute nonviral labyrinthitis or drug toxicity can be diagnosed. As mentioned earlier, a full-scale neurologic evaluation should proceed only after

TABLE 7.3. CLINICAL SIGNS DIFFERENTIATING CENTRAL (BRAINSTEM-CEREBELLUM) FROM PERIPHERAL (VESTIBULAR)

Sign	Peripheral	Central
Spontaneous	Horizontal torsional	Pure horizontal
Nystagmus	Suppressed with visual fixation	Pure vertical
Smooth pursuit	Intact	Broken
Positional nystagmus	Delay, fatigability	No delay or fatigability

Adapted from Seemungal BM, Bronstein AM. A practical approach to acute vertigo. *Pract Neurol* 2008; 8:211–221. With permission of the publisher.

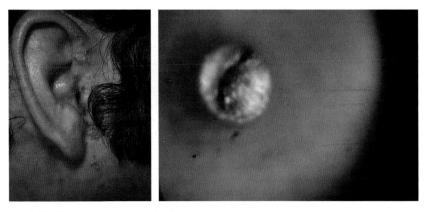

FIGURE 7.1: Otitis due to herpes zoster infection.

otologic emergencies (Figure 7.1) have been considered unlikely explanations. Albeit frequently included in "stroke alerts," most patients with dizziness have no stroke.[5] CT scans have a very low diagnostic value.[20] In a recent population-based study, one-fifth of discharged patients with initial diagnoses of peripheral vertigo underwent head CT imaging during their ED visit (almost all noncontrast), and 17% had more CT imaging in the following year suggesting overuse.[10] One can easily argue that if there are signs and symptoms that point to a central cause of vertigo, it warrants urgent MRI and magnetic resonance angiography. These studies will more clearly image the posterior fossa structures and flow interruptions in the vertebrobasilar circulation, and this should be investigated in patients with warning signs. In one study, 12% of MRIs showed pathology.[1]

A reasonable approach is summarized in Figure 7.2. Cerebrospinal fluid examination may document elevated immunoglobulin G synthesis and oligoclonal bands, thus supporting a first bout of multiple sclerosis, or show pleocytosis, which opens a wide range of diagnostic possibilities, including meningeal carcinomatosis and major CNS infections. Acute vertigo with deafness may indicate Ménière's disease or acute ischemic stroke in the brainstem,[13] or may indicate a tumor in the cerebellopontine angle, such as an acoustic neuroma. Ménière's disease is perhaps

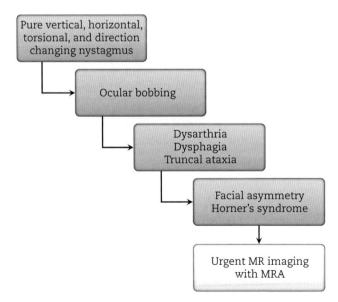

FIGURE 7.2: Critical steps in vertigo evaluation due to a lesion in the central nervous system.

MR, magnetic resonance; MRA, magnetic resonance angiography.

most common with recurrent vertigo attacks of at least 20 minutes. Patients who have nausea and vomiting with hearing loss due to endolymphatic hydrops should be referred to an otolaryngology specialist.[24]

Vestibular migraine (vertigo as the main determinant of a migraine attack) is more difficult to define and separate from basilar migraine.[21] The precipitants of these attacks are quite similar to those of common migraine, but the attack may persist for several days.

CONCLUSIONS
- The type and direction of a newly discovered nystagmus provides clues to the source of vertigo.
- The vestibulo-ocular reflex differentiates between a central and peripheral lesion (abnormal in a peripheral lesion).
- Acute vertigo and deafness may indicate a pontocerebellar lesion.

REFERENCES

1. Ahsan SF, Syamal MN, Yaremchuk K, Peterson E, Seidman M. The costs and utility of imaging in evaluating dizzy patients in the emergency room. *Laryngoscope* 2013;123:2250–2253.
2. Baloh RW. Clinical practice: vestibular neuritis. *N Engl J Med* 2003;348:1027–1032.
3. Baloh RW, Honrubia V. *Clinical Neurophysiology of the Vestibular System.* 3rd ed. New York: Oxford University Press; 2001.
4. Bronstein AM, Lempert T. *Dizziness: A Practical Approach to Diagnosis and Management.* Cambridge: Cambridge University Press; 2007.
5. Chase M, Joyce NR, Carney E, et al. ED patients with vertigo: can we identify clinical factors associated with acute stroke? *Am J Emerg Med* 2012;30:587–591.
6. Cummings CW, Fredrickson JM, Harker LA, et al. *Otolaryngology: Head and Neck Surgery.* 3rd ed. St. Louis: Mosby; 1998.
7. Eagles D, Stiell IG, Clement CM, et al. International survey of emergency physicians' priorities for clinical decision rules. *Acad Emerg Med* 2008;15:177–182.
8. Friedland DR, Wackym PA. A critical appraisal of spontaneous perilymphatic fistulas of the inner ear. *Am J Otol* 1999;20:261–276.
9. Fukuda T. Vertical writing with eyes covered: a new test of vestibulo-spinal reaction. *Acta Otolaryngol* 1959;50:26–36.
10. Grewal K, Austin PC, Kapral MK, Lu H, Atzema CL. Missed strokes using computed tomography imaging in patients with vertigo: population-based cohort study. *Stroke* 2015;46:108–113.
11. Henderson RD, Wijdicks EFM. Downbeat nystagmus associated with intravenous patient-controlled administration of morphine. *Anesth Analg* 2000;91:691–692.
12. Kerber KA, Meurer WJ, West BT, Fendrick AM. Dizziness presentations in U.S. emergency departments, 1995–2004. *Acad Emerg Med* 2008;15:744–750.
13. Lee H, Baloh RW. Sudden deafness in vertebrobasilar ischemia: clinical features, vascular topographical patterns and long-term outcome. *J Neurol Sci* 2005;228:99–104.
14. Lee H, Sohn SI, Jung DK, et al. Sudden deafness and anterior inferior cerebellar artery infarction. *Stroke* 2002;33:2807–2812.
15. Lee MS, Lessell S. Lithium-induced periodic alternating nystagmus. *Neurology* 2003;60:344.
16. Leigh RJ, Zee DS. *The Neurology of Eye Movements.* 4th ed. New York: Oxford University Press; 2006.
17. Magnusson M, Karlberg M. Peripheral vestibular disorders with acute onset of vertigo. *Curr Opin Neurol* 2002;15:5–10.
18. Mandala M, Nuti D, Broman AT, Zee DS. Effectiveness of careful bedside examination in assessment, diagnosis, and prognosis of vestibular neuritis. *Arch Otolaryngol Head Neck Surg* 2008;134:164–169.
19. McShane D, Chapnik JS, Noyek AM, Vellend H. Malignant external otitis. *J Otolaryngol* 1986;15:108–111.
20. Mitsunaga MM, Yoon HC. Journal Club: Head CT scans in the emergency department for syncope and dizziness. *AJR Am J Roentgenol* 2015; 204:24–28.
21. Neuhauser H, Lempert T. Vestibular migraine. *Neurol Clin* 2009;27:379–391.
22. Raupp SF, Jellema K, Sluzewski M, de Kort PL, Visser LH. Sudden unilateral deafness due to a right vertebral artery dissection. *Neurology* 2004;62:1442.
23. Robillard RB, Hilsinger RL, Jr., Adour KK. Ramsay Hunt facial paralysis: clinical analyses of 185 patients. *Otolaryngol Head Neck Surg* 1986;95:292–297.
24. Sajjadi H, Paparella MM. Meniere's disease. *Lancet* 2008;372:406–414.
25. Seemungal BM, Bronstein AM. A practical approach to acute vertigo. *Prac Neurology* 2008;8:211–221.
26. Stone HE. Vertigo: a practical approach. *Emerg Med Australas* 2004;16:13–16.
27. Virre E, Purcell I, Baloh RW. The Dix-Hallpike test and the canalith repositioning maneuver. *Laryngoscope* 2005;115:184–187.

8

Moving, Jerking, and Spasm

Acute movement disorder emergencies need to be separated from movement disorders in an established neurologic disorder. Acute movement disorders may indicate a new lesion to the brain or may be due to drug effect, electrolyte disturbance, or worsening neurologic disorder, particularly Parkinson's disease.

The accurate diagnosis of acute movement disorders remains difficult and is often tentative, but most emergency department (ED) physicians ask neurologists to name and treat the cause. This chapter describes the acute movement disorders occasionally observed in the ED, concentrating on the more serious and those that are drug induced.

CLINICAL ASSESSMENT

Involuntary movements are described using the following characteristics: rhythm, regularity, displacement by movement, generalized or in the same muscle group, presence or absence with relaxation, and whether the movement is fast, slow, flowing, or resembling spasm.[6,8,9] A movement disorder can be very difficult to differentiate from a focal seizure or epilepsia partialis continua. Staring, automatisms, and lip smacking may be absent, and the abnormality may be simply a continuous repetitive jerk in one limb. Clonic jerks can be felt or seen, and may evolve into a generalized seizure. (An electroencephalogram [EEG] may be the only option to differentiate seizures from movement disorders.)

Myoclonus describes muscle contractions that are brief, of small amplitude, and produce shock-like sensations. The movements may be random or rhythmic, generalized or limited to one or multiple groups of muscles. Usually they are chaotic and arrhythmic but, when rhythmic, are called *myorhythmus*. Myoclonus due to lesions in the cortex is touch- and sound-sensitive and, in awake patients, these contractions are caused by attempted motion (action myoclonus) or muscle stretch.[17]

Myoclonus can originate from the cortex, basal ganglia, brainstem, or spinal cord.[6,9] In severe anoxic–ischemic brain injury, all of these locations may be involved. Myoclonus status epilepticus in a comatose patient after cardiac resuscitation is the result of devastating multilayer cortical damage and an indicator of poor prognosis.[29]

Generalized myoclonus is common in acute metabolic derangements, but usually accompanies end-stage organ failure, as in advanced hepatic and renal disease. Myoclonus may occur as a result of selective serotonin reuptake inhibitors (SSRIs), and the elderly are at risk. It may be one of the first considerations in a presenting patient.[30] It has also been observed in hypernatremia, hypomagnesemia, and non-ketotic hyperglycemia. Unusual causes are heat stroke, decompression injury, and pesticide exposure. Toxic exposure may cause permanent damage to the cortex and basal ganglia. Drug-induced myoclonus may involve manifestations of first exposure or much more commonly appears in toxic doses (Table 8.1).[13,15,18,26]

Segmental myoclonus affecting the arm or leg may be due to acute spinal cord injury, including trauma. Segmental myoclonus may closely mimic epilepsia partialis continua, in which the jerking movements are more regular and occur at a repetitive fast rate.

Dystonia describes movements characterized by a persistent posture in one extremity, in which a sustained, patterned spasm occurs, but normal tone is resumed between spasms. The positions of the limbs or trunk may be bizarre.[5,8] In the ED, it is useful to distinguish between a generalized or focal dystonia, and whether the dystonia occurs at rest. Sensory tricks (touching the limb to reduce spasm), also known as *geste antagoniste*, are characteristic in dystonia.

One form of dystonia is ocular deviation (oculogyric crises). Oculogyric crises may be associated with backward or lateral flexion of the neck, and the tongue may protrude. The deviation of the eyes upward, sideways, or downward is held for several minutes and can be corrected by effort, but only for a brief moment. This eye movement

TABLE 8.1. DRUGS CAUSING MYOCLONUS

Drug Type	Drug
Antidepressants	Monoamine oxidase inhibitors
	Tricyclic antidepressants
	Lithium
	Fluoxetine
Antimicrobials	Penicillin
	Ticarcillin
	Carbenicillin
	Cephalosporins
	Acyclovir
	Isoniazid
Anesthetics	Etomidate
	Enflurane
	Isoflurane
	Fentanyl
	Anticonvulsants
	Valproic acid
	Carbamazepine
	Clozapine
	Vigabatrin
Calcium channel–blocking agents	Verapamil
	Nifedipine
	Diltiazem
	Amlodipine
Opiate derivatives	Meperidine
	Methadone
	Morphine
	Oxycodone
	Other drugs
	Bismuth
	Chlorambucil
Overdoses or poisonings	Antihistamines
	Methyl bromide fumes
	Organic mercury
	Gasoline sniffing
	Dichloromethane
	Strychnine
	Chloralose (rodenticide)

Source: Adapted from reference 23.

is commonly drug-induced, and discontinuation of the drug is rapidly successful in reversing the dystonia. Oculogyric crisis does occur in serious neurologic conditions such as bilateral paramedian thalamic infarction, multiple sclerosis, head injury, and tumors in the ventricles. It may also be seen as a manifestation of schizophrenia. Drugs causing oculogyric crisis and oromandibular dyskinesis include phenothiazines and many of the antipsychotic drugs as well as carbamazepine, gabapentin, lithium, ondansetron, and, perhaps best known, metoclopramide (Figure 8.1).[3]

Acute drug-induced dystonia is not only associated with antipsychotic drug use, but other well-established associations have been reported (Table 8.2).[5,16,23]

Dystonia is a common symptom in Parkinson's disease and neurodegenerative disorders associated with extrapyramidal signs, such as progressive supranuclear palsy, multisystem atrophy, corticobasal ganglia degeneration, and inherited movement disorders.[2,8,11] Any physician seeing patients with acute dystonia should consider Wilson's disease, particularly when patients are 20–30 years old. Additional findings are an artificial grin (retracted lips) and brown irides in previously blue-eyed persons. Diagnostic tests include reduced serum ceruloplasmin level (in 5% of patients it is normal), Kayser-Fleischer rings under slit lamp examination, and increased signal in the basal ganglia and cortex on magnetic resonance imaging (MRI).

Acute laryngeal dystonia may occur after recent administration of phenothiazine or other neuroleptic agents.[10,19,25] In describing this condition, one report coined the term *status dystonicus*.[3] Life-threatening complications occurred in these patients with respiratory failure due to upper airway obstruction or decreased respiratory function. Generalized dystonic spasm may impair swallowing and affect the diaphragm. A tracheostomy was needed in more than a third of patients, and rhabdomyolysis from persistent spasm did occur.

Chorea and *athetosis* are movements that are often combined and overlapping. Chorea is arrhythmic, with a jerky, thrusting component that is always purposeless but often incorporated into a voluntary movement. It may include grimacing, respiratory grunts, or a "dance-like" walk. Athetosis involves slow, undulating movements seen with the attempt to sustain a posture. Fairly typical movement patterns are known, such as an alteration between extension—pronation and flexion—supination of arm, flexion and extension of fingers, and foot inversion. Pursing and parting of the lips or side-to-side movements of the neck are observed commonly.

The most likely offending agents in drug-induced chorea are listed in Table 8.3, with a well-established presentation of central nervous system (CNS) stimulants and oral contraceptives.

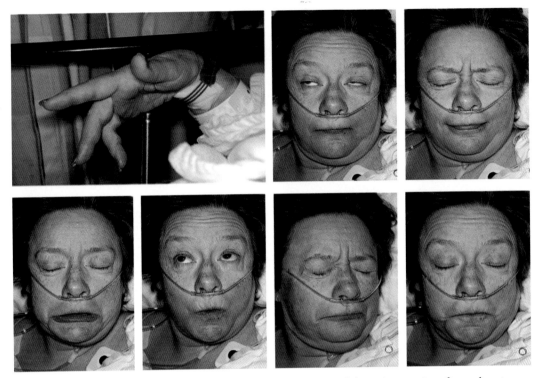

FIGURE 8.1: Patient with oromandibular dystonia, oculogyric crises, and dystonic posturing after ondansetron administration. The facial pictures were made 90 seconds apart.

From Ritter MJ, Goodman BP, Sprung J, Wijdicks EFM. Ondansetron-induced multifocal encephalopathy. *Mayo Clin Proc* 2003;78:1150–1152. With permission of *Mayo Clinic Proceedings*.

Some patients seem highly susceptible to chorea gravidarum and its association with birth control medication, but many others had prior Sydenham's chorea and heart valve damage from streptococcal infection. Chorea is also associated with new-onset hyperthyroidism, polycythemia vera, and systemic lupus erythematosus. Structural CNS lesions commonly involve ischemic or hemorrhagic stroke in the basal ganglia but usually are one-sided, thus producing *hemichorea*.

Tremor is common and diagnosed by synchronous contractions of opposing muscles. Tremor produces rhythmic oscillations. Acute tremors may indicate damage to the red nucleus (Benedikt syndrome) that may produce a rubral tremor with a frequency of 2–5 Hz. This tremor is typically seen in action and with posture holding and not at rest.

TABLE 8.2. DRUG-INDUCED DYSTONIA

Anesthetics
Antiepileptics
Benzodiazepines
Calcium antagonists
Dextromethorphan
Dopamine agonists
Metoclopramide
Monoamine oxidase inhibitors
Ondansetron
Ranitidine
Selective serotonin reuptake inhibitors
Sumatriptan
Amitriptyline

TABLE 8.3. DRUG-INDUCED CHOREA

Amphetamines
Cocaine
Pemoline
Oral contraceptives
Tricyclic antidepressants
Selective serotonin reuptake inhibitors
Theophylline
Lithium
Antiepileptics

TABLE 8.4. DRUG-INDUCED TREMORS
Antiepileptics
Antidepressants
Antihyperglycemics
Calcium channel blockers
Corticosteroids
Dopamine receptor–blocking agents
Lithium
Theophylline
Thyroxine

Drug-induced tremors (Table 8.4) are also usually postural and primarily enhanced physiologic tremors. Withdrawal of alcohol, barbiturates, benzodiazepines, β-blockers, and opioids may produce tremors.

Finally, movement disorders may even be factitious.[9] The similarities between certain acute movement disorders may make a definitive diagnosis elusive. This becomes particularly difficult when the abnormal movement presents less characteristically, so much so that, on first examination, even a seasoned neurologist may say, "I have no idea what this is."

Certain rare entities can be encountered in the ED, and these require prompt action. Acute parkinsonism may be induced by toxins such as 1-methyl-4-phenyl-1,2,3,6-tetrahydropyridine (MPTP), organophosphates, carbon monoxide, carbon disulfide, cyanide, and methanol.[24] It may also be particularly severe in acute withdrawal from dopaminergic drugs in patients with established Parkinson syndrome. Many chemotherapeutic agents have been implicated, including paclitaxel, vincristine, and CHOP (cyclophosphamide, hydroxydaunomycin, vincristine [Oncovin], and prednisone). Response to levodopa or prednisone is potentially successful but not in toxic parkinsonism. Parkinsonism can be part of neuroleptic malignant syndrome; fever, dysautonomia, and elevation of serum creatine kinase usually point in that direction. In addition, there are reasonably well-delineated disorders that include lethal catatonia (due to a prior major lesion to the CNS) and serotonin syndrome (due to serotonin-specific reuptake inhibitors,[4,22] the recreational drug "ecstasy," and a combination of monoamine oxidase inhibitors and meperidine).

Neuroleptic malignant syndrome should be considered when hyperthermia, rigidity, autonomic features, and increased creatine kinase are present. Acute serotonin syndrome has a profile similar to that of any of the acute dysautonomias, but profound myoclonus and shivering may be present.[7,21] Drugs that exacerbate a serotonin syndrome are lithium, valproate, antiemetics such as ondansetron, metoclopramide, and most recently recognized opioids.[14] Other antidepressants such as trazodone or buspirone may worsen serotonin syndrome when symptoms are initially mild.

LINE OF ACTION

Acute movement disorders could point to a structural lesion and justify an MRI scan. Paroxysmal dyskinesias, whether dystonia, chorea, or athetosis, could be due to a secondary cause.

Toxicity from overdose is a common occurrence, and the physician should not be satisfied with other explanations until drug overdose is carefully excluded. All drug-induced movement disorders are self-limiting, but failure to recognize their severity may lead to progression of the disorder, with hypotension and cardiac arrhythmias.

In patients with severe myoclonus, medication to enhance γ-aminobutyric acid (GABA) inhibition may be useful, including lorazepam and valproate. Propofol infusion (titrating to effect) is successful in treating myoclonus status epilepticus.[28]

Acute dystonic reactions are often successfully treated with intravenous or oral administration of anticholinergics (benztropine) or antihistaminic agents (diphenhydramine) or benzodiazepines (lorazepam). In status dystonicus, neuromuscular paralysis and sedation may be needed for several days, followed by benzhexol, tetrabenazine, and pimozide or haloperidol. Intravenous diphenhydramine 25–50 mg dramatically resolved the status in acute laryngeal dystonia.[20]

The first line of action in status dystonicus is intubation and sedation with propofol or IV midazolam, and not to wait when the patient demonstrates diaphragmatic dystonia. Laryngeal spasm or severe trismus may make intubation very difficult and may lead to a difficult airway (*can't intubate can't ventilate*). Fluid resuscitation with multiple boluses of crystalloids and temperature control with cooling pads may be needed. The dystonic contractions are best treated with oral or IV clonidine (3–5 mg/kg) administered every 3 hours. In extreme situations neuromuscular blocking agents may be used initially for 24–48 hours. Intravenous or oral administration of anticholinergics (benztropine) or antihistaminic agents (diphenhydramine) and hydromorphone

CAPSULE 8.1   RIGIDITY AND HYPERTHERMIA

The diagnostic spectrum of this (for the most part) poorly understood disorder includes profuse perspiration, fluctuating pulse rate and blood pressure, and hyperthermia due to impaired thermoregulation. Untreated, the condition leads to rhabdomyolysis and dehydration, and may become lethal due to myocardial stress. This condition may be drug-induced (neuroleptic agents or serotonin syndrome—mostly due to recent use or increase in dose of SSRIs) or due to drug withdrawal (dopamine withdrawal in severe Parkinson's disease or as a result of a major brain injury, encephalitis, or anoxic–ischemic damage). It may also occur in the setting of acute catatonia in prior schizophrenics. The degree of increase in creatine kinase is variable but expected, and produces prolonged symptoms. Therapy is supportive, with oxygenation, rehydration, anticoagulation, and options including dantrolene (1–10 mg/kg), bromocriptine (5 mg), lisuride (0.02–0.25 mg/hr), or, certainly not as a last resort, electroconvulsive therapy.

are early options. Intrathecal baclophen and deep brain stimulation are later options.

Alternative later options for patients with severe dystonia are outside the scope of this chapter but may include deep brain stimulation.[31] Dantrolene, bromocriptine, lisuride, or electroconvulsive therapy is effective in neuroleptic malignant syndrome or lethal catatonia (Capsule 8.1).[1,12,27] Cyproheptadine has shown promise in serotonin syndrome.[12] The management of movement disorders leading to major systemic involvement or airway involvement is summarized in Figure 8.2.[11]

CONCLUSIONS

- Acute movement disorders may be drug-induced or a result of intoxications.
- Acute catatonia is a life-threatening disorder that requires immediate treatment of its dysautonomic features.
- Chorea can be a first manifestation of a systemic medical illness.
- Acute myoclonus may be the first manifestation of a serotonin syndrome and is becoming more common due to the increased use of SSRIs.

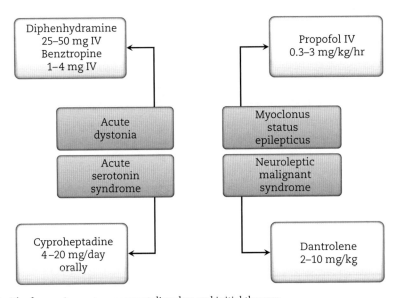

FIGURE 8.2: The four major acute movement disorders and initial therapy.

IV, intravenous.

REFERENCES

1. Addonizio G, Susman VL. ECT as a treatment alternative for patients with symptoms of neuroleptic malignant syndrome. *J Clin Psychiatry* 1987;48:102–105.
2. Ahlskog JE. *Parkinson's Disease Treatment Guide for Physicians*. New York: Oxford University Press; 2009.
3. Blakeley J, Jankovic J. Secondary causes of paroxysmal dyskinesia. *Adv Neurol* 2002;89:401–420.
4. Boyer EW, Shannon M. The serotonin syndrome. *N Engl J Med* 2005;352:1112–1120.
5. Calne DB, Lang AE. Secondary dystonia. *Adv Neurol* 1988;50:9–33.
6. Caviness JN. Parkinsonism and related disorders: myoclonus. *Parkinsonism Relat Disord* 2007;13 Suppl 3:S375–384.
7. Dosi R, Ambaliya A, Joshi H, Patell R. Serotonin syndrome versus neuroleptic malignant syndrome: a challenging clinical quandary. *BMJ Case Rep* 2014 pii: bcr2014204154
8. Fahn S, Bressman SB, Marsden CD. Classification of dystonia. *Adv Neurol* 1998;78:1–10.
9. Fahn S, Jankovic J. *Principles and Practice of Movement Disorders*. New York: Churchill Livingstone; 2007.
10. Flaherty JA, Lahmeyer HW. Laryngeal-pharyngeal dystonia as a possible cause of asphyxia with haloperidol treatment. *Am J Psychiatry* 1978;135:1414–1415.
11. Gasser T, Bressman S, Durr A, et al. State of the art review: molecular diagnosis of inherited movement disorders. Movement Disorders Society task force on molecular diagnosis. *Mov Disord* 2003;18:3–18.
12. Graudins A, Stearman A, Chan B. Treatment of the serotonin syndrome with cyproheptadine. *J Emerg Med* 1998;16:615–619.
13. Hicks CB, Abraham K. Verapamil and myoclonic dystonia. *Ann Intern Med* 1985;103:154.
14. Jhun P, Bright A, Herbert M. Serotonin syndrome and opioids: what's the deal? *Ann Emerg Med* 2015;65:434–435.
15. Klawans HL, Carvey PM, Tanner CM, et al. Drug-induced myoclonus. In: Fahn SC, Marsden D, van Woert M, eds. *Myoclonus*. Vol 43. New York: Raven Press; 1986:251.
16. Koek RJ, Pi EH. Acute laryngeal dystonic reactions to neuroleptics. *Psychosomatics* 1989;30:359–364.
17. Lance JW, Adams RD. The syndrome of intention or action myoclonus as a sequel to hypoxic encephalopathy. *Brain* 1963;86:111–136.
18. Lang A. Miscellaneous drug-induced movement disorders. In: Lang AE, Weiner WJ, eds. *Drug-Induced Movement Disorders*. Mount Kisco, NY: Futura Publishing; 1992:339.
19. Manji H, Howard RS, Miller DH, et al. Status dystonicus: the syndrome and its management. *Brain* 1998;121: 243–252.
20. Marion MH, Klap P, Perrin A, Cohen M. Stridor and focal laryngeal dystonia. *Lancet* 1992;339:457–458.
21. Pedavally S, Fugate JE, Rabinstein AA. Serotonin syndrome in the intensive care unit: clinical presentations and precipitating medications. *Neurocrit Care* 2014;21:108–113.
22. Radomski JW, Dursun SM, Reveley MA, Kutcher SP. An exploratory approach to the serotonin syndrome: an update of clinical phenomenology and revised diagnostic criteria. *Med Hypotheses* 2000;55:218–224.
23. Ritter MJ, Goodman BP, Sprung J, Wijdicks EFM. Ondansetron-induced multifocal encephalopathy. *Mayo Clinic Proc* 2003;78:1150–1152.
24. Savin S, Cartigny B, Azaroual N, et al. 1H NMR spectroscopy and GC-MS analysis of alpha-chloralose: application to two poisoning cases. *J Anal Toxicol* 2003;27:156–161.
25. Vaamonde J, Narbona J, Weiser R, et al. Dystonic storms: a practical management problem. *Clin Neuropharmacol* 1994;17:344–347.
26. Vadlamudi L, Wijdicks EFM. Multifocal myoclonus due to verapamil overdose. *Neurology* 2002;58:984.
27. Weder ND, Muralee S, Penland H, Tampi RR. Catatonia: a review. *Ann Clin Psychiatry* 2008;20:97–107.
28. Wijdicks EFM. Propofol in myoclonus status epilepticus in comatose patients following cardiac resuscitation. *J Neurol Neurosurg Psychiatry* 2002;73:94–95.
29. Wijdicks EFM, Parisi JE, Sharbrough FW. Prognostic value of myoclonus status in comatose survivors of cardiac arrest. *Ann Neurol* 1994;35:239–243.
30. Yee AH, Wijdicks EFM. A perfect storm in the emergency department. *Neurocrit Care* 2010;12:258–260.
31. Yu H, Neimat JS. The treatment of movement disorders by deep brain stimulation. *Neurotherapeutics* 2008;5:26–36.

PART III

Evaluation of Presenting Symptoms Indicating Critical Emergency

9

Can't Walk or Stand

The normal walking pattern can become impaired because of leg weakness. The inability to maintain balance also is reflected in walking and often is clear after a few steps or few minutes of unsupported stance. Differentiating muscle weakness, lack of balance, or even the inability to initiate walking requires careful assessment and, frequently, emergent neuroimaging. Examination of strength, sensation, and coordination should localize the lesion in the nervous system, determine the severity of illness, and provide a likely diagnosis. Statistically, the most serious acute disorders in the emergency department (ED) associated with leg weakness are those due to acute spinal cord compression, acute spinal cord ischemia, and Guillain-Barré syndrome. These disorders are critical neurologic disorders and require a neurologic consultation to get appropriately thought through. In this chapter, the initial considerations in a patient presenting with acute gait difficulties or leg weakness are discussed, but with a focus on the recognition of acute spinal cord compression. Further management of acute spinal cord disorders is discussed in Chapter 36.

CLINICAL ASSESSMENT

If a patient is able to walk, balance and gait can be examined using a simple set of tests. Clinical scales have been developed to assess balance and to better quantify deficiencies and risk of falls.[38]

Normally, during walking or running, the feet pass very close to each other, with minimal distance (a few inches) between them. In cerebellar ataxia, the distance widens and patients have poorly directed foot landing, they are unable to perform a tandem gait and tend to sway and fall in all directions. (Note that keeling over consistently toward the examiner is psychogenic.) Inability to sit without falling over indicates a midline cerebellar vermis lesion.

As the examination continues, failure to initiate walking, "freezing" of gait during walking

through a door, the step and stride, and arm swing (including turns) and tandem gait are all noted.

Failure to initiate gait or lift the feet from the floor ("as if glued to the floor") may be due to acute frontal brain lesions or a more diffuse motor control failure, as seen in patients with profound leukoaraiosis. Parkinsonian gait is usually suspected in the patient with small steps, audible shuffle, en bloc turns, and flexed posture. Freezing is common in parkinsonian[12] syndromes and is more a result of disease progression than of an acute, first prominent manifestation. Freezing may occur in a third of patients with hemiparetic stroke. Unilateral thalamus lesions with sensory loss but no motor weakness may result in falling backward or sideways.[19] The thalamofrontal connections and input from the cerebellum and spinal long tracts are responsible for this gait difficulty.

Gait apraxia is diagnosed when there is difficulty initiating steps (ignition failure). Some have defined this disorder as a "loss of ability to properly use the lower limbs in the act of walking."[25] Gait is counterproductive, with repeated leg movements, crossing of legs while attempting to walk, and inability to march on the spot or wipe feet on an imagined mat.

Spastic gait, with its typical scissoring and increased tone, proportionally involves the extensor muscles in the legs (rapid stretching causes increased resistance). Its presentation implies a much longer process, but patients may more or less acutely notice their symptoms becoming severe. When seen with paraparesis and Lhermitte sign, a cervical myelopathy (e.g., cervical spondylosis or multiple sclerosis) should be considered. Patients may have additionally useless, numb, clumsy hands and may be unable to identify simple objects (e.g., coins) in their hands.

Sensory ataxia may be a consequence of loss of proprioception, the result of a disorder involving dorsal root ganglia cells and large-fiber afferents in the posterior columns. Proprioception after standing is tested by assessing posture with eyes closed. The ability to maintain stance with eyes closed is impaired, with patients veering to one side. Pseudo-athetosis, areflexia, and absent position and vibration sense are hallmarks of sensory ataxia. These "subacute" conditions can be due to prior use of chemotherapeutic agents such as cisplatin (dose > 500 mg/m^2),[10] nitrous oxide (often sniffed from gas propellants or abused by dentists), pyridoxine overdose, or due to paraneoplastic destruction. Key syndromes are paraneoplastic cerebellar degeneration, opsoclonus, myoclonus and ataxia syndrome, and sensory or motor polyneuropathy.[28] These manifestations are probably the result of a rapidly evolving immunologic mechanism and may become dramatically apparent in a matter of weeks. Paraneoplastic cerebellar degeneration associated with anti-Purkinje cell antibodies (PCA-1 or anti-Yo) increases suspicion of breast, ovarian, or genital tract cancer; when associated with antineuronal nuclear autoantibody (ANNA), anti-Ri, or anti-Hu, it predicts small-cell lung cancer. In some patients, anti-Tr antibodies predict Hodgkin's lymphoma. Sensory neuropathies are associated with anti-Hu antibodies, which are rarely found in motor neuropathy. Positive antibodies should prompt a more aggressive search using bronchoscopy, bone marrow aspiration, laparoscopy, or positron emission tomography. The serum antibodies that are found vary in type and detection and do not predict response to therapy, if any. The causes of acute or subacute ataxia are listed in Table 9.1.

The inability to support one's own weight due to leg weakness or the inability to get up from a sitting position, climb stairs, or walk uphill without assistance may eventually evolve into full paraplegia. These symptoms are so prominent that they may obscure equally important complaints of tingling and numbness. Progression may be in the ascending direction or suddenly complete.

TABLE 9.1. ACUTE OR SUBACUTE ATAXIA

Intoxications and poisonings
Acute occlusion of PICA
Acute demyelination or multiple sclerosis
Acute cerebellar ataxia*
(vaccinations, varicella zoster virus)
Normal pressure hydrocephalus
Paraneoplastic disease

---

*Children usually less than 5 years old. PICA, posterior inferior cerebellar artery.

It is important to call attention to the presence of pain. Pain is common in acute spinal cord compression. However, significant destructive and compressive spinal lesions may be virtually painless. Pain that is worse with lying down may signal an epidural spinal tumor and can be explained by additional traction from lengthening of the spine in the supine position.[26] Excruciating pain closely associated in time with the development of acute paraplegia or tetraplegia should suggest intramedullary, subarachnoid, or acute epidural hemorrhage, particularly in patients receiving anticoagulation. Equally important to recognize is a spinal epidural abscess, in which acute paraparesis or tetraparesis can evolve within hours. Acute chest pain followed by paraplegia may be due to aortic dissection. Pain in the lower back area may be referred from a dissecting abdominal aneurysm; it may begin in the lower lumbar spine, followed by acute paraplegia from spinal cord infarction. In young patients, acute low back pain preceding acute paraplegia may indicate fibrocartilaginous emboli to the spinal cord from thoracic disk herniation.[31]

Pain should be classified as local, referred, radicular, or funicular. Local spinal percussion pain (deep, boring) in the thoracolumbar spine should be evaluated by having the patient turn to the side and carefully tapping on the spinous processes with a reflex hammer. Pain referred to the abdomen is often experienced by patients with acute spinal cord lesions, who may feel they are strapped into a corset. Acute radicular pain (sharp, stabbing) should be further confirmed by straight leg testing and a forceful cough or Valsalva maneuver. Funicular pain (burning, stabbing, electrical) is a less clearly characterized pain sensation of burning, jolting, and jabbing without clear localization, often occurring with sudden movements of the spine. The pain may signal intramedullary disease (e.g., tumor or demyelination).

If the patient is wheeled in on a gurney, the differential diagnosis of acute or worsening paraplegia is quite broad, but here is tailored toward those disorders that, when not met with immediate attention, may result in permanent disability, bladder dysfunction, or even compromised respiration (Table 9.2).[4,7,8,10,30,36,37]

The first objective is to determine a pattern of weakness. Proximal involvement favors muscle disease, myasthenia gravis, or myasthenic syndromes, but also spinal cord disease. Purely distal weakness is more typical of peripheral nerve disease. Improving strength with repetitive

TABLE 9.2. ACUTE PARAPLEGIA

Disorder	History	Suggest
Myelitis	Vaccination	Postvaccination myelopathy
	Febrile illness	Postinfectious transverse myelitis
	Optic neuritis	Multiple sclerosis or Devic disease
	Travel	Schistosomiasis, cysticercosis
	Tick bite	Lyme disease
	Immunosuppression, AIDS	Tuberculosis, aspergillosis, coccidioidomycosis, syphilis
Myelopathy	Cancer	Acute necrotic myelopathy
	Aortic aneurysms or recent catheterization, low back pain	Infarction of the cord (thromboemboli, fibrocartilaginous emboli)
	Connective tissue disease (Sjögren syndrome, SLE)	Vasculitis
	Cancer	Radiation myelopathy
	Anticoagulation	Paraneoplastic myelopathy
	Progressive symptoms with occasional exacerbation, profound muscle wasting	Epidural hematoma
		Intramedullary hemorrhage
		Spinal AVM
		Dural AV fistula
Polyradiculopathy	Diarrhea, URI, CMV, HSV, EBV, diabetes mellitus, leukemia, sarcoidosis	Guillain-Barré syndrome
		Acute diabetic polyradiculopathy
Neoplastic meningitis	Carcinoma, lymphoma, or other hematologic-oncologic disease	Leptomeningeal spread
Neuromuscular junction disorders	Dysphagia, diplopia, ptosis, fatigability, small cell lung cancer	Myasthenia gravis
		Lambert-Eaton syndrome
	Dry mouth; sixth nerve palsy; fixed, dilated pupils	Botulism
Myopathy	Autoimmune disorder	Polymyositis
	Malar, perioral skin rash	Dermatomyositis
	Exercise intolerance and myoglobinuria	Metabolic myopathy
	Periodic attacks (minutes to hours)	Hyperkalemia or hypokalemic paralysis
	Thyrotoxicosis	Hypokalemic paralysis

AIDS, acquired immunodeficiency syndrome; AV, arteriovenous; AVM, arteriovenous malformation; CMV, cytomegalovirus; EBV, Epstein-Barr virus; HSV, herpes simplex virus; SLE, systemic lupus erythematosus; URI, upper respiratory infection.

testing argues for a presynaptic defect of the neuromuscular junction (Lambert-Eaton myasthenic syndrome). Worsening strength with repetitive testing argues for a postsynaptic disorder of neuromuscular traffic (myasthenia gravis).[30] Tendon reflexes are lost early in acute polyradiculopathy and in spinal shock, and are reduced in Lambert-Eaton syndrome and severe muscle disorders. Fasciculations and atrophy should be noted and indicate rapid worsening of a chronic neurologic disorder, mostly in those disorders involving the anterior horn cell or peripheral nerve. Muscle tone is flaccid in acute Guillain-Barré syndrome, spinal shock, or cauda equina lesion.

Neurologic examination should localize the lesion in patients with acute paraplegia or tetraplegia. Sensory abnormalities localize in the vertical plane (cervical, lumbar, sacral) and, when combined with other long-tract signs, point to localization in the horizontal plane (extradural, intradural, or intramedullary). The sensory dermatomes are shown in Figure 9.1, and other clinical clues helpful in localization are found in Capsule 9.1. The major spinal cord syndromes are subsequently summarized in Table 9.3.

Diagnoses to consider in paraplegic patients with acute chest or lumbar pain are aortic dissection, epidural hematoma, epidural abscess,

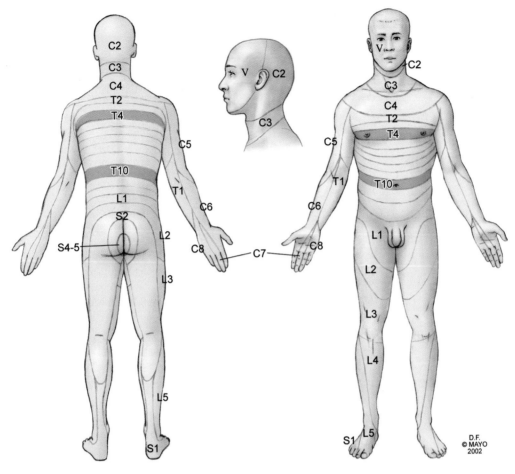

FIGURE 9.1: Sensory dermatomes.

CAPSULE 9.1   LOCALIZING SPINAL CORD LESIONS

FORAMEN MAGNUM SYNDROME AND LESIONS OF THE UPPER CERVICAL CORD

- Suboccipital pain and neck stiffness, Lhermitte sign, occipital and fingertip paresthesias
- Sensory dissociation may be present.
- Sensory findings of posterior column dysfunction may be present.
- High cervical compressive findings (spastic tetraparesis, long-tract sensory findings, bladder disturbance)
- Lower cranial nerve palsies (CN IX–XII) may occur from regional extension of the pathologic process.
- Lesions affecting the C5 segment may compromise the diaphragm.
- With C5 segment lesions, biceps and brachioradialis reflexes are absent or diminished, whereas the triceps reflex and the finger flexor reflex are exaggerated (because of corticospinal tract compression at C5).
- With C6 segment lesions, biceps, brachioradialis, and triceps reflexes are diminished or absent but the finger flexor reflex (C8–T1) is exaggerated.

LESIONS OF THE SEVENTH CERVICAL SEGMENT
- Paresis involves flexors and extensors of the wrists and fingers.
- Biceps and brachioradialis reflexes are preserved, and the finger flexor reflex is exaggerated.
- May result in flexion of the forearm following olecranon tap. (Weakness of the triceps prevents its contraction and elbow extension, whereas muscles innervated by normal segments above the lesion are allowed to contract.)
- Sensory loss at and below the third and fourth digits (including medial arm and forearm) is present.

LESIONS OF THE EIGHTH CERVICAL AND FIRST THORACIC SEGMENTS
- Weakness that predominantly involves the small hand muscles with associated spastic paraparesis
- With C8 lesions, the triceps reflex (C6–C8) and finger flexor reflex (C8–T1) are decreased.
- With T1 lesions, the triceps reflex is preserved, but the finger flexor reflex is decreased.
- Unilateral or bilateral Horner syndrome is possible with C8–T1 lesions.
- Sensory loss involves the fifth digit, medial forearm and arm, and the rest of the body below the lesion.

LESIONS OF THE THORACIC SEGMENTS
- Root pain or paresthesias that mimic intercostal neuralgia
- Segmental lower motor neuron involvement is difficult to detect clinically.
- Paraplegia, sensory loss below thoracic level, and bowel and bladder disturbances occur.
- With a lesion above T5, vasomotor control may be impaired.
- With a lesion at the T10 level, upper abdominal musculature is preserved but lower abdominal muscles are weak. For example, when the head is flexed against resistance with the patient supine, the intact upper abdominal muscles pull the umbilicus upward (Beevor sign).
- If the lesion lies above T6, superficial abdominal reflexes are present.
- If the lesion is at or below T10, upper and middle abdominal reflexes are present.
- If the lesion is below T12, all abdominal reflexes are present

LESIONS OF THE FIRST LUMBAR SEGMENT
- Weakness in all muscles of the lower extremities; lower abdominal muscle paresis
- Sensory loss includes both the lower extremities up to the level of the groin and the back to a level above the buttocks.
- With long-standing lesions, the patellar and ankle jerks are brisk.

LESIONS OF THE SECOND LUMBAR SEGMENT
- Spastic paraparesis but no weakness of abdominal musculature
- Cremasteric reflex (L2) is not elicitable, and patellar jerk may be depressed.
- Ankle jerks are hyperactive.

LESIONS OF THE THIRD LUMBAR SEGMENT
- Some preservation of hip flexion (iliopsoas and sartorius) and leg adduction (adductor longus, pectineus, and gracilis).
- Patellar jerks are decreased or not elicitable.
- Ankle jerks are hyperactive.

(continued)

LESIONS OF THE FOURTH LUMBAR SEGMENT

- Better hip flexion and leg adduction than in L1–L3 lesions
- Knee flexion and leg extension are better performed, and the patient is able to stand by stabilizing the knees.
- Patellar jerks are absent, and ankle jerks are hyperactive.

LESIONS OF THE FIFTH LUMBAR SEGMENT

- Normal hip flexion and adduction and leg extension; patient can extend legs against resistance when extremities are flexed at the hip and knee (normal quadriceps).
- Patellar reflexes are present.
- Ankle jerks are hyperactive.

LESIONS OF THE FIRST SACRAL SEGMENT

- Achilles reflexes are absent, but patellar reflexes are preserved.
- Complete sensory loss over the sole, heel, and outer aspect of the foot and ankle.
- Anesthesia over medial calf, posterior thigh

CONUS MEDULLARIS LESIONS

- Paralysis of the pelvic floor muscles and early sphincter dysfunction
- Disruption of the bladder reflex arc results in autonomous neurogenic bladder characterized by loss of voluntary initiation of micturition, increased residual urine, and absent bladder sensation.
- Constipation
- Impaired erection and ejaculation
- May have symmetric saddle anesthesia
- Pain is uncommon but may involve thighs, buttocks, and perineum.

CAUDA EQUINA LESIONS

- Early radicular pain in the distribution of the lumbosacral roots due to compression below the L3 vertebral level
- Pain may be unilateral or asymmetric and is increased by the Valsalva maneuver.
- With extensive lesions, flaccid, hypotonic, areflexic paralysis develops, affecting the glutei, posterior thigh muscles, and anterolateral muscles of the leg and foot, resulting in a true peripheral type of paraplegia.
- Sensory testing reveals asymmetric sensory loss in saddle region, involving anal, perineal, and genital regions and extending to the dorsal aspect of the thigh, anterolateral aspect of the leg, and outer aspect of the foot.
- Achilles reflexes are absent, and patellar reflexes are variable in response.
- Sphincter changes are similar to those with a conus lesion, but occurrence tends to be late in the clinical course.
- Although it can be concluded that lesions of the conus result in early sphincter compromise, late pain, and symmetric sensory manifestations, whereas cauda lesions have early pain, late sphincter manifestations, and asymmetric sensory findings, this distinction is difficult to establish and is of little practical value.

Source: Data abstracted from The localization of lesions affecting the spinal cord. In Brazis PW, Masdue JC, Biller J, eds. Localization in Clinical Neurology Sixth edition. Philadelphia, Lippincot Williams and Wilkins 2011.

TABLE 9.3. ACUTE SPINAL CORD
SYNDROMES

Complete

All sensory modalities and reflexes impaired below
   level of severance: pinprick loss most valuable
Flaccid, paraplegia, or tetraplegia
Fasciculations
Urinary or rectal sphincter dysfunction
Sweating, piloerection diminished below lesions
Genital reflexes lost, priapism

Central

Vest-like loss of pain and temperature
Initial sparing of proprioception
Sacral sensation spared
Paraparesis or tetraparesis

Hemisection

Loss of pain and temperature opposite to the lesion
Sensory loss two segments below lesion
Loss of proprioception on same side as lesion
Light touch may be normal or minimally decreased
Weakness on same side as lesion

Anterior

Pain and temperature loss below lesion
Proprioception spared
Flaccid, areflexia
Paraparesis or tetraparesis
Fasciculations
Urinary or rectal sphincter dysfunction

intramedullary hematoma, or vertebral collapse from cancer. Acute paraplegia may be an immediate consequence of aortic dissection.[2,11] Acute pain may be associated with a widening mediastinum on chest radiograph. An emergent echocardiogram or magnetic resonance angiogram can confirm the diagnosis. Ischemic myelopathy may be due to reduced spinal blood flow, which in turn is due to increased intraspinal CSF pressure.

Many other neurologic disorders can mimic spinal cord compression. Essential facts in the medical history include recent viral illness, vaccinations, illicit drug use, fever, weight loss, myalgia, severe back pain with radiation, recent tick bite, and skin rash, which may indicate acute myelitis or polyradiculopathy. *Acute transverse myelitis* should be considered in young patients (< 40 years of age) with acute paraplegia but is uncommon. Criteria include the development of sensorimotor or autonomic dysfunction from a cord lesion, defined sensory level, bilateral signs that can be asymmetric, and progression to maximal deficit within hours to 3 weeks. It is very important to

determine whether the patient is immunocompromised, has clinical evidence of human immunodeficiency virus (HIV) infection, or has risk factors for the acquired immunodeficiency syndrome (AIDS) virus, including previous blood or blood-product transfusions (the risks were higher before 1985, when regular HIV screening was not available in blood banks). Recent travel may be relevant and may suggest a myelopathy from *Schistosoma* species (endemic in Brazil) or cysticercosis (any country in Latin America).

Finally, two neurosurgical emergencies need special mention not only because recognition may be difficult but also because presentation mimics common disorders seen in the ED. First, epidural spinal abscess is caused in 50% of the patients by *Staphylococcus aureus* infection.[9,16] Drug use and chronic alcoholism predispose to diskitis and osteomyelitis, which may extend to the epidural space. Recognition is difficult because most patients have signs suggesting sepsis or acute bacterial meningitis, and they may be confused or delirious. Paraparesis and loss of voluntary muscles and sphincters may rapidly become defining features in these patients admitted to the ED. Blood cultures have a much higher yield in identifying the organism than does cerebrospinal fluid (CSF) testing, and the responsible microorganism can be isolated from blood in at least 30% of cases. CSF examination in the ED—done to document or exclude bacterial meningitis—is potentially dangerous, because shifts in CSF pressure that displace the spinal cord may cause sudden worsening of paraparesis.

Second, epidural spinal hematoma may present with acute chest pain or pain between the shoulder blades. The pain has been described as a dagger thrust (*le coup de poignard*) and is rapidly followed by tingling, the development of a sensory demarcation, and often Brown-Séquard syndrome. Acute weakness and pain in combination with the use of any anticoagulant or recent multilevel spine surgery, should immediately point to this possibility.[21] Tetraparesis or paraparesis follows. Spontaneous spinal subarachnoid hematoma, although rare, may lead to paralysis when located dorsally in the spinal cord. A ventral type of spinal subarachnoid hematoma has a much more benign presentation and resolves spontaneously.

LINE OF ACTION

It is imperative to admit any patient with acute severe impairment of gait or balance and to

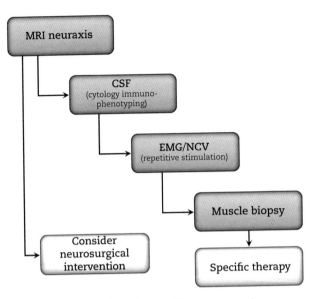

FIGURE 9.2: Critical steps in the evaluation of gait abnormalities or paraparesis.

CSF, cerebrospinal fluid; EMG/NCV, electromyography/nerve conduction velocity; MRI, magnetic resonance imaging.

expedite evaluation. With so many possible levels of involvement in the nervous system, laboratory tests should focus on the most probable localization (Figure 9.2). Magnetic resonance imaging (MRI) is mandatory because compression of the thoracic or lumbar spinal cord or meningeal pathology is common in acute or rapidly worsening weakness (if no further localization can be made).[17,18,27,32] It is not unreasonable to proceed with an MRI of the entire neuraxis to visualize all structures involved in gait initiation.[24] However, there is a low catch rate on MRI (1%–4%) in patients with suspected spinal cord compression. Bowel and urinary symptoms and saddle sensory disturbances increase the probability to approximately 30%. If no structural lesions are found, CSF examination is warranted.

Immediate- or delayed-onset paraplegia from spinal cord ischemia can be a consequence of aortic dissection. It is often inappropriately considered permanent at onset. An acute lumbar puncture may lead to rapid recovery, and a high opening pressure is evident.[2,11,20] Aortic occlusion of the descending aorta and cardiac outflow obstruction increase volume in the intracranial sinuses, translating into increased intraspinal volume and increased CSF pressure. Early spinal cord edema also may cause the CSF pressure to rise. Spinal cord perfusion is reduced, and is equal to spinal arterial pressure minus CSF pressure. Removal of 20–30 mL of CSF followed by continuous CSF drainage at a rate of 5–10 mL per hour

can be dramatically effective, with resolution of symptoms within hours.[2]

Infectious myelitis is the most common alternative diagnosis in acute spinal cord syndromes and often involves viral infections. Viruses affecting spinal gray matter usually include herpes zoster, but other herpes viruses (cytomegalovirus, herpes simplex) may injure nerve roots. CSF in herpes zoster myelitis shows pleocytosis, increased protein levels, and normal glucose values. Viruses with a proclivity for white matter include HIV and human T-cell lymphotropic virus (type I). A viral serologic panel should be obtained in the ED in appropriate cases (HSV-1, HSV-2, HHV-6, VZV, CMV, EBV, HIV, and enteroviruses). In appropriate circumstances, such as in concurrent tuberculosis (TB) infection, CSF and fast bacilli smear and culture should be obtained. A moderate lymphocytic pleocytosis is common in acute transverse myelitis and may be accompanied by increased immunoglobulin G and oligoclonal bands. Cytologic examination of CSF should focus on malignant cells (only 50% positive yield), and flow cytometry is indicated if atypical lymphocytes are found. Flow-cytometric immunophenotyping consists of antibodies against several antigens such as CD19, CD45, and κ and λ immunoglobulin light chains to characterize a possible blast population or monoclonal B-cell population.

Oligoclonal bands in CSF suggest multiple sclerosis, particularly if other white matter lesions are found (up to 80% positive predictive value). Visual evoked potentials can be useful to document optic neuritis, as in Devic disease or multiple sclerosis. Systemic inflammatory disease may be complicated by myelitis, and autoantibodies (ANA [antinuclear antibodies], double-stranded DNA, SS-A [RO], SS-B [La], Sm [Smith], and RNP [ribonucleoprotein]) levels are useful.

More peripherally, other important rapid discriminating tests in the ED are creatine kinase and nerve conduction studies with repetitive stimulation (presynaptic rapid stimulation results in incremental amplitude, postsynaptic decremental amplitude at low stimulation rate). We have seen severe muscle weakness with marked hypokalemia (potassium levels less than 1.5 mmol/L) in the setting of Graves disease, with rapid response to intravenous replacement.[22] Serum antibodies are tested for paraneoplastic syndromes, which can be quite rapid in presentation. Muscle and nerve biopsy may be needed to document inflammatory myopathy.

An expedited evaluation in patients with acute spinal cord compression is paramount because reversal of tetraparesis or paraparesis is time-locked.[5,6] Beyond a certain interval, the symptoms may remain complete, with no prospect of future ambulation or bladder control.

Patients with spinal cord compression from malignant disease often have some degree of ambulation at first evaluation. It has been estimated that 30% of patients with epidural spinal cord compression from metastatic cancer become paraplegic within 1 week.[3,5,10] This observation clearly indicates a dynamic process that possibly can be halted or partly reversed. Unfortunately, unacceptable delay in diagnosis, referral, and investigation occurs in some patients with spinal cord compression.

The approach to acute spinal cord compression is determined by its cause, but immediate surgical management is warranted in patients with an epidural abscess localized at a few levels, epidural hematoma, or extradural metastasis with rapidly evolving neurologic deterioration. Its benefit lies in the preservation of at least partial mobility and, equally important, complete bladder function. Outcome also depends on the ability to prevent complications and treat non-neurologic problems (lungs, skin, bladder) early.

Surgery should be the preferred approach when the primary tumor is unknown and histologic diagnosis is needed. If vertebral collapse coincides with spinal cord compression, the chances for ambulation are lower and the potential for further deterioration after surgery is real.

Epidural metastatic lesions often can be treated effectively only by surgery with anterior-posterior resection with instrumentation. Marginal life expectancy and the degree of metastasis often preclude major surgery.[14,23,33–35]

Dexamethasone is given to all patients with metastatic cord compression (100 mg IV push followed by 16 mg/day PO in divided doses) until definitive management has been determined.

Patients with an epidural hematoma need prothrombin complex concentrate (highly preferred), fresh-frozen plasma and vitamin K for immediate reversal of anticoagulation to international normalized ratio (INR) levels within the normal range.[15] An INR of 1.5 is satisfactory for surgical exploration. (Patients with a high risk for cardioembolization [e.g., metallic heart valve] may tolerate short-term discontinuation of anticoagulation and reversal should not be delayed.)[29]

Two major factors predict favorable postoperative recovery in spontaneous epidural hematoma: decompression within 36 hours in patients with complete cord syndrome, and decompression within 48 hours in patients with incomplete cord syndrome. Rapid onset of paraplegia is not predictive of outcome and should not discourage surgical intervention.[13] Others found that the degree of deficit at the time of intervention was the most important determinant of outcome and not timing of surgery. Sparing of some sensory function despite a complete motor deficit increased the chance of a good outcome.[1]

CONCLUSIONS

- Acute gait disorder may be caused by viral infections or recent vaccination in children and acute cerebellar infarction or medication overdose in the elderly.
- Acute paraplegia may be a consequence of spinal cord compression, and neuroimaging with MRI is urgently needed.
- Acute chest pain and paraplegia requires immediate evaluation for aortic dissection.

REFERENCES

1. Bakker NA, Veeger NJ, Vergeer RA, Groen RJ. Prognosis after spinal cord and cauda compression in spontaneous spinal epidural hematomas. *Neurology* 2015;84:1894–1903.
2. Blacker DJ, Wijdicks EFM, Ramakrishna G. Resolution of severe paraplegia due to aortic dissection after CSF drainage. *Neurology* 2003;61:142–143.

3. Byrne TN, Borges LF, Loeffler JS. Metastatic epidural spinal cord compression: update on management. *Semin Oncol* 2006;33:307–311.

4. Byrne TN, Waxman SG. *Spinal Cord Compression: Diagnosis and Principles of Management.* Philadelphia: FA Davis; 1990.

5. Carlson GD, Gorden CD, Oliff HS, Pillai JJ, LaManna JC. Sustained spinal cord compression: part I: time-dependent effect on long-term pathophysiology. *J Bone Joint Surg Am* 2003;85-A:86–94.

6. Carlson GD, Minato Y, Okada A, et al. Early time-dependent decompression for spinal cord injury: vascular mechanisms of recovery. *J Neurotrauma* 1997;14:951–962.

7. Celesia GG. Disorders of membrane channels or channelopathies. *Clin Neurophysiol* 2001;112:2–18.

8. Criscuolo GR, Oldfield EH, Doppman JL. Reversible acute and subacute myelopathy in patients with dural arteriovenous fistulas: Foix-Alajouanine syndrome reconsidered. *J Neurosurg* 1989;70:354–359.

9. Darouiche RO. Spinal epidural abscess. *N Engl J Med* 2006;355:2012–2020.

10. DeAngelis LM, Posner JB. *Neurologic Complications of Cancer.* 2nd ed. New York: Oxford University Press; 2008.

11. Gaul C, Dietrich W, Erbguth FJ. Neurological symptoms in aortic dissection: a challenge for neurologists. *Cerebrovasc Dis* 2008;26:1–8.

12. Giladi N. Medical treatment of freezing of gait. *Mov Disord* 2008;23 Suppl 2:S482–488.

13. Groen RJ, van Alphen HA. Operative treatment of spontaneous spinal epidural hematomas: a study of the factors determining postoperative outcome. *Neurosurgery* 1996;39:494–508.

14. Helweg-Larsen S, Sorensen PS, Kreiner S. Prognostic factors in metastatic spinal cord compression: a prospective study using multivariate analysis of variables influencing survival and gait function in 153 patients. *Int J Radiat Oncol Biol Phys* 2000;46:1163–1169.

15. Henderson RD, Pittock SJ, Piepgras DG, Wijdicks EFM. Acute spontaneous spinal epidural hematoma. *Arch Neurol* 2001;58:1145–1146.

16. Huang PY, Chen SF, Chang WN, et al. Spinal epidural abscess in adults caused by Staphylococcus aureus: clinical characteristics and prognostic factors. *Clin Neurol Neurosurg* 2012;114:572–576.

17. Husband DJ. Malignant spinal cord compression: prospective study of delays in referral and treatment. *BMJ* 1998;317:18–21.

18. Husband DJ, Grant KA, Romaniuk CS. MRI in the diagnosis and treatment of suspected malignant spinal cord compression. *Br J Radiol* 2001;74:15–23.

19. Karnath HO, Johannsen L, Broetz D, Kuker W. Posterior thalamic hemorrhage induces "pusher syndrome." *Neurology* 2005;64:1014–1019.

20. Killen DA, Weinstein CL, Reed WA. Reversal of spinal cord ischemia resulting from aortic dissection. *J Thorac Cardiovasc Surg* 2000;119:1049–1052.

21. Kou J, Fischgrund J, Biddinger A, Herkowitz H. Risk factors for spinal epidural hematoma after spinal surgery. *Spine (Phila Pa 1976)* 2002;27:1670–1673.

22. Kung AW. Clinical review: thyrotoxic periodic paralysis: a diagnostic challenge. *J Clin Endocrinol Metab* 2006;91:2490–2495.

23. Loblaw DA, Perry J, Chambers A, Laperriere NJ. Systematic review of the diagnosis and management of malignant extradural spinal cord compression: the Cancer Care Ontario Practice Guidelines Initiative's Neuro-Oncology Disease Site Group. *J Clin Oncol* 2005;23:2028–2037.

24. Masdeu JC. Neuroimaging and gait. *Adv Neurol* 2001;87:83–89.

25. Mayer YS, Barron DW. Apraxia of gait: clinico-physiological study. *Brain* 1960;83:261–284.

26. Nicholas JJ, Christy WC. Spinal pain made worse by recumbency: a clue to spinal cord tumors. *Arch Phys Med Rehabil* 1986;67:598–600.

27. O'Phelan KH, Bunney EB, Weingart SD, Smith WS. Emergency neurological life support: spinal cord compression (SCC). *Neurocrit Care* 2012;17 Suppl 1:S96–S101.

28. Pascuzzi RM. Pearls and pitfalls in the diagnosis and management of neuromuscular junction disorders. *Semin Neurol* 2001;21:425–440.

29. Phuong LK, Wijdicks EFM, Sanan A. Spinal epidural hematoma and high thromboembolic risk: between Scylla and Charybdis. *Mayo Clinic Proc* 1999;74:147–149.

30. Sanders DB, Juel VC. The Lambert-Eaton myasthenic syndrome. *Handb Clin Neurol* 2008;91:273–283.

31. Sasaki S, Kaji K, Shiba K. Upper thoracic disc herniation followed by acutely progressing paraplegia. *Spinal Cord* 2005;43:741–745.

32. Schiff D, Batchelor T, Wen PY. Neurologic emergencies in cancer patients. *Neurol Clin* 1998;16:449–483.

33. Siegal T. Spinal cord compression: from laboratory to clinic. *Eur J Cancer* 1995;31A:1748–1753.

34. Sun H, Nemecek AN. Optimal management of malignant epidural spinal cord compression. *Emerg Med Clin N Am* 2009;27:195–208.

35. Sundaresan N, Sachdev VP, Holland JF, et al. Surgical treatment of spinal cord compression from epidural metastasis. *J Clin Oncol* 1995;13:2330–2335.

36. Symon L, Kuyama H, Kendall B. Dural arteriovenous malformations of the spine: clinical features and surgical results in 55 cases. *J Neurosurg* 1984;60:238–247.

37. Tang HJ, Lin HJ, Liu YC, Li CM. Spinal epidural abscess: experience with 46 patients and evaluation of prognostic factors. *J Infect* 2002;45:76–81.

38. Yelnık A, Bonan I. Clinical tools for assessing balance disorders. *Neurophysiol Clin* 2008;38:439–445.

10

Short of Breath

Neurologic disease can impair respiration at multiple levels. The interconnections between cerebral hemispheres, respiratory centers in the brainstem, motor neurons, and the respiratory muscles provide a functional system that moves air in and out of the lungs. If the system fails, hypercapnia results. The alveoli and pulmonary capillaries permit efficient gas exchange by diffusion through a foil-thin barrier; if that fails, hypoxemia results. Both conditions may occur simultaneously, or one disorder may lead to the other when reduced airflow leads to poor alveolar recruitment and collapse.[32]

Any breathless patient is alarming, and this may be the first defining sign of neuromuscular disease. Respiratory distress may not be apparent but may be noticeable only when provoked by a change in position or with testing of respiratory mechanics. In other circumstances, patients may present with impaired consciousness, catching breaths, or even ceasing to breathe.

This chapter provides a discussion of the causes of respiratory failure caused by neurologic disease and the initial airway management in the emergency department (ED) before transfer to the neurosciences intensive care unit (NICU).

CLINICAL ASSESSMENT

A number of steps can be taken to narrow down the diagnostic possibilities in the patient with shortness of breath. In the initial evaluation, consider three main questions: Does the patient generate breaths? Is air getting to where it needs to go? Is the pulmonary apparatus intact?[24,50] The causes of respiratory failure in neurologic disease are illustrated in Figure 10.1 and are summarized in Table 10.1.

Acute lesions of the hemisphere or brainstem affect automatic or voluntary respiratory control (Capsule 10.1). The automatic control of the respiratory drive is generated in the primary ventilatory nuclei in the brainstem. Loss of automatic control (Ondine's curse) has been reported with neuroblastoma and syringobulbia but is extremely rare. The breathing patterns that herald the loss

of automatic control result in hypercapnia, but can rarely be observed well because patients usually have already been placed on a mechanical ventilator.

Voluntary control originates in the cortex and connects to those spinal cord levels, with motor neurons sending connecting fibers to the diaphragm, intercostal muscles, and abdominal muscles. (Impaired voluntary breathing involves a gamut of respiratory disorders and is not discussed further here.)

Failure to maintain a patent airway may originate directly from acute neurologic disease. Breathing may be obstructed at the pharyngeal or laryngeal level due to tongue displacement, vomit, or tooth fragments. Breathing may also be labored from stridor, recognized by a high-pitched noise at inspiration. It is not infrequent after extubation, a procedure that may cause an inadvertent subglottic edema or traumatic epithelial injury. Stridor may also be due to laryngeal dystonia (Chapter 8) or vocal cord paralysis. Failure of gas exchange could be due to profound aspiration or, less commonly, neurogenic pulmonary edema. Frothy sputum and tachypnea often accompany hypoxemia and an increased alveolar–arterial oxygen gradient.

Acute spinal cord lesions affecting higher cervical regions (C3–C5) result in ventilator dependence. Lesions below the level of C5 spare the nerve connections to the diaphragm, but expiratory effort is markedly reduced due to involvement of the abdominal and intercostal muscles. Placing the patient in a supine position improves expiration due to the pressure of abdominal contents in the chest; breathing becomes labored when the patient is placed upright in a chair.

The phrenic nerve may be injured, and unilateral damage could cause marked breathlessness during any form of exercise and prevent the patient from lying flat.[30,31] Many cases of phrenic nerve damage are unexplained, but may be due to neuralgic amyotrophy (associated with intense pain in shoulder muscles), stretch injury, or traumatic brachial plexus injury.[5] Phrenic nerve injury

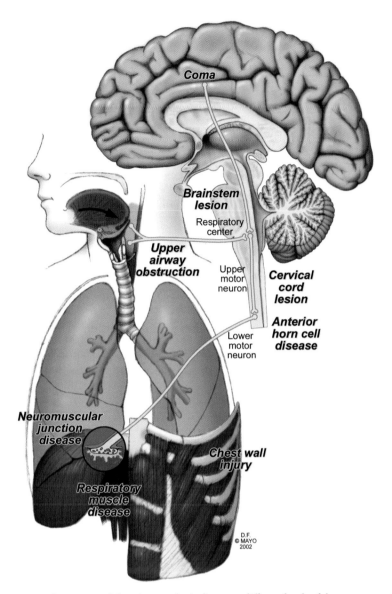

FIGURE 10.1: Causes of respiratory failure in neurologic disease at different levels of the nervous system.

is known to occur in compression of the brachial plexus due to tumor (commonly squamous cell lung carcinoma) or aneurysm (thoracic aorta), prior chest surgery or cannulation of the subclavian or internal jugular vein, herpes zoster infection, or chiropractic manipulation. More chronic progressive disorders of the central nervous system may also affect mechanics of the rib cage. Restricted muscle movements in advanced stages of Parkinson's disease are also reflected in the respiratory muscles by an incoordinated respiratory muscle pump function.[45]

Before clinical features are discussed, a review the normal and pathologic state of respiratory muscles is helpful.[12] The muscles of inspiration are the diaphragm, intercostal muscles, and scalene muscles. Expiration is largely caused by recoil of the lungs, but abdominal muscles also contribute. When ventilatory demand is increased, accessory muscles (such as the sternocleidomastoid, pectoralis major and minor, and latissimus dorsi) are activated. The diaphragm has a central noncontractile tendon (dome), from which muscle fibers radiate to insert to the xiphoid in the front, to the lower ribs, and to the first two or three lumbar vertebral bodies. When the diaphragm contracts, the dome retains its shape but descends in a piston-like action and the rib cage expands. The lower ribs are lifted because the abdominal viscera counter the descent of the diaphragmatic dome

TABLE 10.1. THREE MAJOR CAUSES OF RESPIRATORY FAILURE IN ACUTE NEUROLOGIC DISEASE

Abnormal respiratory drive
Sedatives (e.g., opioids, barbiturates, benzodiazepines, propofol)
Pontomedullary lesion (e.g., hemorrhage, infarct, trauma)
Hypercapnia
Hypothermia
Hypothyroidism

Abnormal respiratory conduit
Upper airway obstruction
Massive aspiration
Neurogenic pulmonary edema
Pneumothorax (e.g., after subclavian catheterization)

Abnormal respiratory mechanics
Spinal cord lesion (e.g., trauma, demyelination, amyotrophic lateral sclerosis)
Absent or decreased neuromuscular junction traffic (e.g., myasthenia gravis, organophosphates, botulism, tick paralysis)
Diaphragm failure (e.g., myopathies, phrenic nerve lesion trauma)

and the costal part of the diaphragmatic fibers is shortened. The remaining rib cage expands as a result of the synchronized contractile force of the parasternal intercostal muscles, which run caudally and laterally between the ribs. Inspiration thus results in an outward movement of chest and abdomen (Figure 10.2). Expiration involves relaxation of the diaphragm and recoil of the lungs. The abdominal muscles lengthen the diaphragm's fibers and assist in the next inspiratory cycle but, most importantly, produce an increase in intra-abdominal pressure. Abdominal muscles are also involved in coughing and clearing of secretions.

When respiratory muscle weakness occurs, pulmonary mechanics change. Ineffective diaphragm contraction results in a pulling up of the rib cage by other inspiratory muscles, resulting in a decrease in intra-abdominal pressure, which leads to inward movement of the anterior abdomen. This is called the *respiratory paradox* (Figure 10.2) or *paradoxical breathing* or *rocking horse breathing*. In addition, the scalene and sternocleidomastoid muscles are recruited. The rhythmic contraction of these muscles, which can be palpated, is known as the respiratory pulse.

CAPSULE 10.1   NEURAL CONTROL OF BREATHING AND ABNORMAL PATTERNS

Two centers in the brainstem generate a respiratory oscillating pattern: the medulla oblongata central pattern generator and the pontine respiratory group. The medulla oblongata center consists of two major respiratory neuron groups with separate tasks. The dorsal respiratory group times inspiration and the respiratory cycle, and the ventral respiratory group is involved with expiration and includes the expiratory neurons of the Bötzinger complex. The nucleus ambiguus, for dilator function of the upper airway during inspiration, and the nucleus paraambigualis, for inspiratory force, are also within this ventral population. When these respiratory neurons in the medulla oblongata fire, specific patterns of the respiratory cycle are identified, suggesting architectural organization. The pontine respiratory neuronal group consists of a medial parabrachial/Kölliker fuse (phase switch between inspiration and expiration) and a lateral parabrachial group (inspiration). The pontine center has a connecting link to the medulla center and functions as a time-tuning controller (e.g., setting lung volumes). Input to these centers comes from nonchemical reflexes (pharyngeal and pulmonary receptors and vagus nerve) and chemoreceptors (hydrogen ion). Stimulation is by decreased PaO_2 (not content such as anemia) and increased $PaCO_2$.[28] The cortex can override these control centers, allowing speech, singing, coughing, and breath holding.

The respiratory pacemaker or rhythmogenesis is likely located in a complex of neurons located in the pre-Bötzinger complex.

Multiple patterns have been recognized and named (see accompanying illustration). These patterns, when present, indicate a structural lesion in the brain but a clinicopathologic correlation is far from established and more likely absent. These patterns may occur in patients with bihemispheric lesions, brainstem lesions or both.

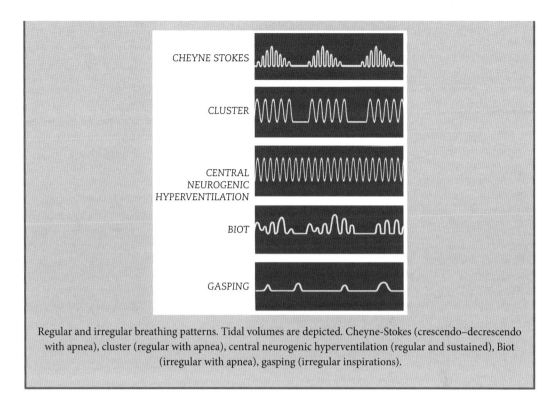

Regular and irregular breathing patterns. Tidal volumes are depicted. Cheyne-Stokes (crescendo–decrescendo with apnea), cluster (regular with apnea), central neurogenic hyperventilation (regular and sustained), Biot (irregular with apnea), gasping (irregular inspirations).

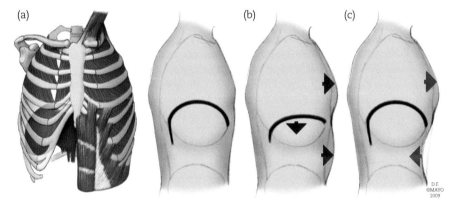

FIGURE 10.2: Anatomy of respiratory muscles. (a) Normal position. (b) Normal breathing. (c) Paradoxical breathing.

When breathing is impaired, not only is pump failure a major concern, but lung function also becomes impaired. This is partly due to the inability to cough, which results in atelectasis, shunting, and hypoxemia. When respiratory muscle weakness occurs, tidal volumes are reduced, and this might reduce surfactant. Surfactant allows oxygen (O_2) and carbon dioxide (CO_2) to diffuse freely across the alveolar membrane. Surfactant reduces the work of breathing, allows the opening of collapsed lung regions with minimal inspiratory pressures, and prevents atelectasis.

The clinical features that should alert one to the possibility of neuromuscular respiratory failure are listed in Table 10.2. The first signs are subtle and typically are not detected by bedside measurements of respiratory mechanics or by pulse oximeter. The arterial blood gas levels can be entirely normal because the patient, due to an increase in breathing frequency, is still able to compensate for a threatening hypoxemia. (The typical response in other medical disorders is increased tidal volume. In this situation, because of respiratory muscle fatigue, tidal volume is reduced.) Hypoxemia

TABLE 10.2. CLINICAL FEATURES OF
NEUROMUSCULAR RESPIRATORY
FAILURE

Restlessness, out of breath sensation
Tachycardia (pulse rate > 100/min)
Tachypnea (respiratory rate > 20/min)
Use of sternocleidomastoid or scalene muscles (by
    palpation alone)
Forehead sweating
Hesitant, constantly interrupting speech
Asynchronous (paradoxical) breathing

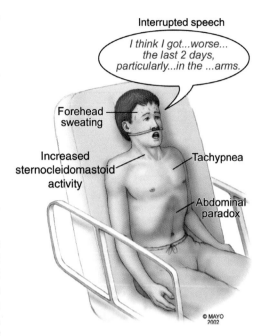

FIGURE 10.3: Bedside assessment of neuromuscular respiratory failure and need for intubation.

occurs due to significant shunting associated with collapse of multiple alveoli that are not recruited from breathing. It is important to note here that normocarbia (or rising $PaCO_2$ still within the normal range) indicates failure in a patient with tachypnea (unable to "blow off" CO_2). Eventually, when pulmonary function tests are markedly reduced, $PaCO_2$ profoundly increases. Moreover, low-flow (1–2 L/min) oxygen administration may worsen hypercarbia substantially.[11]

The focus of examination in patients with breathlessness due to neuromuscular disease should be on oropharyngeal dysfunction, frequent coughing as a sign of inability to clear secretions, and paradoxical breathing.[4,7,9] Paradoxical breathing due to diaphragm weakness reveals itself late in a patient with an acute neuromuscular disorder, and more than likely indicates that an early opportunity for endotracheal intubation has been missed and that the patient is on the verge of major respiratory collapse.

Careful inspection and testing of the oropharyngeal muscles may point to a diagnosis. Long-standing dysfunction, such as in amyotrophic lateral sclerosis (ALS), is often evident by the presence of a wrinkled, fasciculating, slowly moving tongue and a hyperactive jaw reflex. In myasthenia gravis, next to ptosis and ophthalmoparesis, muscle weakness is prominent in the masseter muscles, and repetitive forceful biting on a tongue depressor is soon followed by inability to close the teeth. Passage of air through the nose when asked to blow up the cheek against counterpressure by the examiner's thumb and index finger reveals additional oropharyngeal weakness. These findings hint not only of involvement of the respiratory mechanics but also that ineffective swallowing could lead to aspiration. In a study on predictors of respiratory decline in Guillain-Barré syndrome, oropharyngeal

dysfunction predicted later requirement of mechanical ventilation.[22]

In the more extreme situations Abdominal retraction, sternocleidomastoid contraction, sweating, and interrupted speech is seen and not infrequently accompanied by nasal flaring and sternal retraction.

The symptoms and signs of acute neuromuscular respiratory failure are often far more subtle. After striking up a conversation, it becomes obvious that the patient frequently pauses to take a breath. Sweat is occasionally found at the hairline or has collected in the eyebrows as a sign of the increased work of breathing. Restlessness may be apparent, but other patients are quiet and simply nod "yes" when asked if they are short of breath. Many will feel they are not catching enough air or experience a feeling as if they have "run to catch a train" (Figure 10.3).

Use of accessory muscles is not always recognized through simple observation, and, as mentioned earlier, palpation of the sternocleidomastoid muscles may disclose muscle contractions during breathing. Contraction of the sternocleidomastoid muscles can be palpated long before paradoxical breathing becomes obvious clinically. The rhythmicity of these contractions have been called "respiratory pulse." At night, relaxation of these muscles may result in increased demand for diaphragmatic performance and thus hypoventilation and hypercapnia. Frequent nocturnal awakening may signal respiratory dysfunction that is not yet evident during the daytime.[34] Nonetheless, the clinical hallmark of diaphragmatic fatigue is dyssynchronous movement of the chest cage and abdomen. Dyspnea is much more significant when the patient is supine rather than sitting upright, and this also explains the tendency to worsen overnight.[49]

Patients with signs of diaphragmatic failure invariably have tachycardia and tachypnea.[15] These clinical warning signs are usually associated with some sense of discomfort and anxiety. The tachypnea may be subtle, and the respiratory rate is often increased to 20 breaths per minute and quickly rises. A useful bedside test is to have the patient count to 20 in one breath after maximal inhalation. If the patient can count that far, advancing one per second, the vital capacity is probably still within normal range. In Guillain-Barré syndrome, acute neuromuscular respiratory failure, once present, progresses usually in a day and is typically seen in patients with rapid progression to quadriplegia (1–3 days) and oropharyngeal weakness. Coughing eventually becomes weak and this is best judged by touching the abdominal muscles. Often the abdominal and spinal muscles are affected simultatously and patients may not be able to turn or even sit upright. Recognition of acute respiratory neuromuscular failure and oropharyngeal weakness remains difficult and so is the decision to preemptively intubate. Most of the time, patients say they can hold on to it, but hours later request easily consent to go ahead or even may request a ventilator.

BEDSIDE RESPIRATORY TESTS

Laboratory measurements are very useful, but they must be viewed together with the clinical manifestations of respiratory failure (Table 10.3). All these bedside respiratory tests are effort-dependent and require some training on the part of the examiner. The test results are not infrequently spuriously low from inadequate mouth closure, particularly in patients with bilateral facial palsy.

Pulmonary function tests provide quite useful values and are easy to obtain using non-electrical bedside devices. Commonly used peak flow devices (e.g., for asthma) are unreliable because expiratory peak flow rates can be normal in neuromuscular respiratory failure, as the airway is patent and lung recoil is actually increased. The simplest tests are assessment of vital capacity (VC), maximal inspiratory pressure (PI_{max}), and maximal expiratory pressure (PE_{max}).[6,48] The patient's position when these values are obtained is critical

because clinically relevant diaphragmatic fatigue may become obvious in the supine position.

The technique of obtaining respiratory muscle function values is important. A scuba diving mouthpiece may reduce leakage, particularly when bilateral facial palsy is present. After the patient is connected to this apparatus, a nose clip is placed and the airway is occluded by blocking a port in the valve or by closing a shutter. VC is the volume of gas measured from a slow, complete forced expiration after maximal inspiration. VC can be reduced by additional airway and pulmonary disorders, certainly in patients with prior restricted pulmonary disease. PI_{max} is recorded when a patient forcefully inspires against an occluded device. Typically, PI_{max} is measured near residual volume at the end of maximal expiration and has a negative value as a result of the inspiratory effort in the presence of an occluded airway. PE_{max} measured near total lung capacity is the maximal pressure that can be generated by the patient making a forceful expiratory effort in an occluded airway. The manometer is able to record from 0 to 100 cm H_2O (Figure 10.4). Coaching the patient in these breathing exercises is very important. Many patients have a tendency to produce a Valsalva maneuver, after which the required pressure is not generated, leading to falsely low values. Lack of patient understanding on how to perform this test remains a major problem in obtaining these spirometric values. In patients with substantial leaks from facial diplegia, mask spirometry may substantially improve the numbers and may even avoid triage to the NICU for spurious findings.[17,51]

Pulmonary function tests are useful in GBS. A retrospective analysis of 114 patients with GBS noted possible critical values of vital capacity of less than 20 mL/kg, PI_{max} less than −30 cm H_2O,

TABLE 10.3. PULMONARY FUNCTION TESTS TO MONITOR NEUROMUSCULAR RESPIRATORY FAILURE

Parameter	Normal Value	Critical Value
Vital capacity	40–70 mL/kg	20 mL/kg
Maximum inspiratory pressure	Male ≥ −100 cm H_2O Female ≥ −70 cm H_2O	−30 cm H_2O
Maximum expiratory pressure	Male > 100 cm H_2O Female > 40 cm H_2O	40 cm H_2O

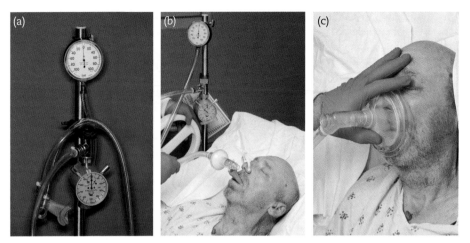

FIGURE 10.4: (a) Bedside device for measurement of maximal inspiratory and expiratory pressures and vital capacity. Upper meter measures pressure in cm H_2O. Sucking in gives a negative reading, and the needle moves to the left (normal, 100 cm H_2O). Blowing out gives a positive reading, and the needle moves to the right. Lower meter (Dräger volumeter) shows the tidal volume (spontaneous breathing) or vital capacity. (b) Typical setup with testing of patient. (c) Use of mask in a patient with marked facial diplegia.

PE_{max} less than 40 cm H_2O (the so-called 20/30/40 rule), but also noted as critical any reduction in vital capacity of more than 30% from baseline.[22] Not unexpectedly, another study found VC at 60% of the predictive value a warning sign of respiratory failure in Guillain-Barré syndrome.[6] A new technique is chest ultrasound, which provides direct visualization of diaphragmatic function.[40] Data are not yet available in the major acute neuromuscular disorders. Muscle thickening is seen with a functioning diaphragm, and diaphragm thickness can be measured (Figure 10.5).

The chest radiograph remains important in assessing pulmonary abnormalities. In neurogenic pulmonary edema, it may show hazy opacities and airspace shadowing indistinguishable from cardiogenic pulmonary edema or aspiration pneumonitis (Figure 10.6).[8] Both acute lung injury and cardiac dysfunction may be present as a result of an adrenergic surge in acute hemispheric lesions or subarachnoid hemorrhage. Suppression of cough reflex by sedatives or antiepileptic agents (e.g., barbiturates) may cause mucus plugging of a main bronchus (Figure 10.7). The chest radiograph may also show indirect signs of phrenic nerve injury (Figure 10.8).

The pulmonary complications associated with acute neurologic disease are discussed in detail in Chapter 55. Arterial blood gas interpretation as a result of hypoxemia, hypercarbia, and respiratory acidosis, is discussed in Chapter 57.

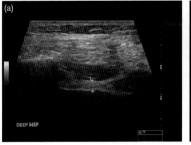
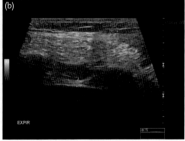

FIGURE 10.5: Chest Ultrasound: Note diaphragm change in thickness with inspiration and expiration.

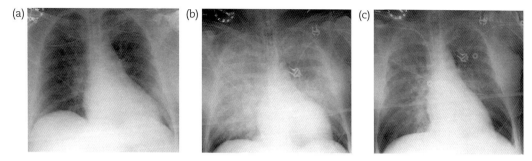

FIGURE 10.6: Serial chest radiographs in a patient with subarachnoid hemorrhage showing acute development of pulmonary edema. (a) Chest radiograph on admission. (b) Acute development of pulmonary infiltrates and enlargement of the heart shadow, indicating pulmonary edema due to cardiac dysfunction. (c) After improvement in cardiac function with use of inotropes, infiltrates remain, suggesting dual injury to lungs and heart.

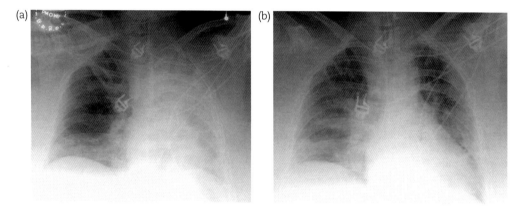

FIGURE 10.7: Acute bronchial occlusion from mucus plug (a), with re-expansion of the lung after bronchoscopic removal (b).

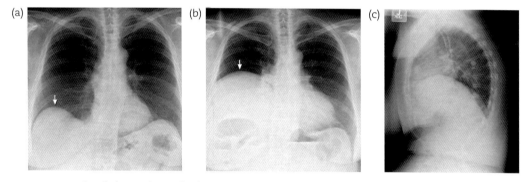

FIGURE 10.8: Serial chest radiographs showing development of hemidiaphragm elevation due to phrenic nerve injury on the right. (a, normal; b and c, abnormal.)

LINE OF ACTION

One of the first decisions is to determine whether the patient might benefit from noninvasive ventilation. In the absence of airway obstruction and pooling of secretions, patients with neuromuscular failure may benefit from a trial of bi-level positive airway pressure (BiPAP).[33,38] A BiPAP has been successful in patients with chronic neuromuscular disease and worsening respiratory mechanics. Myasthenia gravis and ALS are commonly seen in the ED, and these patients could be successfully treated with BiPAP if their arterial blood gas levels do not demonstrate a profound hypercarbia. Patients with an acutely progressive disorder (e.g., Guillain-Barré syndrome) do not have enough reserve to breathe satisfactorily and need full mechanical ventilation after intubation.[23,26,33,39,41–44,50]

Elective endotracheal intubation must be performed in any patient with marginal oxygenation.[47] Patients who have a mild tachycardia, display evidence of hypoxemia on a pulse oximeter, have evidence of increased work of breathing with change in posture, or are simple restless and short of breath must be intubated preemptively.[13]

In comatose patients, obstruction of the airway occurs for several reasons.[14,37,48] First, muscles of the floor of the mouth and tongue become reduced in tone, and this changes their anatomic relationships. The tongue is repositioned to the back wall of the oropharynx and obstructs the airway. This position is even more exaggerated when the head is flexed. The airway can be reopened using a simple technique called the *head-tilt/chin-lift* (Figure 10.9). First, the examiner tilts the patient's head backward to what is often called the "sniffing position." In this position, trachea and pharynx angulation is minimal, thus allowing for air transport. Next, the index and middle fingers of the examiner's hand lift the mandible and bring the tongue forward, thus clearing the airway.

Another technique is the *jaw-thrust/head-tilt*. The examiner places his middle three fingers under the patient's jaw and lifts the chin forward. The examiner's index finger and thumb are free to fit a mask snugly to the face, and the other hand is left free to operate a resuscitation bag.

When the airway appears blocked by foreign material or dentures, this technique is modified by placing the thumb in the mouth, grasping the chin, and pulling it upward, leaving the other hand free to clear obstructing material from the airway (Figure 10.9).

An oropharyngeal airway should be placed in comatose patients, and it is essential in patients who recently had a seizure because it prevents further tongue biting. To place this oral airway device, the mouth is opened, a wooden tongue depressor is placed at the base of the tongue, and downward pressure is applied to displace the tongue from the posterior pharyngeal wall. The oropharyngeal tube is then placed close to the posterior wall of the oropharynx and is moved toward the tongue until the teeth are at the bite-block section.

Alternatively, the jaw is thrust forward and the device is placed in a concave position, toward the palate, and then rotated.

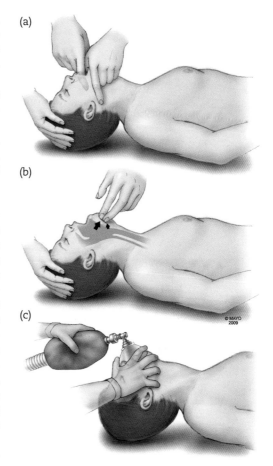

FIGURE 10.9: Techniques of airway management. (a) Tongue jaw lift/finger sweep. (b) Head-tilt/chin-lift. (c) Jaw thrust/mask ventilation.

The proper length of the oropharyngeal tube can be estimated by holding one end to the corner of the mouth and the other to the ear. An airway that is too long pushes the epiglottis down and compresses the larynx, reducing the capacity to ventilate and, worse, increases the risk of gastric insufflation. Too short an airway pushes the tongue posteriorly, aggravating the obstruction.

Hypoxemia is often encountered, and oxygen administration has a high priority in patients with impaired consciousness.

An adequate supply of oxygen can be provided through a large selection of delivery systems. Nasal prongs (flow rate of oxygen of 1–5 L/min) can be inefficient because they provide only 30% oxygen concentrations and often dislodge. A face mask with a flow rate of 6–12 L/min and up to 60% oxygen should be considered.[29] Resuscitation bags are an optimal source of oxygen, and they can deliver a fraction of inspiratory O_2 (FIO_2)

above 0.9 when the oxygen flow in the bag is 10 mL/min. Oxygenation should be monitored with a pulse oximeter (O_2 saturation should exceed 90%) or measurement of an arterial blood gas sample (PaO_2 >100 mm Hg).

An inappropriately secured airway may rapidly result in hypoxemia. The risks of hypoxemia are considerable, even in controlled hospital settings such as EDs and intensive care units, and it is reasonable to assume that improper airway management in patients with a neurologic catastrophe may influence outcome. If ignored, these events may potentially contribute to the initial insult and may lead to a worse outcome than otherwise would be expected.

Jaw thrust and mask ventilation securely maintain an open airway but must be followed by endotracheal intubation, done by an experienced physician. Endotracheal intubation may be complicated in a traumatized patient with possible cervical spine injury. The ideal solution in these patients is to use fiberoptic bronchoscopy, because with this procedure the risk of further neck trauma from neck movement is low.[19] Immediate endotracheal intubation is required in patients with penetrating neck trauma or significant intra-oral bleeding. Complications of airway management remain high, particularly in traumatic head injury, and temporarily, a cricothyrotomy can be made.[20] A 14-gauge needle is inserted through the cricothyroid membrane, followed by insertion of a cannula. (The cricothyroid membrane is located just under the thyroid.) A formal tracheostomy should follow because ventilation through this small, highly flow-resistant tube is compromised.

The technique of intubation should be mastered. Elective intubation is done by an experienced physician, an experienced anesthesia team, or fellows training in neurologic intensive care.[2,3,46] (It is important to maintain the skill of endotracheal intubation. Generally, 50–70 intubations are needed to acquire competency, and simulation training on manikins has been perfected over the years.)

The choice of the intubation route is important. Nasal intubation is rarely done but has some advantages, including improved patient comfort, significantly tighter tube fixation, reduced laryngeal damage, and the possibility for proper mouth care. However, in patients with traumatic brain injury and potential cerebrospinal fluid leak, nasal intubation may lead to contamination. Moreover, it has been well appreciated that nasal intubation produces a transient bacteremia. The infectious risks of prolonged nasotracheal intubation (more than 5 days) from purulent paranasal sinusitis are considerable, and patients with diabetes mellitus or corticosteroid coverage are at increased risk.[10,25] It may also lead to nasal septal necrosis and perforation of the nasal palate. Associated possible cervical spine injury should not necessarily sway the decision toward a nasal route for intubation, because if time allows, fiberoptic intubation more likely minimizes displacement of the unstable cervical spinal column.

The technique of endotracheal intubation begins with recognition of the difficult airway. When a difficult endotracheal intubation is expected (even conservative estimates place this at 1 in 10 critically ill patients), a physician with daily expertise in endotracheal intubation should supervise or, more likely, perform the procedure. Important cues for a difficult intubation include the inability to visualize oral structures (tongue, soft palate, tonsillar fossa, and uvula) when the mouth is wide open, significant facial trauma, cervical spine fracture, mandibular hypoplasia prognathia, history of rheumatoid arthritis, spondylitic ankylosis, morbid obesity, or a short, muscular, thick neck.

The Mallampati's classification of a difficult airway has been modified, which is based on the visibility of the pharyngeal structures due to variation in tongue base. Class I is full exposure of soft palate, uvula, and tonsillar pillars; class II, exposure of the soft palate and base of the uvula with only a portion of the posterior pharyngeal wall visible; class III, visibility of soft palate only; and class IV, no visualization of pharyngeal structures except the hard palate. Its predictive value for a difficult intubation remains limited, and the classification should be incorporated with other physical signs.

Physical examination should at least include an assessment of the temporomandibular joint, length of the mandible, and, most important, extension of the cervical spine. Important bedside estimates are the ability to insert three fingers into the oral cavity and to place three fingers between the thyroid bone and the mandible when the head is extended (Figure 10.10). Patients with long-standing insulin-dependent diabetes mellitus have a major limitation in cervical spine mobility.[36] Difficulty in closing the palms and bowing at the interphalangeal area, creating a "prayer sign," also seem to be correlated with limitations in neck extension.

Elective intubation can proceed if the patient has not taken food for at least 6 hours. The procedure of endotracheal intubation can be accompanied by cricoid pressure (Sellick maneuver). Movement of this circle of cartilage posteriorly occludes the esophagus and may prevent regurgitation (Figure 10.11). However, the maneuver is poorly applied and its effect has been questioned.[27]

Stepwise performance is usually successful. The patient is placed in the sniffing position and

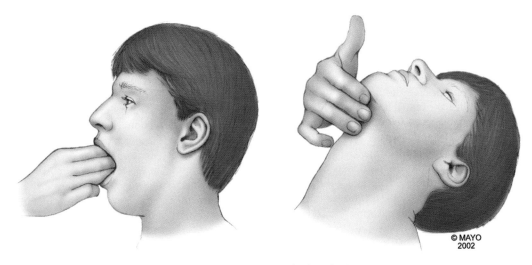

FIGURE 10.10: Bedside estimates of possible difficult endotracheal intubation.

given 100% oxygen through ventilation with a bag and mask. To begin the laryngoscopic initiation of intubation, the physician extends the patient's head and carefully introduces the laryngoscope into the patient's mouth with the left hand. The physician must be careful not to injure the patient's teeth and lips. Dental injury mostly occurs in patients who have significant dental or periodontal disease.

During laryngoscopy, the base of the tongue is seen first. As the laryngoscope is advanced, the epiglottis appears. If the Miller blade is used, the tip is placed under the epiglottis to lift it up and out of the way. At this point, the laryngoscope is lifted in the direction of its handle; pivoting the instrument back onto the upper incisor will injure the patient's teeth.

Lifting the laryngoscope brings the arytenoids, at the most posterior part of the larynx, into view.

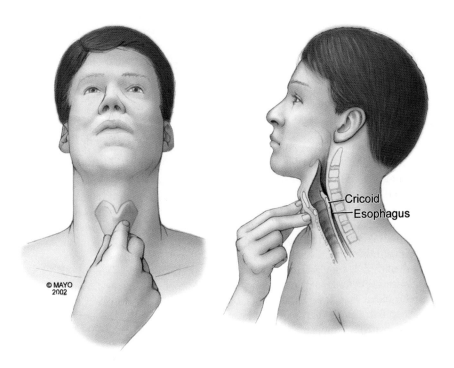

FIGURE 10.11: The Sellick maneuver.

Further lifting exposes the cords. External pressure on the thyroid cartilage or cricoid cartilage by an assistant might help bring the laryngeal structures into view. As the endotracheal tube is advanced, it passes between the cords. After the cuff has passed the cords, advancement of only 3 cm is needed for proper placement. The technique of intubation is depicted in Figure 10.12. The endotracheal tube is shown in Figure 10.13.

The cuff is inflated up to 10–15 cm H_2O or more if a leak is still heard. The physician must auscultate over both lungs to ensure the presence of bilateral breath sounds. The gastric area is also auscultated to rule out esophageal ventilation. A quick method to confirm proper tube placement is to use a disposable capnometer that changes to yellow when exposed to carbon dioxide. The location of the endotracheal tube must be positively confirmed by a routine chest radiograph, which identifies the tip of the tube 5–7 cm above the carina or at the T6 level.

In some circumstances—if the airway is categorized as a *"cannot intubate, cannot ventilate"* situation[13,16,18,21]—cricothyroidotomy is the only option for providing an airway. A horizontal incision is made over the lower part of cricothyroid membrane, followed by insertion of a tube, in some cases over a guidewire.[1]

Alternatively, in patients with difficult airways, a modified laryngeal mask airway can be used, particularly by emergency medical services in the field and non-anesthesiologists.[35] The mask is modified to facilitate tracheal intubation with a tracheal tube. The major incentives for its use are obscured vision of the larynx by blood and secretions and the potential for spinal cord damage when neck injuries are not yet known. Considerable training is required. This technique may be a useful bridging device to a more traditional cuffed tracheal tube in acute trauma care, but it is not particularly useful in the NICU.

Intubation in the ED has evolved into a standardized approach known as *rapid-sequence intubation*, which entails the near-simultaneous administration of an induction agent and a paralytic agent. Preinduction drugs (lidocaine, esmolol, or opioids) have been used, but there is little evidence for their use. The induction agent rapidly causes unconsciousness, and most protocols use etomidate and succinylcholine or rocuronium for this purpose. Rapid-sequence intubation involves "s7 Ps" (preparation, preoxygenation, premedication, paralysis, positioning, placement of the tube, and postintubation care) (Table 10.4).

After endotracheal intubation, virtually all patients are well served with an initial ventilator

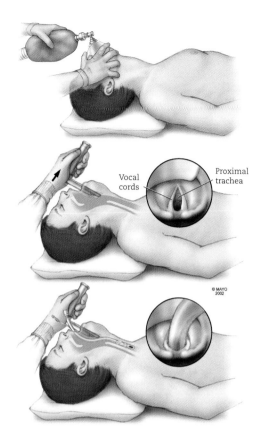

FIGURE 10.12: Technique of endotracheal intubation.

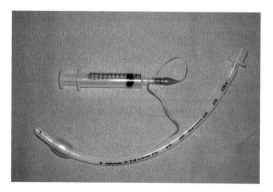

FIGURE 10.13: Endotracheal tube with inflated cuff (usually 10–12 mL of air in the syringe is sufficient).

order that includes rate control in the intermittent mandatory ventilation mode.[45] The positive pressure breaths that are delivered by the mechanical ventilator are triggered by the patient, who has to generate only small pressure differences. The patient is able to breathe between ventilator breaths and has entirely unsupported breaths. This ventilator order is particularly useful in neurologic patients because it allows for spontaneous

TABLE 10.4. RAPID SEQUENCE
INTUBATION

Preinduction agents	Lidocaine 1.5 mg/kg IV
	Fentanyl 2–3 µg/kg IV push
Induction agents	Etomidate 0.3 mg/kg IV push
	Ketamine 2 mg/kg IV push
Paralytic agents	Succinylcholine 1.5 mg/kg IV push
	Rocuronium 1 mg/kg IV push

breathing, and it can deliver hyperventilation if needed. Mechanical ventilation is discussed in Chapter 17.

CONCLUSIONS

- Initial appropriate airway management includes mask ventilation with oxygen (10–15 L/min flow) after the jaw is lifted upward to open the airway. An oropharyngeal airway may facilitate mask ventilation.
- Intubation is needed in patients with acute brain injury who cannot protect their airway, as shown by frequent hypoxic episodes; in patients with tachycardia and tachypnea associated with neuromuscular failure (Guillain-Barré syndrome, myasthenia gravis); and in patients with primary pulmonary disease (pulmonary edema or progressive aspiration pneumonitis).
- Clinical features of imminent neuromuscular respiratory failure are restlessness, asynchronous breathing, use of sternocleidomastoid muscles, and forehead sweating. Pulmonary function tests are of potential use; the critical values are vital capacity, 20 mL/kg; maximum inspiratory pressure, −30 cm H_2O; and maximum expiratory pressure, 40 cm H_2O (the 20-30-40 rule).

REFERENCES

1. Archan S, Prause G, Gumpert R, Seibert FJ, Kugler B. Cricothyroidotomy on the scene in a patient with severe facial trauma and difficult neck anatomy. *Am J Emerg Med* 2009;27:133, e131–e134.
2. Boet S, Naik VN, Diemunsch PA. Virtual simulation training for fibreoptic intubation. *Can J Anaesth* 2009;56:87–88.
3. Boylan JF, Kavanagh BP. Emergency airway management: competence versus expertise? *Anesthesiology* 2008;109:945–947.
4. Braun NM, Arora NS, Rochester DF. Respiratory muscle and pulmonary function in polymyositis and other proximal myopathies. *Thorax* 1983;38:616–623.
5. Chen ZY, Xu JG, Shen LY, Gu YD. Phrenic nerve conduction study in patients with traumatic brachial plexus palsy. *Muscle Nerve* 2001;24:1388–1390.
6. Chevrolet JC, Deleamont P. Repeated vital capacity measurements as predictive parameters for mechanical ventilation need and weaning success in the Guillain-Barre syndrome. *Am Rev Respir Dis* 1991;144:814–818.
7. de Carvalho M, Matias T, Coelho F, et al. Motor neuron disease presenting with respiratory failure. *J Neurol Sci* 1996;139 Suppl:117–122.
8. de Chazal I, Parham WM, 3rd, Liopyris P, Wijdicks EFM. Delayed cardiogenic shock and acute lung injury after aneurysmal subarachnoid hemorrhage. *Anesth Analg* 2005;100:1147–1149.
9. de Troyer A, Estenne M. The respiratory system in neuromuscular disorders. *Lung Biol Health Dis* 1995;85 (Part C):2177–2212.
10. Fassoulaki A, Pamouktsoglou P. Prolonged nasotracheal intubation and its association with inflammation of paranasal sinuses. *Anesth Analg* 1989;69:50–52.
11. Gay PC, Edmonds LC. Severe hypercapnia after low-flow oxygen therapy in patients with neuromuscular disease and diaphragmatic dysfunction. *Mayo Clinic Proc* 1995;70:327–330.
12. Gibson GJ, Pride NB, Davis JN, Loh LC. Pulmonary mechanics in patients with respiratory muscle weakness. *Am Rev Respir Dis* 1977;115:389–395.
13. Green L. Can't intubate, can't ventilate! A survey of knowledge and skills in a large teaching hospital. *Eur J Anaesthesiol* 2009;26:480–483.
14. Heffner JE. Airway management in the critically ill patient. *Crit Care Clin* 1990;6:533–550.
15. Kelly BJ, Luce JM. The diagnosis and management of neuromuscular diseases causing respiratory failure. *Chest* 1991;99:1485–1494.
16. Kheterpal S, Martin L, Shanks AM, Tremper KK. Prediction and outcomes of impossible mask ventilation: a review of 50,000 anesthetics. *Anesthesiology* 2009;110:891–897.
17. Kramer CL, McCullough M, Wijdicks EFM. Teaching video neuroimages: how to unmask respiratory strength confounded by facial diplegia. *Neurology* 2015;84:e57–e58.
18. Langeron O, Semjen F, Bourgain JL, Marsac A, Cros AM. Comparison of the intubating laryngeal mask airway with the fiberoptic intubation in anticipated difficult airway management. *Anesthesiology* 2001;94:968–972.
19. Langford RA, Leslie K. Awake fibreoptic intubation in neurosurgery. *J Clin Neurosci* 2009;16:366–372.

20. Lanza DC, Parnes SM, Koltai PJ, Fortune JB. Early complications of airway management in head-injured patients. *Laryngoscope* 1990;100:958–961.

21. Lavery GG, McCloskey BV. The difficult airway in adult critical care. *Crit Care Med* 2008;36:2163–2173.

22. Lawn ND, Fletcher DD, Henderson RD, Wolter TD, Wijdicks EFM. Anticipating mechanical ventilation in Guillain-Barre syndrome. *Arch Neurol* 2001;58:893–898.

23. Lyall RA, Donaldson N, Fleming T, et al. A prospective study of quality of life in ALS patients treated with noninvasive ventilation. *Neurology* 2001;57:153–156.

24. Maramattom BV, Wijdicks EFM. Neurology of pulmonology and acid-base disturbance. In: Schapira AHV, ed. *Neurology and Clinical Neuroscience.* Philadelphia: Mosby; 2007:1569–1576.

25. Michelson A, Schuster B, Kamp HD. Paranasal sinusitis associated with nasotracheal and orotracheal long-term intubation. *Arch Otolaryngol Head Neck Surg* 1992;118:937–939.

26. Miller RG, Rosenberg JA, Gelinas DF, et al. Practice parameter: the care of the patient with amyotrophic lateral sclerosis (an evidence-based review): report of the Quality Standards Subcommittee of the American Academy of Neurology: ALS Practice Parameters Task Force. *Neurology* 1999;52:1311–1323.

27. Nafiu OO, Bradin S, Tremper KK. Knowledge, attitude, and practice regarding cricoid pressure of ED personnel at a large U.S. teaching hospital. *J Emerg Nurs* 2009;35:11–15.

28. Nogues MA, Benarroch E. Abnormalities of respiratory control and the respiratory motor unit. *Neurologist* 2008;14:273–288.

29. Ooi R, Joshi P, Soni N. An evaluation of oxygen delivery using nasal prongs. *Anaesthesia* 1992;47:591–593.

30. Pandit A, Kalra S, Woodcock A. An unusual cause of bilateral diaphragmatic paralysis. *Thorax* 1992;47:201.

31. Piehler JM, Pairolero PC, Gracey DR, Bernatz PE. Unexplained diaphragmatic paralysis: a harbinger of malignant disease? *J Thorac Cardiovasc Surg* 1982;84:861–864.

32. Pontoppidan H, Geffin B, Lowenstein E. Acute respiratory failure in the adult. 2. N *Engl J Med* 1972;287:743–752.

33. Rabinstein A, Wijdicks EFM. BiPAP in acute respiratory failure due to myasthenic crisis may prevent intubation. *Neurology* 2002;59:1647–1649.

34. Ragette R, Mellies U, Schwake C, Voit T, Teschler H. Patterns and predictors of sleep disordered breathing in primary myopathies. *Thorax* 2002;57:724–728.

35. Reardon RF, Martel M. The intubating laryngeal mask airway: suggestions for use in the emergency department. *Acad Emerg Med* 2001;8:833–838.

36. Reissell E, Orko R, Maunuksela EL, Lindgren L. Predictability of difficult laryngoscopy in patients with long-term diabetes mellitus. *Anaesthesia* 1990;45:1024–1027.

37. Reynolds SF, Heffner J. Airway management of the critically ill patient: rapid-sequence intubation. *Chest* 2005;127:1397–1412.

38. Rumbak MJ, Walker RM. Should patients with neuromuscular disease be denied the choice of the treatment of mechanical ventilation? *Chest* 2001;119:683–684.

39. Samsoon GL, Young JR. Difficult tracheal intubation: a retrospective study. *Anaesthesia* 1987;42:487–490.

40. Sarwal A, Walker FO, Cartwright MS. Neuromuscular ultrasound for evaluation of the diaphragm. *Muscle Nerve* 2013;47:319–329.

41. Sharshar T, Chevret S, Bourdain F, Raphael JC. Early predictors of mechanical ventilation in Guillain-Barré syndrome. *Crit Care Med* 2003;31:278–283.

42. Sivak ED, Shefner JM, Mitsumoto H, Taft JM. The use of non-invasive positive pressure ventilation (NIPPV) in ALS patients: a need for improved determination of intervention timing. *Amyotroph Lateral Scler Other Motor Neuron Disord* 2001;2:139–145.

43. Sivak ED, Shefner JM, Sexton J. Neuromuscular disease and hypoventilation. *Curr Opin Pulm Med* 1999;5:355–362.

44. Slutsky AS. Mechanical ventilation. American College of Chest Physicians' Consensus Conference. *Chest* 1993;104:1833–1859.

45. Soler JJ, Perpina M, Alfaro A. Hemidiaphragmatic paralysis caused by cervical herpes zoster. *Respiration* 1996;63:403–406.

46. Varney SM, Dooley M, Bebarta VS. Faster intubation with direct laryngoscopy vs handheld videoscope in uncomplicated manikin airways. *Am J Emerg Med* 2009;27:259–261.

47. Walz JM, Zayaruzny M, Heard SO. Airway management in critical illness. *Chest* 2007;131:608–620.

48. Wijdicks EFM, Borel CO. Respiratory management in acute neurologic illness. *Neurology* 1998;50:11–20.

49. Wijdicks EFM, Henderson RD, McClelland RL. Emergency intubation for respiratory failure in Guillain-Barre syndrome. *Arch Neurol* 2003;60:947–948.

50. Wijdicks EFM. Short of breath, short of air, short of mechanics. *Practical Neurology* 2002;2:208–213.

51. Wohlgemuth M, van der Kooi EL, Hendriks JC, Padberg GW, Folgering HT. Face mask spirometry and respiratory pressures in normal subjects. *Eur Respir J* 2003;22:1001–1006.

11

Seizing

An unquestionable seizure in an otherwise healthy patient is worrisome and must lead to a comprehensive search for a cause. Recurrent seizures are a neurologic emergency and brings a patient into the ED. Certainly when seizures are de novo a progression as such increases the odds of an underlying neurologic or medical condition for which, rapid therapeutic interventions are urgently needed. The persistence of seizure activity is an important discriminating factor because it is directly linked to the cumulative development of neurologic and medical complications.

Concurrent brain lesions are common in adult status epilepticus and, in most cases, are responsible for morbidity and mortality.[41,46] Status epilepticus lasting 1 hour or more increases morbidity 10-fold.[41,47] Prolonged apnea and anoxia may result in an additional anoxic–ischemic injury and persistent coma, emphasizing the need for early intubation and airway control. Conversely, rapidly treated status epilepticus may have an excellent neurologic outcome.

Long-standing morbidity in patients has been linked to less aggressive control of seizure activity. Therefore, rapid termination of seizures and simultaneous treatment of the underlying illness are of utmost priority, particularly when the disorder evolves into tonic-clonic status epilepticus.[41,46,51]

Status epilepticus in adults can be distinguished in several forms, each of which is discussed in detail. This chapter provides guidance for the recognition and initial management of different types of seizures seen in the ED. Prolonged and advanced care of status epilepticus is discussed in Chapter 40.

CLASSIFICATION AND PRESENTATION OF STATUS EPILEPTICUS

Convulsive status epilepticus can be divided into several major categories (Figure 11.1).[12,30,70,77] The distinction has relevance because the initial choice

of antiepileptic agents may be different, management may not involve antiepileptic agents (as in myoclonus status epilepticus and psychogenic seizures), and outcome may differ from category to category.

Tonic-Clonic Status Epilepticus

Tonic-clonic status epilepticus has typically been defined as repetitive generalized tonic-clonic seizures lasting 30 minutes or longer, or seizures without full return of consciousness between episodes. However, the evolution of seizures into status epilepticus often becomes clinically probable within a matter of minutes.

The tonic phase involves flexion of the axial muscles, upward or sideways eye deviation, and marked widening of the pupil diameter with sluggish light responses. The eyes remain open. The arms and legs are flexed and is soon followed by extension, clenching of teeth, and forced expiration for several seconds. Sweating may be seen and there may be an increase in blood pressure and pulse. The clonic phase begins with a tremor or shivering but gives way to uninterrupted jerking, which dies out gradually and may result in urinary and fecal incontinence after the sphincter muscles relax from a forceful contraction during the clonic phase. Usually, a generalized tonic-clonic seizure lasts 1–2 minutes, resolves with the appearance of labored breathing, and is followed for up to 5 minutes by a dazed state.[19] Some patients in status epilepticus gradually awaken but never to a point at which conversation is understood or simple commands are followed. Then, tonic spasm occurs again with a similar pattern of jerking and resolution.

Electroencephalographic (EEG) recordings, if available, typically show rhythmic spike or sharp-wave complexes or sharp and slow-wave discharges with a generalized distribution. Clinically, the distinction between a postictal confusional state emerging from a generalized tonic-clonic seizure and convulsive status epilepticus is difficult to make in the ED. Subtle eyelid or limb

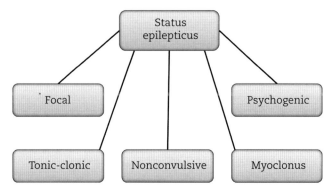

FIGURE 11.1: Classification of status epilepticus.

twitching in a stuporous patient may indicate continuous epileptic activity, but the distinction may require urgent EEG recording.

Typical clinical findings are tongue bite (large purple hematoma or erosion at the lateral border of the tongue, which should be carefully inspected after the tongue is pushed out or sideways with a tongue depressor) (Figure 11.2) and, occasionally, petechial hemorrhages are seen in the conjunctiva, chest, and neck. Other complications are bone fractures, posterior shoulder dislocation, pulmonary aspiration, and, rarely if ever, neurogenic pulmonary edema. Prolonged status epilepticus may produce fever, even on the day after presentation.

The most common causes of convulsive status epilepticus are shown in Table 11.1, but despite an exhaustive search, the cause may remain unknown.[14,18,50,74] Withdrawal of antiepileptic drugs or some other drastic change in patients with established seizure disorder is common.

Nonconvulsive Status Epilepticus

Delayed diagnosis of nonconvulsive status epilepticus is common because the condition may be mistaken for behavioral abnormalities or even a psychiatric disorder.[19,30]

Clinical presentation is diverse, but clinical signs are not always suggestive and may be diagnostically confusing. Consciousness is always impaired. Nonconvulsive status epilepticus results in blank staring, sometimes with tremulousness and subtle periorbital, facial, or limb myoclonus, or eye movement abnormalities such as nystagmus or eye deviation.[6,24] Patients have decreased or rambling speech output or are mute; thus, the distinction from aphasia with a structural lesion can be difficult. Aggressive behavior is uncommon, and more often patients are mildly agitated and easy to restrain. A waxing and waning state alternating between agitation and obtundation is characteristic. Inappropriate laughing, crying, or even singing may occur.

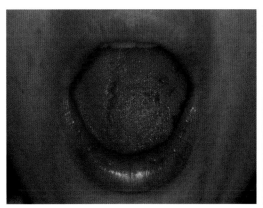 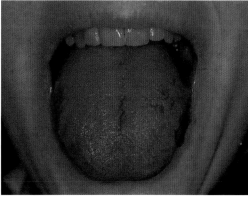

FIGURE 11.2: Tongue bite much more evident when tongue pushed out.

TABLE 11.1. CAUSES OF CONVULSIVE
STATUS EPILEPTICUS

Change in antiepileptic drugs
Bacterial meningitis or intracranial abscess
Encephalitis
Intracranial tumor or metastasis
Stroke
Arteriovenous malformation
Withdrawal of benzodiazepines
Drugs or alcohol withdrawal
Hyperglycemia
Hypoglycemia
Hyponatremia
Preeclampsia

Focal Status Epilepticus

Focal status epilepticus or epilepsia partialis continua involves continuous clonic movements of one or two extremities. Jerking of one arm or leg can be directly observed by the patient, who should be unable to influence its jerking frequency. Hemiparesis (which may last for days) may result if the condition is treated late. The disorder often is related to an acute hemispheric lesion (e.g., contusion, hemorrhage in metastasis). Dyscognitive focal status epilepticus (in the old terminology called complex partial or temporal lobe seizures) is prevalent in adults 20–40 years of age.[12] It may occur after a single seizure, or after replacement of antiepileptic drugs,[76] and it is more likely in patients with prior brain injury. Dyscognitive focal status epilepticus has behavioral disturbances that may resemble a psychotic break, and there may be vivid hallucinations and a temporary alteration of consciousness.

Psychogenic Status Epilepticus

Pseudoseizures can be difficult to differentiate from true seizures and may occur comparatively frequently in patients with proven seizure disorder.[53] The assessment of psychogenic seizures can be complicated because previous indiscriminate administration of a benzodiazepine may cloud the neurologic assessment, and EEG often is not immediately available to verify the psychiatric origin of the convulsions.

Several clinical characteristics should increase the likelihood of a diagnosis of psychogenic status epilepticus. An important discriminating sign is the presence of closed eyelids throughout the major motor manifestations.[63] Jerking movements are characteristically out of phase and asynchronous, with a highly typical forward thrusting of the pelvis. Screaming is common. Tongue biting is less likely, pupils may be dilated but have retained light responses, and the gag reflex is present. Jerking of the extremities may rapidly alternate in tonic-clonic-like movements, and often the arms can be positioned above the patient's face while continuously jerking and without falling on the face.[25,33] The head turns from side to side, and more characteristically, both eyes are consistently deviated from the examiner, occasionally switching with the examiner's position.[68] In between the jerking movements, the patient may speak brief sentences voicing major distress.

All of these manifestations, although very characteristic, can be imitated by nonconvulsive status epilepticus due to a frontal epileptic focus.

Myoclonus Status Epilepticus

Myoclonus status epilepticus is common in ED admitting comatose patients after asphyxia or cardiac arrest.[81] The clinical manifestations of myoclonus status epilepticus are vastly different, but it is still frequently misinterpreted as tonic-clonic seizures.

Myoclonus status epilepticus consists of sustained nearly synchronous brief jerking in the limbs and face and may involve the diaphragm. Touch, intubation, and placement of catheters may provoke the movements, but spontaneous jerking is more commonly the rule. An episodic upward eye position during a series of myoclonic jerks is typical. Myoclonus status epilepticus can be seen moments after cardiac resuscitation when circulation has returned and the patient has failed to awaken. Pathologic withdrawal or extensor motor responses are common. Its presence denotes massive cortical laminar necrosis, often in association with ischemic damage to the thalamus and sometimes even the spinal cord and a poor prognosis. It should be clearly differentiated from a sporadic myoclonic jerk that has a different prognosis even when seen in comatose patients.

Other conditions that cause myoclonus status epilepticus are environmental injuries but again due to anoxia (e.g., electrical injury, decompression sickness). However, profound myoclonus status epilepticus in comatose patients may also be caused by drug intoxication (predominantly lithium but also haloperidol, antiepileptic drugs, tricyclic antidepressants, and cephalosporins), toxic exposure to industrial agents (pesticides) and heavy metals, renal or hepatic failure, or much less common a neurodegenerative condition such as Creutzfeldt-Jakob disease in the final stage.

LABORATORY STUDIES IN STATUS EPILEPTICUS

One may appropriately question if an EEG is truly useful in the ED setting when a seizure seems undisputed by the emergency physician, neurologist, or bystanders. The availability of EEG in the emergency department may detect nonconvulsive status epilepticus in unexplained unresponsiveness or recognize that there are no correlations of the movements with EEG recordings. The yield in the ED for detecting seizures or status epilepticus, however, is very low (3%).[27]

The electrographic patterns of each type of status epilepticus is shown in Figure 11.3. Because withdrawal of antiepileptic drugs remains a commonly recognized cause of status epilepticus in adults with a prior seizure disorder, computed tomography (CT) scan or magnetic resonance imaging (MRI) findings are frequently normal. In refractory epilepsy, the rate of detection of histopathologically proven abnormalities (glioma, hippocampal sclerosis, developmental lesions) is 95% with conventional MRI and much lower with CT scan, with a sensitivity of 32%.[20] However, CT or MRI may show acute lesions, such as stroke or new traumatic contusions, metastatic disease, and glioma. Computed tomographic scanning in myoclonus status epilepticus may show diffuse cerebral edema and, less often, thalamic or cerebral infarcts in watershed territories. Focal hyperintensities on T2-weighted images and decreases in apparent diffusion coefficients in complex partial status epilepticus—all reversible—may be seen as a consequence of cytotoxic edema. Hippocampal or neocortical dropout abnormalities may emerge later and may be a direct correlate of seizures and not of hypoxemia.

In any new-onset status epilepticus, cerebrospinal fluid (CSF) examination should be strongly considered, to exclude acute bacterial meningitis and encephalitis. White blood cell counts in the CSF may increase from seizures, but not above 30 mononuclear cells/mm³, and CSF protein rarely profoundly increases.[3]

MISCELLANEOUS TESTS

Physiologic changes are observed in the aftermath of a seizure. A single generalized tonic-clonic seizure may produce similar laboratory changes to status epilepticus if values are obtained early after presentation. Most laboratory changes directly resulting from seizures or status epilepticus are self-limiting and rarely need intervention. However, abnormal laboratory values may suggest an underlying systemic illness.

White cell counts may increase substantially. Neutrophils usually remain dominant, but equally common is a lymphocyte increase in the differential count. Immature neutrophils can be present. Acute-phase hepatic proteins, glycoproteins, and globulins may transiently increase the erythrocyte sedimentation rate. Plasma glucose concentration may increase but remains in an indeterminate range of approximately 150 mg/dL. Plasma osmolality should be normal or mildly increased in patients with dehydration but is more significantly increased if recent alcohol abuse contributes to status epilepticus. Plasma osmolalities of 400–600 mOsm could be due to nonketotic hyperosmolar hyperglycemia. Hyponatremia may cause status epilepticus only when values are ≤ 110 mmol/L or have decreased at least 20–30 mmol/L within several hours. Spontaneous hypoglycemia possibly indicates a poison or, less commonly, insulinoma. Acute renal failure should point to possible rhabdomyolysis and prompt measurement of serum creatine kinase, which may reach values in the thousands.

Arterial blood gas should be measured. Respiratory acidosis is as common as metabolic lactic acidosis, but the pH is rarely below 7.0. The abnormality is self-limiting and resolves within hours.[80] Cardiac arrhythmias, such as sinus tachycardia, bradycardia, and supraventricular tachycardia, are rarely related to changes in the blood gases.[80]

Laboratory results may be helpful in distinguishing between status epilepticus and pseudoseizures. An entirely normal blood gas value and serum lactate while the patient is having convulsions support pseudoseizures. The serum concentration of prolactin is increased (peak value 15–20 minutes after onset of seizure) after a single epileptic generalized seizure but seldom after pseudoseizures. However, the discriminatory value in pseudo-status epilepticus has been debated, and prolactin may also be increased after syncope.[55]

MANAGEMENT OF RECURRENT SEIZURES

A clinical policy for the initial approach to patients with a seizure who do not have status epilepticus has been published by the American College of Emergency Physicians.[59] Four major issues are highlighted. First, prolonged altered

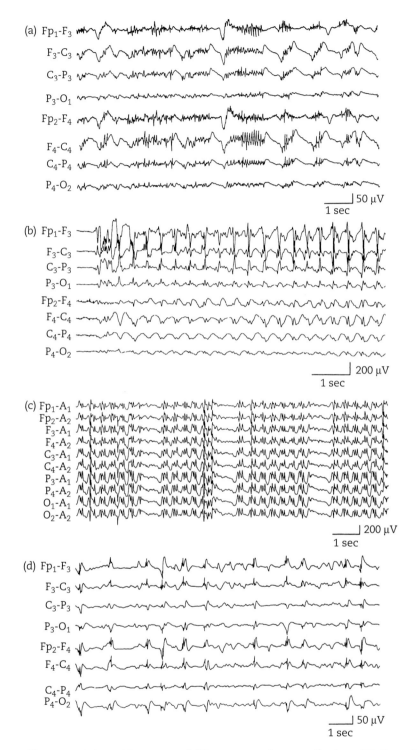

FIGURE 11.3: Electroencephalographic patterns of different types of status epilepticus. (A) Generalized tonic-clonic seizures (generalized high-frequency spikes and spike-and-wave discharges). (B) Focal status epilepticus (rhythmic waves and spikes in one hemisphere). (C) Nonconvulsive status epilepticus (episodes of spike-and-wave discharges coinciding with stupor). (D) Myoclonic status epilepticus (continuous epileptiform discharges with a burst-suppression pattern).

consciousness should not be attributed to a postictal state. Second, patients with prior epilepsy who are alert and have normal findings on neurologic examination do not require aggressive evaluation other than measurement of antiepileptic drug levels. Third, alcohol-related seizures may indicate serious underlying morbidity. Fourth, to prevent major injury, the patient should be implicitly told that driving and operation of machinery should be restricted until a reasonable observation period has passed.

The risk of a second seizure is approximately 35% in the subsequent 3–5 years.[21–23,32,45] Approximately 75% of patients with two or three unprovoked seizures have further seizures within 4 years. The risk of seizure recurrence is substantially increased (probably doubled) when an identifiable brain lesion is found. The risk of recurrent seizures is increased in patients with focal seizures as a result of a greater likelihood of an underlying lesion. The risk may be increased if seizures occur during sleep. The predictive value of an abnormal EEG for recurrence in an unprovoked seizure is uncertain in adults.[5]

Before a patient is dismissed from the ED, several diagnostic tests should be considered (Table 11.2); but in many instances with a single symptomatic or recurrent seizure, admission for IV fosphenytoin loading is advised.

The recommended drugs for primary generalized tonic-clonic seizures or partial seizures with secondary generalization are fosphenytoin (300 mg/day in one dose; therapeutic serum level, 10–20 µg/mL), carbamazepine (300–1,200 mg/day; therapeutic serum level, 4–12 µg/mL), and valproic acid (600–3,000 mg/day; therapeutic serum level, 50–150 µg/mL). Valproic acid has notable side effects, particularly platelet dyscrasias and liver failure (1 in 20,000).[58] The first-line agent for absence seizures is valproic acid (600–3,000 mg/day; therapeutic level, 50–150 µg/mL), ethosuximide (20–30 mg/kg per day; therapeutic level, 40–100 µg/mL), or lamotrigine (100–400 mg/day in two divided doses). A combination of lamotrigine and valproate is often needed to control recurrent absences.[73] Dose reduction of lamotrigine is needed to avoid toxicity.

If seizures continue to occur with first-line agents at therapeutic levels, an alternative medication is gabapentin (900 mg/day in three gradually increasing doses) or other second-line antiepileptic drugs (e.g., lamotrigine, topiramate, or levetiracetam).

Intravenous levetiracetam has become a useful drug in both adults and children.[1] It is largely cleared renally and is associated with very few complications, but dosing has remained poorly defined; usually 1,000–2,000 mg of levetiracetam is administered to treat seizures. Comparative studies with IV loading with fosphenytoin are not available, but its use in the ED is increasing.

Specific concerns may arise when seizures are observed during pregnancy without evidence of eclampsia. Antiepileptic drugs for the brief treatment of recurrent seizures should be well tolerated when pregnancy is beyond the first trimester, and the risk to the infant seems small. Regular use of antiepileptic drugs in pregnancy doubles the risk of congenital malformations, including limb deformities, spina bifida (valproic acid), and growth retardation.[65] Folic acid, 0.4 mg/day, should be added during pregnancy. Monitoring phenytoin levels in pregnancy is complicated by a decrease in serum albumin levels; thus, the unbound fraction should be measured to manage dosage. In addition, the increased volume of distribution and increased clearance by the liver and placenta may result in an increase in the total daily dose.

MANAGEMENT OF STATUS EPILEPTICUS

Prehospital care remains poorly established but clinical trials have shown prehospital care can improve with early administration of drugs.[56] If present, intramuscular (or buccal) midazolam or rectal diazepam are important options.[17,67,71] Not only do patients with status epilepticus urgently need antiepileptic agents to reduce morbidity from injurious seizure activity, but also the systemic effects of prolonged seizures are potentially harmful and may evolve into a complex medical emergency. It is important to immediately ventilate with oxygen, secure instruments to intubate quickly, if needed and obtain IV access. Alternative modes of administration include intranasal and

---

TABLE 11.2. DIAGNOSTIC TESTS IN A PATIENT WITH DE NOVO SEIZURE IN ED

Computed tomographic scan with contrast *
Cervical spine radiograph (if trauma is suspected)
Cerebrospinal fluid (predominantly in immunosuppressed patients, human immunodeficiency virus)
Toxicologic screen, alcohol level
Sodium, calcium, magnesium, blood urea nitrogen, creatinine, complete white blood cell count, glucose

---

* if feasible, MRI

intramuscular administration of antiepileptic drugs.[31,62,78] Intranasal or intramuscular midazolam has rapid absorption and is preferred[48] (Capsule 11.1).

Aspiration is very common in status epilepticus, and may be the overriding cause of hypoxemia at presentation. In patients with altered pulmonary defenses, such as those with chronic obstructive pulmonary disease or alcohol abuse, pneumonia develops rapidly. Food particles may obstruct large airways and cause atelectasis and hypoxemia. Acute respiratory failure may follow rapidly and actually evolve in the ED. Dyspnea can be profound from alveolar flooding and hypoxemia may worsens within minutes. These patients need intubation for airway protection and possibly fiberoptic bronchoscopy if early chest radiographic findings so indicate. Aspiration pneumonitis (Mendelson syndrome) may be due to sterile gastric contents causing chemical injury. Neurogenic pulmonary edema from status epilepticus is uncommon but has been linked to sudden death, mostly in children and young adults. Chest radiographic findings are typically widespread whiteout infiltrates that resolve after several hours of positive end-expiratory pressure (PEEP) ventilation.

Cardiac arrhythmias may appear only if continuous seizures have resulted in prolonged significant lactic acidosis. Many patients have sinus tachycardia from a sympathetic overdrive. Only cardiac arrhythmias causing measurable blood pressure reduction need correction with antiarrhythmic agents and bicarbonate infusion. Creatine kinase should be measured in each patient because rhabdomyolysis may result in acute renal failure, which can be prevented by additional fluid administration.

The sequence of use of antiepileptic agents in status epilepticus continues to evolve[2,7,10,11,28,36,37,44,51,64,66,81] (Capsule 11.2). When patients with status epilepticus are referred to large institutions, approximately 30% have a recurrence of seizure after IV phenytoin loading, and seizures recurred in 40% of patients after a third-line agent.[47] This demonstrates more difficult control with increasing duration.

In the prehospital setting, a large study (RAMPART Rapid Anticonvulsant Medication Prior to Arrival Trial)[71] has shown that IM midazolam is safe and effective when used by first responders. In this study, adults and children with an estimated weight of more than 40 kg received 10 mg midazolam IM followed by IV placebo or IM placebo followed by 4 mg lorazepam IV. The SAMUKeppra trial in France failed to show levetiracetam IV (2500 mg) in addition to clonazepam IV was better than clonazepam alone in the prehospital management of status epilepticus.[52]

Once in the hospital, treatment starts with repeated doses of lorazepam 2 mg every 3 minutes for a total of four doses when seizures are not controlled with a first and second dose, soon followed by phenytoin or fosphenytoin intravenous loading 20–25 mg/kg. In Europe, 1 mg of intravenous clonazepam followed by another 1 mg 5 minutes later is combined with IV phenytoin. Unusual proposals are to use a combination of IV diazepam with ketamine and valproate. The IV dose of diazepam would be 1 mg/kg with ketamine 10 mg/kg and valproic acid 30 mg/kg Sensible. Lorazepam 4 mg bolus is more effective than phenytoin for initial therapy.[8,38,46,49,76] Up to 90% of patients are successfully managed with a combination of benzodiazepines and phenytoin. Failure to control seizures probably is related to inappropriate (fos)phenytoin loading

---

CAPSULE 11.1   NO INTRAVENOUS ACCESS

Best option still is intramuscular use of midazolam and observation for 3 minutes to allow absorption (within minutes, 10 mg). Intravenous access can be difficult in obese patients, long-term users of intravenous drugs and can be anticipated in patients with multiple prior cannulations to treat a major medical illness. Intramuscular administration of fosphenytoin (20 mg/kg phenytoin equivalent) produces plasma concentrations of phenytoin equal to those with the oral dose within 1–2 hours of administration. If intramuscular fosphenytoin is not available, diazepam should be used rectally (0.2 mg/kg repeat in 4 hours).[48] Probably the last resort is a brachial or saphenous vein cutdown. The superficial location of the vein and large diameter make it suitable for placement of a large-bore cannula. IV (fos)phenytoin can then be administered.

CAPSULE 11.2   ANTIEPILEPTIC DRUGS AND SIDE EFFECTS

PHENYTOIN

Phenytoin is rapidly distributed to body tissue and the brain. Respiratory depression does not occur in loading doses of 10–20 mg/kg. Sinus bradycardia is the most common cardiac arrhythmia. Transient diastolic pauses may occur, and the drug may worsen any heart block. Asystole has been reported. Phenytoin can be mixed only in isotonic saline because it precipitates in glucose. Oral dosage should start 6–12 hours after infusion.

FOSPHENYTOIN

Fosphenytoin sodium (Cerebyx) is a prodrug of phenytoin that is rapidly converted by enzymes to phenytoin.[9] Both intravenous and intramuscular administrations of 15–20 mg PE/kg produced therapeutic total (10–20 mcg/mL) and free (1–2 mcg/mL) plasma levels. Intramuscular loading (9–12 mg/kg phenytoin equivalent) produces therapeutic levels in 1–2 hours and can be considered in status epilepticus but only if intravenous access is not available. Fosphenytoin is completely water soluble. Therefore, phlebitis, hypotension, and cardiac arrhythmias, typically associated with propylene glycol–based intravenous phenytoin, are infrequent. However, cardiac arrhythmias may still occur when fosphenytoin is infused at rates > 150 mg PE/min. There is no pharmacokinetic drug interaction with intravenously administered diazepam or lorazepam. Major side effects are nystagmus, headaches, ataxia, and drowsiness. Previously unrecognized and highly typical side effects (up to 30%) are transient but very annoying paresthesias and itching in the groin, genitalia, and head and neck.

MIDAZOLAM

It is not clear why midazolam works when benzodiazepines fail to control seizures.[5,15,54] The half-life of midazolam (1–12 hours) is less than that of lorazepam (10–12 hours), and midazolam produces sedation of short duration in status epilepticus. Hourly infusion of 0.1–0.6 mg/kg should be continued for at least 12 hours before the dose is tapered. The cost, comparable with that of lorazepam, is high, approaching $800 for 24 hours of continuous infusion. The absence of propylene glycol solution in midazolam reduces the risk of hypotension, bradycardia, and electrocardiographic changes, which are more common with diazepam and lorazepam. High rates of infusion may produce cardiac depression and hypotension.[26] Often, the mean dose to abolish seizure activity is three times the starting dose.

PROPOFOL

Propofol has been considered controversial because of its association with myoclonic jerking and opisthotonos in humans. However, several studies have confirmed that it inhibits seizure activity. Propofol has been used in anesthetic doses to control status epilepticus and has reduced the risk of prolonged seizures in electroconvulsive therapy. A bolus of propofol may cause significant hypotension and is ill-advised. Bradycardia, hypotension, and lactic acidosis are side effects. Propofol infusion syndrome (acute hypotension, sudden cardiac arrest, metabolic acidosis) is rare but more common in patients with acute neurologic disease and prolonged infusions of high doses.

BARBITURATES

Phenobarbital is much more potent than pentobarbital. Its major drawbacks are direct myocardial depression and vascular dilatation, but these are not treatment-limiting. Phenobarbital also has a very long elimination half-life (24–140 hours) but zero-order elimination at high doses (constant amount of drug elimination per unit of time). Intravenous pentobarbital (1–3 mg/kg/hr) virtually always controls status epilepticus, but relapse can be substantial,[82] usually preceded by electrographic recurrence of seizure activity. Use of this drug nearly always requires vasopressors to maintain adequate blood pressures.

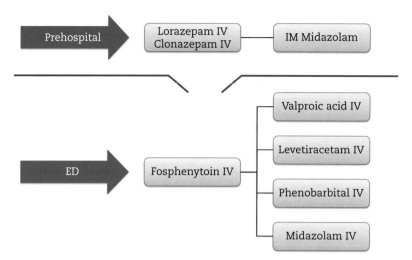

FIGURE 11.4: Algorithm for initial management of convulsive status epilepticus.
IV, intravenous.

(The popular 1 g of phenytoin is almost always inadequate) and failure to appreciate that a second IV bolus of phenytoin may abort status epilepticus. A common sequence is phenytoin, midazolam[26] or propofol, and pentobarbital and phenobarbital.[34,36,39,40,43,57,60,72,79,82] Additional measures include isoflurane, ketamine,[35,69] or topiramate[75] (see Chapter 40 for more details). A sensible algorithm for the management of convulsive status epilepticus is shown in Figure 11.4.

A particularly difficult situation is the treatment of epilepsia partialis continua. One approach is phenytoin loading (20 mg/kg IV) followed by increasing doses of phenobarbital, starting with 1–3 mg/kg/day IV after 20 mg/kg IV loading dose or, in resistant cases, with IV administration of valproic acid (20 mg/kg bolus and 20 mg/min infusion). In our experience, focal seizures are commonly treated well with valproic acid without need for endotracheal intubation due to respiratory depression. If valproic acid fails, additional doses of phenobarbital can be infused to possibly achieve control or at least considerably decrease seizures.

Nonconvulsive status epilepticus, when documented by EEG, can be treated under EEG monitoring with benzodiazepines[61] (lorazepam 4–8 mg, or diazepam 10 mg) or valproic acid.[29]

The management of seizures in patients with preeclampsia is notably different.[4,16] Magnesium sulfate remains the standard in the prevention and treatment of preeclamptic seizures or status epilepticus. Magnesium sulfate is given at a beginning dose of 4–5 g intravenously or 10 g intramuscularly.[42] An IV infusion of 1 g/hr is started. Additional antiepileptic agents are not warranted and may cause respiratory depression in the newborn. Magnesium toxicity may, however, also reduce both maternal and fetal respiration rates. Reduced tendon reflexes may occur and may indicate imminent toxicity; thus, they are a useful monitoring sign during titration of treatment.

Antiepileptic therapy in myoclonus status epilepticus is usually not effective after cardiac arrest. Clonazepam has been advocated for treatment but has not been consistently effective in our experience. There is no rationale to aggressively treat these myoclonic jerks with a series of antiepileptic drugs. When myoclonus causes marked contractions, even hampering normal ventilator cycling, propofol is started (starting dose of 0.5 mg/kg/hr with 0.5 mg/kg/hr increments to effect) and is commonly successful. If myoclonus still cannot be controlled, neuromuscular blocking agents should be considered to eliminate these forceful jerks and until the level of care has been decided upon.

Psychogenic epilepticus typically lasts longer and aborts spontaneously and often instantaneously. The diagnosis can be confirmed by an EEG, but the jerking movements are often so bizarre that the psychogenic cause is clear from the outset. A recent study found that psychogenic status epilepticus could be rapidly induced by administering saline intravenously and telling the patients (some of whom had visited many different EDs) that the saline solution will provoke seizures. However, the use of these deceptive provocative techniques is ethically questionable.[13,53]

CONCLUSIONS

- Different types of status epilepticus require different therapeutic approaches.
- Treatment of tonic-clonic status epilepticus is successful in more than two-thirds of the cases using a combination of adequate doses of IV lorazepam and fosphenytoin.
- Seizure recurrence is substantial in a patient with a new-onset seizure and demonstrable brain lesion and thus requires antiepileptic therapy and often admission.

REFERENCES

1. Abend NS, Monk HM, Licht DJ, Dlugos DJ. Intravenous levetiracetam in critically ill children with status epilepticus or acute repetitive seizures. *Pediatr Crit Care Med* 2009;10:505–510.
2. Arif H, Hirsch LJ. Treatment of status epilepticus. *Semin Neurol* 2008;28:342–354.
3. Barry E, Hauser WA. Pleocytosis after status epilepticus. *Arch Neurol* 1994;51:190–193.
4. Belfort MA, Anthony J, Saade GR, Allen JC, Jr. A comparison of magnesium sulfate and nimodipine for the prevention of eclampsia. *N Engl J Med* 2003;348:304–311.
5. Berg AT. Risk of recurrence after a first unprovoked seizure. *Epilepsia* 2008;49 Suppl 1:13–18.
6. Beyenburg S, Elger CE, Reuber M. Acute confusion or altered mental state: consider nonconvulsive status epilepticus. *Gerontology* 2007;53:388–396.
7. Bleck TP. Intensive care unit management of patients with status epilepticus. *Epilepsia* 2007;48 Suppl 8:59–60.
8. Brophy GM, Bell R, Claassen J, et al. Guidelines for the evaluation and management of status epilepticus. *Neurocrit Care* 2012;17:3–23.
9. Browne TR. Fosphenytoin (Cerebyx). *Clin Neuropharmacol* 1997;20:1–12.
10. Cascino GD. Generalized convulsive status epilepticus. *Mayo Clinic Proc* 1996;71:787–792.
11. Claassen J, Hirsch LJ, Emerson RG, Mayer SA. Treatment of refractory status epilepticus with pentobarbital, propofol, or midazolam: a systematic review. *Epilepsia* 2002;43:146–153.
12. Cockerell OC, Walker MC, Sander JW, Shorvon SD. Complex partial status epilepticus: a recurrent problem. *J Neurol Neurosurg Psychiatry* 1994;57:835–837.
13. Cohen RJ, Suter C. Hysterical seizures: suggestion as a provocative EEG test. *Ann Neurol* 1982;11:391–395.
14. Costello DJ, Kilbride RD, Cole AJ. Cryptogenic New Onset Refractory Status Epilepticus (NORSE) in adults-Infectious or not? *J Neurol Sci* 2009;277:26–31.
15. Crisp CB, Gannon R, Knauft F. Continuous infusion of midazolam hydrochloride to control status epilepticus. *Clin Pharm* 1988;7:322–324.
16. Crowther C. Magnesium sulphate versus diazepam in the management of eclampsia: a randomized controlled trial. *Br J Obstet Gynaecol* 1990;97:110–117.
17. de Haan GJ, van der Geest P, Doelman G, Bertram E, Edelbroek P. A comparison of midazolam nasal spray and diazepam rectal solution for the residential treatment of seizure exacerbations. *Epilepsia* 2010;51:478–482.
18. DeLorenzo RJ, Hauser WA, Towne AR, et al. A prospective, population-based epidemiologic study of status epilepticus in Richmond, Virginia. *Neurology* 1996;46:1029–1035.
19. Fagan KJ, Lee SI. Prolonged confusion following convulsions due to generalized nonconvulsive status epilepticus. *Neurology* 1990;40:1689–1694.
20. Goyal MK, Sinha S, Ravishankar S, Shivshankar JJ. Role of MR imaging in the evaluation of etiology of status epilepticus. *J Neurol Sci* 2008;272:143–150.
21. Group FST. Randomized clinical trial on the efficacy of antiepileptic drugs in reducing the risk of relapse after a first unprovoked tonic-clonic seizure. *Neurology* 1993;43:478–483.
22. Hauser WA, Rich SS, Lee JR, Annegers JF, Anderson VE. Risk of recurrent seizures after two unprovoked seizures. *N Engl J Med* 1998; 338:429–434.
23. Hesdorffer DC, Benn EK, Cascino GD, Hauser WA. Is a first acute symptomatic seizure epilepsy? Mortality and risk for recurrent seizure. *Epilepsia* 2009;50:1102–1108.
24. Husain AM, Horn GJ, Jacobson MP. Nonconvulsive status epilepticus: usefulness of clinical features in selecting patients for urgent EEG. *J Neurol Neurosurg Psychiatry* 2003;74:189–191.
25. Jagoda A, Richey-Klein V, Riggio S. Psychogenic status epilepticus. *J Emerg Med* 1995;13:31–35.
26. Jawad S, Oxley J, Wilson J, Richens A. A pharmacodynamic evaluation of midazolam as an antiepileptic compound. *J Neurol Neurosurg Psychiatry* 1986;49:1050–1054.
27. Kadambi P, Hart KW, Adeoye OM, et al. Electroencephalography findings in patients presenting to the ED for evaluation of seizures. *Am J Emerg Med* 2015;33:100–103.
28. Kälviäinen R. Status epilepticus treatment guidelines. *Epilepsia* 2007;48 Suppl 8:99–102.
29. Kaplan PW. Intravenous valproate treatment of generalized nonconvulsive status epilepticus. *Clin Electroencephalogr* 1999;30:1–4.
30. Kaplan PW. Nonconvulsive status epilepticus in the emergency room. *Epilepsia* 1996;37:643–650.

31. Kendall JL, Reynolds M, Goldberg R. Intranasal midazolam in patients with status epilepticus. *Ann Emerg Med* 1997;29:415–417.

32. Kho LK, Lawn ND, Dunne JW, Linto J. First seizure presentation: do multiple seizures within 24 hours predict recurrence? *Neurology* 2006;67:1047–1049.

33. King DW, Gallagher BB, Murvin AJ, et al. Pseudoseizures: diagnostic evaluation. *Neurology* 1982;32:18–23.

34. Koul RL, Raj Aithala G, Chacko A, Joshi R, Seif Elbualy M. Continuous midazolam infusion as treatment of status epilepticus. *Arch Dis Child* 1997;76:445–448.

35. Kramer AH. Early ketamine to treat refractory status epilepticus. *Neurocrit Care* 2012;16:299–305.

36. Kuisma M, Roine RO. Propofol in prehospital treatment of convulsive status epilepticus. *Epilepsia* 1995;36:1241–1243.

37. Kumar A, Bleck TP. Intravenous midazolam for the treatment of refractory status epilepticus. *Crit Care Med* 1992;20:483–488.

38. Labar DR, Ali A, Root J. High-dose intravenous lorazepam for the treatment of refractory status epilepticus. *Neurology* 1994;44:1400–1403.

39. Lawn ND, Wijdicks EFM. Progress in clinical neurosciences: status epilepticus: a critical review of management options. *Can J Neurol Sci* 2002;29:206–215.

40. LeDuc TJ, Goellner WE, el-Sanadi N. Out-of-hospital midazolam for status epilepticus. *Ann Emerg Med* 1996;28:377.

41. Lowenstein DH, Cloyd J. Out-of-hospital treatment of status epilepticus and prolonged seizures. *Epilepsia* 2007;48 Suppl 8:96–98.

42. Lucas MJ, Leveno KJ, Cunningham FG. A comparison of magnesium sulfate with phenytoin for the prevention of eclampsia. *N Engl J Med* 1995;333:201–205.

43. Mackenzie SJ, Kapadia F, Grant IS. Propofol infusion for control of status epilepticus. *Anaesthesia* 1990;45:1043–1045.

44. Marik PE, Varon J. The management of status epilepticus. *Chest* 2004;126:582–591.

45. Marson AG. When to start antiepileptic drug treatment and with what evidence? *Epilepsia* 2008;49 Suppl 9:3–6.

46. Martin-Gill C, Hostler D, Callaway CW, Prunty H, Roth RN. Management of prehospital seizure patients by paramedics. *Prehosp Emerg Care* 2009;13:179–184.

47. Mayer SA, Claassen J, Lokin J, et al. Refractory status epilepticus: frequency, risk factors, and impact on outcome. *Arch Neurol* 2002;59:205–210.

48. Mayhue FE. IM midazolam for status epilepticus in the emergency department. *Ann Emerg Med* 1988;17:643–645.

49. Meierkord H, Boon P, Engelsen B, et al. EFNS guideline on the management of status epilepticus in adults. *Eur J Neurol* 2010;17:348–355.

50. Millikan D, Rice B, Silbergleit R. Emergency treatment of status epilepticus: current thinking. *Emerg Med Clin North Am* 2009;27:101–113.

51. Mitchell WG. Status epilepticus and acute serial seizures in children. *J Child Neurol* 2002;17 Suppl 1:S36–43.

52. Navarro V, Dagron C, Elie C, et al. Prehospital treatment with levetiracetam plus clonazepam or placebo plus clonazepam in status epilepticus (SAMUKeppra): a randomized, double-blind, phase 3 trial. *Lancet Neurol* 2016;15:47–55.

53. Ney GC, Zimmerman C, Schaul N. Psychogenic status epilepticus induced by a provocative technique. *Neurology* 1996;46:546–547.

54. Nordt SP, Clark RF. Midazolam: a review of therapeutic uses and toxicity. *J Emerg Med* 1997;15:357–365.

55. Oribe E, Amini R, Nissenbaum E, Boal B. Serum prolactin concentrations are elevated after syncope. *Neurology* 1996;47:60–62.

56. Osborne A, Taylor L, Reuber M, et al. Pre-hospital care after a seizure: evidence based and United Kingdom management guidelines. *Seizure* 2015;24:82–87.

57. Parent JM, Lowenstein DH. Treatment of refractory generalized status epilepticus with continuous infusion of midazolam. *Neurology* 1994;44:1837–1840.

58. Perucca E. Pharmacological and therapeutic properties of valproate: a summary after 35 years of clinical experience. *CNS Drugs* 2002; 16:695–714.

59. Physicians ACoE. Clinical policy for the initial approach to patients presenting with a chief complaint of seizure who are not in status epilepticus. *Ann Emerg Med* 1997;29:706–724.

60. Pitt-Miller PL, Elcock BJ, Maharaj M. The management of status epilepticus with a continuous propofol infusion. *Anesth Analg* 1994; 78:1193–1194.

61. Privitera MD, Strawsburg RH. Electroencephalographic monitoring in the emergency department. *Emerg Med Clin North Am* 1994;12:1089–1100.

62. Rey E, Delaunay L, Pons G, et al. Pharmacokinetics of midazolam in children: comparative study of intranasal and intravenous administration. *Eur J Clin Pharmacol* 1991;41:355–357.

63. Rosenberg ML. The eyes in hysterical states of unconsciousness. *J Clin Neuroophthalmol* 1982;2:259–260.

64. Runge JW, Allen FH. Emergency treatment of status epilepticus. *Neurology* 1996;46:S20–23.

65. Samren EB, van Duijn CM, Christiaens GC, Hofman A, Lindhout D. Antiepileptic drug

regimens and major congenital abnormalities in the offspring. *Ann Neurol* 1999;46:739–746.

66. Scholtes FB, Renier WO, Meinardi H. Generalized convulsive status epilepticus: causes, therapy, and outcome in 346 patients. *Epilepsia* 1994;35:1104–1112.

67. Scott RC, Besag FM, Neville BG. Buccal midazolam and rectal diazepam for treatment of prolonged seizures in childhood and adolescence: a randomised trial. *Lancet* 1999;353:623–626.

68. Shen W, Bowman ES, Markand ON. Presenting the diagnosis of pseudoseizure. *Neurology* 1990;40:756–759.

69. Sheth RD, Gidal BE. Refractory status epilepticus: response to ketamine. *Neurology* 1998;51:1765–1766.

70. Shorvon S. What is nonconvulsive status epilepticus, and what are its subtypes? *Epilepsia* 2007;48 Suppl 8:35–38.

71. Silbergleit R, Durkalski V, Lowenstein D, et al. Intramuscular versus intravenous therapy for prehospital status epilepticus. *N Engl J Med* 2012; 366:591–600.

72. Stecker MM, Kramer TH, Raps EC, et al. Treatment of refractory status epilepticus with propofol: clinical and pharmacokinetic findings. *Epilepsia* 1998;39:18–26.

73. Stein MA, Kanner AM. Management of newly diagnosed epilepsy: a practical guide to monotherapy. *Drugs* 2009;69:199–222.

74. Sung CY, Chu NS. Status epilepticus in the elderly: etiology, seizure type and outcome. *Acta Neurol Scand* 1989;80:51–56.

75. Towne AR, Garnett LK, Waterhouse EJ, Morton LD, DeLorenzo RJ. The use of topiramate in refractory status epilepticus. *Neurology* 2003;60:332–334.

76. Treiman DM, Meyers PD, Walton NY, et al. A comparison of four treatments for generalized convulsive status epilepticus. Veterans Affairs Status Epilepticus Cooperative Study Group. *N Engl J Med* 1998;339:792–798.

77. Weise KL, Bleck TP. Status epilepticus in children and adults. *Crit Care Clin* 1997;13:629–646.

78. Wermeling DP. Intranasal delivery of antiepileptic medications for treatment of seizures. *Neurotherapeutics* 2009;6:352–358.

79. Wheless JW, Treiman DM. The role of the newer antiepileptic drugs in the treatment of generalized convulsive status epilepticus. *Epilepsia* 2008;49 Suppl 9:74–78.

80. Wijdicks EFM, Hubmayr RD. Acute acid-base disorders associated with status epilepticus. *Mayo Clinic Proc* 1994;69:1044–1046.

81. Wijdicks EFM, Parisi JE, Sharbrough FW. Prognostic value of myoclonus status in comatose survivors of cardiac arrest. *Ann Neurol* 1994;35:239–243.

82. Yaffe K, Lowenstein DH. Prognostic factors of pentobarbital therapy for refractory generalized status epilepticus. *Neurology* 1993;43:895–900.

12

Comatose

The assessment of comatose patients permeates the practice of all physicians. Finding the cause of coma requires a specific neurologic assessment and considerable deductive effort. The priorities in the evaluation of comatose patients have changed considerably with the arrival of neuroimaging, possibly leading to the misconception that the cause of coma usually is easily established with computed tomography (CT) scan or magnetic resonance imaging (MRI). Relying solely on these tests can be counterproductive and, in some instances, potentially dangerous. Failure to recognize diabetic coma, thyroid storm, acute hypopituitarism, fulminant hepatic necrosis, or any type of poisoning while spending valuable time performing neuroimaging tests may potentially result in a rapidly developing medical fiasco.

The circumstances under which comatose patients are discovered can also be misleading. For example, a patient found next to an empty bottle of analgesic medication may have a painful otitis with fulminant meningitis; traumatic brain injury with skin lacerations may be a consequence of a fall from acute hemiplegia due to a stroke or brief loss of consciousness from cardiac arrhythmia. Another dramatic situation occurs when a patient with diabetes consumes a little alcohol but fails to have dinner and is brought in comatose and smelling of alcohol but also profoundly hypoglycemic. Some comatose patients are not as they seem, and all of these situations have the potential to be misjudged.

The evaluation of comatose patients is best approached systematically, trying to place it in one of the five major categories (Table 12.1): (1) unilateral hemispheric mass lesions that compress or displace the diencephalon and brainstem; (2) bilateral hemispheric lesions that damage or compress the reticular formation in the thalamus, interrupting the projecting fibers of the thalamocortical circuitry; (3) lesions in the posterior fossa that damage or compress the reticular formation in the brainstem; (4) diffuse brain lesions affecting the physiologic processes of the brain; and (5) less commonly, psychiatric unresponsiveness,

mimicking coma.[19,47,79] Accidental and self-inflicted poisoning and illicit drug overdose are common in the emergency department (ED) and thus receive proportionally more attention in this chapter. The management of structural causes of coma is disease-specific and discussed in more detail in Parts V through IX.

Examination of the Comatose Patient

A physical examination that sorts out specific and localizing neurologic findings remains of great importance and is necessary in trying to get to the nature of coma. Equally important is a reliable history. Relatives, bystanders, and police may all provide important information, but personal belongings, medical alert cards, and bracelets can provide invaluable clues. However, the patient's history, particularly of those "wheeled in," is always unclear and fragmentary, and there is often little or no documentary evidence, leaving physicians to work with snippets culled from existing medical records.

One needs to know the onset of coma. Acute onset in a previously healthy person points to aneurysmal subarachnoid hemorrhage (SAH), a generalized tonic-clonic seizure, traumatic brain injury, self-induced drug poisoning, or an environmental injury. Gradual worsening in responsiveness to stupor may indicate an evolving intracranial mass, a diffuse infiltrative neoplasm, or inflammatory neurologic disorder.

GENERAL FEATURES OF CLINICAL EXAMINATION

The general appearance of the patient is noted. Extremely poor hygiene or anorexia may indicate alcohol or drug abuse. A foul breath in most instances means poor dental and periodontal hygiene or alcohol consumption. The classic types of foul breath should be known, but not many physicians are alerted by it. These are "dirty restroom" (uremia), "fruity sweat" (ketoacidosis), "musty or fishy" (acute hepatic failure), "onion" (paraldehyde), and "garlic" (organophosphates, insecticides, thallium).

TABLE 12.1. CLASSIFICATION AND MAJOR CAUSES OF COMA

Structural Brain Injury
Hemisphere
Unilateral (with displacement)
Intraparenchymal hematoma
Middle cerebral artery occlusion
Hemorrhagic contusion
Cerebral abscess
Brain tumor

Bilateral
Penetrating traumatic brain injury
Multiple traumatic brain contusions
Anoxic-ischemic encephalopathy
Aneurysmal subarachnoid hemorrhage
Multiple cerebral infarcts
Bilateral thalamic infarcts
Cerebral venous thrombosis
Lymphoma
Encephalitis
Gliomatosis
Acute disseminated encephalomyelitis
Cerebral edema
Multiple brain metastases
Acute hydrocephalus
Acute leukoencephalopathy

Brainstem
Pontine hemorrhage
Basilar artery occlusion
Central pontine myelinolysis
Brainstem hemorrhagic contusion

Cerebellum (with displacement of brainstem)
Cerebellar infarct
Cerebellar hematoma
Cerebellar abscess
Cerebellar glioma

Acute Metabolic-Endocrine Derangement
Hypoglycemia
Hyperglycemia (nonketotic hyperosmolar)
Hyponatremia
Hypernatremia
Addison's disease
Hypercalcemia
Acute hypothyroidism
Acute panhypopituitarism
Acute uremia
Hyperbilirubinemia
Hypercapnia

Diffuse Physiologic Brain Dysfunction
Generalized tonic-clonic seizures
Poisoning, illicit drug use
Hypothermia
Gas inhalation
Acute (lethal) catatonia, malignant
   neuroleptic syndrome

Psychogenic Unresponsiveness
Hysterical
Malingering[18,41,72]

Fever and particularly hyperthermia (> 40°C) in comatose patients may indicate a fulminant infection, endocarditis with multiple emboli, or a central nervous system (CNS) infection, but can occur in massive pontine hemorrhage, aneurysmal SAH, and traumatic brain injury. It may originate from direct compression, ischemia, or contusion of the hypothalamus. High fever may be part of a hyperthermia syndrome such as serotonin syndrome or neuroleptic malignant syndrome, but both are suggested by the additional presence of rigidity or severe myoclonus (Chapter 8). Hypothermia (≤ 35°C) indicates exposure to a cold environmental temperature, marked hypothyroidism, Addison's disease, hypoglycemia, or intoxication. In patients with a devastating traumatic brain and spine injury, it may be a systemic sign of brain death or acute spinal cord transection.

Examination of the skin may provide important additional findings leading to the cause of coma. Bullous skin lesions ("coma blisters") can be seen at pressure points and are very uncommon at other sites, suggesting skin necrosis from ischemia rather than a specific cutaneous toxicity. These lesions are expected in patients found down after someone was checking up. The acute appearance of blisters may indicate barbiturate, amitriptyline, or theophylline intoxication.[18,41,72]

In a patient with a long-bone fracture, rapidly developing pulmonary edema, acute unresponsiveness, and petechiae in the axilla strongly indicate fat emboli. Skin rash in a comatose patient may indicate a rapidly evolving encephalitis or fulminant meningococcal meningitis (Figure 12.1). Intravenous illicit drug use should be considered when appropriate, and the skin should be carefully inspected for needle marks in multiple sites outside the cubital fossa. (However, scars in the cubital fossa alone often may indicate that the patient is a blood donor or receives regular blood transfusions.) Significant periorbital ecchymosis ("raccoon eyes") and retroauricular ecchymosis

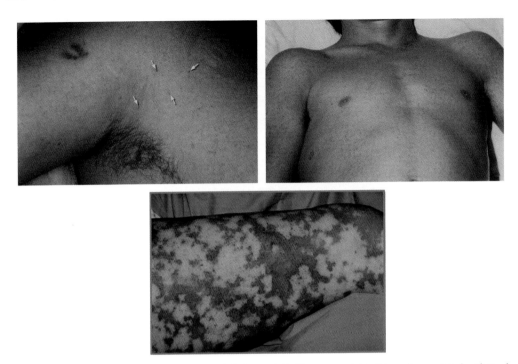

FIGURE 12.1: Skin lesions in coma. Upper row left: Fat emboli. Upper row right: Skin rash associated with Rocky Mountain spotted fever. Lower row: Purpura associated with meningococcal meningitis.

(Battle sign) indicate midface or skull base fractures; they should be carefully looked for but often become apparent much later (Chapter 41). The skin should be touched at different areas to assess its texture; both dry skin and skin drenched in sweat may point to certain intoxications (Table 12.2). Dry skin in a comatose patient (particularly in typically moist areas such as the

TABLE 12.2. IMPORTANT SKIN ABNORMALITIES THAT MAY HAVE DISCRIMINATORY VALUE IN THE ASSESSMENT OF COMA

Sign or Symptom	Meaning
Acne	Long-term antiepileptic drug use
Bullae	Barbiturates, sedative-hypnotic drugs
Butterfly eruption on face	Systemic lupus erythematosus
Cold, malar flush, yellow tinge, puffy face	Myxedema
Dark pigmentation	Addison's disease
Dryness	Barbiturate poisoning, anticholinergic agents
Edema	Acute renal failure
Purpura	Meningococcal meningitis, thrombotic thrombocytopenic purpura, vasculitis, disseminated intravascular coagulation, aspirin intoxication
Rash	Meningitis or seasonal encephalitis
Sweating	Cholinergic poisoning, hypoglycemia, sympathomimetics, malignant catatonia or acute paroxysmal sympathetic hyperactivity, thyroid storm

groin and axilla) points to overdose of anticho- linergic agents (common tricyclic antidepres- sants). Characteristically, these intoxications are associated with tachycardia, fever, and cardiac arrhythmias. As discussed in a later section, because electrocardiographic (EKG) abnormali- ties can be absent early in tricyclic antidepressant overdose, its recognition may thus be extremely difficult. Profuse sweating should always point to severe hypoglycemia or organophosphate pesti- cide poisoning.

Hypertension is a common clinical feature in coma associated with acute structural CNS lesions and therefore has little predictive value. It usually subsides because the sympathetic outburst from the initial insult wanes, but unexplained surges of hypertension could indicate poisoning from cer- tain drugs, such as amphetamines, cocaine, halluci- nogens, and sympathomimetic agents. Conversely, hypertension should be considered a cause of pos- terior reversible encephalopathy syndrome (PRES) in patients with profound hypertension (e.g., mean

arterial pressure > 140 mm Hg), documented sei- zures, papilledema, and retinal hemorrhages—key signs that may be preceded by visual hallucinations.

Hypotension may indicate that coma is a result of severe sepsis or a sign of a rapidly developing meningococcal meningitis. Hypotension may also be due to loss of vascular tone, when all brain func- tion is lost or as a consequence of acute spinal cord injury (Chapter 63).

Combinations of changes in vital signs may suggest certain poisonings.[2] These toxins are sum- marized in Table 12.3 and may be helpful in nar- rowing down the list of possible intoxications.

Neurologic Features of Clinical Examination

The depth of coma should be documented. It should reflect the astuteness of a clinical neurolo- gist to first evaluate whether the patient truly is comatose, in a locked-in syndrome, or even malin- gering. Every physician should appreciate that a major lesion in the brainstem may not necessarily

TABLE 12.3. COMMON CHANGES IN VITAL SIGNS IN COMA FROM POISONING

Toxin	Blood Pressure	Pulse	Respiration	Temperature	Additional Signs
Amphetamines	↑	↑	↑	↑	Mydriasis
Arsenic	↓	↑	~	~	Marked dehydration
Barbiturates	↓	~	↓	↓	Bullae, hypoglycemia
β-adrenergic blockers	↓	↓	~	~	Seizures
Carbon monoxide	~	~	~	~	Seizures
Cocaine	↑	↑	~	↑	Mydriasis, seizures
Cyclic antidepressants	↓	↑	~	↑	Mydriasis
Ethylene glycol	~	↑	↑	~	Anion gap and osmolar gap, metabolic acidosis
Lithium	↓	~	~	~	Seizures, myoclonus
Methanol	↓	~	↓	~	Anion gap and osmolar gap, acidosis
Opioids	↓	↓	↓	↓	Miosis
Organophosphates	↓	↓/↑	↑/↓	~	Fasciculations, bronchospasm, hypersalivation, sweating, miosis
Phencyclidine	↑	↑	~	↑	Miosis, myoclonus
Phenothiazine	↓	↑	~	↓/↑	Dystonia
Salicylates	~	~	↑	↑	Anion gap, metabolic acidosis, respiratory alkalosis
Sedative-hypnotics	↓	~	↓	↓	Bullae

↑ = increase; ↓ = decrease; ~ = no change

cause coma but rather a so-called locked-in syndrome. In locked-in syndrome, an acute structural lesion in the pons (which spares pathways to oculomotor nuclei of the mesencephalon and reticular formation) causes a nearly uncommunicative state. Patients often have eyes partly open but cannot move their limbs or grimace. Before pain stimuli are applied, the patient should be asked to blink and look up and down. (Grim accounts have been published of failure to appreciate this entity.[4]) Psychogenic unresponsiveness is often considered but is rare and requires a skill not only to think about it in the first place but also before ordering a battery of tests.

A neurologic examination often initially starts with an assessment of the patient's response to voice, a prod, or a squeeze. An ideal noxious stimulus in the assessment of comatose patients must respect the patient and not be associated with significant bruising. Proper stimuli are

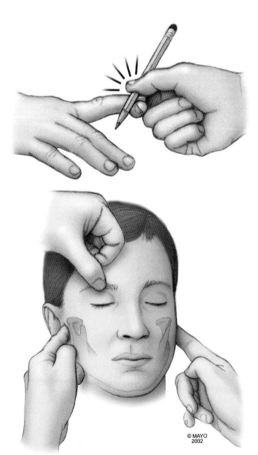

FIGURE 12.2: Methods of pain stimuli in coma: compression of nail bed with pencil; supraorbital nerve compression; compression of temporomandibular joints.

sternal rubbing, rubbing the knuckles against the ribs in the axilla, and pressure on the supraorbital nerve. Deep pressure with a blunt object against the nail bed has become standard but may cause subungual hematoma in anticoagulated patients or those with an underlying coagulopathy.[88] Alternatively, deep pressure on both condyles at the level of the temporomandibular joint can be considered[82] (Figure 12.2).

Coma scales are used to grade the depth of coma. The Glasgow Coma Scale (GCS), introduced in 1974 by Teasdale and Jennett, was originally devised to facilitate communication between nurses, junior inexperienced physicians, and, particularly, non-neurologic staff working in other medical or surgical units.[80] The scale proved to be more useful in communication (e.g., during transfer from another hospital or from the field) than any other previously used descriptive term for decreased level of consciousness (such as "somnolent," "nonarousable," "unresponsive," or "half asleep").[70,71] Subsequent studies, however, emphasized that clinical experience in using the GCS is very important, and substantial errors may occur with inexperienced observers.[59]

The GCS (a combination of the best possible eye, motor, and verbal responses, summarized in Table 12.4) has withstood the test of time and has been tested for its reliability in daily clinical practice. The individual components of the GCS have been graded, most often summed to a score

TABLE 12.4. GLASGOW COMA SCALE

Eye opening

4 Spontaneous
3 To speech
2 To pain
1 None

Best motor response

6 Obeying
5 Localizing pain
4 Withdrawal
3 Abnormal flexing
2 Extensor response
1 None

Best verbal response

5 Oriented
4 Confused conversation
3 Inappropriate words
2 Incomprehensible sounds
1 None

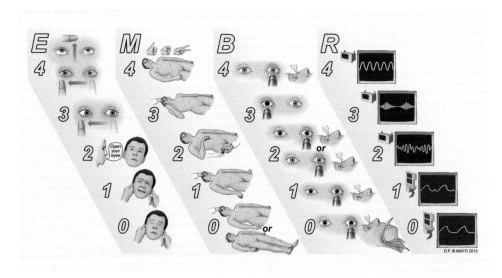

FIGURE 12.3: The FOUR Score.

Eye response

4 = eyelids open or opened, tracking, or
   blinking to command

3 = eyelids open but not tracking

2 = eyelids closed but open to loud voice

1 = eyelids closed but open to pain

0 = eyelids remain closed with pain

Motor response

4 = thumbs-up, fist, or peace sign

3 = localizing to pain

2 = flexion response to pain

1 = extension response to pain

0 = no response to pain or generalized
   myoclonus status

Brainstem reflexes

4 = pupil and corneal reflexes present

3 = one pupil wide and fixed

2 = pupil or corneal reflexes absent

1 = pupil and corneal reflexes absent

0 = pupil, corneal, and cough reflexes absent

Respiration

4 = not intubated, regular breathing

3 = not intubated, Cheyne-Stokes breathing

2 = not intubated, irregular breathing

1 = breathes above ventilatory rate

0 = breathes at ventilator rate or apnea

between 3 and 15, despite the fact that similarly summed scores could represent different levels of decreased consciousness (and individual patients can change but still have the same GCS sum scores).[80] Therefore, in daily practice, the summed scores represent only a crude estimate of the depth of coma. Generally, GCS 3–8 represents coma, 8–12 stupor, and 13–15 drowsiness.

We have devised and extensively tested the Full Outline of Unresponsiveness (FOUR) score, a coma scale that is used in our neurosciences intensive care unit (NICU) and elsewhere (Figure 12.3). The FOUR score has four testable components. The number of components and the maximal grade in each of the categories is four each, which is easy to remember and is reinforced by the acronym. These four components are eye responses (eye opening and eye movements), motor responses (following complex commands

and response to pain stimuli), brainstem reflexes (pupil, corneal, and cough reflexes), and respiration (spontaneous respiratory rhythm or presence of respiratory drive after intubation). The FOUR score can be obtained in a few minutes. The FOUR score not only measures eye opening but also makes an assessment of voluntary horizontal and vertical eye movements. It therefore detects a locked-in syndrome in a patient with a GCS score of 3. It may detect the presence of a vegetative state, in which the eyes can be spontaneously open but do not track the examiner's finger.

The motor category includes the presence of myoclonus status epilepticus, a known poor prognostic sign after cardiac resuscitation (Chapter 48). The motor component combines decorticate (abnormal flexor response) and withdrawal responses, because this difference is often difficult to appreciate. Abnormal extensor response (decerebrate posturing) involves adduction and internal rotation of the shoulder and pronation of the hand. Extreme extensor posturing may cause fist formation or wedging of the thumb between index and middle fingers and is often a sign of major brain injury.

For localization of a pain response, one arm should cross the midline toward the stimulated arm or reach above the shoulder toward the stimulus applied to the supraorbital nerve. The hand position tests (thumbs-up, fist, and peace sign) can further assess alertness. To ask the patient to squeeze a hand may be less valuable because reflex grasping may exist.

Three brainstem reflexes to test mesencephalon, pons, and medulla oblongata functions are used in different combinations. The three important pupil assessments in the FOUR score remain unaffected by any degree of sedation.

Breathing patterns are graded. Cheyne-Stokes respiration and irregular breathing can represent bihemispheric or lower brainstem dysfunction of respiratory control. Cheyne stokes breathing is common in drowsy patients, but when a new short cycle (breathing and apneic phases of several seconds duration) of Cheyne-Stokes breathing occurs, it identifies deterioration. In intubated patients, overbreathing of the mechanical ventilator or spontaneous breaths supported by the ventilator indicates that the patient still has a breathing drive. The FOUR score, unlike the GCS, does not include a verbal response, and thus is more valuable in ED or intensive care unit (ICU) practices that typically have a large number of intubated patients, and it may be useful in young children.

FOUR score assessment in our validation studies was good to excellent.[32,68,83,84,87,90] Patterns of breathing can be easily mastered by physicians and interpreted satisfactorily by neuroscience nurses. The FOUR score has also been successfully validated in the ED and in other ICUs, and data suggest that it can be used by physicians at any level of training and by nursing staff.

Using the FOUR score when confronted with a patient who has impaired consciousness, the examiner is forced to describe essential, clinical features. Changes in the FOUR score are meaningful and imply a deterioration or substantial improvement, unlike the GCS. When all categories are graded 0, the examiner is alerted to consider a brain death examination.

After an assessment of the depth of coma, other neurologic features are examined. Neck stiffness can be assessed but becomes less apparent

in patients with deeper stages of coma (e.g., no eye opening to pain and abnormal motor responses.). Muscle tone can be flaccid (normal in coma but may indicate intoxication with benzodiazepine or tricyclic antidepressant poisoning) or rigid (e.g., neuroleptic agents, etomidate, strychnine, malignant catatonia, or malignant hyperthermia).[89] Abnormal movements such as twitching in the eyelids (may indicate seizures), myoclonus (anoxic–ischemic encephalopathy, lithium intoxication, penicillin intoxication, pesticides),[21] asterixis (acute renal, liver, or pulmonary failure), and shivering (sepsis, hypothermia) should be noted and integrated into the interpretation of the examination.

Neurologic examination proceeds with the cranial nerves. The size of the pupils and whether they are equal, round, oval, or irregular should be noted. It is important to understand the meaning of a unilateral dilated, fixed pupil (traction of the third nerve by brainstem displacement), bilateral fixed, mid-position pupils (may indicate intoxication with scopolamine, atropine, or methyl alcohol, or a mesencephalic lesion); and pinpoint pupils (frequently designate narcotic overdose or an acute pontine lesion). Anisocoria (midposition and pinpoint pupil) often indicates a new brainstem lesion affecting both mesencephalon and pons. The pupillary reactions to a flashlight and preferably under a magnifying glass are studied for both eyes. A magnifying glass may be needed to evaluate questionable or "sluggish" pupillary responses, particularly in patients with small pupils. Pupillary abnormalities and their significance are shown in Figure 12.4.

Funduscopy may reveal new diagnostic findings in comatose patients but rarely so. Subhyaloid hemorrhage is seldom seen in coma, but when present implies aneurysmal SAH or shaken-baby syndrome. Papilledema indicates acutely increased intracranial pressure but also is present in some patients with acute asphyxia and in patients with extreme hypertension (mean arterial pressures over 150 mm Hg).

Absence of spontaneous eye movement should be documented, along with lateral deviation to either side or disconjugate gaze at rest. Forced gaze deviation indicates a large hemispheric lesion at targeted gaze site. Spontaneous eye movements—periodic alternating gaze, ocular dipping, and retractory nystagmus—may be seen in coma but have no localization value other than indicating diffuse brain injury. (However, ocular bobbing—rapid downward, slow return to baseline—is typical for acute pontine lesions.)

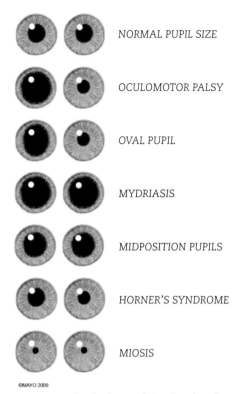

NORMAL PUPIL SIZE

OCULOMOTOR PALSY

OVAL PUPIL

MYDRIASIS

MIDPOSITION PUPILS

HORNER'S SYNDROME

MIOSIS

©MAYO 2009

FIGURE 12.4: Pupil abnormalities in altered consciousness and coma. Top pupils represent normal reference. Unilateral dilated pupil: third-nerve palsy from acute intracranial mass, brainstem contusion, or, rarely, pituitary apoplexy. Oval pupil (often transitory appearance of pupils signaling increased intracranial pressure). Mydriasis (anxiety, delirium, pain, seizures, botulism, atropine, aerosolized albuterol, amyl nitrite, magnesium excess, norepinephrine, dopamine, aminoglycoside, and tetracycline overdose). Pupils fixed in midposition (typical in end-stage brainstem displacement syndromes and brain death). Horner's syndrome (traumatic carotid dissection, brachial plexopathy, trauma from internal jugular vein catheter placement, major thoracic surgery). Miosis (acute pontine lesion, opioids, organophosphate toxicity).

The oculocephalic responses are evaluated with brisk horizontal head turning, and, if appropriate, the response to vertical head movements can be tested. (In patients with any suspicion of head or spine injury, the oculocephalic responses should obviously not be tested because movement may luxate the cervical spine if fractured and immediately cause spinal cord trauma.) Oculovestibular responses are tested by irrigating each external auditory canal with 50 mL of ice water, with the head 30 degrees above the horizontal plane (an intact tympanum needs to be confirmed). Comatose patients exhibit tonic responses with conjugate deviation toward the ear irrigated with

cold water. Bilateral testing can be done by rapidly squirting 50 mL of ice water in each ear, resulting in a forced downward eye movement. Abduction of only the eye on the side being irrigated, with adduction paralysis of the opposite eye, implies a brainstem lesion (internuclear ophthalmoplegia) as a cause of coma.

Finally, corneal responses are tested by drawing a cotton wisp fully across the cornea or by squirting saline. Spontaneous coughing or coughing after tracheal suctioning is recorded (to-and-fro movement of the endotracheal tube is not an adequate stimulus). Absence of coughing may indicate either that the neurologic catastrophe has evolved into brain death or that sedative or anesthetic drugs or neuromuscular blocking agents for emergency intubation have markedly muted the cough reflex.

When all brainstem reflexes are absent in a comatose patient, the clinical diagnosis of brain death is considered, but the cause of the catastrophic event should be known and demonstrated to be irreversible.[81] Brain death often is suspected when patients with fixed pupils stop triggering the ventilator and blood pressure suddenly decreases to low systolic values of around 80–90 mm Hg. Brain death can be considered in the ED but remains a presumptive diagnosis, and final decisions should be postponed. Any physician assessing a patient for brain death should be very sensitive to the possibility that confounding causes may be present, particularly in patients admitted directly to the ED. Even when a catastrophic brain lesion is demonstrated on neuroimaging, the circumstances should be considered ambiguous until the history is complete and, if appropriate, a toxicologic study has ruled out drug ingestion. The clinical criteria for brain death are further discussed in Chapter 63.

MAJOR CATEGORIES AND CAUSES OF COMA

To develop the skills necessary to diagnose the cause of coma, some basic understanding of the anatomical changes that may accompany coma and their consequences is required.[91] This section provides a brief overview; for more detailed accounts, the reader is directed to separate textbooks.[54,89]

Assessment of Structural Causes of Coma

Structural lesions are often acute (hemorrhage, infarct, abscess) or may be a critical extension of an infiltrating tumor, abscess, or giant mass. Structural injury to the brain results in coma

CAPSULE 12.1   ASCENDING RETICULAR ACTIVATING SYSTEM

The role of the ascending reticular activating system (ARAS) is to arouse and maintain alertness. Despite identifiable structures, its definition remains conceptual. Coma is understood as a dysfunction of this anatomic neural network, which spans a large part of the dorsal upper pons, mesencephalon, and thalamus, and projects to the cerebral cortex of both hemispheres.[60] Populations of neurons situated in the tegmentum of the pons and mesencephalon, intralaminar nuclei of the thalamus, and posterior hypothalamus are linked to the basal forebrain and associated cortex (see accompanying illustration). These networks communicate through neurotransmitters, such as acetylcholine, norepinephrine, serotonin, and dopamine, and, through activation of the forebrain, produce wakefulness.

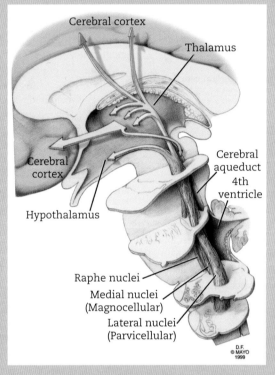

Connections of ARAS with thalamus and cortex.

if it closely follows or directly affects the relay nuclei and connecting fibers that make up the ascending reticular activating system (ARAS). Its connections with the thalamus and both cortices make for a complex network[54,89,91] (Capsule 12.1).

The boundary in the vertical axis is the lower pons. Destructive lesions below this level may lead to acute dysfunction of autonomic nuclei, resulting in failure to drive respiration or vascular tone. Coma or impaired consciousness in localized medulla oblongata lesions therefore is only an indirect consequence of hypercapnia or hypotension-induced global hemispheric injury. These lesions do not involve the ARAS structures and thus, by themselves, do not produce coma or hypersomnia. These medullary structural lesions may involve hemorrhages (often arteriovenous malformation or cavernous hemangioma), metastasis, lateral or medially located medullary infarct, or an inflammatory lesion such as a bacterial or fungal abscess.

Tegmental pontine lesions interrupt the ARAS midway, but result in impaired consciousness only with bilateral injury. The base of the pons does not participate in arousal; therefore, large lesions such as infarcts or central pontine myelinolysis do not impair consciousness but may interrupt all motor output except vertical eye movement and blinking initiated by centers in the mesencephalon.

Mesencephalic damage is seldom seen in isolation and more commonly occurs from the extension of a lesion in the thalamus (e.g., destructive intracranial hematoma) or as a result of occlusion of the tip of the basilar artery, producing simultaneous infarcts in both thalami and in the mesencephalic tegmentum.

Bilateral thalamic damage resulting in coma most often involves the paramedian nuclei, but damage to interlaminar, ventrolateral, or lateral posterior nuclei may impair consciousness by interrupting the thalamocortical projections. Infarcts in the distribution of the penetrating thalamogeniculate or anterior thalamic perforating arteries are the most common causes of bilateral thalamic damage, but an infiltrating thalamic tumor or infiltrative intraventricular masses in the third ventricle can produce sudden coma. Ganglionic hemorrhages may extend into the thalamus and compress the opposite thalamus. Bithalamic hematoma is more commonly seen as an extension of pontine hematoma. Combined thalamic and mesencephalic damage may result

in marked slowing characterized by immobility, voicelessness, flat emotions, and somnolence most of the day. The term *minimally conscious state* is often used.

Bihemispheric Injury

Bihemispheric structural damage may involve the white matter or cortex or both, and a diversity of disorders may produce damage severe enough to reduce arousal. The most notable disorders are anoxic–ischemic encephalopathy from cardiac standstill that destroys most of the cortical lamina, multiple brain metastatic lesions, multifocal cerebral infarcts from isolated CNS vasculitis, multiple emboli from a cardiac source, markedly reduced global cerebral blood flow from acute SAH, cerebral edema, hydrocephalus, traumatic brain injury causing extensive scattered lesions in white and gray matter structures, and encephalitis. Unusual structural causes for coma are bilateral internal carotid occlusions, very commonly leading to loss of all brain function from profound swelling within days.[36] Bihemispheric brain injury may be associated with up- or downward eye deviation, spontaneous eye movements (mostly roving), intact brainstem reflexes (particularly in less severe forms), and variable motor responses (Figure 12.5). Generalized myoclonus may be seen as a result of severe cortical necrosis.[86]

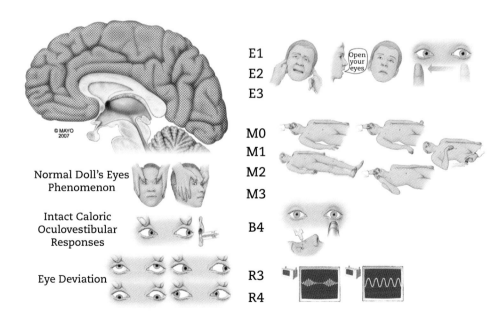

FIGURE 12.5: Bihemispheric injury and key clinical findings.

Acute Unilateral Hemispheric or Cerebellar Mass

Two major clinical manifestations may be observed in patients with an acute hemispheric mass: first, direct destruction of brain tissue, leading to clinical features related to the involved lobe; and, second, remote effects from the displacement of essentially normal tissue.

The quintessential neuropathologic findings associated with brain displacement are (1) displacement of the falx, (2) central brainstem displacement (displacement of the diencephalon structures, such as the thalamus), (3) lateral brainstem displacement, and (4) up- or downward displacement of brain tissue of the posterior fossa.

Displacement of brain tissue under the falx on CT scanning or MRI most frequently is a prelude to further displacement, when masses shift brain tissue even more. The cingulate gyrus is squeezed under the falx, but unless the anterior cerebral artery occludes (producing infarction and edema with frontal release signs and abulia), no major neurologic manifestation can be expected.

The modern view is that horizontal or vertical shift of the brainstem (and not so much herniation of tissue) correlates better with early changes in consciousness in acute unilateral masses. The diencephalic structures are compressed and are dislocated toward the opposite side of the mass lesion. Bilateral masses compress the upper brainstem rather than push it down. In addition, direct destructive damage of the thalamus with compression of the opposite dorsal thalamus may produce in the process bilateral involvement of the ARAS and may cause coma, despite an impressive shift in all directions (e.g., large, destructive ganglionic hemorrhage). Thus clinical features of "herniation or coning" are essentially manifestations of displacement of the thalamus and brainstem.

Lateral brainstem displacement has a more apparent presentation, with the sudden appearance of a wide pupil with loss of light response (Figure 12.6). Level of consciousness is reduced further when brain tissue shifts the brainstem to the opposite direction. Contralateral hemiparesis occurs when the brainstem is nicked against the opposite tentorial edge, damaging the pyramidal long tracts (classically named after the neuropathologist Kernohan; i.e., Kernohan's notch). The midbrain displaces horizontally and may rotate if the compression is off center. The process can progress only more vertically, but more likely the brainstem buckles. Compression of the brainstem causes smaller mid-position pupils (sometimes misinterpreted as "improvement of the blown pupil" after administration of mannitol).

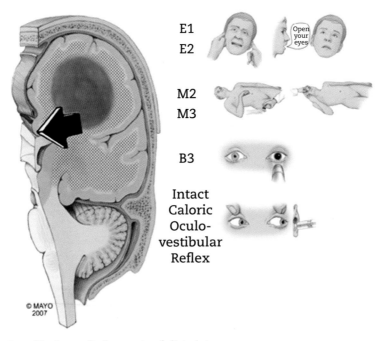

FIGURE 12.6: Lateral brainstem displacement and clinical signs.

From Wijdicks EFM. *The Comatose Patient*. 2nd edition. New York: Oxford University Press, 2014.

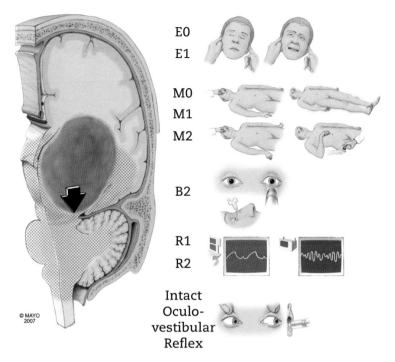

E0
E1

M0
M1
M2

B2

R1
R2

Intact
Oculo-
vestibular
Reflex

FIGURE 12.7: Central brainstem displacement and clinical signs.

From Wijdicks EFM. *The Comatose Patient*. 2nd edition. New York: Oxford University Press, 2014.

Central brainstem displacement occurs when a mass located medially forces the thalamus-midbrain through the tentorial opening. During this downward shift, the brainstem caves in further, and the shearing off of penetrating branches from the basilar artery fixed to the circle of Willis results in irreversible brainstem damage.

Signs of central brainstem displacement have been recognized by the appearance of midposition pupils with sluggish light responses (Figure 12.7). At the same time, respiration becomes rapid, or there is Cheyne-Stokes breathing. Patients barely localize pain stimuli and may fidget with bed linen or show a withdrawal response. Further progression results in extensor or flexor posturing and the development of midposition pupils (diameter 5–6 mm) unresponsive to light, disappearance of oculocephalic reflexes, and irregular gasping. Central brainstem displacement may progress to a midbrain stage in a matter of hours, but then halts or very slowly progresses further.

Acute cerebellar masses (e.g., hematoma) are manifested by vertigo, acute inability to walk, and excruciating headache. Vomiting is common, and many patients can only crawl to the bathroom. Approximately 60% of patients have a noticeable ataxia and nystagmus on examination before level of consciousness deteriorates from upward or downward tissue displacement.

Upward displacement occurs when the brainstem is lifted upward or when cerebellar tissue, particularly the vermis, is squeezed through the tentorial opening into the supracerebellar cisterns. The effects of brainstem compression and upward displacement are almost impossible to distinguish clinically. Patients deteriorate with progressive paralysis of upward gaze and further lapse into a deeper coma. Pupils become asymmetric and finally contract to pinpoint size when pontine compression advances.

Intrinsic Brainstem Injury

Intrinsic brainstem injury is reflected by major changes in pupil size, eye position, or spontaneous eye movement, immediately at onset. Pinpoint pupils, skew deviation, pupil anisocoria, ocular bobbing, and extensor or flexor posturing all are major indications of upper brainstem injury, often due to hemorrhage or infarction (Figure 12.8). As alluded to earlier, a "locked-in syndrome" is often mistaken for unresponsiveness until blinking and repeated up-and-down eye movements seem to coincide with questions posed to the patient. Cognition is intact, and patients may communicate through code systems. Locked-in syndrome

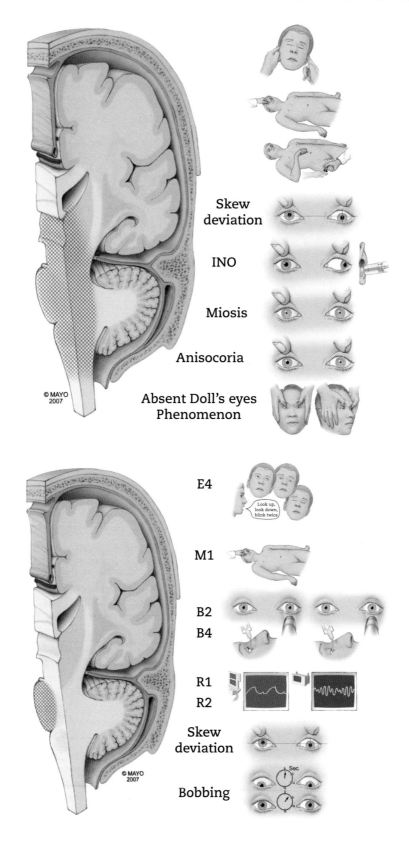

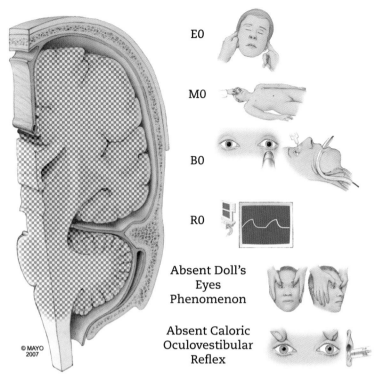

EO

MO

BO

RO

Absent Doll's
Eyes
Phenomenon

Absent Caloric
Oculovestibular
Reflex

© MAYO
2007

FIGURE 12.8: Intrinsic brainstem syndrome with key clinical findings (upper panel) and locked-in syndrome with key clinical findings (middle panel) and brain death (lower panel).

is mostly due to infarction of the pons but may occur with downward brainstem displacement[85] (Figure 12.8).

Assessment of Poisoning or Drug Abuse

Intentional poisoning and drug abuse are common causes of coma in patients admitted to EDs (Capsule 12.2). The distribution of different causes may reflect the geographic location of the hospital. The most common substances used for self-inflicted death by poisoning are tricyclic antidepressants, salicylates (particularly children), and street drugs. In the elderly, suicide attempts and unintentional intoxication through misjudgment of dose remain the leading causes.

This section reviews the most commonly encountered poisonings causing coma.[2,11] It is hardly possible to discuss all drugs that may cause coma; in fact, many do when ingested in enormous quantities. Polydrug abuse or intentional intoxication often results in widely different clinical presentations. Many of the drug overdose cases are so complicated and difficult to diagnose that physicians are left with a dizzying array of possibilities (major textbooks should be consulted).[2,11] There is

a potential flaw in presenting these intoxications in a simplistic fashion, but some clinical patterns are characteristic and should be recognized at first appearance.

Central Nervous System Depressants

CNS depressants first impair vestibular and cerebellar function. Therefore, nystagmus, ataxia, and dysarthria accompany or even precede the first signs of impaired consciousness.

Diagnosing an overdose of CNS depressant agents remains difficult, and one should appreciate the dangerous potential of some agents (e.g., tricyclic antidepressants).

Ethanol

Alcohol intoxication is a frequent cause of reduced arousal.[21,28] Alcohol ingestion can be fatal, but for death to occur, extreme quantities of ethanol will have been consumed, and more often an alcoholic binge is combined with the consumption of other depressant drugs, leading to respiratory arrest or respiratory airway obstruction from vomiting.

The development of acute alcohol intoxication depends not only on the blood alcohol concentration but also on the rapidity of the increase

---

CAPSULE 12.2   MECHANISMS OF TOXIN-INDUCED COMA

Coma induced by poisoning may result from at least five mechanisms. First, a chief factor may be hypoglycemia. Because many toxins cause profound hypoglycemia, early intravenous administration of glucose in any comatose patient has been advocated. Common examples are salicylates, β-adrenergic blockers, and ethanol.

Second, in other toxins, hypoxia is the main mechanism underlying coma and is produced by interference of oxygen transport, tissue utilization of oxygen, or simply displacement of oxygen by another gas, such as an industrial gas. Hypoxia can also be produced by acute pulmonary edema (e.g., cocaine) or aspiration pneumonitis (e.g., after seizures).

Third, a major mechanism of coma is depression of neuronal function involving the γ-aminobutyric acid (GABA)–benzodiazepine chloride iodophor receptor complex. The mechanism of action through GABA, one of the major CNS neurotransmitters, is increased output of GABA, which also leads to reduction of the turnover of acetylcholine, dopamine, and serotonin, culminating in a marked hypnotic-depressant effect. Opioids, however, exert their depressant effects on the CNS through a different set of receptors.

Fourth, toxins may cause seizures, usually as a terminal manifestation, which may be followed by a postictal decreased level of consciousness or nonconvulsive status epilepticus.

Fifth, structural CNS lesions may be caused by the toxin itself or by traumatic head injury. Coma in poisoning or drug abuse may be due to spontaneous intracranial hematoma (e.g., amphetamine or cocaine overdose) or hemorrhagic brain contusions associated with a fall.

---

in blood and on tolerance, which is significantly increased in heavy drinkers (typically, they are able to "drink someone under the table"). The clinical features of alcohol intoxication in relation to blood alcohol level are thus unreliable and apply only to naive drinkers. The clinical presentation of alcohol intoxication is well known and involves ataxia, dysarthria, loss of rapid reaction to sudden danger, and a feeling of high self-esteem that can lead to a series of misjudgments, including driving despite warnings from passengers. Aggression to well-intended restraint may lead to fist fights in susceptible persons and significant head injury or epidural hematoma due to acute skull fracture overlying the middle meningeal artery.

Seizures are uncommon as a direct result of alcohol consumption but may be associated with severe hyponatremia (e.g., after consumption of large quantities of alcohol at "beer fests"). Alcohol intoxication may mimic or coincide with many neurologic disorders, including hepatic encephalopathy, hypoglycemia, subdural hematoma, fulminant bacterial meningitis, and central pontine myelinolysis. Progressive confusion and combativeness in a previously alcoholic person, particularly if associated with tremors, marked (often initially unexplained) hypertension, and tachycardia may indicate alcohol

withdrawal and delirium. Recognition of profound alcohol withdrawal may become difficult, particularly if patients have passed well into a stage of agitation and decreased alertness.

The diagnosis of acute drunkenness seems straightforward, but laboratory confirmation and exclusion of confounding metabolic derangements are needed. Crucial laboratory tests should include measurement of serum alcohol level, arterial blood gases (to exclude hypoventilation), electrolytes, blood glucose (alcohol reduces gluconeogenesis and causes hypoglycemia in a predisposed patient), calcium and magnesium, and serum osmolality. A large osmolar gap is compatible with alcohol intoxication. Routine drug screens should be performed at all times to rule out other ingested drugs of abuse. When truly measured, the legal limit in many states is 80 mg alcohol/100 mL blood, but toxic levels are usually more than 200 mg alcohol/100 mL blood.

The management of patients in stupor or coma from alcohol intoxication consists of endotracheal intubation to protect the airway, thiamine intravenously, rewarming, liberal intravenous fluids, treatment of recurrent seizures, if any, and frequent assessment and management of potential hypoglycemia.

Barbiturates

Barbiturates are hypnotic-sedative agents that should be considered a cause of coma in drug addicts rushed into the ED. It is not surprising to find that barbiturates have been taken with other street drugs, which may considerably deepen the level of coma.

Barbiturates significantly differ in duration of action (Table 12.5). They are very powerful stimulants of the inhibitory neurotransmitter γ-aminobutyric acid (GABA), resulting in early depression of respiratory drive. In the event of overdose, these differences often determine how long the patient will be on the mechanical ventilator. Depending on the degree of CNS depression, barbiturate overdose produces flaccid coma with initially small reactive pupils advancing to light-fixed, dilated pupils in near-fatal doses, often with associated profound hypotension from direct myocardial depression, clammy skin, and hypothermia.[57]

The depth of coma can be estimated by measurement of barbiturate levels and by an electroencephalogram (EEG), which in severe cases may show isoelectric tracing mimicking brain death, but more commonly displays a burst suppression pattern.

Management of barbiturate coma is supportive, with full mechanical ventilation until cough

TABLE 12.5. Classification of Barbiturates

Ultra-short-acting (DA, 0.3 hour)
Thiopental
Thiamylal
Methohexital
Short-acting (DA, 3 hours)
Hexobarbital
Pentobarbital*
Secobarbital†
Intermediate-acting (DA, 3–6 hours)
Amobarbital‡
Aprobarbital
Butabarbital
Long-acting (DA, 6–12 hours)
Barbital
Mephobarbital
Phenobarbital§
Primidone

DA, duration of action
* Also known as "yellow jackets."
† Also known as "red devils."
‡ Also known as "blue heavens."
§ Also known as "purple hearts," "goofballs," and "downs."

reflexes return. Vasopressors are needed to support blood pressure. Forced alkaline diuresis and hemodialysis with high blood flow rate should be considered.

With the improvement in ICU support and hemodialysis, outcome is difficult to predict on the basis of depth of coma.[53]

Tricyclic Antidepressants

The prescription of antidepressant drugs for patients with severe depression may lead to a suicide attempt, possibly related to the observation that it takes 2–3 weeks to achieve the antidepressant effect, and thus patients with suicidal tendencies may take all of their medication at once.[44] Tricyclic overdose is one of the principal causes of death in an ICU series of drug-overdosing surveys. By virtue of the profound cardiac toxicity of the drugs, death can be imminent in some patients on arrival in the ED.

Coma from tricyclic antidepressant toxicity may progress to a loss of most brainstem reflexes, but never exactly mimicking brain death.[78] Coma with no response to painful stimuli occurred in only 13% of 225 patients with tricyclic overdose. Tricyclic overdose may be manifested by delirium from cholinergic blockade, and some patients have other manifestations, such as dry skin, hyperthermia, and dilated pupils. Seizures are common within hours of ingestion, often emerge at peak serum concentration, but seldom evolve into status epilepticus.

A widened QRS interval on the EKG is a common manifestation,[7] but, at least initially, cardiac arrhythmias may be absent. In a significant overdose, the management of cardiac arrhythmia determines care and can involve a temporary pacemaker. Sodium bicarbonate (50 mEq of $NaHCO_3$, 1 mEq/mL) should be administered to produce alkalosis, which inhibits sodium channel blockade by tricyclic antidepressants, a mechanism thought to be responsible for cardiac arrhythmia. Seizures can be managed with intravenous administration of phenytoin or fosphenytoin, but because of its own risk of producing cardiac arrhythmias, this agent probably is indicated only if seizures recur.

Selective Serotonin Reuptake Inhibitors

Tricyclic antidepressants are still used but selective serotonin reuptake inhibitors (SSRIs) are now used far more often. Serotonin syndrome as a result of ingestion of large amounts of SSRIs usually presents with agitation, dysautonomia (diaphoresis, tachycardia, severe unrelenting myoclonus, and hyperreflexia), and seizures; but stupor or deep coma is uncommon. Rhabdomyolysis should be recognized with serial CPK values and adequate hydration should be provided if elevated. Resolution is typically within 24–48 hours.[42] A serotonin syndrome can also occur when a regular dose of SSRI is combined with opioids (e.g., oxycodone). Treatment in comatose patients is with cyproheptadine (histamine H1 antagonist) starting with 12 mg followed by 2 mg every two hours until clinical response is seen. A higher starting dose (20 mg) may be needed in more severe cases.

Lithium
Toxic manifestations of lithium are most often a result of incorrect dosage. Anticholinergic manifestations are common, including flushing of the face, dilated pupils, fever, and dry skin.

With increasing blood levels, a rather slowly progressing clinical picture seems to emerge, characterized by myoclonus, hand tremor, and slurring of speech. This may further progress to delirium, acute mania, dystonic movements, oculogyric crises, facial grimacing, and, finally, stupor. Serum lithium levels are reasonably correlated with the severity of toxicity, which is serious when these levels reach or exceed 2.5 mEq/L.[62]

Restoration of sodium and water balance, which is disturbed by lithium-induced nephrogenic diabetes insipidus, is key in its management. Hemodialysis or peritoneal dialysis should be instituted immediately in most cases.

Benzodiazepines
Patients with a benzodiazepine ("downs," "nerve pills," "tranks") overdose seldom are in need of a long hospital stay unless co-ingestions have occurred. Massive exposure to benzodiazepines results in coma, but with appropriate support, neurologic morbidity is rare. Coma can be profound, but most patients awaken within 2 days; recovery times are longer with increasing age.[26]

The clinical presentation of benzodiazepine poisoning is nonspecific, and coma with extreme flaccidity is common. Respiratory depression may not be evident, and hypoxic respiratory drive often becomes clear only when a pulse oximeter is connected to the patient on arrival in the ED. Not uncommonly, oxygen administration with high flow may then produce hypercarbia and hyperoxemia. Many patients may need to be intubated, but adjustment of the oxygen source and rate-controlled, noninvasive ventilation may be effective in some instances.

The use of flumazenil is controversial because seizures from acute withdrawal have been reported. A more recent study in 110 patients contradicted these risks and demonstrated that flumazenil is safe.[77]

Abuse of Illicit Drugs
It is not possible to gather all illicit drugs under one umbrella and discuss them in a few paragraphs. This section discusses some of the most commonly encountered examples of drug overdose. For complex problems, readers should refer to major toxicology textbooks, available in most EDs, or to a neurology text.[2,11] Not infrequently, these unfortunate, poorly nourished, shelterless patients are found hypothermic or next to an empty syringe, bottle of liquor, or unlabeled pill vial.

Phencyclidine
Phencyclidine ("angel dust") is rising in popularity among illicit drug users and college students, and thus the prevalence of phencyclidine overdose is increasing in EDs. Phencyclidine is usually packed in tablets and sold as powder or mixed with marijuana ("wacky weed").[43]

Phencyclidine is a potent anesthetic agent, acting on both GABA and dopamine systems. Its clinical manifestations are highly unusual, with deep anesthesia and coma but a facial appearance of being fully awake. Typically, a strong pain stimulus is not registered by the patient, and this sign should immediately point to phencyclidine as a toxin. Commonly, phencyclidine produces hypertension, tachycardia, salivation, sweating, and bidirectional nystagmus. Many patients act violently, demonstrate bizarre behavior, and speak endlessly. Distortion of body image and vivid visual hallucinations may occur, and some patients are catatonic, which additionally may lead to rhabdomyolysis. When the patient's condition progresses to coma, cholinergic signs are obvious, with significant frothing, flushing, sweating (often with typical strings of large sweat droplets on the forehead), and miosis.[43]

Many patients recover fully with adequate ventilator support, but some may continue to manifest a schizophrenia-like picture of withdrawal, negativism, and delusions, which suggests chronic use of phencyclidine.

Cocaine
Cocaine ("blow," "snow," "toot," "coke," "rock") blocks the presynaptic uptake of norepinephrine and dopamine and causes excitation.[22] Its

recreational use is widespread, either by intranasal snorting or by smoking after dissolution in water and the addition of a strong base ("crack").[38]

The clinical presentation after inhalation, smoking, or intravenous injection is characteristic. Patients have hypertension, widely dilated pupils, and tachypnea. Seizures often occur after the initial "rush." In severely intoxicated patients, progression to generalized tonic-clonic epilepticus is not unusual.[15,16,40]

Coma from cocaine overdose may have other origins. These are cardiac arrest, producing a profound anoxic–ischemic encephalopathy, intracerebral (ganglionic or pons), or subarachnoid hemorrhage from brief malignant hypertension.[74] Outcome is worse in aneurysmal SAH associated with cocaine. Up to 50% of patients harbor a vascular malformation or aneurysm. Bilateral cerebral infarcts can be a result of diffuse vasoconstriction or long-standing occlusive disease of the major cerebral arteries.[69]

General measures for cocaine overdose often include management of hyperthermia with cooling blankets or fans, α-adrenergic blockade or lidocaine to treat ventricular tachycardia, and careful monitoring for the possible development of acute myocardial infarction and recognition of status epilepticus.

Opiates

Acute opiate overdose may be produced by heroin (diacetylmorphine; "H," "speedball") or deliberate use of massive doses of those narcotic drugs used for pain control. Fentanyl dermal patches, particularly, have become popular for pain control, and the absorption of this very potent opioid is so erratic that rapidly progressive stupor may occur.

The clinical manifestations of opiate overdose include miosis, hypoventilation, and flaccidity. Brainstem reflexes may become lost, and the preserved light reflex in patients with extremely small pupils may be impossible to discern. Severe hypoxia from hypoventilation may be a major contributory factor to coma. Seizures appear more commonly with meperidine and propoxyphene.

The management of opioid poisoning has been facilitated by the use of naloxone. This opiate antagonist is without major adverse effects, and dramatic reversal of coma is seen.

Arterial blood gas values are supportive in opioid overdose, demonstrating marked hypoxia and hypercapnia from hypoventilation. A point that cannot be emphasized strongly enough is that because serum drug screens do not identify opioids, urine samples are needed for detection.

Naloxone is administered in doses of 0.4–2.0 mg, repeated at 1- to 2-minute intervals. The effect is brief. An intravenous drip of naloxone is justified only in patients with a profound overdose resulting in hypotension and ventricular tachyarrhythmias.

Environmental and Industrial Toxins

Exposure to these toxins, whether intentional or accidental, frequently alters consciousness and produces prolonged coma long after the toxin has been eliminated, washed out, or neutralized. Important clues to environmental poisoning are dead pets and distinctive odors (from often-added sulfur-containing compounds) detected by neighbors.

The effect of these toxins on the CNS can be catastrophic, with a high probability of poor neurologic outcomes.

Carbon Monoxide Poisoning

Carbon monoxide remains one of the leading causes of death by poisoning. Exposure to this odorless gas is possible at the time of a fire, from poorly vented fireplaces, from furnaces, and in any closed space where internal combustion engines have been used without ventilation. In most instances, suicide can be implicated, but one-third of admitted patients are victims of accidental circumstances.[35]

Carbon monoxide readily binds to hemoglobin, with a 200 times greater attraction than oxygen. The cerebral injury due to carbon monoxide poisoning, however, is an accumulation of factors. Pathognomonic lesions can be produced only by carbon monoxide and hypotension and not by inhalation of carbon monoxide alone.

Carbon monoxide poisoning causes a shift of the hemoglobin dissociation curve to the left, which reduces oxygen unloading (the Haldane effect). Through binding with myoglobin, carbon monoxide may trigger cardiac arrhythmias, hypotension, and hypoxemia from pulmonary edema, adding to the injury.

The neuropathologic changes (selected from the most severe cases at autopsy) are predominant in the white matter, with demyelination and edema, and in the hippocampus, cerebellum, and globus pallidus.[34] These lesions may be detected on CT scans; they predict a severely disabled state as the best possible outcome.[46] MRI may more clearly delineate these abnormalities, which emerge even within hours of exposure, but only in patients with levels high enough to lead to coma (virtually always more than 50% carboxyhemoglobin levels).

The symptoms preceding coma from carbon monoxide poisoning are nonspecific and vague, including headache, dizziness, and shortness of breath, all suggesting a developing viral illness. A cherry red appearance of the skin is very uncommon and signals a near-fatal exposure. Other clinical findings are retinal hemorrhages, dark color of retinal arteries and veins, and pulmonary edema. Rhabdomyolysis may be related to pressure necrosis in patients immobilized for an unknown length of time.[23]

The most important laboratory test is the determination of a carbon monoxide hemoglobin level, which may be falsely low if oxygen has been administered in the ED or if the time between exposure and blood testing is more than 6 hours, which is approximately the half-life of carboxyhemoglobin (a 5% level of hemoglobin carbon monoxide can be attributed to smoking). Other laboratory test results that are more or less supportive are metabolic acidosis, increased creatine kinase, and myocardial ischemia on EKG.

The management of carbon monoxide poisoning is treatment with 100% oxygen with a sealed face mask. Hyperbaric oxygen increases the amount of dissolved oxygen 10 times and may significantly shorten the duration of coma.[12] Hyperbaric oxygen is not routinely available, but hard data prove a better outcome with this therapy. A recent clinical trial held three sessions within a 24-hour period consisting of 100% oxygen at 3 atmospheres, followed by 2 atmospheres. Cognitive impairment was almost halved, although number of treatments and time window are not exactly known.[76] Benefit may still be possible 6–12 hours after exposure. Additional factors, such as hypotension, are equally important in carbon monoxide's damaging effect. Therefore, hyperbaric oxygen therapy is the preferred approach in nonintubated comatose patients and in patients with significant myocardial ischemia despite initial breathing of 100% oxygen.

Cyanide

Cyanide poisoning should be entertained in any coma of undetermined cause, particularly in laboratory or industrial workers. A well-recognized intentional cause is the ingestion of nail polish removers.[39] Prevalence of cyanide poisoning is low, but its effects can be reversed with antidotes.

Cyanide has an unusual mechanism of action. By interacting with cytochrome oxidase (an essential enzyme in the mitochondrial electron transport chain), it greatly reduces the production of adenosine triphosphate. Consequently,

significant lactic acidosis results from a shift in anaerobic metabolism. Additionally, cyanide, like carbon monoxide, shifts the hemoglobin dissociation curve to the left and directly binds with the iron of hemoglobin, reducing the delivery of oxygen to the brain and other vital organs.

Coma from cyanide poisoning is often accompanied by hypoventilation from central inhibition of the respiratory centers, severe lactic acidosis, bradycardia, hypotension, and rapidly developing pulmonary edema.[75] A bitter almond or musty smell has been linked to cyanide poisoning, but recognition of its odor is impossible for many physicians.

The supportive laboratory finding is metabolic acidosis, which may be combined with respiratory alkalosis from hyperventilation to overcome hypoxia or respiratory acidosis from hypoventilation. Plasma cyanide can be measured, but correlation with the degree of coma is poor, thus making testing impractical.

Cyanide poisoning has a good outcome when treated with the Lilly cyanide antidote kit. This contains amyl nitrite (the pellets are crushed and inhaled by the patient), sodium nitrite, and sodium thiosulfate (intravenous, 50 mL of a 25% solution). The effect is based on the conversion of hemoglobin into methemoglobin, which combines with cyanide but easily breaks down into free cyanide, which then combines with sodium thiosulfate and is eventually eliminated in the urine.

Reliable neurologic data on outcomes are not available. Parkinsonism and dystonia have been reported, with associated lesions in the basal ganglia detected by CT scanning but with improvement in some instances.[13,58]

Toxic Alcohols

Methanol, ethylene glycol, and isopropyl alcohol are used in many commercial products, including antifreeze (ethylene glycol) and solvents (methanol). Isopropyl alcohol is best known as rubbing alcohol. The alcohols produce virtually similar laboratory effects, the most noticeable of which is a high anion gap metabolic acidosis.[45,49]

Methanol infrequently causes coma, but then a fatal outcome is likely. Methanol more commonly produces delirium and blurred vision. Careful examination reveals hyperemia of the optic disk, and blindness may follow as a result of the toxic effect of formaldehyde on retinal ganglion cells. Bilateral necrosis of the putamen is highly characteristic, frequently becoming apparent on neuroimaging studies in comatose patients only after several weeks.[61] However, the brains of patients dying of methanol poisoning may be normal or variably show congestion, edema, petechiae, and necrosis of the cerebellar white matter.

Several features of methanol poisoning are of interest. First, a latent period (up to 12 hours) is typical, making it very difficult for bystanders to understand the sudden occurrence of a lapse into coma. Second, prominent restlessness, with vomiting and doubling over from abdominal cramps, may be followed by seizures before the stage of unresponsiveness. Treatment is focused on correcting the acidosis with bicarbonate, but in comatose patients extracorporeal hemodialysis is imperative. Although the outcome can be very satisfactory, permanent neurologic disability may occur.

Ethylene glycol is most commonly known as a major component of antifreeze and many detergents. Suicide is the most common reason for ingestion, and then mortality is high. The metabolites produce toxicity, and the clinical features preceding coma are dramatic. Marked gait ataxia, nystagmus, and paralysis of the extraocular muscles are followed by generalized tonic-clonic seizures or profound myoclonus and, because of severe hypocalcemia, tetanic contractions. Lactic acidosis and an osmolar gap are characteristic laboratory features, but diagnosis is confirmed with the demonstration of calcium oxalate crystals in the urine.[33,48] Ethylene glycol poisoning is often treated with hemodialysis and has been previously treated with high doses of ethanol. In a recent study, an inhibitor of alcohol dehydrogenase (fomepizole) was successful in preventing renal damage by inhibiting toxic metabolites such as oxalate. Fomepizole is an expensive alternative to ethanol but is without toxic effects. Intravenous loading of 15 mg/kg is followed by 10 mg/kg every 12 hours for 2 days, with a further increase to 15 mg/kg every 12 hours until the plasma ethylene glycol concentration is less than 20 mg/dL.[10]

Finally, isopropyl alcohol is rather potent, producing rapidly developing coma, always with severe hypotension from cardiomyopathy. The typical acetone breath should point to this toxin. The characteristic oxalate crystals in ethylene glycol are not found in isopropyl poisoning. Management involves gastric lavage; because the onset of coma is rapid, recovery of the substance from the stomach can still be substantial.

Miscellaneous Intoxications

This section reviews those poisonings that are of great clinical importance and proportionally frequent or that produce striking clinical features.

Salicylates

As a result of safety packaging, the incidence of accidental salicylate poisoning has substantially decreased, but it is still prevalent in children. Salicylates may take some time to dissolve in the acidic stomach milieu but then are rapidly absorbed, and blood levels are maximal within 1 hour. After exposure to a massive dose, the usual pharmacokinetics of the drug change, and through a complex mechanism the half-life of salicylates increases to 15–20 hours from a baseline level of 2–4 hours in therapeutic doses.[29]

Salicylates equilibrate rapidly with cerebrospinal fluid (CSF), and the levels of salicylates in CSF appear to correlate better with outcome than do serum levels. Determination of salicylate levels in CSF, however, is cumbersome. Salicylates significantly interfere with platelet function and prolong prothrombin time and may preclude lumbar puncture.

The mechanism of action of salicylates is not entirely clear. It may involve (1) uncoupling of the oxidative phosphorylation and blocking of glycolysis, producing a metabolic acidosis; (2) direct stimulation of the brainstem respiratory centers, leading to respiratory alkalosis, independent of an already compensatory response to the induced acidosis; and (3) increased metabolic demand from increased glycolysis to compensate for the aforementioned uncoupling, which may result in profound hypoglycemia. Severe acidemia caused by increased lipid solubility of salicylates in an acidic environment facilitates the entry of salicylates into the brain.

Salicylate poisoning should always be considered in restless, hyperventilating patients. Hyperthermia and purpura in the eyelids and neck may occur, due to platelet dysfunction, and simulate fulminant acute meningococcal meningitis. Pulmonary edema may occur and may become rapidly life-threatening.

The laboratory features of increased anion gap, metabolic acidosis, and respiratory alkalosis are well appreciated and should lead to the measurement of serum salicylate levels or, more practically, ferric chloride testing of the urine. Purple discoloration of the urine is diagnostic, and the test has good predictive value. A plasma salicylate level of 6 mg/dL usually is correlated with seizures and coma.

Management of salicylate poisoning involves gastric lavage, activated charcoal, and forced alkaline diuresis. Alkalization is performed with sodium bicarbonate or, in less severe cases, acetazolamide.

Acetaminophen

Acetaminophen is a component of many nonprescription drugs; as a result, poisoning is common. Usually, however, extremely large doses (plasma level > 800 µg/mL) are required to directly depress consciousness; more likely, the development of acute hepatic necrosis or hepatorenal syndrome causes coma.[20,50]

Overdose of acetaminophen proceeds in phases, but liver damage can occur within 24 hours after ingestion. The biochemical basis for acute liver necrosis has been elucidated and is the rationale for therapy with *N*-acetylcysteine. In normal situations, acetaminophen is metabolized in the liver through either sulfation or glucuronidation, and only a small fraction through the P450 oxidase system, which produces an active metabolite that has the potential for liver necrosis. Overloading of the glucuronidation system by the ingestion of large amounts of acetaminophen increases the formation of toxic metabolites. Decreased glutathione stores, as in patients with long-term antiepileptic drug use or chronic alcoholism, may increase the probability of liver necrosis after acetaminophen intoxication.

Clinical features of acetaminophen overdose are nausea, vomiting, diaphoresis, and abdominal pain in the right upper quadrant, but no depression in consciousness unless hepatic failure develops.[73] Hepatic encephalopathy, with its characteristic asterixis and myoclonus, develops approximately 4 days after ingestion. Brain edema may become a feature in fulminant hepatic failure when patients lapse into stupor.

Together with *N*-acetylcysteine loading, management is largely supportive. *N*-acetylcysteine is metabolized to cysteine, which functions as a precursor for glutathione and restores the glutathione scavenging. Acetaminophen half-lives may vary from 4 to 120 hours, depending on the severity of liver necrosis.[63]

Liver transplantation may be needed, and its consideration leads to an ethical quagmire in patients who used acetaminophen for a suicide attempt.

Antiepileptic Drugs

Overdose with antiepileptic drugs is most often intentional, but every now and then a prescription blunder or drug interaction that reduces metabolism can be implicated. Coma from antiepileptic drug overdose is not common, and most often nonspecific signs, such as dizziness, tremor, nystagmus, and profound ataxia, occur. Paradoxically, antiepileptic drug overdose may produce seizures, and the risk, at least in carbamazepine overdose, is increased in patients with a seizure disorder.

Acute overdose of phenytoin is characterized by rapid ataxia, dysarthria with combative behavior, and hallucinations, very seldom followed by generalized tonic-clonic seizures and progression to flaccid coma. Management is supportive, with mechanical ventilation, charcoal to minimize further absorption, and benzodiazepines (e.g., lorazepam) or barbiturates (e.g., phenobarbital) in the rare event that seizures occur.

Carbamazepine is widely used in neurologic disorders. Its side effects are reminiscent of those of tricyclic antidepressants because of structural similarities, and neurologists, who are usually the primary healthcare providers, should appreciate the potential life-threatening side effects. Respiratory depression is common in carbamazepine overdose, and prospective studies have found a median duration of 18 hours. Coma occurs in 20%–50% of the reported series of carbamazepine overdose.[64,67] Fatal outcome may reach 15% of patients, most often affecting those in coma, with seizures, and with resuscitation for cardiac arrest; ingestion often exceeds 100 tablets. Other manifestations of carbamazepine overdose are hypothermia, hypotension, tachycardia, and a diverse range of cardiac arrhythmias from its anticholinergic properties.[25] Overdose with controlled-release carbamazepine may lead to peak toxicity 4 days postingestion, and whole-bowel irrigation may be needed.[67]

Typically, management is focused on cardiac manifestations, and problems similar to those in tricyclic antidepressant overdose should be anticipated. Recovery from carbamazepine overdose can be protracted, with fluctuating levels of consciousness for many days.

Valproate toxicity is notable for its association with acute liver failure, but this devastating side effect has occurred only in young children and with concomitant use of other antiepileptic agents. Hyperammonemia may be a major mechanism for stupor.[3] Massive ingestions produce coma with pinpoint pupils. As in acetaminophen poisoning, fulminant hepatic failure may produce many of the earlier manifestations of asterixis, myoclonus, and nystagmus. Valproate-associated hyperammonemia is treated with L-carnitine, which could mitigate its effect (50–100 mg/kg IV daily).[8,37,66]

Assessment of Acute Metabolic or Endocrine Causes of Coma

Acute metabolic derangements may produce reduced arousal and, when unrecognized, coma.

Typical examples are hypoglycemia, hyponatremia, acute uremia, and acute liver failure. Overt hemiparesis, pupil abnormalities, and gaze preference are conspicuously absent on neurologic examination, but asterixis, tremor, and myoclonus predominate before deep coma sets in. Hyperglycemic non-ketotic hyperosmolar coma is a notable exception. Focal signs may occur in this condition because of previous strokes in these patients with severe cerebrovascular risk factors. The mechanisms of these conditions causing hypometabolism in the brain are poorly understood, but many of these disorders cause diffuse cerebral edema; seizures intervene or cardiorespiratory resuscitation results in diffuse anoxic–ischemic damage. Endocrine crises, such as rarely encountered Hashimoto thyroiditis (thyroid coma), Addison's disease, and panhypopituitarism, may be responsible for coma; and hormones of the hypothalamic pituitary axis should be measured in unexplained coma. The laboratory values compatible with marked impairment of consciousness are shown in Table 12.6. Coma should be attributed to other causes if the biochemical derangement is less severe.

NEUROIMAGING AND LABORATORY TESTS

Computed tomography scanning of the brain is particularly useful when the neurologic examination reveals localizing symptoms. Acute lesions in the brainstem and cerebellum may not be visualized on CT. Patients with acute basilar artery occlusion or evolving cerebellar infarction often have normal CT findings on admission, and MRI is needed to resolve the cause of the coma. It may also demonstrate sparing of the ARAS in locked-in syndrome.

The CT findings in patients with altered consciousness, hemiparesis, or gaze preference are

TABLE 12.6. Laboratory Values Compatible with Coma in Patients with Acute Metabolic and Endocrine Derangements*

Derangement	Serum
Hyponatremia	≤ 110 mmol/L
Hypernatremia	≥ 160 mmol/L
Hypercalcemia	≥ 15 mg/dL
Hypermagnesemia	≥ 5 mg/dL
Hypercapnia	≥ 70 mm Hg
Hypoglycemia	≤ 40 mg/dL
Hyperglycemia	≥ 800 mg/dL

* Sudden decline in value is obligatory.

often abnormal. One should particularly evaluate whether basal cisterns are present on CT scans because they may be filled in early brain swelling.

A CT of the brain defines the existence of a mass, its remote effect, and edema, and it may hint at a cause. Contralateral hydrocephalus may be present, usually caused by compression at the level of the foramen of Monro. The ambient cistern is usually effaced, and an enlargement of the temporal horn is seen. However, because of multiplanar views, MRI is more sensitive for recording the extension of the mass and may reveal necrosis, pigments (deoxyhemoglobin, melanin), or fat, which may suggest the underlying pathologic condition.

In the ED, the CT scan appearance of a mass is most often characteristic enough to determine an early plan of action. Solitary lesions in nonimmunosuppressed patients most commonly represent intra-axial brain tumors or abscess. On unenhanced images, low density may represent tumor with edema. The degree of edema may reflect the degree of malignancy; rapidly growing tumors, such as glioblastoma, produce much more surrounding edema. Edema is also comparatively common in metastasis.

Most intracranial masses are hypodense, but hyperdense masses may point to a meningioma or lymphoma, or may hemorrhage into a tumor. Speckled calcification inside a mass, an important CT scan finding, is present in more than 50% of patients with an oligodendroglioma but may point to an inflammatory cause, particularly parasite infestation, such as cysticercosis, and less common disorders, such as paragonimiasis and echinococcosis. They are often seen in areas other than the cystic mass, indicating calcium deposits in necrotic brain tissue.

Intracranial mass of inflammatory origin has become a much more common presentation in the ED from the increase in transplantation surgery and the acquired immunodeficiency syndrome (AIDS) epidemic.

Brain abscesses, usually from toxoplasmosis, are very commonly associated with AIDS infection. Toxoplasmosis seldom appears as a single mass, although one large mass may predominate. Basal ganglia localization is typical, and hemorrhage may occur. Tuberculoma or aspergillosis should be considered. Magnetic resonance imaging can be helpful because a dark (hypointense) T2 signal inside the mass is often found. Neuroimaging is an obligatory study in patients who may be brain dead. The results of neuroimaging studies or CSF examination should be generally compatible with the diagnosis of brain death. Thus, one should expect a large mass lesion, producing brain tissue shift with herniation, or an intracranial hemorrhage with enlarged ventricles. Other validating CT scan findings are multiple, large, acute cerebral infarcts; massive cerebral edema; multiple hemorrhagic contusions; and cerebellar-pontine lesions compressing or destroying the brainstem. Normal brain images in brain death can be seen immediately after cardiac arrest, carbon monoxide poisoning, asphyxia, acute encephalitis, and cyanide or other fatal poisoning. The most common CT and MRI findings in comatose patients are summarized in Table 12.7. Functional MRI may provide another level of sophistication in imaging of the comatose patient but is neither yet widely used, nor proven yet to be of practical value (Capsule 12.3). The diagnostic accuracy of functional MRI in predicting recovery remains unknown.

Normal findings on neuroimaging, with no clinical evidence of an acute cerebellar infarction or acute basilar artery occlusion, should prompt immediate examination of the CSF to search for possible CNS infection. Failure to exclude a potentially treatable CNS infection may have devastating consequences. The evaluation of CSF findings in meningitis and encephalitis is further discussed in Chapters 33 and 35.

Abdominal radiographs can be helpful in establishing whether the patient has ingested any tablets or foreign objects. Examples of radiopaque pills are chloral hydrate, trifluoperazine, amitriptyline, and enteric-coated tablets; however, many tablets may have dissolved before the patient is admitted to the ED.

The EKG can be useful, and results are nearly always abnormal if intoxication is due to phenothiazines, quinidine, procainamide, or tricyclic antidepressants. Tricyclic antidepressant overdose characteristically produces widening of the QRS complex and QT prolongation. Widening of the QRS complex considerably increases the risk of seizures associated with tricyclic antidepressant overdose. The EKG findings are also important in confirming hypothermia as a cause of coma (typically, the QRS complex widens and ST elevation occurs, also known as a "camel's hump").

When poisoning is strongly considered as a cause of coma, laboratory tests are essential before

TABLE 12.7. Frequent Abnormalities on Neuroimaging Studies in Coma

Findings	Suggested Disorders
Computed Tomography	
Mass lesion	Hematoma, hemorrhagic contusion, MCA territory infarct
Hemorrhage in basal cisterns	Aneurysmal SAH
Intraventricular hemorrhage	Arteriovenous malformation
Multiple hemorrhagic infarcts	Cerebral venous thrombosis
Multiple cerebral infarcts	Endocarditis, coagulopathy, CNS vasculitis
Diffuse cerebral edema	Cardiac arrest, fulminant meningitis, acute hepatic necrosis, encephalitis
Acute hydrocephalus	Aqueduct obstruction, colloid cyst, pineal region tumor
Pontine or cerebellum hemorrhage	Hypertension, arteriovenous malformation, cavernous malformation
Shear lesions in the white matter	Traumatic brain injury
Magnetic Resonance Imaging	
Bilateral caudate and putaminal lesions	Carbon monoxide poisoning, methanol
Hyperdense signal along sagittal, straight, and transverse sinuses	Cerebral venous thrombosis
Lesions in corpus callosum, white matter	Traumatic head injury
Diffuse confluent hyperintense lesions in white matter	Acute disseminated encephalomyelitis, immunosuppressive agent or chemotherapeutic agent toxicity, metabolic leukodystrophies
Pontine trident-shaped lesion	Central pontine myelinolysis
Thalamus, occipital, pontine lesions	Acute basilar artery occlusion
Temporal, frontal lobe hyperintensities	Herpes simplex encephalitis

CNS, central nervous system; MCA, middle cerebral artery; SAH, subarachnoid hemorrhage.

CAPSULE 12.3   FUNCTIONAL MRI IN COMA

Functional MRI of the brain is able to demonstrate engaged networks after the patient is asked a task. This "default" network is an active system that is present only when individuals are not focused on the external environment. It was discovered when researchers measured activity in humans who had no directed mental state. It is known that the global rate of metabolism in the resting state was as active as when individuals were asked to solve complex mathematical problems. Other studies have suggested that autobiographical memory, remembering the past, and thinking about future events all are activated in this network. These networks thus could represent task-unrelated images and thoughts, or perhaps operation of self-awareness. The system, therefore, is active in passive settings and during tasks that direct attention away from external stimuli (mind-wandering). The network is deactivated with a target-directed and attention-focused processing. This default network includes the precuneus, temporoparietal junction and medial prefrontal cortex, which shows "idling" activity when at rest and deactivation in task. Reduction in the functional connectivity of these brain regions have been prominently seen in patients with altered consciousness and the extremes of abnormal consciousness such as minimally conscious state and vegetative state.

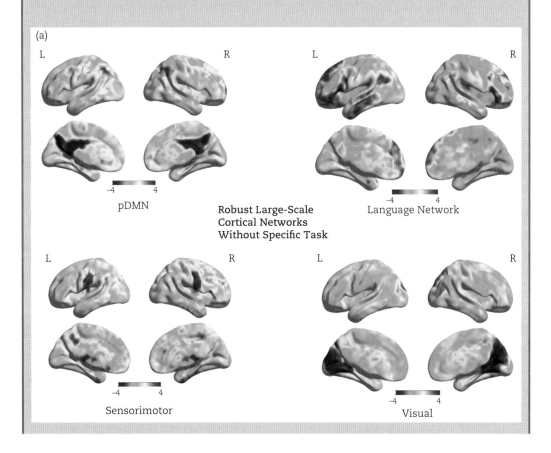

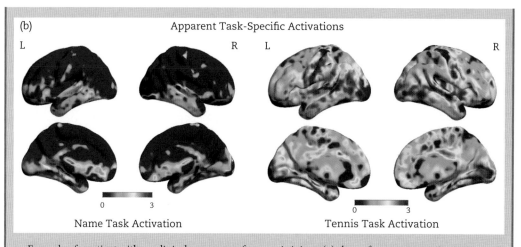

(b)   Apparent Task-Specific Activations

Name Task Activation   Tennis Task Activation

Example of a patient with no clinical awareness after anoxic injury. (a) shows four representative intrinsic connectivity networks identified via independent component analyses of the task-free, or resting state, fMRI. The images are displayed on a surface rendering of the brain. The color bars encode the strength of the positive (red) and negative (blue) synchrony, or connectivity, between the regions on each brain rendering. (b) shows the t-score (blue for low and red for high task activation) for each task. Both tasks have different activation patterns similar in a fully cognitively intact person doing the tennis task or passively listening to his or her name. The findings suggest internal and external awareness.

time-consuming toxicologic screening is performed. However, most poisons and illicit drugs do not cause significant laboratory derangements. In fact, if abnormalities are found in a comatose patient, they may be more representative of poor nutrition, dehydration, or a rapidly developing febrile illness.

Acid–base abnormalities, however, may point to certain toxins. A high anion gap acidosis is most common. The most prevalent toxins are shown in Table 12.8. Often, a high anion gap acidosis indicates ethylene glycol or methanol ingestion. Increased lactate, particularly when venous lactate can entirely account for a decrease in serum bicarbonate, may point to previous, often undetected, seizures, shock, and early sepsis.

The anion gap is calculated from the serum electrolytes. Normally, more cations (sodium and potassium) than anions (chloride and bicarbonate) are present, causing an anion gap of 11–13 mEq/L. Generally, potassium is deleted from the equation because its extracellular contribution in the anion gap is minimal; therefore, the equation becomes as follows: anion gap = $(Na^+ - [Cl^- + HCO_3^-])$. Increases in the anion gap result from the additional presence of an anion. Most of the time, it is lactate that increases in serum and creates an anion gap, often originating from poor tissue perfusion.

Salicylates usually produce a combined acid–base abnormality, and compensatory respiratory alkalosis is often also present. The partial pressure of carbon dioxide ($PaCO_2$) decrease in metabolic acidosis can be calculated ($PaCO_2 = [1.5 \times (HCO_3)] + 8 \pm 2$), and a lower $PaCO_2$ should point to additional respiratory alkalosis.

TABLE 12.8. BLOOD GAS ABNORMALITIES DUE TO TOXINS

Metabolic Acidosis (Anion Gap)	Respiratory Acidosis
Methanol	Barbiturates
Ethanol	Benzodiazepines
Paraldehyde	Botulism toxin
Isoniazid	Opioids
Salicylates	Strychnine
Metabolic Alkalosis	Tetrodotoxin
Diuretics	*Respiratory Alkalosis*
Nonketotic hyperglycemia	Salicylates
Lithium	Amphetamines
	Anticholinergics
	Cocaine
	Cyanide
	Paraldehyde
	Theophylline
	Carbon monoxide

Osmolar gap is a useful test to determine the accumulation of osmotically active solutes. The normal osmolar gap is calculated with the equation $2 \times$ Na (glucose/18) + (blood urea nitrogen/2.8). This calculated osmolality is less than the measured osmolarity (the so-called osmolar gap) and should be less than 10 mOsm/L. Alcohols of any kind increase the osmolar gap, and blood levels can be estimated by multiplying the osmolar gap with the molecular weight of the alcohol (46 for ethanol) and dividing the result by a factor of 10.

Urine testing for salicylates is important and can be done with a 10% ferric chloride solution, which turns urine purple if salicylates are present. Urine should be tested for ketones. Ketones in combination with a marked anion gap immediately suggest salicylate poisoning, but this combination can also be observed in alcohol- or diabetes-induced ketoacidosis. The absence of ketones in a patient with anion gap metabolic acidosis suggests the ingestion of methanol or ethylene glycol. Urinalysis is also important specifically in looking for calcium oxalate crystals associated with ethylene glycol (antifreeze) ingestion. The use of a Wood's lamp (if available) may be important because fluorescein is added to many antifreeze products.

Hospitals have laboratories that can provide drug screens, but their value often lies in the demonstration of the toxin rather than quantification.[52] The blood levels of many sedatives and alcohol correlate poorly with depth of coma, duration of mechanical ventilation, and time in the ICU. This lack of correlation applies particularly to patients who attempt suicide with a medication they have taken long enough to cause tolerance.

Many smaller hospitals use thin-layer chromatography, which is less reliable, operator-dependent, and unable to quantitate the toxin. Most academic centers can measure toxin levels with gas chromatography and mass spectrometry. This laboratory investigative tool is powerful and quantitates the toxin. Physicians assessing patients with poisoning and drug abuse should be well informed about the hospital laboratory methods available. Laboratory confirmation of the clinical diagnosis is often very desirable and may also serve a medicolegal purpose. Delay in the performance of these tests remains a major limitation, and, in daily practice, the information often becomes available too late to be useful in guiding treatment.

Blood tests that should be performed include a full hematologic screen and differential cell count, blood glucose, serum osmolality, liver function panel, electrolytes, and renal function tests (Table 12.9). Arterial blood gas measurements further assist in categorizing the major classes of acid–base imbalance, if present.

CLINCHING THE CAUSE OF COMA

With this armamentarium of knowledge, laboratory availability, and timely neuroimaging, a plan of action can be constructed. The following steps might be useful: (1) Categorize clinical findings (bihemispheric injury, lateral brainstem displacement, central brainstem displacement, and intrinsic brainstem injury); (2) study the interpretation of neuroimaging and, depending on findings of neuroimaging (diffuse injury, mass, hydrocephalus, or even normal findings), a more specific differential diagnosis follows. The algorithms needed are shown in Figures 12.9 and 12.10.

MANAGEMENT OF COMA IN THE FIRST HOUR

The initial management of a comatose patient is to correct abnormal vital signs and laboratory abnormalities. Detailed care is described in part VII, but some guidance may be helpful here.

First, improve oxygenation (face mask with 10-liter oxygen flow aiming at a pulse oximeter of more than 95%).

TABLE 12.9. LABORATORY TESTS IN THE EVALUATION OF COMA

Hematocrit, white blood cell count
Glucose
Electrolytes
Urea, creatinine
Aspartate transaminase (AST) and
    γ-glutamyltransferase (GGT)
Ammonia
Osmolality
Arterial blood gases (optional)
Platelets, smear, fibrinogen degradation products,
    international normalized ratio (optional)
Plasma thyrotropin (optional)
Blood and cerebrospinal fluid cultures (optional)
Toxic screen in blood and urine (optional)
Cerebrospinal fluid (protein, cells, glucose, India
    ink stain, and cryptococcal antigen, viral titers)
    (optional)

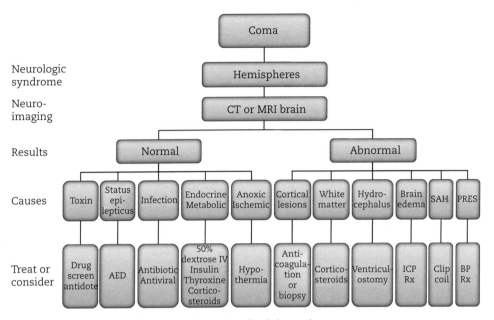

FIGURE 12.9: Algorithm to elucidate cause of coma based on bihemispheric signs.

AED, antiepileptic drugs; BP, blood pressure; CT, computed tomography; HEP, heparin; ICP, intracranial pressure; IV, intravenous; MRI, magnetic resonance imaging; PRES, posterior reversible encephalopathy syndrome; RX, treatment; SAH, subarachnoid hemorrhage; TBI, traumatic brain injury.

From Wijdicks EFM. *The Comatose Patient*. 2nd edition. New York: Oxford University Press, 2014.

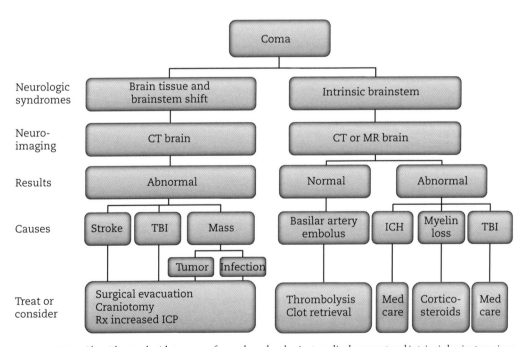

FIGURE 12.10: Algorithm to elucidate cause of coma based on brainstem displacement and intrinsic brainstem signs.

CT, computed tomography; ICH, intracranial hemorrhage; ICP, intracranial pressure; MR, magnetic resonance; TBI, traumatic brain injury.

From Wijdicks EFM. *The Comatose Patient*. 2nd edition. New York: Oxford University Press, 2014.

Second, intubate if patient cannot protect airway (increased work of breathing, pooling secretions, gurgling sounds). Intubate any comatose patient with irregular ineffective breathing drive and poor oxygenation, or consider emergency tracheostomy in any comatose patient with major facial injury.

Third, correct hypotension by placing patient in Trendelenburg and add crystalloids (rapid infusion of 500 cc normal saline followed by 100 cc/hour) and if no response, start vasopressors (use phenylephrine boluses of 100 microgram until central catheter is placed). Correct extreme hypertension (systolic above 250 mm Hg or MAP above 130 mm Hg) with intravenous labetalol 20 mg IV, hydralazine 20 mg IV, or nicardipine 5 mg IV.

Fourth, correct hypothermia with warming blankets. However, consider induced hypothermia (33–34°C) treatment in patients who have been successfully resuscitated for cardiac arrest (patients who had ventricular fibrillation or other shockable rhythms).[5] Correct hyperthermia with cooling blankets, icepacks, and ice water lavage.

Fifth, correct major metabolic derangements. No harm is done if a patient with a high likelihood of hypoglycemia is given 50 mL/50% glucose solution even before the blood sugar is known and is co-administered 100 mg thiamine IV. Treatment of severe hyponatremia involves hypertonic saline (3% hypertonic saline, 0.5 mg per kilogram hourly) or a vaptan. Treatment of hypercalcemia is by saline rehydration infusion, followed by parenteral bisphosphonate pamidronate.

Sixth, consider administering naloxone (0.4 to 2 mg every 3 minutes IV) if opioid intoxication is suspected, and consider administering flumazenil (slow IV administration at 0.2 mg per minute up to 1 mg) to reverse any benzodiazepine toxicity. The drug, however, is contraindicated in patients with a seizure disorder and in whom concomitant tricyclic antidepressant intoxication is suspected.

Seventh, consider elimination of the toxin by hemodialysis or hemoperfusion.

The next phase of management will be disease specific.

Management of Structural Lesions

In the ED, the first priorities when faced with a patient presenting with an acute structural cause of coma can be summarized in three steps:[14]

First, an attempt should be made to reduce presumed increased intracranial pressure (ICP).[56] Mass effect and clinical signs of brainstem injury (abnormal corneal, pupil, or oculocephalic reflexes) should prompt immediate

administration of osmotic agents. Mannitol is best suited to the ED. Hypertonic saline is likely a better osmotic drug, but it requires placement of a central venous catheter first, and valuable time may be lost by placing this catheter first. Mannitol is administered in an initial dose of 1–2 g/kg (often in two repeated doses, 30–45 minutes apart).[17,65] Placement of a ventriculostomy to reduce ICP may not be helpful because acute hydrocephalus is caused by obstruction of a mass and could increase tissue shift when the CSF counterpressure is released. Hyperventilation is a useful simple additional measure in intubated comatose patients, and through this method $PaCO_2$ can be lowered quickly to target levels ($PaCO_2$ of 25–30 mm Hg) (Tables 12.10 and 12.11).

Second, consider evacuation of the mass. The early evacuation of a mass (e.g., traumatic subdural, epidural, or lobar hematoma or contusion) is a definite early option and requires immediate assessment by a neurosurgeon. When performed within 6–12 hours of onset, the clinical improvement following evacuation of such a mass is often impressive.

Third, consider decompressive craniectomy.[1] Diffusely swollen brain may compress the deeper diencephalic structures or may move these

---

TABLE 12.10. MANAGEMENT OF ACUTE SUPRATENTORIAL MASS WITH BRAIN SHIFT

Stabilizing Measures
Intubation and mechanical ventilation
Correct hypoxemia with O_2 nasal catheter, 3–4 L/min, or face mask
Elevate head to 30 degrees
Treat extreme agitation with lorazepam, 2 mg IV, or propofol, 0.3 mg/kg/hr IV
Correct coagulopathy with fresh-frozen plasma, vitamin K (if applicable), PCC or factor VIIa

Specific Medical Measures
Hyperventilation: increase respiratory rate to 20 breaths/minute, aim at $PaCO_2$ of 25–30 mm Hg
Mannitol 20%, 1 g/kg; if no effect, 2 g/kg; aim at plasma osmolality of 310 mOsm/L
Dexamethasone, 100 mg intravenously (in tumors only)

Specific Surgical Measures
Evacuation of hematoma
Placement of drain in abscess
Decompressive craniectomy with brain swelling

$PaCO_2$, partial arterial pressure of CO_2; IV, intravenously; PCC, prothrombin complex concentrate.

TABLE 12.11. MANAGEMENT
OF ACUTE SUBTENTORIAL MASS OR
BRAINSTEM LESION

Stabilizing Measures
Intubation and mechanical ventilation
Correct hypoxemia with 3 L of O_2/min
Flat body position (in acute basilar artery occlusion)
Specific Medical Measures
Intra-arterial tPA (in basilar artery occlusion)
Mannitol 20%, 1 g/kg (in acute cerebellar mass)
Hyperventilation to $PaCO_2$ of 25–50 mm Hg (in
     acute cerebellar mass)
Specific Surgical Measures
Ventriculostomy
Suboccipital craniectomy

$PaCO_2$, partial arterial pressure of CO_2.

structures downward. Pressure relief can rarely be
accomplished with osmotic agents, and removal
of a large bone flap (or flaps) is the only remaining option to salvage the patient with diffuse
cerebral edema.

An acute hydrocephalus documented by the
presence of markedly ballooned ventricles should
be treated immediately by placing a ventriculostomy in the right frontal horn. Patients with
aneurysmal SAH and acute obstructive hydrocephalus may rapidly improve after ventriculostomy placement and CSF drainage. Placement of
a ventriculostomy may be precluded in patients
on anticoagulation or those with an acquired
coagulopathy. Prothrombin complex concentrate,
recombinant factor VIIa, or platelet transfusions
are needed before the drain is placed.

The clinical history may have provided important clues for a CNS infection. It is then appropriate to proceed with a CSF examination. When CSF
is suspicious for an infection, full antibiotic coverage with cefotaxime (2 g every 6 hours), vancomycin (20 mg/kg IV every 12 hours [goal trough level
at 15–20 mcg/mL]), and ampicillin (2 g IV every
4 hours), in combination with antiviral coverage
(acyclovir 10 mg/kg every 8 hours) is needed until
final results become available. A screening CT
scan is preferable when a patient with a suspicion
of bacterial meningitis presents in coma and, in
particular, when CT can be obtained in a matter of
minutes. However, empirical intravenous antibiotic therapy and dexamethasone (10 mg initially)
are administered before transfer to the CT scanner and, if cerebral edema is absent, this initial
treatment is then followed by lumbar puncture
(Chapter 3).

With the emergence of immunosuppression
(particularly in the human immunodeficiency
virus [HIV]–infected population), toxoplasma
encephalitis should be considered. Initial treatment remains empiric and includes pyrimethamine and sulfadiazine, particularly in patients
with multiple abscesses. In endemic areas, patients
in coma may have cysticercosis associated with
Taenia solium infestation, and immediate treatment with praziquantel is required. It is important
to start these treatments early, after consulting an
infectious disease specialist. The initial management in these acute inflammatory conditions of
the CNS is summarized in Table 12.12.

Management of Acute Metabolic Derangements and Intoxications

As alluded to earlier, with 50 mL of a 50% glucose
solution in a suspected hypoglycemic, immediate
awakening during infusion is highly indicative
of severe hypoglycemia. Failure to awaken after
hypoglycemia, however, may indicate that hypoglycemia has been lengthy and has caused significant brain damage, leading to prolonged or no
recovery.

Management of severe hyponatremia involves
hypertonic saline and furosemide (3% hypertonic saline, 0.5 mL/kg hourly) with frequent
serum sodium surveillance. Overcorrection (>
150 mmol/L) and rapid correction (within 12
hours) have been linked to the development of
central pontine myelinolysis.

Hypercalcemia is adequately corrected by
saline rehydration infusion (3–4 L), followed
by the parenteral bisphosphonate pamidronate
(infused at 60 mg over 24 hours).

TABLE 12.12. EMPIRICAL ANTIBIOTIC
AND ANTIVIRAL THERAPY
IN PATIENTS IN COMA ASSOCIATED
WITH INFLAMMATORY CONDITIONS

Antibacterial	Cefotaxime 2 g every 6 hours; Vancomycin 20 mg/kg IV every 12 hours for target trough level at 15–20 mcg/mL
Antiviral	Acyclovir 10 mg/kg every 8 hours
Antiparasitic	Pyrimethamine 50–75 mg per day orally
	Sulfadiazine 2–8 g orally divided every 6 hours
	Praziquantel 75 mg/kg/day orally in 3 divided doses

The use of a "coma cocktail" in assessing and managing a coma of undetermined cause must be questioned.[31] Usually, this cocktail consists of a combination of hypertonic dextrose, thiamine hydrochloride, naloxone hydrochloride, and, recently, flumazenil.[27] Its use must be discouraged simply because of the possible side effects of naloxone and flumazenil. Naloxone has great efficacy but also potentially serious side effects, such as aspiration from rapid arousal and development of a florid withdrawal syndrome characterized by agitation, diaphoresis, hypertension, dysrhythmias, and pulmonary edema.[55] In addition, after 30 minutes, the patient may again lapse into coma, which if unwitnessed may cause significant respiratory depression and respiratory arrest. A more prudent approach is to prophylactically intubate the patient and to gradually reverse the overdose of opiates by use of naloxone, 0.4–2 mg every 3 minutes by incremental doubling. At the first sign of relapse, 0.4–4 mg of naloxone can be given intravenously, or an infusion of 0.8 mg/hour (for 8–12 hours until recovery) can be started.[6,24,30] Failure to reverse coma from alleged opiate overdose has many causes, and they are summarized in Table 12.13.

Flumazenil reverses the effect of any benzodiazepine but has the same major disadvantages as naloxone: rapid arousal and risk of life-threatening aspiration pneumonitis. In addition, when high doses of flumazenil are administered, seizures may occur. Therefore, flumazenil is contraindicated in patients with a seizure disorder and in patients in whom concomitant tricyclic antidepressant intoxication is suspected. When flumazenil is administered, cardiac arrhythmias may occur, and status epilepticus has been reported in patients who had an overdose of tricyclic antidepressants and received treatment with flumazenil.[77] The recommended dose of flumazenil, by slow intravenous administration, is 0.2 mg/min up to a total dose of 1 mg. Benzodiazepine overdose, in general, is not life-threatening and can be managed by supportive care only.[51]

Inducing emesis in a patient who is stuporous from poisoning may be a mistake because of the significant danger of aspiration. Gastric lavage, which is possible if a comatose patient is protected by endotracheal intubation, should be done if the suspicion of a massive overdose is great.[9] Also, activated charcoal (60–100 g) can be delivered through the gastric tube. Placement of the tube in the stomach before administration of charcoal should be confirmed by radiography because charcoal deposition in the lung is often fatal. The technique of gastric lavage includes placement of the patient in the left lateral decubitus position after intubation of the trachea with a cuffed endotracheal tube. This position greatly facilitates drainage. The largest possible gastric tube should be inserted through the nose or mouth into the stomach and checked often with air insufflation while the physician listens over the stomach. The stomach aspirate should be investigated for possible toxins, and activated charcoal should be administered before lavage is started. Charcoal absorbs material that cannot be removed by active suctioning and that may enter the intestine. Lukewarm tap water or saline in 200 mL aliquots up to a total of 2 L is infused and aspirated until no pills or toxic materials are observed.

Elimination of the toxin can also be enhanced by hemodialysis and hemoperfusion, and many drugs and toxins can be cleared (the most common are acetaminophen, amitriptyline, lithium, and salicylates) using these methods.

CONCLUSIONS

- Neurologic examination followed by categorization in bihemispheric, brainstem displacement or intrinsic brainstem injury may be helpful in the focused assessment and evaluation of coma.
- Early stabilizing of the comatose patient may include intubation for airway protection, correction of hypotension and hypovolemia, and correction of acute metabolic derangements.
- Early recognition of increased ICP from mass effect or acute hydrocephalus is essential, and early medical and surgical intervention may reduce morbidity.
- Intoxications are common causes of coma in the ED, and drug screens are mandatory, followed by specific antidotes if indicated.

TABLE 12.13. DIFFERENTIAL DIAGNOSIS IN FAILURE TO REVERSE COMA FROM ALLEGED OPIATE OVERDOSE

Traumatic brain injury
Hypoglycemia
Anoxic–ischemic encephalopathy
Mixed overdose with drug in another category
 (e.g., cocaine, ethanol)
Central nervous system infection, systemic
 infection, sepsis
Seizures, nonconvulsive status epilepticus (rare)

REFERENCES

1. Aarabi B, Hesdorffer DC, Simard JM, et al. Comparative study of decompressive craniectomy after mass lesion evacuation in severe head injury. *Neurosurgery* 2009;64:927–939.

2. Auerbach PS. *Wilderness Medicine.* 6th ed. St. Louis: Mosby; 2011.

3. Barrueto F, Jr, Hack JB. Hyperammonemia and coma without hepatic dysfunction induced by valproate therapy. *Acad Emerg Med* 2001;8:999–1001.

4. Bauby J-D. *The Diving Bell and the Butterfly.* Translated from French by J Leggatt. New York: Alfred A. Knopf; 1997.

5. Bernard SA, Gray TW, Buist MD, et al. Treatment of comatose survivors of out-of-hospital cardiac arrest with induced hypothermia. *N Engl J Med* 2002;346:557–563.

6. Betten DP, Vohra RB, Cook MD, Matteucci MJ, Clark RF. Antidote use in the critically ill poisoned patient. *J Intensive Care Med* 2006;21:255–277.

7. Boehnert MT, Lovejoy FH, Jr. Value of the QRS duration versus the serum drug level in predicting seizures and ventricular arrhythmias after an acute overdose of tricyclic antidepressants. *N Engl J Med* 1985;313:474–479.

8. Bohan TP, Helton E, McDonald I, et al. Effect of L-carnitine treatment for valproate-induced hepatotoxicity. *Neurology* 2001;56:1405–1409.

9. Bond GR. The role of activated charcoal and gastric emptying in gastrointestinal decontamination: a state-of-the-art review. *Ann Emerg Med* 2002;39:273–286.

10. Brent J, McMartin K, Phillips S, Aaron C, Kulig K. Fomepizole for the treatment of methanol poisoning. *N Engl J Med* 2001;344:424–429.

11. Brust JCM. *Neurological Aspects of Substance Abuse.* 2nd ed. Boston: Butterworth-Heinemann; 2004.

12. Buckley NA, Isbister GK, Stokes B, Juurlink DN. Hyperbaric oxygen for carbon monoxide poisoning: a systematic review and critical analysis of the evidence. *Toxicol Rev* 2005;24:75–92.

13. Carella F, Grassi MP, Savoiardo M, et al. Dystonic-Parkinsonian syndrome after cyanide poisoning: clinical and MRI findings. *J Neurol Neurosurg Psychiatry* 1988;51:1345–1348.

14. Chesnut RM. Care of central nervous system injuries. *Surg Clin N Am* 2007;87:119–156, vii.

15. Choy-Kwong M, Lipton RB. Seizures in hospitalized cocaine users. *Neurology* 1989;39:425–427.

16. Dhuna A, Pascual-Leone A, Langendorf F, Anderson DC. Epileptogenic properties of cocaine in humans. *Neurotoxicology* 1991;12:621–626.

17. Diringer MN, Zazulia AR. Osmotic therapy: fact and fiction. *Neurocrit Care* 2004;1:219–233.

18. Dunn C, Held JL, Spitz J, et al. Coma blisters: report and review. *Cutis* 1990;45:423–426.

19. Edlow JA, Rabinstein A, Traub SJ, Wijdicks EFM. Diagnosis of reversible causes of coma. *Lancet* 2014;384:2064–2076.

20. Flanagan RJ, Mant TG. Coma and metabolic acidosis early in severe acute paracetamol poisoning. *Hum Toxicol* 1986;5:179–182.

21. Flomenbaum NE, Goldfrank LR, Hoffman RS, et al. *Goldfrank's Toxicologic Emergencies.* 8th ed. New York: McGraw Hill Professional; 2006.

22. Gawin FH, Ellinwood EH, Jr. Cocaine and other stimulants: actions, abuse, and treatment. *N Engl J Med* 1988;318:1173–1182.

23. Ginsberg MD. Carbon monoxide intoxication: clinical features, neuropathology and mechanisms of injury. *J Toxicol Clin Toxicol* 1985;23:281–288.

24. Goldfrank L, Weisman RS, Errick JK, Lo MW. A dosing nomogram for continuous infusion intravenous naloxone. *Ann Emerg Med* 1986;15:566–570.

25. Graudins A, Peden G, Dowsett RP. Massive overdose with controlled-release carbamazepine resulting in delayed peak serum concentrations and life-threatening toxicity. *Emerg Med* 2002;14:89–94.

26. Greenblatt DJ, Shader RI, Abernethy DR. Drug therapy: current status of benzodiazepines. *N Engl J Med* 1983;309:354–358.

27. Gueye PN, Hoffman JR, Taboulet P, Vicaut E, Baud FJ. Empiric use of flumazenil in comatose patients: limited applicability of criteria to define low risk. *Ann Emerg Med* 1996;27:730–735.

28. Henderson A, Wright M, Pond SM. Experience with 732 acute overdose patients admitted to an intensive care unit over six years. *Med J Aust* 1993;158:28–30.

29. Hill JB. Salicylate intoxication. *N Engl J Med* 1973;288:1110–1113.

30. Hoffman JR, Schriger DL, Luo JS. The empiric use of naloxone in patients with altered mental status: a reappraisal. *Ann Emerg Med* 1991;20:246–252.

31. Hoffman RS, Goldfrank LR. The poisoned patient with altered consciousness: controversies in the use of a "coma cocktail." *JAMA* 1995;274:562–569.

32. Iyer VN, Mandrekar JN, Danielson RD, et al. Validity of the FOUR score coma scale in the medical intensive care unit. *Mayo Clinic Proc* 2009;84:694–701.

33. Jaffery JB, Aggarwal A, Ades PA, Weise WJ. A long sweet sleep with sour consequences. *Lancet* 2001;358:1236.

34. Kondziella D, Danielsen ER, Hansen K, et al. 1H MR spectroscopy of gray and white

matter in carbon monoxide poisoning. *J Neurol* 2009;256:970–979.

35. Krantz T, Thisted B, Strom J, Sorensen MB. Acute carbon monoxide poisoning. *Acta Anaesthesiol Scand* 1988;32:278–282.

36. Kwon SU, Lee SH, Kim JS. Sudden coma from acute bilateral internal carotid artery territory infarction. *Neurology* 2002;58:1846–1849.

37. Leao M. Valproate as a cause of hyperammonemia in heterozygotes with ornithine-transcarbamylase deficiency. *Neurology* 1995;45:593–594.

38. Levine SR, Brust JC, Futrell N, et al. Cerebrovascular complications of the use of the "crack" form of alkaloidal cocaine. *N Engl J Med* 1990;323:699–704.

39. Losek JD, Rock AL, Boldt RR. Cyanide poisoning from a cosmetic nail remover. *Pediatrics* 1991;88:337–340.

40. Lowenstein DH, Massa SM, Rowbotham MC, et al. Acute neurologic and psychiatric complications associated with cocaine abuse. *Am J Med* 1987;83:841–846.

41. Maguiness S, Guenther L, Shum D. Coma blisters, peripheral neuropathy, and amitriptyline overdose: a brief report. *J Cutan Med Surg* 2002;6:438–441.

42. Mason PJ, Morris VA, Balcezak TJ. Serotonin syndrome. Presentation of 2 cases and review of the literature. *Medicine (Baltimore)* 2000;79:201–209.

43. McCarron MM. Phencyclidine intoxication. *NIDA Res Monogr* 1986;64:209–217.

44. McKenzie MS, McFarland BH. Trends in antidepressant overdoses. *Pharmacoepidemiol Drug Saf* 2007;16:513–523.

45. Megarbane B, Borron SW, Baud FJ. Current recommendations for treatment of severe toxic alcohol poisonings. *Intensive Care Med* 2005;31:189–195.

46. Miura T, Mitomo M, Kawai R, Harada K. CT of the brain in acute carbon monoxide intoxication: characteristic features and prognosis. *AJNR Am J Neuroradiol* 1985;6:739–742.

47. Moore SA, Wijdicks EFM. The acutely comatose patient: clinical approach and diagnosis. *Semin Neurol* 2013;33:110–120.

48. Morgan BW, Ford MD, Follmer R. Ethylene glycol ingestion resulting in brainstem and midbrain dysfunction. *J Toxicol Clin Toxicol* 2000;38:445–451.

49. Mutlu GM, Leikin JB, Oh K, Factor P. An unresponsive biochemistry professor in the bathtub. *Chest* 2002;122:1073–1076.

50. Navarro VJ, Senior JR. Drug-related hepatotoxicity. *N Engl J Med* 2006;354:731–739.

51. Ngo AS, Anthony CR, Samuel M, Wong E, Ponampalam R. Should a benzodiazepine antagonist be used in unconscious patients presenting to the emergency department? *Resuscitation* 2007;74:27–37.

52. Nice A, Leikin JB, Maturen A, et al. Toxidrome recognition to improve efficiency of emergency urine drug screens. *Ann Emerg Med* 1988;17:676–680.

53. Palmer BF. Effectiveness of hemodialysis in the extracorporeal therapy of phenobarbital overdose. *Am J Kidney Dis* 2000;36:640–643.

54. Posner JB, Saper CB, Schiff N, Plum F. *Plum and Posner's Diagnosis of Stupor and Coma.* Vol 71. 4th ed. Oxford: Oxford University Press; 2007.

55. Prough DS, Roy R, Bumgarner J, Shannon G. Acute pulmonary edema in healthy teenagers following conservative doses of intravenous naloxone. *Anesthesiology* 1984;60:485–486.

56. Rabinstein AA, Wijdicks EFM. Coma, raised intracranial pressure and hydrocephalus. In: Warlow CP, ed. *The Lancet Handbook of Treatment in Neurology*. London: Elsevier Limited; 2006: 179–200.

57. Reed CE, Driggs MF, Foote CC. Acute barbiturate intoxication: a study of 300 cases based on a physiologic system of classification of the severity of the intoxication. *Ann Intern Med* 1952;37 :290–303.

58. Rosenberg NL, Myers JA, Martin WR. Cyanide-induced parkinsonism: clinical, MRI, and 6-fluorodopa PET studies. *Neurology* 1989;39: 142–144.

59. Rowley G, Fielding K. Reliability and accuracy of the Glasgow Coma Scale with experienced and inexperienced users. *Lancet* 1991;337:535–538.

60. Rubin M, Safdieh J. *Netter's Concise Neuroanatomy*. Philadelphia: Elsevier Health Sciences; 2007.

61. Rubinstein D, Escott E, Kelly JP. Methanol intoxication with putaminal and white matter necrosis: MR and CT findings. *AJNR Am J Neuroradiol* 1995;16:1492–1494.

62. Sansone ME, Ziegler DK. Lithium toxicity: a review of neurologic complications. *Clin Neuropharmacol* 1985;8:242–248.

63. Schiodt FV, Ott P, Christensen E, Bondesen S. The value of plasma acetaminophen half-life in antidote-treated acetaminophen overdosage. *Clin Pharmacol Ther* 2002;71:221–225.

64. Schmidt S, Schmitz-Buhl M. Signs and symptoms of carbamazepine overdose. *J Neurol* 1995;242:169–173.

65. Schrot RJ, Muizelaar JP. Mannitol in acute traumatic brain injury. *Lancet* 2002;359:1633–1634.

66. Schwarz S, Georgiadis D, Schwab S, et al. Fulminant progression of hyperammonaemic encephalopathy after treatment with valproate

in a patient with ureterosigmoidostomy. *J Neurol Neurosurg Psychiatry* 2002;73:90–91.

67. Spiller HA, Krenzelok EP, Cookson E. Carbamazepine overdose: a prospective study of serum levels and toxicity. *J Toxicol Clin Toxicol* 1990;28:445–458.

68. Stead LG, Wijdicks EFM, Bhagra A, et al. Validation of a new coma scale, the FOUR score, in the emergency department. *Neurocrit Care* 2009;10:50–54.

69. Storen EC, Wijdicks EFM, Crum BA, Schultz G. Moyamoya-like vasculopathy from cocaine dependency. *AJNR Am J Neuroradiol* 2000;21: 1008–1010.

70. Teasdale G, Jennett B. Assessment of coma and impaired consciousness: a practical scale. *Lancet* 1974;2:81–84.

71. Teasdale G, Knill-Jones R, van der Sande J. Observer variability in assessing impaired consciousness and coma. *J Neurol Neurosurg Psychiatry* 1978;41:603–610.

72. Tsokos M, Sperhake JP. Coma blisters in a case of fatal theophylline intoxication. *Am J Forensic Med Pathol* 2002;23:292–294.

73. Vale JA, Proudfoot AT. Paracetamol (acetaminophen) poisoning. *Lancet* 1995;346:547–552.

74. Vannemreddy P, Caldito G, Willis B, Nanda A. Influence of cocaine on ruptured intracranial aneurysms: a case control study of poor prognostic indicators. *J Neurosurg* 2008;108:470–476.

75. Vogel SN, Sultan TR, Ten Eyck RP. Cyanide poisoning. *Clin Toxicol* 1981;18:367–383.

76. Weaver LK, Hopkins RO, Chan KJ, et al. Hyperbaric oxygen for acute carbon monoxide poisoning. *N Engl J Med* 2002;347:1057–1067.

77. Weinbroum A, Rudick V, Sorkine P, et al. Use of flumazenil in the treatment of drug overdose: a double-blind and open clinical study in 110 patients. *Crit Care Med* 1996;24:199–206.

78. White A. Overdose of tricyclic antidepressants associated with absent brain-stem reflexes. *CMAJ* 1988;139:133–134.

79. Wijdicks EFM. The bare essentials: coma. *Practical Neurology* 2010;10:51–60.

80. Wijdicks EFM. Clinical scales for comatose patients: the Glasgow Coma Scale in historical context and the new FOUR Score. *Rev Neurol Dis* 2006;3:109–117.

81. Wijdicks EFM. The diagnosis of brain death. *N Engl J Med* 2001;344:1215–1221.

82. Wijdicks EFM. Temporomandibular joint compression in coma. *Neurology* 1996;46:1774.

83. Wijdicks EFM, Bamlet WR, Maramattom BV, Manno EM, McClelland RL. Validation of a new coma scale: the FOUR score. *Ann Neurol* 2005;58:585–593.

84. Wijdicks EFM, Kramer AA, Rohs T, Jr., et al. Comparison of the Full Outline of UnResponsiveness Score and the Glasgow Coma Scale in predicting mortality in critically ill patients. *Crit Care Med* 2015;43:439–444.

85. Wijdicks EFM, Miller GM. Transient locked-in syndrome after uncal herniation. *Neurology* 1999;52:1296–1297.

86. Wijdicks EFM, Parisi JE, Sharbrough FW. Prognostic value of myoclonus status in comatose survivors of cardiac arrest. *Ann Neurol* 1994;35:239–243.

87. Wijdicks EFM, Rabinstein AA, Bamlet WR, Mandrekar JN. FOUR score and Glasgow Coma Scale in predicting outcome of comatose patients: a pooled analysis. *Neurology* 2011;77: 84–85.

88. Wijdicks EFM, Schievink WI. Neurological picture: coma nails. *J Neurol Neurosurg Psychiatry* 1997;63:294.

89. Wijdicks EFM. *The Comatose Patient*. 2nd ed. New York: Oxford University Press; 2014.

90. Wolf CA, Wijdicks EFM, Bamlet WR, McClelland RL. Further validation of the FOUR score coma scale by intensive care nurses. *Mayo Clinic Proc* 2007;82:435–438.

91. Young GB. Coma. *Ann N Y Acad Sci* 2009;1157:32–47.

PART IV

Organization of the Neurosciences Intensive Care Unit

13

The Responsibilities of the Neurointensivist

The essence of critical care neurology lies in acute decision-making and the management of emergent neurologic conditions. New skill sets and support structures are necessary to practice neurologic and neurosurgical intensive care. Anyone setting up a clinical program soon discovers that what is needed is a team: driven and primed physicians who also understand the distinctive features of neurologic critical illness, appreciate the presence of a neurointensivist service and a specialized neurosciences intensive care unit (NICU), and willingly support it. Neurologic critical care is an appealing subspecialty of neurology and a field with status. There are enough days filled with a sense of accomplishments gained from patients recovering with intact or nondisabling neurologic function. The rewards are not simply personal or professional gratification, but the knowledge that a specialized service for the management of neurologic critical illness ultimately benefits patients.[24]

The responsibilities of the neurointensivist are substantial. They involve aspects of acute neurologic care, major elements of medical care, close communication with family members, and joint effort with multiple disciplines, particularly neurosurgery. A major task of the neurointensivist is therefore to orchestrate a cohesive policy of assessment and management, and to prevent fractionation of care. Threats to some of these principles include limited resources and capacity, nursing staff shortage, and excessive expense.

There is an increasing number of NICU beds and an increasing proportion of NICU care in the United States and elsewhere. To put it in perspective, regional differences in general ICU care are substantial. In the United States, physician workforce issues remain—manpower is improving, but about a decade ago, approximately 50% of all ICUs had no intensivists. Some have asserted that the "workforce crisis" in the United States is an "artifact of overestimated demand"[7] and that minimizing unclear benefit and improvement of quality is a better way forward.

Most academically affiliated medical centers have some area of critical care dedicated to neurologic and neurosurgical patients,[13,25] and increasing numbers of neurointensivists are practicing in the United States, Europe, and elsewhere. The field of pediatric neurocritical care is growing within the United States, and some institutions have pediatric neurocritical care consulting services.[14]

This chapter highlights some of the challenges facing those eager to start a new neurointensive care program, and discusses the duties and obligations that affect the practicing neurointensivist.

LEGITIMACY

Generally, neurointensivists are often neurologists with formal training in to practice neurologic intensive care. Some have argued that neurocritical care does not necessarily require a neurologic or neurosurgical background, and such is immediately debatable and worrisome to many of us. However successful programs proved otherwise and over the coming years neurointensivists representing the officialdom may have diverse backgrounds. Fellowship programs are available throughout the United States and in several countries in Europe.[11,12] Neurointensivists have a supportive society (Capsule 13.1).

Complex preconceptions may remain, and beginning neurointensivists find themselves the target of a seemingly endless argument. Critical care physicians may be quick to point out that neurointensivists are not board certified in critical care medicine, do not understand the complexities of the ventilator, and cannot take care of "really sick" patients (known as the "neurocritical care lite" argument). Some medical or surgical intensivists with many years of experience in taking care of critically ill neurologic patients consider it an assault on their autonomy and even prestige (the "turf" argument). Neurosurgeons may argue that neurosurgical emergencies should not be managed by neurologists and perhaps feel justly threatened by losing responsibility after many hours in the operating room. Moreover,

CAPSULE 13.1   THE NEUROCRITICAL CARE SOCIETY

Emerging from an area of interest in neurology, critical care neurology has profiled itself as a full subspecialty. Founded in 2004, the Neurocritical Care Society (NCS) has grown rapidly. As stated, NCS is "a multidisciplinary, international organization whose mission is to improve outcomes for patients with life-threatening neurological illness" (www.neurocriticalcare.org).

The Neurocritical Care Society provides education and training, and promotes its practice. The Leapfrog Group (representing many of the largest US corporations and public agencies that buy health benefits on behalf of their clients) has recognized neurologists and neurosurgeons as intensivists.

The United Council of Neurologic Specialties has worked with the NCS to accredit fellowships and a neurocritical care certification examination.[11,12] Core curricula, with training requirement and procedural competency, have been developed. In the United States, multiple NICUs are led by fellowship-trained neurologists and other physicians.

The Neurocritical Care Society promises a new period in the care of critically ill neurologic patients, and neurointensivists are its most articulate voices. The Neurocritical Care Society is premised on all-inclusiveness rather than orthodoxy, on multidisciplinary cooperation rather than predominance of one specialty, on progress rather than maintaining status quo. The Neurocritical Care Society has grown not only in its membership but also has produced an academic journal, educational material (ENLS and NCS on demand), and guidelines for treatment.[9,20]

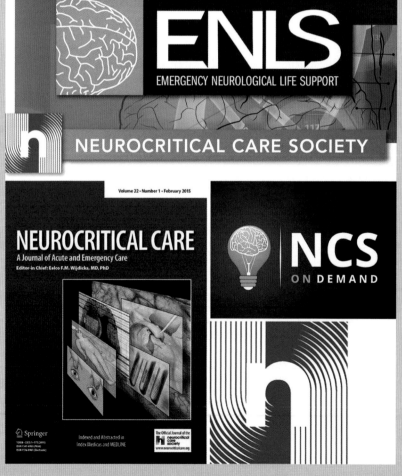

Neurocritical Care Society Educational Programs.

perioperative care is a core requirement for the training of neurosurgery residents and fellows (the "educational" argument). Other subspecialists with overlapping interests may be even more disdainful, believing that neurointensivists are too aggressive and too self-assured, and that a fundamental paradigm shift is not justified.[23] All these arguments on what might be the principal terrain may be superficially understandable—yet they do not help in finding the best patient-care options.

However, as the first part of this book shows, neurological critical care is complex and requires the ability to decide quickly and frequently. The neurointensivist must have training in neurosurgical issues, appreciate the impact of cardiopulmonary changes on central nervous system function, understand secondary deterioration in major catastrophes, integrate systemic illness with neurologic illness, fully manage acute disorders of the nervous system, and also possess core skills in the interpretation of neuroimaging and critical care (Table 13.1). To compare neurologic intensive care with medical or surgical intensive care is to compare incommensurables with the same ruler. Neurointensivists must rise to this challenge, fostering collaborative relationships, convincing skeptics of their complementary expertise, sharing clinical responsibility, and creating opportunities for mutual research. Many NICUs have a shared directorship with neurosurgery, and provide a visible role for consultants from other specialities, such as the critical care infectious disease service. Within such an environment of trust, patient care and education should improve tremendously.

Neurointensivists should try to find the best model in their institution, comply with the requirements of the Joint Commission, and negotiate management strategies. The impact of neurointensivists will remain difficult to prove, and current studies comparing the outcome of patients in two different management trajectories, with or without a neurointensivist, are far from definitive. Prospective studies could potentially demonstrate reduced mortality, shortened stays in the NICU, shorter duration of mechanical ventilation, fewer consultations, reduction in both readmissions to the NICU and inappropriate early dismissals, and, eventually, reduced NICU costs.

MORALE

Critical care neurology deals with human beings and their frailties. It demands professionalism. Neurointensivists must make the care of patients their primary concern and communication with family their next most important concern. Neurointensivists should accept any patient in need of intensive care, without allowing personal beliefs to prejudice the provision of care.

Many physicians describe neurology and neurointensive care as miserabilist. A mixture of feelings and experiences, motivators and discouragements, accompanies any physician faced with acute neurologic disease, but the overriding attitude of the ICU physician must be one of patience and resolve. Hubristic behavior must be recognized and avoided.[15] Some uniformity of thought and habit creates a mindset we could aspire to (Figure 13.1).

A new neurointensivist will have to develop credibility and respect, and this level of performance comes at considerable personal cost. In many institutions, intensive care is a comparatively

---

TABLE 13.1. THE NEUROINTENSIVIST

Is trained in medical management of critically ill
    patients with neurologic or neurosurgical disease
Implements collaborative practices
Has clinical credibility
Makes daily rounds
Develops quality projects and novel research
Spends 30%–50% of professional time in practice

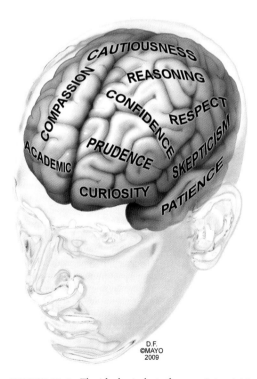

FIGURE 13.1: The ideal mindset of a neurointensivist.

impecunious profession, and this fact may also add to professional frustration.

The NICU invites a psychologic phenomenon called *burnout* among staff, brought about by overwork and lack of downtime. Burnout describes the physical and emotional exhaustion typified by negative self-concept, negative job attitude, and a loss of concern and feeling for patients. Most worrisome for many is a feeling of "being on autopilot" and "just going through the motions."[3,4,8,10,17,22] Other signs of burnout are a run-down feeling, disillusionment, sarcasm and rigidity, and fading enthusiasm. Burnout may largely depend on the individual, but common triggers for burnout are routine in the NICU: physicians are often on call 24 hours a day, 7 days a week; they face high patient mortality rates[19,24] and, more significantly, high rates of damaging morbidity in patients. They are familiar with overwhelming tragedies and constant exposure to grieving families. They often suffer sleep deprivation, and are at times called upon to resolve conflicts between physicians and nursing staff.[16] Maladaptive coping to these stressors may be recognized as loss of humor, displacement of anger, frustration, cynicism, depression, and anxiety, which may lead to use of excessive alcohol and tranquilizer use. Often, neurointensivists have more "nightly neurochecks" than patients, and if not already in house, may be awakened hourly by phone calls and pages at night.

There is a 10% lifetime prevalence for depression in male physicians and a 20% lifetime prevalence for female physicians; rates of suicide are higher among physicians than in the general population. Marital problems, indecision, diminished ability to think or concentrate, diminished interest in work, and depressed mood are strong indicators of clinical depression. Very few studies of depression in ICU physicians are available, but one study in pediatric critical care medicine (comparable to neurologic intensive care because of frequent family interaction and sudden loss) found 50% of physicians at risk.[3] A study in Australia suggested a possible link between excessive workload and mortality in the intensive care unit.[19]

Protection against these stressors may include regular exercise to improve fitness and health, restriction to 1-week shifts, a total of at least three rotating attending neurointensivists, no outpatient responsibilities, few administrative meetings, protected downtime, academic opportunities, and time to write and to have enough fun outside the daily grind.

Finally, because neurologic critical care is a modern and evolving field, there is a great deal of enthusiasm for testing new technologies. Collaborative relationships with the industry can greatly enhance the careers of clinician-scientists, and could result in important innovations.[21] At this intersection of technology and medicine, ethical pitfalls abound: business considers profitability a major objective, and the pressures on the clinician to bias or exaggerate results in the interests of the industry are great. Complicating matters even more, financial inducements are common and could undermine the integrity of professional judgment.[5] The American College of Physicians has published a proposal for controlling these conflict-of-interest issues.[1,2,18]

PROCEDURES

The picture of a scrubs-clad, sneaker-wearing, do-it-all physician swarming around the bedside, putting in central lines, performing emergency tracheostomies and even inserting ventricle and lumbar drain catheters may prove irresistible to some personalities, but this approach may backfire if the neurointensivist tries to usurp turf previously held by trained surgeons and neurosurgeons. In some institutions, the scarcity of specialty care or interdisciplinary cooperation may prompt such a multitasking approach, but in tertiary centers, responsibilities are more clearly defined. As an example, anyone who has seen a neurosurgery resident place a ventriculostomy may think it is easy, and some neurointensivists (and interventional neuroradiologists) may attempt to place ventriculostomies. This is neurosurgery territory, however, and a difficult one to enter—one accompanied by a number of questions, such as who will deal with any complications that arise, and how proficiency will be maintained.

High proficiency sets a tone and a standard, but there is always a job to be done. Many procedures performed in the ICU are now fully trainable in simulation centers—in growing numbers in major US institutions—and many hospitals may feel the need sooner or later. Simulation centers allow the re-creation of an ICU setting and may teach elective or urgent procedures. The placement of intravascular catheters, bronchoscopy, and punctures, including lumbar drain placement, can be taught. Failure to perform a procedure can be remediated, and such an option is appreciated. Critical care neurology is ideally suited for this approach because situations are uncommon and therefore difficult to master (Capsule 13.2).

Currently, procedures do not define the field of neurointensive care, because none of them is specific to the specialty. Finding new procedures that help us monitor the brain and get the data we

CAPSULE 13.2   SIMULATION TRAINING

Simulation-based training has been developed by procedure-based specialties, including surgical, critical care, anesthesia, and emergency medicine, but is increasingly used in nonprocedural specialties during training. Simulation usually involves common clinical situations (such as "running a code" or management of a multi-trauma patient). Simulation of acute neurology or more complex management of neurocritical care is in its infancy. Simulation of acute neurology is particularly well suited for instruction in communication because these conditions are challenging for both neurologists and non- neurologists.[6] There are many conditions that can be written into a scenario, and each may focus on the common pitfalls. Learners may err in a safe environment where feedback can be provided on the spot, enhancing the learning process. This is one of the reasons that these specialties have widely adopted simulation as a method of education. Acute neurology in general, and the determination of brain death in particular, is similar to these specialties, as there is no margin for error. Trained actors may function as patient family members, the registered nurse, attending physician, or respiratory therapist, depending on the design of the scenario. A manikin functions as the patient (see Capsule Figure). Mistakes can be made without harm, and remediation can take place after feedback is provided in order to enhance the learner's confidence. This model may be more effective than the didactic and verbal or written testing model.

(a) (b)

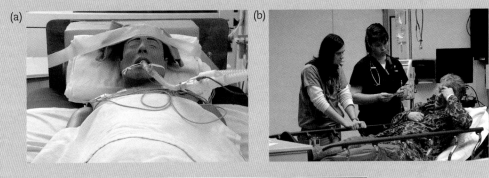

(c)

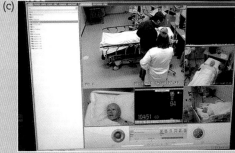

a. A manikin is able to mimic acute medical conditions and some neurologic conditions. b) Actors can be used to provide important history of acute onset of symptoms(e.g thunderclap headache) and mimick signs c) Video recording allows review of learner performance during debriefing.

need to address the questions is a future task for neurointensivists[9] (Chapters 23 and 25).

COMPETENCIES

In the end, the practicing critical care neurology unit concentrates on several major principles, which are summarized in Table 13.2.[25] Many health care workers—having seen critical care neurology in action—will successfully argue that the delivery of care by a neurointensivist is an absolute requirement with an undisputed value for the patient. We must move past the idea that these patients can be managed by generalists, and the only way to achieve this is through integrated care. A well-run neurocritical care program should have several neurointensivists with one physically present at all times. The neurointensivist combines contributions from neuroscience nursing staff, physical therapists, and pharmacists, among many other health professionals. Major neurologic problems occur in many hospital locations, and neurointensivists are also in a good position to expand their role outside the NICU.[24]

It is important to get the little things right—neurocritical care is as much about meticulous systemic physiological optimization as about specific brain-directed therapies. Patients are stable until they are not, and acute brain injury is worsened by ongoing insults. Acute neurosurgical intervention (decompressive craniectomy or mass evacuation) can salvage a patient who rapidly deteriorates from brain tissue shift and brainstem displacement. Organs may fail from a sympathetic surge that can cause neurogenic pulmonary edema, stress cardiomyopathy, gastric erosions, and a more general endocrinopathy.

TABLE 13.2. THE PRACTICE OF NEUROCRITICAL CARE

Create a Core Group

Built a collaborative practice

Minimize secondary brain injury

Recognize the importance of deterioration

Interpret neuroimaging and neuromonitoring

Consult with Neurosurgery and Interventional Neuroradiology

Appreciate the importance of systemic complications

Identify neuroemergencies elsewhere

Look at the quality of survival, not just survival

Connect with the family of the patient

The basic tenet is to treat acute problems as aggressively as possible, since minimizing second insults will minimize residual disability. However, we all expect some proportionality in care and a focus on quality of life. Communication with family members about these matters is a crucial and time-consuming role of the neurointensivist (Chapter 15). It is our responsibility to decidedly convey the clinical picture and what to expect.

ROUNDS

Initial daily rounds are needed to integrate findings at the bedside with laboratory test results, current therapies, and technologic support into a "plan for the day." Intermittent visits to the bedside are frequent, but care is facilitated if responsible team members meet in the morning and late afternoon. Morning rounds may include the respiratory therapist and pharmacist, but the charge nurse, responsible assigned nurse, senior resident, fellow, and consultant should be present. The attending physician is briefed by the residents or fellow. After a detailed overview of the neurologic condition is provided, other specific problems are discussed. These include careful review of systems (cardiac, pulmonary, gastrointestinal, bladder, skin), intercurrent infections, prophylactic medication, and recent institution of drugs. Rates of adverse drug events may be substantially lower when the pharmacist participates. The necessity of catheters (arterial line, central venous catheter, nasogastric tube, ventriculostomy) should be addressed. Neuroimaging studies should be reviewed and, when appropriate, compared.

Major emphasis is placed on causes of deterioration, which require discussion. Monitoring orders that trigger calls to the resident or consultant when a patient's conditions change should be written and the rationale should be explained. Overt laboratory abnormalities are important, but trends also need attention and management. The results of recent discussions with the patient or family members should be communicated. A plan of management should be clear before the next patient is approached. A rounding tool is shown in Table 13.3.

Morning rounds are a fertile ground for teaching and for channeling certain ideas for research to interested residents or fellows. The late afternoon round can be truncated and should typically involve follow-up of earlier plans and reiteration of potential nighttime problems. It is ill advised to use afternoon rounds to discharge or transfer patients, but patients can be identified when such a need arises. Sufficient observation requires at least 24 hours, and transfer of patients from 6 P.M. to 6 A.M. is not good practice. Early communication

---

TABLE 13.3. NEUROSCIENCES INTENSIVE CARE ROUNDING TOOL

General Section
Sedatives and pain control?
- Need to continue?
- Adjustments in dose?

ICP/CPP and hemodynamic goals reviewed?
Antiepileptic medications being given?
- Truly indicated?
- Levels reviewed?

EVD or LD present?
- Should it be kept?
- Should level of drainage be weaned?

EEG monitoring?
- Need to continue?

Need for additional neuroimaging?
Reviewed code status?
Intensive care or progressive care unit status?
Level of activity?
Discharge timing reviewed?
Communication with family or proxy adequate and detailed?

Respiratory Section
Patient on a ventilator
- Head of bed > 30 degrees?
- Chest radiograph reviewed?
- Low tidal volume strategy implemented?
- Ready to wean?

Patient not on a ventilator
- Respiratory care, incentive spirometry?

Cardiovascular Section
Need for cardiac drugs?
Need for vasopressors?
Blood pressure parameters adequate?

Infectious Disease Section
Current antibiotics necessary?
Cultures reviewed?

Gastrointestinal Section
Bowel function normal?
Stress ulcer prophylaxis?

Fluids, Electrolytes, Nutrition Section
Fluid balance and electrolytes reviewed?
Glucose control protocol initiated?
Nutrition adequate?

Prophylaxis Section
DVT prophylaxis?
GI prophylaxis?

Skin Section
Skin issues?
Need for clinical nurse specialist?

Medication Section
Medication reconciled with pharmacy?

Access Section
Intravascular catheters?
Indications and necessity of each have been reviewed?

CPP, cerebral perfusion pressure; DVT, deep vein thrombosis; EEG, electroencephalography; LD, lumbar drain; EVD, external ventricular drain; GI, gastrointestinal; ICP, intracranial pressure.

with the neurosurgical resident or staff is important and may prevent conflicting opinions when triage is needed to accommodate a new patient in greater need of critical care.

CONCLUSIONS

- Neurointensive care is practiced by neurointensivists who manage critically ill patients with acute neurologic disease.
- Neurointensivists have major daily responsibilities and are deciders.
- There are defined core competencies for neurointensivists.
- Daily rounds are best standardized to address specific problems.

REFERENCES

1. Coyle SL. Physician-industry relations: part 1: individual physicians. *Ann Intern Med* 2002;136:396–402.
2. Coyle SL. Physician-industry relations: part 2: organizational issues. *Ann Intern Med* 2002;136:403–406.
3. Embriaco N, Azoulay E, Barrau K, et al. High level of burnout in intensivists: prevalence and associated factors. *Am J Respir Crit Care Med* 2007;175:686–692.
4. Fields AI, Cuerdon TT, Brasseux CO, et al. Physician burnout in pediatric critical care medicine. *Crit Care Med* 1995;23:1425–1429.
5. Hauser SL, Johnston SC. Scripts for science: a new wrinkle on academic ties with industry. *Ann Neurol* 2008;64:A13–15.
6. Hocker S, Wijdicks EFM. The major opportunities in simulation of acute neurology. *Ann Neurol* 2015;78:337–342.
7. Kahn JM, Rubenfeld GD. The myth of the workforce crisis: why the United States does not need more intensivist physicians. *Am J Respir Crit Care Med* 2015;191:128–134.
8. Keidel GC. Burnout and compassion fatigue among hospice caregivers. *Am J Hosp Palliat Care* 2002;19:200–205.

9. Le Roux P, Menon DK, Citerio G, et al. Consensus Summary Statement of the International Multidisciplinary Consensus Conference on Multi-modality Monitoring in Neurocritical Care: a statement for healthcare professionals from the Neurocritical Care Society and the European Society of Intensive Care Medicine. *Neurocrit Care* 2014;21 Suppl 2: S297–S361.

10. Lederer W, Kinzl JF, Traweger C, Dosch J, Sumann G. Fully developed burnout and burnout risk in intensive care personnel at a university hospital. *Anaesth Intensive Care* 2008;36:208–213.

11. Mayer SA, Coplin WM, Chang C, et al. Core curriculum and competencies for advanced training in neurological intensive care: United Council for Neurologic Subspecialties guidelines. *Neurocrit Care* 2006;5:159–165.

12. Mayer SA, Coplin WM, Chang C, et al. Program requirements for fellowship training in neurological intensive care: United Council for Neurologic Subspecialties guidelines. *Neurocrit Care* 2006;5:166–171.

13. Medicine GCSoCC. Guidelines for the definition of an intensivist and the practice of critical care medicine. *Crit Care Med* 1992;20:540–542.

14. Murphy SA, Bell MJ, Clark ME, Whalen MJ, Noviski N. Pediatric neurocritical care: a short survey of current perceptions and practices. *Neurocrit Care* 2015;23:149–158.

15. Owen D, Davidson J. Hubris syndrome: an acquired personality disorder? A study of US presidents and UK prime ministers over the last 100 years. *Brain* 2009;132:1396–1406.

16. Piquette D, Reeves S, LeBlanc VR. Stressful intensive care unit medical crises: how individual responses impact on team performance. *Crit Care Med* 2009;37:1251–1255.

17. Poncet MC, Toullic P, Papazian L, et al. Burnout syndrome in critical care nursing staff. *Am J Respir Crit Care Med* 2007;175:698–704.

18. Rothman DJ, McDonald WJ, Berkowitz CD, et al. Professional medical associations and their relationships with industry: a proposal for controlling conflict of interest. *JAMA* 2009;301:1367–1372.

19. Tarnow-Mordi WO, Hau C, Warden A, Shearer AJ. Hospital mortality in relation to staff work-load: a 4-year study in an adult intensive-care unit. *Lancet* 2000;356:185–189.

20. Torbey MT, Bosel J, Rhoney DH, et al. Evidence-based guidelines for the management of large hemispheric infarction: a statement for health care professionals from the Neurocritical Care Society and the German Society for Neuro-Intensive Care and Emergency Medicine. *Neurocrit Care* 2015;22:146–164.

21. Turton FE, Snyder L. Physician-industry relations. *Ann Intern Med* 2007;146:469.

22. Verdon M, Merlani P, Perneger T, Ricou B. Burnout in a surgical ICU team. *Intensive Care Med* 2008;34:152–156.

23. Wijdicks EFM. Neurocritical Care: It's what we do and what we do best. *Neurocrit Care* 2006;5:81.

24. Wijdicks EFM, Menon DK, Smith M. Ten things you need to know to practice neurological critical care. *Intensive Care Med.* 2015;41:318–321.

25. Yetman L. Caring for families: double binds in neuroscience nursing. *Can J Neurosci Nurs* 2009;31:22–29.

26. Zimmerman JE, Shortell SM, Rousseau DM, et al. Improving intensive care: observations based on organizational case studies in nine intensive care units: a prospective, multicenter study. *Crit Care Med* 1993;21:1443–1451.

14

The Neurosciences Intensive Care Unit

This chapter introduces the types of administrative structures and models in the NICU. Usually, this unit is a combined neurologic and neurosurgical ICU, but some have remained largely neurosurgical or are specifically designated as trauma units. These ICUs—admitting neurologic and neurosurgical patients—are labeled *neurosciences intensive care units* (NICU).

Historically, neurosurgeon Dandy has been credited with opening the first NICU at Johns Hopkins Hospital in 1932. He and his nursing staff knew very well that some neurosurgical patients needed special care, and he refurbished a ward for sicker postoperative neurosurgical patients. Later, as an outgrowth of the poliomyelitis epidemics, respiratory care units emerged, and this marked the beginnings of the critical care specialty. In London, the Batten Respiratory Unit at the Institute of Neurology and National Hospital for Nervous Diseases opened in 1954 to treat mostly patients with acute neuromuscular disease, but also with stroke and spinal cord disorders who required mechanical ventilation. Also in the 1950's Russell and later Spalding (both neurologists) and Crampton Smith (anesthesiologist) did run the respiratory unit of the Churchill hospital in Oxford. The development of the NICU at the Mayo Clinic recently has been reported.[31] This unit, at Saint Marys Hospital, was one of the first newly built combined NICUs in the United States. It started as a unit with predominantly neurosurgical patients, and most of the expertise was developed in the care of neurosurgical patients. Soon acutely ill neurologic patients were admitted. Teaching of nursing staff and the beginnings of administration became part of the NICU responsibilities. Generally, the development of the NICU can clearly be seen as an outgrowth of nursing ingenuity.

Quality improvement may concentrate on improvement in preventive practices—but also reevaluation of the utilization of certain laboratory tests and bedside technology—and some of the more detailed analysis may involve cost–benefit analysis. In a complex NICU environment, where variables are numerous, administrative requirements and checklists can easily become much too much. Moreover, neurointensivists—who have to make very quick decisions on how to move forward and how to treat a patient—are generally less interested in economics or other forms of cost containment that can result in tailoring management and diagnostics.

Over the last decades, NICUs have become modernized, sophisticated environments that have adopted electronic records and systems delivering data instantaneously and efficiently and picked up by mobile devices. This chapter reviews the current locale, its staff, and commonly used protocols to improve care.

DESIGN

The typical floor plan includes single-patient rooms, nursing station, support storage and utility areas, pharmacy, conference rooms, and family waiting rooms. A large space should be allowed for family members, and sleeping facilities should be offered to them in times of crisis. Current NICUs accommodate multiple computer workstations for immediate access to patient data and radiologic studies. In the patient area, a universal bed, a power column, equipment space, and, preferably, mobile monitoring devices should be readily accessible. Our NICU layout is depicted in Figure 14.1. As a rule, the NICU is close to other ICUs, the emergency department (ED), and the radiology department.

Driven by regulations and the need for cost-effectiveness, NICUs have evolved through several models of organization. The main models are open, transitional (semi-open or hybrid), and closed units (Table 14.1).[4,25] In the closed ICU, all patients are cared for by one team of intensivists, and only intensivists have admitting privileges.[10] In an open ICU, any physician can admit patients to the ICU and provide primary service. Others have defined a transitional model (the "choice ICU"), in which the neurointensivist is the responsible person, but allows the attending to choose to see some patients but not others, thus creating an opportunity for

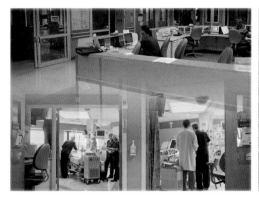
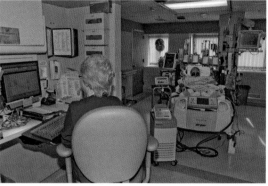

FIGURE 14.1. Layout of a neurosciences intensive care unit. Neurologic intensive care unit rooms with power column and monitors. Patient rooms in the unit should be at least 225 square feet. Natural illumination is important to maintain day and night orientation. Monitors should display electrocardiogram, intracranial pressure, cerebral perfusion pressure, and cardiac and respiratory data. Computer workstation provides electronic medical records, neuroradiologic studies, and other laboratory tests.

TABLE 14.1. NEUROLOGIC-NEUROSURGICAL INTENSIVE CARE UNIT PRACTICE MODELS

Key Features	Model		
	Open	Transitional or Choice	Closed
Hospital type	Nonteaching	Teaching	Teaching
Triage approval	Any neurologist or neurosurgeon	Neurointensivist or unit director	Neurointensivist
Patient care	Any neurologist or neurosurgeon	Neurointensivist	Neurointensivist
Rounds and orders	Each physician separate	Neurointensivist on selected patients	Neurointensivist on all patients
Advantages	Continuity of neurosurgical care	Collaborative practice, nurse satisfaction	Neurointensivist is the responsible person Protocols facilitated Improved efficiency and reduced resources Nurse satisfaction
Disadvantages	Increased subspecialty consultation No team leader	Role of neurointensivist less clear House staff not always present	Physician conflict and alienation

elective consultation. The main feature of the transitional model is that it provides a more active role for the neurointensivist. Recently, however, there has been a major push toward the closed unit model, in which the neurointensivist becomes the team leader with significant administrative powers, but who also makes rounds on every patient, manages their day-to-day care, and forges a collaborative practice with other specialists. Transitional models may be very workable in hospitals where there is uncertainty about relegating total care to one person. Most studies of ICUs suggest that closed units reduce complications and mortality,[19] but these data are not available for NICUs. A recent study suggested that mortality was higher in critically ill patients managed by intensivists in a closed unit, but a plausible mechanism was not identified.[19]

Electronic records have become commonplace in many ICUs, but very few are customized to NICUs. Electronic records—a continuously changing target—have allowed electronic checklists, but most informatics systems have concentrated on general critical illness.

STAFFING

Integrated care is a key principle of a successful NICU. The physicians, nurses, and ancillary staff who determine care in the NICU may include but are not limited to the medical or surgical director (responsible for clinical affairs), the neurointensivist (primary and overseeing care), neurosurgeons, anesthesiologists, neurologic intensive care fellows in training, senior neurology or neurosurgery residents, the nurse manager (responsible for nursing affairs), neuroscience intensive care nurses, and nurses in training (Figure 14.2a). Respiratory therapists (Figure 14.2b) are certified trained professionals in airway and ventilator management and most insert intra-arterial and intravenous catheters, and, in some ICUs, are closely involved in more specialized care (e.g., extracorporeal membrane oxygenation [ECMO]). Respiratory therapists have become crucial in the management of critically ill patients, using efficient strategies to manage these patients.

Consultants, fellows, and residents (mostly in their final years of training) do provide the integral part of care. Physician assistants in critical care units can also be part of an excellent practice model. Other team members may include nutritional consultants, infectious disease consultants, and acute code responders.

Physical therapists and rehabilitation physicians are indispensable in the NICU. A pharmacist who has been linked into a hospital's computerized order system has been shown to improve workflow.[18,21,28] Safe practice standards have been developed that allow a review by the pharmacist of all new orders, and this has increased the impact of the pharmacist on medication reconciliation (Figure 14.2c). Order sets can be made ICU-specific and include electrolyte replacement and medication, as well as intravenous drugs with titration parameters and dose adjustments. Telemedicine has also reached the ICU (Chapter 1), and intensivists have provided round-the-clock monitoring from home and conference through video. TeleNICU is in its infancy and largely nonexisting but is a serious idea. The impact on care is yet uncertain and the impact on costs is small, if present at all.[30]

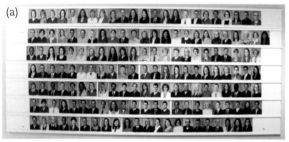
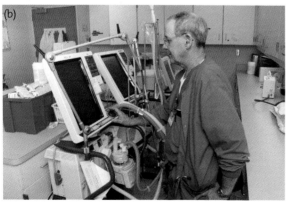
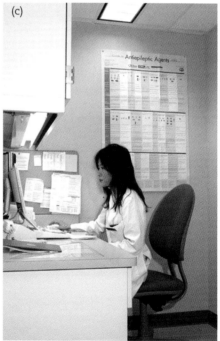

FIGURE 14.2: NICU Staffing. (a) Medical and nursing staff. (b) Respiratory therapist. (c) NICU pharmacist.

QUALITY CONTROL

There is a continuous search for improvement in the quality of NICU care. Regular review of the management of patients and care protocols by the team of healthcare workers functioning in the NICU is useful, and often actions can be improved. The NICU staff should have the ability to provide meaningful input on decisions that affect patient care. Quality improvement and performance benchmarking—two all too familiar buzzwords—actually involve several thought processes and strategies. They are listed in Table 14.2. Since the formation of a coalition of healthcare purchasers by the Leapfrog Group ("dedicated to make great leaps forward";[1] quality improvement projects have been developed for ICUs. These projects have become a staple in medical care; they are now taken for granted and seem self-evident. When judged by auditing agencies, improvement in clinical performance may impact accrediting, but whether or not quality improvement improves outcome is hard to determine. The question is also how to interpret the stream of data. Some have argued that stable mortality in the increasing complexity of patients might already be seen as a positive outcome.

Patient outcome measures of success can be defined and may include NICU readmission rate, ICU mortality, and ICU length of stay, but may also include measures of health-related quality of life after ICU discharge (e.g., SF 36), mental functional status (e.g., Beck Depression Score), recovery (return to work, return to independent living), and patient, family, and staff satisfaction.

Financial measures of success may be addressed by analyzing the cost of testing compared to actual reimbursement, coding and billing efficacy, an analysis of payer mix to ensure that any operational adjustment to bed capacity would result in improved financial performance, and bed occupancy rates (Capsule 14.1).

Cost-effectiveness can even start with transfer to the neurosciences intensive care unit. Several studies involving comprehensive stroke centers and NICUs have found that transferring patients with an intracranial hemorrhage to a specialized NICU is cost-effective. This may even apply to patients with small intracerebral hemorrhages as opposed to larger hemorrhages. Usually these models involve direct costs that are summarized as total costs being the sum of transfer, hospital cost, and caregiver's cost, and quality adjusted life years placed into a decision-making analytic model.[6,17]

The cost of patients in intensive care is enormous. Therefore, expensive treatment in a futile situation—defined as treatment that will never reach patients' goals, or imminent death or inability to survive outside the ICU—is well recognized and has been estimated in at least one study to be nearly $3 million during a 3-month period of assessment.[14] Several studies have found that excessive hospital utilization can be decreased by a palliative care consultation that could identify futility and patient-family goals.[12,13,16]

Quality improvement tools involve checklists such as those that are used in complex industries such as aviation, construction, and nuclear power plants; but they may lead to so-called checklist fatigue, resulting in carelessly filling out checklists. Furthermore, whether or not checklists improve outcome is unclear. Many of the ICU-used checklists improve compliance with best practices.[7–9,29] Quality improvement projects can involve the early recognition and treatment of medical complications such as treatment of sepsis,[15] ventilator-associated pneumonia free time,[22] and enhancing rehabilitation of mechanically ventilated patients in the intensive care unit.[23]

Some of these initiatives include the development of so-called "care bundles" and computerized physician order entry. The Joint Commission has championed ICU care bundles on the prevention and prophylaxis of ventilator-associated pneumonia, stress ulcers, deep vein thrombosis, and central catheter–associated bloodstream infection. Other quality-control measures provide blood product transfusion guidelines and glucose control guidelines. Care bundles can be developed for any major problem and a variety of acute neurologic conditions such as status epilepticus.

Another important improvement are surveillance protocols. The most important surveillance program is deep venous thrombosis (DVT) prophylaxis, and several studies have found that, in trauma, surveillance with ultrasound not only increases DVT detection but also reduces pulmonary embolus incidents and improves the cost in

---

TABLE 14.2. QUALITY IMPROVEMENTS

Diagnostic checklists

Management bundles

Electronic record and smartphone texts

Bedside tests (point of care)

Surveillance programs

Review ICU performance data

Value analysis of utilization/costs of laboratory tests

CAPSULE 14.1   COSTS OF ICU CARE

The costs of intensive care are high ("the expensive care unit") and represent approximately 15% of hospital costs. Fixed overhead, among other costs, will less likely result in a net operating income and more often a net operating loss. Whether it represents good value for money (cost-effectiveness) is dependent on many factors (see accompanying illustration). Some physicians are high spenders, using more monitoring devices and more laboratory values, but specialty may be a factor (costs may be higher with multiple groups with varied training).[3,4,10,11] Higher cost does not improve outcome, and economic endpoints such as length of stay or reduced mortality and quality of life are questionable surrogates of outcome.[14] Outcome perspective is equally important. Saving a life (e.g., emergency craniotomy) may reduce hospital costs but not reduce the costs of a long-term care facility or lost revenue of family members.[6] Hiring a neurointensivist could impact length of stay and complications, but its effect on costs and downstream revenue is unclear, and reduced costs may be only a consequence of reducing medical complications associated with the acute neurologic illness.[13] Interdisciplinary rounds reduce length of stay (e.g., pharmacist recommending drug selection, nursing identification of skin breakdown). Transitioning to intermediate (progressive) care unit, when appropriate, may reduce costs. Identification of patients who are "too well" or "too sick" for the ICU, thus reducing costs, may prove to be a myth.

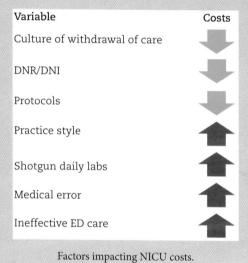

Factors impacting NICU costs.

terms of quality of life gained.[21] These programs are particularly useful in high-risk critical patients but lose their effectiveness in less severely affected patients.[3] Cost–benefit analyses have been performed in delirium prevention strategies[24] and also improvement of intensive care sound environment. Control of sound levels may improve restorative sleep.[26]

Significant improvement has been found with an enteral delivery improvement project. Enteral feeding protocols did help promote compliance and also improved adequacy of calories and proteins and reduction in enteric nutrition–associated diarrhea.[11,27]

Many bedside tests are used for short monitoring (spot EEG) or more prolonged monitoring, but very little evidence exists that continuous use improves outcome. Our value analysis of continuous EEG following cardiac arrest is an example of how these studies can be performed with calculating estimated EEG charges, and we found that these expensive technologies may not improve outcome, although they increased identification of treatable seizures. The costs of expensive monitoring can only be offset by the institution of effective therapies that would improve outcome.[5] Another example of a quality improvement project is the utilization of arterial blood gas analysis in the general intensive care unit, showing that a decrease of the number of studies per patient (from an average of 6 to 2) did actually link to a decrease in a number of ventilator days and a shorter length of stays for ventilator patients in the ICU.[2]

CONCLUSIONS

- NICU practice is collaborative. A closed model is ideal.
- Cost containment of NICU practice requires a multipronged approach.
- The NICU can be used to develop important quality improvement projects.

REFERENCES

1. Ali NA, Mekhjian HS, Kuehn PL, et al. Specificity of computerized physician order entry has a significant effect on the efficiency of workflow for critically ill patients. *Crit Care Med* 2005;33:110–114.
2. Blum FE, Lund ET, Hall HA, et al. Reevaluation of the utilization of arterial blood gas analysis in the intensive care unit: effects on patient safety and patient outcome. *J Crit Care.* 2015:438. e1–e5.
3. Boddi M, Cecchi A, Bonizzoli M, et al. Follow-up after four-year quality improvement program to prevent inferior limb deep vein thrombosis in intensive care unit. *Thromb Res* 2014;134:578–583.
4. Carson SS, Stocking C, Podsadecki T, et al. Effects of organizational change in the medical intensive care unit of a teaching hospital: a comparison of "open" and "closed" formats. *JAMA* 1996;276:322–328.
5. Crepeau AZ, Fugate JE, Mandrekar J, et al. Value analysis of continuous EEG in patients during therapeutic hypothermia after cardiac arrest. *Resuscitation* 2014;85:785–789.
6. Fletcher JJ, Kotagal V, Mammoser A, et al. Cost-effectiveness of transfers to centers with neurological intensive care units after intracerebral hemorrhage. *Stroke* 2015;46:58–64.
7. Gershengorn HB, Kocher R, Factor P. Management strategies to effect change in intensive care units: lessons from the world of business. Part I: targeting quality improvement initiatives. *Ann Am Thorac Soc* 2014;11:264–269.
8. Gershengorn HB, Kocher R, Factor P. Management strategies to effect change in intensive care units: lessons from the world of business. Part II: quality-improvement strategies. *Ann Am Thorac Soc* 2014;11:444–453.
9. Gershengorn HB, Kocher R, Factor P. Management strategies to effect change in intensive care units: lessons from the world of business. Part III: effectively effecting and sustaining change. *Ann Am Thorac Soc* 2014;11:454–457.
10. Ghorra S, Reinert SE, Cioffi W, Buczko G, Simms HH. Analysis of the effect of conversion from open to closed surgical intensive care unit. *Ann Surg* 1999;229:163–171.
11. Heyland DK, Dhaliwal R, Lemieux M, Wang M, Day AG. Implementing the PEP uP protocol in critical care units in Canada: results of a multicenter, quality improvement study. *JPEN J Parenter Enteral Nutr* 2015;39:698–706.
12. Hsu-Kim C, Friedman T, Gracely E, Gasperino J. Integrating palliative care into critical care: a quality improvement study. *J Intensive Care Med* 2015;30:358–364.
13. Huynh TN, Kleerup EC, Raj PP, Wenger NS. The opportunity cost of futile treatment in the ICU. *Crit Care Med* 2014;42:1977–1982.
14. Huynh TN, Kleerup EC, Wiley JF, et al. The frequency and cost of treatment perceived to be futile in critical care. *JAMA Intern Med* 2013;173:1887–1894.
15. Judd WR, Stephens DM, Kennedy CA. Clinical and economic impact of a quality improvement initiative to enhance early recognition and treatment of sepsis. *Ann Pharmacother* 2014;48: 1269–1275.
16. Khandelwal N, Engelberg RA, Benkeser DC, Coe NB, Curtis JR. End-of-life expenditure in the ICU and perceived quality of dying. *Chest* 2014;146:1594–1603.
17. Kramer AH, Zygun DA. Do neurocritical care units save lives? Measuring the impact of specialized ICUs. *Neurocrit Care* 2011;14:329–333.
18. Leape LL, Cullen DJ, Clapp MD, et al. Pharmacist participation on physician rounds and adverse drug events in the intensive care unit. *JAMA* 1999;282:267–270.
19. Levy MM, Rapoport J, Lemeshow S, et al. Association between critical care physician management and patient mortality in the intensive care unit. *Ann Intern Med* 2008;148:801–809.
20. MacLaren R, Bond CA, Martin SJ, Fike D. Clinical and economic outcomes of involving pharmacists in the direct care of critically ill patients with infections. *Crit Care Med* 2008;36:3184–3189.
21. Malhotra AK, Goldberg SR, McLay L, et al. DVT surveillance program in the ICU: analysis of cost-effectiveness. *PLoS One* 2014;9:e106793.
22. Matar DS, Pham JC, Louis TA, Berenholtz SM. Achieving and sustaining ventilator-associated pneumonia-free time among intensive care units (ICUs): evidence from the Keystone ICU Quality

Improvement Collaborative. *Infect Control Hosp Epidemiol* 2013;34:740–743.

23. McWilliams D, Weblin J, Atkins G, et al. Enhancing rehabilitation of mechanically ventilated patients in the intensive care unit: a quality improvement project. *J Crit Care* 2015;30:13–18.

24. Moon KJ, Lee SM. The effects of a tailored intensive care unit delirium prevention protocol: A randomized controlled trial. *Int J Nurs Stud.* 2015;52:1423–1432.

25. Multz AS, Chalfin DB, Samson IM, et al. A "closed" medical intensive care unit (MICU) improves resource utilization when compared with an "open" MICU. *Am J Respir Crit Care Med* 1998;157:1468–1473.

26. Persson Waye K, Elmenhorst EM, Croy I, Pedersen E. Improvement of intensive care unit sound environment and analyses of consequences on sleep: an experimental study. *Sleep Med* 2013;14:1334–1340.

27. Taylor B, Brody R, Denmark R, Southard R, Byham-Gray L. Improving enteral delivery through the adoption of the "Feed Early Enteral Diet Adequately for Maximum Effect (FEED ME)" protocol in a surgical trauma ICU: a quality improvement review. *Nutr Clin Pract* 2014;29:639–648.

28. Weber RJ, Kane SL, Oriolo VA, et al. Impact of intensive care unit (ICU) drug use on hospital costs: a descriptive analysis, with recommendations for optimizing ICU pharmacotherapy. *Crit Care Med* 2003;31:S17–24.

29. Weiss CH, Moazed F, McEvoy CA, et al. Prompting physicians to address a daily checklist and process of care and clinical outcomes: a single-site study. *Am J Respir Crit Care Med* 2011;184:680–686.

30. Wilson LS. Technologies for complex and critical care telemedicine. *Stud Health Technol Inform* 2008;131:117–130.

31. Wijdicks EFM, Worden W, Miers A,Piepgras DG.The early days of the Neurosciences Intensive Care Unit. *Mayo Clinic Proc* 2011;86:903–906.

PART V

General Principles of Management of Critically Ill Neurologic Patients in the Neurosciences Intensive Care Unit

15

General Perspectives of Care

Amid the multiple neurologic and medical complexities of care, neurologists could take general daily matters for granted. The critically ill neurologic patient has vexing needs, and it is conventional wisdom that the daily care of patients with acute neurologic disorders is multipronged. Its scope includes specialized neuroscience nursing care, physical therapy, infection precautions, and other prophylactic measures. Inattention to any of these may potentially result in a less favorable outcome from unnecessary complications. This chapter reviews the principles of supportive care of the critically ill neurologic patient. Communication with family members receives special attention.

GENERAL NURSING CARE AND PHYSICAL THERAPY

Patients admitted to the neurosciences intensive care unit (NICU) have extensive nursing requirements that are expected in critically ill patients. But much more is required. The neurosciences nursing staff routinely evaluates patients every hour to measure their level of alertness, detect new neurologic signs, and recognize subtle seizures, agitation, and pain. They are well aware that changes in neurologic condition may be subtle, and in many instances no exact physiologic measurement is available to confirm a change in neurologic status.

A comprehensive discussion of nursing care of patients with neurologic illness is outside the scope of this book, but several important aspects must be familiar to anyone who manages critically ill neurologic patients. Important categories of nursing care are attention to mouth, eye, and skin care; checking of Foley catheters, nasogastric tubes, and intravascular catheters; dressing changes for monitoring devices; and, most important, adequate body positioning and respiratory care. Equally important in intensive care is the optimization of comfort and, if possible, sleep.

Skin Care

Skin care has a high priority in immobilized patients.[11] Decubital ulcers or, more often, patches of demarcated painful erythema indicative of developing ulcers may appear, even with meticulous care. Pressure ulcers appear in stages, commonly progressing from pressure-produced erythematous blanching to abrasions, shallow ulcers, or full-thickness skin loss. Sores occur mostly over the sacrum, greater trochanter, and heels (Figure 15.1). Heavy smokers, advanced age, and patients with dry skin or hypoalbuminemia are at particularly high risk.[6,42] The risk for ischemic damage over the sacral skin area is most prominent in the supine position and less in the 45-degree position.[62,86] Low body mass, high degree of skin exposure to moisture, and impaired sensory perception contribute considerably to pressure ulcer formation. In a study in the NICU, two-thirds of the patients with pressure sores acquired them within the first week of admission.[35]

On daily rounds, the skin should be inspected carefully at pressure points. Frequent turning in bed, lanolin creams, and dry patting of the skin are essential. Increasing repositioning (from 4 hours to 2 hours) did not reduce decubitus ulcers.[61] Nursing staff assess the patients' risk for pressure ulcers on six indicators of the Braden Scale: sensory perception (patients' responsiveness to verbal or painful stimuli), moisture (from constantly to rarely moist), activity (confined to walking), mobility (immobile to frequent changes in position), nutrition (poor to excellent), and most important, friction and shear (sliding against sheets).[17] Use of air-fluidized mattresses is critical when prolonged immobilization from coma or quadriplegia (e.g., spinal cord injury or Guillain-Barré syndrome) is expected.[44] Without prospective trials, the benefits of medical treatments or even prophylaxis are not known. Constant vigilance is necessary because pressure sores may occur very quickly, within days of admission.[12,20]

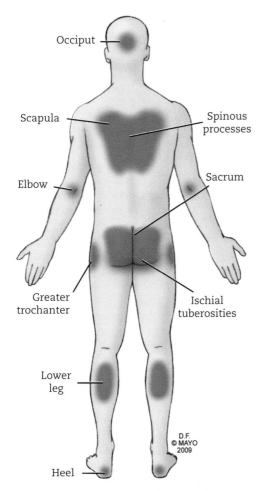

Occiput

Scapula

Spinous
processes

Elbow

Sacrum

Greater
trochanter

Ischial
tuberosities

Lower
leg

D.F.
© MAYO
2009

Heel

FIGURE 15.1: Common areas of pressure ulceration in the supine position.

Modified from Reuler JB, Cooney TG. The pressure sore: pathophysiology and principles of management. *Ann Intern Med* 1981;94:661–666. With permission of the American College of Physicians–American Society of Internal Medicine.

Pressure mapping is a new technology and identifies areas at risk for decubital ulcers.[25,72] Raising the head of the bed by only 30 degrees can increase the sacral pressure above the capillary closing pressure and cause the potential for tissue ischemia. When these abnormal pressures are found, mattress firmness can be set differently to reduce pressure (Figure 15.2).

Avoiding shearing of the skin tissue planes during turning, transfers, and when patients are seated is equally important. In seated patients, leg restraints may markedly reduce shearing and thus skin injury. Repositioning is performed every 2 hours, but must be more frequent if erythema occurs. Medical management of pressure sores

includes topical treatment with hydrocolloid occlusive dressing and polyurethane film dressings, but topical antibiotics such as neomycin and metronidazole may also be needed.

Skin breakdown may also occur from endotracheal tube contact. This can be minimized by adhesive tape and a combination of nystatin and tolnaftate. Protective adhesive tape may reduce pressure on the patient's nares when nasogastric tubes are in place, and these tubes should never be positioned in upward flexion. A known major risk is decubital ulcers with collar placement in patients with presumed cervical injury, and with each day this risk increases substantially. Pressure points include occiput, chin, mandible, ears, shoulders, laryngeal prominence, and sternum. (Waiting for a "clearing" of the cervical spine—which may include magnetic resonance imaging [MRI]—may contribute to this risk.[1])

Eye Care

Eye care is important in comatose patients, and daily application of methylcellulose drops with taping of the eyelids is important to reduce corneal abrasions. One recent study found a risk of exposure keratopathy in 20%–40% of patients.[82] In mechanically ventilated susceptible patients, positive pressure ventilation may cause severe conjunctival edema, resulting in inability to close the eyes.[59] Continuous sedation and muscle relaxation are risk factors for ocular surface disorders, but hypoxemia or hypercapnia may dilate conjunctival vessels (Figure 15.3). Conjunctival edema is self-limiting but can put patients at risk for corneal exposure and drying. Aggressive lubrication may not be effective, and Guibor eye bubbles or temporary tarsorrhaphy (Figure 15.4) may be needed to prevent keratopathy.[46]

Oral Care

Oral care includes the use of lip balm and moistening of the gingiva and mouth. Patients at risk for seizures need adequate protection with mouth guards, but most tongue bites heal spontaneously. Tongue swelling is rare, usually from an anaphylactic reaction (most notably from angiotensin-converting enzyme inhibitors), swelling from hematoma formation (tongue bite and anticoagulation), or angioedema associated with long-term use of barbiturates (Figure 15.5).[49] Oral candidiasis, recognized as creamy white patches on the pharynx or tongue, should be anticipated in patients receiving broad-spectrum antibiotics, corticosteroids, or total parenteral nutrition,

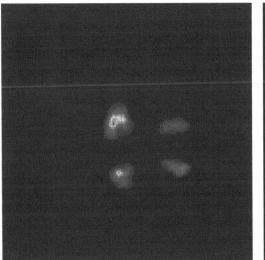

FIGURE 15.2: Pressure mapping of buttocks. Sensor device identifies high (red) pressure (100–200 mm Hg) areas in ischial tuberosities. Change in the bed inflation markedly reduces pressure and may prevent decubital ulcers.

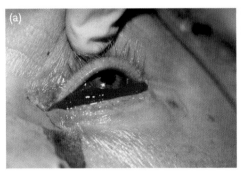
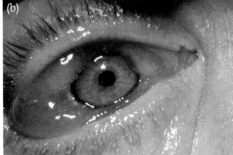

FIGURE 15.3: Chemosis due to accumulation of transudate. (a) Conjunctiva bulges over the cornea or (b) protrudes, between eyelids.

but the probability is increased in any preceding debilitating state. Fluconazole 100 mg/day orally may treat this infection rapidly before it becomes invasive.

Oral care also involves frequent suctioning of secretions. Frequent suctioning (every hour), thick viscosity, and number of passes (> 2) provide some sense of the complexity of airway care. Moreover, many intensive care units have included teeth brushing with chlorhexidine

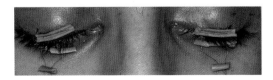

FIGURE 15.4: Closing eyes for keratitis prevention.

(0.2%). Subglottic suctioning in intubated patients results in a nearly 10% reduction in ventilator-associated pneumonia and its associated costs of antibiotics.[28]

Respiratory Care

Atelectasis with stagnant secretions is commonly developing in the left lower lobe because of poor drainage and compression by the heart in prolonged supine positions. Kinetic beds may be considered for comatose patients at high risk, and there is clear benefit above physiotherapy alone.[77]

Physiotherapy is likely to improve atelectasis and may have a short-lived beneficial effect on respiratory function.[22] But whether routine physiotherapy in the NICU (or any other ICU) reduces the chance of nosocomial pneumonia is questionable, and a study that used twice-daily physiotherapy

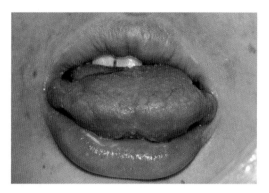

FIGURE 15.5: Tongue and lip swelling associated with prolonged use of barbiturates for treatment of status epilepticus.

suggested no effect.[66] In addition, despite the empirical fact of efficacy, no evidence exists that any of the other techniques avoid atelectasis or decrease the incidence of pulmonary complications.[65,95] Nonetheless, chest physiotherapy is considered important in patients with neurologic critical illness. It involves positioning for postural drainage, suctioning, and, in cooperative patients, breathing exercises and forced expiratory techniques.[48]

Many physical therapists briefly put the patient in a flat position before tracheal suctioning to assess the effect of positional change on intracranial pressure.[38] If intracranial pressure does not return to baseline value after a mild increase from upright into a flat position, brief hyperventilation through a manual resuscitation bag is necessary. Marked intracranial pressure surges or plateau waves can be muted by endotracheal instillation of lidocaine 2 mg/kg[9] and, equally important, by simply limiting the number of tracheal passages. Percussion and vibration are additionally effective in mobilizing retained secretions. However, although the techniques of percussion and vibration reduce atelectasis, they may potentially increase intracranial pressure in susceptible patients with poor brain compliance. Chest percussion generally should not increase intracranial pressure.

Coughing must be stimulated in alert patients with an acute neuromuscular disorder. Huffing (large inspiration followed by short expiratory blasts) may stimulate coughing, and a gentle touch of the oropharynx with an oral suction tube may be helpful as well. The basic requirements for chest physiotherapy are summarized in Table 15.1.

Incentive spirometry (Figure 15.6) could be important in post-neurosurgical patients who have a proclivity for closure of the alveoli in the dependent lung zones. The use of CPAP valves (EzPAP) may be additionally useful (Figure 15.7).[80] Coaching

TABLE 15.1. ESSENTIALS OF CHEST PHYSIOTHERAPY

Percussion and vibration
Coughing exercises (huffing techniques, oropharyngeal stimulation)
Suctioning (preceded by hyperoxygenation, FiO2 1.0, for 15 seconds)
Mucolytic agents, bronchodilators, and nebulizers for humidification

of patients requires an alert and cooperative patient. A reasonable technique is to take 10 maximal inspirations every 2 hours between 8 A.M. and 8 P.M. to allow for a good night's rest. The use of incentive spirometry reduced the postoperative incidence of atelectasis in critically ill patients in some studies, but treatment benefit may be much less than claimed.[71] Systematic studies in patients with acute neurologic illness are not available. It is not expected that aggressive incentive spirometry may prevent mechanical ventilation in patients with Guillain-Barré syndrome (see Chapter 42) and myasthenia gravis (see Chapter 43) and marginal respiratory function. Deterioration in these conditions is too rapid to be averted by this simple measure.

Abdominal Care

Early feeding of the gut to guarantee adequate nutrition is part of daily care. Malnutrition should

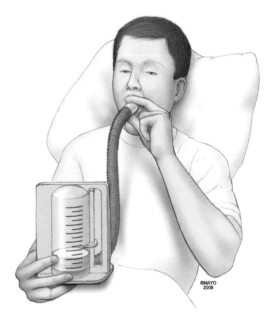

FIGURE 15.6: Incentive spirometry. The patient is encouraged to take a profound inspiratory breath, aiming at elevation of the piston to a set level.

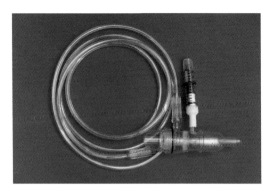

FIGURE 15.7: EzPAP®

be recognized in emergency admission of patients with severe head injury or fulminant meningitis, conditions that are more prevalent in alcoholics and patients with illegal drug use. Vitamin B_1 (thiamine) deficiency is common in these vulnerable patients, and intravenous administration of thiamine is standard (100 mg IV initially, and then 100 mg daily for 5–7 days). The integrity of the gut is maintained by enteral feeding and is greatly challenged by parenteral nutrition. It is prudent to consider postpyloric feeding in patients with neurological catastrophes because gastric atony increases the risk of aspiration. Motility should be checked daily, and several motility drugs are available. Cisapride and erythromycin work best in gastric or small bowel atony, and neostigmine works best on colon.

Bladder Care

Foley catheter placement reduces the chance of retention (if placed correctly). Failure to recognize an extended bladder may to lead to renal failure and rapid rise in serum creatinine and amylase. An unrecognized full bladder can be a major cause of agitation in any neurologic patient and can be due to simple obstruction. In patients with spinal cord injury, urinary bladder may go into spasm during catheter replacement, and the catheter balloon may easily be misplaced. The so-called "positive long catheter" sign has been used to identify the placement of the Foley catheter in the urethra, but this remains subjective. X-ray of the pelvis with contrast may be helpful but practically is less useful than a simple CT scan of the pelvis.

The indications for catheterization are multifold, but the benefits include more accurate urinary output measurement, management of acute urinary retention, and management of a neurogenic bladder. Urinary catheterization improves

patient comfort a great deal. However, placing an indwelling urethral catheter to manage urinary incontinence is an inappropriate indication. After urethral catheter placement, a closed system is attached, and such a system will reduce urinary tract infections. The catheters are left in place and are not frequently changed. Timely removal of the urinary catheter in improving patients is encouraged. Mostly, catheters can be removed after brain or spine surgery. Once an indwelling catheter is placed and a prolonged catheterization is anticipated, a closed system should be maintained at all times. The drainage bay should be placed below the bladder, and the bag should be emptied when two-thirds full and before transport. Management of bladder also includes the management of infections and asymptomatic bacteriuria. Generally, antibiotics are prescribed only if patients become symptomatic in order to avoid drug resistance associated with the use of prophylactic antibiotics. Again, prophylactic antibiotics are associated with reduction of the incidence of asymptomatic bacteriuria, but they increase antibiotic resistance and do not prevent symptomatic infections. Moreover, recurrent upper urinary tract infections may indicate high bladder pressure or bladder stones that may need to be evaluated.

Positioning

Positioning of comatose patients in an appropriate manner may reduce contractures.[21] Irrespective of whether the patient needs to have his or her head elevated (e.g., increased intracranial pressure) or to lie flat (e.g., acute basilar artery occlusion), a neutral or side-lying position should be adopted, with a pillow between the legs to prevent internal rotation, adduction, and inversion of the upper leg. Patients with a flaccid paralysis should have footboards, splinting to prevent contractures, and trochanter towel rolls to prevent entrapment neuropathy of the peroneal nerve. In addition, it is important to avoid compression at the elbows to protect the ulnar nerve. Nonetheless, comatose patients with marked extensor posturing are difficult to position. Footboards and splints in these patients are not useful, because they apply stretch and potentially further increase the tone of the hypertonic muscles. Unfortunately, despite good intent, contractures are mostly observed in patients in a permanent vegetative state when they are re-examined months after the catastrophe.

In the properly aligned patient in a dorsal position, the head is in neutral position in line with the spine in the anteroposterior plane, the arms are flexed at the elbow with the hands resting at the side of the abdomen (pillows may be needed to support this position), and the fingers are extended over the edge of the pillow (Figure 15.8a) (inserting a rolled towel may create normal arching of the fingers). The knees are extended or are slightly flexed, with trochanter rolls folded under the greater trochanter hip joint area to distally reduce pressure on the peroneal nerve at the fibula head caused by external rotation at the hip joint. The feet are ideally at 70–90 degrees to the legs, with the toes pointing upward. The lateral position places the patient on either side without twisting the head. The head is supported by a pillow, and a second pillow is placed between the legs (Figure 15.8b).

Positioning of patients with hemiplegia is different. The head and neck should be in midline or, in patients with considerable hemibody neglect, preferably turned to the affected side. A pillow is placed in the axilla to counter the tendency of the arm to adduct and rotate internally. The paralyzed arm is supported on a pillow with the elbow partially flexed. The leg is placed in a neutral position supported by a trochanter roll. In the lateral position, patients should be turned on the unaffected side without flexion of the trunk and spine. Conventionally, the arm is positioned so that each joint is higher than the preceding one. Generally, extension, adduction, and internal rotation of the shoulder should be avoided. In patients with acute stroke who are lying on the unaffected side, the lower limb should be flexed. It may be beneficial to lift the affected hip forward while the limb is supported by a pillow.

In patients with flaccid quadriplegia a high Fowler's position (semi-upright with head 80–90 degrees) is favored. The shoulders are supported with several pillows in the axilla and under the knees, and the hips are slightly abducted

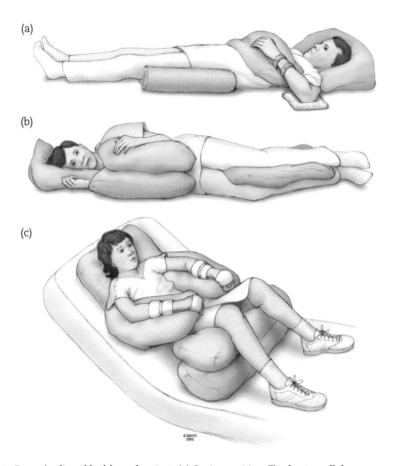

(a)

(b)

(c)

FIGURE 15.8: Properly aligned bed-bound patient. (a) Supine position. Trochanter roll decreases compression on the peroneal nerve, and soft towel or sheepskin reduces pressure at the level of the ulnar nerve. (b) Side-lying position. (c) Semi-upright position in quadriplegic patient. Splints reduce contractures. (Sneakers can be used for splinting of feet.)

(Figure 15.8c). In patients with complete flaccid quadriplegia, splinting of the hands and use of boots (Figure 15.9) are essential in preventing contractures.

Physical Therapy

Most NICUs have specially assigned teams to assist in the care of critically ill patients. Physical therapy should begin virtually immediately; next to appropriate positioning, it includes passive range of motion and chest physiotherapy for postural drainage.[22,34,54,65]

Initially, range-of-motion exercises are passive, consisting of abduction, adduction, flexion, and extension motions.[95] Passive movements of the limbs are focused on the proximal limb muscles, with flexion and extension of the knee while the hip is extended and the foot is held in dorsiflexion. Mild stretching after heat application may be added, but this causes additional discomfort for patients with muscle pain from Guillain-Barré syndrome (see Chapter 42).

Range-of-motion exercises should be done daily and later can be actively performed by the patient. Active exercises should be done gradually, because prolonged bedrest leads to deconditioning, characterized by orthostatic hypotension and loss of muscle mass and contractile strength. Vigorous active range-of-motion exercises may cause oxygen desaturation or may precipitate chest pain if a patient cannot meet the demands of low-level exercises (Capsule 15.1).

A recent national survey of physical therapy in ICUs found that functional mobility retraining and therapeutic exercises were commonly instituted by attending physicians (functional mobility

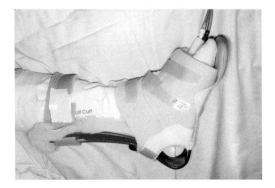

FIGURE 15.9: Boot to prevent contracture. Often one boot is switched from one foot to the other in 4–6 hours to prevent skin breakdown.

retraining helps a patient to regain balance, coordination, and the ability to walk independently).[43] Other studies have investigated the effect of physiotherapy in the ICU. One study found greater functional independence and reduced time on the ventilator when physical therapy was started within 2 days of admission.[87] Physical therapy in the ICU may substantially improve muscle strength.[62]

A major study on very early mobilization in acute stroke unexpectedly found a significant reduction in the odds of good outcome at 3 months after stroke and no evidence of accelerated walking recovery. This protocol started within 24 h of stroke onset and focused on sitting, standing, and walking (i.e., out-of-bed) activity with at least three additional out-of-bed sessions to usual care. Whether early mobilization is useful in other clinical situations is not yet determined but there is a sense among the NICU nursing staff this aggressive approach should at least be studied in a carefully selected patient group.[97]

Thromboembolism Prevention

The actual occurrence of deep vein thrombosis and pulmonary emboli is probably more frequent than the neurologic literature suggests and is, for the most part, preventable. Although the efficacy of heparin in the prevention of deep vein thrombosis is undisputed, in the intensive care unit (ICU), the overall risk of deep vein thrombosis with subcutaneous administration of low-dose heparin remains 5%–15% in the first week.[9] The risk of deep vein thrombosis is determined by the patient mix in the neuroscience intensive care unit (NICU) (trauma or nontrauma and presence of limb weakness). Deep vein thrombosis often develops in a paralyzed leg (or legs in Guillain-Barré syndrome or acute spinal cord disorder).

Simple preventive measures such as thigh-length graduated compression stockings are typically used, but when tested in patients after stroke, these stockings were not sufficient to prevent deep vein thrombosis.[31]

Subcutaneous heparin substantially reduces the risk of deep vein thrombosis and pulmonary embolism when given to patients with ischemic stroke.[2,5,53,63] The presence of an intracerebral hematoma does not necessarily preclude the use of subcutaneous heparin. A study of subcutaneous heparin in patients with intracerebral hematoma found that pulmonary embolism was significantly reduced without increased risk of hemorrhagic

Bedrest has profound effects on the normal physiology of lungs, heart, circulation, and muscles (see accompanying illustration). The effects appear quickly and become more prominent and clinically relevant over time. Lung function changes, with a reduction in vital capacity, forced expiratory volumes, and pulmonary blood flow as a result of unloading of postural muscles in chest and abdomen.[64] Bedrest changes circulation with initially headward redistribution of plasma volume followed by increased diuresis for 3–6 days to a new steady state. This also results in a reduction in left ventricular filling and stroke volume. More specifically, myocardial untwisting is reduced, all leading to orthostatic hypotension. Baroreceptor function declines partly through its gravity-dependent cycles.[60]

Bedrest results in diuresis associated with loss of sodium and potassium and reduced plasma volume in the first 72 hours. Vasopressin aldosterone and renin also rapidly fall concomitantly with a rise in atrial natriuretic peptide.[36] There is a continuing urinary excretion of potassium during bedrest, and this is a major cause for the downward trend of serum potassium. Muscle wasting may decrease plasma potassium and increase urinary concentrations mostly after several weeks of bedrest. The diuretic response is attributed to the Gauer-Henry reflex (increased central blood volume or headward fluid shift increases central venous pressure, thus stimulating atrial mechanoreceptors, vagal stimulation to the thalamus, inhibition of hypothalamus vasopressin release, decreased renal sympathetic nerve activity, and reduced renin aldosterone systems). Initial plasma volume loss may also be directly explained by mechanical atrial stretch not involving vagal pathways (vagotomy does not prevent diuresis).

Cardiac function undergoes minor changes. Heart rate may decrease (or increase) due to decreases in plasma volume. Pulmonary function may be affected by the upward shift of abdominal contents against the diaphragm, but pulmonary volumes do not change with prolonged bedrest.[81] Mild decreases in arterial PO_2 occur, associated with pulmonary circulatory stasis or atelectasis. Gastrointestinal reflux may increase, particularly in patients with a high body mass index.[88] Most prominently, muscle atrophy occurs and may be enhanced by protein undernutrition[55] and may improve with resistance training.[96] Venous compliance is also affected, and venous outflow resistance is increased.

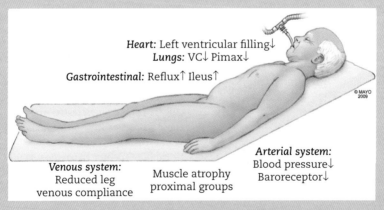

Heart: Left ventricular filling↓
Lungs: VC↓ Pimax↓
Gastrointestinal: Reflux↑ Ileus↑

Arterial system:
Blood pressure↓
Baroreceptor↓

Venous system:
Reduced leg
venous compliance

Muscle atrophy
proximal groups

© MAYO 2009

Physiologic effects of immobilization.

PImax, maximal inspiratory pressure; VC, vital capacity.

complications (pulmonary perfusion scans were only done in instances of clinical suspicion).[15]

Mechanical compression devices compress the calves and markedly increase venous flow velocity. Pneumatic compression devices have significantly reduced the incidence of venous thrombosis postoperatively[23,24,98] but have not been rigorously tested prospectively in the NICU population. Retrospective studies included elective neurosurgical patients and aneurysmal subarachnoid hemorrhage (SAH). In a recently published series,[78] 125 patients with aneurysmal SAH were screened with lower extremity Doppler ultrasonography every 4–7 days to detect asymptomatic deep venous thrombus, and 24% positive studies were reported despite routine use of subcutaneous heparin, thigh-high anti-thrombosis stockings, and mechanical sequential compression boots.

The reduction in deep vein thrombosis and pulmonary embolus with these compression devices is similar to that with low-dose heparin and may be a safer alternative in patients with spontaneous or traumatic hematoma. One study comparing historical controls with stroke patients suggested that these devices should be used in combination with a heparin regimen; with this approach, deep vein thrombosis occurred in 0.2% of 432 patients, and there were no pulmonary emboli.[50]

The current recommendations for the prevention of venous thromboembolism by the American College of Chest Physicians were updated in 2012, and the Neurocritical Care Society issued a statement in 2016 (Part XIV Guidelines).[39] For perioperative neurosurgical patients, intermittent mechanical compression devices are generally reconsidered with postoperative low-molecular-weight heparin (LMWH) in high-risk patients. The risk of intracranial bleeding in postoperative use of low-dose unfractionated heparin is not increased after craniotomy, but there is a serious concern, with use of LMWH showing increased risk of bleeding at any site[39] (Table 15.2).

Generally, venous thromboembolism is most effectively prevented with low doses of unfractionated heparin (5,000 units subcutaneously every 8 hours) until the patient is ambulatory. Patients with a history of recurrent venous thrombosis should receive the LMWH enoxaparin, 30 mg subcutaneously every 12 hours.[3] The LMWHs have better bioavailability, ease of use (once or twice daily subcutaneously), and less binding to platelet factor IV (causing heparin-induced thrombocytopenia).[104] Most importantly reversal of LMWH with protamine is much less effective than in unfractionated heparin. Aspirin, although appealing, or a low dose of warfarin (1 mg) cannot be recommended.[47]

TABLE 15.2. RECOMMENDATIONS FOR DEEP VEIN THROMBOSIS PROPHYLAXIS

Procedure or Diagnosis	Acute Prophylaxis
Polytrauma	Retrievable filter
Craniotomy (general)	Intermittent pneumatic compression device + graduated compression stockings
Craniotomy (malignancy)	Low-dose unfractionated heparin or low-molecular-weight heparin
Acute spinal cord injury	Low-molecular-weight heparin or low-dose unfractionated heparin

Source: Data from Geerts WH, Bergqvist D, Pineo GF, et al. Prevention of venous thromboembolism: American College of Chest Physicians Evidence based Clinical Practice Guidelines. *Chest* 2008;133:381S–453S.

The risk of deep vein thrombosis is increased in patients with previous deep vein thrombosis, skin pigmentation of the legs, and varices. In most of our patients, however, we use mechanical compression devices to prevent deep vein thrombosis. These devices provide more comfort than three times daily subcutaneous heparin injections, but they must remain in place much of the day. (They are disconnected during transport and procedures.) These devices are probably not sufficient in patients with a high risk of venous thromboembolism (previous deep vein thrombosis, underlying malignant disease, or expectation of major surgery; e.g., orthopedic surgery for fractures in patients with multitrauma) or thrombophilia.[89] In these high-risk patients, subcutaneous heparin is warranted.

Thigh-length stockings alone may not be sufficient in immobilized patients, and this measure alone did not prevent proximal deep vein thrombosis in patients after ischemic stroke.[31] The recent CLOTS trial, however, showed benefit of intermittent compression devices to stroke patients when immobilized.[29] Not unexpectedly, functional outcome did not change.[30] In extreme cases of thromboembolic risk, retrievable inferior vena cava filters have been placed in young trauma patients who also have a high risk of bleeding complications (intra-abdominal injury, intracranial injury, pelvic hematoma requiring transfusion, long-bone fractures). The threshold to place these devices in these patients is generally low. Timing and risks of using subcutaneous heparin or low-molecular-weight heparins (LMWH) are shown in Table 15.3.

TABLE 15.3. SUBCUTANEOUS HEPARIN OR LOW-MOLECULAR-WEIGHT HEPARIN

Low risk 48 hours after cerebral hemorrhage
Low risk 24 hours after ischemic stroke
Low risk 12 hours after brain tumor surgery
High risk in unsecured aneurysm
High risk in early traumatic brain injury
Low risk in ventriculostomy (once placed)

Surveillance for asymptomatic venous thrombosis using ultrasound is usually performed randomly and thus, the prevalence varies among series. It is important to estimate the risk of pulmonary emboli when a thrombus is found in the venous system, and this risk is determined by its deep location (Capsule 15.2).

Transfers and Transports

Patients often need to be moved from the NICU to the radiology suite for neuroimaging. In-hospital transport results in a period during which patients are outside a critical care area and monitoring is potentially jeopardized. Safe in-hospital transfer is also among the daily responsibilities of nursing care, residents, and staff.[7,31,84,99]

Adverse events that have been noted during the transport of acutely ill patients and that tentatively may lead to secondary insults to the brain are arterial oxygen saturation of less than 90%, hypoventilation in mechanically ventilated patients, severe hypocapnia by too-frequent manual bagging, cardiovascular changes induced by sudden alteration in the mode of ventilation, and surges of intracranial pressure, all of which may escape detection.[7,91] Catheters and tubes may be pulled, most often during transfer of patients to different beds. The consequences of dislodgment of intravascular catheters are particularly important if patients are receiving vasopressors, inotropic agents, or drugs to control cardiac arrhythmias. For selected patients, it is effective to have mannitol and antiepileptic drugs prepared. Further precautions are listed in Table 15.4. It is important to assess possible change in vital signs after several minutes of manual bagging. This precaution is useful because some patients do not tolerate even this brief intermission. The personnel transferring the patient should include the responsible neurologic critical care nurse most familiar with recent vital signs and should be further accompanied by a respiratory therapist or physician.

ISOLATION AND INFECTION PRECAUTIONS

Strict handwashing between visits to patients, limitation of the use and duration of devices, proper isolation of infected patients, and aseptic techniques reduce nosocomial infections.[32,41] Identification of patients with antimicrobial-resistant strains (e.g., methicillin- and vancomycin-resistant *Staphylococcus aureus*[18]) may control spread. Risk factors are patients admitted from other hospitals, patients staying 4 days or more in the hospital, or prophylactic use of one or more antibiotics for more than 1 day after severe trauma.[99,102] Screening is needed in these patients.[40]

The Centers for Disease Control and Prevention (CDC) have defined categories of isolation: strict isolation, contact isolation, respiratory isolation, tuberculosis isolation, and several other disease-specific isolation precautions.[37] The isolation categories are shown in Table 15.5.

Body-substance isolation implies that gloves should be worn for anticipated contact with blood, secretions, and any moist body substances. Gloves should be changed before contacting another patient. Gowns, plastic aprons, masks, and goggles should be worn when secretions, blood, or body fluid is likely to soil or splash on clothing, skin, or face. Soiled reusable items should be contained. Needles should be placed in rigid containers without recapping.

The main arguments for strict hand hygiene are the following: (a) more than 2 million Americans acquire a healthcare-associated infection each year; (b) 80,000 deaths have been tentatively associated with these infections; (c) pathogens causing these infections are transmitted most often by the hands of healthcare workers; and (d) studies show a temporal relationship between improved hand-hygiene practices and reduced infection rates. The problem is that healthcare provider adherence with hand hygiene recommendations remains low, and even visual displays do not increase compliance.[8,109] Warning labels on mechanical ventilators (wash hands, use gloves) improved handwashing in one study, but others found no measurable effect.[13,68] Most ICUs now use alcohol-based hand rubs for "waterless" hand disinfection.[45] A prospective, randomized trial proved better tolerance and better disinfection with alcohol-based handwashing, but reduction in nosocomial infection was not established.[16,58] Another study found virtually no relationship between handwashing rates and infection rates when two ICUs were

CAPSULE 15.2   PREVENTING DEEP VEIN THROMBOSIS

In the NICU, three major factors increase the risk of thrombus formation in the venous system. The accompanying illustration shows the superficial and deep systems. Bedrest reduces venous flow and promotes the formation of calf thrombi in the valve pockets that may extend into the deep veins. The risk increases after approximately 3 days. Catheter placement in central veins is a common source of thrombus formation. Two-thirds of the deep venous thrombi are located in the calf veins. Isolated calf thrombus is rarely symptomatic and rarely causes clinically important pulmonary emboli.[51] Peripherally inserted central catheters are strongly associated with upper-extremity deep vein thrombosis but the risk of pulmonary emboli is low.

Compression ultrasonography (CUS) is the current technology used to document proximal deep vein thrombosis; it has a sensitivity of 97% and specificity of 95%.[52] The sensitivity for detection of thrombus in the calf veins is lower at 70%, but a CUS is repeated at 5–7 days to detect patients with later extension to the deeper systems. Augmentation methods are used, such as calf squeeze that may show upstroke in venous flow in a proximal deep vein as indication of retained flow, but this method is likely unreliable. Low clinical probability, normal d-dimer test, and a normal compression ultrasound virtually excludes a deep vein thrombosis.

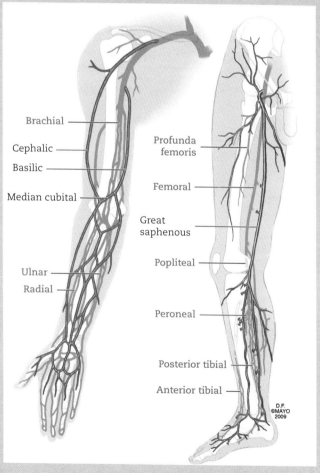

Superficial and deep venous system.

(Blue labels are deep veins; black labels are superficial veins.)

TABLE 15.4. PRECAUTIONS BEFORE IN-HOSPITAL TRANSPORT

Minimum of two persons including neurosciences nurse
Stable vital signs for 1 hour
Tracheal suctioning before transport
Patency of intravenous sites checked
Stable vital signs after manual bagging of the patient for several minutes
SaO₂ > 90%
No recent seizures
Mannitol infusion prepared if needed
When indicated, supplies such as antiepileptic drugs (lorazepam 4 mg)
Sufficient supply of administered fluids and drips
Monitor connected for arterial blood pressure tracings and electrocardiography
Defibrillator

surveyed.[90] Alcohol-based hand rub is easier than washing with soap and water, less irritating, takes less time, and is easily accessible. Users should rub all surfaces of hands and fingers, including fingertips, and it should take 15 seconds of rubbing for hands to dry; otherwise, the amount used is likely not enough. Washing with soap and water is preferred when hands are soiled and after caring for patients with *Clostridium difficile*–associated diarrhea. Handwashing has been well recognized as the most effective method to prevent the spread of infectious agents.[4,79] The type of soap or disinfectant probably is less important than the technique of handwashing. Adequate handwashing should ideally last 20 seconds, and a large volume of soap should be used. The faucet should be closed with a piece of paper towel if a lever is not available. In addition, irritant dermatitis (dry, flaky skin with multiple cracks) may occur with solutions containing chlorhexidine and therefore may discourage handwashing. Care should be taken not

TABLE 15.5. ISOLATION CATEGORIES AND EXAMPLES OF INFECTIOUS DISEASES IN EACH CATEGORY

Category	Requirements
Strict isolation	Private room
Rabies	Negative-pressure ventilation
Varicella	Masks, gowns, and gloves at all times
Hemorrhagic fever	Handwashing after glove removal
Contact isolation	Private room
Adenovirus	Mask when close to patient
Herpes simplex (disseminated)	Gowns if soiling likely
Major staphylococcal infections	Gloves for touching infectious material
	Handwashing after glove removal
Respiratory isolation	Private room
Infectious mononucleosis	Mask when close to patient
	Handwashing
Enteric precautions	Gowns if soiling likely
Enterovirus	Gloves for touching infectious material
Hepatitis A, E	Handwashing after glove removal
Salmonella	
Shigella	
Campylobacter	
Giardia	
Rotavirus	
Drainage and secretion precautions	Gowns if soiling likely
Herpes simplex (local)	Gloves for touching infectious material
Localized herpes zoster	Handwashing after glove removal
Blood and body fluid precautions	Fluid-resistant gowns
Arbovirus	Gloves for touching infectious material
Cytomegalovirus	Mask and glasses with side shields, goggles, or face shield
Hepatitis B, C, D	
Human immunodeficiency virus	Care with needles and sharp instruments

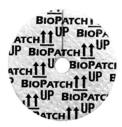

FIGURE 15.10: Biopatch®.

to use over-the-counter hand lotions, which may neutralize the antiseptic effect.

Another important aspect of infection precaution is the protection of patients from infections transmitted by blood or blood products. The most frequent serious transfusion complication is the transmission of hepatitis and human immunodeficiency virus-1 (HIV-1), but these risks are very low (see Chapter 60). In patients with critical neurologic illness, albumin is often used; this is a product of Cohn ethanol fractionation of plasma pools, in which all infectious viral particles should have been inactivated after pasteurization at 60°C for 10 hours.

Many nosocomial infections are associated with specific devices[57,73,110] (Chapter 59), but advice on how to prevent them changes frequently. Current recommendations are (a) maintenance of a sterile urinary closed drainage system and no breaking in to obtain urinary samples or to irrigate the bladder, (b) replacement of intravenous catheters every 2 or 3 days, (c) replacement of central lines every 7 days, and (d) proper handling of condensate in respiratory tubing, dispensing and storage of nebulized solutions, and changing of the tubing (but no more often than every 1–2 weeks). Central line associated bloodstream infections are reportable to the Centers for Medicare & Medicaid Services. Chlorhexidine gluconate impregnated disk are mandatory in many hospitals (Figure 15.10).

THE PATIENT'S FAMILY

More so than in any other type of medical or surgical ICU, the family represents the patient's interests, because patients with acute brain injury may not be able to communicate or comprehend adequately. This fundamentally important responsibility is also what critical care neurology is about, and conversations may occupy large parts of the day. A detailed work on communicating prognosis in critically ill neurologic patients has been recently published.[108]

Neurologists involved in the care of patients with an unexpected acute neurologic condition should foster a close physician–family relationship. The needs of family members are substantial and rather specific. Important predictors of patient family satisfaction have been identified: knowledge of the specific role of the caregiver, avoidance of contradictory information, and adequate time to meet with the attending physician.[10,26,27]

Visits by family members are allowed freely and there should be flexibility.[70] The inability of the ventilated patient to communicate has been identified as a major stressor, but the presence of family may provide calm for the agitated, reassurance for the anxious, and clarification for the overwhelmed. A guide is shown in Table 15.6.

Neurologists should allow families to insert their tragedies into their lives and seize on whatever may comfort them.[101] A positive rapport can only be established with repeated visits and actually taking the time to sit down with family members for more than a few minutes. The main goals are (a) clarification and explanation of the acute neurologic disorder, (b) discussion of the level of responsiveness of the patient, (c) estimation of the expected progression or improvement in the next days, (d) review of possible long-term outcome and expected level of functioning in broad categories of dependence and independence, and (e) establishment of the level of care.[83]

TABLE 15.6. CONVERSATIONS WITH FAMILY

Gather all close members including the person with power of attorney
Spend at least 30 minutes
Have nursing staff, clergy, social work, and other consultants present
Discuss "the big picture"
Discuss what the patient is noticing
Discuss what the patient would want under these circumstances
Discuss current plan
Discuss medical and neurosurgical options
Discuss best estimate of outcome
Discuss timeline of improvement, if any
Discuss code status
Set up follow-up meeting

From Wijdicks EFM, *Communicating Prognosis* (New York: Oxford University Press, 2014).

The ability of family members of patients with acute neurologic disorders to cope with the illness varies from family to family and, more importantly, among individuals. To help families cope with these tragic situations, repeated explanations and encouragement should be provided.[76,105] In most instances, the contacts with families are pleasant and cordial, leading to decisions by consensus. However, the sudden presentation of a very sick family member with a high likelihood of permanent intellectual disability may lead to rapid disintegration of an otherwise very caring family. Acute neurologic catastrophes may cause an acute stress reaction to some family members. Dissociative symptoms are often seen, characterized by depersonalization, crippling panic, and amnesia, which may be accompanied by sleeplessness and restlessness. Parental stress over the sufferings of children, particularly with change in appearance, is considerable. Watching resuscitation efforts, the placement of lines, and physicians rushing in is wrenching and bewildering to family members. Some families may think that "somebody has to be doing something wrong" and continue to display an oppositional mentality. Some families remain opaque in their understanding, and other family members remain mostly quiet, only to explode suddenly in anger and mistrust. Families evolve as they try to cope with a sudden devastating illness, but the evolution of behavior is not well known. (Most likely, the stages are very different from the stages of coping with terminal illness outlined by Kübler-Ross.[56])

Discussion with family members may also become convoluted when religious positions are voiced in such terms as "only He who gave life has the right to take life," and "God may work a miracle if that is His will." These families may continue to believe in dramatic change ("There is always hope"). Nevertheless, religious beliefs must be handled with sensitivity, and consultation with a religious advisor may be considered.

It is useful to have some knowledge of religious positions. The Catholic Church has always held the general view that the medical profession is unable to predict outcome with the utmost certainty except in brain death. The Catholic Church's principal tenet has been to support suffering families and to provide basic care (comfort, nutrition, and hydration) to the sick patient. Islam's traditional teaching is that believers should not give up hope and have no right to determine anyone else's right to die. This implies that the termination of support is not allowed. Devout

Muslims do not accept bad news because it may take away hope, and this can make a conversation addressing future expectations awkward. The Jewish law (Halacha) has accepted futility of care including brain death, although different rabbinic opinions exist.

Very important persons (VIPs) and their families pose a particularly demanding problem in the NICU.[85,92,103] A VIP can be arbitrarily defined as a celebrity, a major political figure, or, closer to home, a department member or board member of a large institution. With a VIP comes the *VIP syndrome*,[103] loosely defined as unusual medical care and unconventional reactions by the attending physician. It is commonplace in tertiary referral hospitals, where the syndrome may be marked by extensive testing for borderline abnormalities or the withholding of necessary procedures that may cause additional discomfort or have potentially major adverse effects.[14] In some attending neurologists, complete paralysis of action may occur.

Families of "VIPs" may have a tendency to raise questions about care more frequently than "non-VIPs." Medical colleagues who are friends of the family member may call, and some may even suggest changes in care. Friends interfere with daily rounds and may potentially reduce the time the treating physician has to spend with other patients and families. It is crucial to limit visits to only persons directly related to the patient, to restrict and concentrate communication with family members to certain time slots (morning and afternoon rounds), and to inform the family and patient that care will follow the same high standards that it does for any and all patients.[92] In these situations, the responsibility of the attending neurologist should be clear, and his decisions should not be diffused by multiple consultations.

The Family Conference

Every attempt should be made to present the clinical condition of the patient to the family in an unambiguous manner, especially to those family members most significant to the patient.[19,94] When appropriate, family members should be encouraged to travel, if necessary, to meet with the clinical staff. Ideally, the nursing staff caring for the patient should be present and should become actively involved in the discussion. The presentation of the clinical neurologic situation should be lucid, and showing family members the lesion on computed tomography (CT) scan often helps to clarify the gravity of the situation. It is important to discuss the level of coma, the patient's experience of pain, why the patient may seem to be fighting the ventilator, the meaning of twitching in the face or limbs, and the cause of agitation. Opening of eyes, blinking, grimacing, grinding of teeth, and sleep–wake cycles could be part of a developing vegetative state and, if this is the case, should be explained.[33,74]

Explaining a locked-in syndrome to family members is particularly difficult. Family members should be made aware that communication is possible only through "yes" and "no" replies conveyed by blinking or vertical eye movements. A simple code, such as one blink for "yes" and three blinks for "no," is helpful and should be posted at the bedside, although responsiveness may wax and wane during the day. The patient and family may want to continue maximal support, including tracheostomy and gastrostomy, but often significant pneumonias intervene, resulting in early death.

Early in the discussion with the family, the actual prospects for recovery must be reviewed. It is important to take time in discussing these matters, realizing that, despite hard evidence to the contrary, the family's initial assessment of prognosis can be more optimistic than the physician's.[67] The attending neurologist should also explain the morbidity if the patient would survive. This, then, could initiate a discussion about quality of life. In this discussion, it is prudent to discuss the possibility of depression, lack of initiative, irritability, disinhibition, and the possibility of being wheelchair bound. Simple explanations such as "survive but handicapped," "survive but walk with a cane," "two-thirds will do poorly," or "cannot tell" are ambiguous and are not helpful in decision-making. To state that a major brain injury with a handicap is worse than death is perhaps a half-truth and has not always been supported by studies that have examined patients surviving this injury. When no improvement in the neurologic deficit is seen and the outlook for a meaningful recovery is remote, withdrawal of treatment and withdrawal of support should be discussed with the family. It may be effective to say, "I wish we could do more to turn things around, and I wish it had been otherwise."[75] One should be aware of each person's right to refuse medical treatment, and some may have legally formalized this right in advance directives. It is imperative to follow these instructions to the fullest extent possible, and the physician should ask family members whether a directive is in effect. Of a number of advance directives, the two most common are the *living will*, which gives specific directions about types of treatment and may appoint a proxy to make decisions on the patient's behalf when a terminal illness exists. The other is a *durable power of attorney*, which authorizes another person to make decisions on the patient's behalf even though the patient is not terminally ill.

An advance directive, however, becomes effective only when patients cannot make and communicate their own decisions. In addition, these documents do not override reasonable medical practice, such as care to provide comfort, to control pain, and to give food and water by mouth when a patient accepts them. The laws regulating advance directives may vary by state, and out-of-state directives may not comply with the laws of the state where the patient is admitted.

No neurointensivist wants to deprive the patient or family of a possible reasonable outcome. No neurointensivist should show a false determined unconquerable spirit when patients are at a breaking point. No neurointensivist should throw in the towel too early. But for some families to demand to have everything done could conflict with the inability to do anything. Many families understand that a perfect prediction is difficult, but optimism and pessimism have no role in straightforward conversations. It does not make sense to withdraw critical care early or move to a DNR status if patients could recover from surgery or other medical measures.

Withdrawal of Care

The decision of families to withdraw care from a patient who has not clearly expressed any wishes in an advance directive or in passing is very difficult, and the burden of responsibility placed on family members is enormous. Some families remain reluctant to accept a grim prognosis, voice distrust, and rationalize the continuation of therapy by recalling examples of acquaintances who "unexpectedly recovered" after long intervals.[106]

When withdrawal is considered, a plan should be discussed with the family.[69] It is useful to state a certain time period in which the next decision is to be made (e.g., no major improvement in a week, do not resuscitate). The decision can be made not to intubate and resuscitate in patients with severe neurologic disability. In these cases, the neurologist must state that resuscitation is likely to bring more suffering than benefit. Withdrawal of treatment may proceed through several levels, from withdrawal from high-technology support (e.g., mechanical ventilation, dialysis, pacemakers, cardiopulmonary resuscitation) to withdrawal of medication (e.g., antibiotics, vasopressors, insulin, antiarrhythmia agents) and withdrawal of hydration and nutrition. Not infrequently, families are themselves immediately convinced of the hopeless situation and can make the decision early to pursue comfort care only.

Another level of withdrawal of support is treatment of infection. Pneumonia and urinary tract infections that develop in many patients can be treated easily and often when treated are not life-threatening. It should be decided whether sepsis or sepsis syndrome is to be treated, because management requires additional hemodynamic monitoring and readmission to the ICU.

Discussion of Brain Death and Organ Donation

Telling a family that a patient fulfills the clinical criteria of brain death is a common task of the neurointensivist (Chapters 63–65). The family should be told in unequivocal terms that brain function has ceased and the patient is no longer here, has passed away, and that there is 100% certainty. Mechanical ventilation and pharmaceutical support are continued in the event the family agrees to the donation of organs and tissue. The initial discussion of organ donation with family members is necessary but potentially threatening, and occasionally the perception of family members is that the physician is rushing from one decision to another. It is helpful, if the opportunity exists, to frequently visit the family briefly before organ donation is discussed. Organ donation saves many lives or dramatically improves the quality of life for many others. A comprehensive discussion of organ donation is done by organ-procurement officers, and their intervention is legally required in the United States. During these meetings, the procedure of organ procurement is described to emphasize that no additional medical costs will be incurred. The charges are the responsibility of the organ procurement agency, which reclaims them from the insurance carrier of the recipients. A follow-up letter on the outcome of donation is sent. The recipients remain anonymous, but occasionally family members have sought contact with them (and the meeting has been comforting). After a decision to donate organs has been made, family members need to visit before organ retrieval. Only a minority of families asks to see the patient after organ retrieval, but if they do, they must be offered this chance to see their loved one.

Family members play an important role in the decision to forgo organ donation, because the patient's preference generally is not known. A recent telephone poll found that only 30% of respondents had decided to donate and that 38% had made their wishes known to family members.[93] Once a patient has given valid consent, it cannot be overridden (under the Uniform Anatomical Gift Act). It is exceedingly rare for family members to disagree with donation if signed consent by the patient is available (usually on a driver's license). Nonetheless, if this situation occurs, it is ill-advised to proceed with organ donation. In all US states, transplant surgeons require the next of kin's permission before removing any organ.

The refusal of families to proceed with donation is based on many reasons, including less rational ones ("came to this life with a complete body and will leave with a complete body"). Refusal of donation removes the need for further support. Most families understand this concept very well. The family must be given adequate time to visit the patient to pay their last respects. It is questionable whether family should be present during discontinuation of ventilation support, because some patients have motor reflex movements. Although these signs are uncommon, considerable effort is required to explain to observing family members that these are reflex movements originating in the spinal cord.

Infrequently, family members want continuation of mechanical ventilation and pharmacologic support because the concept of brain death is not understood. Repeated communication to family members explaining that brain death equates to loss of life is not always helpful and could even result in more distrust. If mechanical ventilation is continued, cardiac arrest usually emerges. In New Jersey and New York, religious exemptions have been added to official statutes, creating possible liability if the mechanical ventilator is disconnected. The important ethical issues surrounding these complex situations have been discussed in a monograph.[107] Hospital ethics committee members may be consulted when this delicate problem occurs.

CONCLUSIONS

- The general aspects of care of critically ill neurologic patients involve eye care, oral care, positioning, and comprehensive monitoring by neurosciences nursing staff.

- Alignment of the body is monitored daily: arms flexed, hands on pillows, and trochanter rolls in place. Compression points are monitored for development of erythema or early decubital ulcers.

- Incentive spirometry (every 2 hours; 6 trials during the day) is begun in patients with neuromuscular respiratory failure and after craniotomy.

- The number of passages during bronchial suctioning must be limited. Evidence of further increase in intracranial pressure should be followed by muting of the response with lidocaine spayed endotracheally.

- Requirements for intrahospital transport are stable vital signs for 1 hour, adequate oxygen saturation, and absence of recent seizures. For patients at risk, albumin 5%, mannitol infusion, and anticonvulsants are prepared for possible use during transport.

- Categories of isolation (Centers for Disease Control and Prevention) are strict control, contact isolation, respiratory isolation, tuberculosis isolation, and specific disease isolation precautions (hepatitis, AIDS).

- Time is taken for detailed communication with the family. Outcome expectations should be explained early, and the purpose of level of care should be clear stated.

REFERENCES

1. Ackland HM, Cooper DJ, Malham GM, Kossmann T. Factors predicting cervical collar-related decubitus ulceration in major trauma patients. *Spine* 2007;32:423–428.
2. Adams HP, Jr., del Zoppo G, Alberts MJ, et al. Guidelines for the early management of adults with ischemic stroke: a guideline from the American Heart Association/American Stroke Association Stroke Council, Clinical Cardiology Council, Cardiovascular Radiology and Intervention Council, and the Atherosclerotic Peripheral Vascular Disease and Quality of Care Outcomes in Research Interdisciplinary Working Groups: The American Academy of Neurology affirms the value of this guideline as an educational tool for neurologists. *Circulation* 2007;115:e478–e534.
3. Agnelli G, Piovella F, Buoncristiani P, et al. Enoxaparin plus compression stockings compared with compression stockings alone in the prevention of venous thromboembolism after elective neurosurgery. *N Engl J Med* 1998;339:80–85.
4. Albert RK, Condie F. Hand-washing patterns in medical intensive-care units. *N Engl J Med* 1981;304:1465–1466.
5. Alhazzani W, Lim W, Jaeschke RZ, et al. Heparin thromboprophylaxis in medical-surgical critically ill patients: a systematic review and meta-analysis of randomized trials. *Crit Care Med* 2013;41: 2088–2098.
6. Andersen KE, Jensen O, Kvorning SA, Bach E. Prevention of pressure sores by identifying patients at risk. *Br Med J* 1982;284: 1370–1371.
7. Andrews PJ, Piper IR, Dearden NM, Miller JD. Secondary insults during intrahospital transport of head-injured patients. *Lancet* 1990;335: 327–330.
8. Assanasen S, Edmond M, Bearman G. Impact of 2 different levels of performance feedback on compliance with infection control process measures in 2 intensive care units. *Am J Infect Control* 2008;36:407–413.
9. Attia J, Ray JG, Cook DJ, et al. Deep vein thrombosis and its prevention in critically ill adults. *Arch Intern Med* 2001;161:1268–1279.
10. Azoulay E, Pochard F, Chevret S, et al. Meeting the needs of intensive care unit patient families: a multicenter study. *Am J Respir Crit Care Med* 2001;163:135–139.
11. Bates-Jensen BM. Pressure ulcers: pathophysiology and prevention. In: Sussman C, Bates-Jensen BM, eds. *Wound Care: A Collaborative Practice Manual for Physical Therapists and Nurses.* Gaithersburg, MD: Aspen Publishers; 1998:235–270.
12. Benoit RA, Jr., Watts C. The effect of a pressure ulcer prevention program and the bowel management system in reducing pressure ulcer prevalence in an ICU setting. *J Wound Ostomy Cont Nurs* 2007;34:163–175.
13. Bischoff WE, Reynolds TM, Sessler CN, Edmond MB, Wenzel RP. Handwashing compliance by health care workers: the impact of introducing an accessible, alcohol-based hand antiseptic. *Arch Intern Med* 2000;160:1017–1021.
14. Block AJ. Beware of the VIP syndrome. *Chest* 1993;104:989.
15. Boeer A, Voth E, Henze T, Prange HW. Early heparin therapy in patients with spontaneous intracerebral haemorrhage. *J Neurol Neurosurg Psychiatry* 1991;54:466–467.
16. Boyce JM, Kelliher S, Vallande N. Skin irritation and dryness associated with two hand-hygiene regimens: soap-and-water hand washing versus hand antisepsis with an alcoholic hand gel. *Infect Cont Hosp Ep* 2000;21:442–448.
17. Braden B, Bergstrom N. A conceptual schema for the study of the etiology of pressure sores. *Rehabil Nurs* 1987;12:8–12.
18. Burton DC, Edwards JR, Horan TC, Jernigan JA, Fridkin SK. Methicillin-resistant Staphylococcus aureus central line-associated bloodstream infections in US intensive care units, 1997–2007. *JAMA* 2009;301:727–736.
19. Campbell ML, Guzman JA. Impact of a proactive approach to improve end-of-life care in a medical ICU. *Chest* 2003;123:266–271.

20. Carlson EV, Kemp MG, Shott S. Predicting the risk of pressure ulcers in critically ill patients. *Am J Crit Care* 1999;8:262–269.

21. Carr EK, Kenney FD. Positioning of the stroke patient: a review of the literature. *Int J Nurs Stud* 1992;29:355–369.

22. Ciesla ND. Chest physical therapy for patients in the intensive care unit. *Phys Ther* 1996;76:609–625.

23. Clarke-Pearson DL, Synan IS, Dodge R, et al. A randomized trial of low-dose heparin and intermittent pneumatic calf compression for the prevention of deep venous thrombosis after gynecologic oncology surgery. *Am J Obstet Gynecol* 1993;168:1146–1153.

24. Coe NP, Collins RE, Klein LA, et al. Prevention of deep vein thrombosis in urological patients: a controlled, randomized trial of low-dose heparin and external pneumatic compression boots. *Surgery* 1978;83:230–234.

25. Compton F, Hoffmann F, Hortig T, et al. Pressure ulcer predictors in ICU patients: nursing skin assessment versus objective parameters. *J Wound Care* 2008;17:417–420, 422–414.

26. Curtis JR, Engelberg RA, Wenrich MD, et al. Missed opportunities during family conferences about end-of-life care in the intensive care unit. *Am J Respir Crit Care Med* 2005;171:844–849.

27. Curtis JR, White DB. Practical guidance for evidence-based ICU family conferences. *Chest* 2008;134:835–843.

28. Damas P, Frippiat F, Ancion A, et al. Prevention of ventilator-associated pneumonia and ventilator-associated conditions: a randomized controlled trial with subglottic secretion suctioning. *Crit Care Med* 2015;43:22–30.

29. Dennis M, Sandercock P, Reid J, et al. Effect of intermittent pneumatic compression on disability, living circumstances, quality of life, and hospital costs after stroke: secondary analyses from CLOTS 3, a randomized trial. *Lancet Neurol* 2014;13:1186–1192.

30. Dennis M, Sandercock P, Reid J, et al. Effectiveness of intermittent pneumatic compression in reduction of risk of deep vein thrombosis in patients who have had a stroke (CLOTS 3): a multicenter randomized controlled trial. *Lancet* 2013;382:516–524.

31. Dennis M, Sandercock PA, Reid J, et al. Effectiveness of thigh-length graduated compression stockings to reduce the risk of deep vein thrombosis after stroke (CLOTS trial 1): a multicenter, randomized controlled trial. *Lancet* 2009;373:1958–1965.

32. Dubbert PM, Dolce J, Richter W, Miller M, Chapman SW. Increasing ICU staff handwashing: effects of education and group feedback. *Infect Cont Hosp Ep* 1990;11:191–193.

33. Engelberg RA, Wenrich MD, Curtis JR. Responding to families' questions about the meaning of physical movements in critically ill patients. *J Crit Care* 2008;23:565–571.

34. Engels PT, Beckett AN, Rubenfeld GD, et al. Physical rehabilitation of the critically ill trauma patient in the ICU. *Crit Care Med* 2013;41:1790–1801.

35. Fife C, Otto G, Capsuto EG, et al. Incidence of pressure ulcers in a neurologic intensive care unit. *Crit Care Med* 2001;29:283–290.

36. Fortney SM, Schneider VS, Greenleaf JE. *The Physiology of Bed Rest*. New York: Oxford University Press; 1996.

37. Garner JS. Guideline for isolation precautions in hospitals. The Hospital Infection Control Practices Advisory Committee. *Infect Cont Hosp Ep* 1996;17:53–80.

38. Garradd J, Bullock M. The effect of respiratory therapy on intracranial pressure in ventilated neurosurgical patients. *Aust J Physiother* 1986;32:107–111.

39. Guyatt GH, Eikelboom JW, Gould MK, et al. Approach to outcome measurement in the prevention of thrombosis in surgical and medical patients: Antithrombotic Therapy and Prevention of Thrombosis, 9th ed: American College of Chest Physicians Evidence-Based Clinical Practice Guidelines. *Chest* 2012;141:e185S–e194S.

40. Girou E, Pujade G, Legrand P, Cizeau F, Brun-Buisson C. Selective screening of carriers for control of methicillin-resistant Staphylococcus aureus (MRSA) in high-risk hospital areas with a high level of endemic MRSA. *Clin Infect Dis* 1998;27:543–550.

41. Graham M. Frequency and duration of handwashing in an intensive care unit. *Am J Infect Control* 1990;18:77–81.

42. Guralnik JM, Harris TB, White LR, Cornoni-Huntley JC. Occurrence and predictors of pressure sores in the National Health and Nutrition Examination survey follow-up. *J Am Geriatr Soc* 1988;36:807–812.

43. Hodgin KE, Nordon-Craft A, McFann KK, Mealer ML, Moss M. Physical therapy utilization in intensive care units: results from a national survey. *Crit Care Med* 2009;37:561–566.

44. Hofman A, Geelkerken RH, Wille J, et al. Pressure sores and pressure-decreasing mattresses: controlled clinical trial. *Lancet* 1994;343:568–571.

45. Hugonnet S, Perneger TV, Pittet D. Alcohol-based handrub improves compliance with hand hygiene in intensive care units. *Arch Intern Med* 2002;162:1037–1043.

46. Imanaka H, Taenaka N, Nakamura J, Aoyama K, Hosotani H. Ocular surface disorders in the critically ill. *Anesth Analg* 1997;85:343–346.

47. Investigators TAiIS. Abciximab in acute ischemic stroke: a randomized, double-blind,

placebo-controlled, dose-escalation study. *Stroke* 2000;31:601–609.

48. Jelic S, Cunningham JA, Factor P. Clinical review: airway hygiene in the intensive care unit. *Crit Care* 2008;12:209.

49. Ji T, Zubkov AY, Wijdicks EFM, et al. Massive tongue swelling in refractory status epilepticus treated with high-dose pentobarbital. *Neurocrit Care* 2009;10:73–75.

50. Kase CS, Albers GW, Bladin C, et al. Neurological outcomes in patients with ischemic stroke receiving enoxaparin or heparin for venous thromboembolism prophylaxis: subanalysis of the Prevention of VTE after Acute Ischemic Stroke with LMWH (PREVAIL) study. *Stroke* 2009;40:3532–3540.

51. Kearon C. Natural history of venous thromboembolism. *Circulation* 2003;107:I22–30.

52. Kearon C, Julian JA, Newman TE, Ginsberg JS. Noninvasive diagnosis of deep venous thrombosis. McMaster Diagnostic Imaging Practice Guidelines Initiative. *Ann Intern Med* 1998;128:663–677.

53. Kelly J, Rudd A, Lewis R, Hunt BJ. Venous thromboembolism after acute stroke. *Stroke* 2001;32:262–267.

54. Klein K, Mulkey M, Bena JF, Albert NM. Clinical and psychologic effects of early mobilization in patients treated in a neurologic ICU: a comparative study. *Crit Care Med* 2015;43:865–873.

55. Kortebein P, Ferrando A, Lombeida J, Wolfe R, Evans WJ. Effect of 10 days of bed rest on skeletal muscle in healthy older adults. *JAMA* 2007;297:1772–1774.

56. Kübler-Ross E. *Death: The Final Stage of Growth.* Englewood Cliffs, NJ: Prentice-Hall; 1975.

57. Labeau SO, Vandijck DM, Rello J, et al. Centers for Disease Control and Prevention guidelines for preventing central venous catheter-related infection: results of a knowledge test among 3405 European intensive care nurses. *Crit Care Med* 2009;37: 320–323.

58. Larson EL, Aiello AE, Bastyr J, et al. Assessment of two hand hygiene regimens for intensive care unit personnel. *Crit Care Med* 2001;29:944–951.

59. Lee TS, Schrader MW, Wright BD. Subconjunctival emphysema as a complication of PEEP. *Ann Ophthalmol* 1980;12:1080–1081.

60. Linnarsson D, Spaak J, Sundblad P. Baroreflex impairment during rapid posture changes at rest and exercise after 120 days of bed rest. *Eur J Appl Physiol* 2006;96:37–45.

61. Manzano F, Colmenero M, Perez-Perez AM, et al. Comparison of two repositioning schedules for the prevention of pressure ulcers in patients on mechanical ventilation with alternating pressure air mattresses. *Intens Care Med* 2014;40: 1679–1687.

62. Martin UJ, Hincapie L, Nimchuk M, Gaughan J, Criner GJ. Impact of whole-body rehabilitation in patients receiving chronic mechanical ventilation. *Crit Care Med* 2005;33:2259–2265.

63. McLeod AG, Geerts W. Venous thromboembolism prophylaxis in critically ill patients. *Crit Care Clin* 2011;27:765–780, v.

64. Montmerle S, Spaak J, Linnarsson D. Lung function during and after prolonged head-down bed rest. *J Appl Physiol* 2002;92:75–83.

65. Norrenberg M, Vincent JL. A profile of European intensive care unit physiotherapists. European Society of Intensive Care Medicine. *Intens Care Med* 2000;26:988–994.

66. Ntoumenopoulos G, Gild A, Cooper DJ. The effect of manual lung hyperinflation and postural drainage on pulmonary complications in mechanically ventilated trauma patients. *Anaesth Intensive Care* 1998;26:492–496.

67. O'Callahan JG, Fink C, Pitts LH, Luce JM. Withholding and withdrawing of life support from patients with severe head injury. *Crit Care Med* 1995;23:1567–1575.

68. O'Donnell A. Handwashing. *Lancet* 2000;355:156.

69. O'Toole EE, Youngner SJ, Juknialis BW, et al. Evaluation of a treatment limitation policy with a specific treatment-limiting order page. *Arch Intern Med* 1994;154:425–432.

70. Olsen KD, Dysvik E, Hansen BS. The meaning of family members' presence during intensive care stay: a qualitative study. *Intens Crit Care Nurs* 2009;25:190–198.

71. Overend TJ, Anderson CM, Lucy SD, et al. The effect of incentive spirometry on postoperative pulmonary complications: a systematic review. *Chest* 2001;120:971–978.

72. Peterson M, Schwab W, McCutcheon K, et al. Effects of elevating the head of bed on interface pressure in volunteers. *Crit Care Med* 2008;36:3038–3042.

73. Pronovost P. Interventions to decrease catheter-related bloodstream infections in the ICU: the Keystone Intensive Care Unit Project. *Am J Infect Control* 2008;36:S171 e171–e175.

74. The Multi-Society Task Force on PVS Medical aspects of the persistent vegetative state (parts 1 and 2). *N Engl J Med* 1994;330:1499–1508; 1572–1579.

75. Quill TE, Arnold RM, Platt F. "I wish things were different": expressing wishes in response to loss, futility, and unrealistic hopes. *Ann Intern Med* 2001;135:551–555.

76. Rabow MW, Hauser JM, Adams J. Supporting family caregivers at the end of life: "they don't know what they don't know." *JAMA* 2004;291:483–491.

77. Raoof S, Chowdhrey N, Feuerman M, et al. Effect of combined kinetic therapy and percussion therapy on the resolution of atelectasis in critically ill patients. *Chest* 1999;115:1658–1666.

78. Ray WZ, Strom RG, Blackburn SL, et al. Incidence of deep venous thrombosis after subarachnoid hemorrhage. *J Neurosurg* 2009;110:1010–1014.

79. Reybrouck G. Handwashing and hand disinfection. *J Hosp Infect* 1986;8:5–23.

80. Rieg AD, Stoppe C, Rossaint R, et al. EzPAP(R) therapy of postoperative hypoxemia in the recovery room: experiences with the new compact system of end-expiratory positive airway pressure. *Anaesthesist* 2012;61:867–874.

81. Rohdin M, Petersson J, Sundblad P, et al. Effects of gravity on lung diffusing capacity and cardiac output in prone and supine humans. *J Appl Physiol* 2003;95:3–10.

82. Rosenberg JB, Eisen LA. Eye care in the intensive care unit: narrative review and meta-analysis. *Crit Care Med* 2008;36:3151–3155.

83. Rubin SB. *When Doctors Say No: The Battleground of Medical Futility*. Bloomington: Indiana University Press; 1998.

84. Sarnaik AP, Lieh-Lai MW. Transporting the neurologically compromised child. *Pediatr Clin N Am* 1993;40:337–354.

85. Schneck SA. "Doctoring" doctors and their families. *JAMA* 1998;280:2039–2042.

86. Schubert V, Heraud J. The effects of pressure and shear on skin microcirculation in elderly stroke patients lying in supine or semi-recumbent positions. *Age Ageing* 1994;23:405–410.

87. Schweickert WD, Pohlman MC, Pohlman AS, et al. Early physical and occupational therapy in mechanically ventilated, critically ill patients: a randomised controlled trial. *Lancet* 2009;373: 1874–1882.

88. Sears VW, Jr., Castell JA, Castell DO. Comparison of effects of upright versus supine body position and liquid versus solid bolus on esophageal pressures in normal humans. *Dig Dis Sci* 1990;35:857–864.

89. Seligsohn U, Lubetsky A. Genetic susceptibility to venous thrombosis. *N Engl J Med* 2001;344:1222–1231.

90. Simmons B, Bryant J, Neiman K, Spencer L, Arheart K. The role of handwashing in prevention of endemic intensive care unit infections. *Infect Cont Hosp Ep* 1990;11:589–594.

91. Smith I, Fleming S, Cernaianu A. Mishaps during transport from the intensive care unit. *Crit Care Med* 1990;18:278–281.

92. Smith MS, Shesser RF. The emergency care of the VIP patient. *N Engl J Med* 1988;319:1421–1423.

93. Spital A. Mandated choice: a plan to increase public commitment to organ donation. *JAMA* 1995;273:504–506.

94. Stapleton RD, Engelberg RA, Wenrich MD, Goss CH, Curtis JR. Clinician statements and family satisfaction with family conferences in the intensive care unit. *Crit Care Med* 2006;34:1679–1685.

95. Stiller K. Physiotherapy in intensive care: towards an evidence-based practice. *Chest* 2000;118:1801–1813.

96. Suetta C, Andersen JL, Dalgas U, et al. Resistance training induces qualitative changes in muscle morphology, muscle architecture, and muscle function in elderly postoperative patients. *J Appl Physiol (1985)* 2008;105:180–186.

97. The Avert study group Efficacy and safety of very early mobilisation within 24 h of stroke onset (AVERT): a randomised controlled trial. *Lancet* 2015;386:46–55

98. Turpie AG, Hirsh J, Gent M, Julian D, Johnson J. Prevention of deep vein thrombosis in potential neurosurgical patients: a randomized trial comparing graduated compression stockings alone or graduated compression stockings plus intermittent pneumatic compression with control. *Arch Intern Med* 1989;149:679–681.

99. Velmahos GC, Toutouzas KG, Sarkisyan G, et al. Severe trauma is not an excuse for prolonged antibiotic prophylaxis. *Arch Surg* 2002;137:537–541.

100. Vernon DD, Woodward GA, Skjonsberg AK. Management of the patient with head injury during transport. *Crit Care Clin* 1992;8:619–631.

101. Wall RJ, Curtis JR, Cooke CR, Engelberg RA. Family satisfaction in the ICU: differences between families of survivors and nonsurvivors. *Chest* 2007;132:1425–1433.

102. Warren DK, Fraser VJ. Infection control measures to limit antimicrobial resistance. *Crit Care Med* 2001;29:N128–N134.

103. Weintraub W. "The VIP syndrome": a clinical study in hospital psychiatry. *J Nerv Ment Dis* 1964;138:181–193.

104. Wells PS, Le Gal G, Tierney S, Carrier M. Practical application of the 10-mg warfarin initiation nomogram. *Blood Coagul Fibrinolysis* 2009;20:403–408.

105. White DB, Braddock CH, 3rd, Bereknyei S, Curtis JR. Toward shared decision making at the end of life in intensive care units: opportunities for improvement. *Arch Intern Med* 2007;167: 461–467.

106. Wijdicks EFM, Rabinstein AA. The family conference: end-of-life guidelines at work for comatose patients. *Neurology* 2007;68:1092–1094.

107. Wijdicks EFM. *Brain Death*. 2nd edition. New York: Oxford University Press; 2011.

108. Wijdicks EFM. *Communicating Prognosis*. New York: Oxford University Press; 2014.

109. Witterick P, Stuart R, Gillespie E, Buist M. Hand hygiene during the intensive care unit ward round: how much is enough? An observational study. *Crit Care Resusc* 2008;10:285–287.

110. Zack J. Zeroing in on zero tolerance for central line-associated bacteremia. *Am J Infect Control* 2008;36:S176. e171–e172.

16

Agitation and Pain

Rapid administration of a sedative may seem appropriate in patients with an acute neurologic illness who are agitated and uncomfortable. It may not only provide proper anxiolysis but may also reduce oxygen consumption and mute the hyperdynamic stress response.[82] It may prevent the pulling of intravascular and bladder catheters and endotracheal and nasogastric tubes, which additionally may pose a danger to the patient.

There are pressing concerns when it comes to administering sedation to patients with acute neurologic disorders. Traditionally, neurologists have bitterly opposed the use of any form of sedation to counter agitation, particularly when administered in an uncertain neurologic condition that has the propensity to worsen. However, this reluctance can be overcome when recovery after discontinuation of sedation is rapid, interaction with other drugs is minimal, or sedation can be reversed with an appropriate antidote.[82] Current examples are propofol and midazolam, both of which have some of these attributes. In addition, patients are benefited greatly by the additional amnestic properties of most anesthetic agents. On the other hand, the common practice of intermittent interruption of sedated patients in medical and surgical intensive care units (ICUs) may be problematic in patients sedated to control increased intracranial pressure.[33,46] Discontinuation of sedation to assess the patient may cause unwanted spikes.[83]

Effective pain management is limited by the poor safety profile of most currently used analgesic agents. Narcotics do not have amnestic or anxiolytic qualities. Furthermore, morphine or fentanyl has a perceptible risk of respiratory depression, an unacceptable situation in patients with neuromuscular respiratory failure and in patients with poor brain compliance, who may not tolerate a relative increase in PCO_2 from hypoventilation. Long-term use of opioids also paralyzes the gut and may come on suddenly.

Newer nonsteroidal anti-inflammatory drugs (NSAIDs) circumvent these concerns but may increase bleeding time and are obviously less suitable, if not contraindicated, for patients with intracranial hemorrhage. Dexmedetomidine is another commonly used drug—if heart rate and blood pressure remain stable—for postoperative sedation and pain control, and it also attenuates cardiovascular responses to endotracheal intubation. Its role in management of agitation, delirium and other feelings of disquiet in very aware mechanically ventilated patients is increasing.[79]

This chapter discusses the assessment and management of agitation and pain, and the pharmacologic choices currently available in the NICU.

CAUSES OF AGITATION

Extreme restlessness, with a mixture of shouting, combative behavior, and disorganized thinking, poses difficulties not only in neurologic assessment but also in management. Self-extubation and the pulling out of central venous access by an agitated patient can cause harm and—at least in one study—in one-third of patients with self-extubation, a potentially life-threatening event may occur.[22] Fairly typical neurologic causes for profound agitation and acute confusional state are bifrontal cerebral infarcts or frontal lobe hematomas in aneurysmal subarachnoid hemorrhage, infarction of the basal ganglia, large infarcts of the middle cerebral artery territory,[59] and involvement of the thalamus, such as occurs in basilar artery occlusion.

The primary central nervous system (CNS) injury can be implicated in many agitated patients, but other causes should be sought. Occasionally, a major withdrawal delirium is the basis of acute confusion. Delirium is typically seen first at night and should be suspected when clinical features such as restlessness, short attention span, perceptional distortions or vivid hallucinations are present.[50,51] Substance withdrawal remains a very important possibility in acute delirium (Table 16.1). Therefore, neurologists should be aware that agitation in any recently hospitalized patient may point to prior substance addiction.[16] In patients with head traumatic brain, ethanol

TABLE 16.1. CAUSES OF DELIRIUM IN THE NEUROSCIENCES INTENSIVE CARE UNIT

Withdrawal syndromes

Alcohol

Benzodiazepines

Barbiturates

Opioids

Central nervous system stimulants

Drug-induced

Antibiotics

Antiarrhythmic agents

Anticholinergic agents

Antihistamines

ß-blockers

Opioids

Metabolic derangements

Hyponatremia

Hyperosmolar hyperglycemia

Endocrine crises

withdrawal is one of the strongest contenders. Alcoholic delirium may be manifested by a generalized tonic-clonic seizure and is a psychiatric emergency. As early as 6–8 hours after stopping drinking, and usually on the day of admission, these patients manifest marked restlessness, disordered perception, shouting at hallucinated objects with lucidity between hallucinations, profound diaphoresis, generalized tremor, sustained tachycardia, respiratory alkalosis, and, often, a significant increase in blood pressure. The prevalence of extreme manifestations or fatal cases is low, possibly because of the increasing use of benzodiazepines for detoxification.

Alcohol-related seizures are often from withdrawal, despite a history of traumatic brain injury. The time to the first seizure from withdrawal varies greatly. More than 50% of patients have multiple seizures, but seizures may be an isolated manifestation because only one-third ultimately have delirium tremens. When seizures occur, it may be prudent to repeat a computed tomography (CT) scan of the brain. However, in a prospective study, the majority of 259 patients with alcohol-withdrawal seizures had normal CT scan findings or cerebral atrophy. In 6% of these patients, a structural lesion was found after the first alcohol-withdrawal seizure, with a potential neurosurgical lesion in half of the cases.[28] When the initial CT is normal, cerebrospinal fluid examination

is mandatory to exclude bacterial meningitis in patients with alcohol abuse. Other considerations in a restless, agitated alcoholic patient are concomitant use of drugs such as cocaine, sepsis, and acute hepatic failure.

Agitation or delirium may be triggered by a toxic response to medication and, less commonly, by acute metabolic derangement. These causes listed in Table 16.1, are not so well defined in the NICU setting, but must be seriously considered in a delirious patient.

Postictal confusion after a seizure or nonconvulsive status epilepticus should be considered. However, nonconvulsive status epilepticus produces a fluctuating twilight state more often than significant combativeness.

Agitation may also have its origin in marginal ventilation and gas exchange. Patients with aspiration pneumonitis or early acute respiratory distress syndrome (ARDS) may become significantly tachypneic and agitated, and oxygenation rapidly becomes insufficient. Mechanical ventilation is often only possible with some degree of sedation (intravenous infusion with lorazepam) and occasionally with use of neuromuscular junction blocking agents. Sedation alone allows positive end-expiratory pressure (PEEP) ventilation and improves gas exchange.

An uncommon cause of agitation is an adverse effect from a contrast agent after cerebral angiography. Acute combativeness, cortical blindness, seizures, nonconvulsive status epilepticus, and even anomic aphasia may occur, but resolve within 24 hours in most patients.[87] This rather dramatic side effect can be managed with mannitol 20% (1 g/kg) to osmotically draw the contrast material out and dexamethasone (10 mg bolus IV, followed by 4 mg every 6 hours) to stabilize the blood–brain barrier. Sedation by repeated boluses of lorazepam (2–4 mg IV) or low doses of propofol per infusion (0.1 mg/kg/hr) is often required.

PHARMACEUTICAL AGENTS FOR SEDATION

Time-honored methods such as company, touch, and a comforting voice are unlikely to be effective in the NICU, and pharmacologic intervention is often considered. The marked autonomic features of delirium warrant immediate treatment.[74] Other (less tested) options include the promotion of sleep, assuming a relation between sleep deprivation and delirium. Music therapy (music through headphones) has not been proven useful in delirium but may reduce anxiety in recovering patients.

The key steps in the treatment of alcohol withdrawal are rehydration, cooling, and prevention of self-harm and harm to others. Lorazepam is a preferred choice in neurologic patients. Haloperidol may reduce the seizure threshold and is a poor choice in susceptible patients. Most experts treat alcohol withdrawal syndrome with intravenous or intramuscular administration of lorazepam, 1–2 mg every 4 hours, avoid phenothiazines and other benzodiazepines, but consider repeated doses of chlordiazepoxide, 50–100 mg intravenously or intramuscularly (up to 300 mg/day).[55] Recurrent seizures are markedly reduced with the use of lorazepam in alcohol withdrawal syndrome.[24] Patients with severe tachycardia, diaphoresis, and hypertension may specifically benefit from oral clonidine (0.2 mg initially, then 0.2 mg three times a day for 2 days, and 0.2 mg on day 4).[6] Alcohol-related seizures may be associated with hypomagnesemia. Although this alleged association has been questioned, hypomagnesemia and other confounding derangements such as hypoglycemia or hypocalcemia should be corrected. Prophylactic antiepileptic medication is not needed, and treatment with fosphenytoin is indicated only for recurrent seizures or patients with prior seizures.

Although sedation in an evolving CNS disorder seems unacceptable, important improvements have been made in the development of short-acting sedating agents and antagonists.[34] Tolerance is excellent in most patients, and side effects are minimal. Propofol has been the preferred drug for the treatment of agitated neurologic patients.[44] Dexmedetomidine has been recently introduced, and may become a preferred agent after craniotomy and in other patients transiently intubated. Currently available studies in ICUs are insufficient to recommend one agent over another.[5,20,65] Continuous infusion of midazolam or propofol may be needed, but daily interruptions in infusion, if tolerated, are important in monitoring the patient's neurologic status.

How to judge ideal sedation is another concern, and levels are defined differently.[65] The sedation-agitation scale (SAS) (Table 16.2) grades patients on three severity levels and has excellent agreement among intensive care nurses, even without extensive training.[12,78] The Richmond Agitation Sedation Scale (RASS) has also been validated (Table 16.3).

A general but quite arbitrary recommendation is to achieve a RASS of –3 (Table 16.3). Movement or eye opening to voice but no eye contact would be the level to achieve, but this may not apply to acute ill neurologic patients, and therefore these scales have limited usefulness in the NICU. Monitoring in the ICU using more objective tools, such as bispectral analysis of the electroencephalogram, could be useful, but early experience in the ICU suggests a poor correlation with depth of sedation.[31] In clinical practice scales are rarely used by physicians and results of treatment is best judged for each patient separately. Protection of the patient is important and includes restraints and Posey mitts. The pharmacologic treatment of extremely agitated patients is summarized in Table 16.4.

Propofol

Propofol is widely used as a sedative drug in adults. Propofol may have a place in the management of increased intracranial pressure and status epilepticus.[21,44,91] In a randomized, controlled trial, the "intensity" of intracranial pressure therapy was

---

TABLE 16.2. RIKER SEDATION-AGITATION SCALE (SAS)

7	Dangerous agitation	Pulling at endotracheal tube (ETT), trying to remove catheters, climbing over bedrail, striking at staff, thrashing side-to-side
6	Very agitated	Does not calm despite frequent verbal reminding of limits, requires physical restraints, biting ETT
5	Agitated	Anxious or mildly agitated, attempting to sit up, calms down to verbal instructions
4	Calm and cooperative	Calm, awakens easily, follows commands
3	Sedated	Difficult to arouse, awakens to verbal stimuli or gentle shaking, but drifts off again, follows simple commands
2	Very sedated	Arouses to physical stimuli, but does not communicate or follow commands, may move spontaneously
1	Unarousable	Minimal or no response to noxious stimuli, does not communicate or follow commands

TABLE 16.3. THE RICHMOND AGITATION SEDATION SCALE (RASS)

Scale	Definitions	Description
+4	Combative	Combative, violent, immediate danger to staff
+3	Very agitated	Pulls or removes tubes or catheters; aggressive
+2	Agitated	Frequent purposeful movement, fights ventilator
+1	Restless	Anxious and apprehensive, but movements not aggressive or vigorous
0	Alert and calm	
−1	Drowsy	Not fully alert but has eye opening and eye contact (< 10 s)
−2	Light sedation	Briefly awakens to voice with eye opening and eye contact (< 10 s)
−3	Moderate sedation	Movement or eye opening to voice (but no eye contact)
−4	Deep sedation	No response to voice but movement or eye opening to physical stimulation
−5	Not arousable	No response to voice or physical stimulation

From Ely EW, Truman B, Shintani A, et al. Monitoring sedation status over time in ICU patients: reliability and validity of the Richmond Agitation-Sedation Scale (RASS). *JAMA* 2003;289:2983–2991.

reduced, but the patients needed a very high dose in order to control intracranial pressure surges.[44] Its use as a third-line drug in status epilepticus is currently questioned (Chapter 40).

Propofol (2, 6-diisopropylphenol) is an anesthetic agent with pharmacologic properties and a chemical structure unrelated to those of any other sedating drug.[43,47] The pharmacokinetics of this drug seems ideal, and rapid crossing of the blood–brain barrier produces a marked hypnotic effect.[4] The major distinguishing feature of propofol is the rate of recovery, which is within minutes in almost all patients when incidentally used. Additionally, clearance of propofol is not altered by hepatic or renal failure,[3] which is a well-recognized limitation to the use of benzodiazepines and opiates. Even after high-dose propofol infusion for almost a full day, awakening after discontinuation is comparatively quick.[45] In our experience, full awakening is prolonged with high doses and infusion lasting several days and may take an hour or so.

TABLE 16.4. TREATMENT OF THE EXTREMELY AGITATED PATIENT

Not intubated
Lorazepam, 1–2 mg slowly IV every 4 hours
Haloperidol, 5 mg IM q2–4h
Quetiapine, 25 mg t.i.d
Chlordiazepoxide, 50–100 mg IV or IM b.i.d.

Intubated
Midazolam, IV infusion of 0.02–0.08 mg/kg/hr
Fentanyl, IV infusion 1.5 mcg/kg/hr
Propofol, IV infusion of 0.1–0.6 mg/kg/hr

Increased fat body mass may also contribute.[4] Antagonists for propofol are not available.

In extremely high doses, brainstem reflexes may become abolished, and only pupil size and light response may remain preserved. The corollary is that this agent is contraindicated in rapidly evolving neurologic catastrophes because infusion of the drug may cause serious difficulties in neurologic assessment.

Propofol for the sedation of agitated patients is given as an intravenous infusion at a low-dose rate of 0.1 mg/kg/hr, with incremental doses at 5-minute intervals until reasonable sedation is achieved. Although the response may vary, continuous sedation can be achieved with a dose of 0.3 to 0.5 mg/kg/hr. In two comparative studies with midazolam, propofol was superior for the sedation of critically ill patients.

Propofol generally has a safe pharmacologic profile in adults. However, with bolus doses it reduces blood pressure by reducing systemic vascular resistance, cardiac contractility, and preload. Hypotension with a low dose of propofol often indicates hypovolemia. Propofol increases serum triglycerides, and, in fact, concentrations of triglycerides can be monitored daily to judge the development of a propofol overdose. The 2% emulsion has reduced the lipid load by 50%. Caloric overload (1 mL equals 1.1 kcal) and possible reactive airway disease in patients sensitive to sulfites are known side effects. Anaphylaxis may occur, predominantly in patients with a history of anaphylaxis to muscle relaxants.[49] When anaphylaxis occurs, it produces the typical symptoms of facial swelling, widespread urticaria, and life-threatening bronchospasm. Anaphylaxis should be managed by immediate intravenous administration of epinephrine (usually 1 mL of 1:1000 solution) or diphenhydramine hydrochloride, 25–50 mg intravenously, and volume resuscitation with 5% albumin. Propofol may reduce blood pressure through multiple mechanisms, but this unwanted effect can be reduced by careful titration. Other short-term side effects of propofol are pain at the site of injection (with use of peripheral veins), bacterial contamination (bottle open for more than 12 hours may lead to serious bacteremia), occasional clonic activity, and involuntary movements such as choreoathetosis and opisthotonos.[56,88] Infusion of propofol at rates >4 mg/kg per hour or >67 mcg/kg per minute has been linked to cardiac failure and cardiac arrest.[23] Propofol in high doses for prolonged time periods may result in rapid cardiovascular collapse and metabolic acidosis. This so-called propofol infusion syndrome (PRIS) is usually seen with levels of more than 10 mg/kg/hr. Cardiac arrest or malignant cardiac arrhythmias may appear as early as 6 hours after the start of infusion.[25,67] Patients may be salvaged using ECMO.[39] Our experience at the Mayo Clinic found a 10% frequency of cardiorespiratory arrest in patients treated with propofol for refractory status epilepticus. Most worrisome was the observation that metabolic acidosis did not herald the development of PRIS.[42] In many protocols for status epilepticus, propofol is currently reconsidered and often withheld (Chapter 40). Its use in children is contraindicated.

Dexmedetomidine

Dexmedetomidine has been used increasingly in the NICU. Dexmedetomidine has a different therapeutic target (α_2 receptors) from benzodiazepines (γ-aminobutyric acid [GABA]) and has a new major role in the treatment of agitation and delirium.[37,41,77,86] In a randomized trial comparing dexmedetomidine to midazolam, the results showed less time on the ventilator, less tachycardia, and less hypertension.[79] Dexmedetomidine usually is started at 0.2 mcg/kg/hr and titrated upward to 1 mcg/kg/hr until adequate sedation is achieved. Most neurointensivists feel that the best treatment for agitated delirium is IV dexmedetomidine. Hypotension remains a concern, and is often a reason to discontinue or replace the drug. Hemodynamic effect of dexmedetomidine may be biphasic with initial hypertension (vasoconstriction peripherally) and hypotension later (usually with a bolus). Short infusion of the loading dose (< 10 minutes) is also a common cause for hypotension. Often it is caused by a bolus of

dexmedetomidine, which might be best avoided. Hypotension without bradycardia responds very well to a fluid bolus during the beginning of the infusion. Bradycardia is, however, a good reason not to continue dexmedetomidine.

Dexmedetomidine prolongs the QT interval (> 450 msec), but major cardiac arrhythmias are unusual. Patients with liver function abnormalities need a dosage reduction, but in most 0.2–0.7 mg/kg/hr is the infusion dose (usually starting at 0.4 mg/kg/hr). More delirium coma–free days and fewer ventilator days were associated with the use of dexmedetomidine when compared with lorazepam. A sedation protocol that dictated minimal use of benzodiazepines and early use of dexmedetomidine found dexmedetomidine problems in one of four patients, due to lack of efficacy, hypotension, or bradycardia.[84]

Midazolam

The relative convenience of midazolam is best illustrated by the availability of an antidote and its distinctive amnestic quality, both characteristics of which are conspicuously absent with propofol.[93,94]

Midazolam is a short-acting benzodiazepine with mostly inactive metabolites.[93] Clearance occurs largely through the liver. Its elimination is rapid, but lipid and active metabolic accumulation may occur after 3 days of continuous intravenous infusion. Tolerance may occur, leading to increasing doses to achieve sedation. A study in critically ill patients, which included patients with multitrauma and respiratory failure, found that in those with renal failure, the mean time to awakening after midazolam administration was stopped was 44 hours.[71] Thus, regardless of its short half-life, midazolam may result in sedation for days in some patients.[71] The clearance of midazolam is reduced even more significantly with concomitant hepatic or renal failure, but both factors are in most instances not relevant in acutely ill patients with neurologic disorders. Sedation with midazolam is initiated with a bolus of 0.01–0.05 mg/kg and is followed by infusion at a rate of 0.02–0.1 mg/kg/hr, but this low maintenance dose should be titrated to the response in the individual patient and may be adjusted up several fold.

Midazolam can be rapidly reversed with flumazenil.[11,14,64,72,81] Flumazenil has a half-life of 60 minutes, and antagonizes any benzodiazepine through its specific action on central benzodiazepine receptors that are part of the $GABA_A$ receptor complex. A dose of 0.2–0.4 mg of flumazenil intravenously over 15 seconds restores consciousness immediately, but resedation may occur, depending largely on the previous dose of benzodiazepines and the dose of flumazenil. Repeat doses of 0.4 mg at 1-minute intervals, up to 3 mg, may be needed for the maximal effect.

Side effects of flumazenil are minor, but seizures have been reported. Seizures occurred almost invariably in patients with preexisting epilepsy, in patients who regularly used benzodiazepines, and in patients using tricyclic antidepressants.[54] In predisposed patients, sudden withdrawal of benzodiazepines may also produce a nonconvulsive status epilepticus. Midazolam may produce withdrawal symptoms after 2–3 weeks of continuous use, but the actual risk is small.

Lorazepam

Lorazepam is often used in critical care units for transient sedation, because it has almost no measurable effect on blood pressure and tidal volume.[57] Nonetheless, patients with chronic obstructive pulmonary disease may be more at risk for hypoventilation. Lorazepam has a long-lasting effect after a single bolus injection and is very suitable in the elderly patient.[27] Its reliable absorption after intramuscular injection is another advantage. The comparatively long half-life of lorazepam (15 hours) makes it less suitable for patients with acute neurologic illness in whom the potential for rapid deterioration is great. Emergence from sedation is much more delayed with lorazepam than with midazolam infusion.[6] Lorazepam is cleared through the liver and excreted by the kidneys. An advantage over midazolam infusion is its considerably lower cost when several days of infusion are anticipated.[17] Lorazepam is usually given intravenously as a single dose of 2 mg. Others have reported a favorable response in extremely agitated patients with an infusion of lorazepam titrated to clinical response.

Haloperidol

Haloperidol has been the drug of choice in psychotic patients with acute disruptive behavior.[95] Approximately 20 minutes after intramuscular injection, a tranquil state can be achieved. The drug undergoes hepatic metabolism and has a half-life of 6–20 hours. Haloperidol may produce marked rigidity. Within days of oral treatment, haloperidol may lead to impressive side effects, such as akathisia (irresistible urge to move about and a feeling that something is crawling under the skin), which may, in fact, suggest ineffective treatment to the novice. This neuroleptic-induced

movement disorder of almost continuous symptoms of restlessness responds to an anticholinergic agent such as benztropine or propranolol, or amantadine.[95] Haloperidol can cause QT prolongation on electrocardiograms and there is a concern it may be more common with IV injections. Extremely high doses of haloperidol have been associated with oculogyral crises, torticollis, trismus, and neuroleptic malignant syndrome. Intravenous administration of haloperidol is problematic, and in one review of neuroleptic malignant syndrome after traumatic brain injury, high doses of intravenous haloperidol could possibly be implicated.[7]

Current recommendations for the use of haloperidol are a starting dose of 2–5 mg intramuscularly, followed by a similar dose 20 minutes later. Agitation can be further controlled by additional doses of 5 mg every 30 minutes until perceptional disturbances subside completely and the patient becomes calm and cooperative. With the emergence of atypical antipsychotic agents, its use has declined.

Atypical Antipsychotics

A new generation of so-called atypical antipsychotics—risperidone (0.5 mg b.i.d. PO, up to 3 mg/day), olanzapine (5–10 mg/day PO), and quetiapine (25 mg b.i.d., up to 300 mg/day)—developed for schizoaffective disorders are also useful in the management of agitation or delirium in patients with prior dementia and Parkinson's disease.[90] Dose adjustment is required in renal disease (risperidone) and liver disease (quetiapine). Clozapine, an alternative agent, can be given orally in a low dose of 6.25 mg/day and increased to 50 mg/day.[34,38,40]

Miscellaneous Pharmacologic Choices for the Management of Agitation

For patients in whom the use of neuroleptic agents must be minimized, thioridazine (100 mg PO three times a day, up to 800 mg/day) can be given, but at the expense of moderate sedation and an increased risk of seizures. Diazepam has been the definitive drug for sedation in agitated patients for years and should not be easily dismissed as obsolete. In intubated patients, a low dose of 5–10 mg results in extremely rapid onset of sedation and can still be given randomly. However, accumulation (half-life, 35–100 hours) is substantial with advancing age and liver disease. This agent, therefore, is far less useful than the newer benzodiazepines.

PAIN MANAGEMENT

Pain is highly prevalent in patients with acute neurologic disorders, and it has widespread consequences. For example, disturbance of sleep from pain is detrimental in patients with increased work of breathing from acute neuromuscular disorders and may prematurely lead to endotracheal intubation. Excruciating head pain in patients with intracranial hemorrhage or after craniotomy may lead to hypertension as part of a complex neuroendocrine response and, more important, may result in myocardial ischemia in patients with underlying coronary artery disease.

Pain is signaled not only by moaning, crying, grimacing, and extreme restlessness, but in some patients also by profuse sweating, sustained tachycardia, blood pressure fluctuations, and dilated pupils. However, one should be sensitive to the fact that lack of expression of pain does not mean lack of pain.[70]

Pain that is insufficiently treated adversely impacts on many physiologic systems (Figure 16.1), and basic principles of compassion require us to treat it.[30] Immediate relief of pain not only results in visible comfort but also may considerably mute these potentially threatening physiologic responses.

Nursing personnel specifically trained in neurologic intensive care have a pivotal role in the recognition and management of pain in various neurologic emergencies. In medical or surgical intensive care units, it has been well appreciated that most patients wait until pain becomes unbearable before they signal for analgesics, but more disturbingly (at least in one survey in Australia), approximately only one-third of nursing personnel honor requests when they are made.[66]

The decision to pursue pain medication depends greatly on whether simple nursing measures (e.g., adequate positioning, catheterization) or use of distraction techniques (music, television, family visits) can reduce pain. When no other obvious cause is apparent, analgesics should be administered. The severity of pain is hard to quantify, but increased agitation with any type of stimulation and change in physiologic functions (e.g., tachycardia, blood pressure surges) are at times helpful indications. Patients who are alert can be asked to rate the pain on a scale of 0 to 10 (0, no pain; 10, excruciating and unbearable pain), but the reliability of this semiquantitative scoring is questionable. Pain can be defined as allodynia (pain with stimulus not usually causing pain) and hyperalgesia (exaggerated pain with a painful

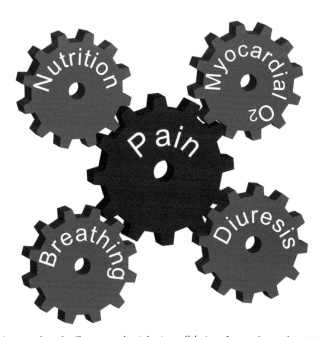

FIGURE 16.1: Pain has profound effects on physiologic well-being. Increasing pain causes low tidal volumes, decreased ventilation, gastric stasis, nausea and vomiting, poor nutritional intake, hypertension, and tachycardia and thus increased myocardial oxygen requirements, and less measurable water and sodium retention due to an increase in antidiuretic hormone.

stimulus), but pain also can be absent in areas that should be normally painful (analgesia).

Nursing rating scales have been used and the Critical-Care Pain Observation Tool (CPOT) is best validated, most reliable, and most in use in major US institutions (Table 16.5).[29,32] The CPOT includes four interpreted behaviors (facial expressions, body movements, muscle tension, compliance with the ventilator for intubated patients or vocalization for nonintubated patients). The CPOT is useful in assessing pain in these patients when they are unable to report pain.

Adequate pain control has a high priority in the management of Guillain-Barré syndrome (GBS). Pain in this disorder may appear in several forms, including hyperalgesia, sciatica, muscle pain and cramps, and joint stiffness. Typical is the nocturnal aggravation of pain that keeps patients from rest and sleep. Positioning, splinting, and use of bed cages, gloves, or cotton socks may reduce burning, needle-like pain and a feeling of skin tightening. Hot or cold packs may be useful as well. Pain is generally managed with opioid analgesics, such as oxycodone, which may have to be administered ad libitum to patients with GBS and severe pain.[69,80] When large doses of opiates are needed to control pain, elective endotracheal intubation should be strongly considered in patients with marginal pulmonary function.

The treatment of pain in GBS can be notoriously difficult and frustrating, and may in certain patients lead to the administration of narcotics into the epidural space,[52,60] a well-accepted treatment of postoperative pain in patients with thoracotomy. A good alternative is tramadol (150 mg, followed by 400 mg/day),[10] and our anecdotal experience in a few cases has been good.

Gabapentin in high doses may be successful (1200–3600 mg). Success has also been claimed with capsaicin, specifically for superficial burning pain,[58] quinine sulfate (300 mg at bedtime) for nocturnal cramping and stiffness,[62] and carbamazepine[92] (400 mg before sleep) for sciatica. Clonidine is an agonist at the alpha 2-adrenergic receptor, and this receptor activation possesses analgesic qualities. Clonidine can be used from

TABLE 16.5. CRITICAL-CARE PAIN OBSERVATION TOOL (CPOT)

Indicator	Description	Score	
Facial expression	No muscular tension observed	Relaxed, neutral	0
	Presence of frowning, brow lowering, orbit tightening, and levator contraction	Tense	1
	All of the above facial movements plus eyelid tightly closed	Grimacing	2
Body movements	Does not move at all (does not necessarily mean absence of pain)	Absence of movements	0
	Slow, cautious movements, touching or rubbing the pain site, seeking attention through movements	Protection	1
	Pulling tube, attempting to sit up, moving limbs/thrashing, not following commands, striking at staff, trying to climb out of bed	Restlessness	2
Muscle tension	No resistance to passive movements	Relaxed	0
Evaluation by passive flexion and extension of upper extremities	Resistance to passive movements	Tense, rigid	1
	Strong resistance to passive movements, inability to complete them	Very tense or rigid	2
Compliance with the ventilator (intubated patients)	Alarms not activated, easy ventilation	Tolerating ventilator	0
	Alarms stop spontaneously	Coughing but tolerating	1
	Asynchrony: blocking ventilation, alarms frequently activated	Fighting ventilator	2
OR	Talking in normal tone or no sound	Talking in normal tone or no sound	0
Vocalization (extubated patients)	Sighing, moaning, crying out, sobbing	Sighing, moaning, crying out, sobbing	1
			2
Total, range			**0–8**

CAPSULE 16.1   PATIENT-CONTROLLED ANALGESIA

Patient-controlled analgesia has been used in the postoperative period but may also be helpful in some patients in the NICU and for those transitioning to a progressive care unit.[36] The patient can titrate the administered medication needed to provide adequate analgesia.

  PCA provides pain relief much quicker than with traditional nurse and pharmacy preparations. Usually fentanyl is administered, started with a 15 mcg/push IV, setting of 10–20 mcg IV every 10 minutes, with maximum lockout administered per 4 hours of 400 µg. Mistakes can be made in programming the pump, and the oversedation that may be seen at the end of a lockout period can cause respiratory depression. Initiation of dose by family members has been observed and should be avoided. Monitoring of the patient involves general ICU care but specific attention is required in five areas: (1) at least 4 hours at stable dose, (2) patient's pain level is 4 or less (on traditional 1–10 scale), (3) oxygen saturations are greater than 90%, (4) respirations are more than 10 per minute, and (5) level of sedation is a RASS score of 0 or –1. Naloxone should be readily available.

---

30 to 300 µg, but with increased sedation, hypotension and bradycardia are noted at the higher doses (temporary, not with long-term use). All these therapeutic measures have often resulted in instant relief after trial and error with other drugs, but they have not been studied in series of patients.

Pharmaceutical Agents for Pain

The choice of pain medication depends on the underlying neurologic condition, the possible interaction with other medication, and the type of pain, as much as on the severity of the pain.[53,61]

Opiates

Opioid analgesics remain the mainstay of pain management in many patients with critical neurologic illness.[2] Opiates are invariably effective.[8,9] Fear of addiction after prolonged hospital use is vastly exaggerated. A survey of 11,882 consecutive patients identified four patients with new opiate dependency, only one of whom had major dependency.[73] Morphine is the prototypical narcotic. Intravenous administration is preferred for acute pain management because transdermal patches delay the analgesic effect. Patient-controlled analgesia (PCA) has not yet found its way into most NICUs because it requires patients to be awake and fully cooperative; however, we have occasionally used it in patients with GBS whose distal muscle power is still preserved. We have also used it in patients with severe subarachnoid hemorrhage unresponsive to a course of corticosteroids (to reduce meningeal inflammation) or repeated CSF drainage (to reduce intracranial pressure). The use

of PCA has been particularly helpful in patients with persistent headache and a good grade subarachnoid hemorrhage. (PCA pump dosing and practical use are shown in Capsule 16.1). However, fentanyl, although commonly used for postoperative pain control in other ICUs, is generally not preferred because of a risk of seizures, an increase in intracranial pressure, and sedation.

  Alternative (but weaker) narcotic analgesics are codeine and meperidine,[35] which may have less severe potential side effects (in particular, less sedation). They must be reserved for patients who cannot tolerate morphine or have mild to moderate pain, and they must be used preferentially in patients with acute CNS injury in whom sedation is unacceptable. Codeine is the agent of choice for relief of severe pain in acute CNS disorders. Codeine and morphine are typically used in the NICU, and dosing is summarized in Table 16.6.

TABLE 16.6. OPIATES FOR PAIN MANAGEMENT IN THE NEUROSCIENCE INTENSIVE CARE UNIT

Agent	Route	Starting Dose (mg)	Peak Effect (hour)	Duration (hour)
Codeine	IM	30	0.5–1	4–6
	PO	30–60	1.5–2	3–4
Morphine	IM	5	0.5–1	3–5
	PO	15	1.5–2	4

Side effects of opiates are considerable. Nausea and vomiting occur in 30% of patients treated with repetitive doses of narcotics, but these are rapidly reversible. Opioids are also known to cause water retention from the suppression of antidiuretic hormone and, combined with excessive vomiting, potentially may lead to profound hyponatremia. Respiratory depression (detected by relative hypercapnia from hypoventilation) occurs in susceptible patients but is dose-dependent and usually appears with the initial doses. This important side effect abates with continuing doses, but hypoventilation remains a major concern in some patients. Constipation and potential for ileus, urinary retention, and itching are equally important side effects (Table 16.7). Inability to temporarily overcome them with measures such as stool softeners and catheterization probably should prompt discontinuation. Meperidine has been linked to seizures, particularly in patients with decreased renal function.

Naloxone reverses opioid toxicity but, like all competitive antagonists, does not produce a long-lasting effect. Repeated intravenous doses of 0.2 mg every 3 minutes (up to 10 mg) are needed to obtain an effect. In addition, naloxone may have side effects of its own. Hypertensive crises, cardiac arrhythmias, and unexplained fatigue 24 hours after administration have been reported.

Corticosteroids

A single dose of 4 mg dexamethasone for several consecutive days may be very successful in severe refractory head pain associated with subarachnoid hemorrhage, in particular if there is associated nausea.[1,89] Continuation of dexamethasone may significantly worsen blood glucose, often requiring the temporary use of insulin sliding scales. Similar empiric effect is found with acute cerebellar hematoma, but its mechanism is not known. An effective drug for associated with GBS is 60 mg methylprednisolone sodium succinate as IV or IM.

Nonsteroidal Anti-inflammatory Agents

Nonsteroidal anti-inflammatory drugs (NSAIDs) are grouped together because of their mode of action, not by their chemical structure. They are used increasingly in surgical ICUs. One of the most recently introduced drugs, ketorolac, is as potent as morphine, and its parenteral form produces faster onset of analgesia, less sedation, and no depressant effect on the ventilatory response to carbon dioxide.[13,15,76] Ketorolac is metabolized by the liver and excreted by the kidneys.

The NSAIDs are promising in patients with acute neurologic illness and severe headaches because they have a minimal effect on the level of consciousness. However, the use of NSAIDs is associated with potentially major side effects. Gastropathy is noticeable in long-term use, typically including mucosal damage, gastrointestinal bleeding, and perforation, but these side effects are less common with brief exposure. Cimetidine and sucralfate are ineffective in protection against gastric ulcers from NSAIDs.[48] The major disadvantage is the risk of hemorrhage or coagulopathy. Therefore, they are contraindicated in patients with intracranial hemorrhage.

Intramuscular administration of 30 mg of ketorolac is comparable to 10 mg of morphine and may be used to complement morphine and to reduce opioid requirements.[63,68] Ketorolac may cause renal vasoconstriction and renal failure through an effect on prostaglandin synthesis. Another agent, parecoxib, a new parenteral-specific inhibitor of cyclooxygenase 2 (COX2), may become a good analgesic agent for postoperative pain control.[19] A single dose of 40 mg is well tolerated, and gastric ulceration may be less than with ketorolac.

Gabapentin

Gabapentin is not an ideal drug for acute severe headache management, but rapid escalation to 1,200 mg daily was successful in SAH.[26] There is also interest in its use in postoperative

---

TABLE 16.7. ADVERSE EFFECTS
OF OPIATES

Respiratory depression
Hypotension
Bronchospasm
Euphoria
Bradycardia
Muscle rigidity
Ileus, impaired gastrointestinal motility
Seizures*
Nausea and vomiting
Urinary retention
Pruritus
Possible withdrawal
Delayed emergence with prolonged infusions or with liver–kidney disease

---

* Meperidine

pain;[85] however, escalating to 1,200 mg daily may cause significant drowsiness.[18,75]

CONCLUSIONS

- Agitation in a patient with an acute neurologic disorder may be from drug or alcohol withdrawal delirium.

- Alcohol-related delirium is best initially treated with repeated doses of intravenous lorazepam 2 mg.

- Extremely agitated patients are best treated with intravenous lorazepam 1–2 mg, given slowly; haloperidol 5 mg intramuscularly; midazolam 0.02–0.1 mg/kg/hr; or propofol 0.1–0.6 mg/kg/hr. Dexmedetomidine may is a useful drug to control agitation.

- Propofol is a potent sedative, but there is a growing concern with a so-called propofol infusion syndrome, particularly in patients with acute neurologic disease.

- Pain relief has a high priority in neurologic intensive care, and opiates are invariably effective. The preferred agent in acute CNS disorders is codeine.

- Pain relief in GBS is crucial to its management. The preferred agents are oxycodone or morphine.

REFERENCES

1. Allen TK, Jones CA, Habib AS. Dexamethasone for the prophylaxis of postoperative nausea and vomiting associated with neuraxial morphine administration: a systematic review and meta-analysis. *Anesth Analg* 2012;114:813–822.
2. Angst MS, Clark JD. Opioid-induced hyperalgesia: a qualitative systematic review. *Anesthesiology* 2006;104:570–587.
3. Bailie GR, Cockshott ID, Douglas EJ, Bowles BJ. Pharmacokinetics of propofol during and after long-term continuous infusion for maintenance of sedation in ICU patients. *Br J Anaesth* 1992;68: 486–491.
4. Barr J, Egan TD, Sandoval NF, et al. Propofol dosing regimens for ICU sedation based upon an integrated pharmacokinetic-pharmacodynamic model. *Anesthesiology* 2001;95:324–333.
5. Battaglia J. Pharmacological management of acute agitation. *Drugs* 2005;65:1207–1222.
6. Baumgartner GR, Rowen RC. Clonidine vs chlordiazepoxide in the management of acute alcohol withdrawal syndrome. *Arch Intern Med* 1987;147:1223–1226.
7. Bellamy CJ, Kane-Gill SL, Falcione BA, Seybert AL. Neuroleptic malignant syndrome in traumatic brain injury patients treated with haloperidol. *J Trauma* 2009;66:954–958.
8. Bernauer EA, Yeager MP. Optimal pain control in the intensive care unit. *Int Anesthesiol Clin* 1993;31:201–221.
9. Black AMS, Alexander JI. Analgesia for postoperative pain. In: Atkinson RS, Adams AP, eds. *Recent Advances in Anesthesia and Analgesia 17.* Edinburgh: Churchill Livingstone; 1992.
10. Bloch MB, Dyer RA, Heijke SA, James MF. Tramadol infusion for postthoracotomy pain relief: a placebo-controlled comparison with epidural morphine. *Anesth Analg* 2002;94:523–528; table of contents.
11. Bodenham A, Park GR. Reversal of prolonged sedation using flumazenil in critically ill patients. *Anaesthesia* 1989;44:603–605.
12. Brandl KM, Langley KA, Riker RR, et al. Confirming the reliability of the sedation-agitation scale administered by ICU nurses without experience in its use. *Pharmacotherapy* 2001;21: 431–436.
13. Bravo LJ, Mattie H, Spierdijk J, Bovill JG, Burm AG. The effects on ventilation of ketorolac in comparison with morphine. *Eur J Clin Pharmacol* 1988;35:491–494.
14. Breheny FX. Reversal of midazolam sedation with flumazenil. *Crit Care Med* 1992;20:736–739.
15. Brown CR, Moodie JE, Wild VM, Bynum LJ. Comparison of intravenous ketorolac tromethamine and morphine sulfate in the treatment of postoperative pain. *Pharmacotherapy* 1990;10:116S–121S.
16. Brust JCM. *Neurological Aspects of Substance Abuse.* Boston: Butterworth-Heinemann; 1993.
17. Cernaianu AC, DelRossi AJ, Flum DR, et al. Lorazepam and midazolam in the intensive care unit: a randomized, prospective, multicenter study of hemodynamics, oxygen transport, efficacy, and cost. *Crit Care Med* 1996;24:222–228.
18. Chang CY, Challa CK, Shah J, Eloy JD. Gabapentin in acute postoperative pain management. *Biomed Res Int* 2014;2014:631756.
19. Cheer SM, Goa KL. Parecoxib (parecoxib sodium). *Drugs* 2001;61:1133–1141.
20. Chevrolet JC, Jolliet P. Clinical review: agitation and delirium in the critically ill—significance and management. *Crit Care* 2007;11:214.
21. Claassen J, Hirsch LJ, Emerson RG, Mayer SA. Treatment of refractory status epilepticus with pentobarbital, propofol, or midazolam: a systematic review. *Epilepsia* 2002;43:146–153.
22. Coppolo DP, May JJ. Self-extubations: a 12-month experience. *Chest* 1990;98:165–169.
23. Cremer OL, Moons KG, Bouman EA, et al. Long-term propofol infusion and cardiac failure in adult head-injured patients. *Lancet* 2001;357:117–118.

24. D'Onofrio G, Rathlev NK, Ulrich AS, Fish SS, Freedland ES. Lorazepam for the prevention of recurrent seizures related to alcohol. *N Engl J Med* 1999;340:915–919.

25. Deer TR, Rich GF. Propofol tolerance in a pediatric patient. *Anesthesiology* 1992;77:828–829.

26. Dhakal LP, Hodge DO, Nagal J, et al. Safety and tolerability of gabapentin for aneurysmal subarachnoid hemorrhage (SAH) headache and meningismus. *Neurocrit Care* 2015;22:414–421.

27. Druckenbrod RW, Rosen J, Cluxton RJ, Jr. As-needed dosing of antipsychotic drugs: limitations and guidelines for use in the elderly agitated patient. *Ann Pharmacother* 1993;27:645–648.

28. Earnest MP, Feldman H, Marx JA, et al. Intracranial lesions shown by CT scans in 259 cases of first alcohol-related seizures. *Neurology* 1988;38:1561–1565.

29. Echegaray-Benites C, Kapoustina O, Gelinas C. Validation of the use of the Critical-Care Pain Observation Tool (CPOT) with brain surgery patients in the neurosurgical intensive care unit. *Intens Crit Care Nurs* 2014;30:257–265.

30. Erstad BL, Puntillo K, Gilbert HC, et al. Pain management principles in the critically ill. *Chest* 2009;135:1075–1086.

31. Frenzel D, Greim CA, Sommer C, Bauerle K, Roewer N. Is the bispectral index appropriate for monitoring the sedation level of mechanically ventilated surgical ICU patients? *Intensive Care Med* 2002;28:178–183.

32. Gelinas C, Puntillo KA, Joffe AM, Barr J. A validated approach to evaluating psychometric properties of pain assessment tools for use in nonverbal critically ill adults. *Semin Respir Crit Care Med* 2013;34:153–168.

33. Girard TD, Kress JP, Fuchs BD, et al. Efficacy and safety of a paired sedation and ventilator weaning protocol for mechanically ventilated patients in intensive care (Awakening and Breathing Controlled trial): a randomised controlled trial. *Lancet* 2008;371:126–134.

34. Glick ID, Murray SR, Vasudevan P, Marder SR, Hu RJ. Treatment with atypical antipsychotics: new indications and new populations. *J Psychiatr Res* 2001;35:187–191.

35. Gottschalk A, Yaster M. The perioperative management of pain from intracranial surgery. *Neurocrit Care* 2009;10:387–402.

36. Grass JA. Patient-controlled analgesia. *Anesth Analg* 2005;101:S44–61.

37. Grof TM, Bledsoe KA. Evaluating the use of dexmedetomidine in neurocritical care patients. *Neurocrit Care* 2010;12:356–361.

38. Group TPS. Low-dose clozapine for the treatment of drug-induced psychosis in Parkinson's disease *N Engl J Med* 1999;340:757–763.

39. Guitton C, Gabillet L, Latour P, et al. Propofol Infusion syndrome during refractory status epilepticus in a young adult: successful ECMO resuscitation. *Neurocrit Care* 2011;15:139–145.

40. Hawkins SB, Bucklin M, Muzyk AJ. Quetiapine for the treatment of delirium. *J Hosp Med* 2013;8:215–220.

41. Hoy SM, Keating GM. Dexmedetomidine: a review of its use for sedation in mechanically ventilated patients in an intensive care setting and for procedural sedation. *Drugs* 2011;71:1481–1501.

42. Iyer VN, Hoel R, Rabinstein AA. Propofol infusion syndrome in patients with refractory status epilepticus: an 11-year clinical experience. *Crit Care Med* 2009;37:3024–3030.

43. Kanto J, Gepts E. Pharmacokinetic implications for the clinical use of propofol. *Clin Pharmacokinet* 1989;17:308–326.

44. Kelly DF, Goodale DB, Williams J, et al. Propofol in the treatment of moderate and severe head injury: a randomized, prospective double-blinded pilot trial. *J Neurosurg* 1999;90:1042–1052.

45. Kress JP, O'Connor MF, Pohlman AS, et al. Sedation of critically ill patients during mechanical ventilation: a comparison of propofol and midazolam. *Am J Respir Crit Care Med* 1996;153:1012–1018.

46. Kress JP, Pohlman AS, O'Connor MF, Hall JB. Daily interruption of sedative infusions in critically ill patients undergoing mechanical ventilation. *N Engl J Med* 2000;342:1471–1477.

47. Langley MS, Heel RC. Propofol: a review of its pharmacodynamic and pharmacokinetic properties and use as an intravenous anaesthetic. *Drugs* 1988;35:334–372.

48. Lanza F, Peace K, Gustitus L, Rack MF, Dickson B. A blinded endoscopic comparative study of misoprostol versus sucralfate and placebo in the prevention of aspirin-induced gastric and duodenal ulceration. *Am J Gastroenterol* 1988;83:143–146.

49. Laxenaire MC, Mata-Bermejo E, Moneret-Vautrin DA, Gueant JL. Life-threatening anaphylactoid reactions to propofol (Diprivan). *Anesthesiology* 1992;77:275–280.

50. Lipowski ZJ. Delirium (acute confusional states). *JAMA* 1987;258:1789–1792.

51. Lipowski ZJ. Delirium in the elderly patient. *N Engl J Med* 1989;320:578–582.

52. Longobardi JJ, Comens R, Jacobs AM. Epidural morphine as an adjuvant to the treatment of pain in a patient with acute inflammatory polyradiculopathy secondary to Guillain-Barre syndrome. *J Foot Surg* 1991;30:267–268.

53. Malchow RJ, Black IH. The evolution of pain management in the critically ill trauma

patient: emerging concepts from the global war on terrorism. *Crit Care Med* 2008;36:S346–357.

54. Marchant B, Wray R, Leach A, Nama M. Flumazenil causing convulsions and ventricular tachycardia. *BMJ* 1989;299:860.

55. Mayo-Smith MF. Pharmacological management of alcohol withdrawal: a meta-analysis and evidence-based practice guideline. American Society of Addiction Medicine Working Group on Pharmacological Management of Alcohol Withdrawal. *JAMA* 1997;278:144–151.

56. Mirenda J, Broyles G. Propofol as used for sedation in the ICU. *Chest* 1995;108:539–548.

57. Modell JG. Further experience and observations with lorazepam in the management of behavioral agitation. *J Clin Psychopharmacol* 1986;6:385–387.

58. Morgenlander JC, Hurwitz BJ, Massey EW. Capsaicin for the treatment of pain in Guillain-Barre syndrome. *Ann Neurol* 1990;28:199.

59. Mori E, Yamadori A. Acute confusional state and acute agitated delirium. Occurrence after infarction in the right middle cerebral artery territory. *Arch Neurol* 1987;44:1139–1143.

60. Moulin DE, Hagen N, Feasby TE, Amireh R, Hahn A. Pain in Guillain-Barre syndrome. *Neurology* 1997;48:328–331.

61. Murray MJ. Pain problems in the ICU. *Crit Care Clin* 1990;6:235–253.

62. Nixon RA. Quinine sulfate for pain in the Guillain-Barre syndrome. *Ann Neurol* 1978;4:386–387.

63. O'Hara DA, Fragen RJ, Kinzer M, Pemberton D. Ketorolac tromethamine as compared with morphine sulfate for treatment of postoperative pain. *Clin Pharmacol Ther* 1987;41:556–561.

64. O'Sullivan GF, Wade DN. Flumazenil in the management of acute drug overdosage with benzodiazepines and other agents. *Clin Pharmacol Ther* 1987;42:254–259.

65. Ostermann ME, Keenan SP, Seiferling RA, Sibbald WJ. Sedation in the intensive care unit: a systematic review. *JAMA* 2000;283:1451–1459.

66. Owen H, McMillan V, Rogowski D. Postoperative pain therapy: a survey of patients' expectations and their experiences. *Pain* 1990;41:303–307.

67. Parke TJ, Stevens JE, Rice AS, et al. Metabolic acidosis and fatal myocardial failure after propofol infusion in children: five case reports. *BMJ* 1992;305:613–616.

68. Peirce RJ, Fragen RJ, Pemberton DM. Intravenous ketorolac tromethamine versus morphine sulfate in the treatment of immediate postoperative pain. *Pharmacotherapy* 1990;10:111S–115S.

69. Pentland B, Donald SM. Pain in the Guillain-Barre syndrome: a clinical review. *Pain* 1994;59:159–164.

70. Petzold A, Girbes A. Pain management in neurocritical care. *Neurocrit Care* 2013;19:232–256.

71. Pohlman AS, Simpson KP, Hall JB. Continuous intravenous infusions of lorazepam versus midazolam for sedation during mechanical ventilatory support: a prospective, randomized study. *Crit Care Med* 1994;22:1241–1247.

72. Pollard BJ, Masters AP, Bunting P. The use of flumazenil (Anexate, Ro 15–1788) in the management of drug overdose. *Anaesthesia* 1989;44:137–138.

73. Porter J, Jick H. Addiction rare in patients treated with narcotics. *N Engl J Med* 1980;302:123.

74. Pun BT, Ely EW. The importance of diagnosing and managing ICU delirium. *Chest* 2007;132:624–636.

75. Rashiq S, Dick BD. Post-surgical pain syndromes: a review for the non-pain specialist. *Can J Anaesth* 2014;61:123–130.

76. Rice AS, Lloyd J, Miller CG, Bullingham RE, O'Sullivan G M. A double-blind study of the speed of onset of analgesia following intramuscular administration of ketorolac tromethamine in comparison to intramuscular morphine and placebo. *Anaesthesia* 1991;46:541–544.

77. Riker RR, Fugate JE. Clinical monitoring scales in acute brain injury: assessment of coma, pain, agitation, and delirium. *Neurocrit Care* 2014;21 Suppl 2:S27–S37.

78. Riker RR, Picard JT, Fraser GL. Prospective evaluation of the Sedation-Agitation Scale for adult critically ill patients. *Crit Care Med* 1999;27:1325–1329.

79. Riker RR, Shehabi Y, Bokesch PM, et al. Dexmedetomidine vs midazolam for sedation of critically ill patients: a randomized trial. *JAMA* 2009;301:489–499.

80. Ropper AH, Wijdicks EFM, Truax BT. *Guillain-Barré Syndrome*. Vol. 34. Oxford University Press; 1991. New York.

81. Sage DJ. Reversal of sedation with flumazenil in regional anaesthesia: a review. *Eur J Anaesthesiol Suppl* 1988;2:201–207.

82. Sessler CN, Varney K. Patient-focused sedation and analgesia in the ICU. *Chest* 2008;133:552–565.

83. Skoglund K, Enblad P, Marklund N. Effects of the neurological wake-up test on intracranial pressure and cerebral perfusion pressure in brain-injured patients. *Neurocrit Care* 2009;11:135–142.

84. Skrupky LP, Drewry AM, Wessman B, et al. Clinical effectiveness of a sedation protocol minimizing benzodiazepine infusions and favoring early dexmedetomidine: a before-after study. *Crit Care* 2015;19:136.

85. Turan A, Kaya G, Karamanlioglu B, Pamukcu Z, Apfel CC. Effect of oral gabapentin on postoperative epidural analgesia. *Br J Anaesth* 2006;96:242–246.

86. Venn M, Newman J, Grounds M. A phase II study to evaluate the efficacy of dexmedetomidine for sedation in the medical intensive care unit. *Intensive Care Med* 2003;29:201–207.
87. Vickrey BG, Bahls FH. Nonconvulsive status epilepticus following cerebral angiography. *Ann Neurol* 1989;25:199–201.
88. Walder B, Tramer MR, Seeck M. Seizure-like phenomena and propofol: a systematic review. *Neurology* 2002;58:1327–1332.
89. Waldron NH, Jones CA, Gan TJ, Allen TK, Habib AS. Impact of perioperative dexamethasone on postoperative analgesia and side-effects: systematic review and meta-analysis. *Br J Anaesth* 2013;110:191–200.
90. Wang PS, Schneeweiss S, Avorn J, et al. Risk of death in elderly users of conventional vs. atypical antipsychotic medications. *N Engl J Med* 2005;353:2335–2341.
91. Wijdicks EFM, Nyberg SL. Propofol to control intracranial pressure in fulminant hepatic failure. *Transplant Proc* 2002;34:1220–1222.
92. Winspur I. Tegretol for pain in the Guillain-Barre syndrome. *Lancet* 1970;1:85.
93. Wright SW, Chudnofsky CR, Dronen SC, et al. Comparison of midazolam and diazepam for conscious sedation in the emergency department. *Ann Emerg Med* 1993;22:201–205.
94. Young C, Knudsen N, Hilton A, Reves JG. Sedation in the intensive care unit. *Crit Care Med* 2000;28:854–866.
95. Ziehm SR. Intravenous haloperidol for tranquilization in critical care patients: a review and critique. *AACN Clin Issues Crit Care Nurs* 1991;2:765–777.

17

Mechanical Ventilation

Managing the mechanical ventilator is different in neurologic critical illness for several reasons. First, patients in the neurosciences intensive care unit (NICU) more likely have normal baseline pulmonary function, unlike medical ICU patients with exacerbation of obstructive respiratory disease or serious newly acquired pulmonary parenchymal disease. Second, the mode of ventilation in acutely ill neurologic patients is often intermittent-mandatory or assisted-control and, much less often, is inverse-ratio prone position ventilation, or high-frequency ventilation used. Third, ventilator dependency is less common, and except for those with cervical spinal cord transection or end-stage amyotrophic lateral sclerosis, most acutely ill neurologic patients can later be successfully weaned from the ventilator.

In many US hospitals, mechanically ventilated patients are seen hourly by respiratory therapists under the supervision of intensivists. It can be confidently said that neurologists with expertise in critical care neurology should have a decisive role in establishing the need for mechanical ventilation, in considering noninvasive ventilation and changing the mode of ventilation, in determining indications for tracheostomy, and in knowing when liberation from the ventilator is appropriate. All these decisions weigh the risks of a brief hypotension and hypoxemia—mostly due to anesthetic drugs—in an already injured brain.

Airway management and indications for intubation were discussed in Chapter 10. The basic principles of mechanical ventilation specifically focused on this patient population are discussed here. The immense subject of mechanical ventilation cannot be captured in a single chapter, and therefore major textbooks on mechanical ventilation can be consulted for more technical aspects.[43,59]

INDICATIONS FOR MECHANICAL VENTILATION

The indications for mechanical ventilation in the heterogencous NICU population can be most effectively discussed in reference to the hemispheres and brainstem (regulation of respiratory drive), peripheral effector organ (the mechanics of the respiratory system),[20] and primary pulmonary causes of inadequate ventilation (intrinsic pulmonary disease).[44]

Changes in respiratory drive may result from acute lesions in the hemispheres or brainstem. Many patients, particularly in the first hour, have marked spontaneous hyperventilation. There is a tendency to assume that the most prominent factor in hyperventilation is sustained resetting of the feedback loops in the respiratory centers, but in daily practice, some patients hyperventilate merely to compensate for considerable hypoxia. Rather than remaining in a marginal situation that, without appropriate intervention, results in ventilatory muscle fatigue, patients with prolonged hyperventilation are probably better served by assisted ventilation with mild sedation. In other patients, tachypnea compensates for metabolic acidosis, which needs correction first. The acute presence of tachypnea may indicate pulmonary embolism, and these patients rarely signal pleuritic pain (Chapter 45). Cheyne-Stokes breathing is relatively frequent in patients in the NICU, but should be left alone. A study found that 50% of patients had Cheyne-Stokes breathing after an acute ischemic stroke, but occasionally this occurred in association with oxygen desaturation below 90 mm Hg.[37] Cheyne-Stokes respiration is recognized by an oscillating cycle (up to 1.5 minutes each) of hyperpnea separated by apnea.[37] Touching the patient in an apneic period can easily start the crescendo hyperventilation phase. (For other less common breathing patterns, see Chapter 10, Capsule 10.1.)

Depression of level of consciousness is not an absolute indication for full mechanical ventilation. Intubated patients with an acute central nervous system (CNS) event are generally well able to maintain efficient gas exchange with some pressure support that can be monitored by pulse oximeter and repeated blood gas determinations. However, patients with abnormal breathing patterns that result in inadequate oxygen delivery and hypercapnia need to be mechanically ventilated. Depending on the type of neurologic disorder, a trial with noninvasive bilevel positive pressure airway (BiPAP) ventilation may be considered.

Intubation and mechanical ventilation are required in patients with acute brainstem or hemispheric stroke, mostly if patients cannot handle secretions.[48] These patients cannot protect the upper airway due to oropharyngeal weakness, decreased level of consciousness, or both.[68,70,71]

Mechanical ventilation is often instituted for patients with poor-grade aneurysmal subarachnoid hemorrhage, particularly in those who have had a rerupture, which often is associated with apnea. Within hours, it should become clear whether apnea persists or if triggering of the ventilator occurs. Rapid-onset diffuse pulmonary edema may coincide with aneurysmal rupture and demand all attention to ensure adequate oxygenation. This may have to be accomplished with high positive end-expiratory pressure (PEEP), high-frequency ventilation, or prone ventilation.

The time course of neuromuscular respiratory failure depends on the underlying disorder. In chronic disorders, progress is comparatively slow and respiratory failure has been anticipated. In acute disorders (mostly Guillain-Barré syndrome and myasthenia gravis), rapid difficulty with clearing secretions and poor mechanical function may occur. Mechanical ventilation to support abnormal pulmonary mechanics and hypoventilation is common,[20] but noninvasive ventilation may be considered first.

Aspiration pneumonitis is a frequent reason for mechanical ventilation. It occurs, for example, in patients with acute oropharyngeal dysfunction, in patients who had seizures, and in vomiting stuporous patients with a diminished response of the pharyngeal reflex. Aspiration is rarely witnessed, but usually after an interval of 6–12 hours, the patient becomes tachypneic with typical harsh bronchial sounds on auscultation.

Chest radiography may show abnormalities in the most dependent part of the lungs, typically including the superior parts of the lower lobes and the posterior segment of the right upper lobe. Mechanical ventilation should be considered if profound hypoxemia develops. Bronchoscopy must be performed when a segmental atelectasis is observed and may locate a large particle that can be removed.

In patients with trauma, pulmonary contusions may become apparent on chest radiographs,

usually within the first hours of admission. Patients with associated flail chest (multiple rib fractures that result in paradoxical chest wall motion during respiration) are at considerable risk for hypoxemia and are best served by stabilization from mechanical ventilation (see Chapter 45).

In occasional patients, underlying pulmonary disease, such as asthma or emphysema, worsens at the time of an acute brain injury. The inability to cough frequently results in mucus plugs that may cause significant oxygen desaturation. Bronchodilators and mild sedation are often needed. In some patients, mechanical ventilation lasting several days is indicated.

More general indications for mechanical ventilation exist. First, mechanical ventilation is indicated when refractory hypoxemia is present, irrespective of the pulmonary insult. Usually, a markedly widened alveolar–arterial oxygen gradient with a maximal FIO_2 of 1.0 or a PO_2 of less than 50 mm Hg, despite 100% oxygen, prompts ventilatory support. This can also be depicted in a PaO_2:FIO_2 ratio of less than 200. Second, inadequate alveolar ventilation is likely with rising $PaCO_2$, usually an acute increase from a patient's baseline or more than 50 mm Hg. Clinically, the work of breathing is assessed as the tidal volume needed to maintain a normal $PaCO_2$. It becomes abnormal at more than 60 L/min.

PHYSIOLOGIC PRINCIPLES AND STANDARD MODES OF MECHANICAL VENTILATION

This section contains common guidelines for setting the ventilator in acutely ill neurologic patients. Modern ICUs are equipped with ventilators and digital touch screens. With changing technology, it makes good sense to become familiar with the commonly used ventilators in the NICU, consult with respiratory therapists, and attend in-service workshops when offered. Usually, general principles pertain to setting the ventilator, and the most important components in setting the ventilator are shown in Figure 17.1. Once on a ventilator, a ventilator bundle is ordered (Capsule 17.1) and noted in the medical record.

Settings of the Ventilator

Traditionally, the initial tidal volume delivered by the ventilator is usually set to be relatively large, ranging from 12 to 15 mL/kg (based on ideal, not actual, body weight).[55,57] However, a tidal volume of more than 15 mL/kg may significantly increase

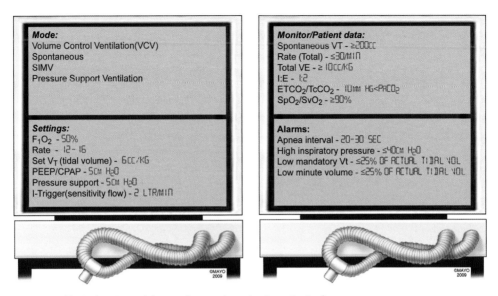

FIGURE 17.1: Typical settings of the ventilator and monitoring criteria alarms.

CPAP, continuous positive airway pressure; E, expiratory; ET, endotracheal; FIO_2, fraction of inspired oxygen; I, inspiratory; PEEP, positive end-expiratory pressure; SIMV, synchronized intermittent-mandatory ventilation; SpO_2, saturation peripheral oxygen; SvO_2, mixed venous saturation; TC, transcutaneous.

the risk of barotrauma. The provided positive pressure breaths to the patient may damage the alveoli. Large tidal volumes do recruit more alveoli by opening them, but stretch injury has been found experimentally and histologically.[32] Another mechanism of mechanical ventilator-induced injury is forceful opening of some airless alveoli, causing repetitive trauma and eventually inflammatory mediators and persistent damage to the surfactant layer.[33,67] If lower tidal volumes improve oxygenation and result in a more stable hemodynamic condition, it can improve cerebral oxygenation. A recent study in a porcine model found significantly worse cerebral oxygenation with implementation of high tidal volume ventilation (12 mL/kg body weight).[4] Therefore, most experts agree that a low tidal volume is most desirable and may reduce ventilation-associated lung injury. Patients with underlying pulmonary disease may need even smaller tidal volumes.

Equally important in reducing strain is measuring the distending pressure of alveoli. Lung protective strategies (mostly developed in clinical protocols on acute respiratory distress syndrome [ARDS] management) involve keeping plateau pressure less than 30 cm H_2O.[23] (The plateau pressure is the pressure measured at the end of inspiration during an inflation hold and a surrogate of elastic threshold stress.)

In some ventilators, the tidal volume is independently controlled. In others, the minute volume is set. (The minute volume is determined by respiratory rate times tidal volume.) The respiratory rate usually ranges from 12 to 16 breaths/min. The respiratory rate must be chosen at the lowest possible setting to reduce the phenomenon of intrinsic PEEP or gas trapping. When rapid rates are set, intrinsic PEEP is created when the time for expiration is diminished. This phenomenon is deleterious because it increases the work of breathing, increases the proximal airway pressures, and may cause hypotension.

Flow rate is set by the inspiratory time in most ventilators, usually through selection by the ratio of inspiration to expiration. This ratio is determined by inspiratory time, pause time, and expiratory time and is expressed in percentages of the total ventilatory cycle. Commonly, the inspiratory time is set for 20% and the pause time for 5%, with the remaining 75% allowed for expiration (inspiration-to-expiration ratio of 1:2).

An important setting is the fraction of inspired oxygen (FIO_2), which is based on the arterial PO_2. High FIO_2 values, those exceeding 0.8 for at least 2 days, are considered toxic (they increased the chance of lung injury in animal experiments). There should be a continuous incentive to decrease FIO_2 in patients receiving mechanical ventilation. However, if reduction of FIO_2 is not tolerated, adequate gas exchange can also be achieved with increasing PEEP. Positive end-expiratory pressure implies a setting that increases the end-expiratory

---

CAPSULE 17.1   VENTILATOR BUNDLE

The ventilator "bundle" is a set of practices to reduce ventilator-associated pneumonia (VAP) and is advocated by the Institute for Healthcare Improvement.[62,64,66] It involves four items: (1) peptic ulcer disease prophylaxis, (2) deep vein thrombosis prophylaxis, (3) elevation of head of the bed, 30–45 degrees, and (4) daily sedation discontinuation and assessment of readiness to wean. Studies found a decrease of VAP ranging from 2.7 to 13.3 cases to 0.0 to 9.3 cases per 1,000 mechanical ventilator days,[75] but none of the studies was blinded. Additions to the main four items have been recently proposed and include use of 2% chlorhexidine antiseptic for oral decontamination and subglottic secretion drainage.[72] Other major preventative measures are tubing changes, appropriate humidification of inspired gases, and closed suctioning of respiratory secretions.

---

pressure to produce a larger functional residual capacity. It maintains alveolar patency throughout respiration, recruits previously collapsed alveoli, and improves ventilation–perfusion matching. Most often, PEEP is indicated when the PO_2 remains less than 60 mm Hg despite an FIO_2 of 0.8. As indicated in cardiogenic pulmonary edema, ARDS, and diffuse bilateral pneumonia, PEEP is often added to ventilation.

Modes of Ventilation

The most frequently used modes in critically ill neurologic patients are controlled mechanical ventilation or assist-control and synchronized intermittent-mandatory ventilation (SIMV), with or without pressure support.[7] In a controlled mode, the ventilator takes over all the work in giving each breath. In SIMV mode, the patient can add breaths spontaneously by triggering the ventilator. Pressure support may be added to reduce the work of breathing on each spontaneous breath.

Current mechanical ventilators provide a graphic display of pressure volume and flow (Figure 17.2). The volume waveform should be scrutinized for possible leaks in the system, which may be caused by an inadequate endotracheal cuff. When such a leak exists, the expired limb of the waveform does not return to baseline (Figure 17.3). The shape of the pressure waveform may indicate flow dyssynchrony. The work of breathing is increased if patient demand exceeds the set flow. The pressure waveform becomes scalloped when the patient's demand exceeds the ventilator output. This anomaly is detected when an assisted patient-triggered breath is compared with an unassisted breath (Figure 17.4).

Controlled Mechanical Ventilation

Controlled-mode ventilation can be used in patients with no breathing drive. Some of these clinical situations result from a severed high cervical cord, treatment with generalized anesthesia (isoflurane or barbiturates) for status epilepticus, or brain death. More often, it is used in mechanically ventilated combative patients treated with neuromuscular blockade, particularly in patients with multitrauma and significant respiratory distress. Its principle is a preset tidal volume with a fixed frequency without any necessary effort by the patient. The timing mechanism determines the delivery of breaths, and the patient is completely dependent on the ventilator.

Controlled mechanical ventilation has many disadvantages, largely related to the use of sedation and neuromuscular blockade. Important risks are disconnection from the machine and the inability to perform any spontaneous breathing. In addition, prolonged controlled mechanical ventilation may cause disuse atrophy and asynchrony of respiratory muscles, creating problems with weaning.

Assist-Control Ventilation

Assist-control ventilation is also a less a frequent initial mode of ventilation in patients with acute neurologic catastrophes. In this mode, the patient is dominant, and the machine takes over if the patient fails to trigger the ventilator. Patients trigger the ventilator by a deflection in a constant flow through the circuit provided by the ventilator ("flowby"). The deflection from patients' inspiration is "read" by the ventilator and provides a breath.

This ventilatory mode is often poorly tolerated by patients who are awake and acutely confused

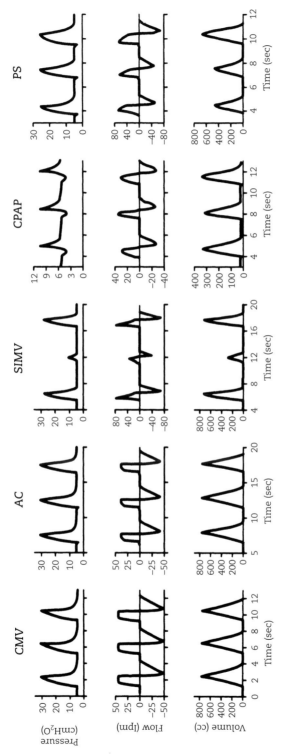

FIGURE 17.2: Modes of mechanical ventilation. Three breaths with pressure curves and accompanying flow and volume waveforms illustrate the most commonly used selections. CMV (continuous mechanical ventilation): All breaths are machine-generated, and a positive end-expiratory pressure of 5 cm H_2O is evident. AC (assist-control): The first two breaths are patient-triggered, as evidenced by a brief negative deflection in airway pressure followed by a machine-triggered breath. SIMV (synchronized intermittent-mandatory ventilation): Two machine-triggered breaths have a spontaneous breath in between. CPAP (continuous positive airway pressure): All breaths are patient-initiated. PS (pressure support): All breaths are patient-initiated. The waveforms of the volume and flow may vary with each breath but have a common rectangular shape.

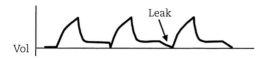

FIGURE 17.3: Cuff leak.

Vol, volume (mL).

and may lead to patient-ventilator dyssynchrony that can be overcome only by additional sedation. The most common side effect of this mode of ventilation is respiratory alkalosis.

Synchronized Intermittent-Mandatory Ventilation

This mode is a combination of machine-initiated breathing at a fixed rate and spontaneous ventilation. Synchronized intermittent mandatory ventilation is the mode chosen for most patients in the NICU after initial stabilization. Again, a preset number of positive-pressure breaths are available for the patient, but they are interrupted by spontaneous breaths. The major shortcoming of positive-pressure ventilation—that ventilator breaths are out of phase with spontaneously generated breaths (stacking)—has been eliminated by synchronization.[31]

This mode has become widely used for weaning, but comparative studies with other regimens (e.g., pressure support, increasing T-piece circuit intervals) are not available in the literature on critical care neurology. The major theoretical disadvantage is that, because spontaneous breaths are not assisted, the mode is not responsive to the patient's needs and therefore may rapidly lead to inadequate ventilation.

Pressure-Support Ventilation

This mode supplies a pressurized breath during spontaneous breathing.[33] The patient generates each breath by triggering the ventilator, again by opening the valve that delivers the breath through creating a negative pressure similar to that in the SIMV mode, but with the important difference of cutoff at a certain flow threshold.

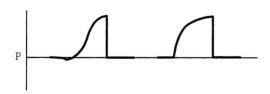

FIGURE 17.4: Dyssynchrony.

P, pressure (cm H_2O).

Pressure-support (PS) ventilation essentially decreases the work of breathing, but the tidal volume and respiration cycle remain controlled by the effort of the patient. Inspiration is terminated when a certain flow threshold is reached. This mode is often used to overcome the resistance of the endotracheal tube and in combination with the SIMV mode.

Continuous Positive Airway Pressure

The continuous positive airway pressure (CPAP) mode assists in spontaneous breathing and may improve oxygenation remarkably. The CPAP mode is often used in patients with sleep apnea, but in the medical ICU, its major goal is to prevent mechanical ventilation. The range of CPAP varies from 0 to 30 cm H_2O.

Pressure-Control Ventilation

This mode of ventilation is essentially the same as controlled mechanical ventilation, but instead of volume limits, a target inspiratory pressure is set. The flow wave characteristics are fairly similar. This mode is often combined with inverse-ratio ventilation, and there is a strong claim of better oxygenation at lower PEEP and peak inspiratory pressure. Many, if not all, patients need additional sedation. Typical indications in the NICU are aspiration pneumonitis and early ARDS.

Noninvasive Ventilation

Noninvasive BiPAP has become an established alternative mode of mechanical ventilation in medical ICUs.[1,8,9,45] Criteria for its use are shown in Table 17.1.[51,65] Typical settings for this ventilatory support system are an inspiratory positive airway pressure (IPAP) of 10 cm H_2O (range, 5–25 cm H_2O) and an expiratory positive airway pressure (EPAP) of 5 cm H_2O (range, 0–30 cm H_2O) (Table

---

TABLE 17.1. INDICATION FOR NONINVASIVE MECHANICAL VENTILATION (BIPAP) IN NICU

Acute (MG) and chronic neuromuscular disease (ALS)
Coma from intoxications
Weaning mode in extubated patients
Supportive mode following craniotomy
Mild (rapid reversible) exacerbation of COPD and cardiogenic pulmonary edema

---

ALS, amyotrophic lateral sclerosis; BiPAP, bilevel positive airway pressure; COPD, chronic obstructive pulmonary disease. MG, myasthenia gravis

17.2). Its major objective is to maintain adequate gas exchange by avoiding intubation. In the general ICU, the procedure is typically used in patients with brief exacerbations of chronic obstructive pulmonary disease and in immunosuppressed patients with acute respiratory failure. It also is an effective weaning mode.[18,24] In the NICU, it has a role in patients with acute neuromuscular disease, and its place in chronic neuromuscular disease, such as amyotrophic lateral sclerosis or muscular dystrophy, has been established.[15] Noninvasive mechanical ventilation is often considered in amyotrophic lateral sclerosis, and patients may be admitted to assess tolerance of the device. Good compliance correlates with preserved upper limb function, less bulbar dysfunction, and the presence of orthopnea. Care is highly specialized and recommendations have been recently published.[36] Experience in Guillain-Barré syndrome (GBS) is concerning with many patients failing due to severe diaphragmatic failure. We have found BiPAP useful in myasthenia gravis exacerbation with respiratory failure and as a weaning device.[51,52] Patients with myasthenia gravis may considerably benefit from noninvasive ventilation using a BiPAP trial, but BiPAP is not likely to be successful if the patient is hypercarbic. Bilevel positive airway pressure could be used while the patient is undergoing plasma exchange, which will often fairly rapidly improve muscle and respiratory weakness. It may not be successful in patients with profound cholinergic symptoms, although BiPAP can dry up secretions. In those patients, endotracheal intubation and CPAP/PS are often a better option, not only to protect the patient from pooling secretions but also to improve respiratory support. Experience with noninvasive mechanical ventilation in spinal cord injury is emerging.

Major limitations of BiPAP include discomfort from the close-fitting mask, failure to rest and sleep, leaks, and gastric distention.[59,73] Patients can be considered only if they do not require vasopressors, are alert and cooperative, can protect the airway, and have hypoxemia of less than 60 mm Hg with an FIO_2 of 50% or hypercapnia of less than 70 mm Hg.

A full-face mask should fit from near the top of the bridge of the nose to just beneath the lower lip (Figure 17.5). Whether the device can prevent intubation or assist in weaning in pulmonary disease remains unclear, and some studies suggest that it does not. Patients who do not tolerate BiPAP may be helped with low-dose dexmedetomidine. A trial of 30 minutes should be sufficient to decide whether intubation can be deferred.

TRACHEOSTOMY

Early tracheostomy should be considered when prolonged mechanical ventilation is anticipated. The main advantages of tracheostomy besides protection from laryngeal injury are improved patient comfort, better mouth care and tracheal suctioning, and a reduced risk of sinusitis and pneumonia. In the general critical care population, the probability of ICU discharge within a month is higher.[3] The main disadvantages are risks with placement, tracheal stenosis, bleeding around the stomal site, and unsatisfactory cosmetic result. Timing remains an unresolved issue. In a recent clinical trial comparing early tracheostomy in 20 medical and surgical ICUs, the comfort level of the patient was significantly different, but there was no effect on other outcome benchmarks such as length of stay or airway or pulmonary complications.[5]

TABLE 17.2. STARTING NONINVASIVE MECHANICAL VENTILATION (BIPAP)

Set pressures starting with low levels (i.e., pressure support 10 cm H_2O and external PEEP 5 cm H_2O).
When patient is tolerant, tighten straps just enough to avoid major leaks, but not too tight.
Set FIO_2 on ventilator or add low-flow oxygen into the circuit, aiming for SO_2 > 90%.
Set alarms; low pressure alarm should be above PEEP level.
Reset pressures (pressure support increased to get expired tidal volume 6 mL/kg or higher; raise PEEP external to get oxygen saturation 90% or higher).
Consider mild sedation if patient is agitated (e.g., dexmedetomidine 0.15 microgram/kg).
Monitor comfort, respiratory rate, oxygen saturation, and dyspnea every 30 minutes for several hours.
Measure arterial blood gases at baseline and within 2 hours from start

BiPAP, bilevel positive airway pressure; FIO_2, fraction of inspired oxygen; NIV, noninvasive ventilation; PEEP, positive end-expiratory pressure; SO_2, oxygen saturation.
Adapted from Nava S, Hill N. Noninvasive ventilation in acute respiratory failure. *Lancet* 2000;374:250–259. With permission.

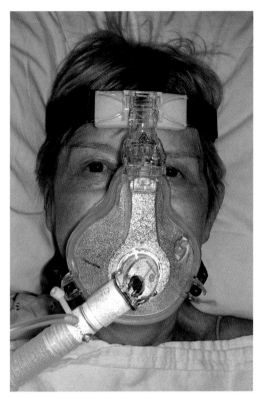

FIGURE 17.5: Noninvasive ventilation. Bilevel positive airway pressure (BiPAP) involves a full-face mask with contoured cushions.

Indications for tracheostomy clearly depend on the clinical course of the acute neurologic illness. A general guideline is to wait 2 weeks to assess the need for tracheostomy but to proceed with tracheostomy earlier in patients who may significantly benefit from the increased comfort. Tracheostomy should probably be considered earlier for comatose patients with head injury who have facial trauma and swelling, because inadvertent extubation may cause major difficulties with reintubation.[27] Early tracheostomy is also reasonable in patients with severe GBS characterized by severe quadriplegia and progressively abnormal results of electrophysiologic studies (inexcitable motor nerves, profuse fibrillations with no voluntary activity). In these unfortunate patients with GBS, prolonged mechanical ventilation is very likely, certainly when no response to plasma exchange or intravenous immunoglobulin has been observed.

Many patients with ischemic or hemorrhagic stroke are weaned from the mechanical ventilator within 2–3 weeks (with the possible exception of patients with pontine hemorrhages or acute basilar artery occlusion), and tracheostomy may be postponed. The need for tracheostomy reflects the need for long-term mechanical ventilation. In many patients, tracheal secretions are better managed with a tracheostomy in place.

Our study of 97 patients refuted the idea that prolonged ventilatory assistance leaves only crippled survivors. Tracheostomy reduced pulmonary complications and provided easier access for pulmonary toilet. In surviving patients, more than a fourth of those with a stroke who required a tracheostomy regained functional independence, and early tracheostomy shortened ICU stay.[46]

Traditional tracheostomy involves a standard elective surgical procedure under general anesthesia.[16] The procedure is usually event-free but may cause postoperative bleeding. Another technique is Ciaglia's percutaneous dilatational tracheostomy.[11–13,39] It is performed by general surgeons in most hospitals, but more recently has also been performed by medical intensivists and neurointensivists.[21] One benefit of this procedure is the use of the smallest possible skin incision, which may reduce scarring.[50,69] Percutaneous dilatational tracheostomy may be preferred in patients with GBS and myasthenia gravis when only comparatively brief periods of ventilation are anticipated.

The technique may include fiberoptic bronchoscopy after the endotracheal tube is deflated and involves needle and Seldinger wire insertion and serial dilatation (Figure 17.6). Insertion is between the second and third tracheal cartilages.

Complications of percutaneous dilatational tracheostomy are inadvertent endotracheal cuff rupture, subcutaneous emphysema, hemorrhage, false passage, pneumothorax, and tracheal stenosis, all with incidences of less than 4%.[5,6,19] Modification of the original technique may cause problems, too. A randomized study of 100 patients documented a much lower surgical complication rate (2%) than that associated with traditional tracheostomy (25%).[56] Contraindications to percutaneous dilatational tracheostomy are obscure anatomical landmarks (goiter, obesity, prior trauma), requirement of an FIO_2 greater than 0.6 to ensure oxygen saturation, and abnormal coagulation.

LIBERATING FROM THE VENTILATOR

Discontinuation from the mechanical ventilator is a major focus of clinical studies, all in an attempt to define variables or indices that predict success. Studies of weaning criteria in patients with CNS injury and neuromuscular weakness are virtually

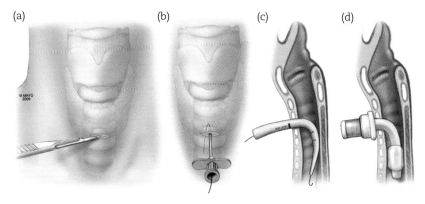

FIGURE 17.6: Procedure of percutaneous dilatory tracheostomy (from left to right): (A) incision, (B) needle puncture, (C) guide wire placement, and (D) introduction of dilators. Most often the Ciaglia Blue Rhino set is used.

unavailable, and the published determinants in critically ill patients with prolonged mechanical ventilation may not apply to the vast majority of patients with acute brain injury.[22,28]

Liberating a patient from the ventilator may be difficult due to decreased respiratory muscle strength and partly due to ventilator-associated respiratory muscle damage, specifically to the diaphragm.[26] A recent pathology study showed marked diaphragm atrophy already after 18 hours of diaphragmatic inactivity.[30] It remains unclear whether axonal injury of the phrenic nerve in a patient with critical illness polyneuropathy—a common complication in any patient with a prolonged stay in the ICU—is a factor in difficulty with weaning. It is common knowledge that liberating the patient from the ventilator can be successful in many of those ventilated for a short time (less than 2 weeks), but weaning of patients with prolonged mechanical ventilation (e.g., after prolonged treatment of refractory status epilepticus) is protracted and often involves many unsuccessful attempts at using spontaneous pressure-supported breathing.[15]

The practice of weaning may differ, but no method should be entertained unless several clinical and laboratory criteria are fulfilled.[38,49] These criteria can be easily assessed at the bedside (Table 17.3).[17,25,47] In addition, weaning should not be entertained in patients who still require PEEP for adequate oxygenation and in patients who have significant chest radiographic abnormalities that do not show considerable improvement (complete clearing on the chest radiograph is ideal but not required in the first attempt at weaning). Weaning should not be started if general anesthesia is planned within 1 or 2 days, the neurologic condition is deteriorating, or active therapy for intracranial pressure is administered. A reduced level of consciousness per se is not a contraindication. Weaning from the ventilator also includes important adjunctive measures, such as correction of electrolyte imbalance, adequate hydration and nutrition, patient in upright position, proper care of secretions, and, perhaps most important, adequate sleep. It is critical that during weaning efforts, patients have effective rest at night. Weaning should be gradual, because a sudden transition may be stressful to patients with underlying cardiovascular disease.

In GBS, a sufficient increase in vital capacity is needed to proceed with a weaning attempt.[10] We devised a pulmonary function ratio (PFR) based on the sum of pulmonary function test results in GBS:

$$PFR = \frac{PFint}{PF2w}$$

in which PF is vital capacity plus PI_{max} plus PE_{max}, int is the value at intubation, and 2w is the value at the second week. Failure of this ratio to improve (< 1) predicted weaning failure and directed the timing of tracheostomy. The potential usefulness

TABLE 17.3. LABORATORY WEANING CRITERIA IN THE ICU

Measurement	Requirement
PaO_2	> 60 mm Hg
Tidal volume	> 5 mL/kg
Vital capacity	> 15 mL/kg
Minute ventilation	< 10 L/kg
Negative inspiratory pressure	≥ −30 mm Hg

of this ratio in GBS implies that pulmonary function tests should continue during mechanical ventilation and may indicate trends in improvement that may initiate an attempt at weaning.

Spontaneous breathing trials are recommended before extubation. This is particularly relevant in patients intubated for acute (and resolving) neuromuscular respiratory failure. I favor both pressure-support weaning trials followed by spontaneous T-piece trials. The "minimal ventilator settings" of PEEP of 5 and PS of 5 have been correctly questioned as criteria for intubation, and it has been pointed out that 30%–60% increase in respiratory load occurs immediately after extubation and demand ischemia is not uncommon in patients with prior cardiovascular disease.[58,60] A T-piece trial of 2 hours may be needed in patients with dubious readiness for extubation. This trial is successful if rapid shallow breathing index remains less than 105 and ABG shows a $PaCO_2$ less than 45 mm Hg.[22]

In most patients with acute CNS lesions who have been intubated for a short time, weaning can be accomplished by gradual T-tube weaning. Before the weaning effort is started, it is important to observe the patient for 5 minutes after placing a T-piece. Next to looking for obvious signs of discomfort, one should specifically watch for an increase in respiratory rate (> 25 breaths/min), a decrease in tidal volume (not below 300 mL), a change in blood pressure (either way), an increase in heart rate (increase of more than 20 beats/min), or the development of premature ventricular contractions or bigeminy. Arterial blood gas values are determined regularly. Common practice is to begin with a trial of 30 minutes; if this is successful, the duration can be rapidly increased to 1–2 hours. Extubation is performed when the arterial blood gas values remain satisfactory and no rapid shallow breathing is observed.[61] If the T-tube trial fails, the patient is given at least 24 hours of rest with mechanical ventilation, and then another attempt is made.[63]

A recent randomized controlled trial on weaning of neurologic and neurosurgical patients documented a decrease in the reintubation rate of 5% versus 13% using a weaning protocol.[40] This weaning protocol included a 1-hour spontaneous breathing trial with 2–3 cm H_2O continuous positive airway pressure. The trial was interrupted when respiratory rate increased to more than 35/min, respiratory distress became apparent, or hypotension, desaturation, or tachycardia occurred. Extubation followed in patients with a respiratory rate/tidal volume ratio of 105 or less, a PaO_2/FIO_2 of 200 or greater, a pH of 7.35 or more,

and a PCO_2 of 50 mm Hg or less. Other studies found that extubation in stuporous patients is feasible when secretions can be handled well.[14,34]

Another approach is to change the settings of the SIMV mode. The frequency is reduced in gradual steps. Arterial blood gas determinations are used to recognize potential trends to respiratory acidosis. SIMV weaning is fairly simple, consisting of gradual reduction with 3 breaths/min starting three times a day. It is prudent to add pressure support at low levels (5–10 cm H_2O) for further comfort. Pressure-support weaning may be preferred to other weaning regimens and may increase synchronicity. Pressure support is set at a level that is comfortable for the patient, usually 15–40 cm H_2O, followed by decrements of 3 cm H_2O. When the pressure support level of 5 cm H_2O is tolerated (pressure just enough to overcome the resistance of the tubing) and the laboratory criteria are fulfilled, extubation can be undertaken.[42,54]

It has been suggested that rapid shallow breathing diagnosed by the ratio of respiratory frequency to tidal volume accurately predicts weaning failure. Patients with a frequency-to-volume ratio of more than 100 had a 95% likelihood of failure in a weaning trial. Patients with a frequency-to-volume ratio of less than 100 had an 80% likelihood of successful weaning[74] (Figure 17.7). A prospective study showed a less optimistic prognostic value[29] (sensitivity, 72%; specificity, 11%). Others have found minute ventilation recovery time a better predictor of successful extubation.[35] The use of the frequency-to-volume ratio may be very helpful as a clinical guide after extubation.

Extubation should be well tolerated, but inspiratory stridor may develop virtually immediately to 1 hour after extubation. There have been attempts to predict airway obstruction from laryngeal edema. A cuff-leak test consists of deflating the balloon cuff of the endotracheal tube and auscultation of flow over trachea or recording of exhaled tidal volumes pre- and post-deflation. A positive cuff-leak test (no leak and thus likely swelling) had a sensitivity of 0.65 and specificity of 0.86.[41]

Most patients have transient hoarseness alone. Topical epinephrine into the hypopharynx is a reasonable option, but reintubation is often necessary. Laryngospasm, however, is less common but life-threatening. It is much more common in children and young adults. Typically, the crowing sound of stridor is absent and strenuous efforts are seen, with significant desaturation.

Lidocaine, 2 mg/kg intravenously, may significantly reduce laryngospasm if used several

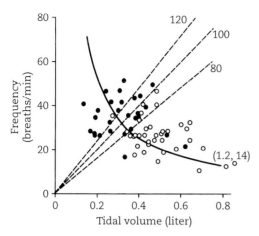

FIGURE 17.7: Rapid shallow breathing index. Weaning success (open circles), weaning failure (solid circles). Patients to the left of the threshold isopleth value of 100 for ratio of frequency to tidal volume had a 95% likelihood of weaning failure. For comparison, the hyperbola represents a minute ventilation of 10 L/min, indicating poor predictive value (minute ventilation of 10 L/min is a frequently used weaning criterion).

From Yang KL, Tobin MJ. A prospective study of indexes predicting the outcome of trials of weaning from mechanical ventilation. *N Engl J Med* 1991;324:1445–1450. With permission of the Massachusetts Medical Society.

minutes before extubation in susceptible individuals. In some patients, reintubation is needed, followed by a 3-day course of dexamethasone 10 mg and another trial of extubation. Laryngoscopy by an ear-nose-throat specialist may be needed to confirm resolution of swelling.

REINTUBATION

Reintubation in critically ill neurologic patients is not uncommon and may reach 25%, dependent on the population.[2] In a neurosurgical population, the risk for reintubation was low (0.4%) and also in patients after craniotomy (0.9%).[53] Not surprisingly, preexisting cardiopulmonary disease and older age increase the probability.

CONCLUSIONS

- Intubation is needed in patients with acute brain injury who cannot protect their airway, as shown by frequent hypoxic episodes; in patients with tachycardia and tachypnea associated with neuromuscular failure (GBS, myasthenia gravis); and in patients with primary pulmonary disease (pulmonary edema or progressive aspiration pneumonitis).

- A typical order for mechanical ventilation in a stable neurologic patient is IMV, 8–12; FIO_2, 0.4–0.9; tidal volume, 5–10 mL/kg; PEEP, 2–5 cm H_2O; and inspiration-to-expiration ratio, 1:2.

- Noninvasive ventilation (BiPAP) is an option in some patients with neuromuscular respiratory weakness (myasthenia gravis; ALS). It may also function as a possible alternative for intubation in patients with less severe pulmonary disease.

- Tracheostomy may provide better comfort to the patient and facilitates bronchial hygiene. The procedure may reduce length of stay in the NICU. It should be postponed until 2 weeks in patients who can potentially be liberated from the ventilator due to early signs of neurologic improvement.

REFERENCES

1. American Thoracic Society tERS, the European Society of Intensive Care Medicine, and the Société de Réanimation de Langue Française. International Consensus Conferences in Intensive Care Medicine: noninvasive positive pressure ventilation in acute Respiratory failure. *Am J Respir Crit Care Med* 2001;163:283–291.

2. Anderson CD, Bartscher JF, Scripko PD, et al. Neurologic examination and extubation outcome in the neurocritical care unit. *Neurocrit Care* 2011;15:490–497.

3. Andriolo BN, Andriolo RB, Saconato H, Atallah AN, Valente O. Early versus late tracheostomy for critically ill patients. *Cochrane Database Syst Rev* 2015;1:CD007271.

4. Bickenbach J, Zoremba N, Fries M, et al. Low tidal volume ventilation in a porcine model of acute lung injury improves cerebral tissue oxygenation. *Anesth Analg* 2009;109:847–855.

5. Blot F, Similowski T, Trouillet JL, et al. Early tracheotomy versus prolonged endotracheal intubation in unselected severely ill ICU patients. *Intens Care Med* 2008;34:1779–1787.

6. Briche T, Le Manach Y, Pats B. Complications of percutaneous tracheostomy. *Chest* 2001;119:1282–1283.

7. Consensus statement on the essentials of mechanical ventilators: 1992. *Respir Care* 1992;37:1000–1008.

8. Carlucci A, Richard JC, Wysocki M, Lepage E, Brochard L. Noninvasive versus conventional mechanical ventilation: an epidemiologic survey. *Am J Respir Crit Care Med* 2001;163:874–880.

9. Chatburn RL. Which ventilators and modes can be used to deliver noninvasive ventilation? *Respir Care* 2009;54:85–101.

10. Chevrolet JC, Deleamont P. Repeated vital capacity measurements as predictive parameters for mechanical ventilation need and weaning success in the Guillain-Barre syndrome. *Am Rev Respir Dis* 1991;144:814–818.

11. Ciaglia P. Percutaneous tracheostomy is really better—if done correctly. *Chest* 1999;116:1138–1139.

12. Ciaglia P. Technique, complications, and improvements in percutaneous dilatational tracheostomy. *Chest* 1999;115:1229–1230.

13. Ciaglia P, Firsching R, Syniec C. Elective percutaneous dilatational tracheostomy: a new simple bedside procedure; preliminary report. *Chest* 1985;87:715–719.

14. Coplin WM, Pierson DJ, Cooley KD, Newell DW, Rubenfeld GD. Implications of extubation delay in brain-injured patients meeting standard weaning criteria. *Am J Respir Crit Care Med* 2000;161:1530–1536.

15. De Jonghe B, Bastuji-Garin S, Durand MC, et al. Respiratory weakness is associated with limb weakness and delayed weaning in critical illness. *Crit Care Med* 2007;35:2007–2015.

16. Dulguerov P, Gysin C, Perneger TV, Chevrolet JC. Percutaneous or surgical tracheostomy: a meta-analysis. *Crit Care Med* 1999;27:1617–1625.

17. Epstein SK. Weaning from ventilatory support. *Curr Opin Crit Care* 2009;15:36–43.

18. Ferrer M, Valencia M, Nicolas JM, et al. Early noninvasive ventilation averts extubation failure in patients at risk: a randomized trial. *Am J Respir Crit Care Med* 2006;173:164–170.

19. Freeman BD, Isabella K, Cobb JP, et al. A prospective, randomized study comparing percutaneous with surgical tracheostomy in critically ill patients. *Crit Care Med* 2001;29:926–930.

20. Gibson GJ, Pride NB, Davis JN, Loh LC. Pulmonary mechanics in patients with respiratory muscle weakness. *Am Rev Respir Dis* 1977;115:389–395.

21. Hoekema D. Percutaneous tracheostomy coming of age for the neurointensivist? *Neurocrit Care* 2009;10:261–263.

22. Jeganathan N, Kaplan CA, Balk RA. Ventilator liberation for high-risk-for-failure patients: improving value of the spontaneous breathing trial. *Respir Care* 2015;60:290–296.

23. Kapinos G, Chichra A. Lung-protective ventilation for SAH patients: are these measures truly protective? *Neurocrit Care* 2014;21:175–177.

24. Keenan SP, Powers C, McCormack DG, Block G. Noninvasive positive-pressure ventilation for postextubation respiratory distress: a randomized controlled trial. *JAMA* 2002;287:3238–3244.

25. Khamiees M, Raju P, DeGirolamo A, Amoateng-Adjepong Y, Manthous CA. Predictors of extubation outcome in patients who have successfully completed a spontaneous breathing trial. *Chest* 2001;120:1262–1270.

26. Laghi F, Tobin MJ. Disorders of the respiratory muscles. *Am J Respir Crit Care Med* 2003;168:10–48.

27. Lanza DC, Koltai PJ, Parnes SM, et al. Predictive value of the Glasgow Coma Scale for tracheotomy in head-injured patients. *Ann Otol Rhinol Laryngol* 1990;99:38–41.

28. Lazaridis C, DeSantis SM, McLawhorn M, Krishna V. Liberation of neurosurgical patients from mechanical ventilation and tracheostomy in neurocritical care. *J Crit Care* 2012;27:417 e411–e418.

29. Lee KH, Hui KP, Chan TB, Tan WC, Lim TK. Rapid shallow breathing (frequency-tidal volume ratio) did not predict extubation outcome. *Chest* 1994;105:540–543.

30. Levine S, Nguyen T, Taylor N, et al. Rapid disuse atrophy of diaphragm fibers in mechanically ventilated humans. *N Engl J Med* 2008;358:1327–1335.

31. Luce JM, Pierson DJ, Hudson LD. Intermittent mandatory ventilation. *Chest* 1981;79:678–685.

32. MacIntyre NR. Current issues in mechanical ventilation for respiratory failure. *Chest* 2005;128:561S–567S.

33. MacIntyre NR. Respiratory function during pressure support ventilation. *Chest* 1986;89:677–683.

34. Manno EM, Rabinstein AA, Wijdicks EFM, et al. A prospective trial of elective extubation in brain injured patients meeting extubation criteria for ventilatory support: a feasibility study. *Crit Care* 2008;12:R138.

35. Martinez A, Seymour C, Nam M. Minute ventilation recovery time: a predictor of extubation outcome. *Chest* 2003;123:1214–1221.

36. Miller RG, Jackson CE, Kasarskis EJ, et al. Practice parameter update: the care of the patient with amyotrophic lateral sclerosis: drug, nutritional, and respiratory therapies (an evidence-based review): report of the Quality Standards Subcommittee of the American Academy of Neurology. *Neurology* 2009;73:1218–1226.

37. Nachtmann A, Siebler M, Rose G, Sitzer M, Steinmetz H. Cheyne-Stokes respiration in ischemic stroke. *Neurology* 1995;45:820–821.

38. Namen AM, Ely EW, Tatter SB, et al. Predictors of successful extubation in neurosurgical patients. *Am J Respir Crit Care Med* 2001;163:658–664.

39. Nates JL, Cooper DJ, Myles PS, Scheinkestel CD, Tuxen DV. Percutaneous tracheostomy in critically ill patients: a prospective, randomized comparison of two techniques. *Crit Care Med* 2000;28:3734–3739.

40. Navalesi P, Frigerio P, Moretti MP, et al. Rate of reintubation in mechanically ventilated neurosurgical and neurologic patients: evaluation of a systematic approach to weaning and extubation. *Crit Care Med* 2008;36:2986–2992.

41. Ochoa ME, Marin Mdel C, Frutos-Vivar F, et al. Cuff-leak test for the diagnosis of upper airway obstruction in adults: a systematic review and meta-analysis. *Intens Care Med* 2009;35:1171–1179.

42. Perren A, Domenighetti G, Mauri S, Genini F, Vizzardi N. Protocol-directed weaning from mechanical ventilation: clinical outcome in patients randomized for a 30-min or 120-min trial with pressure support ventilation. *Intens Care Med* 2002;28:1058–1063.

43. Pilbeam SP, Cairo JM. Pilbeam's *Mechanical Ventilation: Physiological and Clinical Applications*. 5th ed. St. Louis: Mosby; 2015.

44. Pontoppidan H, Geffin B, Lowenstein E. Acute respiratory failure in the adult: 2. *N Engl J Med* 1972;287:743–752.

45. Poponick JM, Renston JP, Bennett RP, Emerman CL. Use of a ventilatory support system (BiPAP) for acute respiratory failure in the emergency department. *Chest* 1999;116:166–171.

46. Rabinstein AA, Wijdicks EFM. Outcome of survivors of acute stroke who require prolonged ventilatory assistance and tracheostomy. *Cerebrovasc Dis* 2004;18:325–331.

47. Sahn SA, Lakshminarayan S. Bedside criteria for discontinuation of mechanical ventilation. *Chest* 1973;63:1002–1005.

48. Salam A, Tilluckdharry L, Amoateng-Adjepong Y, Manthous CA. Neurologic status, cough, secretions and extubation outcomes. *Intens Care Med* 2004;30:1334–1339.

49. Scheinhorn DJ, Artinian BM, Catlin JL. Weaning from prolonged mechanical ventilation: the experience at a regional weaning center. *Chest* 1994;105:534–539.

50. Schwann NM. Percutaneous dilational tracheostomy: anesthetic considerations for a growing trend. *Anesth Analg* 1997;84:907–911.

51. Seneviratne J, Mandrekar J, Wijdicks EFM, Rabinstein AA. Noninvasive ventilation in myasthenic crisis. *Arch Neurol* 2008;65:54–58.

52. Seneviratne J, Mandrekar J, Wijdicks EFM, Rabinstein AA. Predictors of extubation failure in myasthenic crisis. *Arch Neurol* 2008;65: 929–933.

53. Shalev D, Kamel H. Risk of reintubation in neurosurgical patients. *Neurocrit Care* 2015;22:15–19.

54. Shapiro M, Wilson RK, Casar G, Bloom K, Teague RB. Work of breathing through different sized endotracheal tubes. *Crit Care Med* 1986;14:1028–1031.

55. Slutsky AS. Mechanical ventilation. American College of Chest Physicians' Consensus Conference. *Chest* 1993;104:1833–1859.

56. Stock MC, Woodward CG, Shapiro BA, et al. Perioperative complications of elective tracheostomy in critically ill patients. *Crit Care Med* 1986; 14:861–863.

57. Tobin MJ. Advances in mechanical ventilation. *N Engl J Med* 2001;344:1986–1996.

58. Tobin MJ. Extubation and the myth of "minimal ventilator settings." *Am J Respir Crit Care Med* 2012;185:349–350.

59. Tobin MJ. *Principles and Practice of Mechanical Ventilation*. 3nd ed. New York: McGraw-Hill; 2012.

60. Tobin MJ, Laghi F, Jubran A. Ventilatory failure, ventilator support, and ventilator weaning. *Compr Physiol* 2012;2:2871–2921.

61. Tobin MJ, Perez W, Guenther SM, et al. The pattern of breathing during successful and unsuccessful trials of weaning from mechanical ventilation. *Am Rev Respir Dis* 1986;134:1111–1118.

62. Tolentino-DelosReyes AF, Ruppert SD, Shiao SY. Evidence-based practice: use of the ventilator bundle to prevent ventilator-associated pneumonia. *Am J Crit Care* 2007;16:20–27.

63. Tomlinson JR, Miller KS, Lorch DG, et al. A prospective comparison of IMV and T-piece weaning from mechanical ventilation. *Chest* 1989;96:348–352.

64. Torres A. The new American Thoracic Society/Infectious Disease Society of North America guidelines for the management of hospital-acquired, ventilator-associated and healthcare-associated pneumonia: a current view and new complementary information. *Curr Opin Crit Care* 2006;12:444–445.

65. Tromans AM, Mecci M, Barrett FH, Ward TA, Grundy DJ. The use of the BiPAP biphasic positive airway pressure system in acute spinal cord injury. *Spinal Cord* 1998;36:481–484.

66. Westwell S. Implementing a ventilator care bundle in an adult intensive care unit. *Nurs Crit Care* 2008;13:203–207.

67. Whitehead T, Slutsky AS. The pulmonary physician in critical care 7: ventilator induced lung injury. *Thorax* 2002;57:635–642.

68. Wijdicks EFM, Borel CO. Respiratory management in acute neurologic illness. *Neurology* 1998; 50:11–20.

69. Wijdicks EFM, Lawn ND, Fletcher DD. Tracheo-stomy scars in Guillain-Barre syndrome: a reason for concern? *J Neurol* 2001;248:527–528.

70. Wijdicks EFM, Scott JP. Causes and outcome of mechanical ventilation in patients with hemi-spheric ischemic stroke. *Mayo Clinic Proc* 1997;72:210–213.

71. Wijdicks EFM, Scott JP. Outcome in patients with acute basilar artery occlusion requiring mechani-cal ventilation. *Stroke* 1996;27:1301–1303.

72. Wip C, Napolitano L. Bundles to prevent ventilator-associated pneumonia: how valu-able are they? *Curr Opin Infect Dis* 2009;22:159–166.

73. Yamada S, Nishimiya J, Kurokawa K, Yuasa T, Masaka A. Bilevel nasal positive airway pres-sure and ballooning of the stomach. *Chest* 2001;119:1965–1966.

74. Yang KL, Tobin MJ. A prospective study of indexes predicting the outcome of trials of wean-ing from mechanical ventilation. *N Engl J Med* 1991;324:1445–1450.

75. Zilberberg MD, Shorr AF, Kollef MH. Implementing quality improvements in the intensive care unit: ventilator bundle as an exam-ple. *Crit Care Med* 2009;37:305–309.

18

Nutrition

Early feeding to guarantee adequate nutrition is fundamental in patients with any type of acute neurologic illness. To be more precise, feeding prevents gastrointestinal mucosal atrophy, whereas a lag in nutritional support may create a situation in which patients become too weak to effectively cough up secretions or even maximally fend off looming bacterial infections.[53] Outcome studies in general ICU populations emphasize a relation between outcome and caloric intake.[81] Outcome studies in patients with traumatic brain injury and stroke suggest that when nutritional support is prompt, mortality is reduced and the number of nosocomial infections is significantly lower.[41,83–85] Early feeding may be particularly mandatory in mechanically ventilated patients.[3] In contrast, early nasogastric tube feeding in patients with acute gastroparesis increases the risk of aspiration of retained solutions and gastric acid, both extremely damaging to the lung, increasing mortality in some units.[56] Ventilator-associated pneumonia and *Clostridium difficile* infection were shown to be more common in patients fed immediately.[35]

Nutritional support practices vary, and a prospective study in a medical intensive care unit (ICU) suggested underutilization, with half of the patients receiving suboptimal caloric intake[21] and failing to reach targeted nutritional goals. There is also a delay in initiation of enteral feeding when physicians are surveyed.[6] Gradual increase in infusion rates to reduce gastric distention may also be one of the explanations for not meeting goals. Randomized studies have been published in traumatic brain injury, but not in many other conditions, and nutritional support remains based on empirical evidence.[45,83]

Nutritional support in the neurosciences intensive care unit (NICU) has distinctive characteristics, and critical care neurologists must be comfortable with administering various tube feedings and determining the indications for percutaneous endoscopic gastrostomy.[87] Daily care is focused on countering the effects of hypermetabolism and acute gastroparesis and to ward off complications associated with enteral nutrition.[60,61,65,67] Nutritional care, the details of monitoring the adequacy of nutritional support tailored toward specific acute neurologic disorders, and the handling of devices that deliver nutrition form the major focus of this chapter.

NUTRITIONAL NEEDS AND MAINTENANCE

As a matter of principle, and seemingly obvious, a consensus statement from the American College of Chest Physicians emphasizes that doses of nutrients provided should be compatible with the existing metabolism.[14] The main goals of nutritional support are to preserve muscle mass (lean body mass) and to provide adequate fluids, vitamins, minerals, and fats.[10,48]

Any patient transferred to the NICU needs a full assessment of nutritional status. One of the first objectives is to estimate nutritional needs. The components of clinical nutritional assessment should be partitioned into the evaluation of possible underlying malnutrition and the estimation of nutritional needs in a patient in a hypermetabolic state. For example, a common misconception is that obese patients should be able to tolerate intervals without feeding (Capsule 18.1).[52]

There is a fundamental difference between starvation and the much more common hypermetabolic state. In starvation, the major physiologic changes are characterized by decreased energy expenditure and the utilization of alternative fuel sources. Patients can tolerate extended periods of semistarvation because the body responds to decreased energy intake by a reduction of the basal metabolic rate and favors a state in which the fat supplies are used as primary fuel. Patients with a neurologic catastrophe respond differently. The metabolic rate is dramatically increased (hypermetabolism), and rather than depletion of fat, protein stores from lean body mass are rapidly mobilized.[23] The major physiologic changes that are characterized by increased

CAPSULE 18.1   OBESITY AND CRITICAL ILLNESS

It has been estimated that approximately one-third of critically ill patients are obese.[33] Severe (morbid) obesity is defined by usually more than a 20% increase above a normal body mass index (BMI). Comparative studies in critically ill patients with obesity have been insufficient and flawed (comparing results with underweight patients), but risk assessment is important due to obesity's associated comorbidities.

Obesity increases the risk of complications and may require more attentive routine management, but mortality is not increased.[38] The management problems associated with obesity are shown in the accompanying illustration. Aspiration is increased due to high gastric volume and lower pH of gastric fluid in obese patients fasting during critical illness. Nonetheless, insufficient evidence links longer ventilator stays to obesity. Decreased mobility lowers levels of antithrombin III and actually contributes to an increased chance of deep vein thrombosis.[1,8] The volume of distribution of drugs is markedly increased with lipophilic drugs such as propofol, fentanyl, benzodiazepines, and antibiotics such as aminoglycosides and quinolones. Nutritional requirements mostly involve hypocaloric high-protein nutrition in patients with a BMI over 27.[52,64]

On a positive note, it has been speculated that high cholesterol and lipid levels may reduce the effects of sepsis owing to binding of endotoxins.[33]

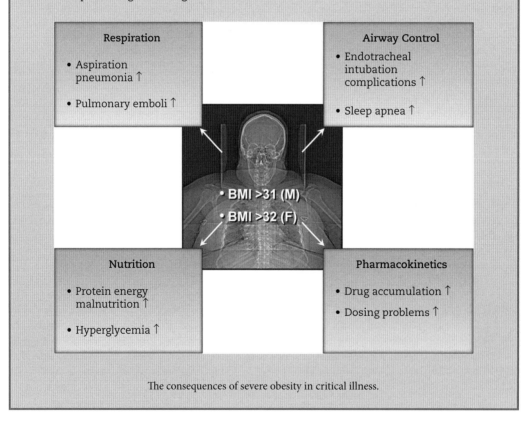

The consequences of severe obesity in critical illness.

metabolic rate are fever, leukocytosis, hyperglycemia, hypoalbuminemia, and increased blood urea nitrogen.

The physical examination should focus specifically on features of underlying malnutrition. Besides the visible appearance of severe wasting, subtler clinical features may indicate malnutrition. Typical clinical signs associated with malnutrition are shown in Table 18.1. Many of these signs may suggest deficiency of a specific nutrient. Awareness of the possibility of malnutrition should be very high in emergency admissions of

TABLE 18.1. PHYSICAL SIGNS
OF MALNUTRITION

Disorder	Deficiency
Generalized muscle wasting	Any
Easily plucked, thin, dyspigmented hair	Zinc
Nasolabial seborrhea	Any
Fissuring of eyelid corners	Vitamin B_2
Angular stomatitis, cheilosis	Vitamin B_{12}
Periodontal disease, mottled enamel, and caries	Any
Raw and swollen tongue	Niacin and folate
Spoon-shaped nails	Iron
Hyperkeratosis and petechial hemorrhages of the skin	Vitamin C or K

patients with traumatic brain injury and fulminant bacterial meningitis, conditions that are considerably more common in alcoholics. Vitamin B_1 (thiamine) deficiency should be anticipated not only because intake is poor but also because alcohol reduces thiamine absorption. Reduced erythrocyte transketolase levels can be diagnostic (thiamine deficiency deranges glucose metabolism, and in the pentose phosphate pathway, transketolase is the thiamine-dependent step). Large doses of parenteral thiamine (50 mg intravenously [IV] initially and 50–100 mg intramuscularly [IM] for 5–7 days) must be administered to prevent a lapse into a Wernicke-Korsakoff syndrome in thiamine-deficient patients, particularly before intravenous carbohydrate loads are administered. Magnesium (1 g as undiluted 50% solution IM) acts as a cofactor for transketolase activity and may have to be additionally administered.[55] Wernicke-Korsakoff syndrome can be recognized by a confusional state, horizontal or vertical nystagmus, gaze palsy, and ataxia of gait or limbs, but is seldom manifested by coma. The dose of thiamine in an established Wernicke-Korsakoff syndrome should be 100–200 mg IV for 5 days, depending on severity and response to therapy. The symptoms, particularly the ophthalmic manifestations, typically disappear within this time period.

Other laboratory values may also help in the interpretation of underlying malnutrition. Hypoalbuminemia is an important marker for malnutrition at the initial presentation. Decrease in plasma albumin in critical illness is a result of decreased hepatic production during the acute-phase response. The daily production rate may be substantially decreased, certainly in patients with continuing bacteremia. Cytokines such as interleukin-1 and tumor necrosis factor decrease food intake and have a direct down-regulating effect on the albumin gene. Surveys in surgical intensive care units have emphasized a significantly higher mortality among patients with serum albumin levels below 3.5 g/L from malnutrition. Decreased transferrin and total lymphocyte count—but also albumin-bound calcium, magnesium, and zinc—may indicate protein wasting, but these values are not very reliable in the NICU. Measurement of triceps skin-fold thickness remains difficult to perform and is less practical.

Malnutrition has a strikingly adverse effect on lung function by impairing respiratory muscles, decreasing ventilatory drive, and diminishing the lung defense mechanism. These effects become important in patients with acute neuromuscular failure and could hamper weaning efforts. However, a fine line may exist here, because overfeeding with excess carbohydrate calories (> 3,000/day) may lead to hypercapnia, which also reduces the success of weaning.

Caloric needs can be estimated by weight and approximate 25–30 kcal/kg/day. The Harris-Benedict formulas, however, are more accurate in determining caloric needs,[61,70] and the nutritional needs of patients with neurologic critical illness should be calculated with this equation to obtain the basal energy expenditure (BEE) in calories. The Harris-Benedict formulas are based on kilograms of weight (W), centimeters of height (H), and years of age (A). For men, the formula is BEE = 66.5 + 13.8W + 5H – 6.8A, and for women, BEE = 655 + 9.6W + 1.8H – 4.7A. This method, although introduced in healthy persons, remains the most practical means of obtaining daily caloric needs. Correcting factors for specific critical disease states, which primarily add a certain percentage to the calculated value, have been proposed, but they increase the inaccuracy of the estimate. More specifically, no correcting factors are known in acute brain injury. It is, however, common practice to add a "stress factor" in patients with an acute central nervous system (CNS) catastrophic event and marked sympathetic manifestations, such as profuse sweating, hyperthermia, hypertension, and tachycardia. Total calories are then calculated by BEE plus 20%. In obese patients, 75% of the basal Harris-Benedict calculation based on obese weight seems reasonable.

More accurate measurements can be obtained by indirect calorimetry, which is based on the calculation of energy expenditure through the measurement of respiratory gas exchange. Metabolism is expressed as oxygen (O_2) consumption and carbon dioxide (CO_2) production. With the use of portable devices (metabolic carts), the resting energy expenditure can be calculated from (oxygen consumption in liters per minute) and (carbon dioxide production in liters per minute). The metabolic cart that measures the concentration of O_2 and CO_2 can be connected to the ventilator tubing. (Resting energy expenditure = 3.94 [] + 1.1[] × 1,440 = kcal in 1 day.) Although metabolic carts are expensive to use and calibration is at times questionable, they can be of value in patients who have difficulty in weaning, are morbidly obese, or have been treated with prolonged volume expansion, which makes the estimation of "dry weight" cumbersome.

The estimated energy expenditure subsequently is divided into proteins of 1.5 g/kg/day, and the remaining calories are evenly divided between carbohydrates and lipids. The simplest way to monitor nutritional support, however, is to weigh patients regularly. A severe catabolic state can be further monitored by nitrogen balance. This can be calculated at intervals of several days, provided that renal function is not changing. Urinary nitrogen is measured in a 24-hour urine collection. The nitrogen balance is calculated as follows: nitrogen balance (grams) = (protein intake/6.25) − (urinary nitrogen + 4). Increased nitrogen secretion results in negative nitrogen balance, and more protein must be delivered. The glucose targets are discussed in Chapter 57.

ASSESSMENT OF ASPIRATION RISK

Patients with traumatic brain injury may be intoxicated from alcohol or other substances at the time of injury, and swallowing mechanics may be disturbed in patients with a brainstem or hemispheric stroke and in patients with acute neuromuscular disease.[43,72,77] The most important risk factors for aspiration are impaired level of consciousness, vomiting, seizures, obesity, nasogastric feeding, and diabetes-associated gastrointestinal motility disorder (Chapter 55).[80] Possibly, acid-suppressive use in acute stroke may lead to increased hospital-acquired pneumonia.[32] Aspiration is markedly increased in patients requiring emergency intubation. A similar risk occurs with extubation, and aspiration is increased immediately after a procedure in which anesthetic agents have been used. Premature extubation postoperatively may be hazardous, because many anesthetic agents reduce laryngeal closure.

Aspiration pneumonia can possibly be prevented if patients with abnormal swallowing mechanisms are identified early. The result of any bedside test of swallowing that suggests an abnormal mechanism should prompt a more formal evaluation.[16,19,26] The gag reflex has a low predictive value and is absent in at least one-third of the normal population. Testing of pharyngeal sensation may be more useful,[20] and studies have confirmed increased risks of aspiration in patients with pharyngeal sensory deficits (Table 18.2). Alternative but more complicated techniques include the assessment of laryngeal adductor reflex with air pulse stimulation. Its absence predicts aspiration.[4]

Patients with a high probability of swallowing difficulties should be evaluated with videofluoroscopy (Figure 18.1).[16] Interpretation requires significant skill. Features, which can be assessed, are bolus formation, residue in oral cavity, oral transit time, triggering of pharyngeal swallowing, laryngeal elevation and epiglottic closure, nasal penetration, vallecular residue, pharyngeal wall coating, and pharyngeal transit time.[30] Videofluoroscopy may also predict long-term difficulties. A study in 128 patients after stroke found that delayed oral transit and penetration into the laryngeal vestibule predicted poor outcome and failure to resume oral feeding.[51] The incidence of aspiration tends to be higher in patients with nondominant hemispheric ischemic stroke (labeled *quiet aspirators*), explained by ineffective throat clearing, possible neglect, and prolonged pharyngeal response (time between initiation of hyoid excursion and return to rest). However, patients with dominant hemispheric stroke typically have an abnormal oral stage, with uncoordinated labial, lingual, and mandibular movements from apraxia of swallowing and prolonged pharyngeal transit times (arrival of the bolus head at the ramus of the mandible before complete passage through the upper esophageal sphincter opening).[39,50,66]

TABLE 18.2. FEATURES SUGGESTING ABNORMAL SWALLOWING MECHANISM

Abnormal laryngeal rise
Abnormal throat clearing
Abnormal volitional and reflexive cough
Abnormal gag reflex
Abnormal pharyngeal sensation
Abnormal oral motor rapid movement and strength
Abnormal vocal clarity
Abnormal sipping of water and eating of crackers

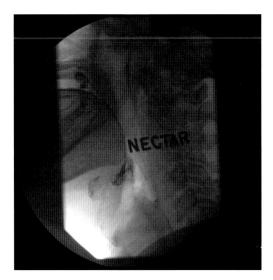

FIGURE 18.1: Video of swallowing, showing nectar overspill.

Patients who, in addition, have aphonia are at particularly high risk. Multiple additional techniques to predict aspiration have been developed and include the 3-ounce water swallow test (an indicator of tolerance for thin liquids, but with a false positive rate of 51%).[75]

The immediate consequences of a high risk of aspiration are clear. However, nil per os may not have any measurable influence on gastric volume or pH and therefore should not substantially reduce aspiration. An H_2-antagonist should be administered to patients at high risk of aspiration, but protein-pump inhibitors may be equally effective. Both agents may reduce gastric volume and increase pH. Positioning the bed at a 45-degree head elevation is an important additional measure.

ENTERAL NUTRITION

The integrity of the gastrointestinal system is maintained by enteral feeding, but the best timing of enteral nutrition is not known. Enteral nutrition is probably required early in most patients in the NICU.[84,85] Enteral feeding not only provides adequate calories and proteins, but luminal feeding maintains intestinal epithelial function. How rapidly the microbiome changes with "starvation" is not known in this category of patients, but the normal commensal flora remains with feeding.[2,53] In the general critical care population, early mortality and time on the ventilator are reduced with each additional 1,000 kcal and 30 g protein daily.[27] Clinical complexity increases the complexity of feeding access from nasogastric to nasoenteric to percutaneous gastrotomy PEG to jejunal extension to PEG.

An 8- or 16-French gauge tube should be inserted and the patient is positioned sitting with the head of the bed elevated to 45 degrees. One end of the tube is held with thumb and index finger behind the ear. The length of the nasogastric tube is estimated by measuring from the ear to the tip of the nose and from the tip of the nose to the xiphoid process. After patency is checked by having the patient breathe through the nose (with one nostril occluded), the feeding tube can be placed. Many techniques may greatly facilitate placement. They include flexion of the neck, generous lubrication of the tube, placement of the tube in an ice water bath to increase rigidity, the Jarmon technique (filling the nostril with lidocaine jelly, which enters the posterior pharynx and relaxes the nasal constrictors), and, as a last resort, direct visualization with a laryngoscope and advancement with a forceps.[5,11] Alert patients can be asked to swallow water through a straw while the tube is advanced.

The technique of advancing the tube consists of a gentle motion with advancement of at least 3 inches each time the patient swallows. Auscultation of a gurgling sound after pushing air through the tube may not be very reliable,[69] and only aspiration of the gastric contents confirms location within the stomach. Correct placement of a nasogastric tube must be checked by radiography before feeding is started[57] (Figure 18.2). It was surprisingly low—5 of 100 placements—in one recent study.[26] In combative, agitated patients, the risk of misplacement is obviously higher,

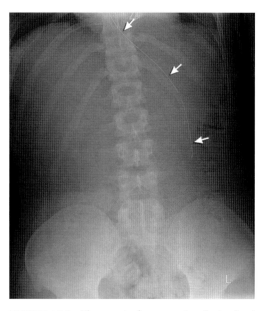

FIGURE 18.2: Placement of nasogastric tube in distal stomach (arrows).

and the risk of aspiration is significant from self-extubation. In addition, intracranial placement has been repeatedly reported in patients with extensive facial trauma.[22,47]

Complications of placement of the nasogastric tube are rare.[22] Occasionally, a feeding tube is placed in the bronchial tree, and if this error is not recognized, a potentially fatal chemical pneumonitis results. One study suggested that connection to a handheld end-tidal carbon dioxide device can identify false placement (presence of a carbon dioxide waveform) and reduce discomfort or formation of an iatrogenic bronchopleural fistula from manipulation.[12] However, a chest radiograph is always needed to confirm adequate placement.

It is prudent to consider postpyloric feeding in patients with CNS catastrophes, because gastric atony increases the risk of aspiration. However, drug absorption in the jejunum may be unreliable. Gastric atony or impaired gastric motility can be anticipated in patients with subarachnoid hemorrhage of poor grade or severe traumatic brain injury.[40] The use of nasoduodenal or nasojejunal tubes may reduce the risk of aspiration. Duodenal placement can be tried by inserting a coiled tube that is at least 10 cm more than the calculated length into the stomach and then waiting 24 hours to allow spontaneous advancement past the pylorus. The right lateral decubitus position may facilitate the motion. Another helpful bedside technique, with a 75% success rate, is air insufflation. A 60 mL syringe is used to pump 500 mL of air into the stomach. There are, however, conflicting data on postpyloric (duodenal) feeding versus gastric feeding. A recent evidence-based guideline of the European Society for Clinical Nutrition and Metabolism found no evidence of improved outcome or aspiration frequency.[49] A prospective trial in critically ill patients found reduced vomiting and reduced ventilator-associated pneumonia, but no effect on ICU days, diarrhea, ventilator days, and outcome (this study included only nine patients with stroke).[34]

Tubes that fail to pass may be placed fluoroscopically, and this technique is very successful.[29] Additionally, metoclopramide or erythromycin elixir facilitates transpyloric passage.[74] Erythromycin (200 mg) given intravenously in patients with a gastric feeding tube may improve nutritional intake, similar to that in patients fed through a tube placed transpylorically,[9,15] and could be considered in appropriate patients. Residual volumes, however, poorly predict risk of aspiration.[54]

Enteral feeding should preferably be done by continuous infusion with a volumetric pump.[17] Continuous tube feedings have been associated with a positive nitrogen balance and weight gain more often than intermittent tube feedings.[78] A recent successful protocol started feeding at 25 mL/hr and increased the volume by 25 mL/hr every 4 hours until the goal of nutrition was achieved.[62] When a gastric residual volume of more than 250 mL was detected, feeding was held for 4 hours and was restarted at the same rate but with a more gradual increase in rate. A prokinetic agent (metoclopramide, cisapride, or domperidone) was mandated. If this approach is not tolerated and residuals are significant, the tube should be relocated into the jejunum. This can be done on a tilting fluoroscopic table with placement beyond the ligament of Treitz. Continuous administration is essential in jejunal feeding because a rapidly formed bolus of a hyperosmolar solution may cause serious cramps and diarrhea.

Feeding can be started with any of the standard commercially available enteral nutrition products. The available formulas provide approximately 1 kcal/mL. However, fluid intake and total volume load could become substantial, and maintenance fluids should be adjusted. We have been using Osmolite and Promote in most patients admitted to the NICU. The enteral formulas should be used as directed and not diluted. Bacterial contamination has been reported with non-sterile handling of the formula. A recent evidence-based feeding guideline has been published.[25]

Problems with enteral feeding are frequent.[7,13] The most common is diarrhea, which can be associated with rapid infusion rates and the use of hyperosmolar formulas (Chapter 48). It is less often due to intolerance to fat, lactulose, and bacterial overgrowth. Nausea, cramps, and abdominal distention are often associated with rapid feeding. Causes in the NICU are shown in Table 18.3. Decreased gastric emptying can be demonstrated if residuals exceed 50% of the amount delivered in the last feeding or are 50% above the flow rate per hour. Prokinetics may significantly reduce gastric volume, and in one study 50% reduction was demonstrated.[63] Intravenously administered metoclopramide (antagonizes dopamine and sensitizes acetylcholine), 10 mg every 6 hours, may be effective in persistent cases that cannot be resolved with changes in the method of delivery.[44] Liver and renal failure should prompt dose adjustment. Erythromycin (acts on motilin receptors), 200 mg intravenously every 8 hours, is the preferred

TABLE 18.3. FACTORS ALTERING
GASTRIC EMPTYING IN THE
NEUROSCIENCES INTENSIVE CARE UNIT

TABLE 18.3. FACTORS ALTERING
GASTRIC EMPTYING IN THE
NEUROSCIENCES INTENSIVE CARE UNIT

Diabetes mellitus

Prior vagotomy

Electrolyte abnormalities (e.g., hyperglycemia,
    hypokalemia)

Drugs (opiates, atropine, cephalosporins)

Sepsis or other major systemic infection

TABLE 18.4. COMPLICATIONS
OF ENTERAL FEEDING

Cause	Events
Mechanical	Misplacement
	Tube clogging
	Nasal mucosal ulceration
	Otitis media
	Pharyngitis
	Pneumothorax
	Reflux esophagitis
Gut	Aspiration of stomach contents
	Bloating, constipation
	Diarrhea, vomiting
Metabolic	Liver function abnormalities
	Dehydration
	Hyperglycemia
	Micronutrient deficiency

promotility agent.[15,86] Renal failure requires dose adjustment.

A consistent problem of enteral feeding is tube obstruction, most commonly in tubes of smaller French size. Clogging of the tube can be resolved by frequent flushing with 50 mL of fluid, but cranberry juice often loosens the residuals within the tube.

Medication can be administered by this route, and absorption should be sufficient. Mortars and pestles are needed to thoroughly crush tablets. Problems arise with sustained-action release and enteric-coated tablets, which lose their intended function by crushing. Specific absorption problems have been noted with warfarin, fosphenytoin, and carbamazepine. Absorption of fosphenytoin with tube feeding is poor, in some patients virtually immeasurable. One method is to hold feeding 2 hours before and after dose administration. This should result in adequate absorption and therapeutic fosphenytoin plasma levels, but the total dose may still need to be increased. Parenteral administration of fosphenytoin, however, is then preferable.

In summary, enteral nutrition is not without complications, and the most common are aspiration and diarrhea. Tube dislodging in a confused patient is the most encountered practice problem—the others are shown in Table 18.4. Repeated placement is not unusual. PEG placement with protective padding covers may be needed to avoid constant interruption. Nasal bridles are very successful, and their effect has been tested (less than 20% of bridled patients dislodged nasogastric tube, reduced from 60% in control patients).[71] Diarrhea often is related to enteral formulation, and reducing the flow rate probably is more effective than changing to another formula[56] (Chapter 58). Nosocomial infections (e.g., *Clostridium difficile*) should be considered, particularly when antibiotics are similarly administered (Chapter 59).

INDICATIONS FOR GASTROSTOMY

The indications for surgical placement of a feeding tube have not been clearly delineated in the patient with critical neurologic illness. The advantages of percutaneous endoscopic gastrostomy (PEG) are great in patients who cannot tolerate nasogastric tubes, who frequently extubate themselves, or who may need long-term enteral feeding largely because of defective swallowing mechanisms.[28,42,43,46,59,82] However, nasogastric tubes can be tolerated for weeks in many patients.

The placement of gastrostomy with the use of endoscopic guidance is often considered in patients with debilitating neurologic disease, particularly when dysphagia persists beyond 2–3 weeks. A PEG placement seems much less attractive in patients with a high probability of death or who are severely disabled. It is very important to note that PEG placement should be postponed if withdrawal of support is anticipated. One should seriously weigh the risks and benefits of gastrostomy, choose wisely, and carefully use this resource.

Patients with anticipated prolonged enteral feeding typically have major hemispheric or, more often, brainstem ischemic stroke or are in prolonged coma from any cause.[42] Early placement may be useful; in many patients, nitrogen loss was reduced, and complications from having the tube in situ were not noted.[43] Whether this aggressive approach can resolve the caloric loss associated with hypermetabolism is very uncertain. More

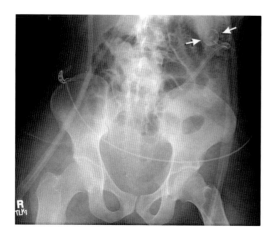

FIGURE 18.3: Percutaneous endoscopic gastrostomy (arrows).

recently, in 30 patients with acute stroke and persistent dysphagia randomized to PEG or nasogastric tube feeding, gastrostomy tube feeding 2 weeks after acute stroke significantly reduced

mortality and aspiration pneumonia.[59] In our study, however, patients who received PEG after acute stroke remained severely disabled, with at least one-third dying from systemic complications of stroke.[79]

Many techniques of PEG placement have been developed.[24] Antibiotic prophylaxis to reduce peristomal infection is standard before placement (cefotaxime 2 g or ceftriaxone 750 mg IV 30 minutes prior to procedure).[37,68] The percutaneous method begins with an endoscope into a stomach distended with air. An introducer catheter is inserted where the light beam from the endoscope can be seen. The procedural steps of introducing the catheter are shown in Figure 18.3 and will project on X-ray (Figure 18.4). Several other techniques are practiced but are outside the scope of this chapter.[5] Complications of PEG are rare (Table 18.5), but bleeding from submucosal vessels of the stomach may occur. Fortunately, iced saline lavage stops the bleeding. Other procedure-related complications are local

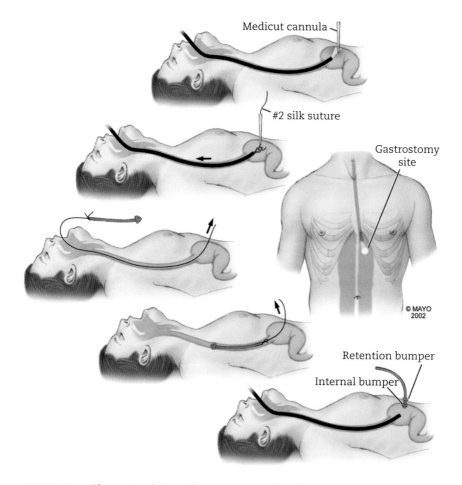

FIGURE 18.4: Placement technique of percutaneous endoscopic gastrostomy.

TABLE 18.5. COMPLICATIONS
OF PERCUTANEOUS ENDOSCOPIC
GASTROSTOMY AND JEJUNOSTOMY
PLACEMENT*

Colocutaneous fistula
Gastric outlet obstruction
Bleeding from submucosal lesions
Ileus
Necrotizing fasciitis
Stoma leakage
Wound and skin infection
Volvulus

*Most complications are minor and occur within the first 3 months of placement.

infection and necrotizing fasciitis, but the morbidity associated with this procedure remains low (less than 10%). Pneumoperitoneum, occurring in 40% of patients, often has no clinical significance. Medical complications (particularly pneumonia) remain more common in patients with PEG in rehabilitation facilities.[36] In our study, aspiration pneumonia occurred in 1 of 10 patients who had a PEG placement, but occlusion or accidental removal was uncommon. Removal of the PEG tube and oral feeding were possible in one of four patients with acute stroke and equally common in those with hemispheric or brainstem lesions.[82]

PARENTERAL NUTRITION

Parenteral nutrition is not a common procedure in the NICU, although some investigators in clinical nutrition favor early initiation of total parenteral nutrition.[18] The decision depends on the underlying nutritional state and metabolic rate and whether enteral nutrition is poorly tolerated.[73] Parenteral nutrition is complex, carries many more complications, and requires close monitoring of laboratory variables. Early parenteral nutrition does not improve outcome in critically ill patients.[31]

Subclavian vein cannulation is the preferred access when parenteral nutrition is considered. Many institutions use triple-lumen catheters. The care of these catheters must include changing over a guidewire regularly to minimize the risk of catheter-related sepsis. Although recorded data are conflicting on the increased risk of infection in triple-lumen catheters over that in single-lumen catheters, colonization remains low (4%–5%). (Catheter sepsis is further discussed in Chapter 59.) Maintenance of the catheter includes

heparin flushes (10 units/mL), frequent change of transparent adherent dressings, and meticulous skin antisepsis with povidone-iodine.

The composition of a parenteral formula requires consultation from nutritional support services. However, parenteral nutritional solutions are easily available to meet individual patient needs.

Energy requirements are again calculated from the total daily calories estimated by the Harris-Benedict equation or indirect calorimetry. Protein requirements are typically about 1.5 g/kg/day, but in patients with an acute devastating CNS disorder, a hypermetabolic state, and insufficient caloric intake by enteral nutrition, protein in doses of 2.0–3.5 g/kg/day should be recommended. Fat must be provided in 500 mL aliquots of 10% emulsion, and the total dose of calories must be less than 60% of the total non-protein calories. The basic components are dextrose 50%, which provides 250 g in a 500 mL solution; amino acid mixture of 8.5% in 500 mL bottles; and 10% fat emulsion in 500 mL bottles. The formula is supplemented with standard electrolyte solutions, daily multivitamins, and trace elements. A basic formula is provided in Table 18.6.

A mechanical or metabolic complication is estimated to occur in approximately 50% of

TABLE 18.6. FORMULATION OF TOTAL
PARENTERAL NUTRITION SOLUTION

Base solution	
40%–70% dextrose	500–1,500 mL
8.5%–15% crystalline amino acids	500–1,500 mL
Intravenous fat emulsion 10%	20–100 g
(200–500 mL 2–7 times/week)	
Add to each 1,000 mL	
Sodium chloride	40–50 mEq
Potassium chloride	20–30 mEq
Potassium or sodium acid	15–30 mEq
phosphate (10–20 mm	
phosphorus)	
Magnesium sulfate	15–18 mEq
Calcium gluconate	4.6–9.2 mEq
Add to daily formulation	
Zinc sulfate, copper sulfate,	5–10 mg; 1–2 mg
selenium, chromium chloride,	60 µg; 10–20 µg
manganese chloride, iron dextran,	0.5 mg; 5 mg
and multivitamin infusion	
Add to any 1 liter 2 times a week	
Vitamin K	10 mg

patients with prolonged parenteral nutrition.[58] The mechanical complications are often associated with placement of the catheter. The most important are pneumothorax, hemothorax, hydrothorax, chylothorax, and air embolism. Complex metabolic problems may arise. The most anticipated complication is hyperglycemia, often manifested as nonketotic hyperosmolar hyperglycemia. Well-established triggers of hyperglycemia are rapid infusion, decreased insulin output from diabetes, transient glucose resistance, and medication, particularly the use of corticosteroids. Coma from nonketotic hyperglycemia is expected when the serum glucose value reaches 1,000 mg/dL and serum osmolarities approach values of 350 mOsm/L. Treatment includes insulin and, more important, rehydration and eventually change into a larger proportion of lipids. Hypophosphatemia occasionally occurs, but rarely produces generalized muscle weakness respiratory failure from diaphragmatic dysfunction. The most common electrolyte abnormality, however, is hyponatremia associated with large infusions of free water. This can be overcome simply by tailoring glucose infusions.[76]

CONCLUSIONS

- Energy requirement in the NICU is calculated by the Harris-Benedict formula, and is based on weight, height, and age. Energy expenditure for men = 66.5 + 13.8W + 5H – 6.8A, and for women = 655 + 9.6W +1.8H – 4.7A. Increased caloric needs in critically ill patients may justify a stress factor of 20%.

- Abnormal swallowing during evaluation is characterized by abnormal laryngeal rise, abnormal throat clearing, inefficient coughing, weak tongue protrusion, and abnormal vocal clarity.

- Enteral nutrition with nasogastric or duodenal placement is recommended. Continuous infusion is started at the rate of 25 mL/hr, the rate is gradually increased, and commercially available enteral formulas providing 1 kcal/mL are used.

- PEG is indicated in patients with persistent dysphagia for 2–3 weeks. The procedure can be considered for patients with repeated nasogastric tube extubations, patients with persistent coma from any cause, and patients with a severe brainstem stroke.

- Parenteral nutrition should be initiated in patients who do not tolerate enteral nutrition.

REFERENCES

1. Almer LO, Janzon L. Low vascular fibrinolytic activity in obesity. *Thromb Res* 1975;6:171–175.
2. Alverdy J, Gilbert J, DeFazio JR, et al. Proceedings of the 2013 A.S.P.E.N. Research workshop: the interface between nutrition and the gut microbiome: implications and applications for human health [corrected]. *JPEN J Parenter Enteral Nutr* 2014;38:167–178.
3. Artinian V, Krayem H, DiGiovine B. Effects of early enteral feeding on the outcome of critically ill mechanically ventilated medical patients. *Chest* 2006;129:960–967.
4. Aviv JE, Spitzer J, Cohen M, et al. Laryngeal adductor reflex and pharyngeal squeeze as predictors of laryngeal penetration and aspiration. *Laryngoscope* 2002;112:338–341.
5. Baskin WN. Advances in enteral nutrition techniques. *Am J Gastroenterol* 1992;87:1547–1553.
6. Behara AS, Peterson SJ, Chen Y, et al. Nutrition support in the critically ill: a physician survey. *JPEN J Parenter Enteral Nutr* 2008;32:113–119.
7. Benya R, Mobarhan S. Enteral alimentation: administration and complications. *J Am Coll Nutr* 1991;10:209–219.
8. Bern MM, Bothe A, Jr., Bistrian B, et al. Effects of low-dose warfarin on antithrombin III levels in morbidly obese patients. *Surgery* 1983;94:78–83.
9. Boivin MA, Levy H. Gastric feeding with erythromycin is equivalent to transpyloric feeding in the critically ill. *Crit Care Med* 2001;29:1916–1919.
10. Bower RH. Nutritional and metabolic support of critically ill patients. *JPEN J Parenter Enteral Nutr* 1990;14:257S-259S.
11. Boyes RJ, Kruse JA. Nasogastric and nasoenteric intubation. *Crit Care Clin* 1992;8:865–878.
12. Burns SM, Carpenter R, Truwit JD. Report on the development of a procedure to prevent placement of feeding tubes into the lungs using end-tidal CO_2 measurements. *Crit Care Med* 2001;29:936–939.
13. Cabre E, Gassull MA. Complications of enteral feeding. *Nutrition* 1993;9:1–9.
14. Cerra FB, Benitez MR, Blackburn GL, et al. Applied nutrition in ICU patients: a consensus statement of the American College of Chest Physicians. *Chest* 1997;111:769–778.
15. Chapman MJ, Fraser RJ, Kluger MT, Buist MD, De Nichilo DJ. Erythromycin improves gastric emptying in critically ill patients

intolerant of nasogastric feeding. *Crit Care Med* 2000;28:2334–2337.

16. Chen MY, Peele VN, Donati D, et al. Clinical and videofluoroscopic evaluation of swallowing in 41 patients with neurologic disease. *Gastrointest Radiol* 1992;17:95–98.

17. Ciocon JO, Galindo-Ciocon DJ, Tiessen C, Galindo D. Continuous compared with intermittent tube feeding in the elderly. *JPEN J Parenter Enteral Nutr* 1992;16:525–528.

18. Cook D, Arabi Y. The route of early nutrition in critical illness. *N Engl J Med* 2014;371:1748–1749.

19. Daniels SK, Ballo LA, Mahoney MC, Foundas AL. Clinical predictors of dysphagia and aspiration risk: outcome measures in acute stroke patients. *Arch Phys Med Rehabil* 2000;81:1030–1033.

20. Davies AE, Kidd D, Stone SP, MacMahon J. Pharyngeal sensation and gag reflex in healthy subjects. *Lancet* 1995;345:487–488.

21. De Jonghe B, Appere-De-Vechi C, Fournier M, et al. A prospective survey of nutritional support practices in intensive care unit patients: what is prescribed? What is delivered? *Crit Care Med* 2001;29:8–12.

22. Dees G. Difficult nasogastric tube insertions. *Emerg Med Clin N Am* 1989;7:177–182.

23. Deutschman CS, Konstantinides FN, Raup S, Thienprasit P, Cerra FB. Physiological and metabolic response to isolated closed-head injury. Part 1: basal metabolic state: correlations of metabolic and physiological parameters with fasting and stressed controls. *J Neurosurg* 1986;64:89–98.

24. DiSario JA, Baskin WN, Brown RD, et al. Endoscopic approaches to enteral nutritional support. *Gastrointest Endosc* 2002;55:901–908.

25. Doig GS, Simpson F, Finfer S, et al. Effect of evidence-based feeding guidelines on mortality of critically ill adults: a cluster randomized controlled trial. *JAMA* 2008;300:2731–2741.

26. Dziewas R, Warnecke T, Hamacher C, et al. Do nasogastric tubes worsen dysphagia in patients with acute stroke? *BMC Neurol* 2008;8:28.

27. Elke G, Wang M, Weiler N, Day AG, Heyland DK. Close to recommended caloric and protein intake by enteral nutrition is associated with better clinical outcome of critically ill septic patients: secondary analysis of a large international nutrition database. *Crit Care* 2014;18:R29.

28. Gencosmanoglu R. Percutaneous endoscopic gastrostomy: a safe and effective bridge for enteral nutrition in neurological or non-neurological conditions. *Neurocrit Care* 2004;1:309–317.

29. Gutierrez ED, Balfe DM. Fluoroscopically guided nasoenteric feeding tube placement: results of a 1-year study. *Radiology* 1991;178:759–762.

30. Han TR, Paik NJ, Park JW. Quantifying swallowing function after stroke: a functional dysphagia scale based on videofluoroscopic studies. *Arch Phys Med Rehabil* 2001;82:677–682.

31. Harvey SE, Parrott F, Harrison DA, et al. Trial of the route of early nutritional support in critically ill adults. *N Engl J Med* 2014;371:1673–1684.

32. Herzig SJ, Doughty C, Lahoti S, et al. Acid-suppressive medication use in acute stroke and hospital-acquired pneumonia. *Ann Neurol* 2014;76:712–718.

33. Hogue CW, Jr., Stearns JD, Colantuoni E, et al. The impact of obesity on outcomes after critical illness: a meta-analysis. *Intensive Care Med* 2009;35:1152–1170.

34. Hsu CW, Sun SF, Lin SL, et al. Duodenal versus gastric feeding in medical intensive care unit patients: a prospective, randomized, clinical study. *Crit Care Med* 2009;37:1866–1872.

35. Ibrahim EH, Mehringer L, Prentice D, et al. Early versus late enteral feeding of mechanically ventilated patients: results of a clinical trial. *JPEN J Parenter Enteral Nutr* 2002;26:174–181.

36. Iizuka M, Reding M. Use of percutaneous endoscopic gastrostomy feeding tubes and functional recovery in stroke rehabilitation: a case-matched controlled study. *Arch Phys Med Rehabil* 2005;86:1049–1052.

37. Jain NK, Larson DE, Schroeder KW, et al. Antibiotic prophylaxis for percutaneous endoscopic gastrostomy: a prospective, randomized, double-blind clinical trial. *Ann Intern Med* 1987; 107:824–828.

38. Joffe A, Wood K. Obesity in critical care. *Curr Opin Anaesthesiol* 2007;20:113–118.

39. Johnson ER, McKenzie SW, Rosenquist CJ, Lieberman JS, Sievers AE. Dysphagia following stroke: quantitative evaluation of pharyngeal transit times. *Arch Phys Med Rehabil* 1992;73:419–423.

40. Kao CH, ChangLai SP, Chieng PU, Yen TC. Gastric emptying in head-injured patients. *Am J Gastroenterol* 1998;93:1108–1112.

41. Kirby DF. As the gut churns: feeding challenges in the head-injured patient. *JPEN J Parenter Enteral Nutr* 1996;20:1–2.

42. Kirby DF. Decisions for enteral access in the intensive care unit. *Nutrition* 2001;17:776–779.

43. Kirby DF, Clifton GL, Turner H, et al. Early enteral nutrition after brain injury by percutaneous endoscopic gastrojejunostomy. *JPEN J Parenter Enteral Nutr* 1991;15:298–302.

44. Kittinger JW, Sandler RS, Heizer WD. Efficacy of metoclopramide as an adjunct to duodenal placement of small-bore feeding tubes: a randomized, placebo-controlled, double-blind study. *JPEN J Parenter Enteral Nutr* 1987;11:33–37.

45. Klein S, Kinney J, Jeejeebhoy K, et al. Nutrition support in clinical practice: review of published

data and recommendations for future research directions. Summary of a conference sponsored by the National Institutes of Health, American Society for Parenteral and Enteral Nutrition, and American Society for Clinical Nutrition. *Am J Clin Nutr* 1997;66:683–706.

46. Koc D, Gercek A, Gencosmanoglu R, Tozun N. Percutaneous endoscopic gastrostomy in the neurosurgical intensive care unit: complications and outcome. *JPEN J Parenter Enteral Nutr* 2007;31:517–520.

47. Koch KJ, Becker GJ, Edwards MK, Hoover RL. Intracranial placement of a nasogastric tube. *AJNR Am J Neuroradiol* 1989;10:443–444.

48. Koretz RL. Nutritional supplementation in the ICU: how critical is nutrition for the critically ill? *Am J Respir Crit Care Med* 1995;151:570–573.

49. Kreymann KG, Berger MM, Deutz NE, et al. ESPEN guidelines on enteral nutrition: intensive care. *Clin Nutr* 2006;25:210–223.

50. Mann G, Hankey GJ, Cameron D. Swallowing disorders following acute stroke: prevalence and diagnostic accuracy. *Cerebrovasc Dis* 2000;10:380–386.

51. Mann G, Hankey GJ, Cameron D. Swallowing function after stroke: prognosis and prognostic factors at 6 months. *Stroke* 1999;30:744–748.

52. Marik P, Varon J. The obese patient in the ICU. *Chest* 1998;113:492–498.

53. Martindale RG, Warren M. Should enteral nutrition be started in the first week of critical illness? *Curr Opin Clin Nutr Metab Care* 2015;18:202–206.

54. McClave SA, Lukan JK, Stefater JA, et al. Poor validity of residual volumes as a marker for risk of aspiration in critically ill patients. *Crit Care Med* 2005;33:324–330.

55. McLean J, Manchip S. Wernicke's encephalopathy induced by magnesium depletion. *Lancet* 1999;353:1768.

56. Mentec H, Dupont H, Bocchetti M, et al. Upper digestive intolerance during enteral nutrition in critically ill patients: frequency, risk factors, and complications. *Crit Care Med* 2001;29:1955–1961.

57. Metheny N. Minimizing respiratory complications of nasoenteric tube feedings: state of the science. *Heart Lung* 1993;22:213–223.

58. Mughal MM. Complications of intravenous feeding catheters. *Br J Surg* 1989;76:15–21.

59. Norton B, Homer-Ward M, Donnelly MT, Long RG, Holmes GK. A randomised prospective comparison of percutaneous endoscopic gastrostomy and nasogastric tube feeding after acute dysphagic stroke. *BMJ* 1996;312:13–16.

60. Norton JA, Ott LG, McClain C, et al. Intolerance to enteral feeding in the brain-injured patient. *J Neurosurg* 1988;68:62–66.

61. Oertel MF, Hauenschild A, Gruenschlaeger J, et al. Parenteral and enteral nutrition in the management of neurosurgical patients in the intensive care unit. *J Clin Neurosci* 2009;16:1161–1167.

62. Payne-James J. Enteral nutrition: accessing patients. *Nutrition* 1992;8:223–231.

63. Pinilla JC, Samphire J, Arnold C, Liu L, Thiessen B. Comparison of gastrointestinal tolerance to two enteral feeding protocols in critically ill patients: a prospective, randomized controlled trial. *JPEN J Parenter Enteral Nutr* 2001;25:81–86.

64. Ray DE, Matchett SC, Baker K, Wasser T, Young MJ. The effect of body mass index on patient outcomes in a medical ICU. *Chest* 2005;127:2125–2131.

65. Ritz MA, Fraser R, Tam W, Dent J. Impacts and patterns of disturbed gastrointestinal function in critically ill patients. *Am J Gastroenterol* 2000;95:3044–3052.

66. Robbins J, Levine RL, Maser A, Rosenbek JC, Kempster GB. Swallowing after unilateral stroke of the cerebral cortex. *Arch Phys Med Rehabil* 1993;74:1295–1300.

67. Roubenoff RA, Borel CO, Hanley DF. Hypermetabolism and hypercatabolism in Guillain-Barre syndrome. *JPEN J Parenter Enteral Nutr* 1992;16:464–472.

68. Saadeddin A, Freshwater DA, Fisher NC, Jones BJ. Antibiotic prophylaxis for percutaneous endoscopic gastrostomy for non-malignant conditions: a double-blind prospective randomized controlled trial. *Aliment Pharmacol Ther* 2005;22:565–570.

69. Salasidis R, Fleiszer T, Johnston R. Air insufflation technique of enteral tube insertion: a randomized, controlled trial. *Crit Care Med* 1998;26:1036–1039.

70. Schlichtig R, Sargent SC. Nutritional support of the mechanically ventilated patient. *Crit Care Clin* 1990;6:767–784.

71. Seder CW, Stockdale W, Hale L, Janczyk RJ. Nasal bridling decreases feeding tube dislodgment and may increase caloric intake in the surgical intensive care unit: a randomized, controlled trial. *Crit Care Med* 2010;38:797–801.

72. Sellars C, Bowie L, Bagg J, et al. Risk factors for chest infection in acute stroke: a prospective cohort study. *Stroke* 2007;38:2284–2291.

73. Skaer TL. Total parenteral nutrition: clinical considerations. *Clin Ther* 1993;15:272–282; discussion 215.

74. Stern MA, Wolf DC. Erythromycin as a prokinetic agent: a prospective, randomized, controlled study of efficacy in nasoenteric tube placement. *Am J Gastroenterol* 1994;89:2011–2013.

75. Suiter DM, Leder SB. Clinical utility of the 3-ounce water swallow test. *Dysphagia* 2008;23:244–250.

76. Sunyecz L, Mirtallo JM. Sodium imbalance in a patient receiving total parenteral nutrition. *Clin Pharm* 1993;12:138–149.

77. Teasell RW, Bach D, McRae M. Prevalence and recovery of aspiration poststroke: a retrospective analysis. *Dysphagia* 1994;9:35–39.

78. Tepaske R, Binnekade JM, Goedhart PT, et al. Clinically relevant differences in accuracy of enteral nutrition feeding pump systems. *JPEN J Parenter Enteral Nutr* 2006;30:339–343.

79. Trapl M, Enderle P, Nowotny M, et al. Dysphagia bedside screening for acute-stroke patients: the Gugging Swallowing Screen. *Stroke* 2007;38:2948–2952.

80. Wakasugi Y, Tohara H, Hattori F, et al. Screening test for silent aspiration at the bedside. *Dysphagia* 2008;23:364–370.

81. Wei X, Day AG, Ouellette-Kuntz H, Heyland DK. The association between nutritional adequacy and long-term outcomes in critically ill patients requiring prolonged mechanical ventilation: a multicenter cohort study. *Crit Care Med* 2015;43:1569–1579.

82. Wijdicks EFM, McMahon MM. Percutaneous endoscopic gastrostomy after acute stroke: complications and outcome. *Cerebrovasc Dis* 1999;9:109–111.

83. Yanagawa T, Bunn F, Roberts I, Wentz R, Pierro A. Nutritional support for head-injured patients. *Cochrane Database Syst Rev* 2000:CD001530.

84. Young B, Ott L, Phillips R, McClain C. Metabolic management of the patient with head injury. *Neurosurg Clin N Am* 1991;2:301–320.

85. Young B, Ott L, Yingling B, McClain C. Nutrition and brain injury. *J Neurotrauma* 1992;9 Suppl 1: S375–383.

86. Zaloga GP, Marik P. Promotility agents in the intensive care unit. *Crit Care Med* 2000; 28:2657–2659.

87. Zarbock SD, Steinke D, Hatton J, et al. Successful enteral nutritional support in the neurocritical care unit. *Neurocrit Care* 2008;9:210–216.

19

Volume Status and Blood Pressure

Hemodynamics is a clinical concern in every patient with acute brain and spine injury, and when abnormal, requires corrective measures without delay. Intravascular volume and blood pressure reflect hemodynamic status and are tightly correlated.

A current paradigm of fluid management has taken shape. Once common orders by physicians for fluid restriction in patients with acute neurologic catastrophic events have now been modified into a more skillful limitation of free water, with maintenance of euvolemic fluid status and permitting some hypervolemia knowing a ceiling may exist.[67,69]

Coinciding with this diametrical change in patient fluid management has been a change in the management of acutely increased blood pressure.[35,36,48,50] Careful titration of antihypertensive drugs has been a standard approach in the immediate aftermath of acute neurologic disorders, but more aggressive blood pressure control in recent intracerebral hemorrhage, in order to reduce expansion, may become a new approach. This chapter also makes several arguments for the judicious use of antihypertensive medications in the acute phase of ischemic stroke. A clear understanding of how to govern volume status is necessary, but changes in volume and pressure must be interpreted in light of the underlying neurologic disorder. Both these parameters may significantly fluctuate and even become erratic.

REGULATION OF BODY WATER

The compartments in which body water settles are defined as the intracellular volume, and the extracellular space determined by the interstitial and intravascular volumes. Although not fixed, the complex mechanisms that control homeostasis locate two-thirds of the body water in this extracellular space. The translocation of body water across these compartments is largely determined by osmotic forces. Solutes that cannot freely cross the cell membrane may produce an osmotic gradient and thus influence the distribution of body water between compartments. This active osmotic state (usually between intracellular and extracellular fluids separated by cell membrane) is called *effective osmolality* or *tonicity*. Sodium is a typical example of a solute that cannot move freely across the cellular membrane and thus increases tonicity. The primary determinant of plasma osmolality is plasma sodium concentration, which is thus a major factor in fluid shifts across the compartments.

Hypovolemia triggers at least three physiologic pathways: antidiuretic hormone, renin, and norepinephrine, all enhancers of sodium reabsorption. At the collecting duct, antidiuretic hormone increases water and sodium absorption by binding to its receptor and activating water channel protein (aquaporin 2). In the proximal tubule cells, sodium absorption is increased by the activation of the renin-angiotensin-aldosteron (RAAS) system increasing reabsorption of sodium at the distal tubule and collection duct. Finally, norepinephrine and epinephrine decrease the glomerular filtration rate and enhance sodium reabsorption at the proximal tubule.

Hypervolemia, in contrast, stimulates sodium excretion through natriuretic peptides and suppression of the vasopressor hormones mentioned earlier. The natriuretic peptides have variable natriuretic, diuretic, and vasorelaxant activities[70] (Chapter 57). However, they also suppress sympathetic tone and RAAS and block the renal effects of antidiuretic hormone. Atrial natriuretic peptide inhibits thirst and the appetite for salt and has another central effect due to decreasing sympathetic tone at the brainstem level. Management of hypertonic and hypotonic states is discussed in Chapter 57. Further analysis of this complex regulating system can be found in major texts on renal disorders.

REQUISITES FOR ADEQUATE FLUID BALANCE

Maintenance fluids can be estimated with a precise patient history and clinical examination.

A key assumption must be that most patients with an acute intracranial injury of any sort tend to have a certain degree of dehydration. The initial "stress response" and pain can stimulate the release of antidiuretic hormone, which theoretically may result in volume expansion, but later the circumstances for hypovolemia are much more favorable. This disproportionately increased risk of dehydration in patients before they enter the NICU has several causes. First, failure to recognize the inability to signal thirst in many patients with impaired consciousness may lead to rapid loss in intravascular volume. Second, insensible losses associated with fever are invariably underestimated. Third, profound emesis may contribute. The most compelling reason for dehydration, however, is that daily data on fluid intake and output are often inaccurate, sometimes are mere estimations, and are not adjusted to the patient's needs. These factors may all lead to accruing fluid losses. This relative hypovolemia may not be reflected by abnormal laboratory markers, but it may come to bear when these patients are placed on mechanical ventilators. The sudden introduction of positive-pressure ventilation decreases venous return and thus cardiac output, resulting in hypotension.

The regimen for normal maintenance of fluid intake is based on an estimation of fluid losses and must be carefully monitored by laboratory measurements. These laboratory investigations should include daily serum electrolytes, osmolality, creatinine, blood urea nitrogen, serum glucose, and, when indicated, arterial blood gases.

The typically used crystalloid is 0.9% sodium chloride Glucose-based solutions should have no place in patients with acute neurologic disorders unless severe hypernatremia needs correction. In an injured or ischemic brain, glucose infusions may worsen stress hyperglycemia and anaerobic cerebral glucose metabolism. This may further produce toxic accumulation of lactate and create intracellular acidosis, which in turn may set off lipid peroxidation and free radical formation. Excitatory amino acids such as glutamate may increase, and edema formation may be exaggerated. [31]

A recent elegant study using perfusion- and diffusion-weighted magnetic resonance imaging documented that nonfasting hyperglycemia may reduce penumbral salvage and increase final infarct size after ischemic stroke.[45] Normoglycemia did result in considerable salvage, and the increase in infarct size quickly became apparent with mild increases in blood glucose. This correlation may

indicate that intensive insulin therapy could improve outcome. The clinical implications of hyperglycemia and treatment goals are further discussed in Chapter 57.

The next step in the computation of maintenance fluid is to approximate insensible losses from lungs and skin. Insensible fluid loss is often underestimated. Gastrointestinal losses average 250 mL/day, and evaporative fluid loss through the skin and lungs easily amounts to 750 mL; together they easily account for 1 L of unmeasured fluid loss. In addition, the increased evaporation with fever ranges widely and can mount to 500 mL per degree Celsius. A thermal stimulus drives sweating, but it is dependent on ambient conditions (e.g., humidity) and the state of hydration. Diarrhea associated with gut feeding may result in additional imperceptible losses. Hyperventilation may increase fluid requirements, but when humidified gases are provided in patients on mechanical ventilators, the increase in fluid requirement becomes insignificant. Sweating can be profuse in patients with traumatic brain injury, typically occurring in association with tachycardia, hyperthermia, and tachypnea (paroxysmal sympathetic hyperactivity; Chapter 41).

Guidelines for maintaining volume status in patients with acute neurologic illness are summarized in Table 19.1. Typically we would start with 80-cc/hr of normal saline but would adjust upward to 100–120 cc/hr if there is a likelihood of dehydration. Serial body weight and fluid balance remain the most practical clinical indicators. The laboratory test results that indicate adequate volume status are normal values of hematocrit, serum osmolality, and serum sodium.

TABLE 19.1. CLINICAL INDICATORS OF VOLUME STATUS IN PATIENTS WITH ACUTE NEUROLOGIC ILLNESS

Urinary output of 1 mL/kg/hr
Fluid intake of 30 mL/kg/day
Fluid balance of 500 to 750 mL/day
Maintenance of body weight
Serum hematocrit
Serum sodium
Creatinine, blood urea nitrogen
Serum glucose
Serum osmolality
Urine osmolality
Urine specific gravity

Representative values for adequate fluid status are hematocrit of less than 55%, osmolality of less than 350 mOsm, and serum sodium of less than 150 mEq/L. Any higher value indicates dehydration and should result in more fluid intake. Ultrasound is used more frequently to assess inferior vena cava diameter and collapsibility as measures of hypovolemia (and explanation for hypotension) and possible success of fluid challenge (Chapter 51).[47,65]

Early signs of volume depletion can be detected by other laboratory measurements that may further guide adjustments. Free water deficit can be calculated by assuming that the total body deficit equals the increase in plasma sodium. The formula for the calculation of water deficit is $0.6 \times$ body weight $\times$ (plasma sodium/140) – 1 in liters. Urine output remains the pivotal variable by which one should measure the effectiveness of correction of fluid balance. Urine output must total at least 1 mL/kg/hr. In contrast, urine output greater than 2 mL/kg may indicate large amounts of fluid intake, but other causes must be considered, particularly diabetes insipidus (Chapter 57). Fluid intake should be adjusted accordingly when a patient is receiving enteral feeding. Aggressive fluid replacement may replete volume compartments, and the heart may eject these increasing volumes. The limits of volume expansion have been physiologically determined by ventricular contractility and filling volumes (Capsule 19.1).

FLUID REPLACEMENT PRODUCTS AND STRATEGY

Several types of replacement fluids are available, each with their own set of characteristics. The use of crystalloids generally is preferred in patients with acute neurologic disorders, and these fluids may increase plasma osmolality and reduce

---

CAPSULE 19.1   THE FRANK-STARLING CURVE

Studies of the isolated mammalian heart (by Ernest Starling in 1914) and frog heart (by Otto Frank in 1895) led to the definition of the relationship between systolic pressure in the heart and volume in ventricles at time of contraction (end-diastolic volume)[32] (see accompanying figure). With increasing end-diastolic volumes, the heart generates more pressure in a linear relationship (ascending limb of the Starling curve). The heart responds to increasing end-diastolic volumes with increasing ejection pressure or stroke volume, and then reaches a plateau. The descending limb of the curve is a nonphysiologic situation in which the heart cannot eject what it receives at diastole. This results in increased end-diastolic volume and pulmonary edema. Diuretics to reduce preload and vasodilation to reduce afterload will reduce end-diastolic volume and will produce a return to the plateau or ascending limb. The stroke volume can also be increased with inotropes. Sympathetic stimulation increases calcium influx and increases systolic contraction.

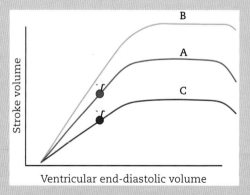

Starling curve. Normal situation in (A) and change after use of inotropes in (B) and cardiac failure such as in stress cardiomyopathy in (C).

cerebral edema if it exists.[11] There is no difference in the incidence of pulmonary edema between crystalloids and colloids, but there is clearly more risk in elderly patients.[15] Crystalloids are solutions in which sodium is the major osmotically active particle (e.g., isotonic saline, lactated Ringer's solution, hypertonic saline). The most commonly used crystalloid is 0.9% sodium chloride (normal saline). This solution is slightly hypertonic to plasma (308 mOsm/kg, as opposed to plasma osmolality of 289 mOsm/kg). Lactated Ringer's solution, an electrolyte solution used frequently in patients with polytrauma, is slightly hypotonic (273 mOsm/kg). The major drawback of using isotonic saline and Ringer's solution is redistribution. These fluids remain intravascular for a maximum

of 2 hours, barely enough time to have a major effect on volume status, and are clearly insufficient when a sustained effect is warranted. The effect of crystalloids on total body water distribution is marginal.[64] Infusion of normal saline or 5% dextrose in water (D5W) results in only a very modest increase in intravascular volume. Figure 19.1 shows these changes: with 3 L of D5W and normal saline, only 250 mL and 750 mL, respectively, briefly remain in the intravascular space. The effect of hypertonic saline is much more significant by means of recruiting fluid from the intracellular space but, again, is transient.[55] Colloid replacement is more effective in situations requiring the rapid correction of intravascular volume. In short, 0.9% sodium chloride accomplishes a

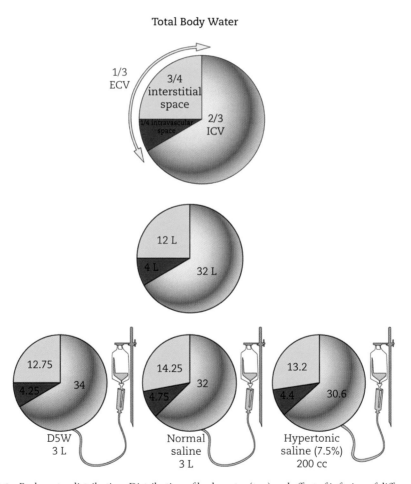

FIGURE 19.1: Body water distribution. Distribution of body water (top) and effect of infusion of different solutions on intravascular volume (bottom).

D5W, 5% dextrose in water; ECV, extracellular volume; ICV, intracellular volume. Note only 200 mL in hypertonic saline and 3 L in other infusions to result in same effect.

Modified from Rainey TG, Read CA. Pharmacology of colloids and crystalloids. In Chernow B, ed., *The Pharmacologic Approach to the Critically Ill Patient*, 3rd ed. Baltimore: Williams & Wilkins, 1994:272–290. With permission of the publisher.

satisfactory physiologic state in most critically ill patients in NICUs. Hypertonic saline is more effective in repleting intravascular volume, but the response is brief.

The characteristics of colloids are different. The major advantages of fluid replacement with colloids are a smaller infused volume, prolonged plasma expansion, and minimal peripheral edema. Colloids are solutions in which substances of large molecular weight are the major osmotically active particles, and these do not easily pass capillary walls. The disadvantages of colloids are greater expense, a reduction in ionized calcium, and a small risk of anaphylactoid reactions. Other colloids such as dextran, gelatin, and hydroxyethyl starch may produce clinically relevant coagulopathy by inhibiting platelet aggregation and reducing activation of factor VIII (e.g., dextran 40) after large-volume infusions.[28]

Albumin is a very effective solution.[21] Albumin 5% expands intravascular volume by only 15 mL of water per gram, but albumin 25% expands intravascular volume five times more than the infused volume. This difference is explained by a much higher colloid osmotic pressure, the major determinant of fluid distribution. The effect of both types of albumin lasts at least 24 hours.

Hetastarch (HES, hydroxyethyl starch, pentastarch) with sodium chloride (Hespan) is an alternative colloid and is much less costly.[29,39] Hetastarch is available in the United States and has a median molecular weight of 450 kd. (In Europe and the United Kingdom, different preparations are available.) Hetastarch may affect platelet function through reduced glycoprotein IIb–IIIa expression and may prolong activated partial thromboplastin time and prothrombin time. Low-molecular-weight hetastarch (70 kd) appears to have a less significant effect on platelet function.[20,60] The reported bleeding complications may be due to hemodilution and inhibition of factor VIII. Contraindications to hetastarch—if used at all—are severe congestive heart failure, renal failure, and hypersensitivity to the agent (e.g., pruritus).[39]

The characteristics of the available plasma expanders are shown in Table 19.2. Fluid replacement is best first accomplished by increasing the rate of maintenance infusion. When blood pressure is reduced (systolic pressure less than 100 mm Hg), a bolus of 500 mL normal saline should be administered. A pressure bag will increase infusion rate. The initial effect should become clear within minutes. This fluid challenge is validated by changes in blood pressure (increase), heart rate (decrease), and urine production (increase). Lack of a persistent effect in hypovolemic patients can be managed with infusion of hypertonic saline 3%, with a suggested rate of 4 mL/kg over 3 minutes into a centrally placed venous catheter.[52] Blood transfusion must be considered if hemorrhage caused the hypovolemic state. Judicious use of small, incremental quantities may reduce the risk of pulmonary edema in patients who have poor underlying cardiac function.

The choice of colloids over crystalloids in acute resuscitation of traumatic brain injury has remained arbitrary until a large prospective trial (Albumen Fluid Evaluation Study, SAFE) uncovered major concerns with colloid infusions. Post hoc analysis of this subgroup found increased risk of mortality with colloids, possibly as a result of worsening intracranial pressure through worsening brain edema.[41] Crystalloids therefore remain a preferred resuscitation fluid.

REGULATION OF BLOOD PRESSURE

The major components of blood pressure are the steady-state part of resistance (mean arterial pressure) and the pulsatile component of impedance (pulse pressure equals systolic blood pressure minus diastolic blood pressure). Neither threshold of normal has been defined in acute neurologic conditions.[1]

Vasomotor control is centered in the central nervous system (CNS). The peripheral sympathetic nerves and the adrenal medulla, also known as the sympathetic nervous system, are the primary operators in acute hypertension. Acute stimulation of the sympathetic system may cause a sudden increase in systemic vascular resistance and an increase in vasoconstrictor substances, including endothelin.

The central adrenergic efferent impulse follows tracts from the hypothalamus to the medulla and spinal cord, and switches to second neurons in the sympathetic ganglia. Norepinephrine is the major neurotransmitter, causing adrenergic receptor stimulation. Stimulation of the α-adrenergic receptor produces vasoconstriction of the arterioles and venules. Stimulation of the β-adrenergic receptor causes vasodilatation, tachycardia, and increased myocardial contractility and metabolism.

Hypertension after acute CNS lesions historically has been attributed to ischemia in the pontomedullary region and is termed the *Cushing reflex*.[17,18] This response consists of an acute surge

TABLE 19.2. VOLUME-EXPANDING AGENTS

Agent	Sodium (mEq/L)	Cost*	T ½	Side Effects
Isotonic saline	154	D	Minutes	None
Albumin 5%	130–160	20D	5–6 hours	Anaphylaxis, pulmonary edema
Albumin 25%	130–160	20D	5–6 hours	Anaphylaxis, pulmonary edema
Lactated Ringer's solution	130	2D	Minutes	Hypo-osmolar state
Hypertonic saline	513	D	Minutes	Hypernatremia, hyperchloremia, hypokalemia, pulmonary edema
Fresh frozen plasma	170	30D	5–6 hours	Hepatitis, human immunodeficiency virus, anaphylaxis
Dextran 70	154	10D	6 hours	Renal failure, anaphylaxis, pseudohyperglycemia, coagulopathy
Hetastarch	130	10D	12 hours	Coagulopathy, congestive heart failure, vomiting, mild hepatotoxicity

*D is the hospital base price in dollars per purchasing contract. The remaining indicators are compared with this price (e.g., 20D = 20 times more expensive).

in blood pressure associated with bradycardia and a change in rhythmic breathing, including apnea. The anatomic location of the hypertensive response is presumptively in the caudal portion of the ventral medulla. The classic explanation is increased intracranial pressure associated with a decrease in cerebral perfusion pressure, resulting in brainstem ischemia. This reflex or response occurs most commonly in patients with acute lesions in the posterior fossa and in patients with very marginal brain compliance from increased intracranial pressure. Hypertension from the Cushing reflex is not always associated with bradycardia. Whether a bradycardic response can be mounted depends on whether the vagal nuclei are ischemic as well. In addition, the hypertensive response can be fluctuating and not sustained.[14,15] Hypertension is common in patients with acute cerebellar hemorrhage or infarct. Distortion of the brainstem is the most probable mechanism.

BLOOD PRESSURE MANAGEMENT

Increase in blood pressure is common in acute CNS lesions.[62] Causes for increased blood pressure may include pain, agitation, intolerance to the mechanical ventilator, and more mundane causes such as acute bladder retention. In every patient with uncontrollable hypertension in the first hours after admission, the use of street drugs must be considered (amphetamines, cocaine), certainly in young patients with an acute stroke. However, when confounding factors have been excluded, the treatment of hypertension in acute CNS lesions

is controversial, surprisingly little is known and could be detrimental in certain disorders.[1] The effects of the treatment of hypertension on outcome in patients with acute neurologic illness have rarely been studied prospectively. The effects of blood pressure modulation are unknown in the very early hours after intracerebral hematoma and in patients with large cerebral arterial occlusion in a compensatory state requiring recruitment of collaterals and maximal vasodilatation.[19,24]

There are three immediate concerns. First, the definition of hypertension occurring after acute brain injury is difficult. Second, the natural history is favorable, with normalization after 24 hours in a large proportion of patients with acute CNS lesions.[7,8,14,16,30] Third, the weight assigned to the risks and benefits of blood pressure treatment in acute CNS catastrophes varies widely.[1,9,10,26,27,34,36,43,56,71,73]

A tendency to immediately control acute hypertension is theoretically linked to the possibility of uncontrolled hypertension causing rebleeding (aneurysmal subarachnoid hemorrhage [SAH]), promoting edema in a lesion with an acutely opened blood–brain barrier (hemispheric stroke), facilitating extension of the volume of intracerebral hematoma (putamen or cerebellum hemorrhage), and possibly causing deterioration from hemorrhagic transformation (hemispheric stroke). An additional reason for the treatment of hypertension is impending cardiac failure, a definite concern in elderly patients with prior coronary artery disease and an often relevant concern in traditional hypertensive emergencies.[6,63,74]

Concerns about sustained hypertension in patients with acute hemorrhagic or ischemic stroke exist. However, a study from Stockholm of patients with untreated very high blood pressures (systolic > 200 mm Hg, diastolic > 115 mm Hg) could not identify an increased risk of progression of symptoms in acute stroke, although mortality was higher.[7] In a post hoc analysis of the International Stroke Trial, outcome was worse when systolic blood pressures fell outside the 120–140 mm Hg range, but the explanation or the practical implications of this association remain uncertain.[34] Although there seems to be no evidence of a periclot ischemic zone in either human or animal experiments,[51,54,75] some concern remains that treatment of increased blood pressure may cause global ischemia or an increased zone of ischemia surrounding the clot. This complication is particularly important in patients with ganglionic hemorrhages who have longstanding hypertension that has resulted in narrowing of the lower limit of the auto-regulation curve (Chapter 27). Untreated hypertension may increase the volume of ganglionic hemorrhages.

The management of hypertension after recent use of thrombolytic agents is important, and failure to do so has been linked to hemorrhagic conversion. In a recently published rat model, increased blood pressure correlated with hemorrhagic transformation, which also could be reduced in incidence after treatment with hydralazine.[61] In the National Institute of Neurological Disorders and Stroke (NINDS) trial, the lower rate of intracerebral hemorrhage than that in other thrombolytic trials has been tentatively linked to the aggressive management of hypertension.[10]

Several studies with retrospective analyses of early rebleeding in putaminal hemorrhages could not demonstrate a relationship with hypertension, but the issue remains unsettled. Extravasation of contrast medium during computed tomographic (CT) angiography has been linked to increased blood pressure, hematoma size, and coma. Contrast material extravasation (which was interpreted as continuing hemorrhage) was more common in patients with a mean arterial pressure (MAP) of more than 120 mm Hg.[5] These findings have been confirmed in a separate CT angiogram study, and the extravasate has been identified as "spot" signs.[66]

Prospective data in acute stoke are emerging. A recent large multicenter randomized study in China found that "intensive" blood pressure management (target systolic blood pressure of 140 mm Hg within 6 hours of onset) reduced volume expansion, although minimally so (mean 1.7 mL). The control group in this study had systolic blood pressures controlled to around 160 mm Hg. Outcome was not substantially improved with intensive control therapy, and a large proportion of these patients were treated with unusual agents such as furosemide (35%), urapidil (47%), and phentolamine (16%)[3] (Chapter 27).

A recent pilot trial randomized patients with ischemic and hemorrhagic stroke and systolic blood pressure increase of more than 160 mm Hg into treatment of systolic blood pressure to 145–155 mm Hg or at least a decrease of 15 mm Hg. Patients were treated with lisinopril, labetalol, or placebo, but again outcome was not significantly different. However, clinical trials with a mix of patients with acute stroke may be very difficult to interpret for efficacy.[49,57,59]

Lowering of the blood pressure could result in a considerable decrease in cerebral perfusion pressure. Some studies suggested that a reduction of MAP by more than 20% could reduce cerebral blood flow, but one prospective study of 14 patients with largely ganglionic hematomas showed no appreciable reduction in cerebral blood flow when positron emission tomography studies were done an average of 15 hours after the ictus and MAP was reduced to 120 mm Hg. The number of patients was limited, blood pressure reduction was small, and the effect of changes in blood pressure in the most critical physiologic period of the first hours after onset of cerebral hemorrhage was not studied.[51] A more recent study of treatment within 24 hours of cerebral hemorrhage found no reduction of cerebral blood flow surrounding hematoma, including in patients with systolic blood pressures < 150 mm Hg.[12]

Acute lowering of blood pressure to systolic blood pressure of < 140 mm Hg (INTERACT-2) after cerebral hemorrhage did not result in significant difference in primary outcome measures such as death and severe disabilities, except for some improved measures of quality of life by modified Rankin scales.[2] Hematoma expansion was not significantly different in patients with systolic blood pressures < 140 mmHg as compared to < 180 mmHg. Therefore how aggressive blood pressure lowering results in slightly better outcomes on modified Rankin scales is not known. (In this study the benefit, however was more pronounced in patients without a history of hypertension). In a post-hoc analysis blood pressure swings in the immediate days after cerebral hemorrhage—spontaneous or rebounds after treatments—correlated better with worse outcome and thus strongly argues for measures to maintain a stable blood pressure control to avoid either surges or hypotension.[37] It is a common error to stop antihypertensives abruptly after initial control has been established leading to resurgence of high systolic or mean arterial pressures. Several days of control with IV antihypertensives and careful weaning is needed in some situations with marked hypertensive response.

The treatment of hypertension in aneurysmal SAH is equally controversial.[68] A recent study claimed that systolic arterial blood pressure of more than 160 mm Hg increased the risk of early rebleeding in aneurysmal SAH, but as it often is, there were serious definitional problems with rebleeding criteria—as it often is in so many studies.[42]

Postoperative hypertension (for example, in patients with coiling or clipping of an aneurysm or craniotomy for cerebellar hemorrhage) is best managed by relief of pain, hypoxemia, and excessive volume overload, if present. In postoperative patients, blood pressure can be normalized by adjusting the ventilation settings to a more comfortable mode by sedating the patient with low doses of propofol, and by use of opioids such as fentanyl for pain management. The treatment of postoperative hypertension after carotid endarterectomy—a consequence of stripping of baroreceptor nerve endings in the atheromatous plaque—is discussed in Chapter 45.

Until the results of prospective studies become available, increased blood pressure after acute brain injury probably should be left alone or treated judiciously.[1,53] Treatment is reasonable with CT scan evidence of rapidly worsening brain edema and certainly with the use of thrombolytic agents. The cutoff point in the treatment of hypertension is very difficult to define because of lack of hard data on any disorder.[1] It is reasonable to gradually decrease blood pressure with rapid-acting antihypertensive drugs when the MAP reaches 120 mm Hg or cerebral perfusion pressure is higher than 85 mm Hg. These values closely correspond with the upper limit of autoregulation, and higher pressures may further increase brain edema, if present. These goals should be higher in chronically hypertensive patients (mean arterial pressure > 130 mm Hg). Treatment of hypertension should also proceed if myocardial ischemia occurs or congestive heart failure develops from significantly increased systemic vascular resistance.[6,13,23,25]

Other attempts to reconcile differences of opinion have been made by the American Heart Association/American Stroke Association (AHA/ASA). In a consensus statement, the AHA/ASA has arbitrarily set for patients with cerebral hemorrhage a systolic blood pressure of more than 200 mm Hg or MAP of more than 150 mm Hg as target levels for "aggressive" management, and more "modest" reduction when systolic blood pressure is more than 180 mm Hg or the MAP is more than 130 mm Hg. Most neurointensivists have changed their parameters to rapidly reduce systolic blood pressure of 130 mm Hg or less in the first hours of cerebral hemorrhage and keeping it there for at least several days. For patients with ischemic stroke, the AHA/ASA has arbitrarily set systolic blood pressure of 220 mm Hg or diastolic blood pressure more than 120 mm Hg, but with lowering of blood pressure by approximately 15% in the first 24 hours after stroke. The blood pressure targets for patients eligible for thrombolytic therapy have been arbitrarily set at systolic blood pressure less than 180 mm Hg and diastolic blood pressure less than 105 mm Hg in the first 24 hours after use of intravenous or intra-arterial thrombolysis (see Guidelines).

PHARMACOLOGIC CHOICES

The pros and cons of the currently available antihypertensive agents are discussed in this section, and the most pertinent characteristics relevant for clinical practice are summarized in Table 19.3. There are many IV drugs available to acutely manage a hypertensive surge, and labetalol, esmolol, nicardipine, or hydralazine can be used. With these drugs I apply a rule of 10 meaning 10 mg IV as a starting dose and this dose will show if the drug is effective or whether more doses are needed.

β- and α-Blocking Agents

Agents with combined α- and β-adrenergic receptor blocking properties are preferred in the management of acute hypertension. Most experience has been gained with labetalol.[38,46,72] Although labetalol is a combined α- and β-blocker, the potency of β-blockade is seven times greater with increasing intravenous doses. Its effect results from a decrease in systemic vascular resistance without measurable effect on cardiac output. The absence of an associated tachycardia is caused by β-adrenergic receptor blockade.

Treatment is started with a bolus of 20 mg of labetalol given in 5 minutes, and this may be followed by a double dose of 40 mg or further increase to 80 mg. A bolus of 40 mg may be repeated every 15 minutes, but when a total dose of 300 mg is reached, no further benefit should be expected. Continuous intravenous infusion is

TABLE 19.3. BLOOD PRESSURE MANAGEMENT IN ACUTE BRAIN INJURY

Drug	Dose†	Onset	Duration	Adverse Effects	Not Recommended
			Action		
Esmolol	500 µg/kg bolus, then infusion of 50–300 mg/kg per min IV	1–2 min	10–30 min	Hypotension, nausea, bronchospasm	Asthma, COPD
Labetalol	20 mg IV bolus, slow 2 min, then every 10 min 40–80 mg injections	5–10 min	3–6 hours	Vomiting, scalp tingling, burning in throat, dizziness, nausea, heart block, liver damage, bronchospasm	Asthma, COPD, ventricular failure
Enalaprilat	0.625 mg IV Slow 5 min, then 1.25 mg q6h	15–30 min	6 hours	Response variable	
Nitroprusside	0.3–10 µg/kg per min as IV infusion	Immediate	3–4 min	Nausea, vomiting, muscle twitching, sweating, thiocyanate intoxication with prolonged use	Coronary artery disease
Diazoxide	1–3 mg/kg (150 mg max dose), repeat 5–15 min	2–4 min	6–12 hours	Nausea, flushing, tachycardia, chest pain	Coronary artery disease
Nicardipine	5 mg/hr infusion IV, to maximum 15 mg/hour	5–10 min	1–4 hours	Tachycardia, headache, flushing	Ventricular failure
Hydralazine	10–20 mg IV every 10 min until effect	10–20 min	1–4 hours	Tachycardia, flushing, headache	
Fenoldopam	0.1 µg/kg per minute; increase 0.05 µg/kg per min every 15 min until effect	5–15 min	1–4 hours	Electrocardiographic changes, reflex tachycardia, hypokalemia, headache	Hepatic cirrhosis

COPD, chronic obstructive pulmonary disease; min, minutes.
† Ranges given are lowest preferred dose until desired pressure is achieved.

seldom needed as intervention but, if desired, can be started in the range of 50–200 mg given at an infusion rate of 2 mg/min.

Labetalol is relatively easy to use, and an unexpected decrease in blood pressure should not occur in patients whose intravascular system is adequately filled. Side effects, including vomiting, scalp itching, lichenoid skin eruptions, and hepatic failure, are rare but are more common with long-term use.

Labetalol is not recommended for patients with asthma, chronic obstructive pulmonary artery disease, or severe left ventricular failure. In these patients, an angiotensin-converting enzyme (ACE) inhibitor or calcium-channel blocker should be the preferred agent.

β-Adrenergic Blockade

The rationale for use of β-blockers is a decrease in central sympathetic nervous activity. (Vasodilatation may be another mechanism by which these agents work.) Use of β-blockade has been considered controversial in acute neurologic injury simply because of the preconceived idea that β-blockers produce sedation. This side effect, however, is extremely rare.

Esmolol is useful in the NICU because of its short half-life (minutes) and ease of intravenous administration. Its effect is easily titrated, and is lost within 15 minutes after administration. Esmolol is cardioselective, producing negative inotropic effects and peripheral vasodilatation. The loading dose is 500 µg/kg in a 1-minute bolus. A maintenance dose of 50 µg/kg/min may be sufficient, but infusion rates to 300 µg/kg/min may be needed to control hypertension surges. (One should be aware of the considerable free water load, because esmolol is administered in D5W instead of isotonic saline.) Again, β-blockers are contraindicated in patients with chronic obstructive pulmonary disease.

Calcium-Channel Blockers

Short-acting calcium-channel blockers have been increasingly used in the NICU as an alternative to β-blockers and are probably the very next option if extremes of blood pressures cannot be controlled. Nicardipine has a long half-life, but an infusion is needed when a rapid onset of action is desired. It is started with a dose of 5 mg/hr and increased with increments of 2.5 mg/hr every 5 minutes to maximum 15 mg/hr. After adequate control of blood pressure, the infusion is then tapered by 1 mg/hr.[52,56] Nicardipine remains a superior drug for long-term control of blood pressure. Infusions starting at 10 mg/hr are successful but may be titrated to 15 mg/hr. Post-craniotomy hypertension was adequately controlled in a series of 52 patients much better than with esmolol infusion.[4] A recently approved drug for intravenous use is Clevidipine, a third-generation IV calcium-channel blocker.[33] It is started in a 1–2 mg/hr infusion (to maximum of 21 mg/hr in 24 hours), but there is yet little experience with this agent in the NICU. Both these calcium-channel blockers are contraindicated in patients with aortic stenosis and liver failure. Sublingual nifedipine has been associated with a precipitous decline in blood pressure and is ill-advised in any patient with severe acute hypertension.

Angiotensin-Converting Enzyme Inhibitors

With the introduction of enalaprilat (Vasotec IV), angiotensin-converting enzyme (ACE) inhibitors can be used in hypertensive emergencies in the NICU.[22] This prodrug has important advantages over many other vasodilators. The ACE inhibitors do not produce a reflex sympathetic stimulation. Their major drawbacks are a peak plasma concentration of 3–4 hours and an early effect after 15–30 minutes, considerably longer than those with intravenously administered β-blockers. A unique effect of ACE inhibitors is the ability to reset the autoregulatory curve to lower pressure levels, so that the risk of diffuse cerebral ischemia from lowering blood pressure is reduced.[58] This attribute may make enalaprilat an interesting drug in patients with acute neurologic illness who have marked treatment-refractory hypertension. The starting dose of enalaprilat is 0.625 mg, followed by repeat doses of 1.25 mg every 6 hours.

Miscellaneous Agents

In most instances, hypertension is well controlled with the agents just mentioned. Recently, a dopamine D_1–like receptor agonist, fenoldopam, was introduced for the treatment of acute hypertension. Because of rapid onset and short duration of action, absence of coronary artery steal, minimal hypotension overshoot, easy titration, and lack of thiocyanate toxicity, it is a reasonable alternative agent to nitroprusside in hypertensive crises. The initial dose is 0.1 µg/kg/min, which is increased by 0.05–0.1 µg/kg/min every 15 minutes to a maximum of 1.6 µg/kg/min.[40,44]

Nitroprusside (starting dose of 0.3 µg/kg/min), however, may be the agent of last resort when any other type of medication fails and regulation of blood pressure is needed. If the dose reaches 10 µg/kg/min, thiocyanate toxicity may occur within hours, and other drugs should be tried.[23] Nitroprusside remains a preferred drug in patients with hypertension from the use of cocaine, crack, and amphetamines who are admitted with traumatic brain injury.

Nitroprusside decreases cerebral blood flow and increases intracranial pressure. It is a potent vasodilator that decreases both afterload and preload. Nitroprusside contains cyanide 44% by weight, and cyanide toxicity (cyanide is metabolized to thio cyanide, which is less toxic) is a true concern. Nitroprusside infusion rates of more than 4 mcq/kg/min for 2 hours or more increases the risk substantially. Nitroprusside is not commonly used and, not infrequently, is discontinued. However, when compared with nicardipine, nitroprusside appeared equally safe.[55]

Hydralazine is another commonly used drug in the NICU. It is a direct-acting vasodilator that may cause hypotension and, due to the drug's half-life of 3 hours, may be prolonged and difficult to correct. The effects of hydralazine on cerebral hemodynamics (increased cerebral blood flow after cerebral vasodilation) are unclear but are rarely of clinical concern. Hydralazine is an alternative drug in patients with bradycardia.

With the availability of transdermal patches, clonidine has been used more frequently, but its rebound effect is a major concern. A review of a large series of patients with aneurysmal SAH treated with clonidine in an attempt to control surges of systolic blood pressure found average blood pressures to be higher than in patients not treated with clonidine.[69] Clonidine, however, may have a role when hypertension is related to opiate and alcohol withdrawal.

CONCLUSIONS

- Minimal initial fluid intake in patients with acute brain injury is 200 mL/hr. The goal is a positive fluid balance of approximately 500–750 mL to correct for insensible loss.

- Water deficit in hypovolemic patients can be calculated as follows: $0.6 \times$ body weight $\times$ (serum sodium/140) – 1 in liters.

- Crystalloids are preferred over colloids. Hypotonic fluids or fluids that cause a hypotonic state must be avoided such as 0.45% saline, 5% Dextrose in water and perhaps Lactated Ringer's.

- Treatment of hypertension after acute CNS injury is debatable. Treatment is indicated in patients with persistent extreme surges in blood pressure, or impending congestive heart failure.

- Preferred agents for the treatment of an acute hypertensive response in patients with acute neurologic illness are IV labetalol, nicardipine, or hydralazine.

REFERENCES

1. Aiyagari V, Gorelick PB. Management of blood pressure for acute and recurrent stroke. *Stroke* 2009;40:2251–2256.
2. Anderson CS, Heeley E, Huang Y, et al. Rapid blood-pressure lowering in patients with acute intracerebral hemorrhage. *N Engl J Med* 2013;368:2355–2365.
3. Anderson CS, Huang Y, Wang JG, et al. Intensive blood pressure reduction in acute cerebral haemorrhage trial (INTERACT): a randomised pilot trial. *Lancet Neurol* 2008;7:391–399.
4. Bebawy JF, Houston CC, Kosky JL, et al. Nicardipine is superior to esmolol for the management of postcraniotomy emergence hypertension: a randomized open-label study. *Anesth Analg* 2015;120:186–192.
5. Becker KJ, Baxter AB, Bybee HM, et al. Extravasation of radiographic contrast is an independent predictor of death in primary intracerebral hemorrhage. *Stroke* 1999;30:2025–2032.
6. Blumenfeld JD, Laragh JH. Management of hypertensive crises: the scientific basis for treatment decisions. *Am J Hypertens* 2001;14:1154–1167.
7. Britton M, Carlsson A. Very high blood pressure in acute stroke. *J Intern Med* 1990;228:611–615.
8. Britton M, Carlsson A, de Faire U. Blood pressure course in patients with acute stroke and matched controls. *Stroke* 1986;17:861–864.
9. Broderick J, Brott T, Barsan W, et al. Blood pressure during the first minutes of focal cerebral ischemia. *Ann Emerg Med* 1993;22:1438–1443.
10. Brott T, Lu M, Kothari R, et al. Hypertension and its treatment in the NINDS rt-PA Stroke Trial. *Stroke* 1998;29:1504–1509.
11. Bunn F, Roberts I, Tasker R, Akpa E. Hypertonic versus isotonic crystalloid for fluid resuscitation in critically ill patients. *Cochrane Database Syst Rev* 2002:CD002045.
12. Butcher KS, Jeerakathil T, Hill M, et al. The Intracerebral Hemorrhage Acutely Decreasing Arterial Pressure Trial. *Stroke* 2013;44:620–626.
13. Calhoun DA, Oparil S. Treatment of hypertensive crisis. *N Engl J Med* 1990;323:1177–1183.
14. Carlberg B, Asplund K, Hägg E. Course of blood pressure in different subsets of patients after acute stroke. *Cerebrovasc Dis* 1991;1:281–287.
15. Choi PT, Yip G, Quinonez LG, Cook DJ. Crystalloids vs. colloids in fluid resuscitation: a systematic review. *Crit Care Med* 1999;27:200–210.
16. Cumbler E, Glasheen J. Management of blood pressure after acute ischemic stroke: an evidence-based guide for the hospitalist. *J Hosp Med* 2007;2:261–267.
17. Cushing H. Concerning a definite regulatory mechanism of the vasomotor centre which controls blood pressure during cerebral compression. *Johns Hopkins Hosp Bull* 1901;12:290–292.
18. Cushing H. Some experimental and clinical observations concerning states of increased intracranial tension. *Am J Med Sci* 1902;124:375–400.
19. Davalos A, Cendra E, Teruel J, Martinez M, Genis D. Deteriorating ischemic stroke: risk factors and prognosis. *Neurology* 1990;40:1865–1869.
20. de Jonge E, Levi M. Effects of different plasma substitutes on blood coagulation: a comparative review. *Crit Care Med* 2001;29:1261–1267.
21. Erstad BL, Gales BJ, Rappaport WD. The use of albumin in clinical practice. *Arch Intern Med* 1991;151:901–911.

22. Fagan SC, Robert S, Ewing JR, et al. Cerebral blood flow changes with enalapril. *Pharmacotherapy* 1992;12:319–323.

23. Feldstein C. Management of hypertensive crises. *Am J Ther* 2007;14:135–139.

24. Fisher M. *Stroke Therapy*. 2nd ed. Boston: Butterworth-Heinemann; 2001.

25. Gifford RW, Jr. Management of hypertensive crises. *JAMA* 1991;266:829–835.

26. Graham DI. Ischaemic brain following emergency blood pressure lowering in hypertensive patients. *Acta Med Scand Suppl* 1983;678:61–69.

27. Hachinski V. Hypertension in acute ischemic strokes. *Arch Neurol* 1985;42:1002.

28. Huettemann E. Hetastarch and hydroxyethyl starch are not the same. *Anesth Analg* 2000;91:1561.

29. Jamnicki M, Bombeli T, Seifert B, et al. Low- and medium-molecular-weight hydroxyethyl starches: comparison of their effect on blood coagulation. *Anesthesiology* 2000;93:1231–1237.

30. Jansen PA, Schulte BP, Poels EF, Gribnau FW. Course of blood pressure after cerebral infarction and transient ischemic attack. *Clin Neurol Neurosurg* 1987;89:243–246.

31. Kagansky N, Levy S, Knobler H. The role of hyperglycemia in acute stroke. *Arch Neurol* 2001;58:1209–1212.

32. Katz AM. *Physiology of the Heart*. 4th ed. Philadelphia: Lippincott Williams & Wilkins; 2006.

33. Kenyon KW. Clevidipine: an ultra short-acting calcium channel antagonist for acute hypertension. *Ann Pharmacother* 2009;43:1258–1265.

34. Leonardi-Bee J, Bath PM, Phillips SJ, Sandercock PA. Blood pressure and clinical outcomes in the International Stroke Trial. *Stroke* 2002;33:1315–1320.

35. Lisk DR, Grotta JC, Lamki LM, et al. Should hypertension be treated after acute stroke? A randomized controlled trial using single photon emission computed tomography. *Arch Neurol* 1993;50:855–862.

36. Loyke HF. Lowering of blood pressure after stroke. *Am J Med Sci* 1983;286:2–11.

37. Manning L, Hirakawa Y, Arima H, et al. Blood pressure variability and outcome after acute intracerebral hamorrhage: a post-hoc analysis of INTERACT 2, a randomized controlled trial. *Lancet Neurol* 2014;13:364–373.

38. Marik PE, Varon J. Hypertensive crises: challenges and management. *Chest* 2007;131:1949–1962.

39. Murphy M, Carmichael AJ, Lawler PG, White M, Cox NH. The incidence of hydroxyethyl starch-associated pruritus. *Br J Dermatol* 2001;144:973–976.

40. Murphy MB, Murray C, Shorten GD. Fenoldopam: a selective peripheral dopamine-receptor agonist for the treatment of severe hypertension. *N Engl J Med* 2001;345:1548–1557.

41. Myburgh J, Cooper DJ, Finfer S, et al. Saline or albumin for fluid resuscitation in patients with traumatic brain injury. *N Engl J Med* 2007;357:874–884.

42. Ohkuma H, Tsurutani H, Suzuki S. Incidence and significance of early aneurysmal rebleeding before neurosurgical or neurological management. *Stroke* 2001;32:1176–1180.

43. Ohwaki K, Yano E, Nagashima H, et al. Blood pressure management in acute intracerebral hemorrhage: relationship between elevated blood pressure and hematoma enlargement. *Stroke* 2004;35:1364–1367.

44. Oparil S, Aronson S, Deeb GM, et al. Fenoldopam: a new parenteral antihypertensive: consensus roundtable on the management of perioperative hypertension and hypertensive crises. *Am J Hypertens* 1999;12:653–664.

45. Parsons MW, Barber PA, Desmond PM, et al. Acute hyperglycemia adversely affects stroke outcome: a magnetic resonance imaging and spectroscopy study. *Ann Neurol* 2002;52:20–28.

46. Patel RV, Kertland HR, Jahns BE, et al. Labetalol: response and safety in critically ill hemorrhagic stroke patients. *Ann Pharmacother* 1993;27:180–181.

47. Peterson D, Arntfield RT. Critical care ultrasonography. *Emerg Med Clin N Am* 2014;32:907–926.

48. Phillips SJ. Pathophysiology and management of hypertension in acute ischemic stroke. *Hypertension* 1994;23:131–136.

49. Potter JF, Robinson TG, Ford GA, et al. Controlling hypertension and hypotension immediately post-stroke (CHHIPS): a randomised, placebo-controlled, double-blind pilot trial. *Lancet Neurol* 2009;8:48–56.

50. Powers WJ. Acute hypertension after stroke: the scientific basis for treatment decisions. *Neurology* 1993;43:461–467.

51. Powers WJ, Zazulia AR, Videen TO, et al. Autoregulation of cerebral blood flow surrounding acute (6 to 22 hours) intracerebral hemorrhage. *Neurology* 2001;57:18–24.

52. Prough DS, Johnson JC, Stump DA, et al. Effects of hypertonic saline versus lactated Ringer's solution on cerebral oxygen transport during resuscitation from hemorrhagic shock. *J Neurosurg* 1986;64:627–632.

53. Qureshi AI, Harris-Lane P, Kirmani JF, et al. Treatment of acute hypertension in patients with intracerebral hemorrhage using American Heart Association guidelines. *Crit Care Med* 2006;34:1975–1980.

54. Qureshi AI, Wilson DA, Hanley DF, Traystman RJ. No evidence for an ischemic penumbra in massive experimental intracerebral hemorrhage. *Neurology* 1999;52:266–272.

55. Roitberg BZ, Hardman J, Urbaniak K, et al. Prospective randomized comparison of safety and efficacy of nicardipine and nitroprusside drip for control of hypertension in the neurosurgical intensive care unit. *Neurosurgery* 2008;63:115–120.

56. Rose JC, Mayer SA. Optimizing blood pressure in neurological emergencies. *Neurocrit Care* 2004;1:287–299.

57. Rothwell PM. Blood pressure in acute stroke: which questions remain? *Lancet* 2014.

58. Schmidt JF, Andersen AR, Paulson OB, Gjerris F. Angiotensin converting enzyme inhibition, CBF autoregulation, and ICP in patients with normal-pressure hydrocephalus. *Acta Neurochir (Wien)* 1990;106:9–12.

59. Sheth KN, Sims JR. Neurocritical care and periprocedural blood pressure management in acute stroke. *Neurology* 2012;79:S199–204.

60. Stogermuller B, Stark J, Willschke H, et al. The effect of hydroxyethyl starch 200 kD on platelet function. *Anesth Analg* 2000;91:823–827.

61. Tejima E, Katayama Y, Suzuki Y, Kano T, Lo EH. Hemorrhagic transformation after fibrinolysis with tissue plasminogen activator: evaluation of role of hypertension with rat thromboembolic stroke model. *Stroke* 2001;32:1336–1340.

62. Varon J. Diagnosis and management of labile blood pressure during acute cerebrovascular accidents and other hypertensive crises. *Am J Emerg Med* 2007;25:949–959.

63. Varon J. Treatment of acute severe hypertension: current and newer agents. *Drugs* 2008;68:283–297.

64. Virgilio RW, Rice CL, Smith DE, et al. Crystalloid vs. colloid resuscitation: is one better? A randomized clinical study. *Surgery* 1979;85:129–139.

65. Volpicelli G, Lamorte A, Tullio M, et al. Point-of-care multiorgan ultrasonography for the evaluation of undifferentiated hypotension in the emergency department. *Intensive Care Med* 2013;39:1290–1298.

66. Wada R, Aviv RI, Fox AJ, et al. CT angiography "spot sign" predicts hematoma expansion in acute intracerebral hemorrhage. *Stroke* 2007;38:1257–1262.

67. Wijdicks EFM, Vermeulen M, Hijdra A, van Gijn J. Hyponatremia and cerebral infarction in patients with ruptured intracranial aneurysms: is fluid restriction harmful? *Ann Neurol* 1985;17:137–140.

68. Wijdicks EFM, Vermeulen M, Murray GD, Hijdra A, van Gijn J. The effects of treating hypertension following aneurysmal subarachnoid hemorrhage. *Clin Neurol Neurosurg* 1990;92:111–117.

69. Wijdicks EFM, Vermeulen M, ten Haaf JA, et al. Volume depletion and natriuresis in patients with a ruptured intracranial aneurysm. *Ann Neurol* 1985;18:211–216.

70. Wilkins MR, Redondo J, Brown LA. The natriuretic-peptide family. *Lancet* 1997;349:1307–1310.

71. Willmot M, Leonardi-Bee J, Bath PM. High blood pressure in acute stroke and subsequent outcome: a systematic review. *Hypertension* 2004;43:18–24.

72. Wilson DJ, Wallin JD, Vlachakis ND, et al. Intravenous labetalol in the treatment of severe hypertension and hypertensive emergencies. *Am J Med* 1983;75:95–102.

73. Yatsu FM, Zivin J. Hypertension in acute ischemic strokes: not to treat. *Arch Neurol* 1985;42:999–1000.

74. Zampaglione B, Pascale C, Marchisio M, Cavallo-Perin P. Hypertensive urgencies and emergencies: prevalence and clinical presentation. *Hypertension* 1996;27:144–147.

75. Zazulia AR, Diringer MN, Videen TO, et al. Hypoperfusion without ischemia surrounding acute intracerebral hemorrhage. *J Cereb Blood Flow Metab* 2001;21:804–810.

20

Anticoagulation and Thrombolysis

Therapeutic use of anticoagulants is of importance in only a few acute neurologic conditions. The evidence of its effect in acute ischemic stroke is weak—to say the least—although it is an absolute necessity in cerebral venous thrombosis (Chapter 32). Intravenous and intra-arterial thrombolytic agents are generally accepted interventions within hours of acute ischemic stroke. Several thrombolytic drugs have been tested in the past (urokinase and streptokinase),[30,32,36] but current clinical experience is with intravenous or intra-arterial recombinant tissue plasminogen activator (tPA).[2,50] Intra-arterial thrombolysis has been largely replaced by stent clot retrieval over the years and recent clinical trials have shown 70%–94% recanalization (Chapter 29).[10,14,37,88]

This chapter briefly reviews the clinical guidelines for anticoagulation, the daily management of intravenous heparin, the use of oral anticoagulants, and the indications for use of thrombolysis. Adequate knowledge of the concepts underpinning the use of these agents is needed before they are administered.

INDICATIONS FOR THERAPEUTIC ANTICOAGULATION

In any patient with ischemic stroke intravenous heparin is considered only if the patient is not a candidate for thrombolysis or neurointervention. The effectiveness of heparin in evolving acute ischemic hemispheric stroke or in acute basilar artery occlusion remains unclear.[67] In approximately 25% of patients, further progression of hemiparesis occurs despite prolongation of the activated partial thromboplastin time (APTT).[34] In fact, one critical overview of antithrombotic therapy in acute ischemic stroke did not indicate that heparin is sufficiently effective to prevent further deterioration.[85] The evidence is also less conclusive about the target of APTT.

Few patients with an acute ischemic stroke need to be treated with intravenous heparin, and treatment depends on the underlying mechanism. Patients with a high likelihood of a cardiogenic embolus are at significant risk for recurrence. Typically, this pertains to patients with atrial fibrillation, acute myocardial infarction, evidence of intracardiac thrombus, or a large akinetic ventricular segment. If there is no large territorial involvement—usually a third of middle cerebral artery territory or a watershed infarct—the risk of causing symptomatic hemorrhagic conversion is low.

Heparin can be considered in patients with a critical stenosis or near occlusion of the carotid or vertebral artery. Acute carotid occlusion has a risk of embolization from the carotid stump and may justify anticoagulation.[75] For high-grade stenosis of the basilar artery or recent acute basilar artery occlusion in association with recent ischemic stroke in the posterior circulation, heparin administration is considered by many to be standard therapy, but there is virtually no evidence of a beneficial effect. A clinical trial of treatment in dissection comparing aspirin, clopidogrel, dipyridamole (alone or in combination) did not achieve a better or worse outcome than with anticoagulants; but the number of secondary events were low (6% in patients presenting with dissection and stroke).[57]

Suggested indications for intravenous heparin in acute ischemic stroke are summarized in Table 20.1.

HEPARIN

The main mechanism of action of heparin is binding with antithrombin III. This binding enhances its inhibiting activity of not only thrombin and factor Xa but also factors IXa, XIa, and XIIa.

Intravenous administration of heparin results in an anticoagulant response that is variable and unpredictable. In the conventional approach, an intravenous bolus of 5,000 units is followed by continuous intravenous infusion of heparin (maintenance dose range of 20,000–40,000 units per 24 hours). It is universally recommended that heparin be monitored by APTT, with a predefined range of 1.5–2.0 times the mean control value. (In most laboratories, this is equivalent to 50–75 seconds.)

TABLE 20.1. INDICATIONS
FOR INTRAVENOUS HEPARIN
IN PATIENTS WITH ACUTE STROKE
ADMITTED TO THE NEUROSCIENCE
INTENSIVE CARE UNIT

Cardiogenic ischemic stroke
Acute carotid artery occlusion (or high-grade critical
 stenosis)
Acute basilar artery occlusion (or high-grade critical
 stenosis)
Crescendo transient ischemic attacks
Cerebral venous thrombosis

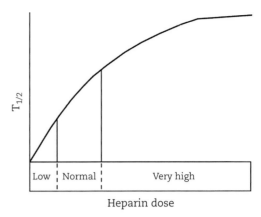

FIGURE 20.1: Clearance of heparin. Half-time
increases with increasing doses.

From Hirsh J, Fuster V. Guide to anticoagulant therapy.
Part 1: heparin. *Circulation* 1994;89:1449–1468. With permission
of the American Heart Association.

The most important concerns in the use
of heparin are the time required to reach this
therapeutic range and the bleeding complications that result from excessive anticoagulation.
Nomograms for the adjustment of heparin dose
have been suggested. Raschke and colleagues[83]
found that a weight-based nomogram was superior to any other standard care nomogram. In the
weight-based nomogram, tested in patients with a
wide variety of diagnoses, the mean time to reach
the therapeutic range was 8 hours, whereas this
time was 20 hours in the standard nomogram. The
therapeutic threshold was achieved in 86% of
the patients on the first drawn sample for APTT,
compared with 32% in the standard group. Major
bleeding complications did not occur in this comparatively small series of 62 patients treated using
this protocol. Confirmatory studies are required
in the ICU patient population.

It is well known from hospital audits that heparin dosage is often inadequate. The bioavailability of heparin is poor through its rapid clearance
and binding to many plasma proteins when initial
therapeutic doses are administered.[23] However,
with the use of an intravenous bolus, the biologic half-life increases significantly (Figure 20.1).
Thus, when immediate anticoagulation must be
achieved (e.g., pulmonary embolus), it is important to initiate heparin with an intravenous bolus.
An example of a dosing regimen is shown in
Table 20.2.[22] (An alternative protocol is described
by Hirsh et al.[51,52])

The major risk of heparin is hemorrhage, at
any site, which can be fatal. It has not been consistently found that excessive prolongation of
APTT exclusively increases this risk. Additional
predictive factors of heparin-induced bleeding
are serious underlying illness, chronic alcohol
abuse, renal failure, and administration of heparin

by intermittent doses. Bleeding from heparin is
possible at any location, but often occurs in the
gastrointestinal tract. However, acute gastrointestinal bleeding is often associated with ulcers, and
endoscopic evaluation may reveal a significant
gastrointestinal lesion. A less common, but life-
threatening, complication is bilateral adrenal hemorrhage,[48,89] which unfortunately has also been

TABLE 20.2. WEIGHT-BASED HEPARIN
NOMOGRAM*

Start: Bolus of heparin, 80 units/kg IV
  Heparin infusion, 18 units/kg/hr (20,000
  units in 500 mL of D5W = 40 units/mL)
Measure: APTT 6 hours after bolus

Adjust:	APTT, second	Bolus, U/kg	New infusion rate, U/kg/hr
	< 35	80	22
	35–45	40	20
	46–70	No	18
	71–90	No	16
	> 90	No	15 (stop for 1 hour)

* Some institutions have adopted a low-intensity nomogram (e.g.,
in ischemic stroke) This includes no loading dose and starts at
12 units/kg/hr.
Administration of warfarin, 10 mg, can be started on the second
day of heparin therapy if long-term anticoagulation is warranted.
Complete blood cell count with platelet count is done every 3 days.
APTT, activated partial thromboplastin time; D5W, 5% dextrose
in water.
Modified from Raschke RA, Reilly BM, Guidry JR, et al. The weight-
based heparin dosing nomogram compared with a "standard care"
nomogram. *Ann Intern Med* 1993;119:874–881. With permission of
the American College of Physicians.

reported with the prophylactic use of subcutaneous heparin. It must be considered when shock suddenly develops without evidence of blood loss in any anticoagulated patient. Retroperitoneal hemorrhage should be considered in patients with a rapid decrease in hematocrit and no other explanations for labile blood pressure. Retroperitoneal hemorrhage can be spontaneous or associated with cerebral angiography. An abdominal computed tomography [CT] scan usually demonstrates a large-volume hematoma (Figure 20.2).

Equally serious hemorrhages may be located in the brain and spinal cord. In acute ischemic stroke, intracranial hemorrhage has most often been associated with large middle cerebral artery territory involvement, occurring within 24 hours after the initiation of intravenous heparin and at times with excessive prolongation of APTT (> 150 seconds).[92] Cerebral amyloid angiopathy, may be a predisposing factor.[66,84] We have also seen heparin-associated intracranial hematomas in patients with evidence of cavernous angioma at other locations on magnetic resonance imaging (MRI), which may suggest that in some patients an underlying lesion is present under these circumstances.

The safety profile of intravenous heparin in ischemic stroke, particularly the danger of hemorrhagic conversion with clinical progression or the development of intracerebral hematoma, has not been well studied. Prior studies have suggested that this risk is low. The outcome of hemorrhagic conversion of brain infarcts in anticoagulated patients did not differ significantly from that in non-anticoagulated patients.[5,74,82] Discontinuation of therapy or adjustment of the heparin dose to a level lower than that aimed at originally is probably already appropriate when ischemic infarcts convert to petechial infarcts.

Thrombocytopenia induced by heparin (HIT) due to an immunologic drug reaction, another well-established complication of IV heparin treatment, is can be mild but when serious typically there is a 75% platelet count drop.[9] This complication can occur solely with flushing of an intravenous access with heparin. HIT is rare with subcutaneous administration of heparin.[53] The incidence of thrombocytopenia associated with therapeutic use of heparin is approximately 2%. It occurs 5–10 days after heparin treatment and more often in patients with previous heparin treatment. HIT can be confirmed with anti-PF4/heparin EIA-IgG or platelet serotonin-release essay. Heparin should be replaced by hirudin (lepirudin) in a loading dose of 0.4 mg/kg by intravenous bolus (44 mg maximum), followed by 0.15 mg/kg/hr (16.5 mg/hr maximum), intravenously to reach an APTT 1.5–2.5 times the normal range.[51]

Although anticoagulation can be greatly simplified with low-molecular-weight heparin (LMWH), the three products (dalteparin, enoxaparin, and ardeparin) available in the United States have been approved only for prophylaxis of deep vein thrombosis.[21,61,69,72] One study showed that the rate of deep vein thrombosis was 59% less with enoxaparin than with compression stockings alone.[3] The recommended dose of enoxaparin is 30 mg subcutaneously twice daily for prophylaxis of deep vein thrombosis. All three LMWH products have different pharmacologic effects because the methods of preparation and molecular structures differ.[11,81] The primary mechanism of action of LMWH is binding to antithrombin III. One of the fundamental differences between LMWH and standard heparin is less significant neutralization by platelet factor IV, which is released after platelet activation. (Platelet factor IV competitively inhibits the binding to antithrombin III, and this effect reduces the anticoagulant effect.)

Low-molecular-weight heparin has greater bioavailability, indicated by longer plasma half-life, less variability in the anticoagulant response, and fewer or equally frequent hemorrhagic complications.[71] Side effects of LMWH are thrombocytopenia (which may be related to the nature of each individual LMWH), transient increase in liver enzymes, and skin necrosis that has been interpreted as toxic epidermal neurolysis.[73] LMWH is much easier to use than heparin because single daily doses are sufficient, and monitoring is not necessary. Currently, its use in the treatment of deep vein thrombosis and various other cardiovascular diseases, including stroke,

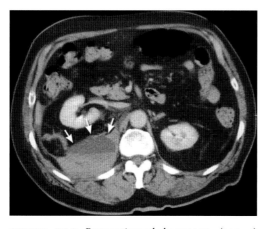

FIGURE 20.2. Retroperitoneal hematoma (arrows) after heparin use, causing a marked decline in hematocrit and blood pressure.

is under investigation.[29,80,86] Enoxaparin compared with unfractioniated heparin did increase extracranial hemorrhage rates.[58] Although a large randomized study of Org-10172 in acute ischemic stroke did not show a benefit, a subgroup of patients with large-artery atherosclerosis seemed to benefit.[1] The LMWH certoparin did not improve outcome in ischemic stroke.[28] In a recent study, high-dose tinzaparin was not superior to aspirin and resulted in a higher incidence of intracerebral hematomas.[7] With these credible trials of different LMWHs, these agents have no role in the treatment of stroke. For now, the main objection to LMWH is cost (three times more expensive than standard heparin) unless it can be offset by reduced hospital and ICU stay. Another potential problem is reversal if it is urgently needed. Protamine reverses unfractionated heparin fully but only 60% of LMWH. There is only protamine effect when administered with 12 hours of subcutaneous injection of enoxaparin. Serum anti-factor Xa—this factor is inhibited directly or indirectly by LMWH—can be measured but takes time and thus is not useful in acute situations which need immediate action.

Finally, a commonly asked question is when heparin can be started in a patient with prior cerebral hemorrhage (spontaneous or traumatic). Little information is available, but the risk seems small when restarted after 2 weeks and preferably in patients with marked resolution of the hemorrhage.[12,15,16]

WARFARIN

Anticoagulation with warfarin is usually started 2 or 3 days after initiation of heparin therapy. Coumadin acts by inhibiting the synthesis of factors II, VII, IX, and X, but several days are required for these vitamin K–dependent anticoagulants to clear from the plasma. When the international normalized ratio (INR) is therapeutic, an overlap of 2 days with heparin is recommended before the administration of heparin is discontinued.

The first- and second-day doses of warfarin are 10 mg and 5 mg, respectively, and subsequent oral doses are adjusted to achieve the desired INR (Table 20.3). Other than patients with a metallic valve, the risk of thromboembolism in patients with atrial fibrillation is usually assessed using the so-called CHADS2 score. (The CHADS2 score is made up by congestive heart failure [1 point], hypertension [1 point], age > 75 years [1 point], diabetes mellitus [1 point], and prior stroke [2 points].) A CHADS2 score of 5–6 has a high risk of arterial or venous thromboembolism when anticoagulation is discontinued. The risk is low with a CHADS2 score of 0–2. A consensus meeting concluded that in patients with small- to moderate-sized ischemic strokes, an INR of 2.0–3.0 was reasonable, but the recommendation for this range of prothrombin time prolongation is derived from expert opinion only. When ischemic strokes are associated with antiphospholipid antibody syndrome, higher INRs (3.0–3.5) are recommended,[59] because the risk of recurrence is high with lower INRs. An INR of 2.5–3.5 is recommended in ischemic stroke associated with mechanical valves.[52]

The risk that bleeding will develop in patients receiving warfarin who have an INR of 3.0 or higher is 1 in 14 per year (serious hemorrhage, 1 in 50 per year). Age is not an important determinant of bleeding until 80 years of age or older.[35] Intensity of anticoagulation is a strong predictor of warfarin-associated bleeding, again most commonly in the gastrointestinal tract. A rare complication of warfarin is warfarin-induced skin necrosis, with onset usually 3 days after initiation. This localized patch of tissue necrosis, often in thighs, breasts, and buttocks, may need skin grafting.[18,73] Another rare complication is "purple toe syndrome" from embolization of microemboli in patients with ulcerated aortic plaques. In occasional patients, a new livedo reticularis is seen.[56]

TABLE 20.3. INTERNATIONAL NORMALIZED RATIO RECOMMENDATIONS FOR VARIOUS INDICATIONS

Indication	International Normalized Ratio
Prophylaxis of deep vein thrombosis	2.0–3.0
Treatment of venous thrombosis	2.0–3.0
Treatment of pulmonary embolism	2.0–3.0
Atrial fibrillation	2.0–3.0
Tissue heart valve	2.0–3.0
Acute ischemic stroke or transient ischemic attacks	2.0–3.0
Antiphospholipid antibody syndrome	3.0–3.5
Mechanical prosthetic valve	2.5–3.5

Antithrombotic Therapy and Prevention of Thrombosis, 9th ed: American College of Chest Physicians Evidence-Based Clinical Practice Guidelines.
Guyatt GH, Akl EA, Crowther M, Gutterman DD, Schuünemann HJ; American College of Chest Physicians Antithrombotic Therapy and Prevention of Thrombosis Panel. Chest. 2012;141(2 Suppl):7S-47S.

TABLE 20.4. COMMONLY USED DRUGS THAT POTENTIATE OR INTERFERE WITH THE ACTION OF WARFARIN

Potentiator	Inhibitor
Acetaminophen	Barbiturates
Amiodarone	Carbamazepine
Anesthetics	Chlordiazepoxide
Chloramphenicol	Cholestyramine
Cimetidine	Corticosteroids
Diazoxide	Griseofulvin
Erythromycin	Haloperidol
Fluconazole	Meprobamate
Indomethacin	Nafcillin
L-Methyldopa	Rifampin
Metronidazole	Sucralfate
Miconazole	Tetracyclines
Omeprazole	
Phenylbutazone	
Phenytoin	
Piroxicam	
Propranolol	
Tolbutamide	
Trimethoprim- Sulfamethoxazole	

Excessive INRs with warfarin use most commonly indicate vitamin K deficiency or interaction with pharmaceutical agents. Drug interactions with warfarin are numerous, and the most relevant are summarized in Table 20.4.

NEW ORAL ANTICOAGULANTS

Direct thrombin inhibitors are the newer oral anticoagulation drugs.[62] These anticoagulants inhibit thrombin factor (factor IIa or factor Xa). Dabigatran, which targets factor II, is currently approved in the United States; and the oral factor Xa inhibitor rivaroxaban is approved for venous thromboembolism after orthopedic surgery and for stroke prevention and atrial fibrillation. Apixaban is an oral Xa inhibitor and is approved in Europe for venous thromboembolism and will likely be approved for atrial fibrillation in the United States.[27,68,79] The problem with these new anticoagulants is that none of the current used methods to reverse anticoagulation could possibly have an effect because these drugs inhibit a single clotting factor (IIa or Xa). Vitamin K administration also has no role. There are significant concerns with the emergent reversal of these new oral anticoagulants (Figure 20.3).

The reversal of thrombin inhibitors has not been clearly established. Recent guidance has been published that suggests a combination of supportive care, discontinuation of the drug, and possible prothrombin complex concentrate or hemodialysis. Supportive care would imply blood transfusions in patients who are actively bleeding, maintenance of renal function, identification of the bleeding source, and possible surgical intervention if needed. The drug should be discontinued, and the anticoagulant effect is absent after 2 days. Activated charcoal (1-2 g/kg) should be administered if the drug was taken within hours of presentation. Hemodialysis and hemoperfusion can be considered in patients with impaired renal function that will cause more difficulty with clearing of the drug; however, it is not effective with apixaban or rivaroxaban because they are highly protein bound. Factor VIIa does not reverse the anticoagulant effect, but PCC has been shown to normalize the prothrombin time (PT) in normal volunteers. It is unclear whether it is effective to stop bleeding but has been used in emergency situations.

A few practical tips are in order. We measure thrombin time with dabigatran (thrombin inhibitor). If normal, then there is no hemostatically meaningful dabigatran present. We measure heparin levels with apixaban, rivaroxaban and edoxaban (direct Factor Xa inhibitors). If normal, then most likely no hemostatically meaningful Factor Xa inhibitor is present. Iraducimab is a new antidote for dabigatran[78] and has been recently approved by the FDA and will enter hospital formularies soon. (Andexanet alpha, antidote for Xa inhibitors, is expected to be approved in 2016.) Reversal strategies are discussed in more detail in Chapter 27.

THROMBOLYTIC THERAPY

Thrombolysis has many applications and has included acute myocardial infarction, massive pulmonary embolus, and peripheral arterial thrombi.[38,39,60]

Thrombolytic therapy can induce complete dissolution of emboli. The mechanism of action is activation of the proteolytic enzyme plasminogen followed by fibrin dissolution and increasing fibrinogen degradation products (Capsule 20.1). Intravenous alteplase is used in acute stroke. The drug has a high fibrin selectivity (higher than previously used urokinase, lower than the newer drug tenecteplase) and a half-life of 4–8 minutes. Tenecteplase (0.25 mg/kg) may be safer and

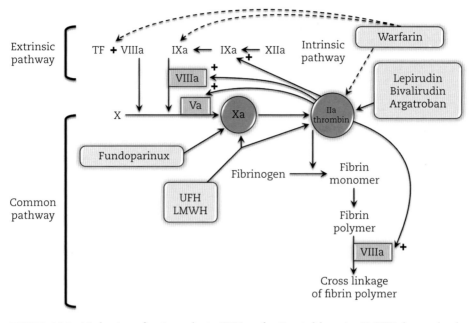

FIGURE 20.3. Mechanism of anticoagulants. UFH, unfractionated heparin; LMWH, low molecular weight heparin.

CAPSULE 20.1   THE FIBRINOLYTIC SYSTEM

Major activators and inhibitors have been identified and have resulted in manufacturing of thrombolytic agents. The fibrinolytic system is shown in the accompanying figure. In brief, the major source of tPA is vascular endothelium, and tPA has a high affinity for plasminogen. Plasminogen is activated by tissue-type plasminogen activator (t-PA) or urokinase-type plasminogen activator (u-PA). Plasminogen activator inhibitor-1 (PAI-1) restricts the activity of tPA and is an important regulator present in plasma and platelets. Plasma degrades intact fibrin and results in degradation products (FDP). This process is regulated by α_2-antiplasmin (α_2-AP). Thrombin converts fibrinogen into fibrin and activates thrombin-activatable fibrinolysis inhibitor (TAFI), which inhibits fibrinolysis.

Adapted from Rijken DC, Lijnen HR. New insights into the molecular mechanisms of the fibrinolytic system. J Thromb Haemost 2009;7:4–13. Used with permission.

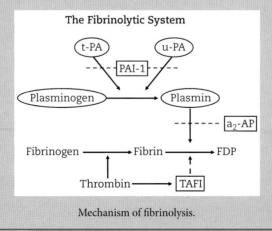

Mechanism of fibrinolysis.

faster (bolus only) and perhaps more effective, but the first trial (ATTEST) with 104 patients found no difference in outcome or radiologic features between tenecteplase and alteplase. Future trials are underway.[54,64,95]

The initial results with intravenous thrombolytic agents in acute carotid territory stroke were far from satisfactory because of recanalization in only one-third of the patients and a 10% incidence of clinical deterioration associated with hemorrhagic conversions, including intracerebral hematoma.[25,47,49,70,93,96] However, intravenous thrombolysis has been studied in several clinical trials, and these have yielded important clinically relevant information. Three studies with streptokinase were discontinued prematurely because of a high frequency of bleeding complications and mortality in treated patients.[30,40,41] Early European studies (European Cooperative Acute Stroke Study and Second European-Australasian Acute Stroke Study) found a threefold increase in parenchymal hemorrhage but improvement in functional disability.[44,45]

A study of recombinant tPA in stroke from the National Institute of Neurological Disorders and Stroke further defined the role of tPA in acute stroke.[42] Within 3 hours of onset of stroke, tPA (Activase) was administered intravenously in a dose of 0.9 mg/kg (maximum, 90 mg), 10% of the total dose in a bolus over 1 minute and 90% in a constant infusion for 1 hour. In the second part of the study (333 patients), there was a 10%–13% absolute increase in improvement at 3 months on several disability and handicap scales. Mortality was similar between the groups, but symptomatic intracerebral hematoma within 36 hours occurred significantly more often in the treated group (6.4%) than in the placebo group (0.6%).[6] These results were confirmed by the European Cooperative Acute Stroke Study (ECASS) I and II trials. Intravenously administered tPA significantly increased intracerebral hemorrhage when administered more than 3 hours after onset.[17] A meta-analysis for the Cochrane Stroke Group concluded that, taking into account fatal cerebral hemorrhage, the overall net benefit of intravenous tPA was very significant. It was summarized elegantly: "For every 1,000 patients treated with i.v. rt-PA, 57 avoided death or dependence when treated up to 6 hours after stroke, and 140 when treated within 3 hours of stroke."[94]

ECASS-3 investigated intravenous tPA (similar dosing regimen of 0.9 mg/kg) administered up to 4.5 hours after onset ($n = 418$) and compared with placebo ($n = 403$) treatment. The trial excluded patients older than 80 years, NIHSS of more than 25, any use of oral anticoagulants irrespective of INR, and prior stroke and diabetes mellitus. Outcome improved significantly, but symptomatic intracranial hemorrhage increased from 3.5% in placebo to 9% in the treated tPA group.[43] This extension of the intravenous tPA window has been endorsed by the American Heart Association/American Stroke Association (AHA/ASA).[26]

Another attractive therapy is intra-arterial infusion of a thrombolytic agent aimed directly at the clot.[20,33,65,76,77,87,90,98] The cerebral angiogram allows for clear visualization of the obstructing clot and thus provides an additional justification for thrombolytic agents. Theoretically, the risk of hemorrhage should be lower in intra-arterial thrombolysis because uninvolved vessels are not infused, but in 5%–17% of the patients, an intracerebral hematoma (and not petechial hemorrhagic conversion) complicated the procedure.[19] Intra-arterial (IA) thrombolysis is administered by neurointerventionalists. With the rapid development of stent retrieval of clots, intra-arterial thrombolysis is currently an adjuvant therapy. As a general guideline, IA thrombolysis should be started before 6 hours in the carotid artery territory[4,24,31,34,63,91,97] and 12 hours in the vertebrobasilar artery territory.[8,13,46,55,76,90]

The new contraindications for thrombolysis are listed in Table 20.5.[2] A comprehensive AHA/ASA scientific statement published in 2016 reviewed the inclusion and exclusion criteria for intravenous alteplase and suggested several modifications (Part XIV guidelines).

CONCLUSIONS

- Indications for intravenous heparin in acute ischemic stroke are cardiogenic ischemic stroke (assuming a small territorial stroke), acute carotid or basilar artery occlusion or high-grade critical stenosis, crescendo transient ischemic attacks, and cerebral venous thrombosis.

- Heparin therapy is begun with 80 units/kg intravenously and is continued with 18 units/kg/hr. Activated partial thromboplastin time is determined 6 hours after an initial bolus, and the dose is adjusted.

TABLE 20.5. SUGGESTED CONTRAINDICATIONS FOR THROMBOLYTIC THERAPY

Interval from onset of stroke: intravenous $\geq$ 4.5 hours; intra-arterial $\geq$ 6 hours in anterior circulation and $\geq$ 12 hours in posterior circulation

Rapidly resolving nondisabling neurologic signs

Treatment-refractory hypertension (inability to maintain a stable blood pressure of < 185/110 mmHg)

Diffuse swelling and hypodensity of affected hemisphere[†]

Computed tomographic evidence of hemorrhagic conversion

Heparin or LMWH within 48 hours

APTT > upper limit of normal

INR > 1.7

Prothrombin time < 15 seconds

Blood glucose $\leq$ 50 mg/dL

Platelets $\leq$ 100,000/mm^3

Recent severe Gastrointestinal or genitourinary bleeding

Pregnancy or lactation[‡]

Severe traumatic brain injury within 3 months

Stroke associated with infective endocarditis

Stroke due to suspected aortic arch dissection

Stroke and prior intracranial neoplasm

Stroke within past 3 months

Surgical procedure or major trauma within 14 days (consider risk in each individual case after consulting with surgeon)

[†] The size of the hypodensity is a matter of debate.

[‡] With early pregnancy, may be given on a compassionate basis. Abortion may have to be granted (for more details consult the 2016 AHA/ASA scientific statement published in Stroke).

- When indicated, administration of warfarin (10 mg) can be started on the second day of heparin therapy, and the dose is usually adjusted to an INR of 2.0–3.0. An INR of 3.0–4.5 is recommended in ischemic stroke associated with mechanical prosthetic valves. An INR of 3.0–3.5 is recommended in patients with antiphospholipid antibody syndrome associated with ischemic stroke.

- IV thrombolysis can be considered in patients seen with ischemic stroke with 3 hours of onset. Expansion of the 3-hour time window to 4.5-hour can be considered for most patients.

REFERENCES

1. Adams HP, Jr., Bendixen BH, Leira E, et al. Antithrombotic treatment of ischemic stroke among patients with occlusion or severe stenosis of the internal carotid artery: a report of the Trial of Org 10172 in Acute Stroke Treatment (TOAST). *Neurology* 1999;53:122–125.

2. Adams HP, Jr., del Zoppo G, Alberts MJ, et al. Guidelines for the early management of adults with ischemic stroke: a guideline from the American Heart Association/American Stroke Association Stroke Council, Clinical Cardiology Council, Cardiovascular Radiology and Intervention Council, and the Atherosclerotic Peripheral Vascular Disease and Quality of Care Outcomes in Research Interdisciplinary Working Groups: The American Academy of Neurology affirms the value of this guideline as an educational tool for neurologists. *Circulation* 2007;115:e478–e534.

3. Agnelli G, Piovella F, Buoncristiani P, et al. Enoxaparin plus compression stockings compared with compression stockings alone in the prevention of venous thromboembolism after elective neurosurgery. *N Engl J Med* 1998;339:80–85.

4. Arnold M, Schroth G, Nedeltchev K, et al. Intra-arterial thrombolysis in 100 patients with acute stroke due to middle cerebral artery occlusion. *Stroke* 2002;33:1828–1833.

5. Babikian VL, Kase CS, Pessin MS, Norrving B, Gorelick PB. Intracerebral hemorrhage in stroke patients anticoagulated with heparin. *Stroke* 1989;20:1500–1503.

6. Barber PA, Zhang J, Demchuk AM, Hill MD, Buchan AM. Why are stroke patients excluded from TPA therapy? An analysis of patient eligibility. *Neurology* 2001;56:1015–1020.

7. Bath PM, Lindenstrom E, Boysen G, et al. Tinzaparin in acute ischemic stroke (TAIST): a randomized aspirin-controlled trial. *Lancet* 2001;358:702–710.

8. Becker KJ, Monsein LH, Ulatowski J, et al. Intraarterial thrombolysis in vertebrobasilar occlusion. *AJNR Am J Neuroradiol* 1996;17: 255–262.

9. Becker PS, Miller VT. Heparin-induced thrombocytopenia. *Stroke* 1989;20:1449–1459.

10. Berkhemer OA, Fransen PS, Beumer D, et al. A randomized trial of intraarterial treatment for acute ischemic stroke. *N Engl J Med* 2015;372:11–20.

11. Bick RL, Fareed J. Low molecular weight heparins: differences and similarities in approved preparations in the United States. *Clin Appl Thromb Hemost* 1999;5 Suppl 1:S63–66.

12. Boeer A, Voth E, Henze T, Prange HW. Early heparin therapy in patients with spontaneous intracerebral haemorrhage. *J Neurol Neurosurg Psychiatry* 1991;54:466–467.

13. Brandt T, von Kummer R, Muller-Kuppers M, Hacke W. Thrombolytic therapy of acute basilar artery occlusion: variables affecting recanalization and outcome. *Stroke* 1996;27:875–881.

14. Campbell BC, Mitchell PJ, Kleinig TJ, et al. Endovascular therapy for ischemic stroke with perfusion-imaging selection. *N Engl J Med* 2015;372:1009–1018.

15. Chalela JA, Katzan I, Liebeskind DS, et al. Safety of intra-arterial thrombolysis in the postoperative period. *Stroke* 2001;32:1365–1369.

16. Claassen DO, Kazemi N, Zubkov AY, Wijdicks EFM, Rabinstein AA. Restarting anticoagulation therapy after warfarin-associated intracerebral hemorrhage. *Arch Neurol* 2008;65:1313–1318.

17. Clark WM, Albers GW, Madden KP, Hamilton S. The rtPA (alteplase) 0- to 6-hour acute stroke trial, part A (A0276g): results of a double-blind, placebo-controlled, multicenter study. Thromblytic therapy in acute ischemic stroke study investigators. *Stroke* 2000;31:811–816.

18. Cole MS, Minifee PK, Wolma FJ. Coumarin necrosis: a review of the literature. *Surgery* 1988;103:271–277.

19. Cross DT, 3rd, Derdeyn CP, Moran CJ. Bleeding complications after basilar artery fibrinolysis with tissue plasminogen activator. *AJNR Am J Neuroradiol* 2001;22:521–525.

20. Cross DT, 3rd, Moran CJ, Akins PT, Angtuaco EE, Diringer MN. Relationship between clot location and outcome after basilar artery thrombolysis. *AJNR Am J Neuroradiol* 1997;18:1221–1228.

21. Cziraky MJ, Spinler SA. Low molecular weight heparins for the treatment of deep-vein thrombosis. *Clin Pharm* 1993;12:892–899.

22. Davydov L, Dietz PA, Lewis P, Twichell ML, Bertino JS, Jr. Outcomes of weight-based heparin dosing based on literature guidelines and institution individualization. *Pharmacotherapy* 2000;20:1179–1183.

23. de Swart CA, Nijmeyer B, Roelofs JM, Sixma JJ. Kinetics of intravenously administered heparin in normal humans. *Blood* 1982;60:1251–1258.

24. del Zoppo GJ, Ferbert A, Otis S, et al. Local intra-arterial fibrinolytic therapy in acute carotid territory stroke: a pilot study. *Stroke* 1988;19:307–313.

25. del Zoppo GJ, Poeck K, Pessin MS, et al. Recombinant tissue plasminogen activator in acute thrombotic and embolic stroke. *Ann Neurol* 1992;32:78–86.

26. Del Zoppo GJ, Saver JL, Jauch EC, Adams HP, Jr. Expansion of the time window for treatment of acute ischemic stroke with intravenous tissue plasminogen activator: a science advisory from the American Heart Association/American Stroke Association. *Stroke* 2009;40:2945–2948.

27. Di Nisio M, Middeldorp S, Buller HR. Direct thrombin inhibitors. *N Engl J Med* 2005;353: 1028–1040.

28. Diener HC, Ringelstein EB, von Kummer R, et al. Treatment of acute ischemic stroke with the low-molecular-weight heparin certoparin: results of the TOPAS trial. Therapy of Patients with Acute Stroke (TOPAS) Investigators. *Stroke* 2001;32:22–29.

29. Dolovich LR, Ginsberg JS, Douketis JD, Holbrook AM, Cheah G. A meta-analysis comparing low-molecular-weight heparins with unfractionated heparin in the treatment of venous thromboembolism: examining some unanswered questions regarding location of treatment, product type, and dosing frequency. *Arch Intern Med* 2000;160:181–188.

30. Donnan GA, Davis SM, Chambers BR, et al. Streptokinase for acute ischemic stroke with relationship to time of administration: Australian Streptokinase (ASK) Trial Study Group. *JAMA* 1996;276:961–966.

31. Edwards MT, Murphy MM, Geraghty JJ, Wulf JA, Konzen JP. Intra-arterial cerebral thrombolysis for acute ischemic stroke in a community hospital. *AJNR Am J Neuroradiol* 1999;20: 1682–1687.

32. Ezura M, Kagawa S. Selective and superselective infusion of urokinase for embolic stroke. *Surg Neurol* 1992;38:353–358.

33. Ferguson RD, Ferguson JG. Cerebral intraarterial fibrinolysis at the crossroads: is a phase III trial advisable at this time? *AJNR Am J Neuroradiol* 1994;15:1201–1216.

34. Fieschi C, Argentino C, Lenzi GL, et al. Clinical and instrumental evaluation of patients with ischemic stroke within the first six hours. *J Neurol Sci* 1989;91:311–321.

35. Fihn SD, Callahan CM, Martin DC, et al. The risk for and severity of bleeding complications in elderly patients treated with warfarin. The National Consortium of Anticoagulation Clinics. *Ann Intern Med* 1996;124:970–979.

36. Furlan A, Higashida R, Wechsler L, et al. Intra-arterial prourokinase for acute ischemic stroke. The PROACT II study: a randomized controlled trial. Prolyse in Acute Cerebral Thromboembolism. *JAMA* 1999;282:2003–2011.

37. Goyal M, Demchuk AM, Menon BK, et al. Randomized assessment of rapid endovascular treatment of ischemic stroke. *N Engl J Med* 2015;12;372:1019–1030.

38. Granger CB, Califf RM, Topol EJ. Thrombolytic therapy for acute myocardial infarction: a review. *Drugs* 1992;44:293–325.

39. Grines CL. Thrombolytic, antiplatelet, and antithrombotic agents. *Am J Cardiol* 1992;70:18I-26I.

40. Group MAST—IM-I. Randomised controlled trial of streptokinase, aspirin, and combination of both in treatment of acute ischaemic stroke. *Lancet* 1995;346:1509–1514.

41. Group TMAST—ES. Thrombolytic therapy with streptokinase in acute ischemic stroke. *N Engl J Med* 1996;335:145–150.

42. Group TNIoNDaSr-PSS. Tissue plasminogen activator for acute ischemic stroke. *N Engl J Med* 1995;333:1581–1587.

43. Hacke W, Kaste M, Bluhmki E, et al. Thrombolysis with alteplase 3 to 4.5 hours after acute ischemic stroke. *N Engl J Med* 2008;359:1317–1329.

44. Hacke W, Kaste M, Fieschi C, et al. Intravenous thrombolysis with recombinant tissue plasminogen activator for acute hemispheric stroke. The European Cooperative Acute Stroke Study (ECASS). *JAMA* 1995;274:1017–1025.

45. Hacke W, Kaste M, Fieschi C, et al. Randomised double-blind placebo-controlled trial of thrombolytic therapy with intravenous alteplase in acute ischemic stroke (ECASS II). Second European-Australasian Acute Stroke Study Investigators. *Lancet* 1998;352:1245–1251.

46. Hacke W, Zeumer H, Ferbert A, Bruckmann H, del Zoppo GJ. Intra-arterial thrombolytic therapy improves outcome in patients with acute vertebrobasilar occlusive disease. *Stroke* 1988;19:1216–1222.

47. Haley EC, Jr., Levy DE, Brott TG, et al. Urgent therapy for stroke. Part II: pilot study of tissue plasminogen activator administered 91–180 minutes from onset. *Stroke* 1992;23:641–645.

48. Hardwicke MB, Kisly A. Prophylactic subcutaneous heparin therapy as a cause of bilateral adrenal hemorrhage. *Arch Intern Med* 1992;152:845–847.

49. Higashida RT, Halbach VV, Barnwell SL, Dowd CF, Hieshima GB. Thrombolytic therapy in acute stroke. *J Endovasc Surg* 1994;1:4–15.

50. Hill MD, Barber PA, Demchuk AM, et al. Acute intravenous–intra-arterial revascularization therapy for severe ischemic stroke. *Stroke* 2002;33:279–282.

51. Hirsh J, Anand SS, Halperin JL, Fuster V. Guide to anticoagulant therapy: heparin: a statement for healthcare professionals from the American Heart Association. *Circulation* 2001;103:2994–3018.

52. Hirsh J, Dalen J, Anderson DR, et al. Oral anticoagulants: mechanism of action, clinical effectiveness, and optimal therapeutic range. *Chest* 2001;119:8S–21S.

53. Horellou MH, Conard J, Lecrubier C, et al. Persistent heparin induced thrombocytopenia despite therapy with low molecular weight heparin. *Thromb Haemost* 1984;51:134.

54. Huang X, Cheripelli BK, Lloyd SM, et al. Alteplase versus tenecteplase for thrombolysis after ischaemic stroke (ATTEST): a phase 2, randomised, open-label, blinded endpoint study. *Lancet Neurol* 2015;14:368–376.

55. Huemer M, Niederwieser V, Ladurner G. Thrombolytic treatment for acute occlusion of the basilar artery. *J Neurol Neurosurg Psychiatry* 1995;58:227–228.

56. Hyman BT, Landas SK, Ashman RF, Schelper RL, Robinson RA. Warfarin-related purple toes syndrome and cholesterol microembolization. *Am J Med* 1987;82:1233–1237.

57. Investigators TCt. Antiplatelet treatment compared with anticoagulation treatment for cervical artery dissection (CADISS): a randomized trial. *Lancet Neurol* 2015;14:361–367.

58. Kase CS, Albers GW, Bladin C, et al. Neurological outcomes in patients with ischemic stroke receiving enoxaparin or heparin for venous thromboembolism prophylaxis: subanalysis of the Prevention of VTE after Acute Ischemic Stroke with LMWH (PREVAIL) study. *Stroke* 2009;40:3532–3540.

59. Khamashta MA, Cuadrado MJ, Mujic F, et al. The management of thrombosis in the antiphospholipid-antibody syndrome. *N Engl J Med* 1995;332:993–997.

60. Kucinski T, Koch C, Grzyska U, et al. The predictive value of early CT and angiography for fatal hemispheric swelling in acute stroke. *AJNR Am J Neuroradiol* 1998;19:839–846.

61. Lensing AW, Prins MH, Davidson BL, Hirsh J. Treatment of deep venous thrombosis with low-molecular-weight heparins: a meta-analysis. *Arch Intern Med* 1995;155:601–607.

62. Levine M, Goldstein JN. Emergency reversal of anticoagulation: novel agents. *Curr Neurol Neurosci Rep* 2014;14:471.

63. Lindley RI. Is intraarterial tPA within 3 hours the treatment of choice for selected stroke patients? No. *Stroke* 2009;40:2613–2614.

64. Marshall RS. Progress in intravenous thrombolytic therapy for acute stroke. *JAMA Neurology* 2015;72:928–934.

65. Matsumoto K, Satoh K. Topical intra-arterial urokinase infusion for acute stroke. In: Hacke W, del Zoppo GJ, Hirschberg M, eds. *Thrombolytic Therapy in Acute Ischemic Stroke*. Berlin: Springer-Verlag; 1991:207–215.

66. Melo TP, Bogousslavsky J, Regli F, Janzer R. Fatal hemorrhage during anticoagulation of cardioembolic infarction: role of cerebral amyloid angiopathy. *Eur Neurol* 1993;33:9–12.

67. Miller VT, Hart RG. Heparin anticoagulation in acute brain ischemia. *Stroke* 1988;19:403–406.

68. Miyares MA, Davis K. Newer oral anticoagulants: a review of laboratory monitoring options and reversal agents in the hemorrhagic patient. *Am J Health Syst Pharm* 2012;69:1473–1484.

69. Mori E, Tabuchi M, Yoshida T, Yamadori A. Intracarotid urokinase with thromboembolic occlusion of the middle cerebral artery. *Stroke* 1988;19:802–812.

70. Mori E, Yoneda Y, Tabuchi M, et al. Intravenous recombinant tissue plasminogen activator in acute carotid artery territory stroke. *Neurology* 1992;42:976–982.

71. Nieuwenhuis HK, Albada J, Banga JD, Sixma JJ. Identification of risk factors for bleeding during treatment of acute venous thromboembolism with heparin or low molecular weight heparin. *Blood* 1991;78:2337–2343.

72. Noble S, Peters DH, Goa KL. Enoxaparin. A reappraisal of its pharmacology and clinical applications in the prevention and treatment of thromboembolic disease. *Drugs* 1995;49:388–410.

73. Ojeda E, Perez MC, Mataix R, et al. Skin necrosis with a low molecular weight heparin. *Br J Haematol* 1992;82:620.

74. Pessin MS, Estol CJ, Lafranchise F, Caplan LR. Safety of anticoagulation after hemorrhagic infarction. *Neurology* 1993;43:1298–1303.

75. Pessin MS, Hinton RC, Davis KR, et al. Mechanisms of acute carotid stroke. *Ann Neurol* 1979;6:245–252.

76. Phan TG, Wijdicks EFM. Intra-arterial thrombolysis for vertebrobasilar circulation ischemia. *Crit Care Clin* 1999;15:719–742, vi.

77. Pillai JJ, Lanzieri CF, Trinidad SB, et al. Initial angiographic appearance of intracranial vascular occlusions in acute stroke as a predictor of outcome of thrombolysis: initial experience. *Radiology* 2001;218:733–738.

78. Pollack CV Jr, Reilly PA, Eikelboom J, et al. Idarucizumab for dabigatran reversal. *N Engl J Med* 2015;373:511–520.

79. Poulsen BK, Grove EL, Husted SE. New oral anticoagulants: a review of the literature with particular emphasis on patients with impaired renal function. *Drugs* 2012;72:1739–1753.

80. Prins MH, Gelsema R, Sing AK, van Heerde LR, den Ottolander GJ. Prophylaxis of deep venous thrombosis with a low-molecular-weight heparin (Kabi 2165/Fragmin) in stroke patients. *Haemostasis* 1989;19:245–250.

81. Racine E. Differentiation of the low-molecular-weight heparins. *Pharmacotherapy* 2001;21:62S–70S.

82. Ramirez-Lassepas M, Quinones MR. Heparin therapy for stroke: hemorrhagic complications and risk factors for intracerebral hemorrhage. *Neurology* 1984;34:114–117.

83. Raschke RA, Reilly BM, Guidry JR, Fontana JR, Srinivas S. The weight-based heparin dosing nomogram compared with a "standard care" nomogram: a randomized controlled trial. *Ann Intern Med* 1993;119:874–881.

84. Rosand J, Hylek EM, O'Donnell HC, Greenberg SM. Warfarin-associated hemorrhage and cerebral amyloid angiopathy: a genetic and pathologic study. *Neurology* 2000;55:947–951.

85. Sandercock PA, van den Belt AG, Lindley RI, Slattery J. Antithrombotic therapy in acute ischaemic stroke: an overview of the completed randomised trials. *J Neurol Neurosurg Psychiatry* 1993;56:17–25.

86. Sandset PM, Dahl T, Stiris M, et al. A double-blind and randomized placebo-controlled trial of low molecular weight heparin once daily to prevent deep-vein thrombosis in acute ischemic stroke. *Semin Thromb Hemost* 1990;16 Suppl:25–33.

87. Sasaki O, Takeuchi S, Koike T, Koizumi T, Tanaka R. Fibrinolytic therapy for acute embolic stroke: intravenous, intracarotid, and intra-arterial local approaches. *Neurosurgery* 1995;36:246–252.

88. Saver JL, Jahan R, Levy EI, et al. Solitaire flow restoration device versus the Merci Retriever in

patients with acute ischemic stroke (SWIFT): a randomized, parallel-group, non-inferiority trial. *Lancet* 2012;380:1241–1249.

89. Stead LG, Vaidyanathan L. Evidence-based emergency medicine/systematic review abstract. Role of abciximab in the management of acute ischemic stroke. *Ann Emerg Med* 2009;53:392–394.

90. Suarez JI, Sunshine JL, Tarr R, et al. Predictors of clinical improvement, angiographic recanalization, and intracranial hemorrhage after intra-arterial thrombolysis for acute ischemic stroke. *Stroke* 1999;30:2094–2100.

91. Theron J, Courtheoux P, Casasco A, et al. Local intraarterial fibrinolysis in the carotid territory. *AJNR Am J Neuroradiol* 1989;10:753–765.

92. Toni D, Fiorelli M, Bastianello S, et al. Hemorrhagic transformation of brain infarct: predictability in the first 5 hours from stroke onset and influence on clinical outcome. *Neurology* 1996;46:341–345.

93. von Kummer R. Intravenous tissue plasminogen activation in acute stroke. In: Hacke W, del Zoppo GJ, Hirschberg M, eds. *Thrombolytic Therapy in Acute Ischemic Stroke.* Berlin: Springer-Verlag; 1991:161–174.

94. Wardlaw JM. Overview of Cochrane thrombolysis meta-analysis. *Neurology* 2001;57:S69–76.

95. Wechsler LR. Intravenous thrombolytic therapy for acute ischemic stroke. *N Engl J Med* 2011;364:2138–2146.

96. Wechsler LR, Jungreis CA. Intra-arterial thrombolysis for carotid circulation ischemia. *Crit Care Clin* 1999;15:701–718, vi.

97. Weitz JI. Unanswered questions in venous thromboembolism. *Thromb Res* 2009;123 Suppl 4:S2–S10.

98. Wijdicks EFM, Nichols DA, Thielen KR, et al. Intra-arterial thrombolysis in acute basilar artery thromboembolism: the initial Mayo Clinic experience. *Mayo Clinic Proc* 1997;72:1005–1013.

21

Fever and Cooling

Fever and its febrile response are not only commonly expected in acutely ill neurologic patients but its physiology demands specific attention.[14,16,17,36] As in any critically ill patient, the appearance of fever mostly signals an infectious cause but there are striking differences in the neurocritically ill.

Acute brain injury is a strong and protracted stimulus to the temperature regulatory center. This type of fever—conveniently called "central fever"—has now been recognized as an important prognostic sign in acute brain injury and, more important, when unchecked may raise intracranial pressure. Seizures may also be more difficult to control without lowering core temperature. Furthermore, high fever reduces a patient's responsiveness or, less commonly, may cause agitated delirium. Convincing studies have demonstrated that there is a deleterious effect of high fever on outcome,[2,4,16,34] but there are also data on possible beneficial effects of fever, such as possibly increasing the activity of antimicrobial agents,[17] and fever may have—at least with moderate levels—some effect on immunomodulation,[12] resulting in improved lymphocyte and phagocyte recruitment. Moreover, side effects of aggressive use of antipyretic drugs are potentially concerning. Cooling of patients with fever from sepsis reduces the vasopressor requirements but also improves the hemodynamic balance. Other studies have not reduced the need for renal replacement therapies and improved sequential organ failure assessment score.[30] (Any of these clinical trials may be hampered by heterogeneity of antibiotics, timing of antibiotics, and nature of the infection.) Nonetheless, there is a broad clinical consensus that fever in any critically ill patient requires control, and the control of fever has become a mainstay of neurocritical care.

There is no reliable way to sort out "infectious" from a "central" or "noninfectious" cause of fever. Even more important, the absence of a source of infection cannot be used as a reliable indicator of noninfectious cause. Central fever may be more likely only after cultures are negative or imaging fails to show a source. This chapter, therefore, first provides insight into the urgent evaluation of new onset fever. Evaluation of fever should be comprehensive each time. The chapter then will discuss methods of fever control in the overall management of a critically ill neurologic patient and how to achieve effective cooling.

PHYSIOLOGIC EFFECTS AND CONSEQUENCES OF FEVER

There is the physiology of fever first. Fever (core temperature > 38.5° C) increases the metabolic demand, resulting in rapid insensible fluid loss, and quickly doubles oxygen consumption. This may not be necessarily harmful when there is yet no evidence of organ dysfunction, and patients may fend off these insults. However, when other organs start to fail, fever may further cascade the patient into a downward vortex, which is characterized by increased glucocorticosteroids, reduced vasopressin, increased carbon dioxide production, and overall substantial increase in energy expenditure. An important part of the febrile response is vasodilatation and sweating, resulting in marked hypovolemia and hypotension. Second, there is the effect on the brain. The protective effect of hypothermia to the brain might have complex mechanisms that include the prevention of apoptosis, reduced mitochondrial dysfunction, reduction of excessive free radical production, mitigation of reperfusion injury, reduction of oxygen and glucose requirements, as well as suppression of epileptic activity and seizures.

Looking at it from the other side, experimental studies have shown that increase in brain temperature can worsen prior brain injury. The operational mechanism is likely through increased level of excitatory amino acids that will eventually lead to breakdown of the blood–brain barrier and cerebral edema. How fever is generated is shown in Capsule 21.1.

EVALUATION OF FEVER

Fever in an acutely ill neurologic patient probably indicates an infection. Unavoidably, because many

CAPSULE 21.1   ORIGIN OF FEVER

Body core temperature is maintained by a functional neuronal system that includes the medial preoptic anterior hypothalamic area, dorsomedial nucleus of the hypothalamus midbrain peri-aqueductal gray matter of the midbrain, and nucleus raphe pallidus in the medulla. Several signals trace back to the center, and this may be the result of an immune system generating pyrogenetic mediators. The impact of brain injury on fever and cytokine production in cerebro-spinal fluid and blood is known. Cytokines can be both protective and damaging to the brain, depending on the cytokine and the quantity produced. Environmental change can be sensed by the skin, and both warm and cool receptors stimulate the preoptic area. Afferent information from the skin and viscera activate so-called warm sensitive neurons and results in heat loss (vasodilation and sweating) or heat gain (vasoconstriction shivering), as "set point" (an unproven concept) can be reached by balancing the activation of heat loss neurons with the inhibition of heat gain neurons. Hypothalamic stimulation in experimental studies has shown that warm sensitive neurons display spontaneous membrane depolarization and are considered "pace-makers." Therefore, hypothermia can be seen in practically any territory involving this "center." Lesions of the dorsomedial region of the posterior hypothalamus prevent shivering. General anesthesia or the use of potent anesthetic drugs decreases the threshold for vasoconstriction and shivering, and in some instances, causes transient poikilothermia. Sweating and active vasodilation remain intact.

In summary, cutaneous warm and cool receptors activate sensory neurons that innervate neurons in spinal and trigeminal maxillary dorsal horn. Through spinal thalamic tracts, connections are made with the somatosensory cortex, which helps in signaling. The normal autonomic response to heat is sweating and vasodilatation. The normal autonomic response to cold is vasoconstriction and shivering.

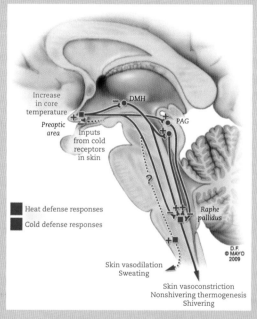

Thermoregulatory pathways.

Adapted from Benarroch EE. Thermoregulation: a recent concept and remaining questions. *Neurology* 2007;69:1293–1297, with permission.

critically ill neurologic patients have dysphagia—due to any level of diminished alertness—acute aspiration pneumonia is a frequent cause of infectious fever. Next comes urinary tract infections, and scrupulous attention to asepsis significantly reduces the risk. Noninfectious causes that can result in increased body temperature must be considered. A fairly common cause of fever in patients with aneurysmal or traumatic subarachnoid hemorrhage is blood disintegration and resorption. As early as the second day after admission to the unit, a low-grade fever, almost never much higher than 39°C, can appear sometimes with short spikes. A typical feature of fever from blood absorption is relative bradycardia, but this is not a strong discriminative clinical feature (some patients may be on beta blockade which blunts tachycardia with fever).[37]

Other major diagnostic categories, aside from infectious causes, are deep venous thrombosis, drug fever, and atelectasis. An important cause for unexplained fever to consider in the intensive care unit is deep venous thrombosis, which may be associated with small subsegmental pulmonary emboli. Careful examination of patients' calves should be part of a daily routine during rounds, but regular ultrasound surveillance of legs (and arms if peripherally inserted central catheter [PICC] has been placed in situ) is much more diagnostic (Chapter 15).

Drug fever is commonly associated with tachycardia and chills, typically appears on the seventh to tenth day after continuous administration of a drug, and is often characterized by a stepwise increase in fever after an initial low-grade fever. An accelerated reaction, instead of an incremental progression, may be seen in patients known to be sensitized to the drug. Fever promptly resolves in 1 to 2 days after the responsible drug is stopped.[30] Virtually any drug can cause fever in a susceptible patient, and in some patients the additional appearance of a skin rash, eosinophilia (only 20% of patients), or abnormal liver function tests are helpful diagnostic signs (Chapter 62).

Postoperative fever has traditionally been linked with atelectasis. Atelectasis may follow early after any type of craniotomy and in any patient with prolonged bedrest. (The mechanism is explained by the appearance of alveolar macrophages producing IL-1 or tumor necrosis factor, causing the febrile response.) Attributing fever to atelectasis found on chest radiographs is potentially troublesome, and a careful search for possibly overlooked infections remains important.

The core temperature may become extremely high, with temperatures reaching 40°C. This is obviously the result of thermoregulatory failure and is seen in a lesion where the ambient temperature—in combination with dehydration—limits sweating and subsequently results in excessive heat production. This may occur with very unusual clinical syndromes such as malignant hyperthermia or neuroleptic malignant syndrome, but in addition to neuroleptics there are other drugs that can generate hyperthermia; these are atropine, amphetamine, SSRI's and cocaine. Large destructive hemorrhages in the pons may be associated with hyperthermia (Chapter 28).

The various causes of fever are listed in Table 21.1. The initial workup for infectious causes of fever is summarized in Table 21.2. Comprehensive laboratory testing for causes of new-onset fever should include full hematologic evaluation, including smear and differential count, routine cultures (blood, sputum, urine, and stool), chest and sinus radiography, and bronchoscopy, definitively in immunosuppressed patients with pulmonary infiltrates.[19,22] Throat and rectal swabs may further identify methicillin-resistant staphylococcus aureus. Any patient with a lumbar drain or ventriculostomy and fever needs CSF cultures. Cerebrospinal fluid examination (presence of β2-transferrin) must be strongly considered in any patient with traumatic brain injury to detect meningitis associated with a possible cerebrospinal fluid leak. Early sepsis should be recognized and biomarkers may be helpful. Procalcitonin level increase (> 0.5 ng/ml) may indicate the beginnings of sepsis. Higher levels (> 10 ng/ml) indicate septic shock (Chapter 51).

MANAGEMENT OF FEVER
Treatment of the source of infection and identification of noninfectious causes of fever and subsequent management will eventually reduce or eliminate febrile responses. Fever may additionally damage the brain, but the mechanisms underlying this additional injury are speculative. Pathways to injury may include revving up the inflammatory cascades with an increase in pro-inflammatory cytokines and the appearance of leukocytes in the injured tissue. Cerebral oxygen utilization may also increase with fever, and supply may be insufficient.

Fever, particularly when sustained and high (39°–40°C), may increase neuronal excitotoxicity. It also has been recognized that fever in any patient with acute brain injury increases morbidity and mortality.[34] However, no study has yet documented that the control of fever improves outcome in critically ill neurologic patients.

TABLE 21.1. CAUSES OF FEVER IN ACUTE NEUROLOGIC ILLNESS

Cause	Characteristics and circumstances
Nosocomial pneumonia	Pulmonary infiltrates Marginal oxygenation Ventilation-perfusion mismatch (increased alveolar-arterial gradient)
Atelectasis	Plate-like collapse of pulmonary parenchyma
Sepsis	Fever and hypotension Increase in leukocyte counts with shift to immature polynuclear cells Respiratory alkalosis (early sepsis)
Urinary tract infection	100,000 colony-forming units White blood cell casts Recent "difficult" catheterization
Decubitus ulcer infection	Preexisting spinal cord injury Preexisting prolonged coma
Resorption of blood	Subarachnoid hemorrhage Traumatic brain injury Traumatic muscle hematomas
Thromboembolism	Persistent tachycardia Painful calves, calf edema, arm-hand swelling Increased alveolar-arterial gradient
Sinusitis	Endotracheal intubation and mechanical ventilation
Meningitis/ventriculitis	Cerebrospinal fluid leak, hematotympanum, ventriculostomy
Drug fever	New introduction (< 5 days) of drugs (e.g., penicillin, phenytoin, amphotericin B, sulfa preparations)

However, a recently completed trial of high doses of acetaminophen (6,000 mg/day) in acute stroke found improved outcome in a selected patient group with temperatures of 37°–39°C. Overall, there is a paucity of effective antipyretics, or their use may cause unnecessary side effects such as gastric bleeding or platelet dysfunction (e.g., NSAIDs such as ibuprofen or diclofenac sodium).

Any neurointensivist will proceed with a cooling method that maintains temperature around 37°C to avoid shivering (expected with temperatures below 35.5°–36°C). Part of management is the assessment of the severity of fever. A simple protocol for fever control can be followed (Table 21.3). Some have suggested calculating the so-called fever burden, defined as a maximal

TABLE 21.2. FEVER EVALUATION FOR INFECTIOUS CAUSES

Fever ≥ 38.3° (≥ 101°F) for > 1 hour*
Examine access sites and catheters for inflammation or purulence
Examine surgical wounds
3–4 blood cultures within 24 hours (venipuncture rather than through device)
Chest radiograph/CT scan or consider bronchoscopy
Sputum cultures
Stool sample for *C. difficile* culture and enzyme immunoassay
Urine sample from sampling port of catheter for gram stain and microscopy
CT facial sinuses (consider aspiration or puncture sinus)
CSF (gram stain, culture, glucose, cell count), preferably from ventricular or lumbar catheter

* definition arbitrary and may be lower in elderly or immunosuppressed patients.
From O'Grady NP, Barie PS, Bartlett JG, et al. Guidelines for evaluation of new fever in critically ill adult patients: 2008 update from the American College of Critical Care Medicine and the Infectious Diseases Society of America. *Crit Care Med* 2008;36:1330–1349. With permission of the publisher.

temperature of 38°C summed over the days it is present. Using this criterion, a high fever burden has been related to poor outcome in subarachnoid hemorrhage and ischemic stroke.[11,21,26]

Any fever spike can be followed and evaluated but does not necessarily have to trigger more complex intervention.

Cooling success can be defined as a markedly defined fever burden; cooling failure could be set at is not reaching control within 24 hours of taking measures. Cooling failure is usually a consequence of a potent persistent stimulus such as serious infection or abscess. Moreover, if drug fever is not appreciated and the responsible drug is not discontinued, fever may not subside.

Shivering continues to be a major issue, and protocols have been developed (Table 21.4).[3,6,25] In most patients, the combination of dexmedetomidine or opioids will provide a good control of shivering. Buspirone (30 mg every 8 hours) has been helpful in treating shivering as well.

Fever control to normal temperature is the main goal.[27] Therapeutic hypothermia is generally used in control of status epilepticus, control of refractory intracranial pressure, and in patients following cardiac arrest. Most evidence has shown that moderate hypothermia is not proven to be effective in traumatic brain injury, ischemic stroke, or hemorrhagic stroke; and even temperature goal in survivors of cardiac arrest is unclear.[24,29,32–34] (Chapter 49) Generally, therapeutic hypothermia is maintained for 24 hours with gradual rewarming 0.2°–0.5° per hour.

METHODS OF COOLING

Cooling blankets or cooling pads that keep a stationary temperature are currently standard.[1] Transnasal cooling devices are in development, but there is no temperature feedback mechanism[5] (e.g., The RhinoChill system evaporates perfluorocarbon gas that cools the nasal cavity). Rapid cooling can be achieved 30 cc/kg of 4°C normal saline infused over 30 minutes through a central catheter.[10] If there is no effect on the maintenance of normal temperature, it is necessary either to repeat the infusion, or to proceed to a more controlled cooling device. Cooling systems provide cooling rates that vary from 1°C/hr to 3°C/hr. Endovascular catheters are connected with temperature feedback control mechanisms and have an even better cooling rate that is between 2°C and 4°C per hour. Adequate maintenance of target temperature is provided by the surface cooling device and is preferred because of its ease of

TABLE 21.3. PROTOCOL FOR FEVER CONTROL

Fever spike	WBC, cultures, lactate
Fever spike with transient hypotension	Fluid challenge (500 mL crystalloid)
Persistent fever after spike	Cooling techniques (cooling device)
Persistent fever with persistent hypotension	Sepsis management bundle

Adapted from reference 6.

application. Poorly controlled temperature and the need for aggressive temperature control might be more successful in devices in which a heat exchange catheter is placed in the inferior vena cava; however, the risk of thromboembolic events with endovascular cooling catheters is significant, even if subcutaneous heparin is used.[18,20,28] However, IV heparin use has improved the number of catheter-associated thrombi. Commonly seen cardiac arrhythmias are bradycardia and new atrial fibrillation and may prompt discontinuation. Pressors are rarely needed and hypertension due to vasocontriction is more common. Skin integrity under the pads should be inspected every 6 hours. The choice of endovascular versus superficial cooling is personal preference; far more endovascular cooling is used in European countries. Both methods may work equally well.[13,31]

To maintain a constant temperature, a feedback-control mechanism is needed; and several devices are on the market. Surface cooling devices circulate cool air or cooled fluids (Blanketrol® III, Arctic Sun® 5000, InnerCool).

TABLE 21.4. TREATMENT OPTIONS IN SHIVERING

Intervention	Dose
Acetaminophen	650–1000 mg q 4–6 h
Buspirone	30 mg q 8 h
Magnesium sulfate	0.5–1 mg/h IV (Goal 3–4 mg/dL)
Dexmedetomidine	0.2–1.5 mcg/kg/h
Opioids	Fentanyl 100 mcg/h
	Meperidine 50–100 mg IM or IV
Propofol	50–75 mcg/kg/min
Vecuronium	0.1 mg/kg IV bolus (rarely)

Adapted from reference 6.

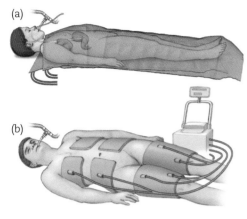

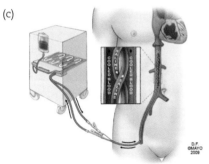

FIGURE 21.1. Methods of cooling of patients in the NICU: (a) sandwich cooling blankets with cold packs in axilla and cold gastric lavage; (b) surface cooling; (c) endovascular cooling system.

Usually pads cover parts of the body, and covered surface area varies.

Endovascular devices[9] (InnerCool, ZOLL CoolGard Alsius®) work through a heat-exchange catheter and are placed in the inferior vena cava. Less temperature fluctuations and better control of rewarming are main advantages. Peritoneal lavage and esophageally placed devices are in clinical trials.[7,15,35] Surface devices may not be much better than simply sandwiching the patient with close contact cooling sheets (Figure 21.1), but hour to hour control of temperature is better; and this mostly applies to both degree of hypothermia and pace of rewarming. In general, surface cooling may not be more effective than endovascular devices when outcome is concerned.[23]

CONCLUSIONS

- New-onset fever often indicates infection but may be caused by resorption of subarachnoid blood, any other major traumatic tissue hematoma, thromboembolism (persistent tachycardia,

swollen calves), or drugs (incremental increase in temperature within several days).

- Antipyretic drugs are rarely successful and cooling devices are needed for sustained control of fever.

- Fever may prevent adequate control of seizures, intracranial pressure, and delirium.

- Fever and hypotension should initiate a sepsis management protocol.

REFERENCES

1. Badjatia N. Fever control in the NICU: is there still a simpler and cheaper solution? *Neurocrit Care* 2011;15:373–374.
2. Badjatia N. Hyperthermia and fever control in brain injury. *Crit Care Med* 2009;37:S250–257.
3. Badjatia N, Strongilis E, Gordon E, et al. Metabolic impact of shivering during therapeutic temperature modulation: the Bedside Shivering Assessment Scale. *Stroke* 2008;39:3242–3247.
4. Bohman LE, Levine JM. Fever and therapeutic normothermia in severe brain injury: an update. *Curr Opin Crit Care* 2014;20:182–188.
5. Castren M, Nordberg P, Svensson L, et al. Intra-arrest transnasal evaporative cooling: a randomized, prehospital, multicenter study (PRINCE: Pre-ROSC IntraNasal Cooling Effectiveness). *Circulation* 2010;122:729–736.
6. Choi HA, Ko SB, Presciutti M, et al. Prevention of shivering during therapeutic temperature modulation: the Columbia anti-shivering protocol. *Neurocrit Care* 2011;14:389–394.
7. de Waard MC, Biermann H, Brinckman SL, et al. Automated peritoneal lavage: an extremely rapid and safe way to induce hypothermia in post-resuscitation patients. *Crit Care* 2013;17:R31.
8. den Hertog HM, van der Worp HB, van Gemert HM, et al. The Paracetamol (Acetaminophen) In Stroke (PAIS) trial: a multicentre, randomized, placebo-controlled, phase III trial. *Lancet Neurol* 2009;8:434–440.
9. Erlinge D, Gotberg M, Lang I, et al. Rapid endovascular catheter core cooling combined with cold saline as an adjunct to percutaneous coronary intervention for the treatment of acute myocardial infarction. The CHILL-MI trial: a randomized controlled study of the use of central venous catheter core cooling combined with cold saline as an adjunct to percutaneous coronary intervention for the treatment of acute myocardial infarction. *J Am Coll Cardiol* 2014;63:1857–1865.

10. Fink EL, Kochanek PM, Clark RS, Bell MJ. Fever control and application of hypothermia using intravenous cold saline. *Pediatr Crit Care Med* 2012;13:80–84.

11. Greer DM, Funk SE, Reaven NL, Ouzounelli M, Uman GC. Impact of fever on outcome in patients with stroke and neurologic injury: a comprehensive meta-analysis. *Stroke* 2008;39:3029–3035.

12. Hasday JD, Singh IS. Fever and the heat shock response: distinct, partially overlapping processes. *Cell Stress Chaperones* 2000;5:471–480.

13. Kasner SE, Wein T, Piriyawat P, et al. Acetaminophen for altering body temperature in acute stroke: a randomized clinical trial. *Stroke* 2002;33:130–134.

14. Kilpatrick MM, Lowry DW, Firlik AD, Yonas H, Marion DW. Hyperthermia in the neurosurgical intensive care unit. *Neurosurgery* 2000;47:850–855.

15. Kulstad E, Metzger AK, Courtney DM, et al. Induction, maintenance, and reversal of therapeutic hypothermia with an esophageal heat transfer device. *Resuscitation* 2013;84:1619–1624.

16. Laupland KB. Fever in the critically ill medical patient. *Crit Care Med* 2009;37:S273–278.

17. Mackowiak PA, Marling-Cason M, Cohen RL. Effects of temperature on antimicrobial susceptibility of bacteria. *J Infect Dis* 1982;145:550–553.

18. Maze R, Le May MR, Froeschl M, et al. Endovascular cooling catheter related thrombosis in patients undergoing therapeutic hypothermia for out of hospital cardiac arrest. *Resuscitation* 2014;85:1354–1358.

19. Mourad O, Palda V, Detsky AS. A comprehensive evidence-based approach to fever of unknown origin. *Arch Intern Med* 2003;163:545–551.

20. Muller A, Lorenz A, Seifert B, Keller E. Risk of thromboembolic events with endovascular cooling catheters in patients with subarachnoid hemorrhage. *Neurocrit Care* 2014;21:207–210.

21. Naidech AM, Bendok BR, Bernstein RA, et al. Fever burden and functional recovery after subarachnoid hemorrhage. *Neurosurgery* 2008;63:212–217.

22. O'Grady NP, Barie PS, Bartlett JG, et al. Guidelines for evaluation of new fever in critically ill adult patients: 2008 update from the American College of Critical Care Medicine and the Infectious Diseases Society of America. *Crit Care Med* 2008;36:1330–1349.

23. Oh SH, Oh JS, Kim YM, et al. An observational study of surface versus endovascular cooling techniques in cardiac arrest patients: a propensity-matched analysis. *Crit Care* 2015;19:85.

24. Oliveira-Filho J, Ezzeddine MA, Segal AZ, et al. Fever in subarachnoid hemorrhage: relationship to vasospasm and outcome. *Neurology* 2001;56:1299–1304.

25. Olson DM, Grissom JL, Williamson RA, et al. Interrater reliability of the bedside shivering assessment scale. *Am J Crit Care* 2013;22:70–74.

26. Phipps MS, Desai RA, Wira C, Bravata DM. Epidemiology and outcomes of fever burden among patients with acute ischemic stroke. *Stroke* 2011;42:3357–3362.

27. Provencio JJ, Badjatia N. Monitoring inflammation (including fever) in acute brain injury. *Neurocrit Care* 2014;21 Suppl 2:S177–178.

28. Reccius A, Mercado P, Vargas P, Canals C, Montes J. Inferior vena cava thrombosis related to hypothermia catheter: report of 20 consecutive cases. *Neurocrit Care.* 2015;23:72–77.

29. Scaravilli V, Tinchero G, Citerio G. Fever management in SAH. *Neurocrit Care* 2011;15:287–294.

30. Schortgen F, Clabault K, Katsahian S, et al. Fever control using external cooling in septic shock: a randomized controlled trial. *Am J Respir Crit Care Med* 2012;185:1088–1095.

31. Schwab S, Kollmar R. Rise of the machines: controlling the body temperature of critically ill patients by endovascular catheters. *Neurocrit Care* 2004;1:127–130.

32. Schwab S, Schwarz S, Spranger M, et al. Moderate hypothermia in the treatment of patients with severe middle cerebral artery infarction. *Stroke* 1998;29:2461–2466.

33. Schwab S, Spranger M, Aschoff A, Steiner T, Hacke W. Brain temperature monitoring and modulation in patients with severe MCA infarction. *Neurology* 1997;48:762–767.

34. Schwarz S, Hafner K, Aschoff A, Schwab S. Incidence and prognostic significance of fever following intracerebral hemorrhage. *Neurology* 2000;54:354–361.

35. Seder DB, Van der Kloot TE. Methods of cooling: practical aspects of therapeutic temperature management. *Crit Care Med* 2009;37:S211–222.

36. Stocchetti N, Rossi S, Zanier ER, et al. Pyrexia in head-injured patients admitted to intensive care. *Intensive Care Med* 2002;28:1555–1562.

37. Wittesjo B, Bjornham A, Eitrem R. Relative bradycardia in infectious diseases. *J Infect* 1999;39:246–247.

22

Increased Intracranial Pressure

The bony skull does not allow for expansion, and too much water in brain tissue, a sizable blood clot, or obstructed CSF flow may eventually not be compensated for. Intracranial pressure (ICP) accordingly rises quickly, resulting in brainstem displacement from brain tissue compression and eventually ischemia to the brainstem. A point may be reached beyond which the patient cannot recover from brainstem damage caused by displacement from encroaching tissue.

The availability of reliable ICP monitoring devices has facilitated management and often dictates therapies that may become potentially harmful if used indiscriminately and not directed by measurements (Chapter 23). For example, uncontrolled use of hyperventilation and osmotic diuretics without laboratory or ICP monitoring may potentially compromise cerebral blood flow and possibly produce cerebral ischemia.

The complex interactions among cerebrospinal fluid (CSF) flow and pressure regulation, blood volume, and other hydrodynamic relationships are discussed in this chapter. The pathophysiologic principles of increased ICP in patients with acute brain injury are known, but some of the feedbacks and couplings remain unexplored. The main objective of this chapter is to introduce the physiologic consequences of increased ICP and the essentials of management.

THE INTRACRANIAL COMPARTMENTS: BASIC PRINCIPLES

The relationships of cerebral blood flow, cerebral blood volume, cerebral perfusion pressure (CPP), increased ICP, and mean arterial pressure (MAP) to one another are complex and vexing. A useful starting point is the Monro-Kellie doctrine, which states that although intracranial volume relationships may vary, the total volume is constant. The intracranial volume is determined by the sum of the volumes of brain tissue, CSF, and blood. The volume of the brain parenchyma is 1,900 mL in adults, filling approximately 80% of the space. Blood and CSF

each contribute 10% of the total volume within the skull. This volume is constant because, in adults, the skull is rigid and tissues are incompressible, with little elasticity. The ICP at equilibrium is less than 10 mm Hg, and usually no pressure differences exist between regions of the brain.

The introduction of an additional volume in brain parenchyma (e.g., a mass from an intracranial hematoma or swollen, infarcted brain tissue) must, by necessity, be compensated for by changes in the blood or CSF compartment for intracranial volume to remain constant. It is clear that the brain may not be able to swell much more than 10% before compliance becomes compromised (Figure 22.1). The same reasoning applies to change in the CSF compartment (e.g., due to an increase in the CSF from hydrocephalus)[59] or blood compartment, which is largely the venous system (e.g., cerebral venous sinus thrombosis) (Table 22.1). Again, these changes increase the total volume and therefore must be counterbalanced by a reduction in volume in the other compartments. Total intracranial volume may increase diffusely from brain edema. Brain edema has three major causes, summarized in Capsule 22.1.

Several compensatory mechanisms keep ICP within normal limits. An important mechanism is a shift of CSF from the ventricular or subarachnoid space into the spinal compartment. However, the volume distensibility at the spinal compartment is small and may not provide a sufficient escape route for changes in intracranial volume.[68] Cerebral blood volume is accommodated mostly in the triangular-shaped dural sinuses and venules, with one-third of the total volume in arterioles. Cerebral blood volume is regulated by changes in the inflow tract (mechanisms that determine cerebral blood flow) and changes in the outflow tract (determined by jugular venous pressure and, eventually, intrathoracic venous pressure). Cerebral blood volume is effectively determined by the caliber of the intracranial vessels, cerebral blood flow, and venous outflow resistance. Thus, the second compensatory mechanism, most likely

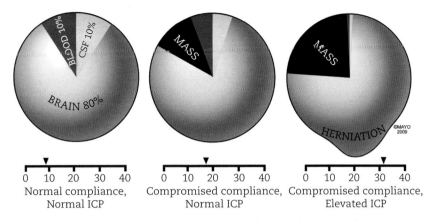

FIGURE 22.1: Illustration of compartments and compensation of increased intracranial pressure.

CSF, cerebrospinal fluid; ICP, intracranial pressure.

equally important, is reduction of the intracranial blood volume by collapsing of veins and dural sinuses and by changes in the diameter of cerebral vessels. The diameter in arterioles significantly determines the cerebral blood volume, and changes can be brought on rapidly. These changes in vessel caliber (particularly arterioles) can result in a wide range of total intravascular blood volume (15–70 mL), and with introduction of a new volume mass, this mechanism may entirely compensate for the increase in volume. The most important regulator of vessel diameter is carbon dioxide tension in arterial blood.

On the whole, the major mechanisms that compensate for an increase in ICP are movement of CSF into the spinal subarachnoid space and removal of blood from the cerebral venous vessels. Cerebrospinal fluid volume may also decrease from increased CSF absorption, largely caused by the low outflow resistance of the arachnoid villi.

TABLE 22.1. CAUSES OF INCREASED INTRACRANIAL PRESSURE

Intracranial mass
Cerebral edema
Cytotoxic (intracellular)
Vasogenic (extracellular)
Increased cerebrospinal fluid volume
Decreased absorption
Obstructed outflow
Increased production
Increased intracranial blood volume
Cerebral vasodilatation (hypoxia, hypercapnia)
Obstructed venous outflow

If the limits of these compensatory mechanisms are exceeded, the ICP begins to rise. Usually, initially a 50–100 mL increase in volume increases ICP. The pressure–volume curve of the intracranial compartment, shown in Figure 22.2, is biexponential. Displacement of CSF and blood represents the horizontal part. The intracranial compliance, defined as a measure of the distensibility of the intracranial cavity, $\Delta V/\Delta P$, decreases rapidly, however. This results in a substantial increase in pressure with any subtle increase in volume. In the steep part of the curve, the compliance is poor, but differences may exist. The curve may be shifted more to the right in patients with more reserve to compensate for increases in volume (mostly due to cerebral atrophy).

In an intact pressure regulation system, cerebral blood flow is constant, with a CPP between 50 and 150 mm Hg or MAP between 60 and 160 mm Hg.[22] The main operators of cerebral autoregulation are pressure and resistance; blood flow itself is guided by the changes in pressure. A marked decrease in CPP results in a similar decrease in cerebral blood flow, but in an autoregulating system, vasodilatation decreases resistance, maintaining cerebral blood flow despite lower pressures. Conversely, a marked rise in CPP results in increased cerebral blood flow, which is corrected by decreasing arteriolar diameter.

Autoregulation is often impaired in patients with acute brain injury, but impairment is highly variable in different regions of the brain. Diffuse head injury, aneurysmal subarachnoid hemorrhage, and any type of global bihemispheric brain damage may virtually abolish autoregulation. In other clinical situations, focal edema surrounding

CAPSULE 22.1   BRAIN EDEMA: PHYSIOLOGY AND PATHOLOGY

In vasogenic edema, the breakdown of the blood–brain barrier results in fluid accumulation into the white matter. Myelin sheets are swollen and filled with vacuoles, which may further result in myelin breakdown. The astrocytes are swollen at a later stage. The breakdown of the blood–brain barrier is most illustrative in vasogenic edema. Whatever disorder triggers the insult, the result is transudation of plasma into the extracellular white matter space. With this flooding of the white matter, however, cerebral blood flow remains unaffected, and cellular mechanisms remain intact.

In cytotoxic or cellular edema, a preferential astrocyte swelling is observed, often maximal in the astrocyte foot processes. Because cytotoxic edema represents intracellular swelling, gray matter is more involved than white matter (see accompanying illustration).

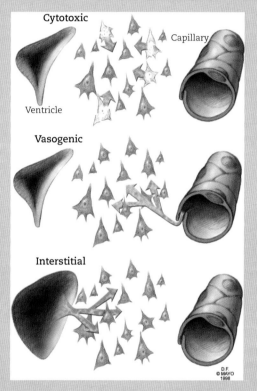

	Vasogenic	Cytotoxic	Interstitial
Pathophysiologic mechanism	Proteinaceous plasma filtrate in extracellular space	Cellular swelling from influx of water and sodium	Cerebrospinal fluid from increased ventricular pressure
Location	Preferentially white matter (often sparing gray matter)	Preferentially gray matter (often adjacent white matter)	Preferentially periventricular white matter
Disorders	Primary or metastatic brain tumor Inflammation Traumatic Brain Injury	Cerebrovascular disorders Global anoxic-ischemic injury Fulminant hepatic failure Water intoxication, dysequilibrium syndrome	Obstructive hydrocephalus
Capillary permeability	Increased	Normal	Normal

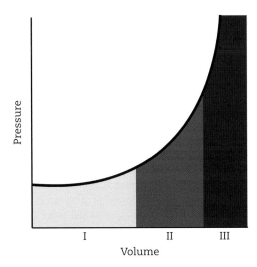

FIGURE 22.2: Intracranial pressure-volume curve. Zone I, compensatory mechanisms are optimal. Zone II, compensatory mechanisms fail. There is a slow rise (partial compensation). Zone III, virtually irreversible increased intracranial pressure and herniations occur. There is a rapid rise (complete decompensation).

masses or increased ICP alone may impair the normal regulation between cerebral blood flow and CPP. Marginal blood flow may cause ischemia, but this can be compensated for by increased oxygen extraction of the blood. Further reduction in cerebral blood flow leads to ischemia and infarction.

Basically, autoregulation is mediated through changes in cerebrovascular resistance (cerebral blood flow is CPP divided by cerebrovascular resistance). Disruption of autoregulation results in a linear relation between cerebral blood flow and CPP. Hypercapnia and hypoxemia both cause cerebral vasodilatation, and may lower the upper limit of autoregulation. The cerebral vessels, however, are less responsive to changes in Po_2 than to those in Pco_2. Little change can be expected in cerebral blood flow until a marked decrease in arterial Po_2 occurs, usually to less than 50 mm Hg, a level found almost exclusively in patients with neurogenic pulmonary edema or massive pulmonary emboli. At that breakpoint, cerebral blood flow increases, almost doubling at a Po_2 of 30 mm Hg. Hyperoxemia does not produce marked changes in cerebral blood flow.

The reactivity with Pco_2 is as follows: In patients with Pco_2 levels above 80 mm Hg, maximal vasodilatation occurs up to 100% of the baseline value, and no significant increase in cerebral blood flow can be expected beyond this point. At the other end of this spectrum, lowering of the

Pco_2 below 20 mm Hg does not cause any further decrease in cerebral blood flow, but flow may actually increase when tissue ischemia causes vasodilatation. Cerebral blood flow generally changes by 2%–3% for each change in Pco_2 within the range of 20–80 mm Hg. An example of the changes associated with Po_2 and Pco_2 is depicted in Figure 22.3.

Many drugs may profoundly alter cerebral blood flow and ICP. Barbiturates, for example, are potent vasoconstrictors, in addition to their characteristic of protecting against ischemic insults, but the reduction in ICP may only be partly explained by vasoconstrictive effects. More likely, the reduction in blood flow is due to reduced neuronal metabolism from coupling. Many inhalation anesthetics and antihypertensive drugs cause a change in autoregulation by dilatation of cerebral vessels (Table 22.2). Muscle relaxants do not affect cerebral circulation nor does ketamine which is often used for induction.[95]

Cerebral blood flow increases in patients who have fever or seizures, and this increase in susceptible patients may trigger marked sustained surges in ICP.

Cerebral blood flow autoregulation in patients with acute intracranial hypertension changes significantly; in particular, the lower limit of autoregulation shifts toward lower CPP levels.[27] This shift is seen only in patients with a marked

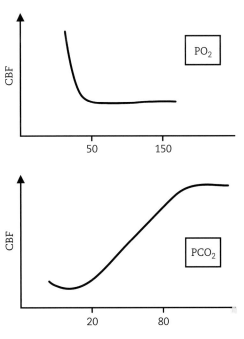

FIGURE 22.3: Effect of changes in arterial Po_2 and arterial Pco_2 in cerebral blood flow (CBF).

TABLE 22.2. DRUG EFFECTS
ON INTRACRANIAL PRESSURE

Anesthetics and sedatives

Halothane	++
Enflurane	++
Isoflurane	++
Desflurane	++
Dexmedetomidine	±
Propofol	±
Midazolam	±

Narcotics

Morphine	0
Alfentanil	±

Vasodilators and calcium-channel blockers

Sodium nitroprusside	+
Hydralazine	+
Nitroglycerin	+
Nifedipine	+
Nicardipine	+
Nimodipine	0

++ = significant and clinically relevant; + = potentially significant; + = not clinically relevant; 0 = no change.

From Artru AA. Intracranial volume/pressure relationship during desflurane anesthesia in dogs: comparison with isoflurane and thiopental/halothane. *Anesth Analg* 1994;79:751–760; Hadley MN, Spetzler RF, Fifield MS, et al. The effect of nimodipine on intracranial pressure: volume-pressure studies in a primate model. *J Neurosurg* 1987;67:387–393; Michenfelder JD, Milde JH. The interaction of sodium nitroprusside, hypotension, and isoflurane in determining cerebral vasculature effects. *Anesthesiology* 1988;69:870–875; Papazian L, Albanese J, Thirion X, et al. Effect of bolus doses of midazolam on intracranial pressure and cerebral perfusion pressure in neurosurgical patients with severe head injury. *Br J Anaesth* 1993;71:267–271; Scheller MS, Todd MM, Drummond JC, et al. The intracranial pressure effects of isoflurane and halothane administered following cryogenic brain injury in rabbits. *Anesthesiology* 1987;67:507–512; Tateishi A, Sano T, Takeshita H, et al. Effects of nifedipine on intracranial pressure in neurosurgical patients with arterial hypertension. *J Neurosurg* 1988;69:213–215; Watts AD, Eliasziw M, Gelb AW. Propofol and hyperventilation for the treatment of increased intracranial pressure in rabbits. *Anesth Analg* 1998;87:564–568; Zornow MH, Scheller MS, Sheehan PB, et al. Intracranial pressure effects of dexmedetomidine in rabbits. *Anesth Analg* 1992;75:232–237. With permission of the publishers.

increase in ICP. The autoregulation curve with moderately increased ICP (approximately 30 mm Hg) remains unchanged. The possible cause of the downward shift of the lower limit of the autoregulation is dilatation of small resistant vessels.

Longstanding hypertension produces a profound change in cerebral autoregulation, resulting in a rightward shift of the entire curve (approximately 20–30 mm Hg) (Figure 22.4). (This compensation is clinically relevant to counter large increases in blood pressure that would otherwise lead to hypertensive encephalopathy from compromise of the blood–brain barrier.) Again, this shift in the lower limit of autoregulation is important when antihypertensive drug therapy is instituted. Carbon dioxide reactivity in patients with chronic hypertension, however, remains intact.

The ICP waveform is shown in Figure 22.5. Typical features of this waveform, which is of vascular origin, are the first peak (percussion wave), most likely originating from the pulsation of the choroid plexus, and a tidal wave (a dicrotic wave) transmitted from pulsations of the major cerebral arteries. The first peak is most prominently displayed, but in conditions of decreased brain compliance, the second wave increases in amplitude. This increase may be due to an increase in transmission of pressure caused by compensatory arterial dilatation. With increasing ICP values, the amplitude of the second and third waves increases without concomitant increases in the first wave, so that the waveform assumes a more rounded configuration. (The three components of the ICP waveform, however, remain distinctively present.)

Next to interpretation of the ICP waveform is interpretation of the trend of the ICP over time. The trend data for ICP values are obtained over hours and may display marked increases in ICP. The most important pressure changes are the so-called plateau waves (Lundberg A waves). Sudden increases in ICP of 50–80 mm Hg that may last for 5–20 minutes and often decrease rapidly create the plateau (Figure 22.6). The origin of the plateau is most likely defined by elevation of the ICP at the beginning of the plateau because of dilatation of the cerebral vessels, and reduction of the ICP because of constriction of the cerebral vessels.[15,65] Marked sluggishness of CSF flow and abnormal CSF absorption may contribute as well to the development of greatly increased ICP during plateau waves.[28,29] Plateau waves must be regarded as strong indicators of failing brain compliance, and they reflect cerebral ischemia.[28,29] Any type of manipulation of the patient may readily trigger these plateau waves. Prevention of these particularly dangerous surges in ICP is an essential part of management. Tracheal suctioning, repositioning and daily hygiene of the patient, replacement and flushing of indwelling bladder catheters, and changing of central venous catheters over a guidewire in a flat position are well-known triggers. The mechanism of triggering these plateau waves is not always clear from careful scrutiny of the daily chart, but in many patients the manipulations mentioned here cause surges in systolic blood pressure that can be implicated as the main instigators. Preemptive treatment with intravenously

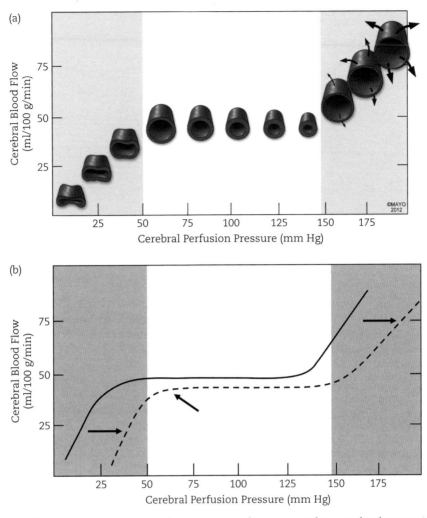

FIGURE 22.4: The autoregulation curve and change in autoregulation curve in long-standing hypertension (right shift).

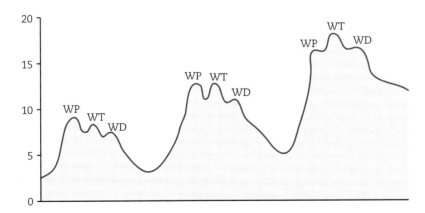

FIGURE 22.5. Components of the intracranial pressure waveform; ICP waveforms and change with increasing ICP.

WP = percussion wave representing arterial pressure and transmitted at systole; WT = tidal wave representing relative brain volume or compliance increases with expanding masses and becomes higher than WP with increasing ICP. WD = dicrotic wave representing venous pulsation and aortic closure.

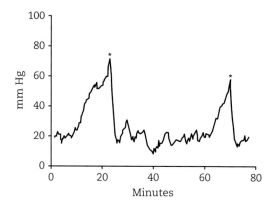

FIGURE 22.6: Example of plateau waves (asterisks).

From Chesnut RM, Marshall LF. Treatment of abnormal intracranial pressure. *Neurosurg Clin N Am* 1991;2:267–284. With permission of WB Saunders Company.

administered lidocaine or pentobarbital may considerably mute these responses.[4]

These waves should not be confused with so-called Lundberg B waves, pressure increases that are seldom higher than 20 mm Hg and that occur one or two times a minute. However, these pressure waves are not innocuous and may be harbingers of plateau waves.

MANAGEMENT OF INCREASED INTRACRANIAL PRESSURE

The indications for placement of monitoring devices are described in Chapter 23. Many consider placement of an ICP monitor in comatose patients with traumatic brain injury, ganglionic hemorrhage with ventricular trapping, cerebral edema from any cause except anoxic-ischemic injury, or after a recent craniotomy to remove contusions. However, when ICP monitoring is tested prospectively in traumatic brain injury, outcome was not better if all patients were treated with a guideline-based management protocol[12] It has been argued that additional use of microdialysis or brain tissue oxygen monitoring may provide compelling information other than a simple pressure but usage varies considerably around the world and within countries.[89] (Chapter 23 for more details.)

In the management of increased ICP, CPP (CPP = MAP − ICP) must be considered another important guide for further titration of treatment.

Reduction of increased ICP is governed by attempts to reduce the total intracranial volume. This involves (a) CSF withdrawal by ventricular drain, (b) reduction of the cerebral tissue volume (e.g., osmotic dehydration), (c) reduction of the cerebral blood volume by reduction of cerebral blood flow or by enhancement of cerebral venous drainage, and (d) removal or decompression of a mass. If left untreated, the consequences are substantial (Capsule 22.2).

The management of increased ICP involves general measures and more specific treatment modalities. General measures should receive great emphasis before more traditional therapies, such as osmotic diuresis, are started.

Strong arguments have been put forward to place greater emphasis on the management of CPP than on the management of ICP. This controversial management pertains only to patients with severe traumatic brain injury. Two opposing protocols (Lund and Rosner) exist. The crux of CPP management techniques, devised by Rosner, is the preservation of cerebral blood flow to prevent cerebral ischemia.[69,72] Cerebral perfusion is set at a minimum of 70 mm Hg, and to finally arrive at that value, one may need to place a ventricular catheter to drain CSF and use a combination of vasopressors, volume expansion, and nursing of the patient in a flat position. This method posits that decreased cerebral perfusion due to increased ICP or decreased blood pressure will lead to increased vasodilatation, increased cerebral blood volume, and a further increase in ICP. Increased ICP reduces CPP, creating a cycle further reducing CPP. Increasing blood pressure breaks the cycle.[69] However, with a high CPP, an abnormal blood–brain barrier may facilitate cerebral edema by driving additional fluids into brain tissue.

The post hoc analysis of the International Selfotel Trial in traumatic brain injury clearly discounted this management protocol. Subsets of patients were compared, and patients with an ICP greater than 20 had a much worse outcome

CAPSULE 22.2   BRAIN COMPARTMENTS AND CONSEQUENCES

The falx and tentorium divide the brain into several compartments (see accompanying illustration) but leave openings through which tissue can wedge. The end result of increased ICP is brain tissue shift with displacement under the falx cerebri, central brainstem compression, lateral displacement of the brainstem with later herniation of brain tissue over the lateral edge of the tentorium, and, in a number of cases, herniation through a craniotomy defect.

Displacement may occur under the falx, tentorium, and foramen magnum. When ICP increases, brain tissue drifts toward a compartment of lower pressure. Unilateral supratentorial lesions force the thalamus and upper brainstem to the opposite side, opening up the ipsilateral cisterna ambiens, a buffer zone between the midbrain and tentorial free edge. The crowding of the tentorial opening involves herniation of uncus of the temporal lobe, either passively or forcefully wedged into the opening. It causes compression and elongation of the ipsilateral cerebral peduncle and hemorrhages.[90]

When both hemispheres swell or a mass is located medially, the cerebral convolutions become flattened and drive brain tissue through the hiatus of the cerebellar tentorium and the brainstem may move down.

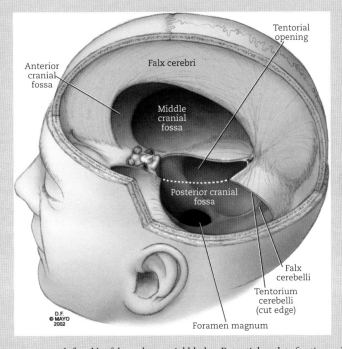

Intracranial compartments defined by falx and tentorial blades. Potential outlets for tissue shift are shown.

than patients with lower ICP recordings, irrespective of CPP. The same investigators reported prolonged brain swelling in patients with artificially increased CPPs greater than 90 mm Hg.[34]

The crux of ICP management, devised by Lund, is to facilitate interstitial fluid reabsorption by preservation of normal osmotic pressure, to reduce intracapillary hydrostatic pressures, and to reduce cerebral blood volume.[19,56] This novel but unusual approach turns to those forces that move fluids out of the capillaries. First, colloid osmotic pressure is maintained by transfusion of albumin, thus maintaining a normovolemic state. Second, hydrostatic pressure is reduced by the reduction of MAP with intravenous metoprolol and clonidine. Third, cerebral blood volume is further reduced by vasoconstriction of the precapillary resistance vessels (using a low dose of thiopental sodium) and veins (using dihydroergotamine, up to 0.9 µg/kg/hr). In both protocols, ICP is not managed traditionally with hyperventilation, CSF drainage, or osmotherapy. Neither the Lund nor the Rosner protocol has shown better outcome than traditional ICP management (aiming at ICP < 20 mm Hg, CPP 60–70 mm Hg).

General Measures of ICP Management

Every patient should be adequately oxygenated, and normal mean arterial pressure should be maintained. Mechanical ventilation may be indicated in patients with marginal gas exchange and inability to protect the airway. Fortunately, the mode of mechanical ventilation does not significantly influence ICP. High levels of positive end-expiratory pressure (PEEP; 15–20 cm H$_2$O) may not markedly influence cerebral venous return. Reduction of pulmonary compliance in patients with acute respiratory distress syndrome (ARDS)—the typical situation in which PEEP is indicated—does not appear to influence ICP. Nonetheless, PEEP may interfere with systemic arterial pressure by causing arteriolar vasodilatation.

Fever, after being investigated thoroughly, should be treated aggressively with cooling blankets or cooling devices. In patients with paroxysmal sympathetic hyperactivity (sudden episodes of tachycardia, tachypnea, increase in temperature up to 41°C, and marked shivering), a combination of morphine, gabapentin (preferred) and clonidine may be indicated.

Head position should be neutral to reduce any possible compression of the jugular veins that could lead to a decrease in intracranial venous outflow.[67,71] Whether the head should be elevated remains somewhat controversial, but many intensive care neurologists consider head elevation of 30 degrees standard. This position is further supported by a careful study in 22 patients with head injury, most of whom had marked reduction in ICP.[21] Elevation of the head, however, may cause a reduction in arterial pressure, particularly if the patient has orthostatic hypotension from diabetes mellitus or has marked hypovolemia or orthostasis from psychotropic drugs used to counter agitation (e.g., phenothiazines). The Trendelenburg position should be avoided, except in overt life-threatening shock. Intracranial pressure should be monitored closely in patients in the supine position at the time of procedures such as placement of a catheter in the jugular or subclavian vein or fiberoptic bronchoscopy.[37]

Any patient with increased ICP should be made calm. Pain, bladder distention, and agitation should be minimized by codeine, placement of a Foley catheter and maintenance of unobstructed urine flow, and small doses of propofol. Episodes of agitation may be caused by "fighting the ventilator," and the mode of ventilation may need to be adjusted. Bronchial suctioning should be performed regularly, but the number of passages through the endotracheal tube should be limited to one, if any. Control of ICP surges during cough and suctioning is important and often overlooked. When a marked increase in ICP is observed during bronchial suctioning, aerosolized lidocaine (1–2 mg/kg) can be blended through the endotracheal tube to mute this response.[46] Endotracheal spraying with lidocaine may not sufficiently mute the response.[6]

One should identify possible, seemingly trivial, triggers in the ICU that may increase ICP. Pain and frequent stimulation by such maneuvers as washing and change of position are factors that may contribute to agitation and increased ICP.

In patients with increased ICP, a euvolemic state is preferred. Fluid restriction is not a recognized treatment of increased ICP. Moreover, dehydration associated with fluid restriction causes hypotension and hemoconcentration with increased viscosity and may for that reason have a deleterious effect.

Seizures are associated with hypoxemia and hypercapnia and may greatly increase ICP through cerebral vasodilatation. Seizures may result in respiratory acidosis, aspiration, and prolonged hypoxemia. Prophylaxis with antiepileptic drugs in patients treated for increased ICP is debatable, but intravenous loading with fosphenytoin or intravenous levetiracetam should be strongly considered in patients assumed to have a marginally compliant brain parenchyma and in patients at comparably high risk for seizures. Finally, vasodilators such as nitroprusside, which may increase ICP to unacceptable levels, should be avoided.[26]

Cerebrospinal Fluid Drainage

Ventricular drainage remains a very rational solution to increased ICP and is perhaps the best option. Its use is predominantly focused on patients with acute obstructive hydrocephalus after aneurysmal subarachnoid hemorrhage or acute expanding cerebellar masses. In traumatic brain injury, however, its use is very controversial, but some trauma centers almost routinely insert ventricular catheters.[69] In patients with head injury, drainage can be significantly compromised by a large volume of intraventricular blood and compression of the frontal horns to slitlike proportions from surrounding edema.

Cerebrospinal fluid drainage may also potentially facilitate bulk flow from edematous brain tissue, moving fluid from an area of high pressure to one of low pressure. Whether drainage of CSF improves CPP or has any effect on ICP reduction remains very uncertain, because most of the increase in ICP is from cerebrovascular compartments. In a study of patients with traumatic brain injury, CSF drainage produced a transient decrease in ICP but no change in cerebral blood flow velocities on regional cerebral oximetry.[36] The use of ventricular catheters is discussed in more detail in Chapter 23.

Hyperventilation

Use of hyperventilation after any injury to the central nervous system, and particularly after traumatic brain injury, has been criticized for its potential long-term adverse effects.[58] Nonetheless, acute hyperventilation remains a very effective way of reducing ICP. Acute hyperventilation causes a reduction in ICP by cerebral vasoconstriction, which in turn reduces cerebral blood flow. Vasoconstriction is mediated by a change in the pH of CSF, and a narrow response to hyperventilation exists. Cerebral blood flow decreases 40% approximately 30 minutes after reduction of the $PaCO_2$ by approximately 20 mm Hg. After several hours, an increase in cerebral blood flow to approximately 90% of the baseline value is seen, with a potential overshoot of cerebral blood flow. The effects of hyperventilation on cerebral blood flow and ICP are therefore not significant after several hours. Bicarbonate is predominantly responsible for the rapid buffering of alkalotic CSF.[68]

The true effect of acute hyperventilation in the setting of severe traumatic brain injuries had not been studied carefully.[80,81] A major question is whether hyperventilation is potentially harmful. In one classic study, patients with severe traumatic brain injury were randomized to treatment with prophylactic hyperventilation for 5 days after the injury with an average $PaCO_2$ of 25 mm Hg or to management without hyperventilation with $PaCO_2$ goals of 35 mm Hg.[49] At 3 and 6 months, comatose patients in the hyperventilation group had significantly worse outcomes. A recent study that monitored brain tissue oxygen found that even a small reduction in $PaCO_2$ caused a decrease in cerebral oxygenation in comatose patients with traumatic brain injury and also minimal cerebral vessel reactivity to $PaCO_2$ in the early days after

the insult.[8,11] It appears that aggressive hyperventilation can cause cerebral blood flow to closely approach an ischemic threshold, and this may explain a potentially more harmful outcome.

Other studies on the effect of hyperventilation[17,33] found contradictory results. Both studies were limited by the small number of patients, but the resulting data were novel. One study found that when a brief period of hyperventilation was introduced, cerebral blood flow, as expected, was reduced substantially.[17] However, in most of these tested patients, cerebral metabolism was not impaired because of increased oxygen extraction. With the use of positron emission tomography (PET) technology for the first time in this particular setting, a $PaCO_2$ of 30 mm Hg did not change global or regional cerebral metabolism. Similar results were obtained in a small subset of patients with more aggressive hyperventilation ($PaCO_2$ < 25 mm Hg). These investigators found that even when cerebral blood flow decreased to only 10 mL per 100 g per minute, cerebral metabolism was still preserved.[17] In contrast, another group of investigators studied in a more indirect way the consequences of hyperventilation using a measurement of cerebral tissue PO_2 and jugular venous oxygen saturation.[33] Both brain tissue PO_2 and the jugular vein oxygenation were reduced with hyperventilation. Whether brain tissue PO_2 and metabolic rate are directly correlated remains uncertain. Other studies have found that moderate hyperventilation may significantly increase the accumulation of lactate and extracellular fluid.[8]

This data indicates that the consequence of hyperventilation may be deleterious to the already injured brain, but it is difficult to define a safe threshold. It has been demonstrated that hyperoxia during acute hyperventilation may further improve oxygen delivery to the brain, and this may be the best compromise.[80] If necessary, hyperventilation to a $PaCO_2$ of 30 mm Hg, with preoxygenation or increasing the oxygen delivery, may protect the brain in certain areas, but a risk of ischemia remains.

Hyperventilation can also be potentially harmful in patients with emphysema and marked obesity associated with carbon dioxide retention. Sudden reduction in $PaCO_2$ may cause very significant hypotension. Other adverse effects of hypocapnia are decreased myocardial oxygen supply and increased myocardial oxygen demand. Hypocapnia may promote the development of cardiac arrhythmia.[40]

Most of the available recommendations are based on work in severe traumatic brain injury, and best practices in other conditions are not exactly known. There is a growing consensus that osmotic agents mostly should be used first and that hyperventilation should be used only if brief, rapid reduction of ICP is necessary.

When hyperventilation is instituted, the change in ventilation should be derived largely from a change in respiratory rate. The respiratory rate can be increased to approximately 20 breaths per minute while a normal tidal volume of 12 mL/ kg is maintained. Increasing minute ventilation by changing both components may potentially lead to high airway pressures, barotrauma, and, at the extreme, pneumothorax. End-tidal carbon dioxide can be used to approximate $PaCO_2$, but arterial blood gas is more reliable, and $PaCO_2$ may remain relatively stable after a certain mode of ventilation is set.

Weaning the patient from hyperventilation should be gradual; minute ventilation is reduced by two breaths per minute during careful monitoring of ICP. An increase in or, less likely, a rebound of ICP occurs in some patients with normalization of $PaCO_2$, but in many instances is simply not distinguishable from increase due to progressive clinical neurologic deterioration. Cerebral vessels adapt in patients with prolonged hyperventilation.[50] Experimental animal studies have found that eventually normalization of the vessel diameter occurs. Restoration of $PaCO_2$ to normocapnia, therefore, can be "read" as relative hypercapnia and may induce vasodilatation with a subsequent increase in both cerebral blood volume and ICP. This increase in ICP can be associated with marked clinical deterioration.

Jugular venous oxygen saturation can be monitored (Chapter 23) to titrate the depth of hyperventilation (cerebral ischemia from vigorous hyperventilation is reflected in increased oxygen extraction and increased arteriovenous oxygen saturation difference).

Osmotic Diuresis

The basic principle of osmotherapy is the decrease of brain water. For osmotic agents to work, an osmotic gradient and intact blood–brain barrier are needed. Consequently, osmotic agents shrink mostly brain tissue that has not been damaged. Brain water filters from a compartment with low osmolality to a compartment with high osmolality. The available diuretic agents for the treatment of increased ICP are mannitol, hypertonic saline, albumin, glycerol and urea, and furosemide.[63,85,91,94] In most institutions, either mannitol or hypertonic saline is used to decrease ICP. The

mechanism of mannitol has traditionally been attributed to the movement of brain water into the vascular space. This osmotic gradient remains the overriding principle, but other mechanisms of action are increased cerebral blood flow from transient hypervolemia and hemodilution resulting in a decrease in blood viscosity.[9,48,51] Cerebral blood volume, however, remains much the same from a compensatory reflex vasoconstriction of the cerebral arterioles. Mannitol also probably increases CSF absorption.[63] Cerebrospinal fluid production is reduced by a high dose (2 g/kg) and continuous infusion.[18] Trials are lacking that compare different doses of mannitol or modes of administration such as bolus versus continuous infusion.[75] Nonetheless, the effect of mannitol in pathologic areas with a breached blood–brain barrier is not known and is not necessarily absent. Mannitol may enter damaged brain tissue and decrease the osmotic gradient; it may, in fact, reverse the osmotic gradient, causing worsening of swelling. An animal study found that a single dose of mannitol was very effective, but administration of multiple doses reversed the blood–brain barrier gradient and increased cerebral edema by 3%.[35]

However, the potential of mannitol for an increasing shift from reducing counterpressure from the unaffected compartment has not been demonstrated.[24,84] A study with serial magnetic resonance imaging (MRI) in patients with hemispheric stroke did not document increased brain shift.[44] A follow-up study, however, found that noninfarcted brain tissue shrank more, and the difference was sufficient to determine a measurable shift on MRI.[84] No clinical deterioration was noted after the use of mannitol.

Mannitol may exert its effect through free radical scavenging capabilities rather than through reduction of edema. An experimental study in rats found that mannitol administered at 6-hour intervals of ischemia reduced the number of histologically apparent ischemic neurons.[41]

Mannitol is typically used in its 20% solution. Elimination follows first-order kinetics (estimated half-life between 30 and 60 minutes), no metabolism occurs, and the agent is excreted entirely through the kidneys. Proportionally more water is lost than sodium, and profound diuresis may result in hypovolemia and hypernatremia. Mannitol should be administered in an initial dose of 1 g/kg over 30–60 min infusion, which can be tapered to various amounts for maintenance (0.25–0.50 g/kg). Rarely, higher doses (up to 2 g/kg) are needed to reduce ICP. The reduction in ICP with mannitol administration should be apparent after 15 minutes, and failure of ICP to respond to mannitol should be considered a poor prognostic sign. The maximum effect approximates 60 minutes. The goal for serum osmolarity should be 310–320 mOsm/L.[68,70] An increase in serum osmolarity of more than 340 mOsm/L ultimately could lead to renal failure from dehydration and renal vasoconstriction. The total dose of mannitol in grams (200 g) may be more important.[66] Dosing of mannitol may be inaccurate and was found erroneous in nearly one in four patients in a study in Canada particularly when patients were transported to other facilities.[20]

Osmolality can be calculated, and a difference of less than 10 mOsm/kg between measured and calculated osmolality (osmolality = 2 Na + glucose/18 + blood urea nitrogen/2.8) can be used to guide the need for an additional bolus of mannitol. An additional dose of mannitol is warranted if osmolar gap is less than 10 or Na less than 160, or serum osmol less than 340. The adverse reactions of mannitol, including congestive heart failure and profound pulmonary edema, are a result of rapid intravascular expansion. Hypotension is due to the rate of infusion and can be avoided. The movement of intracellular water to the extracellular space may cause hyponatremia, but typically this occurs only if mannitol is administered to patients with renal failure. Hyperkalemia may become significant only after infusion of high doses; the underlying physiologic mechanism is unknown.[43]

Rebound after mannitol use has been considered a possible concern. Rebound after mannitol is tentatively explained by the influx of mannitol into brain tissue, reversing osmosis. A "rebound" to higher ICP values after discontinuation of mannitol was found in 12% of 65 patients but could not be explained by higher doses or rapid infusion rates. In addition, factors such as changed fluid management and worsening brain contusion have confounded the results.[57] No rebound effect was found in a study of ischemic infarction in a rat model.[57] Moreover, the ICP-reducing activity of mannitol diminishes over time and becomes ineffective, and cumulatively higher doses are needed to keep the ICP within acceptable limits. The rebound effect of mannitol thus remains an imprecisely defined condition.

If there is no response to mannitol treatment with 2 g/kg, and enlargement of a potentially removable mass on computed tomography (CT) scan is excluded, another treatment should be tried. Studies of combined mannitol and furosemide have been done, but the risk of significant reduction of blood pressure from dehydration is great.[60,91] However, 40 mg of furosemide can be administered to patients with severe congestive heart failure who may not tolerate this volume load from mannitol.

Hypertonic Saline

There has been renewed interest in the use of hypertonic saline as a hyperosmolar solution. The osmolarity of 3% saline is approximately similar to that of 20% mannitol, and it is considerably higher in 7.5% saline and 23.4% saline[2,31,45,62,83,86,87,94] (Table 22.3). This characteristic may be responsible for a much stronger fluid shift directed toward the capillaries and reversal of brain swelling. Despite promising animal experiments, it remains uncertain whether hypertonic saline has more benefits than a possibly prolonged duration of action.[74] A recent small study suggested that repeated bolus infusions of 7.5% saline at a dose of 2 mL/kg of body weight and an infusion over 1–2 hours decreased ICP in patients with traumatic brain injury.[32] In none of these patients could ICP be lowered with mannitol or other common measures. In another study, 75 mL of hypertonic saline (this time 10%) reduced ICP in patients failing to respond to mannitol.[77] Thus, hypertonic saline could be reserved for use in these circumstances.

Many neurosciences intensive care unit practices use a single bolus of 30 mL of 23% saline over 10 minutes (Figure 22.7).[61,62] Alternatively, lower concentrations can be used (e.g., 75 ml of 10% saline over 10 minutes; 150 ml of 7.5% saline in 20 minutes). Hypertonic saline can thus be administered in a small volume while creating a substantial intravascular osmolar gradient. Even if equimolar doses of hypertonic saline and mannitol are compared, ICP is lowered more quickly in hypertonic solutions, and there is a more sustained effect.[23,38,39] Additional effects are achieved by increases in MAP and increased cardiac output and are explained by rapid infusion. These

TABLE 22.3. OSMOLALITY OF OSMOTIC DIURETICS COMPARED TO NORMAL SALINE

Agent	Osmolality (mOsm/kg)
0.9% saline	308
3% saline	1026
7.5% saline	2566
23.4% saline	8008
20% mannitol	1245

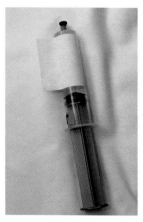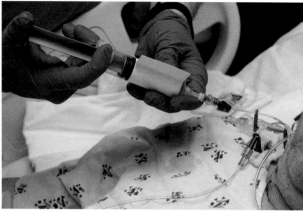

FIGURE 22.7: Left: 30 ml syringe filled with hypertonic 23.4% sodium chloride solution ("saline bullet").
Right: Administration through a central venous catheter.

important hemodynamic effects may improve cerebral blood flow and may be responsible for improving flow to a compressed brainstem rather than the extraction of brain water and diuresis that comes later.[82] A major limitation of hypertonic saline is that it can only be administered through a central venous catheter because severe phlebitis has been seen with peripheral administration. It is therefore not a first-choice agent in most patients worsening in a stroke unit or those urgently admitted to the emergency department.

Slow (10–15 minutes) infusion may reduce the initial blood pressure decrease as a result of acute plasma expansion and reduced peripheral vascular resistance. This blood pressure decrease responds quickly to vasopressors or even a fluid bolus. Other effects of hypertonic saline are acute renal failure, decreased platelet aggregation, coagulopathy, decrease in hemoglobin, fluid overload, hypernatremia, acidosis, hyperkalemia, and rebound increase in ICP, but there is little difficulty expected.[25] Hyperchloremic acidosis is common with prolonged use of hypertonic saline solutions. There is some uncertainty about its harmful effect, but it is prudent to replace sodium chloride with sodium acetate in a similar solution if repeated use is anticipated.

Hypertonic saline has been considered superior to mannitol, but evidence remains weak.[47] However, when equiosmolar doses are used, differences in the efficacy of ICP control between mannitol and hypertonic saline are not apparent.[73] A recent study in traumatic brain injury defined an ICP burden (number of days and number of hours of ICP > 25 mm Hg) and found hypertonic saline superior to mannitol.[42] Randomized trials are not available. Management in daily ICU practice may vary considerably,[30] but most experts would agree that serum sodium should be between 150 and 160 mmol/L and osmolality around 320 mOsm/L. Continuous infusion of hypertonic saline (3%–10%) will produce a steady osmolar state that may not be easily overcome when a hypertonic bolus is administered and should be avoided.[16] Hypertonic saline will markedly increase serum sodium and serum chloride, and these effects linger. Repeated use of hypertonic saline requires change to sodium acetate to prevent hyperchloremic acidosis.[53]

Tromethamine

Tromethamine (THAM) has been introduced as an agent to control increased ICP. Tromethamine is a buffer that is commonly used to correct metabolic acidosis associated with cardiac bypass surgery or cardiac arrest. The advantage of tromethamine is that it alkalizes without increasing $PaCO_2$ and plasma sodium. The dose of tromethamine is 1 mL/kg/hr. In addition to local tissue irritation and necrosis, respiratory depression and hypoglycemia have been described. Tromethamine has been compared with mannitol for ICP control, and one small, nonrandomized trial found it to be at least as effective. Larger studies in patients with traumatic brain injury found that fluctuations in ICP could be better controlled, but the outcome was similar.[92] Tromethamine should be used for patients in whom mannitol is contraindicated (e.g., renal failure). Tromethamine may also have a place in countering rebound from hyperventilation.

Barbiturates

The use of barbiturates has been proposed, particularly in severe traumatic brain injury, as a last resort for patients with refractory intracranial hypertension.[55,64,93] Unfortunately, barbiturates often have been used in patients close to meeting clinical criteria of brain death, making later organ retrieval very problematic, if not impossible. Barbiturate therapy could be useful in the reduction of ICP and may certainly decrease mortality in patients with uncontrollable ICP refractory to all other standard medical and surgical treatments. The position of the American Association of Neurosurgeons joint session on neurotrauma and critical care underscores extreme caution with its use.[10] The number of patients eventually considered for barbiturate treatment is very small, because usually standard therapies or removal of a mass reduces ICP. Moreover, treatment with barbiturates is a challenge. Myocardial depression and hypotension are a major concern. Approximately 50% of the patients treated with barbiturates need inotropic agents to control hypotension.[64,93] In many patients, combinations of dobutamine and epinephrine are needed, as well as additional fluids. There is an increased risk of nosocomial infections,[54] particularly pneumonia, from depression of mucociliary clearance in patients receiving barbiturate treatment.

If barbiturate treatment is considered the very last option, treatment is started with pentobarbital, 10 mg/kg intravenously over 60 minutes.[3] The maintenance dose is generally 1–3 mg/kg/hr by constant intravenous infusion. A higher dose (5 mg/kg/hr) can be used initially for several hours to obtain adequate loading. Suppression of the electroencephalogram is usually seen when serum barbiturate levels are approximately 30–40 mcg/mL. Serum levels should be checked regularly, and one should aim at the lowest possible dose for control of ICP. It is not necessary to proceed to a burst-suppression pattern. The dose of barbiturates that produces a burst-suppression pattern is typically associated with hypotension; therefore, a lower dose may reduce the need for vasopressors and still control ICP. Common practice is to maintain barbiturate treatment for several days. When CT scanning does not show any new findings or progression of findings and ICP is well controlled, barbiturate therapy can be withdrawn slowly by reduction of the infusion rate by 50% each day.

Hypothermia

An important adjunctive measure to reduce ICP is the induction of moderate hypothermia (core temperature, 33°C). In an elegant study, ICP was reduced (mean, 10 mm Hg) and CPP increased (mean, 14 mm Hg) in 16 patients. No increase in bacterial infection was found, but premature ventricular contractions occurred in 40% of the hypothermic patients. Moreover, one patient had hypovolemic shock, and another had a rapid increase in ICP during rewarming.[78]

Moderate hypothermia has been studied in traumatic brain injury but has not been effective in improving outcome.[13] Analysis of its effect on ICP and CPP did not show a significant difference from that of normothermia. Absence of a major effect on outcome was corroborated by a Japanese study of mild hypothermia, which also found significant systemic complications, including pneumonia, leukocytopenia, thrombocytopenia, hyponatremia, hypokalemia, and increased amylase.[79]

Its effect in stroke is not known, although early experience suggests that cerebral swelling can be abated. A carefully studied cohort showed a possible effect on ICP in patients with infarction of the middle cerebral artery distribution, but ICP increased after rewarming.[76]

Miscellaneous Options

The use of corticosteroids has been tested in large prospective trials. In patients with severe traumatic brain injury, high-dose dexamethasone (100 mg/day) and methylprednisolone (30 mg/kg) did not improve outcome.[7] The adverse effects of corticosteroids are significant and include hyperglycemia, sepsis, and an increased risk of gastrointestinal bleeding. High doses of corticosteroids may only be helpful in patients with a malignant brain tumor or metastases and could reduce swelling and intracranial pressure (dexamethasone, 4–6 mg PO or IV q.i.d.).

Many alternative anesthetic agents, including lidocaine and propofol, have been tried to control the increase in ICP.[14] As noted earlier, lidocaine can be used in a dose of 1 mg/kg, given slowly over 3 minutes, to blunt ICP response in patients with marked surges of ICP during nursing care, nasotracheal suctioning, or procedures such as fiberoptic bronchoscopy.[37] An alternative option, treatment with a lidocaine spray, is also successful in reducing ICP.[37]

The use of propofol as a sedative has been accepted as effective, but the reduction in blood pressure and associated decrease in CPP when higher doses are needed may seriously limit its use for ICP control. Propofol administration can begin with an infusion of 1–3 mg/kg/hr. A bolus of 1 mg/kg may transiently lower the ICP without the marked change in blood pressure typically

TABLE 22.4. TREATMENT OF INCREASED INTRACRANIAL PRESSURE

Method	Procedure	Monitoring
Ventricular catheter	Ventricular right frontal placement with subcutaneous tunneling	CSF pressures, changes in waveform Daily calibration Drip chamber at 5–10 cm H_2O Consider prophylactic antibiotics
Hyperventilation	Increase respiratory rate to 20 breaths/min	Pco_2, 25–30 mm Hg Daily chest radiograph
Osmotic diuresis	Mannitol 20%, 1 g/kg Hypertonic saline 23%, 30 mL	Plasma osmolarity, 310–320 mOsm/L BUN, creatinine, sodium, potassium arterial blood gas, urine output
Surgical decompression	Bifrontal craniotomies Suboccipital decompression	CT scanning ICP monitor

BUN, blood urea nitrogen; CSF, cerebrospinal fluid.

observed with propofol infusion. Rates higher than 5 mg/kg/hr may cause propofol infusion syndrome (Chapter 16).

A preliminary study suggested considerable success with a bolus of indomethacin (a cyclooxygenase inhibitor; 50 mg in 20 minutes) in patients with increased ICP refractory to therapy. Sudden discontinuation, however, led to a marked rebound effect.[5]

Surgical management of increased ICP has come into vogue, especially in patients with swelling from large middle cerebral artery infarcts. Interest in decompressive craniotomy in traumatic brain injury has been recently rekindled.[1,52,88] The procedure may reduce ICP and reopen compressed basal cisterns, and some early data suggest improved outcome and increased compensatory reserve. The results of the RESCUEicp decompressive craniectomy trial are eagerly awaited particularly after the DECRA trial was negative (Chapter 41). Suboccipital decompressive craniotomy and ventriculostomy for hydrocephalus—both highly effective therapies for mass lesions in the posterior fossa—are discussed in Part VII of this book. Salvage has also been claimed with extensive craniotomy in subarachnoid hemorrhage associated with massive cerebral edema, but the operation is hard to defend in these cases. The options of management of increased ICP are summarized in Table 22.4.

CONCLUSIONS

- Intracranial pressure must be monitored for recognition of plateau waves—sudden increases in ICP of 50–80 mm Hg lasting several minutes—which indicate failing brain compliance. Plateau waves can be muted by a change in nursing techniques and by increasing depth of sedation or intravenous administration of lidocaine or pentobarbital.

- Hypercapnia, hypoxemia, inhalation anesthetics, fever, and seizures all may increase ICP.

- The first measures to decrease ICP are head elevation to 30 degrees, treatment of agitation, and maintenance of patient comfort during mechanical ventilation.

- Traditional measures for treatment of increased ICP are CSF drainage in patients with obstructive hydrocephalus, administration of mannitol, and hyperventilation. Osmotic diuresis is the preferred first treatment. Administration of mannitol 20% is started with 1 g/kg, repeated in doses 0.5–1 g/kg, aiming at a serum osmolarity of 310 mOsm/L

- In equiosmolar doses, hypertonic saline is equally effective to mannitol.

REFERENCES

1. Aarabi B, Hesdorffer DC, Simard JM, et al. Comparative study of decompressive craniectomy after mass lesion evacuation in severe head injury. *Neurosurgery* 2009;64:927–939.
2. Battison C, Andrews PJ, Graham C, Petty T. Randomized, controlled trial on the effect of a 20% mannitol solution and a 7.5% saline/6% dextran solution on increased intracranial pressure after brain injury. *Crit Care Med* 2005;33:196–202.
3. Bayliff CD, Schwartz ML, Hardy BG. Pharmacokinetics of high-dose pentobarbital in severe

head trauma. *Clin Pharmacol Ther* 1985;38: 457–461.

4. Bedford RF, Persing JA, Pobereskin L, Butler A. Lidocaine or thiopental for rapid control of intracranial hypertension? *Anesth Analg* 1980;59: 435–437.

5. Biestro AA, Alberti RA, Soca AE, et al. Use of indomethacin in brain-injured patients with cerebral perfusion pressure impairment: preliminary report. *J Neurosurg* 1995;83:627–630.

6. Bilotta F, Branca G, Lam A, et al. Endotracheal lidocaine in preventing endotracheal suctioning-induced changes in cerebral hemodynamics in patients with severe head trauma. *Neurocrit Care* 2008;8:241–246.

7. Braakman R, Schouten HJ, Blaauw-van Dishoeck M, Minderhoud JM. Megadose steroids in severe head injury. Results of a prospective double-blind clinical trial. *J Neurosurg* 1983;58:326–330.

8. Bullock R. Hyperventilation. *J Neurosurg* 2002; 96:157–159.

9. Burke AM, Quest DO, Chien S, Cerri C. The effects of mannitol on blood viscosity. *J Neurosurg* 1981;55:550–553.

10. Brain Trauma Foundation. The American Association of Neurological Surgeons. The Joint Section on Neurotrauma and Critical Care. Use of barbiturates in the control of intracranial hypertension. *J Neurotrauma* 2000;17:527–530.

11. Carmona Suazo JA, Maas AI, van den Brink WA, et al. CO2 reactivity and brain oxygen pressure monitoring in severe head injury. *Crit Care Med* 2000;28:3268–3274.

12. Chesnut RM, Temkin N, Carney N, et al. A trial of intracranial-pressure monitoring in traumatic brain injury. *N Engl J Med* 2012;367: 2471–2481.

13. Clifton GL, Miller ER, Choi SC, et al. Lack of effect of induction of hypothermia after acute brain injury. *N Engl J Med* 2001;344:556–563.

14. Cremer OL, Moons KG, Bouman EA, et al. Long-term propofol infusion and cardiac failure in adult head-injured patients. *Lancet* 2001;357:117–118.

15. Czosnyka M, Smielewski P, Piechnik S, et al. Hemodynamic characterization of intracranial pressure plateau waves in head-injury patients. *J Neurosurg* 1999;91:11–19.

16. Diringer MN. New trends in hyperosmolar therapy? *Curr Opin Crit Care* 2013;19:77–82.

17. Diringer MN, Videen TO, Yundt K, et al. Regional cerebrovascular and metabolic effects of hyperventilation after severe traumatic brain injury. *J Neurosurg* 2002;96:103–108.

18. Donato T, Shapira Y, Artru A, Powers K. Effect of mannitol on cerebrospinal fluid dynamics and brain tissue edema. *Anesth Analg* 1994;78:58–66.

19. Eker C, Asgeirsson B, Grande PO, Schalen W, Nordstrom CH. Improved outcome after severe head injury with a new therapy based on principles for brain volume regulation and preserved microcirculation. *Crit Care Med* 1998;26:1881–1886.

20. Elliot CA, MacKenzie M, O'Kelly CJ. Mannitol dosing error during interfacility transfer for intracranial emergencies. *J Neurosurg* 2105; 123:1166–1169.

21. Feldman Z, Kanter MJ, Robertson CS, et al. Effect of head elevation on intracranial pressure, cerebral perfusion pressure, and cerebral blood flow in head-injured patients. *J Neurosurg* 1992;76:207–211.

22. Florence G, Seylaz J. Rapid autoregulation of cerebral blood flow: a laser-Doppler flowmetry study. *J Cereb Blood Flow Metab* 1992;12:674–680.

23. Francony G, Fauvage B, Falcon D, et al. Equimolar doses of mannitol and hypertonic saline in the treatment of increased intracranial pressure. *Crit Care Med* 2008;36:795–800.

24. Frank JI. Large hemispheric infarction, deterioration, and intracranial pressure. *Neurology* 1995;45:1286–1290.

25. Froelich M, Ni Q, Wess C, Ougorets I, Hartl R. Continuous hypertonic saline therapy and the occurrence of complications in neurocritically ill patients. *Crit Care Med* 2009;37:1433–1441.

26. Gopinath SP, Robertson CS. Management of severe head injury. In: Cottrell JE, Smith DS, eds. *Anesthesia and Neurosurgery*. 3rd ed. St. Louis: Mosby-Year Book; 1994:661–684.

27. Hauerberg J, Juhler M. Cerebral blood flow autoregulation in acute intracranial hypertension. *J Cereb Blood Flow Metab* 1994;14:519–525.

28. Hayashi M, Handa Y, Kobayashi H, et al. Plateau-wave phenomenon (I): correlation between the appearance of plateau waves and CSF circulation in patients with intracranial hypertension. *Brain* 1991;114:2681–2691.

29. Hayashi M, Kobayashi H, Handa Y, et al. Plateau-wave phenomenon (II): occurrence of brain herniation in patients with and without plateau waves. *Brain* 1991;114:2693–2699.

30. Hays AN, Lazaridis C, Neyens R, et al. Osmotherapy: use among neurointensivists. *Neurocrit Care* 2011;14:222–228.

31. Hinson HE, Stein D, Sheth KN. Hypertonic saline and mannitol therapy in critical care neurology. *J Intensive Care Med* 2013;28:3–11.

32. Horn P, Munch E, Vajkoczy P, et al. Hypertonic saline solution for control of elevated intracranial pressure in patients with exhausted response to mannitol and barbiturates. *Neurol Res* 1999; 21:758–764.

33. Imberti R, Bellinzona G, Langer M. Cerebral tissue PO2 and SjvO2 changes during moderate hyperventilation in patients with severe traumatic brain injury. *J Neurosurg* 2002;96:97–102.

34. Juul N, Morris GF, Marshall SB, Marshall LF. Intracranial hypertension and cerebral perfusion pressure: influence on neurological deterioration and outcome in severe head injury. The Executive Committee of the International Selfotel Trial. *J Neurosurg* 2000;92:1–6.

35. Kaufmann AM, Cardoso ER. Aggravation of vasogenic cerebral edema by multiple-dose mannitol. *J Neurosurg* 1992;77:584–589.

36. Kerr EM, Marion D, Sereika MS, et al. The effect of cerebrospinal fluid drainage on cerebral perfusion in traumatic brain injured adults. *J Neurosurg Anesthesiol* 2000;12:324–333.

37. Kerwin AJ, Croce MA, Timmons SD, et al. Effects of fiberoptic bronchoscopy on intracranial pressure in patients with brain injury: a prospective clinical study. *J Trauma* 2000;48:878–882.

38. Khanna S, Davis D, Peterson B, et al. Use of hypertonic saline in the treatment of severe refractory posttraumatic intracranial hypertension in pediatric traumatic brain injury. *Crit Care Med* 2000;28:1144–1151.

39. Koenig MA, Bryan M, Lewin JL, 3rd, et al. Reversal of transtentorial herniation with hypertonic saline. *Neurology* 2008;70:1023–1029.

40. Laffey JG, Kavanagh BP. Hypocapnia. *N Engl J Med* 2002;347:43–53.

41. Luvisotto TL, Auer RN, Sutherland GR. The effect of mannitol on experimental cerebral ischemia, revisited. *Neurosurgery* 1996;38:131–138.

42. Mangat HS, Chiu YL, Gerber LM, et al. Hypertonic saline reduces cumulative and daily intracranial pressure burdens after severe traumatic brain injury. *J Neurosurg* 2015;122:202–210.

43. Manninen PH, Lam AM, Gelb AW, Brown SC. The effect of high-dose mannitol on serum and urine electrolytes and osmolality in neurosurgical patients. *Can J Anaesth* 1987;34:442–446.

44. Manno EM, Adams RE, Derdeyn CP, Powers WJ, Diringer MN. The effects of mannitol on cerebral edema after large hemispheric cerebral infarct. *Neurology* 1999;52:583–587.

45. Marko NF. Hypertonic saline, not mannitol, should be considered gold-standard medical therapy for intracranial hypertension. *Crit Care* 2012;16:113.

46. Mathieu A, Guillon A, Leyre S, et al. Aerosolized lidocaine during invasive mechanical ventilation: in vitro characterization and clinical efficiency to prevent systemic and cerebral hemodynamic changes induced by endotracheal

47. Mortazavi MM, Romeo AK, Deep A, et al. Hypertonic saline for treating raised intracranial pressure: literature review with meta-analysis. *J Neurosurg* 2012;116:210–221.

48. Muizelaar JP, Lutz HA, 3rd, Becker DP. Effect of mannitol on ICP and CBF and correlation with pressure autoregulation in severely head-injured patients. *J Neurosurg* 1984;61:700–706.

49. Muizelaar JP, Marmarou A, Ward JD, et al. Adverse effects of prolonged hyperventilation in patients with severe head injury: a randomized clinical trial. *J Neurosurg* 1991;75:731–739.

50. Muizelaar JP, van der Poel HG, Li ZC, Kontos HA, Levasseur JE. Pial arteriolar vessel diameter and CO2 reactivity during prolonged hyperventilation in the rabbit. *J Neurosurg* 1988;69:923–927.

51. Muizelaar JP, Wei EP, Kontos HA, Becker DP. Cerebral blood flow is regulated by changes in blood pressure and in blood viscosity alike. *Stroke* 1986;17:44–48.

52. Münch E, Horn P, Schurer L, et al. Management of severe traumatic brain injury by decompressive craniectomy. *Neurosurgery* 2000;47:315–322.

53. Neavyn MJ, Boyer EW, Bird SB, Babu KM. Sodium acetate as a replacement for sodium bicarbonate in medical toxicology: a review. *J Med Toxicol* 2013;9:250–254.

54. Neuwelt EA, Kikuchi K, Hill SA, Lipsky P, Frenkel E. Barbiturate inhibition of lymphocyte function: differing effects of various barbiturates used to induce coma. *J Neurosurg* 1982;56:254–259.

55. Nordby HK, Nesbakken R. The effect of high dose barbiturate decompression after severe head injury: a controlled clinical trial. *Acta Neurochir (Wien)* 1984;72:157–166.

56. Nordstrom CH. Physiological and biochemical principles underlying volume-targeted therapy—the "Lund concept." *Neurocrit Care* 2005;2:83–95.

57. Paczynski RP, He YY, Diringer MN, Hsu CY. Multiple-dose mannitol reduces brain water content in a rat model of cortical infarction. *Stroke* 1997;28:1437–1443.

58. Patel PM. Hyperventilation as a therapeutic intervention: do the potential benefits outweigh the known risks? *J Neurosurg Anesthesiol* 1993;5:62–65.

59. Penn RD, Linninger A. The physics of hydrocephalus. *Pediatr Neurosurg* 2009;45:161–174.

60. Pollay M, Fullenwider C, Roberts PA, Stevens FA. Effect of mannitol and furosemide on blood-brain osmotic gradient and intracranial pressure. *J Neurosurg* 1983;59:945–950.

61. Qureshi AI, Suarez JI. Use of hypertonic saline solutions in treatment of cerebral edema and

intracranial hypertension. *Crit Care Med* 2000;28:3301–3313.

62. Qureshi AI, Wilson DA, Traystman RJ. Treatment of elevated intracranial pressure in experimental intracerebral hemorrhage: comparison between mannitol and hypertonic saline. *Neurosurgery* 1999;44:1055–1063.

63. Ravussin P, Abou-Madi M, Archer D, et al. Changes in CSF pressure after mannitol in patients with and without elevated CSF pressure. *J Neurosurg* 1988;69:869–876.

64. Rea GL, Rockswold GL. Barbiturate therapy in uncontrolled intracranial hypertension. *Neurosurgery* 1983;12:401–404.

65. Risberg J, Lundberg N, Ingvar DH. Regional cerebral blood volume during acute transient rises of the intracranial pressure (plateau waves). *J Neurosurg* 1969;31:303–310.

66. Ropper AH. Management of raised intracranial pressure and hyperosmolar therapy. *Practical Neurology* 2014;14:152–158.

67. Ropper AH, O'Rourke D, Kennedy SK. Head position, intracranial pressure, and compliance. *Neurology* 1982;32:1288–1291.

68. Ropper AH, Rockoff MA. Physiology and clinical aspects of raised intracranial pressure. In: Ropper AH, ed. *Neurological and Neurosurgical Intensive Care.* 3rd ed. New York: Raven Press; 1993:11–27.

69. Rosner MJ. Pathophysiology and management of increased intracranial pressure. In: Andrews BT, ed. *Neurosurgical Intensive Care.* New York: McGraw-Hill; 1993:57–112.

70. Rosner MJ, Coley I. Cerebral perfusion pressure: a hemodynamic mechanism of mannitol and the postmannitol hemogram. *Neurosurgery* 1987;21:147–156.

71. Rosner MJ, Coley IB. Cerebral perfusion pressure, intracranial pressure, and head elevation. *J Neurosurg* 1986;65:636–641.

72. Rosner MJ, Rosner SD, Johnson AH. Cerebral perfusion pressure: management protocol and clinical results. *J Neurosurg* 1995;83:949–962.

73. Sakellaridis N, Pavlou E, Karatzas S, et al. Comparison of mannitol and hypertonic saline in the treatment of severe brain injuries. *J Neurosurg* 2011;114:545–548.

74. Saltarini M, Massarutti D, Baldassarre M, et al. Determination of cerebral water content by magnetic resonance imaging after small volume infusion of 18% hypertonic saline solution in a patient with refractory intracranial hypertension. *Eur J Emerg Med* 2002;9:262–265.

75. Schierhout G, Roberts I. Mannitol for acute traumatic brain injury. *Cochrane Database Syst Rev* 2000:CD001049.

76. Schwab S, Schwarz S, Spranger M, et al. Moderate hypothermia in the treatment of patients with severe middle cerebral artery infarction. *Stroke* 1998;29:2461–2466.

77. Schwarz S, Georgiadis D, Aschoff A, Schwab S. Effects of hypertonic (10%) saline in patients with raised intracranial pressure after stroke. *Stroke* 2002;33:136–140.

78. Shiozaki T, Hayakata T, Taneda M, et al. A multicenter prospective randomized controlled trial of the efficacy of mild hypothermia for severely head injured patients with low intracranial pressure. Mild Hypothermia Study Group in Japan. *J Neurosurg* 2001;94:50–54.

79. Shiozaki T, Sugimoto H, Taneda M, et al. Effect of mild hypothermia on uncontrollable intracranial hypertension after severe head injury. *J Neurosurg* 1993;79:363–368.

80. Thiagarajan A, Goverdhan PD, Chari P, Somasunderam K. The effect of hyperventilation and hyperoxia on cerebral venous oxygen saturation in patients with traumatic brain injury. *Anesth Analg* 1998;87:850–853.

81. Thomas SH, Orf J, Wedel SK, Conn AK. Hyperventilation in traumatic brain injury patients: inconsistency between consensus guidelines and clinical practice. *J Trauma* 2002;52:47–52.

82. Tseng MY, Al-Rawi PG, Czosnyka M, et al. Enhancement of cerebral blood flow using systemic hypertonic saline therapy improves outcome in patients with poor-grade spontaneous subarachnoid hemorrhage. *J Neurosurg* 2007;107: 274–282.

83. Tyagi R, Donaldson K, Loftus CM, Jallo J. Hypertonic saline: a clinical review. *Neurosurg Rev* 2007;30:277–289.

84. Videen TO, Zazulia AR, Manno EM, et al. Mannitol bolus preferentially shrinks noninfarcted brain in patients with ischemic stroke. *Neurology* 2001;57:2120–2122.

85. Wald SL, McLaurin RL. Oral glycerol for the treatment of traumatic intracranial hypertension. *J Neurosurg* 1982;56:323–331.

86. Ware ML, Nemani VM, Meeker M, et al. Effects of 23.4% sodium chloride solution in reducing intracranial pressure in patients with traumatic brain injury: a preliminary study. *Neurosurgery* 2005;57:727–736.

87. White H, Cook D, Venkatesh B. The use of hypertonic saline for treating intracranial hypertension after traumatic brain injury. *Anesth Analg* 2006;102:1836–1846.

88. Whitfield PC, Patel H, Hutchinson PJ, et al. Bifrontal decompressive craniectomy in the management of posttraumatic intracranial hypertension. *Br J Neurosurg* 2001;15: 500–507.

89. Wijayatilake DS, Talati C, Panchatsharam S. The monitoring and management of severe traumatic brain injury in the United Kingdom: is

there a consensus? A national survey. *J Neurosurg Anesthesiol*. 2015 Jul;27(3):241–245.

90. Wijdicks EFM. Uncal herniation in acute subdural hematoma: point of no return. *Arch Neurol* 2002;59:305.

91. Wilkinson HA, Rosenfeld SR. Furosemide and mannitol in the treatment of acute experimental intracranial hypertension. *Neurosurgery* 1983;12:405–410.

92. Wolf AL, Levi L, Marmarou A, et al. Effect of THAM upon outcome in severe head injury: a randomized prospective clinical trial. *J Neurosurg* 1993;78:54–59.

93. Woodcock J, Ropper AH, Kennedy SK. High dose barbiturates in non-traumatic brain swelling: ICP reduction and effect on outcome. *Stroke* 1982;13:785–787.

94. Worthley LI, Cooper DJ, Jones N. Treatment of resistant intracranial hypertension with hypertonic saline. Report of two cases. *J Neurosurg* 1988;68:478–481.

95. Zeller FA, Teitelbaum J, West M, et al. The ketamine effect on ICP in traumatic brain injury. *Neurocrit Care* 2014;21:163–173.

PART VI

Technologies in the Neurosciences Intensive Care Unit

23

Monitoring Devices

Patients in the NICU are monitored differently from those in other medical or surgical ICUs. The emphasis should remain on the clinical neurologic examination and knowledge of the causes of clinical deterioration in any acute central nervous system (CNS) injury. Monitoring of critically ill neurologic patients requires the correct interpretation of changes in brainstem reflexes and motor responses to pain and an awareness of the early signs of brainstem displacement. Any of these changes may have immediate clinical relevance.

Devices can be used to assist in intracranial pressure management and to monitor brain oxygen. These devices may be even more useful if patients need heavy sedation or even paralytic agents rendering neurologic examination nearly useless. There is a major opportunity to better monitor neuronal pathophysiology as it develops. However, there are few ways to measure neuronal changes other than in small at random areas. Devices are available that may provide measurements of brain oxygenation, cerebral blood flow (CBF), and certain elements of metabolism, particularly when these systems are stressed to their limits. Before it carves out a niche in the NICU, the performance of any new device should demonstrate that the expected benefits are balanced against the costs and the possible risks of monitoring, and it should be validated for its predictive value. Technology-driven neurologic intensive care or multimodal monitoring is of considerable interest,[3,32,40,42] but the applications in clinical practice may be questionable if the thresholds of interventions have not been defined. Moreover, a high level of monitoring creates a great number of alarms.[24] Labor-intensive analysis of continuous data is problematic, reimbursement of expense is not yet expected for many new devices, and they are therefore largely used as research tools.[12,13] Chapter 24 addresses some of these limitations, as well as major opportunities to allow major technology in the NICU. This chapter discusses the most frequently used monitoring devices

in the NICU. Monitoring changes in ICP is the main theme of the chapter, but other technologies are discussed as well.

MONITORING OF INCREASED INTRACRANIAL PRESSURE

Several good ways exist to invasively measure ICP. However, monitoring of changes in ICP and, equally important, calculated cerebral perfusion pressure (CPP) has been criticized because few studies show improved outcome in monitored patients.[23,47,78,93] Important in this debate is whether the observed change is accurate, whether the observed variable leads to a therapeutic intervention, whether this therapeutic intervention favorably changes the clinical course, and whether placement of this monitoring device is potentially associated with major complications such as hemorrhage, or later, infection.

Guidelines for monitoring ICP in neurologic critical care practice are summarized in Table 23.1. Intracranial pressure monitoring is considered in comatose patients with a high probability of increased ICP, and often is anticipated on the basis of initial readings of computed tomography (CT) images (edema, mass with shift of midline structures). Intracranial pressure monitoring is also used in patients who have had large cerebral tumors removed or frontal lobectomy for seizure control, because of the risk of postoperative swelling. The rationale for ICP monitoring is further detailed in the chapters on specific clinical entities.

In most patients, a fiberoptic parenchymal monitor of ICP is placed, but ventriculostomy is needed if obstructive hydrocephalus is present. Epidural or subdural monitors are far less reliable than intraparenchymal monitors.[6,100] In the past, they have been preferred over parenchymal or ventricular catheters in patients with a need for ICP monitoring but with underlying coagulopathy that cannot be easily reversed with platelets or fresh frozen plasma (e.g., cerebral hematomas

TABLE 23.1. CONDITIONS THAT MAY REQUIRE MONITORING INTRACRANIAL PRESSURE

Disorder	Specific Indications
Traumatic brain injury	Any comatose patient
	Bifrontal lobe contusions and edema
	Temporal lobe contusion and edema
	Polytrauma and need for neuromuscular blockade
Aneurysmal subarachnoid hemorrhage	Acute hydrocephalus
Cerebellar stroke	Acute hydrocephalus
Encephalitis	Diffuse brain edema
Fulminant hepatic failure	Diffuse brain edema

associated with hematologic malignant lesions or head injury in patients with chronic liver failure).[14] Subdural or epidural ICP monitors are now rarely used also because of common spurious readings. Monitoring devices currently available for clinical use and research are shown in Figure 23.1.

INTRAPARENCHYMAL MONITORS

Fiberoptic, transducer-tipped monitors (Camino Laboratories) are used in most NICUs.[17,19,25,36,69,82] Experience with this device is broad. Its easy maintenance, reliable waveforms, lack of significant drift, and simple insertion techniques at the bedside have added to its popularity and have convinced many skeptics to use ICP monitoring. The disadvantages of this system are sizable costs from investment in equipment, fragility of the fiberoptic device, and, most important, inability to withdraw cerebrospinal fluid (CSF). The monitor is calibrated before insertion, and resetting is not possible after placement. The monitor is advanced toward the white matter, 2–3 cm into the brain parenchyma, after a very small burr hole is placed in the right frontal area. The correct distance is indicated on the probe itself, and the bolt can be tightly screwed when this indicator line touches the outside of the bolt. Placement of ICP monitors is by the neurosurgeon and neurosurgical residents, or assisted by neurosurgical nurse practitioners. Whether neurosurgeons would allow neurointensivists to develop expertise in placement is unknown, but one large level I trauma center reported experience with 38 placements with no technical or patient complications.[80]

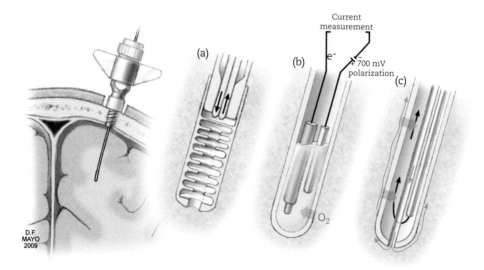

FIGURE 23.1: Three currently used monitoring devices using light, electrochemical probes, and dialysis. (a) Intraparenchymal placement of fiberoptic intracranial pressure monitor. Metal pleated-like tip bounces light and transduces pressure wave. (b) A schematic diagram of a polarographic oxygenation probe. The components of the diagram are polyethylene tube diffusion membrane, polarographic gold cathode and silver anode, and cell filled with electrolytes. (c) A catheter with a polyamide dialysis membrane. The catheter is perfused and dialysate is collected that contains substances such as glucose, lactate, and pyruvate.

The monitor with its metal transducer is shown in Figure 23.2. Light is transmitted by one of the fiberoptic bundles and is reflected by a metal probe. The change in this metal configuration from brain tissue pressure is transduced in a pressure reading and displayed as a typical waveform (see Chapter 22 for interpretations of waveform). The waveform can be displayed through hardware provided by the manufacturer, but most modern bedside monitors should have the capability to enter the ICP recordings and also calculate the CPP. The accuracy of the system was tested by comparison with ventricular catheters, and most studies found acceptable variations over a range of 2–5 mm Hg in both directions. The monitor could drift after approximately 5 days (actual daily drift of 2–3 mm Hg). It must be replaced if large variations occur while monitoring is still indicated, but there is minimal under-reading and over-reading.[7,65,69] The metallic fixation bolt causes a substantial magnetic resonance artifact, and the monitor may move in magnetic resonance fields.[101] Technical complications are unusual, including dislocation of the probe screw and breakage of the optic fiber, mostly after prolonged monitoring. One case of cerebral abscess is on record.[61]

INTRAVENTRICULAR MONITORING

Intraventricular pressure monitoring devices have been used less frequently since the introduction of intraparenchymal fiberoptic devices. Currently, the indications for placement of intraventricular catheters are conditions in which decompression of the ventricular system is urgently indicated. Examples are acute hydrocephalus in aneurysmal subarachnoid hemorrhage and obstructive hydrocephalus in ischemic or hemorrhagic stroke in the cerebellum obliterating the fourth ventricle. Insertion of the ventriculostomy is shown in Figure 23.3a. In most patients, neurosurgeons use antibiotic-coated catheters (Figure 23.3b and c). The ventricular catheters are connected to an external transducer that allows continuous ICP readings. We and others[6] use the Becker intraventricular external drainage and monitoring system

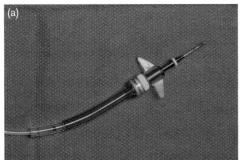
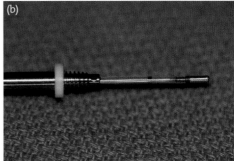
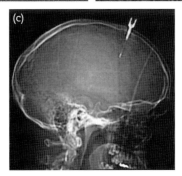

FIGURE 23.2: Intraparenchymal fiberoptic ICP monitor. (a) Intraparenchymal monitor (Camino Laboratories) showing placement in a bolt and (b) close-up view of metal tip. (c) Skull radiograph showing fiberoptic monitor in situ.

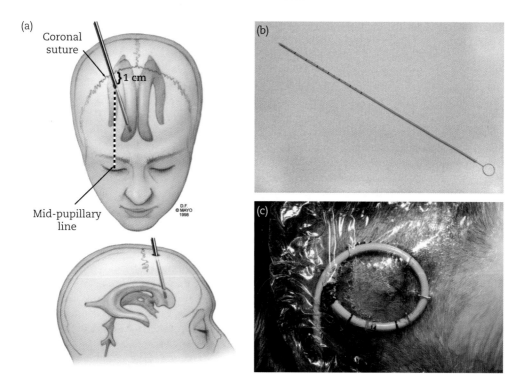

FIGURE 23.3: Ventriculostomy. (a) Technique of ventriculostomy showing landmarks and approach. A ventricular catheter is inserted in the right (nondominant) frontal region. The patient is fully supine. In many instances, the burr hole is placed 1 cm anterior to the coronal suture in the midpupillary line. The catheter is directed to the middle of the nose. The ventricular system (particularly when dilated) is reached at 5–7 cm below the skin. After insertion, the tube is subcutaneously tunneled far from the incision and secured. (b) Ventricular catheter containing clindamycin and rifampin identified by orange color (Codman Bactiseal; Ryanham, MA). (c) catheter secured in situ (different technigues are used by different neurosurgeons and each claim pullout proof with their method of attachment).

(PS Medical, Goleta, CA). One side-port is used for continuous drainage and sampling. The external pressure transducer can be connected to the main system stopcock, which is level with the patient's ear; this provides a zero reference level that approximates the catheter tip location at the foramen of Monro. The drip chamber can be moved up and down and placed at a desired level against the zero reference level stopcock. The drip chamber at the end of the drain line empties into a removable bag (Figure 23.4).

As a practical rule, abnormal resorption of CSF can be assumed when the daily yield approximates 200 mL with a drip chamber at a level of 20 cm H_2O.

An intraventricular catheter based on a fluid-filled system has the major disadvantage of system damping, which makes readings less reliable. This may become a problem when progressive cerebral edema collapses the ventricles, positioning the catheter against the ventricular wall. More commonly, the system becomes blocked when filled with blood. An occluded catheter can be irrigated with small amounts of sterile isotonic saline. Frequently, however, damping of the waveform suggests an air bubble. Air bubbles in the system can be eliminated by withdrawing air from the monitoring line, but only after the system to the patient is closed.

Antibiotic prophylaxis should certainly be considered in patients with a ventriculostomy. The benefit of this prophylactic measure is not exactly known, but it should be emphasized that ventriculitis is associated with considerable morbidity and mortality.[102] The risk of infection with a therapy-resistant infectious agent seems low. However, in a randomized study in 228 patients, the infection rate was reduced from 11% to 3%, but emergence of methicillin-resistant *Staphylococcus aureus* and *Candida* pathogens increased.[71] Long duration antibiotics (weeks) may lead to an increased incidence of Clostridium difficile colitis, but this association is not found in several studies (Part XIV Guidelines).   Subcutaneous tunneling may

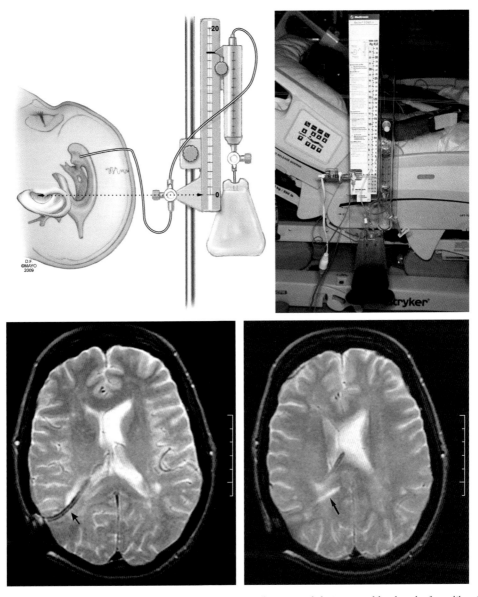

FIGURE 23.4: Intraventricular drainage. Becker intraventricular external drainage and landmarks for calibrating. The stopcock is leveled at the ear, and the drip chamber is fixed at a desired level (usually 10–15 cm H$_2$O). Left MRI shows ventriculostomy in situ (arrow), Right MRI shows effect of prior attempt (arrow).

also considerably reduce the risk of ventriculitis. Intravenous administration of antibiotics cefazolin IV, 2g q8h is preferred while the ventricular catheter is in situ and for up to 3 days after removal. However, it is unclear if prophylaxis is needed with the newer antibiotic-coated catheters, and practices vary, but many neurosurgeons continue antibiotics.

If CSF yield is low in the collecting bag, clamping of the catheter for 24 hours can be tried. The catheter is pulled when no clinical change is observed and when repeat CT scanning does not show a significant increase in ventricular size. If continuous ventricular drainage is indicated, because either weaning or clamping fails or the cause of obstruction in the ventricular system is not expected to reverse within 10 days, a permanent ventricular–peritoneal shunt is considered, preferably if no blood sediments are observed. The risk of ventriculitis is too high (despite subcutaneous tunneling of the catheter and prophylactic antibiotics) to permit long-term external drainage.[91] In one study, these catheters caused ventriculitis in 3% of patients when still in place after 10 days.[54]

BRAIN TISSUE OXIMETRY

The general indications for brain tissue oximetry monitoring are (a) recognition of ischemia thresholds (assuming the sensor measures a damaged area), (b) assessment of autoregulation, and (c) as a tool for prognosis.[55,90] More specific possible applications are shown in Table 23.2.

The microsensor can be placed through a bolt or through a craniotomy site, which makes it easier to use in patients with traumatic brain injury who had a subdural hematoma or contusions removed.

The measurement of brain tissue oxygenation is based on the Clark principle (use of electrochemical properties of noble metals to measure oxygen content in brain tissue) or by using fiberoptic technology to measure brain tissue oxygen partial pressure (PbO_2), brain tissue carbon dioxide partial pressure ($PbCO_2$), and pH (Figure 23.1(b)).[18,26–29,36,39,46,48,51,56,57,64]

In the United States, two probes are available commercially, and they are largely used in specialized trauma units. These probes are the LICOX (Integra Neurosciences, San Diego, CA) and the Neurotrend (Godman, Raynham, MA). The probes read approximately 7–17 mm^2 and extrapolate data from the microvessels (both arteries and veins) in that area. Cerebral oxygen tension probes have been used on the assumption that oxygen levels decrease in parenchyma at risk for ischemia. These probes monitor only small areas and do not provide a global view—total oxygen delivery—of the parenchyma. The brain oxygen pressure has been correlated to CBF, and certain thresholds for ischemia may exist.[81] The ischemic threshold of CBF is 18 mL/100 gram/minute and has been associated with values of brain PO_2 of less than 22 mm Hg[31] (Capsule 23.1). Patients with persistent low brain tissue PO_2 values were at high risk of poor outcome, but trends do appear more reliable. Hyperventilation has shown to decrease brain tissue oxygenation

as much as 40% from baseline, and brain tissue oxygen may therefore be a helpful guide in titrating this measure.[50]

Clinical data are emerging, but two recent studies in traumatic brain injury using brain tissue monitoring found opposing results.[55,66] A retrospective study of 122 patients compared combined brain tissue monitoring and ICP monitoring with ICP monitoring alone and found unexpectedly higher mortality, increased hospital cost, and length of hospital stay in the brain tissue oxygen-monitored group.[55] The therapeutic interventions (sedation, analgesia, osmotic diuretics, and hyperventilation) were significantly more common in the brain tissue oxygen-monitored group, but the differences could be explained by mismatch between study groups. A recent prospective study of 139 patients with traumatic brain injury found reduced mortality and morbidity when compared to historical controls. This study found that persistently low brain tissue oxygen (< 20 mm Hg) and elevated ICP despite "maximal therapy intensity" resulted in high probability of death or poor outcome.[66] It is self-evident that a randomized prospective study may be able to provide a better rationale for its use.

Experience with brain tissue oxygen-based therapy is growing,[11] and a recent detailed study found increased favorable outcome in oxygen-guided intervention. Better outcome was seen in patients with shorter durations of compromised brain oxygen, less episodes of compromised brain oxygen, and more often successful treatment of brain oxygen—all pointing to a possible effect of these interventions. A flowchart on how to manage abnormal cerebral oxygenation is shown in Figure 23.5.[87]

MICRODIALYSIS

Another relatively new option is the detection of ischemic neuronal compromise by a microdialysis catheter.[1,9,25] The principle of microdialysis—an expensive and labor-intensive monitoring device—is a catheter with a polyamide dialysis membrane that allows diffusion of molecules below 20,000 DA. The catheter is perfused and the dialysate that is collected contains energy-related substances such as glucose, lactate, and pyruvate (Figure 23.1). The lactate-to-pyruvate ratio is calculated, and increased ratios are an indicator of ischemia.[10,13,89,95] Glycerol can be measured, and an increase may indicate permanent tissue damage. Episodes of hypotension, hypoxemia and increased intracranial hypertension correlated reasonably well with changes in glucose, lactate,

TABLE 23.2. INDICATIONS FOR CEREBRAL OXYGENATION MONITORING

Monitoring of brain tissue exposed to ischemia

To guide hyperventilation and other measures to decrease intracranial pressure

Recognition of delayed cerebral vasospasm

Monitoring peri hematoma brain tissue exposed to mass effect

CAPSULE 23.1:   CEREBRAL BLOOD FLOW AND BRAIN TISSUE OXYGEN

Cerebral metabolic requirements are coupled to cerebral blood flow (CBF). Cerebral metabolism is decreased in many disorders with a global injury, including traumatic brain injury, and may not be compensated for by an increase in CBF, thus leading to further ischemia. Persistently decreased CBF leads to ischemia and neuronal death.

In times of plenty, CBF decreases; in times of shortage, CBF increases. Brain tissue oxygen is closely related to CBF, and its relation is shown in the accompanying illustration. The CBF threshold of ischemia has been traditionally placed at 18 mL/100 g/min, but this is not well supported by human data. Monitoring of brain tissue oxygen and cerebral perfusion pressure may provide an indication of cerebral autoregulation. When brain tissue oxygen is not affected by changes in cerebral perfusion pressure, it can be assumed that autoregulation is intact.

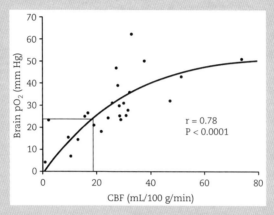

Regression plot between cerebral blood flow and brain tissue PO_2 at the ischemic threshold of CBF (18 mL/100 g/min). Brain PO_2 is 22 mm Hg.

Used with permission from Doppenberg EMR, Zauner A, Bullock R, et al. Correlations between brain tissue oxygen tension, pH, and cerebral blood flow—a better way of monitoring the severely injured brain? *Surg Neurol* 1998;49:630–634.

and lactate/pyruvate. Microdialysis has been studied in aneurysmal subarachnoid hemorrhage, traumatic head injury, and fulminant hepatic failure.[10,13,95]

JUGULAR VENOUS OXYGEN SATURATION

A technique made possible by the introduction of fiberoptic catheters may be useful in monitoring cerebral metabolism through jugular venous oxygen saturation.[4] (In many ways, this measurement technique is similar to the operation of oximetric Swan-Ganz catheters.) It has been claimed that the monitoring of jugular venous deterioration may identify secondary insults to the brain. Most of the studies have been performed in a few centers, specifically in patients with traumatic brain injury and in patients with subarachnoid hemorrhage and intracerebral hematomas.[35,37,97]

This monitoring device may be able to provide a more global picture of brain tissue oxygenation than the brain tissue oxygen monitor. The high number of false alarms and technical difficulties has, however, reduced enthusiasm for this device. The physiologic assumptions for the monitoring of jugular venous deterioration are that CBF is closely linked to the cerebral metabolic rate of oxygen, and its relationship is determined by the Fick equation.[45] The Fick equation defines the oxygen uptake as the product of cardiac output (substituted by CBF) and the arteriovenous difference in oxygen content. Studies showed a close relationship between CBF and jugular venous saturation ($SjvO_2$).[74–76] When CBF falters, it is compensated by increasing cerebral oxygen extraction, which results in a decrease in $SjvO_2$. Cerebral blood flow is significantly reduced when one or more episodes of jugular desaturation of oxygen are

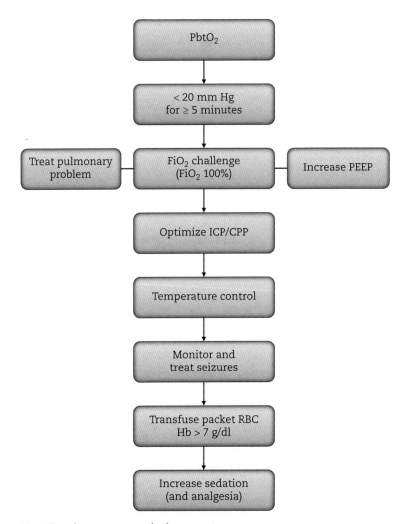

FIGURE 23.5: Clinical guide to improve cerebral oxygenation.

recorded. The normal $SjvO_2$ is 50%–65%, and values below 50% for 15 minutes indicate ischemia. Cerebral blood flow can be reduced by many causes, including cerebral vasospasm, intracranial hypertension, induced hypocapnia, and hypotension, all of which reduce oxygen delivery to the brain. In addition, reduced hemoglobin may further reduce oxygen delivery.

The monitoring device is placed inside the jugular bulb. The catheter is preferably placed at the site of the largest jugular foramen (Figure 23.6) (dominance of venous flow) on CT scan. Its position should ideally be cranial to a line connecting the mastoid processes on a plain anteroposterior skull radiograph.[5]

In previous studies, many abnormal readings were false alarms, with the potential to encourage nursing staff and attending physicians to ignore abnormal values. In one study, the sensitivity for detection of jugular bulb saturation was 45%–50%, with a specificity of 98%–100%, but only after repositioning or flushing.[21] The monitoring technique, however, should not be easily discarded as unreliable and may still have considerable promising value. A significant limitation is that a low-intensity reading ($SjvO_2$ < 50%) may have its origin in poor positioning of the probe against the wall as a result of collapse of the internal jugular vein. One study confirmed false-positive findings in more than half of these measurements.[85] The observed oxygen desaturation must therefore be confirmed by measurement of blood withdrawn from the catheter, and unfortunately this may be necessary with every other saturation measurement. In addition, arterial hypoxemia or anemia from whatever source should be excluded as a

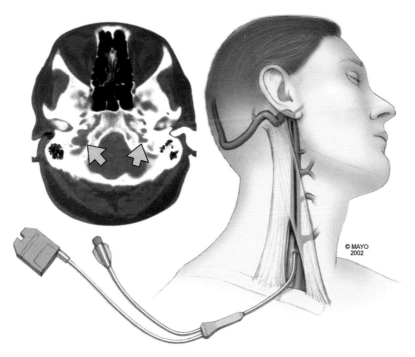

FIGURE 23.6: Jugular oxygen saturation catheter. Placement of catheter, and jugular foramen on computed tomography scan. Right is typically larger than left (*arrows*).

possible cause of oxygen desaturation. It is also important to calculate the arteriovenous difference in oxygen, which should move in the opposite direction[85] (Part XIV Guidelines). Trends may be more important (Figure 23.7).

Complications such as infections, accidental misplacement, and carotid puncture were very uncommon, whereas jugular bulb venous thrombosis was found in 40% of 44 monitored patients.[20]

The therapeutic interventions in patients with markedly decreased SjvO$_2$ are adjustment of the depth of hypocapnia, more frequent administration of mannitol boluses, correction of anemia, and adjustment of mean arterial pressure. A guideline is shown in Figure 23.8. No study has determined the effect of these corrections on outcome in those patients considered for monitoring, but repeated SjvO$_2$ desaturation has been correlated with poor outcome in head injury.[26-29]

NEAR-INFRARED SPECTROSCOPY

Near-infrared spectroscopy can monitor changes in cerebral oxygenation and blood volume by measuring concentrations of oxyhemoglobin and deoxyhemoglobin.[67,98] Although superficially similar to pulse oximetry, near-infrared spectroscopy is fundamentally different because of different wavelengths and greater tissue penetration. The principle is shown in Figure 23.9. The absorbance measured by detectors is predominantly that of venous blood, and the findings would thus be equivalent to, for example, those of jugular bulb saturation.

The main assumption is that concentrations of oxyhemoglobin and hemoglobin and oxidized cytochrome oxidase (considered negligible) change with changes in cerebral perfusion and oxygenation. Near-infrared light (650–1,000 nm) penetrates the scalp to a depth of 2.5 cm. The path of the photons is parabolic, and the depth of the tissue penetrated is related to the distance between limited light and detector. The proximal receiver thus detects light passed through tissue outside the cortex. Both signals (proximal and distal detectors) are subtracted, and the ratio gives a value for cerebral oxygen saturation.[8,43,44,63,72]

Major problems are unreliability due to extracerebral blood (e.g., subdural hematoma), difficulty in establishing criteria of ischemia by comparative methods such as electroencephalography and somatosensory evoked potentials, and general problems with replication of results.[92] Only a few pilot studies have been published. With further generations, the device may become clinically useful.[96]

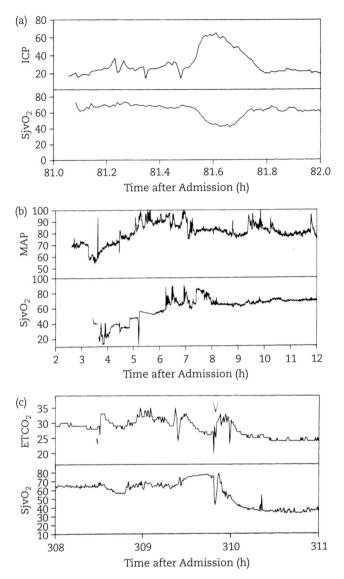

FIGURE 23.7: Example of trend recordings of jugular venous oxygen saturation ($SjvO_2$). Marked decline correlates with known triggers. (a) Increased intracranial pressure. (b) Hypotension. (c) Hypocapnia.

$ETCO_2$, end-tidal carbon dioxide concentration; ICP, intracranial pressure; MAP, mean arterial pressure.

From Feldman Z, Robertson CS. Monitoring of cerebral hemodynamics with jugular bulb catheters. *Crit Care Clin* 1997;13:51–77. With permission of WB Saunders Company.

ULTRASOUND OF THE OPTIC NERVE SHEATH

There is considerable interest in finding a correlation between sonographic optic nerve sheath diameter (ONSD) and ICP, and accuracy seems consistent among centers.[31,73,86,92,99] Measurements of ONSD by magnetic resonance imaging correlate with ICP measurements.[41] Most notable, its reliability was strengthened by reductions of the ocular nerve sheath diameter after mannitol infusion.[49] This monitoring device has not yet been introduced in major neurocritical care units in the United States, nor is its value undisputedly established, but ONSD is the most promising. It has been tested in the emergency department and there is good interobserver agreement between emergency physicians who were able in normals to find normal values (usually 5–6 mm).[38] Most studies have considered 5 mm as a cutoff value with increasing values as high as 7 mm soon after

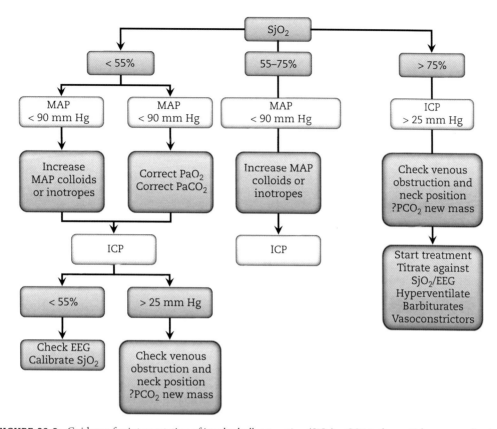

FIGURE 23.8: Guidance for interpretation of jugular bulb saturation (SjO$_2$). pCO2 is the partial pressure of carbon dioxide.

EEG, electroencephalogram; ICP, intracranial pressure; MAP, mean arterial pressure.

Modified from Macmillan CS, Andrews PJ. Cerebrovenous oxygen saturation monitoring: practical considerations and clinical relevance. *Intensive Care Med* 2000;26:1028–1036. With permission of Springer-Verlag.

tracheal suctioning in some when measured serially.[49] ONSD measurement with ultrasonography has a median intraobserver variability of 0.2 mm (range 0.1–0.5 mm).

MONITORING OF HEMODYNAMIC AND OXYGENATION PARAMETERS

Invasive monitoring devices can access the arterial or venous circulatory system and provide the potential for optimization of treatment. None of this equipment is without risk or procedural complications. Use of pulmonary artery catheters has virtually disappeared in the ICUs. The pulmonary catheter requires considerable skill and knowledge of the engineering principles—from basic zeroing and leveling of the transducer to understanding of the dynamic responses. (The reader is referred to

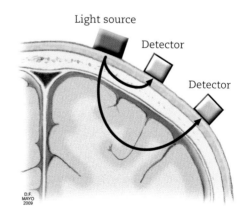

FIGURE 23.9: The principle of near-infrared spectroscopy (see text for explanation). Illumination of the head (usually left and right), using infrared light, diffuses through tissue and is detected by photodiode detectors.

critical care textbooks and a handbook.[68]) Its efficacy and safety in surgical and medical ICUs have been seriously questioned.[30,34,70,88]

PULSE OXIMETRY

Pulse oximetry is based on spectrophotometric principles. Emitted light is reflected by hemoglobin; different hemoglobin configurations reflect different wavelengths. With pulse oximetry, two wavelengths are used to determine the relative concentration of oxyhemoglobin and reduced hemoglobin. Several factors, such as anemia, nail polish, hypothermia, and dark-pigmented skin, can produce inaccurate results.[84] Pulse oximetry is accurate in patients with dysrhythmias and a pulse deficit.

Noninvasive oximetry is widely considered to be one of the most important technical advances in monitoring respiratory status and has reduced the number of arterial blood gas determinations. Prospective studies have clearly demonstrated a multifold increase in the detection of hypoxemia (pulse oximeter saturation of oxygen < 90%) in postoperative patients.[84] However, when audited, pulse oximetry appeared less useful in certain studies. One study found that the number of arterial blood gas measurements decreased by only 3% in mechanically ventilated patients monitored by pulse oximetry.[2] In another study, no mention of hypoxemic episodes was made in clinical notes in many patients with desaturation values below 85%.[15] In the NICU, we routinely use pulse oximetry and find it particularly useful in monitoring of patients in need of intermediate care or overnight observation, such as after trauma, any type of acute ischemic or hemorrhagic stroke, Guillain-Barré syndrome (GBS), or myasthenic gravis. Pulse oximetry has repeatedly guided us to increase oxygen intake or to proceed with intubation.[59,60]

RADIAL ARTERY CATHETER

Radial artery catheterization is considered in patients with unstable blood pressure and thus is much more common in general medical and surgical ICUs.[33] In the NICU, common indications are use of vasoactive drugs, anesthetic agents that potentially lower blood pressure (such as midazolam or propofol in status epilepticus), and the need for multiple blood sampling in, for example, mechanically ventilated patients. Oscillometric blood pressure measurements are quite unreliable, and typically the displayed blood pressure is 15–30 minutes old (frequency of measurement is arbitrarily set from 1 minute to 1 hour).[16,103] A recent study with different cuff sizes found a discrepancy of more than 20 mm Hg in one-third of almost 1,500 measurement pairs, a result favoring radial artery cannulation.[16]

The technique of arterial cannulation is simple and in the United States is often performed by respiratory therapists. Generally, an 85% success rate is achieved with attempted cannulation. Catheter colonization is low, but radial artery thrombosis (often asymptomatic) is high with long-term use.[53] Frequent changing of arterial cannulas does not prevent these complications, and the cannulas may remain in place for a week or longer. Patency is maintained by flushing with small volumes of saline for 5 seconds.

FUTURE DIRECTIONS

The availability of reliable ICP monitors has changed the monitoring of patients in the NICU. However, noninvasive monitoring of cerebral well-being remains elusive. New noninvasive approaches have included cerebrovenous oxygen monitoring,[48] venous transcranial Doppler ultrasonography for increased ICP (venous blood is pooled to larger venous vessels, and venous maximal blood flow velocity increases),[83] measurement of tympanic membrane pressure (changes in ICP change the hydrostatic pressure of the cochlea and displace the tympanic membrane),[73] ophthalmodynamometry (pressure in the central retinal vein correlates linearly with ICP),[52,62] pupillometry ("sluggish pupil" reduction in constriction velocity may herald an increase in ICP), and tissue resonance analysis (ultrasonography obtains echopulsograms from the third ventricle, equivalent to ICP waves).[58] The role of the industry is substantial, and enthusiasts of each new device will continue to promote its merits.[22,77,79,94] In this age of technology, it is perhaps a travesty that neurointensivists involved with the care of acute brain injury still lack a tool to monitor brain injury or neuronal compromise. Such a reliable and workable parameter would be not only practically useful but a major innovation.

CONCLUSIONS

- Fiberoptic monitors are the most contemporary and reliable devices for intraparenchymal monitoring of ICP. Ventriculostomy should be reserved for patients with acute hydrocephalus.
- Continuous brain oxygen monitoring and microdialysis are research tools with the

potential to become invasive monitoring devices used in daily practice. Both monitors may allow identification of brain tissue at risk.

- Jugular venous oxygen saturation may identify further insults to the brain, monitor depth of hypocapnia, and could lead to adjustment of mean arterial pressure.

REFERENCES

1. Afinowi R, Tisdall M, Keir G, et al. Improving the recovery of S100B protein in cerebral microdialysis: implications for multimodal monitoring in neurocritical care. *J Neurosci Methods* 2009;181:95–99.
2. Alford PT, Hawkins P, Sherrill TR, al. e. Impact of pulse oximetry on demand for arterial blood gases in an ICU. [Abstract]. *Chest* 1989;96 (Suppl):288S.
3. Andrews PJ, Citerio G, Longhi L, et al. NICEM consensus on neurological monitoring in acute neurological disease. *Intens Care Med* 2008;34:1362–1370.
4. Andrews PJ, Dearden NM, Miller JD. Jugular bulb cannulation: description of a cannulation technique and validation of a new continuous monitor. *Br J Anaesth* 1991;67:553–558.
5. Bankier AA, Fleischmann D, Windisch A, et al. Position of jugular oxygen saturation catheter in patients with head trauma: assessment by use of plain films. *AJR Am J Roentgenol* 1995;164:437–441.
6. Barnett GH. Intracranial pressure monitoring devices: principles, insertion, and care. In: Ropper AH, ed. *Neurological and Neurosurgical Intensive Care*. 3rd ed. New York: Raven Press; 1993:53–68.
7. Bavetta S, Norris JS, Wyatt M, Sutcliffe JC, Hamlyn PJ. Prospective study of zero drift in fiberoptic pressure monitors used in clinical practice. *J Neurosurg* 1997;86:927–930.
8. Beese U, Langer H, Lang W, Dinkel M. Comparison of near-infrared spectroscopy and somatosensory evoked potentials for the detection of cerebral ischemia during carotid endarterectomy. *Stroke* 1998;29:2032–2037.
9. Bellander BM, Cantais E, Enblad P, et al. Consensus meeting on microdialysis in neurointensive care. *Intens Care Med* 2004;30: 2166–2169.
10. Belli A, Sen J, Petzold A, et al. Extracellular N-acetylaspartate depletion in traumatic brain injury. *J Neurochem* 2006;96:861–869.
11. Beynon C, Kiening KL, Orakcioglu B, Unterberg AW, Sakowitz OW. Brain tissue oxygen

monitoring and hyperoxic treatment in patients with traumatic brain injury. *J Neurotrauma* 2012;29:2109–2123.
12. Bhatia A, Gupta AK. Neuromonitoring in the intensive care unit. I: intracranial pressure and cerebral blood flow monitoring. *Intens Care Med* 2007;33:1263–1271.
13. Bhatia A, Gupta AK. Neuromonitoring in the intensive care unit. II: cerebral oxygenation monitoring and microdialysis. *Intens Care Med* 2007;33:1322–1328.
14. Blci AT, Olafsson S, Webster S, Levy R. Complications of intracranial pressure monitoring in fulminant hepatic failure. *Lancet* 1993;341:157–158.
15. Bowton DL, Scuderi PE, Harris L, Haponik EF. Pulse oximetry monitoring outside the intensive care unit: progress or problem? *Ann Intern Med* 1991;115:450–454.
16. Bur A, Hirschl MM, Herkner H, et al. Accuracy of oscillometric blood pressure measurement according to the relation between cuff size and upper-arm circumference in critically ill patients. *Crit Care Med* 2000;28:371–376.
17. Chambers KR, Kane PJ, Choksey MS, Mendelow AD. An evaluation of the camino ventricular bolt system in clinical practice. *Neurosurgery* 1993;33:866–868.
18. Charbel FT, Du X, Hoffman WE, Ausman JI. Brain tissue PO(2), PCO(2), and pH during cerebral vasospasm. *Surg Neurol* 2000;54: 432–437.
19. Chesnut RM, Marshall LF. Management of head injury: treatment of abnormal intracranial pressure. *Neurosurg Clin N Am* 1991;2:267–284.
20. Coplin WM, O'Keefe GE, Grady MS, et al. Accuracy of continuous jugular bulb oximetry in the intensive care unit. *Neurosurgery* 1998;42:533–539.
21. Coplin WM, O'Keefe GE, Grady MS, et al. Thrombotic, infectious, and procedural complications of the jugular bulb catheter in the intensive care unit. *Neurosurgery* 1997;41:101–107.
22. Coyle SL. Physician-industry relations. Part 1: individual physicians. *Ann Intern Med* 2002;136:396–402.
23. Cremer OL, van Dijk GW, van Wensen E, et al. Effect of intracranial pressure monitoring and targeted intensive care on functional outcome after severe head injury. *Crit Care Med* 2005;33: 2207–2213.
24. Cropp AJ, Woods LA, Raney D, Bredle DL. Name that tone: the proliferation of alarms in the intensive care unit. *Chest* 1994;105:1217–1220.
25. Crutchfield JS, Narayan RK, Robertson CS, Michael LH. Evaluation of a fiberoptic

intracranial pressure monitor. *J Neurosurg* 1990;72: 482–487.

26. Cruz J. Combined continuous monitoring of systemic and cerebral oxygenation in acute brain injury: preliminary observations. *Crit Care Med* 1993;21:1225–1232.

27. Cruz J. On-line monitoring of global cerebral hypoxia in acute brain injury: relationship to intracranial hypertension. *J Neurosurg* 1993;79: 228–233.

28. Cruz J, Miner ME, Allen SJ, Alves WM, Gennarelli TA. Continuous monitoring of cerebral oxygenation in acute brain injury: injection of mannitol during hyperventilation. *J Neurosurg* 1990;73:725–730.

29. Cruz J, Raps EC, Hoffstad OJ, Jaggi JL, Gennarelli TA. Cerebral oxygenation monitoring. *Crit Care Med* 1993;21:1242–1246.

30. Dalen JE. The pulmonary artery catheter-friend, foe, or accomplice? *JAMA* 2001;286:348–350.

31. Dunham CM, Sosnowski C, Porter JM, Siegal J, Kohli C. Correlation of noninvasive cerebral oximetry with cerebral perfusion in the severe head injured patient: a pilot study. *J Trauma* 2002; 52:40–46.

32. Dunn IF, Ellegala DB, Kim DH, Litvack ZN. Neuromonitoring in neurological critical care. *Neurocrit Care* 2006;4:83–92.

33. Frezza EE, Mezghebe H. Indications and complications of arterial catheter use in surgical or medical intensive care units: analysis of 4932 patients. *Am Surg* 1998;64:127–131.

34. Gnaegi A, Feihl F, Perret C. Intensive care physicians' insufficient knowledge of right-heart catheterization at the bedside: time to act? *Crit Care Med* 1997;25:213–220.

35. Gopinath SP, Robertson CS, Contant CF, et al. Jugular venous desaturation and outcome after head injury. *J Neurol Neurosurg Psychiatry* 1994;57:717–723.

36. Grant SA, Bettencourt K, Krulevitch P, Hamilton J, Glass R. Development of fiber optic and electrochemical pH sensors to monitor brain tissue. *Crit Rev Biomed Eng* 2000;28:159–163.

37. Gupta AK, Zygun DA, Johnston AJ, et al. Extracellular brain pH and outcome following severe traumatic brain injury. *J Neurotrauma* 2004;21:678–684.

38. Hassen GW, Bruck I, Donahue J, et al. Accuracy of optic nerve sheath diameter measurement by emergency physicians using bedside ultrasound. *J Emerg Med* 2015;48:450–457.

39. Kett-White R, Hutchinson PJ, Al-Rawi PG, et al. Adverse cerebral events detected after subarachnoid hemorrhage using brain oxygen and microdialysis probes. *Neurosurgery* 2002;50:1213–1221.

40. Kett-White R, Hutchinson PJ, Czosnyka M, et al. Multi-modal monitoring of acute brain injury. *Adv Tech Stand Neurosurg* 2002;27: 87–134.

41. Kimberly HH, Noble VE. Using MRI of the optic nerve sheath to detect elevated intracranial pressure. *Crit Care* 2008;12:181.

42. Kirkpatrick PJ, Czosnyka M, Pickard JD. Multimodal monitoring in neurointensive care. *J Neurol Neurosurg Psychiatry* 1996;60:131–139.

43. Kirkpatrick PJ, Lam J, Al-Rawi P, Smielewski P, Czosnyka M. Defining thresholds for critical ischemia by using near-infrared spectroscopy in the adult brain. *J Neurosurg* 1998;89:389–394.

44. Kirkpatrick PJ, Smielewski P, Czosnyka M, Menon DK, Pickard JD. Near-infrared spectroscopy use in patients with head injury. *J Neurosurg* 1995;83:963–970.

45. Lang EW, Lagopoulos J, Griffith J, et al. Cerebral vasomotor reactivity testing in head injury: the link between pressure and flow. *J Neurol Neurosurg Psychiatry* 2003;74:1053–1059.

46. Lewis SB, Myburgh JA, Thornton EL, Reilly PL. Cerebral oxygenation monitoring by near-infrared spectroscopy is not clinically useful in patients with severe closed-head injury: a comparison with jugular venous bulb oximetry. *Crit Care Med* 1996;24:1334–1338.

47. Mack WJ, King RG, Ducruet AF, et al. Intracranial pressure following aneurysmal subarachnoid hemorrhage: monitoring practices and outcome data. *Neurosurg Focus* 2003;14:e3.

48. Macmillan CS, Andrews PJ. Cerebrovenous oxygen saturation monitoring: practical considerations and clinical relevance. *Intens Care Med* 2000;26:1028–1036.

49. Maissan IM, Dirven PJ, Haitsma IK, et al. Ultrasonographic measured optic nerve sheath diameter as an accurate and quick monitor for changes in intracranial pressure. *J Neurosurg* 2015;1–5.

50. Manley GT, Hemphill JC, Morabito D, et al. Cerebral oxygenation during hemorrhagic shock: perils of hyperventilation and the therapeutic potential of hypoventilation. *J Trauma* 2000;48:1025–1032.

51. Manley GT, Pitts LH, Morabito D, et al. Brain tissue oxygenation during hemorrhagic shock, resuscitation, and alterations in ventilation. *J Trauma* 1999;46:261–267.

52. Marshall LF. Head injury: recent past, present, and future. *Neurosurgery* 2000;47:546–561.

53. Martin C, Saux P, Papazian L, Gouin F. Long-term arterial cannulation in ICU patients using the radial artery or dorsalis pedis artery. *Chest* 2001;119:901–906.

54. Martinez-Manas RM, Santamarta D, de Campos JM, Ferrer E. Camino intracranial pressure monitor: prospective study of accuracy and complications. *J Neurol Neurosurg Psychiatry* 2000;69:82–86.

55. Martini RP, Deem S, Yanez ND, et al. Management guided by brain tissue oxygen monitoring and outcome following severe traumatic brain injury. *J Neurosurg* 2009;111:644–649.

56. McLeod AD, Igielman F, Elwell C, Cope M, Smith M. Measuring cerebral oxygenation during normobaric hyperoxia: a comparison of tissue microprobes, near-infrared spectroscopy, and jugular venous oximetry in head injury. *Anesth Analg* 2003;97:851–856.

57. Menon DK, Coles JP, Gupta AK, et al. Diffusion limited oxygen delivery following head injury. *Crit Care Med* 2004;32:1384–1390.

58. Michaeli D, Rappaport ZH. Tissue resonance analysis; a novel method for noninvasive monitoring of intracranial pressure. Technical note. *J Neurosurg* 2002;96:1132–1137.

59. Moller JT, Johannessen NW, Espersen K, et al. Randomized evaluation of pulse oximetry in 20,802 patients. II: perioperative events and postoperative complications. *Anesthesiology* 1993;78:445–453.

60. Moller JT, Pedersen T, Rasmussen LS, et al. Randomized evaluation of pulse oximetry in 20,802 patients. I: design, demography, pulse oximetry failure rate, and overall complication rate. *Anesthesiology* 1993;78:436–444.

61. Morton R, Lucas TH, 2nd, Ko A, et al. Intracerebral abscess associated with the Camino intracranial pressure monitor: case report and review of the literature. *Neurosurgery* 2012;71:E193–E198.

62. Motschmann M, Muller C, Kuchenbecker J, et al. Ophthalmodynamometry: a reliable method for measuring intracranial pressure. *Strabismus* 2001;9:13–16.

63. Muellner T, Schramm W, Kwasny O, Vecsei V. Patients with increased intracranial pressure cannot be monitored using near infrared spectroscopy. *Br J Neurosurg* 1998;12:136–139.

64. Mulvey JM, Dorsch NW, Mudaliar Y, Lang EW. Multimodality monitoring in severe traumatic brain injury: the role of brain tissue oxygenation monitoring. *Neurocrit Care* 2004;1:391–402.

65. Munch E, Weigel R, Schmiedek P, Schurer L. The Camino intracranial pressure device in clinical practice: reliability, handling characteristics and complications. *Acta Neurochir (Wien)* 1998;140:1113–1119.

66. Narotam PK, Morrison JF, Nathoo N. Brain tissue oxygen monitoring in traumatic brain injury and major trauma: outcome analysis of a brain tissue oxygen-directed therapy. *J Neurosurg* 2009;111:672–682.

67. Owen-Reece H, Smith M, Elwell CE, Goldstone JC. Near infrared spectroscopy. *Br J Anaesth* 1999;82:418–426.

68. Perret C, Tagan D, Feihl F, Marini JJ. *The Pulmonary Artery Catheter in Critical Care: A Concise Handbook*. New York: Oxford, Blackwell Science; 1996.

69. Poca MA, Sahuquillo J, Arribas M, et al. Fiberoptic intraparenchymal brain pressure monitoring with the Camino V420 monitor: reflections on our experience in 163 severely head-injured patients. *J Neurotrauma* 2002;19:439–448.

70. Polanczyk CA, Rohde LE, Goldman L, et al. Right heart catheterization and cardiac complications in patients undergoing noncardiac surgery: an observational study. *JAMA* 2001;286:309–314.

71. Poon WS, Ng S, Wai S. CSF antibiotic prophylaxis for neurosurgical patients with ventriculostomy: a randomised study. *Acta Neurochir Suppl* 1998;71:146–148.

72. Prough DS, Pollard V. Cerebral near-infrared spectroscopy: ready for prime time? *Crit Care Med* 1995;23:1624–1626.

73. Reid A, Marchbanks RJ, Burge DM, et al. The relationship between intracranial pressure and tympanic membrane displacement. *Br J Audiol* 1990;24:123–129.

74. Robertson CS, Contant CF, Gokaslan ZL, Narayan RK, Grossman RG. Cerebral blood flow, arteriovenous oxygen difference, and outcome in head injured patients. *J Neurol Neurosurg Psychiatry* 1992;55:594–603.

75. Robertson CS, Grossman RG, Goodman JC, Narayan RK. The predictive value of cerebral anaerobic metabolism with cerebral infarction after head injury. *J Neurosurg* 1987;67:361–368.

76. Robertson CS, Narayan RK, Gokaslan ZL, et al. Cerebral arteriovenous oxygen difference as an estimate of cerebral blood flow in comatose patients. *J Neurosurg* 1989;70:222–230.

77. Robertson JH. Neurosurgery and industry. *J Neurosurg* 2008;109:979–988.

78. Rosner MJ, Daughton S. Cerebral perfusion pressure management in head injury. *J Trauma* 1990;30:933–940.

79. Rothman DJ, Chimonas S. New developments in managing physician-industry relationships. *JAMA* 2008;300:1067–1069.

80. Sadaka F, Kasal J, Lakshmanan R, Palagiri A. Placement of intracranial pressure monitors by neurointensivists: case series and a systematic review. *Brain Inj* 2013;27:600–604.

81. Scheufler KM, Rohrborn HJ, Zentner J. Does tissue oxygen-tension reliably reflect cerebral oxygen delivery and consumption? *Anesth Analg* 2002;95:1042–1048.

82. Schickner DJ, Young RF. Intracranial pressure monitoring: fiberoptic monitor compared with the ventricular catheter. *Surg Neurol* 1992;37:251–254.

83. Schoser BG, Riemenschneider N, Hansen HC. The impact of raised intracranial pressure on cerebral venous hemodynamics: a prospective venous transcranial Doppler ultrasonography study. *J Neurosurg* 1999;91:744–749.

84. Severinghaus JW, Kelleher JF. Recent developments in pulse oximetry. *Anesthesiology* 1992;76:1018–1038.

85. Sheinberg M, Kanter MJ, Robertson CS, et al. Continuous monitoring of jugular venous oxygen saturation in head-injured patients. *J Neurosurg* 1992;76:212–217.

86. Soldatos T, Chatzimichail K, Papathanasiou M, Gouliamos A. Optic nerve sonography: a new window for the non-invasive evaluation of intracranial pressure in brain injury. *Emerg Med J* 2009;26:630–634.

87. Spiotta AM, Stiefel MF, Gracias VH, et al. Brain tissue oxygen-directed management and outcome in patients with severe traumatic brain injury. *J Neurosurg* 2010;113:571–580.

88. Squara P, Bennett D, Perret C. Pulmonary artery catheter: does the problem lie in the users? *Chest* 2002;121:2009–2015.

89. Stahl N, Schalen W, Ungerstedt U, Nordstrom CH. Bedside biochemical monitoring of the penumbra zone surrounding an evacuated acute subdural haematoma. *Acta Neurol Scand* 2003;108:211–215.

90. Stiefel MF, Spiotta A, Gracias VH, et al. Reduced mortality rate in patients with severe traumatic brain injury treated with brain tissue oxygen monitoring. *J Neurosurg* 2005;103:805–811.

91. Sundbarg G, Nordstrom CH, Soderstrom S. Complications due to prolonged ventricular fluid pressure recording. *Br J Neurosurg* 1988;2:485–495.

92. Tateishi A, Maekawa T, Soejima Y, et al. Qualitative comparison of carbon dioxide-induced change in cerebral near-infrared spectroscopy versus jugular venous oxygen saturation in adults with acute brain disease. *Crit Care Med* 1995;23:1734–1738.

93. Thees C, Scholz M, Schaller MDC, et al. Relationship between intracranial pressure and critical closing pressure in patients with neurotrauma. *Anesthesiology* 2002;96:595–599.

94. Turton FE, Snyder L. Physician-industry relations. *Ann Intern Med* 2007;146:469.

95. Vespa P, Bergsneider M, Hattori N, et al. Metabolic crisis without brain ischemia is common after traumatic brain injury: a combined microdialysis and positron emission tomography study. *J Cereb Blood Flow Metab* 2005;25:763–774.

96. Villringer A, Steinbrink J, Obrig H. Editorial comment—cerebral near-infrared spectroscopy: how far away from a routine diagnostic tool? *Stroke* 2004;35:70–72.

97. von Helden A, Schneider GH, Unterberg A, Lanksch WR. Monitoring of jugular venous oxygen saturation in comatose patients with subarachnoid haemorrhage and intracerebral haematomas. *Acta Neurochir Suppl (Wien)* 1993;59:102–106.

98. Wahr JA, Tremper KK, Samra S, Delpy DT. Near-infrared spectroscopy: theory and applications. *J Cardiothorac Vasc Anesth* 1996;10:406–418.

99. Watanabe A, Kinouchi H, Horikoshi T, Uchida M, Ishigame K. Effect of intracranial pressure on the diameter of the optic nerve sheath. *J Neurosurg* 2008;109:255–258.

100. Weinstabl C, Richling B, Plainer B, Czech T, Spiss CK. Comparative analysis between epidural (Gaeltec) and subdural (Camino) intracranial pressure probes. *J Clin Monit* 1992;8:116–120.

101. Williams EJ, Bunch CS, Carpenter TA, et al. Magnetic resonance imaging compatibility testing of intracranial pressure probes. Technical note. *J Neurosurg* 1999;91:706–709.

102. Wright K, Young P, Brickman C, et al. Rates and determinants of ventriculostomy-related infections during a hospital transition to use of antibiotic-coated external ventricular drains. *Neurosurg Focus*. 2013;34:E12.

103. Young CC, Mark JB, White W, et al. Clinical evaluation of continuous noninvasive blood pressure monitoring: accuracy and tracking capabilities. *J Clin Monit* 1995;11:245–252.

24

Transcranial Doppler Ultrasound and Neurophysiology

Neurologists who care for patients with a critical neurologic illness commonly order and interpret neuroimaging studies, particularly computed tomography (CT) angiograms and CT perfusion, magnetic resonance imaging (MRI), magnetic resonance angiography (MRA), and cerebral angiography. These technologies remain the daily tools of the trade. The most pertinent neuroradiologic features in acute neurologic conditions are discussed and illustrated in the chapters of Part VII of this book. Transcranial Doppler ultrasonography (TCD) and electrodiagnostic tests such as electroencephalography (EEG) or continuous video electroencephalographic monitoring are just as common diagnostic tests in the neurosciences intensive care unit (NICU). This chapter discusses the value of transcranial Doppler ultrasound, EEG, and evoked potentials. Neurointensivists should have a thorough knowledge of these diagnostic studies.

TRANSCRANIAL DOPPLER ULTRASONOGRAPHY

The use of TCD in the NICU has generated both enthusiasm and criticism. The precise clinical implications of results obtained by TCD are not always clear. Currently, data are obtained with a single examination. Continuous TCD monitoring (using a probe cradled in a tight headset) may increase its practical use but is not commonplace.

General Principles of Transcranial Doppler Ultrasonography Examination

The technique of TCD is easy to master, but requires that the examiner be familiar with the three-dimensional planes of the circle of Willis.[59,68] Insonation from a temporal window is started first. Several strategies can be tried to obtain adequate TCD signals. The probe is positioned directly above the zygomatic arch, with the transducer often resting on the zygomatic

arch midway from the helix of the ear to the orbital rim. A reliable signal can be obtained by coating the transducer with acoustic gel and pressing it to the temporal bone. A slow circular movement of the end of the transducer without a change in contact may help in finding a signal. A signal identifying the middle cerebral artery (MCA) can be obtained at a starting depth of 55 mm. If a signal is not found, the probe is shifted more anteriorly toward the orbital rim. If a signal is still not found, the probe is moved upward at the crossing of the zygomatic bone and the lateral orbital margin. Approximately 10% of patients do not have a temporal window, and failure to find a signal cannot be attributed to technique. (Two major reviews can be consulted for further refinements in the examination technique.[3,50]) Doppler examination can proceed only when a reliable signal is identified. No particular prerequisites are necessary. The patient must be immobilized and not continuously moving or speaking. Hyperventilation decreases the mean MCA velocities by 5 cm/sec, an amount often too small to measure.

The typical Doppler waveform (Figure 24.1) shows the peak systolic velocity (PSV) and end-diastolic velocity (EDV) needed to measure the mean velocity (PSV – EDV/3 + EDV). The pulsatility index indicates the resistance in the system.

An obstructive lesion proximal to the point of insonation has a lengthened rise time and dampening of the peak systolic and end-diastolic components from loss of pressure across the proximal obstruction. Increased pulsatility index typically occurs proximal to the lesion, because maximal vasodilatation from intact autoregulation produces less resistance and therefore increased pulsation. Abnormalities in absolute values, relative difference of more than 50% from each side, and turbulence, if present, producing a cracked or harsh sound and localized focal reversal of the signal, should be noted.

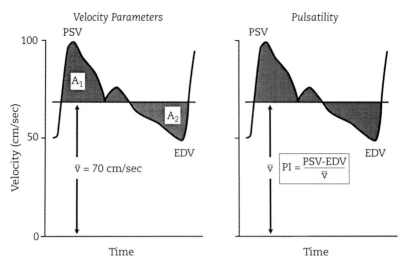

FIGURE 24.1: Typical Doppler waveform and measurement of mean velocity ($\bar{v}$) and pulsatility index (PI). *Left panel:* A cursor is placed so that the area above the cursor (A_1, defined by the peak velocity display) is equal to the area below the cursor (A_2, defined by the diastole display). *Right panel:* The PI, usually automatically calculated on transcranial Doppler machines, is the difference between the maximal and the minimal velocities, divided by the mean velocity.

EDV, end-diastolic velocity; PSV, peak systolic velocity.

Again, a common technique is to start by identifying the MCA signal at 55 mm (Figure 24.2a). Flow is directed toward the probe, and typical mean velocities are in the range of 50–60 cm/sec. Next, the probe is held constant while the depth is advanced incrementally to 60–65 mm. A bidirectional signal becomes apparent, identifying the bifurcation of the MCA and the anterior cerebral artery (ACA) (Figure 24.2b). The ACA signal is further investigated by minor repositioning of the probe upward and anteriorly and by an increase in depth to 70–80 mm. The ACA velocities (50 cm/sec) are slightly lower than the MCA velocities (Figure 24.2c).

Subsequently, the internal carotid artery (ICA) is identified by reducing the depth of the probe to 60–65 mm and adjusting the angle of the probe to relocate the MCA–ACA signal (Figure 24.2d). From this important landmark, the probe is angulated downward, but this time without any change in depth. The ICA is characterized by flow directed toward the probe. The velocities of the terminal part of the ICA are lower (40 cm/sec) (Figure 24.2e).

The last vessel to be insonated, the posterior cerebral artery (PCA), is found by again relocating the bifurcation signal, MCA–ACA (Figure 24.2f), and angling the probe downward and toward the occiput, with only minimal increments (5 mm) in depth but to a total depth of up to 80 mm. The PCA signal can be confused with the MCA because of its similar characteristics, but the sound of the PCA signal is lower pitched (Figure 24.2g). When the result is in doubt during bedside examination, compression of the carotid artery often dampens the MCA signal, or use of a very bright light can reveal increased flow in the PCA signal.

Although less in vogue, examination of the carotid siphon is done through the orbit. The signal of the siphon can provide additional information when no signal can be found through temporal windows. For example, this may be of benefit in patients with acute carotid artery occlusion (to estimate the extent of the thrombus) and in brain dead patients (when no second window is available). The probe is placed over the closed eyelid and against the glabella. Information can be obtained from the ophthalmic artery at a depth of 35 mm (Figure 24.3a) and of the siphon at 50–70 mm (Figure 24.3b).

Examination of the posterior circulation by TCD is useful in patients with acute basilar artery occlusion and in those with ruptured basilar aneurysm with vasospasm. The probe is placed just under the occipital crest in the midline with the patient in the side-lying position. The posterior window through the foramen magnum can be opened only with considerable head flexion, which is limited in patients with neck stiffness

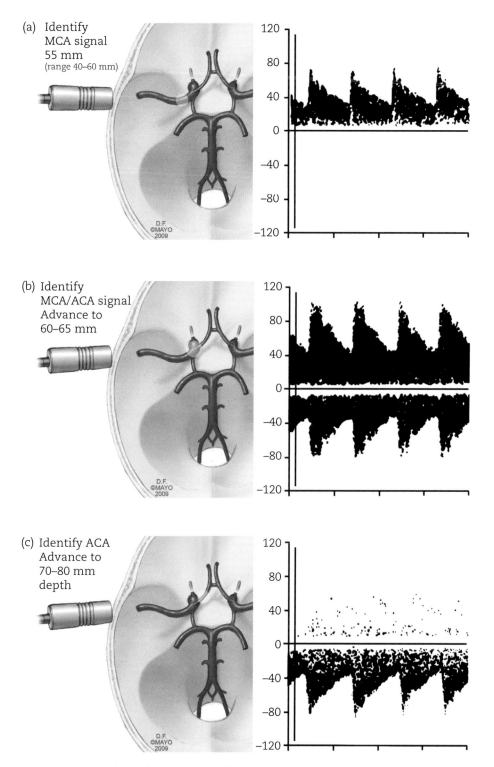

FIGURE 24.2: Transcranial Doppler ultrasonography: temporal window technique. (a) Middle cerebral artery (MCA) signal. (b) Bifurcation of the MCA and anterior cerebral artery (ACA) signal. (c) ACA signal.

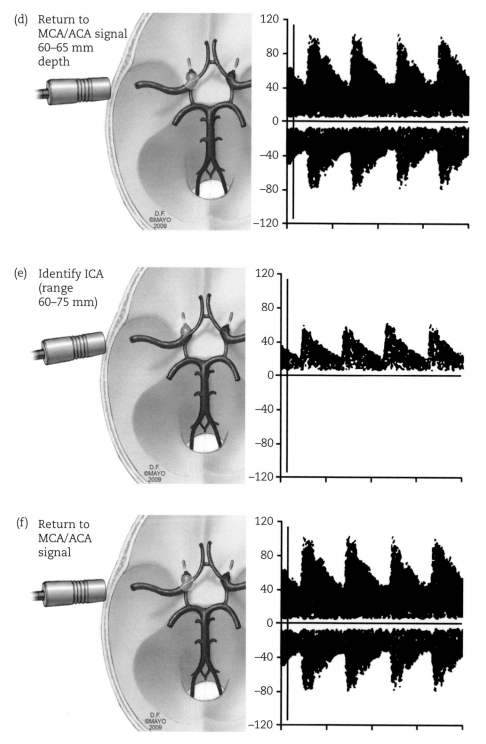

FIGURE 24.2: (d) Relocation of the MCA–ACA signal. (e) Internal carotid artery (ICA) signal. (f) Relocation of the MCA–ACA signal.

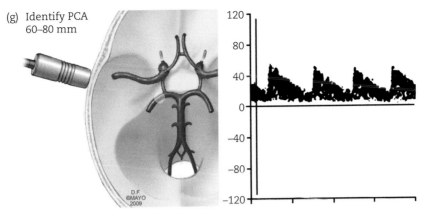

FIGURE 24.2: (g) Posterior cerebral artery (PCA) signal.

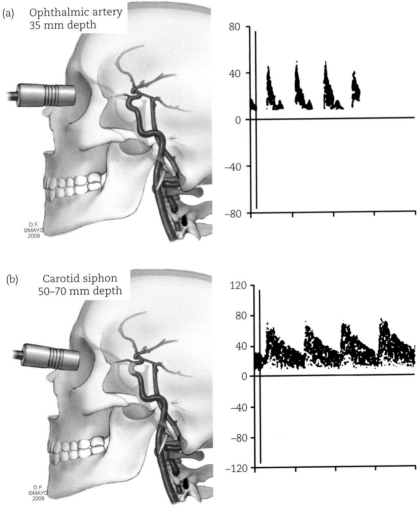

FIGURE 24.3: Transcranial Doppler ultrasonography through the orbital window. (a) Ophthalmic artery. (b) Carotid siphon.

from subarachnoid hemorrhage (SAH). The probe is advanced to a depth of 60 mm, where the vertebral artery is identified (Figure 24.4a). As expected, flow is away from the probe on both sides. Advancing the depth to 120 mm insonates the major part of the basilar artery (Figure 24.4b).

Carotid artery dissection can be investigated by TCD as well. The technique with a submandibular approach is demonstrated in Figure 24.5.

Transcranial Doppler Ultrasonography in Acute Neurologic Conditions

There is sufficient evidence that TCD findings complement clinical assessment in acute neurologic conditions.[50,58] This section describes the usefulness and limitations of TCD in specific clinical neurologic disorders.

Aneurysmal Subarachnoid Hemorrhage

Cerebral vasospasm is very common after SAH, and angiographic studies have reported incidences of up to 50%. By TCD criteria, vasospasm has been reported in 30% of patients with SAH.[22–24,29,51] This marked difference in frequency has been explained by the inability of TCD to assess the distal vasculature, but in some studies may also reflect a selection of patients with SAH at low risk of delayed cerebral ischemia. The sensitivity

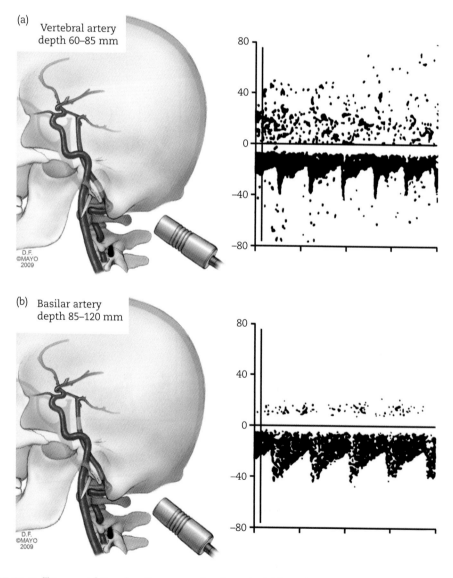

FIGURE 24.4: Transcranial Doppler ultrasonography of vertebral (a) and basilar artery (b) through the occipital window.

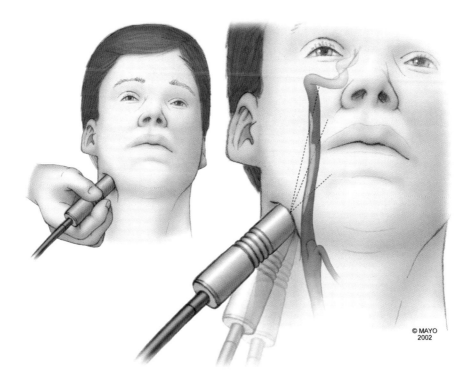

© MAYO
2002

FIGURE 24.5: Submandibular technique. Insonation at the mandibular angle may identify increased flow velocities in patients with carotid artery stenosis and in patients with carotid artery dissection.

of TCD for vasospasm in the middle cerebral artery is 60%–80%, with virtually 95% specificity in several studies.[7,41,43,65,67,73] The sensitivity for vasospasm in the ACA in SAH is only approximately 20%.[41] Sensitivities of TCD for the basilar and vertebral arteries are 77% and 44%, respectively, and specificities, 79% and 88%, respectively.[43] One study suggested that age may affect mean flow velocity, and thus older patients may have comparatively lower thresholds for TCD-associated vasospasm.[67]

Unfortunately, strict criteria for cerebral vasospasm have not been clearly established and may be difficult to define anyway. Most laboratories accept the following criteria: MCA mean velocity of ≥ 120 cm/sec, Lindegaard MCA–ICA velocity ratio of > 3 or marked turbulence. Turbulence is recognized as brief low frequency components in the mirror image of the TCD spectrum located close to the zero line, and musical sounds in the insonated arteries with increased velocities. With a higher cutoff of at least 130 cm/sec, others have found that the specificity is 100% in ICA and 87% in MCA.[7] At the extreme, one group believes that only flow velocities of more than 200 cm/sec reliably predict angiographically significant vasospasm (positive predictive value of 87%).[73]

Increased flow velocities on TCD strongly indicate cerebral vasospasm on angiography, but their presence often does not precede clinical deterioration from cerebral vasospasm.[39] It has been suggested, however, that a relative increase in MCA velocities in the first days has some predictive value for the development of symptomatic vasospasm. A study from Southern General Hospital in Glasgow found that delayed cerebral ischemia developed in more than 60% of patients with a relative velocity increase of 50 cm/sec in the MCA segment within 24 hours. A typical example of developing cerebral vasospasm in SAH on TCD is shown in Figure 24.6.

Important practical questions remain on how to use TCD in the daily assessment of patients with SAH. Routine TCD may lead to a change in management in almost half of the cases,[29,74,75] but its effect on outcome is not clear. It is not known exactly whether TCD reduces the need for angiography. This has become an important issue because the use of cerebral angiography has increased in the management of SAH since the introduction of interventional neuroradiologic procedures. Angioplasty has been advocated for patients with focal vasospasm and intra-arterial papaverine for those with diffuse vasospasm. The predictive value

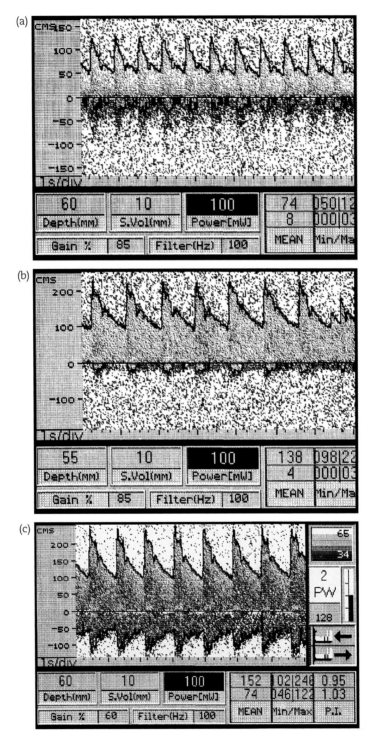

FIGURE 24.6: Sequential transcranial Doppler ultrasonography in subarachnoid hemorrhage. (a) Normal velocities in middle cerebral artery (MCA). (b) Two days later, mean velocities are increased. (c) Further increases in velocities. (The patient remained asymptomatic during all three recordings.)

of TCD in focal symptomatic vasospasm is not known, although one small series suggested a possible connection.[29] Unfortunately, angiographic studies in several of our patients with a suggestion of unilateral ACA or MCA spasm on TCD found diffuse cerebral vasospasm without any clear focal segments that could be eligible for angioplasty.

Another important clinical question is whether initial TCD findings of cerebral vasospasm should call for more aggressive fluid management. Although this approach is unproven and potentially leads to more complications associated with hypervolemia, we often feel the need to deliberately increase fluid intake in patients with large amounts of cisternal blood on CT and a recent increase in MCA velocities (more than 50 m/sec between studies). The manipulation of blood pressure may increase TCD velocities in the insonated MCA segment, and this effect should not be misinterpreted as worsening vasospasm. In one study, 53% of patients had an increase in TCD velocities of more than 15%.[44]

Transcranial Doppler ultrasonographic findings of cerebral vasospasm theoretically may influence the timing of surgery. Some neurosurgeons are reluctant to clip an aneurysm if TCD supports cerebral vasospasm, and others ignore the findings. However, the timing of surgery remains dependent on the World Federation of Neurological Surgeons' clinical grade at admission. The findings on TCD alone probably should not influence planning of aneurysmal clipping or coil placement.

Rebleeding in SAH has been diagnosed by TCD. In extreme circumstances, a patient rebleeds during a routine TCD study. Rebleeding results in a massive surge in intra-cranial pressure (ICP) and produces a reversible TCD pattern with small systolic peaks and diastolic reversal, findings that strongly mimic patterns seen in brain death. (In some patients with rebleeding, these brain death patterns on TCD may be real and remain.)

Transcranial Doppler ultrasonographic findings in postoperative patients with successful clipping of an aneurysm are notoriously difficult to interpret. Postoperative TCD may demonstrate increased velocities from hyperemia or aggressive hypervolemic treatment. On the other hand, the effect of surgery alone has been studied, and only minor increases in velocity may be seen, rarely above 120 cm/sec. Therefore, in postoperative patients with secondary deterioration in the first 24 hours, swelling from prolonged retraction is difficult to differentiate from cerebral vasospasm by TCD. Normal TCD values or improved velocities (if results of previous studies are available for

comparison) preclude vasospasm and may defer cerebral angiography; but in any other patient with a decreased level of consciousness or new focal signs and increased TCD velocities, a confirmatory cerebral angiography may be indicated.

Traumatic Brain Injury

Studies of TCD in traumatic brain injury (TBI) have shown potential usefulness.[21] However, the experience with TCD in TBI is very limited, and in most instances the diagnosis of vasospasm by TCD criteria has been made in patients with large amounts of traumatic subarachnoid blood.[46,64] One study in 66 patients with TBI showed an increase in MCA velocities at a maximum of 5–7 days after the impact. In this study, cerebral angiographic confirmation of possible cerebral vasospasm was not available and, more important, clinical deterioration from cerebral infarction did not follow.[64]

Noninvasive measurement of ICP by TCD in traumatic brain injury has been a disappointing experience. Only in patients with a considerable increase in ICP (more than 60 mm Hg) are changes expected in the TCD waveform configuration. These changes include a decrease in cerebral perfusion pressure resulting in an increase in PSV and a decrease in diastolic velocity. The pulsatility index increases, but the relationship between pulsatility index and ICP is weak.[64] Transcranial Doppler ultrasonography is of value only in a patient with a steep systolic fall-off and marked reduction in diastolic flow, but again this situation usually occurs at a point when ICP equals diastolic blood pressure (Figure 24.7). Transcranial Doppler ultrasonography, therefore, may have limited value in the assessment of comatose patients with TBI to determine in which patient an intracranial monitoring device is placed. Transcranial Doppler ultra-sonography has been used in experimental settings, however, to study defective autoregulation.[13] Transcranial Doppler ultrasonography in TBI could even be diagnostic for development of swollen contusional masses. Reduced velocities and high pulsatility index were found in a small series of patients with TBI, and these findings require further study using continuous TCD monitoring.[46]

Thus, in clinical practice, TCD has very limited value in patients with severe TBI. Its use is justified in those at risk for cerebral vasospasm; but when increased values are found, it is virtually impossible to distinguish between cerebral vasospasm and hyperemia from vasomotor paralysis.[21] In research projects, TCD has value in estimating ICP and autoregulation.

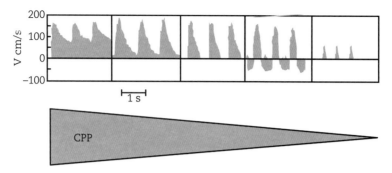

FIGURE 24.7: Progressive transcranial Doppler changes in patients with increased intracranial pressure. CPP, cerebral perfusion pressure; V, velocity; s, second.

Acute Ischemic Stroke

Transcranial Doppler ultrasonography can be used to demonstrate intracranial ICA stenosis (70%–90% sensitivity), MCA main stem obstructions (70%–100% sensitivity), and vertebral artery stenosis (70% sensitivity).[8,10,38,42] In these patients, TCD demonstrates significantly increased velocities on the side of the stenosis, with a decreased pulsatility index at the level of the stenosis. The normal physiologic direction should be maintained. In general, a marked increase in velocity indicates a focal intracranial stenosis. Lesions producing greater than 60% stenosis should be detectable by TCD. Middle cerebral artery stenosis in general produces velocities greater than 100 cm/sec; a basilar artery stenosis is within the range of 50–150 cm/sec.

The diagnostic capability of TCD in vertebral and carotid dissection is promising. (In one study, 8 of 10 patients with vertebral dissection had abnormalities, largely a high-resistance signal.[28]) However, in many of these patients, MRA is indicated. Transcranial Doppler ultrasonography may also have a role in monitoring and facilitating thrombolysis.[34] Transcranial Doppler ultrasonography in acute MCA occlusion may document recanalization during intravenous tPA. A combination of TCD and infusion of microbubbles accelerating clot dissolution with sonic energy is currently being tested.[48]

Brain Death

Patients who fulfill the clinical criteria of brain death have waveforms similar to those in patients with markedly increased ICP. TCD is less reliable in patients with surgical skull defects due to lower ICPs, again emphasizing the mere fact that TCD is simply representing increased intracranial pressure.[66] Insonation of both MCA segments is required. The TCD criteria for brain death were summarized in a consensus statement of the World Federation of Neurology.[18] Typical brain death patterns are reversal of flow in diastole with a sharp systolic upstroke, systolic spike waveforms (Figure 24.8), and occasionally complete absence of flow in a patient with previously demonstrated TCD signal through the same temporal window.[4,17,18,57,60,63]

ELECTRODIAGNOSTIC STUDIES

Divergent opinions exist on the best way to monitor patients with an acute neurologic disorder. On the presumption that clinical features of deterioration are less reliable, several investigators examined continuous EEG monitoring in the NICU.[12,14,32,33,56,71,81,83] Intraoperative EEG monitoring is common practice during carotid endarterectomy, but the predictive value of intraoperative changes for perioperative stroke is quite poor, with a sensitivity of 50% and specificity of 70%.[30,45] Electrodiagnostic

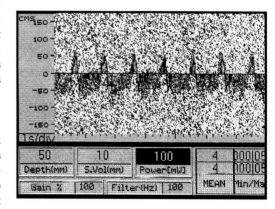

FIGURE 24.8: Transcranial Doppler ultrasonography in brain death. Typical tiny systolic peaks on transcranial Doppler ultrasonography are compatible with a clinical diagnosis of brain death.

monitoring undoubtedly has potential value in critically ill neurologic patients.[54,81,82] Most pioneering work has been performed at Columbia University, New York. An example of its value is demonstrated in Capsule 24.1. It is possible that EEG is underutilized, particularly in patients worsening from aneurysmal SAH or massive hemispheric stroke and in patients with fluctuating level of consciousness after a single seizure.

The possibility that a relatively simple technique of continuous EEG monitoring may increase the early recognition of nonconvulsive status epilepticus and confirm worsening of cerebral blood flow and ischemia is understandably important.[37] Unfortunately, hard data of a major role of EEG in monitoring patients in the NICU are lacking. Moreover, in monitored patients with a wide spectrum of acute neurologic disorders, EEG may not contribute to an already clinically evident changing situation. In addition, enthusiasm must be tempered because some of the EEG abnormalities may not have clinical relevance. A recent review pointed out the major problems in standardization and interpretation of EEGs.[52] The American Clinical Neurophysiology Society ICU continuous EEG (cEEG) standardized terminology is one attempt at ICU cEEG terminology standardization.[27] Many of us have struggled differentiating between nonconvulsive status epilepticus and triphasic waves. One of the most interesting patterns are periodic lateralized epileptiform discharges (PLEDS) and generalized periodic epileptiform discharges (GPEDS). PLEDS are morphologically sharp waves, spikes, slow waves, or combinations. They can be seen in any new structural lesion, but these morphologies should not be considered seizures if they do not progress to low-amplitude rhythmic discharges.

Continuous EEG monitoring may only be helpful in patients who had earlier seizures recognized clinically or during management of status epilepticus. In our unit, we have the capability of video monitoring of patients at risk for seizures, and we found that cEEG monitoring is useful in selected patients. In a recent study cEEG of 625 monitored patients (with multiple clinical diagnosis or no clinical diagnoses such "altered mental status"), seizures were found in 27%. (The first seizure occurred within 30 min of monitoring in 58% of monitored patients.) In 3 days the risk of seizures declined below 5% if no epileptiform abnormalities were present in the first two hours, whereas 16 hours of monitoring were required when epileptiform discharges were present. Only 4% of monitored patients experienced a seizure without preceding epileptiform abnormalities.[77]

Serial EEGs or evoked potentials may continue to have significant value in a variety of acute neurologic disorders.[61] The use of cEEG monitoring has increased our awareness of the possibility of nonconvulsive status epilepticus in patients with acute neurologic catastrophes. In addition, EEG may have some prognostic value.[71] In this section, EEGs and evoked potentials are discussed as useful diagnostic tests, rather than as means for monitoring. A recent consensus on the applicability of electrophysiology in the ICU has been published, but a critical evidence-based evaluation of these modalities has not been performed.[25] Electrocorticography is an area which has become an interesting research field to study changes in a variety of pathologies (Capsule 24.2).

Electroencephalography

In patients with critical neurologic illness, the EEG continues to be a useful adjunct to clinical observation and, in the proper situation, supports the clinical diagnosis.

Encephalitis

The EEG has an important role in the early diagnosis of encephalitis, particularly herpes simplex encephalitis. Most patients with a presumed diagnosis of viral encephalitis are admitted to the NICU with impaired level of consciousness or coma, often unable to protect their airway and in need of intubation and mechanical ventilation. Magnetic resonance imaging cannot be performed easily in these patients, and in some patients cerebrospinal fluid (CSF) findings are nondiagnostic or equivocal. Fairly early in herpes simplex encephalitis, the EEG shows polymorphic δ activity over the temporal lobes, which suggests preferential involvement of these regions.[63] Although nonspecific for herpes simplex encephalitis, focal or lateralized sharp- or slow-wave complexes emerge early and eventually become periodic, usually after 1 or 2 days of illness (Figure 24.9). Sharp waves may occur almost continuously or several seconds apart, and may evolve into more distinctive seizure discharges, recognized by repetitive sharp and slow waves or bursts of spike waves. Periodic complexes in the acute phase may indicate a more severe involvement.[63]

Many other encephalitides have diffuse slow-wave abnormalities, and the degree of slowing is often directly related to the severity of the infection.

The main arguments for using continuous EEG monitoring are (1) increase in seizure detection,[2,19,55,56] (2) the value of predicting poor outcome in certain EEG patterns,[37,71] (3) a quantification with compressed spectral array that may correlate with abnormal cerebral blood flow,[78] and (4) the monitoring of cerebral vasospasm in SAH and titration of hemodynamic augmentation using EEG charges.[12]

The main drawbacks are cost (equipment, staffing, time-consuming evaluation), artifacts, and less-than-perfect interrater reliability when tested.[37]

The accompanying figure shows the capability of detecting changes in EEG spectral power.

A plot of the average hemispheric spectral power for each frequency (0–20) versus time for 12 hours or recording depicts several neurologic events in a 76-year-old patient with a small right subdural hematoma and an altered consciousness. Transient increases of power, especially in the higher frequencies (black arrows), indicate brief right hemisphere nonconvulsive seizures (see b_1 for example raw EEG tracing). The patient was being maintained on multiple antiepileptic drugs but nonconvulsive seizures persisted. Seizures then resolved without further treatment (dotted black line and b_2). This turned out to be due to acidosis from CO_2 retention. The patient was then tracheally intubated (blue arrow), and seizures returned approximately 2 hours later (just before the solid black line). Afterward, the patient progressed to nonconvulsive status epilepticus (NCSE), which appears as a prolonged period of escalating spectral power on quantitative EEG (qEEG) analysis (solid line, b_3). Finally, the patient was given an IV bolus (red arrow) and continuous infusion of midazolam, which lead to suppression of most EEG frequencies (b_4).

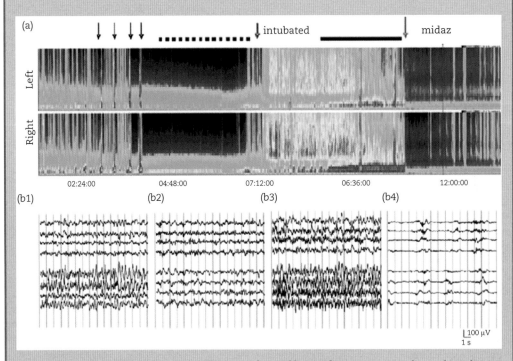

Quantitative electroencephalogram (EEG) review of several hours of continuous EEG data and trending of pathological changes in brain function.

From Friedman D, Claassen J, Hirsch LJ. Continuous electroencephalogram monitoring in the intensive care unit. Anesth Analg 2009;109:506–523. Used with permission.

CAPSULE 24.2   SPREADING DEPOLARIZATION

Another way of evaluating neuronal distress is monitoring patients for the appearance of spreading depolarization.[16,26,31] The basic premise behind this concept is that spreading depolarization of neurons reflects the breakdown of ion gradients. Mostly the sodium and calcium pumps provide insufficient outward current to balance the inward current of sodium and potassium, leading to inactivation of action potentials at the membrane channels. During spreading depolarization, neuronal signaling is markedly depressed; and this mechanism may play a role in anoxic ischemic injury, hypoglycemia, status epilepticus, or traumatic brain injury.[40,72,79] These abnormalities can only be detected using subdural electrodes providing an electrocorticography and, therefore, only in selected patients. It is assumed that these repetitive spreading depolarizations are indicative of neuronal injury and could also be used to monitor the development of cerebral ischemia. When this depolarization occurs, the circulation either becomes hyperdynamic or hypodynamic, which may further progress the ischemia and neuronal distress; hence, the spreading of depolarization. The study of spreading depression is organized through the COSBID group.

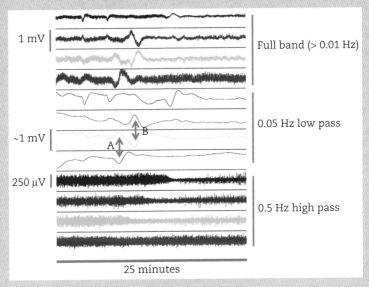

Example of a single spreading depolarization event following craniotomy for a traumatic intracerebral hematoma. A Wyler 6-contact subdural electrode strip was placed on cortex judged salvageable, and adjacent to the location of the core lesion. A sequential bipolar montage was used, such that each trace is the voltage recorded between a pair of adjacent electrodes. Preamplifier input frequency range extended down to approximately 0.01 Hz. Time and voltage scales are illustrative only: note the time compression used for display. With low pass filtering, the typical slow potential change (SPC) of a spreading depolarization is seen first on cortex corresponding to the lowest two traces (A), as illustrated by the phase inversion on the electrode shared by the two traces. As the depolarization spreads along the electrode strip, phase inversion is seen at cortex corresponding to the next electrode (B). In traces filtered at 0.5 Hz high pass, typical of "standard" EEG recording filter settings, low-pass event A is associated with barely perceptible loss of EEG amplitude, but this becomes progressively more apparent as the wave moves along the contact strip. In some 20%–30% of cases, sequences of multiple, stereotyped events are observed, often recurring at remarkably constant intervals of between 20 and 50 minutes: this recurrent activity is believed to represent the repetitive cycling of a single depolarization around the entire perimeter of a focus of permanently depolarized and unsalvageable cortex.[49] The highest total number of SPCs recorded from a single patient during a 4-day monitoring is approximately 100 events.

Kindly provided by Dr. Martin Fabricius, Rigshospitalet Copenhagen.

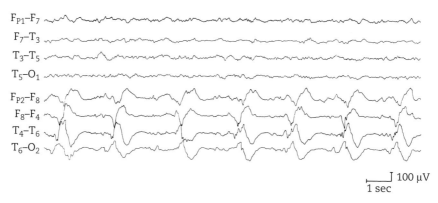

FIGURE 24.9: Typical periodic lateralized sharp waves in herpes simplex encephalitis. Courtesy of Dr. B. F. Westmoreland.

Stroke

A preliminary study found deterioration in EEG patterns before clinical deterioration in patients with ischemic stroke.[47] These EEG abnormalities consisted of increasing focal slow activity, onset of epileptiform activity, or appearance of generalized slowing. The nature of these abnormalities was not clear, although they were tentatively attributed to worsening ischemia. Indeed, earlier studies suggested that an increase in mean arterial pressure to the extreme value of 150 mm Hg resulted in clinical and EEG improvement. This observation needs further refinement and confirmation before EEG abnormalities prompt the additional use of vasopressors in stroke.[80]

Electroencephalography, however, has some use in prognostication. A study found that prominent continuous and polymorphic δ activity, together with slowing or depression of the α or β activity in the ischemic hemisphere, predicted poor functional outcome[11] (Figure 24.10). Recovery was more likely with absence of slow activity and no decrease in α frequency or μ rhythm.

Seizures and Status Epilepticus

Acute structural lesions of the central nervous system may be accompanied by or present with seizures. Focal seizures are somewhat more common and may be therapy-resistant.

At the time of recording of status epilepticus, most EEG tracings show continuous epileptic discharges (Figure 24.11a) or periodic lateralized epileptiform discharges (PLEDs). These periodic discharges may be associated with focal twitches in the eyelids, face, arm, or leg, but more often PLEDs are interictal phenomena.

Patients with generalized tonic-clonic seizures that evolve into status epilepticus and that are not controlled with intravenous fosphenytoin loading alone are often further managed with midazolam, or barbiturates. During this episode, EEG recording is very helpful in titrating the antiepileptic agent. These drugs generally are titrated to seizure-free EEG recordings rather than to a burst-suppression pattern. Further titrating to a burst-suppression (Figure 24.11b) or isoelectric EEG is indicated only when clinical seizures persist, but it may seriously complicate hemodynamic stability.

Breakthrough seizures during treatment of status epilepticus may be very subtle and may not be recognized clinically. Patients may display brief forced gaze that is not appreciated with the eyelids closed or barely noticeable eyelid twitching.

Recurrence of electrographic status epilepticus after at least two trials of midazolam, propofol, or barbiturates is associated with a poor outcome. In many of these patients, electrographic seizures are not associated with clinical manifestations, and they remain comatose, only to later awaken severely disabled.

Traumatic Brain Injury

A single EEG has limited value in patients with severe closed head injury.[5,6,15] Earlier studies of EEG in head injury commonly showed a generalized widespread slowing (θ and δ range of frequencies) that was associated with poor outcome if it persisted in the first 2 days after injury. The EEG has some prognostic value in comatose survivors of severe head injury but no clear pattern has emerged which could strongly indicate poor prognosis or could even be used to limit

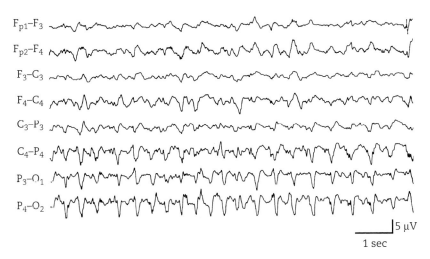

FIGURE 24.10: Seizure discharge associated with middle cerebral artery occlusion.

Courtesy of Dr. B. F. Westmoreland.

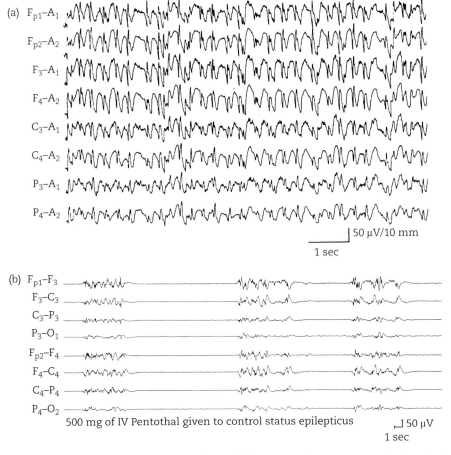

FIGURE 24.11. (a) Typical status epilepticus. (b) 500 mg of IV pentothal given to control epilepticus showing now burst-suppression.

Courtesy of Dr. B. F. Westmoreland.

care. *Spindle coma*—characterized by paroxysmal activity in the vertex and rolandic regions, but also more widespread, on a background of θ and δ waves—may potentially indicate a favorable outcome. However, α coma, burst-suppression, triphasic waves, and reduced α variability within 5 days of injury are electrographic patterns that indicate significant damage.[70]

In 22% of 94 patients, continuous EEG monitoring (from admission to 2 weeks) detected convulsive and nonconvulsive status epilepticus that was not recognized clinically in more than half the patients. All patients with status epilepticus after traumatic brain injury died; therefore, the value of monitoring for therapeutic intervention is very uncertain.[62] The EEG features in these patients may reflect severe brain injury rather than a treatable disorder.[71]

Brain Death

Many countries in the world mandate EEG or even serial EEG recordings to confirm brain death. In the United States, confirmatory tests in adults are considered only when certain components of clinical testing are less reliable.

Electroencephalography remains a useful test, and the long-term experience with interpretation in brain death is a major advantage over other tests.

Electrocerebral silence is defined as no electrical activity when high instrument activity is used (Figure 24.12). The recording should be done by an experienced technician.

The current recommendations published by the American Electroencephalographic Society are the following:

1. A minimum of eight scalp electrodes
2. Interelectrode impedances between 100 and 10,000 V
3. Interelectrode distance of at least 10 cm
4. Sensitivity increase up to 2 μV and time constant of 0.3–0.4 seconds
5. Recording of 30 minutes
6. Testing of EEG reactivity to pain stimuli and flashlight.

Noise signals on EEG in the NICU are significant because recordings are made with the sensitivity set high. These artifacts are associated with many electrical devices, such as mechanical ventilators, heating blankets to correct hypothermia, and intravenous infusion equipment.

Persistent EEG activity is still compatible with the clinical diagnosis of brain death, and residual activity may be observed in 20% of patients. In patients with brain death from a destructive pontine hemorrhage or acute basilar artery occlusion, a typical α coma (8–10 Hz; 15–50 μV) occurs, with widely distributed activity but little spontaneous variability and no response to pain or visual stimuli.[76] In other patients with destructive brainstem lesions, spindle and diffuse δ activity alternating with α coma is observed.[53,76]

Evoked Potentials

Evoked potentials are used sparingly in critically ill patients with neurologic disorders but there may be a renewed interest.[35] Future developments may make continuous monitoring possible, with a potentially promising application for somatosensory potentials.[1] Of the available techniques, somatosensory evoked potential (SSEP) is most often used; the additional value of brainstem auditory evoked potential (BAEP) and visual evoked potential in the clinical assessment of patients with acute neurologic illness has been disappointing. Currently, SSEPs are most often used for prognosis in traumatic brain injury and anoxic–ischemic encephalopathy. The recent development of motor evoked potentials may have promise, although currently no studies in critically ill patients are available.

Auditory stimulation to the acoustic nerve (usually clicks through headphones) generates BAEPs with a typical waveform. The wave I latency (distal portion of the acoustic nerve), wave I–III interpeak latency (tract of the proximal eighth nerve to the inferior pons), and wave III–IV interpeak latency (tract between caudal pons and midbrain) are used for interpretation (Figure 24.13).

The applications of BAEPs in patients with acute neurologic illness are limited to head injury and confirmation of the clinical diagnosis of brain death. Brainstem auditory-evoked potentials have recently been explored in patients with brainstem compression from a large supratentorial mass. Several studies, however, have suggested that BAEPs can be useful in testing brainstem integrity. Whether BAEPs provide important information not already known from the clinical examination or intracranial monitoring remains to be investigated. Indeed, one study in patients with deteriorating hemispheric mass lesions suggested marginal additional predictive value.[36]

Another potential use is the assessment of brainstem function in patients with traumatic brain injury who are comatose and who

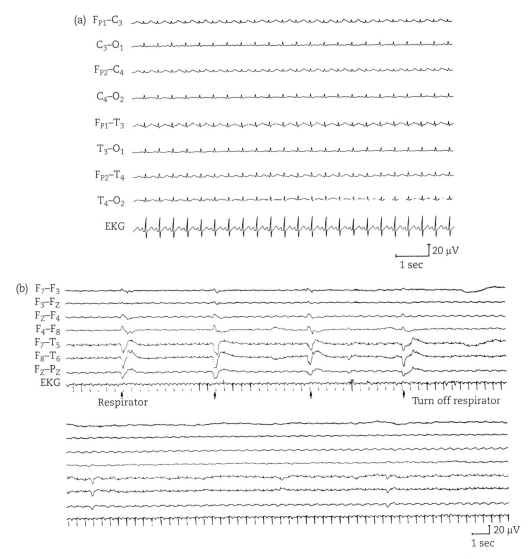

FIGURE 24.12: Electroencephalograms in brain death. Note (a) electrocardiographic artifact and (b) respirator artifact disappearing after briefly shutting off ventilator.

Courtesy of Dr. B. F. Westmoreland.

need barbiturate treatment for control of ICP. Brainstem auditory evoked potentials can also be helpful in patients who have lost most of their clinical brainstem function from presumed intoxication, in which case the results of BAEP studies are normal.

The prognostic value of BAEPs has been studied in large series of patients with traumatic brain injury. Abnormalities are usually signaled by complete absence of the late responses. Wave I must remain identifiable, because deafness from damage to the cochlea or peripheral nerve at the temporal bone may eliminate the potential. One study[69] claimed that patients who lost waves III and IV died or remained in a persistent vegetative state. Two other studies found less accurate results but claimed that patients with bilaterally absent BAEP responses had a much higher likelihood of poor outcome and death.[38] (It should be noted that most patients in a persistent vegetative state have normal BAEP responses.)

Brainstem auditory evoked potential testing has also been examined in patients who fulfill the clinical criteria for brain death. Abnormal BAEP findings, however, may also be seen in patients

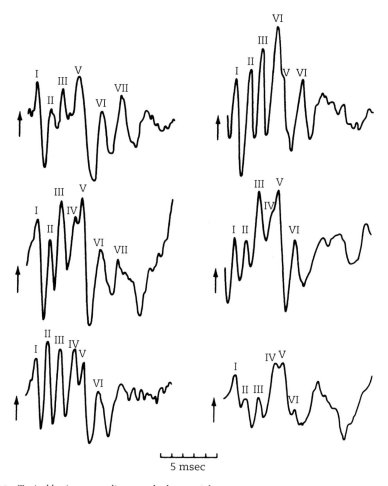

FIGURE 24.13: Typical brainstem auditory evoked potential response.

From Chiappa KH, Gladstone KJ, Young RR. Brain stem auditory evoked responses: studies of waveform variations in 50 normal human subjects. *Arch Neurol* 1979;36:81–87. With permission of the American Medical Association.

with a central nervous system catastrophe who do not yet fulfill the clinical criteria for brain death. A combined examination with SSEP may have more confirmatory value, particularly in patients with preserved EEG activity, but these studies are rarely used for this indication.[32]

In a study from the Massachusetts General Hospital, 27 patients who fulfilled the clinical criteria for brain death were tested with both SSEP and BAEP. In 16 patients, BAEP and central conduction responses were absent on SSEP; two patients had only BAEP wave I and no SSEP; one patient had BAEP waves I and II and no SSEP; and the remaining patients had no identifiable waves at all.[20]

Somatosensory evoked potentials may have more practical value in the NICU. Electrical stimulation of the median or tibial nerve results in an afferent volley that can be recorded at the cortex. Median nerve stimulation is easier to perform

and generally provides the information needed. The electrodes record from Erb's point, over the cervical spine process at C6, and over the scalp. The typical waveform is shown in Figure 24.14. It is assumed that the N13 waveform identifies the dorsal columns and nuclei and that the scalp potentials are correlated with the thalamocortical radiations. An advantage of SSEP recordings is that the waveforms could be recorded unchanged in patients in whom barbiturate treatment is producing suppressed EEGs.

The bilateral absence of N20 scalp potentials is a measure of poor prognosis.[9] In coma after cardiac resuscitation and traumatic head injury (both conditions often appear together in resuscitated trauma patients), this finding has been associated with a permanent vegetative state. Surprisingly, in a systematic review of SSEP in traumatic brain injury, 12 of 777 patients with

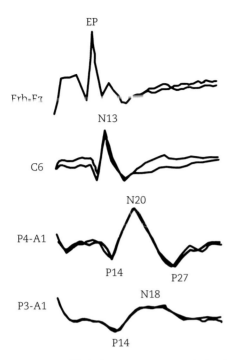

FIGURE 24.14: Typical somatosensory evoked potential (EP) with normal responses.

Erb's point, cervical spine, and bilateral scalp recordings represent the thalamocortical components from upper to lower tracings. Electrode positions: Erb, Erb's point (shoulder); Fz, midfrontal; C6, middle back of neck over C6 cervical vertebra; P4–A1 and P3–A1, scalp overlying the parietal cortex (odd numbers are left); A, earlobe.

bilaterally absent scalp potentials had a favorable outcome.[9]

CONCLUSION

- Transcranial Doppler ultrasound is most useful in the detection of cerebral vasospasm in SAH and in the diagnosis of brain death. Typical features of cerebral vasospasm are increased mean velocities ($\geq$ 120 cm/sec) and turbulence.
- Electroencephalogram is most useful in the NICU for the diagnosis of herpes simplex encephalitis, monitoring in status epilepticus, and guidance in therapy.
- Evoked potentials currently can be used only for prognostication. Poor outcome can be expected in patients with characteristic BAEP (III and IV waves absent) and SSEP (N20 potentials absent) abnormalities.
- Continuous EEG monitoring is commonly used to monitor for seizures and to assess effect of antiepileptic drugs.

REFERENCES

1. Amantini A, Amadori A, Fossi S. Evoked potentials in the ICU. *Eur J Anaesthesiol Suppl* 2008;42:196–202.
2. Andre-Obadia N, Parain D, Szurhaj W. Continuous EEG monitoring in adults in the intensive care unit (ICU). *Neurophysiol Clin* 2015;45:39–46.
3. Arnolds BJ, von Reutern GM. Transcranial Doppler sonography: examination technique and normal reference values. *Ultrasound Med Biol* 1986;12:115–123.
4. Azevedo E, Teixeira J, Neves JC, Vaz R. Transcranial Doppler and brain death. *Transplant Proc* 2000;32:2579–2581.
5. Bickford RG, Klass DW. Acute and chronic EEG findings after head injury. In: Caveness WF, Walker AE, eds. *Head Injury: Conference Proceedings.* Philadelphia: J. B. Lippincott; 1966:63–88.
6. Bricolo AP, Turella GS. Electrophysiology of head injury. In: Vinken PJ, Bruyn GW, Klawans HL, eds. *Handbook of Clinical Neurology.* Vol. 57; Revised Series 13. Amsterdam: Elsevier Science; 1990:181–206.
7. Burch CM, Wozniak MA, Sloan MA, et al. Detection of intracranial internal carotid artery and middle cerebral artery vasospasm following subarachnoid hemorrhage. *J Neuroimaging* 1996;6:8–15.
8. Camerlingo M, Casto L, Censori B, et al. Transcranial Doppler in acute ischemic stroke of the middle cerebral artery territories. *Acta Neurol Scand* 1993;88:108–111.
9. Carter BG, Butt W. Review of the use of somatosensory evoked potentials in the prediction of outcome after severe brain injury. *Crit Care Med* 2001;29:178–186.
10. Cher LM, Chambers BR, Smidt V. Comparison of transcranial Doppler with DSA in vertebrobasilar ischaemia. *Clin Exp Neurol* 1992;29:143–148.
11. Cillessen JP, van Huffelen AC, Kappelle LJ, Algra A, van Gijn J. Electroencephalography improves the prediction of functional outcome in the acute stage of cerebral ischemia. *Stroke* 1994;25:1968–1972.
12. Claassen J, Hirsch LJ, Frontera JA, et al. Prognostic significance of continuous EEG monitoring in patients with poor-grade subarachnoid hemorrhage. *Neurocrit Care* 2006;4:103–112.
13. Czosnyka M, Smielewski P, Piechnik S, Steiner LA, Pickard JD. Cerebral autoregulation following head injury. *J Neurosurg* 2001;95:756–763.
14. Daube JR, Rubin DI. *Clinical Neurophysiology.* 4th edition, New York: Oxford University Press; 2016.

15. Dawson RE, Webster JE, Gurdjian ES. Serial electroencephalography in acute head injuries. *J Neurosurg* 1951;8:613–630.
16. Dreier JP, Major S, Manning A, et al. Cortical spreading ischaemia is a novel process involved in ischaemic damage in patients with aneurysmal subarachnoid haemorrhage. *Brain* 2009;132:1866–1881.
17. Ducrocq X, Braun M, Debouverie M, et al. Brain death and transcranial Doppler: experience in 130 cases of brain dead patients. *J Neurol Sci* 1998;160:41–46.
18. Ducrocq X, Hassler W, Moritake K, et al. Consensus opinion on diagnosis of cerebral circulatory arrest using Doppler-sonography: Task Force Group on cerebral death of the Neurosonology Research Group of the World Federation of Neurology. *J Neurol Sci* 1998;159:145–150.
19. Gavvala J, Abend N, LaRoche S, et al. Continuous EEG monitoring: a survey of neurophysiologists and neurointensivists. *Epilepsia* 2014;55:1864–1871.
20. Goldie WD, Chiappa KH, Young RR, Brooks EB. Brainstem auditory and short-latency somatosensory evoked responses in brain death. *Neurology* 1981;31:248–256.
21. Gomez CR, Backer RJ, Bucholz RD. Transcranial Doppler ultrasound following closed head injury: vasospasm or vasoparalysis? *Surg Neurol* 1991;35:30–35.
22. Grosset DG, Straiton J, du Trevou M, Bullock R. Prediction of symptomatic vasospasm after subarachnoid hemorrhage by rapidly increasing transcranial Doppler velocity and cerebral blood flow changes. *Stroke* 1992;23:674–679.
23. Grosset DG, Straiton J, McDonald I, Bullock R. Angiographic and Doppler diagnosis of cerebral artery vasospasm following subarachnoid haemorrhage. *Br J Neurosurg* 1993;7:291–298.
24. Grosset DG, Straiton J, McDonald I, Cockburn M, Bullock R. Use of transcranial Doppler sonography to predict development of a delayed ischemic deficit after subarachnoid hemorrhage. *J Neurosurg* 1993;78:183–187.
25. Guerit JM, Amantini A, Amodio P, et al. Consensus on the use of neurophysiological tests in the intensive care unit (ICU): electroencephalogram (EEG), evoked potentials (EP), and electroneuromyography (ENMG). *Neurophysiol Clin* 2009;39:71–83.
26. Hartings JA, Bullock MR, Okonkwo DO, et al. Spreading depolarisations and outcome after traumatic brain injury: a prospective observational study. *Lancet Neurol* 2011;10:1058–1064.
27. Hirsch LJ, LaRoche SM, Gaspard N, et al. American Clinical Neurophysiology Society's Standardized Critical Care EEG Terminology: 2012 version. *J Clin Neurophysiol* 2013;30:1–27.
28. Hoffmann M, Sacco RL, Chan S, Mohr JP. Noninvasive detection of vertebral artery dissection. *Stroke* 1993;24:815–819.
29. Hurst RW, Schnee C, Raps EC, Farber R, Flamm ES. Role of transcranial Doppler in neuroradiological treatment of intracranial vasospasm. *Stroke* 1993;24:299–303.
30. Illig KA, Burchfiel JL, Ouriel K, et al. Value of preoperative EEG for carotid endarterectomy. *Cardiovasc Surg* 1998;6:490–495.
31. Jeffcote T, Hinzman JM, Jewell SL, et al. Detection of spreading depolarization with intraparenchymal electrodes in the injured human brain. *Neurocrit Care* 2014;20:21–31.
32. Jordan KG. Continuous EEG and evoked potential monitoring in the neuroscience intensive care unit. *J Clin Neurophysiol* 1993;10:445–475.
33. Jordan KG. Neurophysiologic monitoring in the neuroscience intensive care unit. *Neurol Clin* 1995;13:579–626.
34. Karnik R, Stelzer P, Slany J. Transcranial Doppler sonography monitoring of local intra-arterial thrombolysis in acute occlusion of the middle cerebral artery. *Stroke* 1992;23:284–287.
35. Koenig MA, Kaplan PW. Clinical applications for EPs in the ICU. *J Clin Neurophysiol* 2015;32:472–480.
36. Krieger D, Jauss M, Schwarz S, Hacke W. Serial somatosensory and brainstem auditory evoked potentials in monitoring of acute supratentorial mass lesions. *Crit Care Med* 1995;23:1123–1131.
37. Kurtz P, Hanafy KA, Claassen J. Continuous EEG monitoring: is it ready for prime time? *Curr Opin Crit Care* 2009;15:99–109.
38. Kushner MJ, Zanette EM, Bastianello S, et al. Transcranial Doppler in acute hemispheric brain infarction. *Neurology* 1991;41:109–113.
39. Laumer R, Steinmeier R, Gonner F, et al. Cerebral hemodynamics in subarachnoid hemorrhage evaluated by transcranial Doppler sonography. Part 1: reliability of flow velocities in clinical management. *Neurosurgery* 1993;33:1–8.
40. Lauritzen M, Dreier JP, Fabricius M, et al. Clinical relevance of cortical spreading depression in neurological disorders: migraine, malignant stroke, subarachnoid and intracranial hemorrhage, and traumatic brain injury. *J Cereb Blood Flow Metab* 2011;31:17–35.
41. Lennihan L, Petty GW, Fink ME, Solomon RA, Mohr JP. Transcranial Doppler detection of anterior cerebral artery vasospasm. *J Neurol Neurosurg Psychiatry* 1993;56:906–909.
42. Ley-Pozo J, Ringelstein EB. Noninvasive detection of occlusive disease of the carotid siphon

and middle cerebral artery. *Ann Neurol* 1990;28: 640–647.

43. Lysakowski C, Walder B, Costanza MC, Tramer MR. Transcranial Doppler versus angiography in patients with vasospasm due to a ruptured cerebral aneurysm: a systematic review. *Stroke* 2001;32:2292–2298

44. Manno EM, Gress DR, Schwamm LH, Diringer MN, Ogilvy CS. Effects of induced hypertension on transcranial Doppler ultrasound velocities in patients after subarachnoid hemorrhage. *Stroke* 1998;29:422–428.

45. McCarthy WJ, Park AE, Koushanpour E, Pearce WH, Yao JS. Carotid endarterectomy: lessons from intraoperative monitoring—a decade of experience. *Ann Surg* 1996;224:297–305.

46. McQuire JC, Sutcliffe JC, Coats TJ. Early changes in middle cerebral artery blood flow velocity after head injury. *J Neurosurg* 1998;89:526–532.

47. Mecarelli O, Pro S, Randi F, et al. EEG patterns and epileptic seizures in acute phase stroke. *Cerebrovasc Dis* 2011;31:191–198.

48. Molina CA, Barreto AD, Tsivgoulis G, et al. Transcranial ultrasound in clinical sonothrombolysis (TUCSON) trial. *Ann Neurol* 2009;66:28–38.

49. Nakamura H, Strong AJ, Dohmen C, et al. Spreading depolarizations cycle around and enlarge focal ischaemic brain lesions. *Brain* 2010;133:1994–2006.

50. Newell DW, Aaslid R. *Transcranial Doppler.* New York: Raven Press; 1992.

51. Newell DW, Winn HR. Transcranial Doppler in cerebral vasospasm. *Neurosurg Clin N Am* 1990;1:319–328.

52. Ng MC, Gaspard N, Cole AJ, et al. The standardization debate: a conflation trap in critical care electroencephalography. *Seizure* 2015;24: 52–58.

53. Niedermeyer E, Lopes da Silva FH. *Electroencephalography: Basic Principles, Clinical Applications, and Related Fields.* 5th ed. Baltimore: Williams & Wilkins; 2004.

54. Nuwer MR. Continuous EEG monitoring in the intensive care unit. *Electroencephalogr Clin Neurophysiol Suppl* 1999;50:150–155.

55. Nuwer MR, Hovda DA, Schrader LM, Vespa PM. Routine and quantitative EEG in mild traumatic brain injury. *Clin Neurophysiol* 2005; 116:2001–2025.

56. Pandian JD, Cascino GD, So EL, Manno E, Fulgham JR. Digital video-electroencephalographic monitoring in the neurological-neurosurgical intensive care unit: clinical features and outcome. *Arch Neurol* 2004;61:1090–1094.

57. Petty GW, Mohr JP, Pedley TA, et al. The role of transcranial Doppler in confirming brain death: sensitivity, specificity, and suggestions for performance and interpretation. *Neurology* 1990; 40:300–303.

58. Petty GW, Wiebers DO, Meissner I. Transcranial Doppler ultrasonography: clinical applications in cerebrovascular disease. *Mayo Clinic Proc* 1990;65:1350–1364.

59. Purkayastha S, Sorond F. Transcranial Doppler ultrasound: technique and application. *Semin Neurol* 2012;32:411–420.

60. Ropper AH, Kehne SM, Wechsler L. Transcranial Doppler in brain death. *Neurology* 1987;37:1733–1735.

61. Rosenthal ES. The utility of EEG, SSEP, and other neurophysiologic tools to guide neurocritical care. *Neurotherapeutics* 2012;9:24–36.

62. Schmitt S, Dichter MA. Electrophysiologic recordings in traumatic brain injury. *Handb Clin Neurol* 2015;127:319–339.

63. Siren J, Seppalainen AM, Launes J. Is EEG useful in assessing patients with acute encephalitis treated with acyclovir? *Electroencephalogr Clin Neurophysiol* 1998;107:296–301.

64. Steiger HJ, Aaslid R, Stooss R, Seiler RW. Transcranial Doppler monitoring in head injury: relations between type of injury, flow velocities, vasoreactivity, and outcome. *Neurosurgery* 1994;34:79–85.

65. Suarez JI, Qureshi AI, Yahia AB, et al. Symptomatic vasospasm diagnosis after subarachnoid hemorrhage: evaluation of transcranial Doppler ultrasound and cerebral angiography as related to compromised vascular distribution. *Crit Care Med* 2002;30:1348–1355.

66. Thompson BB, Wendell LC, Potter NS, et al. The use of transcranial Doppler ultrasound in confirming brain death in the setting of skull defects and extraventricular drains. *Neurocrit Care* 2014;21:534–538.

67. Torbey MT, Hauser TK, Bhardwaj A, et al. Effect of age on cerebral blood flow velocity and incidence of vasospasm after aneurysmal subarachnoid hemorrhage. *Stroke* 2001;32:2005–2011.

68. Totaro R, Marini C, Cannarsa C, Prencipe M. Reproducibility of transcranial Dopplersonography: a validation study. *Ultrasound Med Biol* 1992;18:173–177.

69. Tsubokawa T, Nishimoto H, Yamamoto T, et al. Assessment of brainstem damage by the auditory brainstem response in acute severe head injury. *J Neurol Neurosurg Psychiatry* 1980;43:1005–1011.

70. Vespa PM, Boscardin WJ, Hovda DA, et al. Early and persistent impaired percent alpha variability on continuous electroencephalography monitoring as predictive of poor outcome after traumatic brain injury. *J Neurosurg* 2002;97:84–92.

71. Vespa PM, Nuwer MR, Nenov V, et al. Increased incidence and impact of nonconvulsive and convulsive seizures after traumatic brain injury as detected by continuous electroencephalographic monitoring. *J Neurosurg* 1999;91:750–760.

72. von Oettingen G, Bergholt B, Gyldensted C, Astrup J. Blood flow and ischemia within traumatic cerebral contusions. *Neurosurgery* 2002;50:781–788.

73. Vora YY, Suarez-Almazor M, Steinke DE, Martin ML, Findlay JM. Role of transcranial Doppler monitoring in the diagnosis of cerebral vasospasm after subarachnoid hemorrhage. *Neurosurgery* 1999;44:1237–1247.

74. Wardlaw JM, Offin R, Teasdale GM, Teasdale EM. Is routine transcranial Doppler ultrasound monitoring useful in the management of subarachnoid hemorrhage? *J Neurosurg* 1998;88:272–276.

75. Westermaier T, Pham M, Stetter C, et al. Value of transcranial Doppler, perfusion-CT and neurological evaluation to forecast secondary ischemia after aneurysmal SAH. *Neurocrit Care* 2014;20:406–412.

76. Westmoreland BF, Klass DW, Sharbrough FW, Reagan TJ. Alpha-coma. Electroencephalographic, clinical, pathologic, and etiologic correlations. *Arch Neurol* 1975;32:713–718.

77. Westover MB, Shafi MM, Bianchi MT, et al. The probability of seizures during EEG monitoring in critically ill adults. *Clin Neurophysiol* 2015;126: 463–471.

78. Williamson CA, Wahlster S, Shafi MM, Westover MB. Sensitivity of compressed spectral arrays for detecting seizures in acutely ill adults. *Neurocrit Care* 2014;20:32–39.

79. Woitzik J, Dreier JP, Hecht N, et al. Delayed cerebral ischemia and spreading depolarization in absence of angiographic vasospasm after subarachnoid hemorrhage. *J Cereb Blood Flow Metab* 2012;32:203–212.

80. Wood JH, Polyzoidis KS, Epstein CM, Gibby GL, Tindall GT. Quantitative EEG alterations after isovolemic-hemodilutional augmentation of cerebral perfusion in stroke patients. *Neurology* 1984;34:764–768.

81. Young GB. Continuous EEG monitoring in the ICU. *Acta Neurol Scand* 2006;114:67–68.

82. Young GB. The EEG in coma. *J Clin Neurophysiol* 2000;17:473–485.

83. Young GB, Doig GS. Continuous EEG monitoring in comatose intensive care patients: epileptiform activity in etiologically distinct groups. *Neurocrit Care* 2005;2:5–10.

25

Multimodal Monitoring and Biomarkers

Multimodal monitoring has been a major focus in the management of severe brain injury, primarily of traumatic brain injury. The underlying premise is that more is better, more is more detailed, more is more informative. This remains to be demonstrated. A recent study using ICP, microdialysis, and brain oxygenation showed good correlation of global CBF with regional CBF, but discordant values were found, suggesting that the different values can be complementary but also confusing.[3] As expected, monitoring of ICP alone did not sufficiently predict cerebral hypoperfusion.[3] Similar findings were reported by several study groups.[2,7,22]

This chapter comments briefly on current interest and emerging research. There is no need for a condescending attitude and much of it is definitively promising. There is no question that technology could help the field of neurocritical care greatly if studied rigorously and with a healthy dose of skepticism. However, in the words of Robert Wachter, "computers and medicine are awkward companions."[26] But it looks that an ultrasound in critical care may "replace" the stethoscope, and intracranial probes or grids may suggest that they tell us much more than static neuroimages or clinical assessment. We must remain defenders of a good neurologic examination. Furthermore, it is not disingenuous to suggest that advances in medical and neurosurgical management may have a larger impact on outcome than brain monitoring.

Multimodal monitoring has been subjected to a consensus meeting of a group of investigators reviewing available material and rating it for quality of evidence. A consensus was reached in multiple areas, although most of the recommendations were based on weak or basically no evidence. The consensus statement concluded that several monitoring devices are available that can address several important physiological parameters. Some of the monitoring devices have been used predominantly in traumatic brain injury and subarachnoid hemorrhage, and extrapolation to other causes of acute brain injury cannot be easily justified. The consensus statement recognized a considerable number of shortcomings that perhaps could question the foundation of multimodal monitoring. Very few studies purport to show that outcome is improved with knowledge of certain physiological data, and a number of significant flaws were found in published material.

It is a given fact that neurologic examination may lag behind physiological findings, particularly if gross scales are used. More detailed aspects of neurologic examination have to be compared with changes in physiological data. There are several important reasons to monitor patients who require neurocritical care. These are summarized in Table 25.1. An ideal neuromonitor has been identified as providing noninvasive and reliable and reproducible data, no operator dependency, spatial and temporal resolution, and requiring little training to use it. The current most important

TABLE 25.1	RATIONALE FOR MONITORING
Detect early neurological worsening before irreversible brain damage occurs	
Individualize patient care decisions and guide patient management	
Monitor the physiologic response to treatment and to avoid any adverse effects	
Allow clinicians to better understand the pathophysiology of complex disorders	
Design and implement management protocols	
Improve neurological outcome and quality of life in survivors of severe brain injuries	
Develop new mechanistically oriented therapies where treatments currently are lacking or are empiric in nature	

Adapted from Le Roux et al. (2014).[11]

CAPSULE 25.1.   REQUIREMENTS FOR MONITORING

What is the device (i.e., what exactly does it measure)?
Are there complimentary monitors that can be used in the same pathophysiologic process?
How to use it and in whom to use it
Are we measuring what we think we are measuring (accuracy, precision, sensitivity, and specificity)?
Define limitations, technical problems, troubleshooting, and safety
Define the limiting conditions in which accuracy or precision are lost
Reproducibility of measurements
Effects of observer bias
Does data from a device (or of monitoring a specific pathophysiological process) make a contribution to
    patient care?
Cost-effectiveness and justification in clinical care

adapted from reference 25.

---

questions that need to be considered when evaluating neuromonitors are summarized in Capsule 25.1.[25] Several monitoring modalities may become useful and are shown in Table 25.2.

Tremendous challenges come with multimodal informatics. Many relate to volume and resolution of data,[5] the reliability of automated artifact detection, cleaning of acquired data before analysis and the effort of real-time analysis and feedback to the bedside.[25] It is evident that very few neurocritical care-specific monitors are available, and much of the hemodynamic monitoring uses general critical care monitoring devices. ICP monitoring through an ICP monitor or ventriculostomy, monitoring of brain oxygenation, assessment of cerebral blood flow by transcranial Doppler, and cerebral metabolism with microdialysis remain the best options. All of them are not widely available, nor is there sufficient expertise interpreting the acquired data. Research collaborations and improvement in standardization are required. The current options are shown in Figure 25.1.

BIOMARKERS

Biomarkers are typically used as determinants of prognosis or in assessing the risk of developing disease. There are many candidate biomarkers but there is interest in ischemic stroke, in particular to find a potential application in large infarction and swelling.[20] Biomarkers for cerebral swelling can be broadly categorized into specifics of neuroimaging, specific circulating substances, or continuous neuromonitoring. Blood-based biomarkers, if translated into routine clinical practice, are generally envisioned as an adjunct to the overall clinical assessment.

Several biomarkers are of interest but none has entered clinical practice. Future work in biomarkers for acute brain injury will need to focus on prospective validation in independent cohorts and the development of rapid and reliable testing methodologies. One review of 58 single biomarkers and seven panels consisting of several biomarkers reveals high sensitivity and specificity, but none was used clinically. Clinical

TABLE 25.2. RECOMMENDATIONS FROM CONSENSUS CONFERENCE ON MULTIMODALITY MONITORING IN NEUROCRITICAL CARE

What to Monitor	How to Monitor
Neurologic exam	GCS, FOUR Score
Pain/agitation	NRS, SAS, RASS
Hemodynamics	Arterial catheter, echocardiogram, transpulmonary hemodilution
Intracranial pressure	ICP monitor, EVD
Brain oxygenation	PbtO₂, SjvO₂
Cerebral blood flow	TCD, TCCS
Cerebral metabolism	Microdialysis
Hemostasis	POCT
Temperature	BSAS
Biomarkers	NSE

GCS, Glasgow Coma Scale; FOUR Score, Full Outline of UnResponsiveness Scale; NRS, Numeric Rating Scale; SAS Sedation-agitation scale, RASS: Richmond Area Sedation Scale; $PbtO_2$, brain oximetry; SjO_2, jugular bulb oximetry; TCD, Transcranial Doppler; TCCS, Transcranial Color-Coded Doppler; POCT, point of care; BSAS, Bedside Shivering Scale; NSE, neuron-specific enolase.

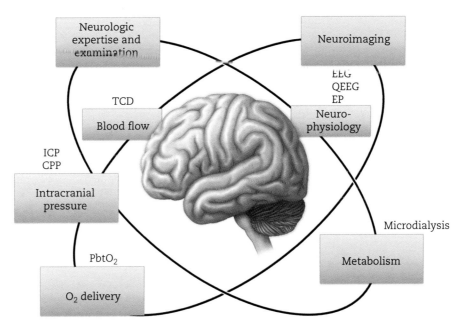

FIGURE 25.1: The current options in multimodal monitoring of the critically ill neurologic patient.

TCD: transcranial Doppler; ICP: intracranial pressure; CPP: cerebral perfusion pressure; PbtO2: partial pressure of oxygen in brain tissue; EEG: electroencephalography; Q: quantitative; EP: Evoked potentials.

TABLE 25.3. BIOMARKERS IN TRAUMATIC BRAIN INJURY

Biochemical markers	Location	Results	References
S100B	Astrocytes, fat, bone marrow, skeletal muscle	Correlation between serum S100B level and the patient outcome. S100B positively correlated with the injury severity and negatively correlated with outcome.	9,23,28
NSE	Neurons, platelets, red blood cells, neuroendocrine cells	Increased NSE is found in TBI correlating with injury severity. In severe TBI, NSE correlated with clinical outcome.	1,19
MBP	Myelin	MBP levels were significantly higher in patients who died.	8,9,14
GFAP	Glial cells	High levels of GFAP were strongly predictive of death or a poor outcome.	10,12,16
CKBB	Astrocytes, glial cells	Severity of the damage correlated with serum of CKBB.	9,24
Plasma DNA	Blood plasma or serum	Higher DNA concentrations were significantly associated with fatal outcome.	4,17,21
BDNF	Neurons, glial cells	A correlation between the brain injury severity and BDNF serum has been demonstrated.	18
UCH-L1	Neurons	UCH-L1 was significantly elevated in severe TBI patients. Levels of UCH-L1 were associated with injury severity, complications, and outcome.	13,15

TBI, traumatic brain injury; S100B S100, calcium binding protein B; NSE, neuron-specific enolase; MBP, myelin basic protein; GFAP, glial fibrillary acidic protein; CKBB, creatine kinase brain isoenzyme; DNA, desoxyribonucleic acid; BDNF, brain-derived neurotrophic factor; UCH-L1, ubiquitin carboxy-terminal hydrolase-L1.

validation of these biomarkers is insufficient and this include unknown reference standards.[27]

Some are of future interest. In swollen stroke, circulating markers that relate to the blood–brain barrier (BBB) have been studied, because the integrity of the BBB may play a role in the development of cerebral edema. A key BBB-degrading enzyme, matrix metalloproteinase-9 (MMP-9), has been associated with malignant edema, with one study reporting that a concentration of ≥ 140 ng/mL has a 64% sensitivity and 88% specificity for predicting malignant infarction. Elevated MMP-9 is also associated with an increased risk of hemorrhagic conversion, in accord with the high rates of hemorrhagic conversion found in this population.

Other reports to predict malignant edema include cellular fibronectin, a constituent of the basal lamina, of which elevations > 16.6 ug/mL predict malignant edema with 90% sensitivity and 100% specificity. The glial marker S100B is released into the bloodstream after ischemic stroke, with increasing amounts correlating with infarct size. Serum levels > 1.03ug/L at 24 hours are also associated with malignant infarction.

Microdialysis probe placements adjacent to hemispheric infarcts have revealed decrements in extracellular amino acids in malignant infarction compared to non-malignant edema. Though none of these biomarkers has reached usefulness in clinical practice, they may offer insights into the pathophysiology of malignant brain edema and warrant further investigation.

Biomarkers have been investigated in traumatic brain injury also to improve outcome; but apart from prognostication of elevated levels in more severely injured patients (and mortality), its clinical use is doubtful as a monitoring parameter or as a marker of adequate management (Table 25.3). Combinations of biomarkers may increase prediction.[6]

CONCLUSIONS

- One monitor may not change management or outcome. Multiple monitors may impact both, but it is not known how.
- Ideal setups for multimodal monitoring can be defined, and research may provide valid data.
- We have an obligation to monitor the patient, not only the brain.
- Biomarkers could help in assessment of the severity of damage when not otherwise known.

REFERENCES

1. Berger RP, Dulani T, Adelson PD, et al. Identification of inflicted traumatic brain injury in well-appearing infants using serum and cerebrospinal markers: a possible screening tool. *Pediatrics* 2006;117:325–332.
2. Bhatia A, Gupta AK. Neuromonitoring in the intensive care unit. II: cerebral oxygenation monitoring and microdialysis. *Intens Care Med* 2007;33:1322–1328.
3. Bouzat P, Marques-Vidal P, Zerlauth JB, et al. Accuracy of brain multimodal monitoring to detect cerebral hypoperfusion after traumatic brain injury. *Crit Care Med* 2015;43:445–452.
4. Campello Yurgel V, Ikuta N, Brondani da Rocha A, et al. Role of plasma DNA as a predictive marker of fatal outcome following severe head injury in males. *J Neurotrauma* 2007;24:1172–1181.
5. Citerio G, Park S, Schmidt JM, et al. Data collection and interpretation. *Neurocrit Care* 2015;22:360–368.
6. Diaz-Arrastia R, Wang KK, Papa L, et al. Acute biomarkers of traumatic brain injury: relationship between plasma levels of ubiquitin C-terminal hydrolase-L1 and glial fibrillary acidic protein. *J Neurotrauma* 2014;31:19–25.
7. Eriksson EA, Barletta JF, Figueroa BE, et al. Cerebral perfusion pressure and intracranial pressure are not surrogates for brain tissue oxygenation in traumatic brain injury. *Clin Neurophysiol* 2012;123:1255–1260.
8. Gale SD, Johnson SC, Bigler ED, Blatter DD. Nonspecific white matter degeneration following traumatic brain injury. *J Int Neuropsychol Soc* 1995;1:17–28.
9. Ingebrigtsen T, Romner B. Biochemical serum markers of traumatic brain injury. *J Trauma* 2002;52:798–808.
10. Lam NY, Rainer TH, Chan LY, Joynt GM, Lo YM. Time course of early and late changes in plasma DNA in trauma patients. *Clin Chem* 2003;49:1286–1291.
11. Le Roux P, Menon DK, Citerio G, et al. Consensus Summary Statement of the International Multidisciplinary Consensus Conference on Multimodality Monitoring in Neurocritical Care: a statement for healthcare professionals from the Neurocritical Care Society and the European Society of Intensive Care Medicine. *Neurocrit Care* 2014;21 Suppl 2:S297–361.
12. McAllister AK, Katz LC, Lo DC. Neurotrophins and synaptic plasticity. *Annu Rev Neurosci* 1999;22:295–318.
13. Mondello S, Papa L, Buki A, et al. Neuronal and glial markers are differently associated with

computed tomography findings and outcome in patients with severe traumatic brain injury: a case control study. *Crit Care* 2011;15:R156.

14. Nylen K, Ost M, Csajbok LZ, et al. Increased serum-GFAP in patients with severe traumatic brain injury is related to outcome. *J Neurol Sci* 2006;240:85–91.

15. Papa L, Akinyi L, Liu MC, et al. Ubiquitin C-terminal hydrolase is a novel biomarker in humans for severe traumatic brain injury. *Crit Care Med* 2010;38:138–144.

16. Rainer TH, Wong LK, Lam W, et al. Prognostic use of circulating plasma nucleic acid concentrations in patients with acute stroke. *Clin Chem* 2003;49:562–569.

17. Riley CP, Cope TC, Buck CR. CNS neurotrophins are biologically active and expressed by multiple cell types. *J Mol Histol* 2004;35:771–783.

18. Rodrigues E, Oliveira C, Cambrussi A, et al. Increased serum brain derived neurotrophic factor (BDNF) following isolated severe traumatic brain injury in humans [Abstract]. *Brain Inj* 2008;22 (Suppl 1):165.

19. Ross SA, Cunningham RT, Johnston CF, Rowlands BJ. Neuron-specific enolase as an aid to outcome prediction in head injury. *Br J Neurosurg* 1996;10:471–476.

20. Saenger AK, Christenson RH. Stroke biomarkers: progress and challenges for diagnosis, prognosis, differentiation, and treatment. *Clin Chem* 2010;56:21–33.

21. Saha RN, Liu X, Pahan K. Up-regulation of BDNF in astrocytes by TNF-alpha: a case for the neuroprotective role of cytokine. *J Neuroimmune Pharmacol* 2006;1:212–222.

22. Sala N, Suys T, Zerlauth JB, et al. Cerebral extracellular lactate increase is predominantly nonischemic in patients with severe traumatic brain injury. *J Cereb Blood Flow Metab* 2013;33:1815–1822.

23. Savola O, Pyhtinen J, Leino TK, et al. Effects of head and extracranial injuries on serum protein S100B levels in trauma patients. *J Trauma* 2004;56:1229–1234.

24. Tyler WJ, Alonso M, Bramham CR, Pozzo-Miller LD. From acquisition to consolidation: on the role of brain-derived neurotrophic factor signaling in hippocampal-dependent learning. *Learn Mem* 2002;9:224–237.

25. Vespa P, Menon D, Le Roux P. The International Multi-disciplinary Consensus Conference on Multimodality Monitoring: future directions and emerging technologies. *Neurocrit Care* 2014;21 Suppl 2:S270–281.

26. Wachter R. *The Digital Doctor: Hope, Hype, and Harm at the Dawn of Medicine's Computer Age.* New York: McGraw-Hill; 2015.

27. Whiteley W, Tseng MC, Sandercock P. Blood biomarkers in the diagnosis of ischemic stroke: a systematic review. *Stroke* 2008;39:2902–2909.

28. Woertgen C, Rothoerl RD, Metz C, Brawanski A. Comparison of clinical, radiologic, and serum marker as prognostic factors after severe head injury. *J Trauma* 1999;47:1126–1130.

PART VII

Management of Specific Disorders in Critical Care Neurology

26

Aneurysmal Subarachnoid Hemorrhage

Major medical institutions may admit 50–75 patients with an aneurysmal subarachnoid hemorrhage (SAH) a year. A multidisciplinary team is required to respond to the immediate needs of the patient and to plan for repair of the aneurysm.[8,42,101,154,175] Expertise may prevent poor outcome.[25,47,133]

After aneurysmal rupture, 10% of patients die suddenly or within the first hours before ever receiving adequate medical attention. Many of these patients had marked intraventricular extension of the hemorrhage and acute pulmonary edema, both reasons for sudden death.[144] Of those most severely affected who reach the emergency department (ED) or neurosciences intensive care unit (NICU), half die within 3 months. Some of these patients may have been found pulseless and required prolonged cardiopulmonary resuscitation. Patients who survive a major first rupture face the immediate risk of catastrophic rebleeding, rapidly developing hydrocephalus, potentially life-threatening pulmonary edema, and cardiac arrhythmias. Presentation in a poor clinical condition often indicates that the hemorrhage is not confined to the subarachnoid space but rather there is intraventricular and intraparenchymal extension. Many have additional large ventricles and are in need of CSF diversion with a ventriculostomy.

The critical steps in managing SAH are to surgically clip the aneurysm or occlude the sac by inserting platinum coils, to treat clinical neurologic deterioration early, and to manage major systemic complications.[169]

Aneurysmal subarachnoid hemorrhage is a prime example of a neurocritical and neurosurgical disorder where outcome in the first days after presentation cannot be judged adequately and care of the initially comatose patient can lead to a satisfactory outcome.

Fortunately, a considerable proportion of patients with SAH present with severe headache and are alert with little other findings. Early repair of the aneurysm may result in an excellent outcome.

CLINICAL RECOGNITION

The incidence of aneurysmal SAH varies, but overall is 10 cases per 100,000 persons per year (doubled in Finland and Japan).[112] The risk is nearly two times higher in women (particularly with smoking history) than in men and in blacks than in whites. Subarachnoid hemorrhage is more common in patients with a family history of SAH,[101] polycystic kidney disease, systemic lupus erythematosus, or Ehlers-Danlos disease (Capsule 26.1).[60,61]

Aneurysmal SAH may be manifested in many ways. Typically, an unexpected instantaneous headache warns the patient of a very serious disorder and is often described as excruciating and overwhelming[113] (Chapter 4).

Vomiting may occur several minutes into the ictus as a result of further distribution of blood throughout the subarachnoid space. Profuse vomiting may override the headache and has been mistaken for a "gastric flu" by the patient or initially consulted physician.

With an incomplete medical history and no inquiry about acute headache, patients may be wrongly transferred to a medical ICU (cardiac resuscitation and pulmonary edema), gastrointestinal service (vomiting), or coronary care unit (cardiac arrhythmias with new electrocardiographic [EKG] changes). Other unusual clinical presentations have included acute paraplegia (anterior cerebral artery aneurysm rupture into frontal lobes) and severe thoracic and lumbar pain caused by meningeal irritation. These presentations may have resulted in a delay in cranial computed tomography (CT) scan imaging.

The abruptness of the headache is not specific for SAH; it may occur in conditions such as arterial dissection, pituitary apoplexy, hypertensive encephalopathy, spontaneous intracranial hypotension, and cerebral venous thrombosis[43,44,143] (Chapter 4). Some patients briefly lose consciousness. Inappropriate behavior and agitation or drowsiness may follow. Localizing neurologic findings, although transient, may indicate the

CAPSULE 26.1   ANEURYSMAL RUPTURE

What causes aneurysms to rupture is puzzling. Risk factors have included recently documented enlargement (rupture of aneurysms < 4 mm is uncommon; most ruptured aneurysms are 7–8 mm, and risk of rupture increases significantly in aneurysms of ≥ 10 mm),[88] hypertension, cigarette smoking, and family history of aneurysms and SAH. Aneurysmal rupture has been reported to have occurred during weightlifting, sexual orgasm, and brawling, events that suggest acute hypertensive stress on a thin aneurysmal wall.[160] However, at least 50% of patients have SAH while at rest. Seasonal changes have been implicated with increased rupture rate during colder temperatures and influenza peaks. An association between a recent infection and aneurysmal rupture has not been definitively established, but is plausible.

Intracranial pressure rises dramatically to at least the level of the diastolic blood pressure, causing cerebral perfusion standstill. The increase in intracranial pressure decreases within 15 minutes but may persist if acute hydrocephalus or a shift from intracerebral hematoma has occurred. Rupture stops within 3–6 minutes after ejection of up to 15–20 mL/min into the basal cistern.

Hemodynamic variables have been tested on cadaver and computer models. Variables that may determine rupture are wall shear stress, intra-aneurysmal flow velocity, and inflow jet and angles of entry and vortexes. Wall sheet stress is caused by the frictional force of blood, and areas with high forces may fragment the internal elastic lamina and cause blebs and aneurysms.[56,148]

Hemodynamic stress may cause morphologic changes involving the endothelial lining of the walls, with intimal hyperplasia, and organizing thrombosis. Many ruptured vacular aneurysms show inflammatory changes, with infiltrating leukocytes and macrophages promoting fibrosis. Other theories focus on the multitudes of vortices or unstable flow. High inflow jets with large impact zones may result in thrombus or daughter sac formation.[20,21]

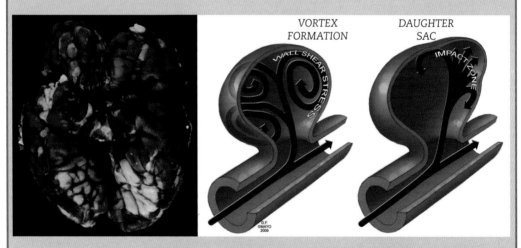

Subarachnoid hemorrhage. *Left*: aneurysmal rupture causing diffuse subarachnoid hemorrhage. *Right*: Vortex formation in aneurysm.

site of the ruptured aneurysm. For example, patients with a ruptured middle cerebral artery (MCA) aneurysm may have transient or persistent aphasia. In patients with a ruptured MCA aneurysm and intraparenchymal extension, hemiparesis often is found. Abulia most often occurs as a complication of a rupture of an aneurysm of the anterior cerebral artery (ACA). Generalized

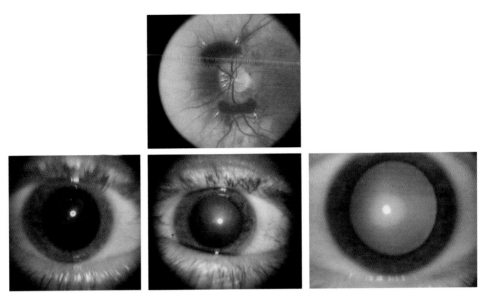

FIGURE 26.1: Subhyaloid and vitreous hemorrhages. *Top*: Subhyaloid hemorrhage in subarachnoid hemorrhage. *Bottom left*: Red reflex is absent from vitreous hemorrhage also known as Terson syndrome. *Bottom middle*: Improvement in vision. *Bottom right*: Normal red reflex as shown by retro illumination with fundus camera.

tonic-clonic seizures are not quite so often seen at the time of rupture, and it is possible that extensor posturing or brief myoclonic jerks with syncope at onset may be mistaken for a seizure. These clinical features in SAH are identical whether or not an aneurysm is detected. Different presentation is expected, however, in an established benign variant of nonaneurysmal SAH, so-called pretruncal or perimesencephalic SAH. The patients are almost exclusively alert. Loss of consciousness is seldom observed and seizures are absent, and the onset of headache is less acute—in minutes rather than a second.

Neurologic examination reveals neck stiffness in most patients, except those seen early after the initial event and those who are comatose. Nuchal rigidity can be demonstrated by failure to flex the neck in the neutral position and failure of the neck to retroflex when both shoulders are lifted. Retinal subhyaloid hemorrhages are present in approximately 25% of the patients (Figure 26.1). (This syndrome is more often observed in comatose patients and after rebleeding.) These flat-topped hemorrhages occur when outflow in the optic nerve venous system is suddenly obstructed by the intracranial pressure (ICP) wave.[55] Visual loss may be severe, with perception of light or hand motion only, if the hemorrhage expands and ruptures into the vitreous (Terson syndrome).[131] Cranial nerve abnormalities occur infrequently in SAH unless a giant basilar artery aneurysm (third- or

sixth-nerve palsy) or a large carotid artery aneurysm (chiasmal syndromes) directly compresses surrounding structures. The pupil is dilated and unreactive to light in a third-nerve palsy because of compression of the exteriorly located fibers that form the light reflex. However, up to 15% of posterior communicating artery aneurysms may occur with a pupil-sparing third-nerve palsy. Aneurysm of the basilar artery may produce unilateral or bilateral third- or sixth-nerve palsy.[87] If the basilar artery aneurysm enlarges and progressively compresses the oculomotor nuclei of the pons, horizontal gaze paralysis, skew deviation, internuclear ophthalmoplegia, and nystagmus occur, commonly in association with long-tract signs such as hemiparesis and ataxia. Occlusion of the proximal posterior cerebral artery, often encased in a giant aneurysm, may occur, causing either classic Weber syndrome (Chapter 30) due to mesencephalon infarction (third-nerve palsy with opposite hemiparesis) or homonymous hemianopia due to occipital lobe infarction.

In comatose patients, a certain eye position may be localizing. These forced gaze positions include downward gaze and wall-eyed bilateral internuclear ophthalmoplegia, and are characteristically seen with acute hydrocephalus (Figure 26.2).[90]

Hemiparesis that usually involves the face, arm, and leg should point to an intracranial hematoma in SAH. An anteriorly placed intracranial

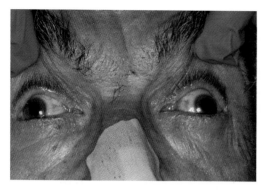

FIGURE 26.2: Wall-eyed bilateral internuclear ophthalmoplegia with acute hydrocephalus in patient with aneurysmal subarachnoid hemorrhage.

hematoma in the frontal lobe may not produce motor weakness but may be associated with agitation and bizarre behavior. Many patients are confused, and may ramble nonsensically. Korsakoff syndrome with impaired recall and fabrications may occur in ruptured anterior communicating aneurysm. Abulia, a general sense of disinterest, and lackluster attention are also features, becoming apparent days later.[62] Temporal lobe hematoma in the dominant hemisphere may produce aphasia, but often associated mass effect and brainstem displacement decrease the level of consciousness and word output.

Generalized tonic-clonic seizures are accompanied by aneurysmal rupture in 10% of patients, or these appear during rebleeding. These "seizures" are likely ischemic in nature and a result of a major increase in ICP. Nonconvulsive status epilepticus may occur, and the clinical signs are difficult to differentiate from the effects of initial rupture. However, in our experience, electroencephalography (EEG) has rarely documented nonconvulsive status epilepticus. Epilepsia partialis continua is equally uncommon in aneurysmal SAH. It is more common in patients with additional subdural hematoma and when delayed cerebral infarction occurs.

Systemic manifestations may include respiratory failure and oxygen desaturation from aspiration, pulmonary edema, or obstruction of the airway. Cardiac arrhythmias may involve the entire spectrum of supraventricular and ventricular arrhythmias. Most of the time they are associated with EKG changes, which may simulate or indicate acute myocardial infarction. Elevated troponin I levels may occur in approximately 25% of the cases seen on the first day. Major cardiac arrhythmias may lead to cardiac resuscitation

after SAH and generally portend poor outcome, but patients may improve substantially.[152]

When patients are comatose at presentation, it is largely due to the initial rise in ICP with reduction of cerebral blood flow and, as a consequence, diffuse bihemispheric ischemia.[79] However, one should try to make a distinction between the direct effects of the initial impact and early neurologic deterioration due to other causes. Acute hydrocephalus may have developed in the interim, and placement of a ventricular drain could markedly improve the level of consciousness. Patients admitted days after the ictus may have symptomatic cerebral vasospasm, and focal signs and symptoms may not be present. Coma may be caused by brain tissue shift from a large expanding hematoma in the sylvian fissure. Removal of the hematoma and repair of the aneurysm may result in marked improvement.

The clinical course in poor-grade aneurysmal SAH is unpredictable in the first 24–48 hours. Patients moribund at presentation may improve in a matter of hours without much neurosurgical or medical intervention, although the prognosis may remain guarded.

Systemic metabolic factors may contribute, and each of them should be excluded. Measurements of arterial blood gas, electrolytes, and serum glucose must be obtained rapidly in every patient with SAH who enters the NICU.

A simple clinical grading system proposed by the World Federation of Neurological Surgeons (WFNS) introduced the Glasgow Coma Scale in SAH grading[46,139] (Table 26.1), and for practical reasons the severity is graded as good (WFNS I–III) or poor (WFNS IV or V). A correlation between outcome and initial grading level exists. This rather crude scale may also guide the timing

TABLE 26.1. GRADING SYSTEM PROPOSED BY THE WORLD FEDERATION OF NEUROLOGICAL SURGEONS FOR THE CLASSIFICATION OF SUBARACHNOID HEMORRHAGE

WFNS Grade	Glasgow Coma Scale Score	Motor Deficit
I	15	Absent
II	14–13	Absent
III	14–13	Present
IV	12–7	Present or absent
V	6–3	Present or absent

WFNS, World Federation of Neurological Surgeons.

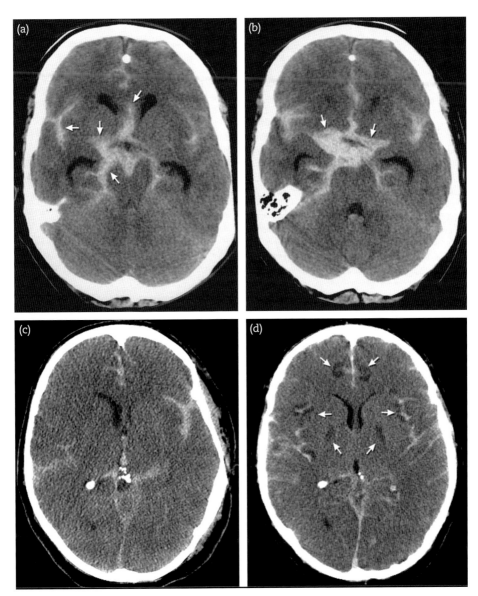

FIGURE 26.3: Subarachnoid hemorrhage. (a, b) Subarachnoid hemorrhage with complete filling of the basal cisterns and fissures (*arrows*), creating a "crab-like" cast. (c) Global cerebral edema. (d) Extensive low-attenuation changes (*arrows*) in frontal and insular cortex.

of surgery. Some neurosurgeons defer craniotomy for aneurysmal clipping in patients with WFNS V, but coiling may proceed. Improvement in grade may make the patient eligible for aneurysmal clipping.

NEUROIMAGING AND LABORATORY TESTS

Subarachnoid hemorrhage shows on CT scan (Figure 26.3a and b). Some patients show CT scans with massive SAH and early global edema (Figure 26.3c and d).[27] CT perfusion may show reduced blood flow. These findings are more common in patients who remain comatose after cardiopulmonary resuscitation. When CT scan is done within hours after the event, the sensitivity in aneurysmal SAH is very high and may approach 95%. In 2%–5% of the patients, subarachnoid blood has completely "washed out" on CT scans within 24 hours, but more likely, CT may have missed a thin layer of blood. Repeat CT scan in patients with initial "negative CT" and xanthochromia often documents traces of SAH in sulci or ventricles.[54]

Fisher developed one of the first grading systems for SAH. The *Fisher scale*, although deeply ingrained in neurological practice, remains a gross estimate of the amount of subarachnoid blood, and it has significant inter-observer variability. This scale, currently modified (Table 26.2), emphasizes the presence or absence of a thick clot and the presence of intraventricular hemorrhage, and predicts the development of delayed cerebral ischemia.[53]

Another grading system was developed by Hijdra and colleagues[78] (Table 26.2). A sum score

TABLE 26.2. COMPUTED TOMOGRAPHY FINDINGS IN THE MODIFIED FISHER AND HIJDRA SCALE

Grade	Finding
1	Focal or diffuse thin SAH without IVH
2	Focal or diffuse thin SAH with IVH
3	Thick SAH present without IVH
4	Thick SAH present with IVH

SAH: subarachnoid hemorrhage; IVH: intraventricular hemorrhage. Data from Kistler JP, Crowell RM, Davis KR, et al. The relation of cerebral vasospasm to the extent and location of subarachnoid blood visualized by CT scan: a prospective study. *Neurology* 1983;33:424–436; and Frontera J, Claassen J, Schmidt JM, et al. Prediction of symptomatic vasospasm after subarachnoid hemorrhage: the modified Fisher scale. *Neurosurgery* 2006;59:21–27.

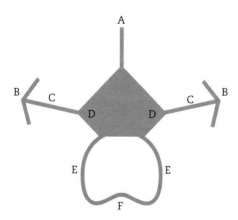

Hijdra method of grading subarachnoid hemorrhage identifies 10 basal cisterns and fissures: (A) frontal interhemispheric fissure; (B) sylvian fissure, lateral parts both sides; (C) sylvian fissure, basal parts both sides; (D) suprasellar cistern both sides; (E) ambient cisterns both sides; and (F) quadrigeminal cistern. The amount of blood in each cistern and fissure is graded 0, no blood; 1, small amount of blood; 2, moderately filled with blood; and 3, completely filled with blood. The sum score is 0 to 30 points.[78]

of greater than 20 is considered predictive of cerebral vasospasm. In our recent study of different scales, we found the Hijdra scale superior to other scales in prediction of cerebral vasospasm.[49] Quantification of SAH and calculation of volume may remain a useful alternative, but the applicability of this method remains unknown. Grading after "resuscitation" correlates better with outcome.[59]

Important information can be gathered by careful inspection of CT scans. The distribution of the subarachnoid blood on CT scan may suggest the location of the aneurysm, but despite subtle differences, CT scanning often cannot reliably predict the location of the aneurysm. There is no correlation between the size of the aneurysm and the amount of SAH.[140] Generally, patients with diffuse distribution of blood in cisterns and fissures often have a basilar artery or ACA aneurysm. However, patients with a concentration of blood in the interhemispheric fissure may have an aneurysm of the anterior cerebral artery, and patients with cisternal blood surrounding the perimesencephalic cisterns most likely harbor a basilar artery aneurysm. Likewise, sylvian fissure hemorrhages are mostly from an aneurysm of the MCA.

The additional presence of an intracerebral hematoma, however, has more localizing value. Hematomas may be found in the frontal lobe (anterior communicating artery aneurysm), in the medial part of the temporal lobe (internal carotid artery aneurysm), and within the sylvian fissure extending into the temporal lobe (MCA aneurysm) (Figure 26.4).[73]

As alluded to earlier a benign form of SAH has been reported in which bleeding is confined to the cisterns in front of the brainstem without evidence of an aneurysm in the posterior cerebral circulation—so-called *pre-truncal SAH*[141,142,170] (also called perimesencephalic hemorrhage)[159] (Figure 26.5a). True perimesencephalic hemorrhages are purely traumatic, due to either a P2 aneurysm or spinal dural arteriovenous fistula.[141,146] Typically, in these variants, blood clots do not extend to the lateral sylvian fissures or to the anterior interhemispheric fissure. Some extension to the basal part of the sylvian fissure is possible when CT scanning is performed very early. Intraventricular hemorrhage is absent except for some sedimentation in the posterior horns. Magnetic resonance imaging (MRI) is helpful in localizing the blood clot in front of the brainstem, and no cause has been found with this modality (Figure 26.5b). MRI of the cervical spine has also been unrevealing.[170]

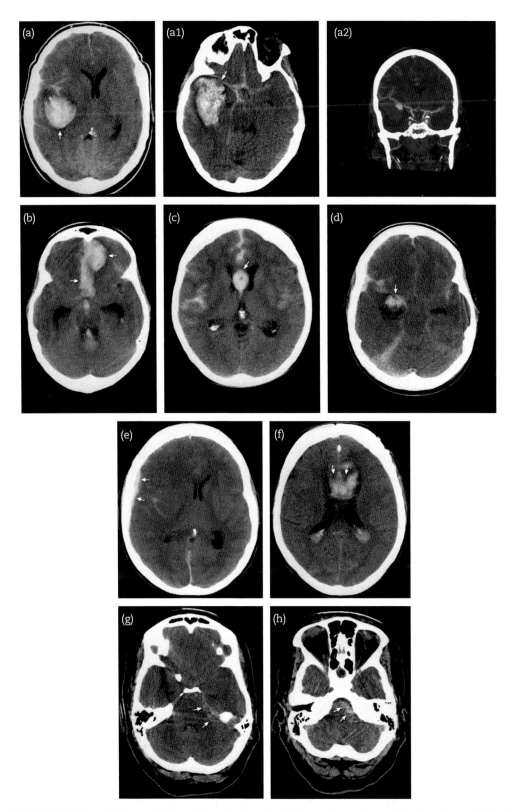

FIGURE 26.4: Computed tomographic patterns of subarachnoid hemorrhage with associated hematomas indirectly localizing ruptured aneurysms. Temporal lobe and sylvian fissure hematoma (a, a1) (middle cerebral artery aneurysm on CTA (a2)). Frontal hematoma (anterior cerebral artery) (b). Hematoma in cavum septum pellucidum (c). Medial temporal lobe hematoma (d). Subdural hematoma (carotid artery, mostly ophthalmic artery) (e). Corpus callosum (pericallosal artery) (f). Cerebellopontine angle hematoma with posterior inferior cerebellar artery aneurysm (g, h).

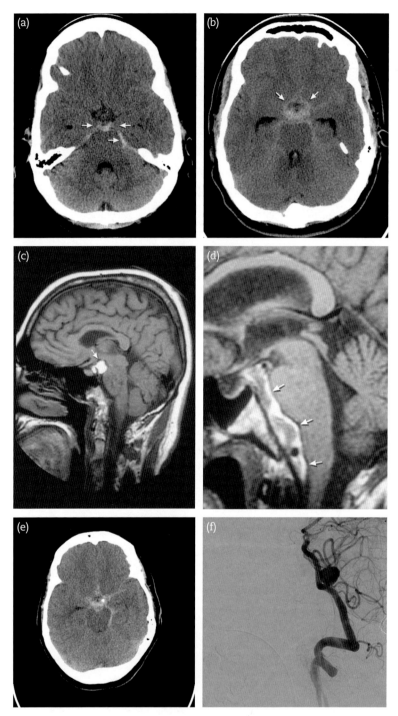

FIGURE 26.5: Nonaneurysmal pretruncal (perimesencephalic) subarachnoid hemorrhage. (a, b) Computed tomographic scan patterns of pretruncal nonaneurysmal subarachnoid hemorrhage in different patients. The spectrum includes complete filling of suprasellar cisterns to more restricted clots and subtle interpeduncular hematoma. The amount of blood is not critical in its recognition. However, the distribution of blood is limited and should not involve the entire lateral part of the sylvian fissure or the anterior hemisphere and ventricles. (c, d) Magnetic resonance imaging patterns of pretruncal nonaneurysmal subarachnoid hemorrhage. Blood may involve all or part of the cisterns in front of the brainstem. (e) Typical pretruncal CT pattern, but PICA aneurysm (f) proving a detailed vascular study is needed.

The cause of this perplexing benign form of nonaneurysmal SAH remains unclear. Prior speculative explanations have included spinal dural arteriovenous fistula, rupture of a dilated vein in the prepontine cistern, and intramural dissection,[72,141,171] but there is accumulating evidence that a small blister-like aneurysm of the posterior circulation may be implicated. Recent 3D cerebral angiograms have been able to document these small lesions.[166]

Pretruncal hemorrhage may closely mimic a ruptured basilar artery or dissecting P1–P2 aneurysm, and therefore a four-vessel cerebral angiogram is warranted.[93] In our experience and that of others,[126] we have found small (dissecting) aneurysms occasionally on repeat studies; and repeat cerebral angiograms on CTA may remain warranted in this subset.

Localized blood in the sulci alone is unusual in aneurysmal SAH and often indicates trauma coagulopathy or, much less common, vasculitis.[104,136] Subarachnoid blood caused by trauma is most often confined to the vertex and superficial cortical sulci or accumulates in the ambient cisterns at the level of the tentorium.[40] Computed tomography scans should be scrutinized for fractures on bone windows when physical examination shows other signs of trauma, for example, skin bruising or a soft-tissue swelling. When blood is in the sylvian fissure, a reliable distinction from a ruptured middle cerebral aneurysm cannot be made on clinical grounds or by CT scan, and cerebral angiography is needed.

Intraventricular blood on CT scans signals a severe SAH. Aneurysms of the ACA have a proclivity to perforate the lamina terminals and enter the ventricular system. Massive intraventricular hemorrhage in patients with SAH may also suggest rerupture. Subdural hematomas are seen in 1% of patients with SAH, often with cisternal blood, and very rarely in isolation. Most often, a carotid artery (ophthalmic or posterior communicating) aneurysm can be demonstrated on the angiogram.

An important feature on CT scanning is acute hydrocephalus. Enlargement of the lateral ventricles is often asymptomatic in acute SAH, and acute hydrocephalus as an explanation for drowsiness is more convincing if progression on sequential CT scans can be demonstrated or if the ventricles are very plump (Chapter 36).

Cerebral angiography remains the unchallenged gold standard for the diagnosis of cerebral aneurysm. One can argue for early four-vessel cerebral angiography in every patient, including those with poor-grade SAH. These patients may have aneurysms that can be occluded through endovascular techniques.

Before cerebral angiography is undertaken, serum creatinine concentration should be determined. The risk for neurologic deficit associated with the procedure is 0.07%.[29] The most important risk factor for contrast-induced nephrotoxicity is preexisting renal failure. The risk is also increased in patients with reduced intravascular volume and in patients using drugs that impair renal responses, such as angiotensin-converting enzyme inhibitors and nonsteroidal anti-inflammatory drugs. In patients with preexisting renal impairment, defined as a creatinine value of more than 1.8 mg/dL, 0.45% saline should be given intravenously at a rate of 1 mL/kg of body weight per hour beginning 12 hours before the scheduled angiography.[29,74]

Cerebral angiography may demonstrate aneurysms at typical locations (Figure 26.6). Standard examination should include anteroposterior and lateral views, but because overlapping is significant, oblique views are often necessary. The neuroradiologist may be guided by the findings on CT scan and should frequently use additional oblique views in evaluating the circle of Willis. Important additional views are submentovertex views (particularly useful for demonstrating the neck of an anterior communicating aneurysm) and transorbital projection (neck of the MCA). Towne's projection is important to visualize the tip of the basilar artery. Failure to demonstrate an aneurysm may be related to inadequate projection or incomplete study (three-vessel study), and a second angiogram at a slightly different angle may uncover an aneurysm. Three-dimensional image volume generated by digital fluorography with rotational image acquisition has improved detection. Multiple aneurysms may be found, and it is virtually impossible to predict which aneurysm has bled. However, additional clues (next to CT scan patterns) may be present, such as irregularity of the wall of the aneurysm produced by the sealing clot, vasospasm in the vicinity of the aneurysm, and size between 5 and 15 mm.

When an angiogram is negative, a second cerebral angiogram may demonstrate an aneurysm in approximately 10% of cases. The second cerebral angiogram should be particularly carefully scrutinized for a posterior circulation aneurysm, which could have been "missed" on the first angiogram.

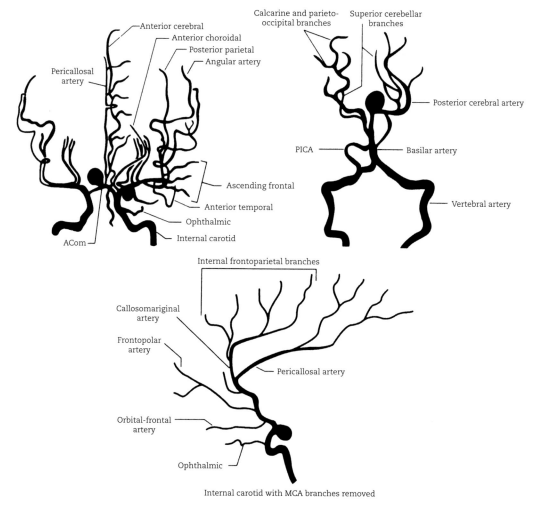

FIGURE 26.6: Anterior cerebral artery, middle cerebral artery, basilar artery tip, and posterior communicating artery aneurysms on cerebral angiogram in their optimal projections.

ACom, anterior communicating artery; MCA, middle cerebral artery; PICA, posterior inferior cerebellar artery.

Whether exploratory craniotomy is needed in patients with a high suspicion of an aneurysm (presence of subarachnoid blood and intracranial hematoma) is very unclear and this is rarely done, even though some explorations have been successful in detecting the ruptured aneurysm.[41]

CT angiogram has been used in patients with large aneurysms to better document anatomical configuration,[71,176] in patients with an initial negative cerebral angiogram (as a means of follow-up), and as the only additional diagnostic test in patients with pretruncal SAH in some European centers.[162] Its place in the diagnostic evaluation of patients with an SAH is unclear. Moreover, the less than perfect sensitivity of 97% (87% in aneurysms, 3 mm) and specificity of 86% may have medicolegal implications if it is

the only study done. Moreover, anatomic bulges of the basilar tip and pituitary stalk mistaken for aneurysms and incorrect three-dimensional reconstruction of overlapping MCAs are some of the reasons for false-positive results. The role of CT angiogram largely is as a simple and quick (but also expensive) method to demonstrate or exclude an aneurysm. CT angiogram, therefore, has been performed during night hours while waiting for a more definitive study in the morning.

Magnetic resonance imaging is usually not sensitive for SAH but may be able to show SAH when fluid attenuation inversion recovery (FLAIR) sequences are used. Recirculation of bloody cerebrospinal fluid (CSF) over the convexity is commonly seen as well. MRI may be important in demonstrating an acute SAH in the posterior fossa, which, as mentioned previously, may be difficult to detect on CT scan because of beam-hardening artifacts. Often, in retrospect, CT scans showed a similar blood clot. Sometimes a small deposit of blood in the sylvian fissure not visualized on CT scans can be demonstrated on MRI.

Magnetic resonance angiography (MRA) is equally useful in demonstrating the aneurysm, and with three-dimensional time-of-flight MRA, aneurysms 3 mm in diameter and larger can be demonstrated.

FIRST STEPS IN MANAGEMENT

Initial management in patients with aneurysmal SAH can be adapted to the initial grade. Subarachnoid hemorrhage of WFNS grade I to III should be differentiated from poor-grade SAH (WFNS grade IV or V), assuming that the poor clinical grade is caused by the initial impact alone.

The initial management in aneurysmal SAH is summarized in Table 26.3. Continuous assessment of alertness and performance remains important. Experienced nurses in neurologic intensive care usually are familiar with the peak time of cerebral ischemia and the first clinical signs of acute hydrocephalus.

An important component of management in SAH is the relief of pain. Severe headache is best treated by acetaminophen with codeine. Many patients benefit from the calming effect of these agents, but others do not tolerate opioids and may vomit excessively. Codeine remains effective in many patients. Tramadol (usually only in its maximal dose of 400 mg/day) may be helpful in this situation but should be avoided if the patient had a seizure at onset. In patients with marked neck stiffness and severe unrelenting headache, 4 mg of dexamethasone for a few days may do wonders in some.

Respiratory care is largely supportive, and serial chest radiographs should be reviewed for signs of gastric aspiration or pulmonary edema. Intubation and mechanical ventilation are often indicated in poor-grade SAH. The ventilatory mode chosen should provide adequate

TABLE 26.3. INITIAL MANAGEMENT OF ANEURYSMAL SUBARACHNOID HEMORRHAGE

Airway management	Intubation if patient has hypoxemia despite facemask with 10 L of 60%–100% oxygen/minute, if abnormal respiratory drive or if abnormal protective reflexes (likely with motor response of withdrawal or worse)
Mechanical ventilation	IMV/PS
	AC with aspiration pneumonitis, ARDS or early neurogenic pulmonary edema
Fluid management	2–3 L of 0.9% NaCl per 24 hours
	Fludrocortisone acetate, 0.2 mg b.i.d. orally, if patient has hyponatremia
Blood pressure management	Aim at SBP of < 160 mm Hg
	IV labetalol 10–15 mg every 15 min if needed
	Hydralazine 10–20 mg IV if bradycardia
Nutrition	Enteral nutrition with continuous infusion (on day 2)
	Blood glucose control (goal 140–180 mg/dL)
Prophylaxis	DVT prophylaxis with pneumatic compression devices
	SC heparin 5,000 U t.i.d. after clipping or coiling of aneurysm
	GI prophylaxis: pantoprazole 40 mg IV daily or lansoprazole 30 mg orally through nasogastric tube.
Other measures	Nimodipine, 60 mg six times a day orally for 21 days
	Tranexamic acid 1 gram IV, second dose 2 hours later, third dose 6 hours later if delayed clipping or coiling
	Codeine 30–60 mg orally every 4 hours as needed
	Tramadol, 50–100 mg orally q4h, for pain management
	Levetiracetam 20 mg/kg IV over 60 minutes; 1,000 mg b.i.d. maintenance (if seizures have occurred)
Access	Arterial catheter to monitor blood pressure (if IV antihypertensive drugs anticipated)
	Peripheral venous catheter or peripheral inserted central catheter

ARDS, acute respiratory distress syndrome; DVT, deep vein thrombosis; GI, gastrointestinal; IMV, intermittent mandatory ventilation; IV, intravenously; MAP, mean arterial pressure; NaCl, sodium chloride; PS, pressure support; SBP, systolic blood pressure; SC, subcutaneously.

minute ventilation at the lowest possible airway pressure—in most instances, an intermittent mandatory ventilation mode.

Stress cardiomyopathy tends to develop in patients with poor-grade SAH, and it can be observed clinically and on repeat echocardiograms. It may be a cause for the development of pulmonary edema (Chapter 46).

To provide adequate fluid intake is an essential part of the management of SAH. Approximately one-third of the patients have a decrease in plasma volume of more than 10% in the first days, often detected by negative fluid balance.[173] Initially, most patients are probably best managed with 3 L of isotonic saline (or infusion of 125 mL/hr). Fever (> 38.5°C) is more common in poor-grade intubated patients, but fever is also associated, in the absence of any infection, with the development of cerebral vasospasm after other causes have been excluded. Fever is typically controlled aggressively, and different methods are available[3] (Chapter 21).

The management of acute hypertension after SAH is uncertain[18] (Chapter 19). When using antihypertensive treatment, a fine line separates necessity from harm. A retrospective study suggested that the incidence of cerebral infarction is increased in patients treated with antihypertensive drugs (largely clonidine).[172] On the other hand, earlier studies suggested that rebleeding and death from rebleeding are increased in patients with persistently increased systolic blood pressures (Chapter 19). Given the lack of evidentiary data, there is insufficient guidance for antihypertensive management soon after aneurysmal subarachnoid hemorrhage.

Most practicing neurointensivists and neurosurgeons decrease blood pressure with intravenous labetalol when a mean arterial pressure of approximately 120 mm Hg or systolic blood pressure of 180 mm Hg persists.

Patients with SAH may be combative and may require sedation. Agitation may be directly related to placement of the endotracheal tube and to inappropriate mechanical ventilator settings (e.g., high-frequency assist-control in an alert patient). Not infrequently, these patients can be extubated without any difficulty, which resolves the distress and agitation. Combative and agitated patients can be best treated with low-dose midazolam or propofol infusion.

Nutrition can usually be deferred until the second day. Enteral feedings in patients with critical neurologic illness are not always tolerated, and poor gastric emptying may lead to aspiration. However, placement of a nasoenteric feeding tube

into the duodenum or jejunum may overcome these problems. Usually, concentrated commercial solutions infused at a low rate are administered (see Guidelines).

Stool softeners are prescribed, particularly for patients who regularly require opiates. Prophylaxis of deep vein thrombosis is provided by stockings and pneumatic compression devices. Proton-pump inhibitors are provided only for patients who have a history of gastric ulcers or who have been using nonsteroidal anti-inflammatory agents or aspirin and in patients on the mechanical ventilator. Patients who have a decreased level of consciousness need an indwelling bladder catheter. The use of intermittent catheterization may decrease the incidence of urinary tract infection, but the procedure is too stressful for patients with acute SAH.

Nimodipine is administered in all patients with SAH to prevent delayed cerebral ischemia.[2,5,130] It can be crushed and applied through the nasogastric tube.[2] A regimen of nimodipine (60 mg orally every 4 hours) is instituted for 21 days on the basis of significant reduction in the incidence of delayed cerebral ischemia and mortality.[2,132] A review of 90 patients treated with nimodipine for 15 days or less did not suggest an increase in delayed cerebral ischemia, but there is no reason to shorten the period of administration.[153] Nimodipine can be discontinued when cerebral angiogram shows no aneurysm. No other agents have been found to reduce cerebral ischemia.[66,67] There was interest in the use of statins following SAH. Cholesterol-lowering agents may also prevent thrombogenesis, increase cerebral arterial diameter, and reduce inflammation. Only small studies have been performed, and there were early indications of a possible benefit.[116,149,155] The Simvastatin in Aneurysmal Subarachnoid Hemorrhage (STASH) trial, however found no benefit.[98]

The use of prophylactic antiepileptic medication is very questionable. The incidence of seizures after acute SAH is low, and most seizures recur during re-rupture. The risk of late seizures may theoretically be increased in patients who have a temporal lobe or frontal lobe hematoma and large amounts of blood on CT, but again, no hard data are available to specifically justify prophylactic antiepileptic agents. Newer studies raised the possibility of worse cognitive outcome after the use of phenytoin.[127] The underlying mechanism is unclear and could be related to a pharmaceutical interaction between phenytoin and nimodipine (phenytoin may reduce bioavailability of nimodipine through induction of the hepatic cytochrome P450 isoenzymes).

Currently, antifibrinolytic therapy is not used routinely. Antifibrinolytic therapy is very effective in preventing rebleeding and significantly reduces the risk of rebleeding.[83] However, when used for prolonged periods of time, a reciprocal increase in delayed cerebral ischemia is observed and results in no overall benefit.[163] A pilot study in which tranexamic acid was given for only 4 days produced the reverse of the desired result, with no effect on the incidence of rebleeding and an increase in the incidence of cerebral ischemia.[168]

Use of antifibrinolytic agents varies among institutions and among neurosurgeons. There is a tendency to use a few doses of antifibrinolytic drugs in recently admitted patients while they await the planning of surgical repair or endovascular coiling.[26]

Emergency or early surgery is indicated in patients with evidence of rebleeding or intracerebral hematoma in the temporal lobe and tissue shift[12] and, at the opposite end of the spectrum, any patient in good prior health with WFNS grade I–III.[13] Surgery can be temporarily withheld in patients in WFNS grade IV or V with packed intraventricular hemorrhage and hydrocephalus. Ventriculostomy could produce improvement in such patients. Surgery may also be postponed in patients with early symptomatic vasospasm, but the timing of surgery has always remained contentious.

For eligible patients, cerebral angiography should be performed as soon as feasible and should be followed by surgical clipping of the aneurysm (operative techniques and neuro-anesthesia are beyond the scope of this book). A cooperative study group found in a large survey that no major differences existed between early and late surgery but that outcome was worse when surgery was performed between days 7 and 10.[95]

The development of detachable coils (Guglielmi detachable platinum coils) has dramatically modified practices.[14,19,38,107,123,152,165] A direct electrical current disconnects the coil, and the positive electrical charge increases thrombus formation. The procedure of multiple coil placement is time-consuming, taking several hours, and needs general anesthesia monitoring. Coil placement has become the first consideration in most patients with a ruptured aneurysm, irrespective of the WFNS grade.[7,11,100] It is often the first choice of treatment in basilar artery apex aneurysms because clipping is more complicated and risky.[64] In the International Subarachnoid Aneurysm

Trial (ISAT) study,[96,122] results found benefit from the use of coils in good-grade patients with small anterior circulation aneurysms, but no sufficient proof in other patients with SAH. At 1 year, coiling was superior, with a 7.4% absolute risk reduction in mortality and major disability. At 5 years, mortality in the endovascularly treated group was lower than in the surgically treated patients (11% versus 14%). There was no difference in disability between the groups.[121]

Large series of patients from France reported good outcomes in endovascularly treated patients, many with poor-grade SAH.[11] The generalizability of the ISAT trial has been questioned, most recently by a study from the University of Toronto that suggested worse hemorrhage-free survival of coiling compared with clipping.[127] Long-term outcome is not yet available, and concern about imperfect repair with coiling remains. A review of 509 patients with treated ruptured aneurysms found ischemic complications in 7% and aneurysm perforation in 3%, with procedure-related mortality of 1%.[14] The estimated morbidity related to the technique was 9%, with an overall mortality of 6%, but these numbers are now likely lower with improved skills.[14] A considerable drawback of endovascularly treated patients is rebleeding from a remnant aneurysm, with reported rebleeding rates of 6%–25%.

Experience with endovascular coil placement in acute ruptured aneurysm is currently substantial, but the decision to "clip or coil" remains arbitrary. In the ISAT trial, the inclusion of patients required that both the neurosurgeon and neuro-interventionalist considered the patients eligible for both treatments. However, in this trial[122] the involved physicians did not agree with each other in more than two-thirds of cases. Currently it can be estimated that more than 70% of ruptured aneurysms are treated endovascularly in US referral centers.

Certain criteria have emerged that are based on the width of the neck and the size and location of the aneurysm. Selection for coiling is often determined by location of the aneurysm in the posterior circulation, width of neck less than 5 mm, and a dome-to-neck ratio greater than 2 (Figure 26.7). There is a sharp reduction in the rate of complete persistent occlusion for aneurysms greater than 10 mm in diameter and in aneurysms with broad necks. However, some of these aneurysms with complex anatomy can be treated with stent-assisted coiling or balloon-modeling techniques in which a soft balloon is temporarily inflated in the parent artery to

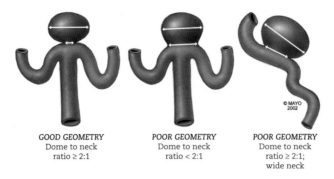

GOOD GEOMETRY
Dome to neck
ratio ≥ 2:1

POOR GEOMETRY
Dome to neck
ratio < 2:1

POOR GEOMETRY
Dome to neck
ratio ≥ 2:1;
wide neck

FIGURE 26.7: Assessment of the geometry of cerebral aneurysm. Using the neck: dome ratio to assess the feasibility of coil placement.

hold coils within the aneurysm cavity.[105,167] The endovascular techniques are evolving (hydrogel-coated and bioactive coils[106]), but the rate of complete occlusion (50%–70%) remains frustratingly low. The current coiling materials have been recently reviewed,[105,167] but a comprehensive discussion is outside the scope of this chapter. Many types of cerebral aneurysms can be coiled, but middle cerebral bifurcation aneurysms often have arterial branches arising from the sac, making coiling hazardous. The neurosurgeon is able to avoid these branches by carefully modeling and clipping the aneurysm (Figure 26.8). Platinum coil placement is illustrated in Figure 26.9, and clipping is shown in Figure 26.10. More recently, a pipeline embolization device has been used in complex (dissecting, blister, or dysplastic) aneurysms; but to use this technology (and

its complications) in acute aneurysmal sub-arachnoid hemorrhage is not fully known, and many neurointerventionalists would use it later for secondary repair of partially occluded giant aneurysms. Clopidogrel and aspirin are needed to avoid occlusion of the device and massive cerebral infarction.[24,36]

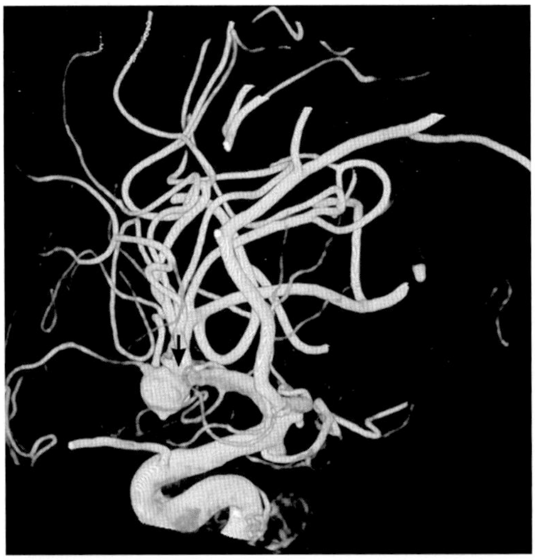

DETERIORATION: CAUSES AND MANAGEMENT

Most often, patients with SAH are prone to deterioration from delayed cerebral ischemia,[68] rebleeding, acute hydrocephalus, and enlargement of a temporal lobe hematoma.[164]

Delayed cerebral ischemia or symptomatic vasospasm is manifested by a gradual decrease in the level of consciousness in most patients,[77,80] and in some is associated with hemiparesis, mutism, and, less frequently, apraxia. Unusual presentations, such as paraparesis, have been described.[62] Patients with delayed cerebral ischemia may become apathetic, cut short answers to questions, and have initial weakness of one leg or both legs, indicating infarction in both territories of the anterior cerebral arteries.[62] However, cerebral infarcts may appear without appreciable clinical signs.[147] Delayed cerebral ischemia may cause sudden deterioration and coma, and then often massive brain swelling, and bihemispheric infarction is detectable on a repeat CT scan. Early recognition of the decrease in level of consciousness remains crucial. Patients have a fluctuating level of consciousness: days with daytime sleep and being barely arousable, intermingled with days of appropriate behavior and better responsiveness. Risk factors for delayed cerebral ischemia include a large number of cisternal and ventricular clots (mostly on the first CT scan),[15,48] poor WFNS clinical grade, hyperglycemia, and early surgery.[34] The incidence of

FIGURE 26.8: Middle cerebral artery aneurysm (*arrow*) with multiple branches.

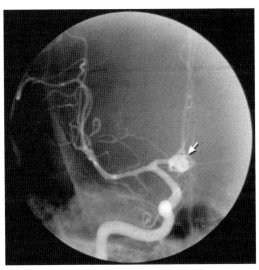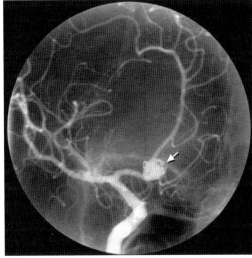

FIGURE 26.9: Successful endovascular coil placement in anterior cerebral artery (ACOM complex) aneurysm (*arrow*).

cerebral vasospasm in patients who have endovascular treatment is not known exactly, but our review suggests significantly less symptomatic vasospasm than that which occurs with clipping of the aneurysm.[134] Additional laboratory testing (e.g., transcranial Doppler ultrasonography, CT perfusion, or cerebral angiography) may confirm cerebral vasospasm.

Diffusion-weighted MRI can detect abnormalities and a reduction in diffusion coefficients. It is unknown whether these abnormalities are potentially reversible with therapeutic intervention.

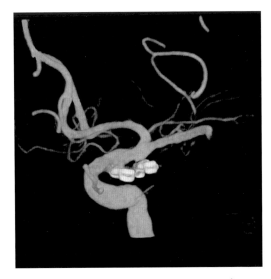

FIGURE 26.10: Aneurysmal clip. Clipping of aneurysm on 3D cerebral angiogram.

Currently, limited experience suggests a role in the diagnosis of delayed cerebral ischemia. Studies have shown scattered multiple hyperintense signals highly consistent with the diffuse nature of cerebral vasospasm.

One study reported the use of diffusion-weighted MRI in patients with vasospasm. All 10 patients with Doppler-confirmed vasospasm had diffusion-weighted imaging abnormalities, whereas four control patients without vasospasm had no such abnormalities. Interestingly, seven of the 10 patients with vasospasm were asymptomatic, and some of the diffusion-weighted abnormalities were reversible.[32] Another modality that may become clinically useful is CT perfusion.[37] However, the definition of hypoperfusion, despite use of color maps, remains unclear. There is insufficient data to use CT perfusion as guidance for hemodynamic augmentation. We recognize the difficulties in the timely acquisition of these tests.

The management of cerebral vasospasm has been guided by a medical attempt first and then, almost simultaneously, a cerebral angiogram and endovascular intervention if severe vasospasm can be demonstrated. Current published data on the best approach are unconvincing because systematic measurements of variables are lacking, with different methods used in each of the cohorts. The areas of uncertainty are the timing of hemodynamic augmentation, the variable to be augmented (perfusion pressure or cardiac

TABLE 26.4. PROTOCOL FOR EUVOLEMIC HYPERTENSION IN THE TREATMENT OF CEREBRAL VASOSPASM IN ANEURYSMAL SUBARACHNOID HEMORRHAGE

SAH, clinically asymptomatic but TCD or CT (angiogram or perfusion) evidence of diffuse cerebral vasospasm
Obtain hourly readings of fluid balance and body weight
Accomplish volume repletion with crystalloids
Avoid antihypertensive and diuretic agents
SAH, secured aneurysm, clinical evidence of cerebral vasospasm
Notify neurointerventionalist for possible cerebral angiography
Give crystalloid bolus or albumin 5%
Match fluid input with urine output
When urine output is > 250 mL/hr, start administration of fludrocortisone acetate, 0.2 mg b.i.d.
Concurrently start administration of IV phenylephrine, 10–30 µg/min, with increase in MAP 25% above
    baseline or > 120 mm Hg (a central access is secured).
Start administration of IV dobutamine, 5–15 µg/kg/min if no response.
Consider replacing phenylephrine with norepinephrine if no response.
Perform cerebral angiography for angioplasty or intra-arterial infusion with verapamil.

CT, computed tomography; MAP, mean arterial pressure; SAH, subarachnoid hemorrhage; TCD, transcranial Doppler ultrasonography.

output), the management of a concomitant cerebral salt-wasting syndrome,[172,173] and the timing of endovascular procedures.[109-111,119] One such protocol is outlined in Table 26.4, and we summarize our approach with euvolemic hypertension. Maintenance of intravascular volume expansion can be enhanced by fludrocortisone acetate 0.2 mg orally twice a day. The fluid balance is carefully calculated every hour and scrutinized for changes in urinary output. Weight change is essentially equivalent to change in body water, and therefore the daily availability of body weight is useful in adjusting fluid intake. Commonly used hemodynamic agents are shown in Table 26.5.

Particular care is warranted in patients with significant EKG changes, and induced hypertension may possibly trigger cardiac arrhythmias.

When patients do not rapidly improve with these measures, we proceed with a cerebral angiogram. Angioplasty can be considered if adequate volume expansion has not resulted in marked clinical improvement. Cerebral vasospasm can be arbitrarily categorized as mild, moderate, or severe with 50% luminal narrowing. Focal cerebral vasospasm indicates vasospasm in one cerebral artery; in diffuse cerebral vasospasm, multiple vessels are involved. Angioplasty of focal spastic segments is a potentially effective treatment for cerebral vasospasm. Neurologic

TABLE 26.5. COMMONLY USED HEMODYNAMIC AGENTS IN SUBARACHNOID HEMORRHAGE

Agent	Action	Dose	Side Effect
Dobutamine	β_1 agonist ($\uparrow$CO) β_2 stimulation ($\downarrow$SVR)	5–40 µg/kg/min	Tachycardia (often when hypovolemic)
Dopamine	Low dose (0.5–3 µg/kg/min) →renal vasodilatation →small decrease in BP High dose (10–20 µg/kg/min) ($\uparrow\beta_2$ receptors) $\uparrow$increase in CO $\uparrow$increase in BP	1–20 µg/kg/min	Tachyarrhythmia (common)
Phenylephrine	agonist ($\uparrow$SVR) No effect on CO	10–30 µg/min	Reflex bradycardia

BP, blood pressure; CO, cardiac output; SVR, systemic vascular resistance. (Also see appendix for titration schedule.)

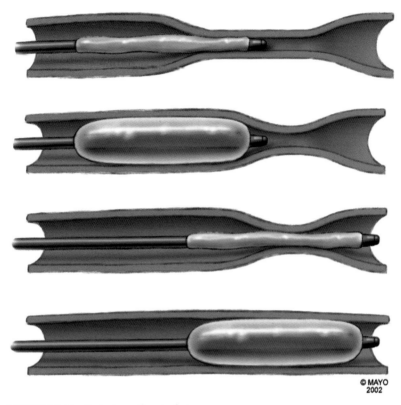

© MAYO
2002

FIGURE 26.11: Technique of angioplasty.

improvement has been reported in 60%–70% of patients who did not have a response to hypervolemic hypertensive treatment, but these results seem too optimistic.

Angioplasty of the major cerebral arteries is performed with a silicone balloon catheter.[33,50,51,91,102,108] After proper placement, the balloon is gently inflated to one atmosphere and almost immediately deflated and advanced 1 cm to the next segment. The technique most commonly used is shown in Figure 26.11. The middle cerebral, anterior cerebral, posterior cerebral, and vertebral arteries are eligible for angioplasty. More distal arteries are technically accessible, but the risk of rupture from overextension is real. Angioplasty of a feeding artery of a recently ruptured aneurysm is contraindicated unless the aneurysm is secured first with coils or clips. Risk of rupture of the artery itself is low, but rupture may occur with overdistention or distal placement in the artery.[114] Except for this caveat, most neurointerventionalists treat all accessible vasospastic arteries at once.[178]

Histopathologic studies showed that compression and expansion of the intima caused considerable stretching of the vessel to diameters larger than original.[86] Intimal damage appeared minimal. Angioplasty can be performed without major complications. Virtually no patients have subsequent infarcts in the territory of the perforators of the MCA, most likely because there is no intimal damage.

Several intra-arterial agents have been used in small groups of patients and have shown variable success (Table 26.6). The main objective against its use is a temporary effect (not more than 24 hours) of any of the vasodilating agents and safety concerns, particularly papaverine,[31,76] resulting in myocardial depression and suppression of

TABLE 26.6. INTRA-ARTERIAL AGENTS TO IMPROVE CEREBRAL VASOSPASM

Agent	t1/2	Improvement Arteries vs. Clinical
Papaverine[85]	2 hours	43% vs. n/a
Verapamil[52]	7 hours	44% vs. 33%
Nicardipine[4,150]	16 hours	60% vs. 91%
Nimodipine[9]	9 hours	43% vs. 76%

n/a = not available.

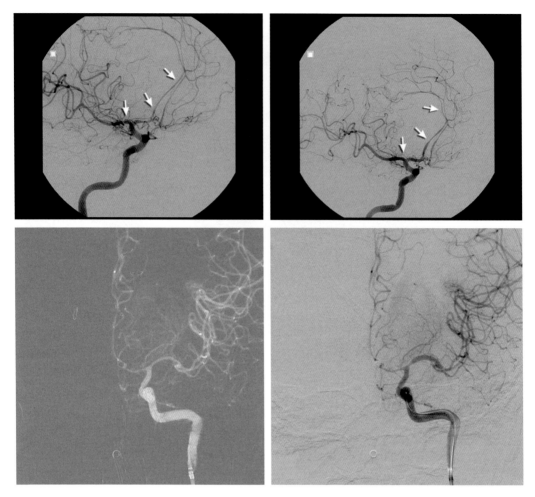

FIGURE 26.12: Two patients with symptomatic cerebral vasospasm. *Upper row*: Some improvement of cerebral vasospasm with intra-arterial verapamil. *Lower row*: Marked improvement with angioplasty.

the AV and SA node. Most institutions now use intra-arterial verapamil or nicardipine, either selectively or in the carotid artery (Figure 26.12). Some groups[92] have advocated multiple papaverine infusions with a follow-up angiogram 24 hours later, followed by repeat infusions (up to three infusions on consecutive days), but papaverine is out of favor with most interventional neuroradiologists.[6,30,94,115]

Failure to reverse clinical deficits most commonly indicates cerebral infarction. Computed tomography scanning may be helpful but, if done early, may give only a limited view of the area that is infarcted. Not infrequently, only a single arterial territory appears affected, but multifocal infarction may become apparent on subsequent CT scans or at autopsy.[135] (One should be aware that multiple small hypodensities on CT scan, particularly in the cerebellum, thalamus, and cortical

areas, may be related to complications from cerebral angiography.[89]) Mass effect from large hemispheric infarction may occur and often is fatal. Temporal lobectomy may salvage the patient but at the price of severe disability. It may be an option only in young patients.

The risk of rebleeding after the first rupture is approximately 30% in the first month. Larger aneurysms are at higher risk for rebleeding (possible cutoff of 10 mm).[10] Early placement of ventriculostomy in patients not treated with antifibrinolytics[157] was a major risk factor in one study not ours.[120] Many patients rebleed within hours after the first bleeding.[58,81,97] The clinical presentation of re-rupture can be dramatic and could involveare loss of consciousness associated with loss of several brainstem reflexes, including pupillary light response and oculocephalic responses. In most patients, respiratory arrest or

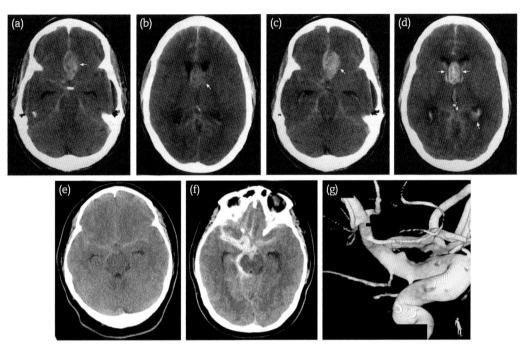

FIGURE 26.13: Two examples of rebleeding. Initial hemorrhage (a, b). Rebleeding (c, d); note new blood in ventricles (*arrows*). Initial SAH with worsening hemiparesis soon after admission. (e) Contrast CTA shows contrast leakage. (f) Cerebral angiogram shows carotid artery blister (1 mm by 2.5 mm) aneurysm (g).

gasping breathing occurs, necessitating immediate endotracheal intubation and mechanical ventilation.[82] Computed tomography scanning very often demonstrates fresh blood, more common in the ventricular system (Figure 26.13), or less often a new intracerebral hematoma that causes marked brain tissue shift. Recovery from rebleeding is difficult to predict, but many patients begin to trigger the ventilator within hours, and recovery is also signaled by a return of brainstem reflexes. These patients may improve rapidly, up to the point of self-extubation. Rebleeding can be much less dramatic in patients presenting with acute headache alone. In some fortunate patients, rebleeding begins with sudden emergence of fresh blood in the collection bag of the ventricular drain, and rapid evacuation of intraventricular blood is often life-saving. More subtle presentation are possible with patients complaining of a worsening headache after headache had subsided or became more tolerable. New onset and transient focal signs maybe observed.

Management of rebleeding is essentially supportive. Emergency clipping or coiling of the aneurysm must be strongly considered, since most patients will have a second rebleed, which is associated with high mortality. The initial mortality of rebleeding is 50%. The total mortality from rebleeding and from complications associated with persistent coma is 80% in 3 months.[81] Patients with a devastating rebleed may progress to brain death. This clinical course is most likely in patients with massive hydrocephalus and ventricles packed with blood clots.

The clinical presentation of acute hydrocephalus is characterized by progressive impairment of consciousness.[45,70,158] Patients become much more drowsy, tachypneic, and may not be able to protect the airway or cough up secretions. Most patients cannot follow complex commands, and only vigorous pain stimuli will open the eyes and cause localization of a pain stimulus. Pinpoint pupils and downward deviation of the eyes may develop, most often in patients with dramatic enlargement of the ventricular system. The diagnosis of acute hydrocephalus becomes clear when serial CT scans show further enlargement of the ventricular system.

Placement of a ventricular drain is indicated in patients with intraventricular blood and clinical deterioration. It has been suggested that the risk of rebleeding is increased in patients with ventricular drainage. Our study in SAH failed to show an increased incidence of rebleeding when

TABLE 26.7. CONTRAINDICATIONS FOR LUMBAR DRAIN PLACEMENT
IN ANEURYSMAL SUBARACHNOID HEMORRHAGE

Any hemispheric or extracranial hematoma with mass effect or shift of midline structures
Effacement of the basilar cisterns
Obstructive clot in third or fourth ventricle
Coagulopathy (INR > 1.4)

preoperative ventriculostomy was done within 24 hours after SAH before aneurysmal repair.[120]

Ventriculostomy is often performed when enlarged hemoventricles are present in comatose patients, but we have not often seen dramatic improvement in patients with loss of upper brainstem reflexes. Late hydrocephalus may be more common in patients with intraventricular casts, and 20%–50% may need a permanent shunt.[23] The external ventricular drainage (EVD) is kept open at 10 cm above the external auditory canal or lower if no clinical improvement is seen after CSF drainage the first day of placement.

Increased intracranial pressure is common in SAH from edema in severe cases or due to acute hydrocephalus.[177] Acute hydrocephalus may also be managed with placement of a lumbar drain.[84,117] Contraindications are summarized in Table 26.7. Placement is simple through a lumbar puncture needle, but may need fluoroscopy[84] (Figure 26.14). The collection chamber is placed at the level of the shoulder and CSF of 20 mL or less is drained per hour. The collection chamber can be raised to reduce CSF collection. It is unresolved whether lumbar drainage provides better clot removal than ventriculostomies, but one retrospective study found a dramatic threefold reduction in cerebral vasospasm using a lumbar drain. However, differences in cerebral vasospasm may be related to better ICP control and not blood washout.[99] A prospective study using lumbar drain versus standard therapy reduced ischemia but did not improve outcome.[1] We found aggressive CSF diversion improved CBF after lumbar drainage.[57] Higher complications were found in one study.[128]

There are different practices of weaning of the ventriculostomy. It can be convincingly argued

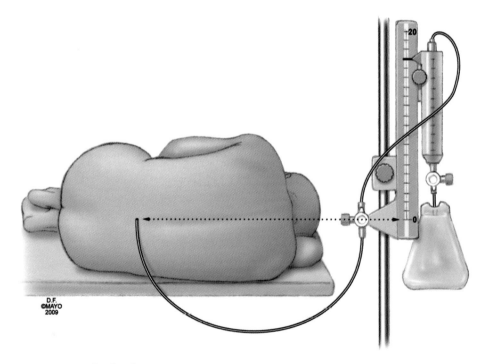

FIGURE 26.14: Lumbar drain in situ.

that patients with high risk of cerebral vasospasm should continue to drain CSF to reduce ICP and to enhance clot removal. Acute hydrocephalus may also reduce cerebral perfusion in the periventricular white matter and basal ganglia and somewhat less in cortical areas.[156] Therefore, weaning should be considered in patients only after 7–10 days in situ. Patients with CSF red blood cell counts of less than 10,000 cells/mL, CSF protein levels less than 40 mg/dL, and normal or improving bicaudate and third ventricle size after 24 hours clamping can be weaned successfully. In some patients, raising the EVD to 20 cm will develop headaches and increasing ICP, but multiple attempts in the following days may still be successful. We have used acetazolamide to reduce CSF production because it inhibits carbonic anhydrase mediated CSF production and this can be substantial, up to 50% of normal CSF production. Rapid or slow weaning does not predict ventricular peritoneal shunt placement. Some studies found a higher incidence of shunt dependency in coiled patients versus clipped patients, a finding tentatively explained by clot removal during surgery.[39,161] Shunt valves maintain an instant flow of CSF. Flow control valves with low settings may cause overdrainage, in particular if it lowers CSF below the physiologic limits (<5 cm H_2O). Valve settings can be programmed (from 3–20 cm H_2O pressures). In some patients normal pressure hydrocephalus may occur weeks after subarachnoid hemorrhage and low ventriculostomy levels are needed to maintain drainage. Low valve settings or no valve may be needed to avoid post ventriculoperitoneal hydrocephalus.

Subarachnoid hemorrhage in a patient admitted with a temporal lobe hematoma, almost invariably associated with an MCA aneurysm, is relatively unusual but potentially life-threatening. The hematoma usually is large, and virtually no blood is present in the cisterns other than the suprasellar cistern.

Acute deterioration with massive enlargement of the hematoma may occur with rebleeding, most often diagnosed when additional intraventricular hemorrhage is found. Early neurosurgical intervention is indicated and, in addition to evacuation of the clot, includes repair of the aneurysm.[75] It is difficult to decide whether patients with drowsiness alone should have emergency neurosurgical evacuation, but one may opt for emergency angiography in this situation and proceed with clipping of the aneurysm soon after presentation. A study of intracerebral

hematoma in aneurysmal SAH showed that intracranial hemorrhage on CT scan alone was more often associated with a poor outcome. In another study, rebleeding occurred statistically more often in patients with SAH-associated intracranial hematomas. Therefore, patients with intracerebral hemorrhage should be scheduled for early angiographic study and emergency surgery. The management of temporal lobe hematoma in the current endovascular era has become more difficult. Patients may have the aneurysm secured, but clinical improvement may stall due to mass effect. In some of these patients, later evacuation of the temporal hematoma is performed.

Subarachnoid hemorrhage may be the first manifestation of a ruptured giant aneurysm. Sudden deterioration in a patient with a giant aneurysm may indicate thrombus formation, and extension to the parent vessel may cause infarction.[97] Timing of surgery and planning of techniques, including hypothermic cardiopulmonary bypass, may take additional days after admission. The management mortality has been estimated to be about 21%, with perioperative mortality reaching 10%. Temporary occlusion of a patent vessel is needed in two-thirds of the cases.

A particularly difficult problem arises when a patient's condition deteriorates in the days after clipping of the aneurysm. Drowsiness is common in patients who have had early surgery, and whether lifting and retraction causing swelling of the brain or vasospasm is the cause of neurologic deterioration is clinically difficult to determine. Transcranial Doppler ultrasonography or perfusion CT scan may distinguish between the two possibilities. In patients with postoperative swelling, transcranial Doppler ultrasonography findings are within normal limits, and most of these patients improve over days.

Of all possible systemic complications, hyponatremia is the most common but is seldom a cause of deterioration. It is more common in patients with hydrocephalus, particularly enlargement of the third ventricle. A mild degree of hyponatremia (125–134 mmol/L) is asymptomatic and self-limiting. Severe hyponatremia (< 120 mmol/L) requires urgent treatment with 3% saline but is very rare after SAH. If hyponatremia is persistent, fludrocortisone can be added (Chapter 57).[68,174] Pituitary dysfunction is more common than appreciated.[63]

An unusual but well-documented cause of sudden deterioration is acute cardiac arrhythmia with a significant decrease in blood pressure.[118] Well-known life-threatening cardiac arrhythmias are brief ventricular tachycardia, asystole, and torsades de pointes (Chapter 56).

Seizures may cause sudden deterioration, but most are observed at the initial rupture or during rebleeding.[69] Failure to fully awaken after a generalized tonic-clonic seizure may point to nonconvulsive status epilepticus, but again, this cause of deterioration is very unusual.[17]

An uncommon cause of sudden deterioration is pulmonary embolism. The risk is increased after craniotomy and in patients who have leg paralysis predisposing to deep vein thrombosis (often after clipping of the ACA aneurysm). Sudden death from pulmonary embolism may occur in the first 2 weeks after successful clipping of the aneurysm.

In summary, acute, often transient, deterioration in SAH remains unexplained in 20%–30% of patients. It is certainly possible that unwitnessed seizures, drug effects (e.g., from large doses of opioids for pain management), or swelling surrounding a parenchymal hematoma can be implicated in some instances, but the cause often remains elusive.

OUTCOME

Several outcome studies have shown that, in patients with SAH who reach the hospital, the initial grade and coma on admission determine outcome

(Figure 26.15).[22,132,145] Failure to improve in neurologic grade within 48 hours in poor-grade SAH (IV or V) despite ventriculostomy is associated with a high likelihood of poor outcome, particularly in patients with intraventricular hemorrhage and ventriculomegaly. Many of these patients die from systemic complications if they do not awaken from coma 2–3 weeks after admission.[35] Many other factors also contribute, such as amount of blood on CT scan, aneurysm site (particularly the posterior circulation), and size, age, and further neurologic deterioration, all of which determine a less satisfactory outcome. Poor outcome is likely in patients with early or delayed cerebral edema, but reasonably good outcome is found in approximately 40% of patients.[27] In several studies, seizures at onset emerged as an independent risk factor for late seizures and poor outcome.[16,28]

Lower hemoglobin concentrations may be associated with worse outcome. This association can be explained by more blood samples in poor-grade SAH patients and possibly more aggressive fluid management. However, microdialysis and brain tissue oxygen tension data suggest increased brain tissue hypoxemia and a higher lactate/pyruvate ratio (indicative of cell energy dysfunction) in patients already with hemoglobin levels of less than 9 gr/dL.[103]

Good clinical grade at presentation, no cerebral hematoma on CT or later cerebral infarction,

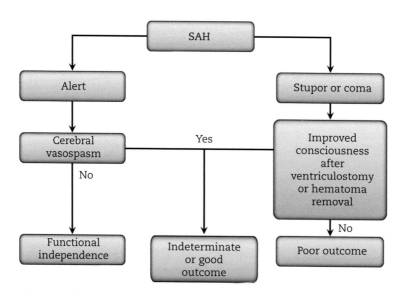

FIGURE 26.15: Outcome algorithm. Functional independence: No assistance needed, minor handicap may remain. Indeterminate: Any statement would be a premature conclusion. Poor outcome: Severe disability, persistent vegetative state, or death.

SAH, subarachnoid hemorrhage.

and absence of severe anemia requiring blood transfusion all increased the likelihood of excellent functional outcome.[129] Patients who have a supposedly good outcome after SAH could have neuropsychologic deficits characterized by disturbed concentration, disturbed mood, short-term memory lapses, and difficulty with information processing.[65] This condition may be more prevalent in patients with surgery for anterior circulation aneurysms. In many of these patients, extensive neuropsychologic battery tests are needed to demonstrate these findings. Mood changes may remain at 1 year after SAH.

Patients with normal angiograms have a much better outcome, but only if they have a pretruncal pattern on CT scan.[138,159] One study found that patients with normal angiograms and so-called aneurysmal patterns on CT scan (diffuse localized blood in all cisterns rather than more focal perimesencephalic hemorrhage) did as poorly as patients with aneurysmal hemorrhage, whereas patients with pretruncal nonaneurysmal hemorrhage did not have any major cognitive deficits, rebleeding, or delayed cerebral ischemia.[137]

Recent follow-up data of the ISAT trial revealed after 1 year higher mortality in coiling (10% coiling vs. 8% clipping) and more disability in the surgical treated patients (21% clipping vs. 15% coiled).[125] Rebleeding rates were substantial—and unacceptable for some critics—with 2.9% for coiling and 0.9% for surgery. A statistical model using the ISAT data also projected that the lifetime rebleeding rate may be unacceptably high in young patients (< 40 years).[121] Better coiling techniques and less "redos" may change these projections.

Recurrence of SAH after satisfactory obliteration of the aneurysm by surgical clipping is low. In a large study from Japan with a median follow-up of 11 years, recurrence approximated 3%. The risk of regrowth of a previously clipped aneurysm was 0.26% annually. De novo formation of aneurysms after clipping was 0.89% annually and, as expected, was more common in patients with prior multiple aneurysms.

CONCLUSIONS

- Basic management in SAH consists of (a) endotracheal intubation if patients cannot protect their airway, have aspirated, or have acquired neurogenic pulmonary edema; (b) adequate fluid management with 2 or 3 L of 0.9% sodium chloride; (c) no antihypertensive agents unless mean arterial pressure is more than 120 mm Hg or 160 mm Hg systolic; (d) nimodipine, 60 mg every 4 hours; and (e) pneumatic compression devices and pain management with codeine.
- The management of rebleeding consists of mechanical ventilation, antiepileptic agents if seizures occurred and emergency angiography on recovery, and early clipping or coiling.
- Delayed cerebral ischemia is managed by hemodynamic augmentation and, if this is unsuccessful, angioplasty or intra-arterial administration of verapamil or nicardipine.
- Ventriculostomy is indicated in acute hydrocephalus and hemoventricles.
- Lumbar drain placement may decrease subarachnoid blood and control ICP.

REFERENCES

1. Al-Tamimi YZ, Bhargava D, Feltbower RG, et al. Lumbar drainage of cerebrospinal fluid after aneurysmal subarachnoid hemorrhage: a prospective, randomized, controlled trial (LUMAS). *Stroke* 2012;43:677–682.
2. Allen GS, Ahn HS, Preziosi TJ, et al. Cerebral arterial spasm: a controlled trial of nimodipine in patients with subarachnoid hemorrhage. *N Engl J Med* 1983;308:619–624.
3. Badjatia N, O'Donnell J, Baker JR, et al. Achieving normothermia in patients with febrile subarachnoid hemorrhage: feasibility and safety of a novel intravascular cooling catheter. *Neurocrit Care* 2004;1:145–156.
4. Badjatia N, Topcuoglu MA, Pryor JC, et al. Preliminary experience with intra-arterial nicardipine as a treatment for cerebral vasospasm. *AJNR Am J Neuroradiol* 2004;25:819–826.
5. Barker FG, 2nd, Ogilvy CS. Efficacy of prophylactic nimodipine for delayed ischemic deficit after subarachnoid hemorrhage: a metaanalysis. *J Neurosurg* 1996;84:405–414.
6. Barr JD, Mathis JM, Horton JA. Transient severe brain stem depression during intraarterial papaverine infusion for cerebral vasospasm. *AJNR Am J Neuroradiol* 1994;15:719–723.
7. Bavinzski G, Killer M, Gruber A, et al. Treatment of basilar artery bifurcation aneurysms by using Guglielmi detachable coils: a 6-year experience. *J Neurosurg* 1999;90:843–852.
8. Bederson JB, Connolly ES, Jr., Batjer HH, et al. Guidelines for the management of aneurysmal subarachnoid hemorrhage: a statement for healthcare professionals from a special writing group of the Stroke Council, American Heart Association. *Stroke* 2009;40:994–1025.

9. Biondi A, Ricciardi GK, Puybasset L, et al. Intra-arterial nimodipine for the treatment of symptomatic cerebral vasospasm after aneurysmal subarachnoid hemorrhage: preliminary results. *AJNR Am J Neuroradiol* 2004;25:1067–1076.

10. Boogaarts HD, van Lieshout JH, van Amerongen MJ, et al. Aneurysm diameter as a risk factor for pretreatment rebleeding: a meta-analysis. *J Neurosurg* 2015;122:921–928.

11. Bracard S, Lebedinsky A, Anxionnat R, et al. Endovascular treatment of Hunt and Hess grade IV and V aneuryms. *AJNR Am J Neuroradiol* 2002;23:953–957.

12. Brandt L, Sonesson B, Ljunggren B, Saveland H. Ruptured middle cerebral artery aneurysm with intracerebral hemorrhage in younger patients appearing moribund: emergency operation? *Neurosurgery* 1987;20:925–929.

13. Brilstra EH, Rinkel GJ, Algra A, van Gijn J. Rebleeding, secondary ischemia, and timing of operation in patients with subarachnoid hemorrhage. *Neurology* 2000;55:1656–1660.

14. Brilstra EH, Rinkel GJ, van der Graaf Y, van Rooij WJ, Algra A. Treatment of intracranial aneurysms by embolization with coils: a systematic review. *Stroke* 1999;30:470–476.

15. Brouwers PJ, Wijdicks EFM, Van Gijn J. Infarction after aneurysm rupture does not depend on distribution or clearance rate of blood. *Stroke* 1992;23:374–379.

16. Butzkueven H, Evans AH, Pitman A, et al. Onset seizures independently predict poor outcome after subarachnoid hemorrhage. *Neurology* 2000;55:1315–1320.

17. Byrne JV, Boardman P, Ioannidis I, Adcock J, Traill Z. Seizures after aneurysmal subarachnoid hemorrhage treated with coil embolization. *Neurosurgery* 2003;52:545–552.

18. Calhoun DA, Oparil S. Treatment of hypertensive crisis. *N Engl J Med* 1990;323:1177–1183.

19. Casasco AE, Aymard A, Gobin YP, et al. Selective endovascular treatment of 71 intracranial aneurysms with platinum coils. *J Neurosurg* 1993;79:3–10.

20. Cebral JR, Castro MA, Burgess JE, et al. Characterization of cerebral aneurysms for assessing risk of rupture by using patient-specific computational hemodynamics models. *AJNR Am J Neuroradiol* 2005;26:2550–2559.

21. Cebral JR, Hendrickson S, Putman CM. Hemodynamics in a lethal basilar artery aneurysm just before its rupture. *AJNR Am J Neuroradiol* 2009;30:95–98.

22. Cesarini KG, Hardemark HG, Persson L. Improved survival after aneurysmal subarachnoid hemorrhage: review of case management during a 12-year period. *J Neurosurg* 1999;90:664–672.

23. Chan M, Alaraj A, Calderon M, et al. Prediction of ventriculoperitoneal shunt dependency in patients with aneurysmal subarachnoid hemorrhage. *J Neurosurg* 2009;110:44–49.

24. Chan RS, Mak CH, Wong AK, Chan KY, Leung KM. Use of the pipeline embolization device to treat recently ruptured dissecting cerebral aneurysms. *Interv Neuroradiol* 2014;20:436–441.

25. Chang TR, Kowalski RG, Carhuapoma JR, Tamargo RJ, Naval NS. Impact of case volume on aneurysmal subarachnoid hemorrhage outcomes. *J Crit Care* 2015;30:469–472.

26. Chwajol M, Starke RM, Kim GH, Mayer SA, Connolly ES. Antifibrinolytic therapy to prevent early rebleeding after subarachnoid hemorrhage. *Neurocrit Care* 2008;8:418–426.

27. Claassen J, Carhuapoma JR, Kreiter KT, et al. Global cerebral edema after subarachnoid hemorrhage: frequency, predictors, and impact on outcome. *Stroke* 2002;33:1225–1232.

28. Claassen J, Peery S, Kreiter KT, et al. Predictors and clinical impact of epilepsy after subarachnoid hemorrhage. *Neurology* 2003;60:208–214.

29. Cloft HJ, Joseph GJ, Dion JE. Risk of cerebral angiography in patients with subarachnoid hemorrhage, cerebral aneurysm, and arteriovenous malformation: a meta-analysis. *Stroke* 1999;30:317–320.

30. Clouston JE, Numaguchi Y, Zoarski GH, et al. Intraarterial papaverine infusion for cerebral vasospasm after subarachnoid hemorrhage. *AJNR Am J Neuroradiol* 1995;16:27–38.

31. Clyde BL, Firlik AD, Kaufmann AM, Spearman MP, Yonas H. Paradoxical aggravation of vasospasm with papaverine infusion following aneurysmal subarachnoid hemorrhage: case report. *J Neurosurg* 1996;84:690–695.

32. Condette-Auliac S, Bracard S, Anxionnat R, et al. Vasospasm after subarachnoid hemorrhage: interest in diffusion-weighted MR imaging. *Stroke* 2001;32:1818–1824.

33. Coyne TJ, Montanera WJ, Macdonald RL, Wallace MC. Percutaneous transluminal angioplasty for cerebral vasospasm after subarachnoid hemorrhage. *Can J Surg* 1994;37:391–396.

34. Crobeddu E, Mittal MK, Dupont S, et al. Predicting the lack of development of delayed cerebral ischemia after aneurysmal subarachnoid hemorrhage. *Stroke* 2012;43:697–701.

35. Cross DT, 3rd, Tirschwell DL, Clark MA, et al. Mortality rates after subarachnoid hemorrhage: variations according to hospital case volume in 18 states. *J Neurosurg* 2003;99:810–817.

36. Cruz JP, O'Kelly C, Kelly M, et al. Pipeline embolization device in aneurysmal subarachnoid hemorrhage. *AJNR Am J Neuroradiol* 2013;34:271–276.

37. Dankbaar JW, de Rooij NK, Velthuis BK, et al. Diagnosing delayed cerebral ischemia with different CT modalities in patients with subarachnoid hemorrhage with clinical deterioration. *Stroke* 2009;40:3493–3498.

38. Debrun GM, Aletich VA, Kehrli P, et al. Selection of cerebral aneurysms for treatment using Guglielmi detachable coils: the preliminary University of Illinois at Chicago experience. *Neurosurgery* 1998;43:1281–1295.

39. Dehdashti AR, Rilliet B, Rufenacht DA, de Tribolet N. Shunt-dependent hydrocephalus after rupture of intracranial aneurysms: a prospective study of the influence of treatment modality. *J Neurosurg* 2004;101:402–407.

40. Demircivi F, Ozkan N, Buyukkececi S, et al. Traumatic subarachnoid haemorrhage: analysis of 89 cases. *Acta Neurochir (Wien)* 1993;122:45–48.

41. Di Lorenzo N, Guidetti G. Anterior communicating aneurysm missed at angiography: report of two cases treated surgically. *Neurosurgery* 1988;23:494–499.

42. Diringer MN. Management of aneurysmal subarachnoid hemorrhage. *Crit Care Med* 2009;37:432–440.

43. Dodick DW. Thunderclap headache. *J Neurol Neurosurg Psychiatry* 2002;72:6–11.

44. Dodick DW, Wijdicks EFM. Pituitary apoplexy presenting as a thunderclap headache. *Neurology* 1998;50:1510–1511.

45. Dorai Z, Hynan LS, Kopitnik TA, Samson D. Factors related to hydrocephalus after aneurysmal subarachnoid hemorrhage. *Neurosurgery* 2003;52:763–769.

46. Drake CG. Report of World Federation of Neurological Surgeons Committee on a universal subarachnoid hemorrhage grading scale. *J Neurosurg* 1988;68:985–986.

47. Dupont SA, Wijdicks EFM, Lanzino G, Rabinstein AA. Aneurysmal subarachnoid hemorrhage: an overview for the practicing neurologist. *Semin Neurol* 2010;30:545–554.

48. Dupont SA, Wijdicks EFM, Manno EM, et al. Timing of computed tomography and prediction of vasospasm after aneurysmal subarachnoid hemorrhage. *Neurocrit Care* 2009;11:71–75.

49. Dupont SA, Wijdicks EFM, Manno EM, Lanzino G, Rabinstein AA. Prediction of angiographic vasospasm after aneurysmal subarachnoid hemorrhage: value of the Hijdra sum scoring system. *Neurocrit Care* 2009;11:172–176.

50. Eddleman CS, Hurley MC, Naidech AM, Batjer HH, Bendok BR. Endovascular options in the treatment of delayed ischemic neurological deficits due to cerebral vasospasm. *Neurosurg Focus* 2009;26:E6.

51. Elliott JP, Newell DW, Lam DJ, et al. Comparison of balloon angioplasty and papaverine infusion for the treatment of vasospasm following aneurysmal subarachnoid hemorrhage. *J Neurosurg* 1998;88:277–284.

52. Feng L, Fitzsimmons BF, Young WL, et al. Intraarterially administered verapamil as adjunct therapy for cerebral vasospasm: safety and 2-year experience. *AJNR Am J Neuroradiol* 2002;23:1284–1290.

53. Fisher CM, Roberson GH, Ojemann RG. Cerebral vasospasm with ruptured saccular aneurysm: the clinical manifestations. *Neurosurgery* 1977;1:245–248.

54. Foot C, Staib A. How valuable is a lumbar puncture in the management of patients with suspected subarachnoid hemorrhage? *Emerg Med (Fremantle)* 2001;13:326–332.

55. Frizzell RT, Kuhn F, Morris R, Quinn C, Fisher WS, 3rd. Screening for ocular hemorrhages in patients with ruptured cerebral aneurysms: a prospective study of 99 patients. *Neurosurgery* 1997;41:529–533.

56. Frosen J, Piippo A, Paetau A, et al. Remodeling of saccular cerebral artery aneurysm wall is associated with rupture: histological analysis of 24 unruptured and 42 ruptured cases. *Stroke* 2004;35:2287–2293.

57. Fugate JE, Rabinstein AA, Wijdicks EFM, Lanzino G. Aggressive CSF diversion reverses delayed cerebral ischemia in aneurysmal subarachnoid hemorrhage: a case report. *Neurocrit Care* 2012;17:112–116.

58. Fujii Y, Takeuchi S, Sasaki O, et al. Ultra-early rebleeding in spontaneous subarachnoid hemorrhage. *J Neurosurg* 1996;84:35–42.

59. Giraldo EA, Mandrekar JN, Rubin MN, et al. Timing of clinical grade assessment and poor outcome in patients with aneurysmal subarachnoid hemorrhage. *J Neurosurg* 2012;117:15–19.

60. Goodman BP, Wijdicks EFM, Schievink WI. Systemic lupus erythematous and intracranial aneurysms [Abstract]. *Ann Neurol* 2001;50 (Suppl):S1–S5.

61. Graf S, Schischma A, Eberhardt KE, et al. Intracranial aneurysms and dolichoectasia in autosomal dominant polycystic kidney disease. *Nephrol Dial Transplant* 2002;17:819–823.

62. Greene KA, Marciano FF, Dickman CA, et al. Anterior communicating artery aneurysm paraparesis syndrome: clinical manifestations and pathologic correlates. *Neurology* 1995;45:45–50.

63. Gross BA, Laws ER. Pituitary dysfunction after aneurysmal subarachnoid hemorrhage. *World Neurosurg* 2015;83:1039–1040.

64. Gruber DP, Zimmerman GA, Tomsick TA, et al. A comparison between endovascular and surgical management of basilar artery apex aneurysms. *J Neurosurg* 1999;90:868–874.

65. Hackett ML, Anderson CS. Health outcomes 1 year after subarachnoid hemorrhage: an international population-based study. The Australian Cooperative Research on Subarachnoid Hemorrhage Study Group. *Neurology* 2000;55:658–662.

66. Haley EC, Jr., Kassell NF, Apperson-Hansen C, Maile MH, Alves WM. A randomized, double-blind, vehicle-controlled trial of tirilazad mesylate in patients with aneurysmal subarachnoid hemorrhage: a cooperative study in North America. *J Neurosurg* 1997;86:467–474.

67. Hansen-Schwartz J. Cerebral vasospasm: a consideration of the various cellular mechanisms involved in the pathophysiology. *Neurocrit Care* 2004;1:235–246.

68. Hasan D, Lindsay KW, Wijdicks EFM, et al. Effect of fludrocortisone acetate in patients with subarachnoid hemorrhage. *Stroke* 1989;20:1156–1161.

69. Hasan D, Schonck RS, Avezaat CJ, et al. Epileptic seizures after subarachnoid hemorrhage. *Ann Neurol* 1993;33:286–291.

70. Hasan D, Vermeulen M, Wijdicks EFM, Hijdra A, van Gijn J. Management problems in acute hydrocephalus after subarachnoid hemorrhage. *Stroke* 1989;20:747–753.

71. Hashimoto H, Iida J, Hironaka Y, Okada M, Sakaki T. Use of spiral computerized tomography angiography in patients with subarachnoid hemorrhage in whom subtraction angiography did not reveal cerebral aneurysms. *J Neurosurg* 2000;92:278–283.

72. Hashimoto H, Iida J, Shin Y, Hironaka Y, Sakaki T. Spinal dural arteriovenous fistula with perimesencephalic subarachnoid haemorrhage. *J Clin Neurosci* 2000;7:64–66.

73. Hauerberg J, Eskesen V, Rosenorn J. The prognostic significance of intracerebral haematoma as shown on CT scanning after aneurysmal subarachnoid haemorrhage. *Br J Neurosurg* 1994;8:333–339.

74. Heiserman JE, Dean BL, Hodak JA, et al. Neurologic complications of cerebral angiography. *AJNR Am J Neuroradiol* 1994;15:1401–1407.

75. Heiskanen O, Poranen A, Kuurne T, Valtonen S, Kaste M. Acute surgery for intracerebral haematomas caused by rupture of an intracranial arterial aneurysm: a prospective randomized study. *Acta Neurochir (Wien)* 1988;90:81–83.

76. Hendrix LE, Dion JE, Jensen ME, Phillips CD, Newman SA. Papaverine-induced mydriasis. *AJNR Am J Neuroradiol* 1994;15:716–718.

77. Heros RC, Zervas NT, Varsos V. Cerebral vasospasm after subarachnoid hemorrhage: an update. *Ann Neurol* 1983;14:599–608.

78. Hijdra A, Brouwers PJ, Vermeulen M, van Gijn J. Grading the amount of blood on computed tomograms after subarachnoid hemorrhage. *Stroke* 1990;21:1156–1161.

79. Hijdra A, van Gijn J. Early death from rupture of an intracranial aneurysm. *J Neurosurg* 1982;57:765–768.

80. Hijdra A, Van Gijn J, Stefanko S, et al. Delayed cerebral ischemia after aneurysmal subarachnoid hemorrhage: clinicoanatomic correlations. *Neurology* 1986;36:329–333.

81. Hijdra A, Vermeulen M, van Gijn J, van Crevel H. Rerupture of intracranial aneurysms: a clinicoanatomic study. *J Neurosurg* 1987;67:29–33.

82. Hijdra A, Vermeulen M, van Gijn J, van Crevel H. Respiratory arrest in subarachnoid hemorrhage. *Neurology* 1984;34:1501–1503.

83. Hillman J, Fridriksson S, Nilsson O, et al. Immediate administration of tranexamic acid and reduced incidence of early rebleeding after aneurysmal subarachnoid hemorrhage: a prospective randomized study. *J Neurosurg* 2002;97:771–778.

84. Hoekema D, Schmidt RH, Ross I. Lumbar drainage for subarachnoid hemorrhage: technical considerations and safety analysis. *Neurocrit Care* 2007;7:3–9.

85. Hoh BL, Ogilvy CS. Endovascular treatment of cerebral vasospasm: transluminal balloon angioplasty, intra-arterial papaverine, and intra-arterial nicardipine. *Neurosurg Clin N Am* 2005;16:501–516.

86. Honma Y, Fujiwara T, Irie K, Ohkawa M, Nagao S. Morphological changes in human cerebral arteries after percutaneous transluminal angioplasty for vasospasm caused by subarachnoid hemorrhage. *Neurosurgery* 1995;36:1073–1080.

87. Horikoshi T, Nukui H, Yagishita T, et al. Oculomotor nerve palsy after surgery for upper basilar artery aneurysm. *Neurosurgery* 1999;44:705–710.

88. Investigators ISoUIA. Unruptured intracranial aneurysms: risk of rupture and risks of surgical intervention. *N Engl J Med* 1998;339:1725–1733.

89. Jackson A, Stewart G, Wood A, Gillespie JE. Transient global amnesia and cortical blindness after vertebral angiography: further evidence for the role of arterial spasm. *AJNR Am J Neuroradiol* 1995;16:955–959.

90. Jacob JT, Burns JA, Dupont SA, Lanzino G, Wijdicks EFM. Wall-eyed bilateral internuclear ophthalmoplegia after ruptured aneurysm. *Arch Neurol* 2010;67:636–637.

91. Jestaedt L, Pham M, Bartsch AJ, et al. The impact of balloon angioplasty on the evolution of vasospasm-related infarction after aneurysmal subarachnoid hemorrhage. *Neurosurgery* 2008;62:610–617.

92. Kaku Y, Yonekawa Y, Tsukahara T, Kazekawa K. Superselective intra-arterial infusion of papaverine for the treatment of cerebral vasospasm after subarachnoid hemorrhage. *J Neurosurg* 1992;77:842–847.

93. Kallmes DF, Clark HP, Dix JE, et al. Ruptured vertebrobasilar aneurysms: frequency of the non-aneurysmal perimesencephalic pattern of hemorrhage on CT scans. *Radiology* 1996;201:657–660.

94. Kassell NF, Helm G, Simmons N, Phillips CD, Cail WS. Treatment of cerebral vasospasm with intra-arterial papaverine. *J Neurosurg* 1992;77:848–852.

95. Kassell NF, Torner JC, Jane JA, Haley EC, Jr., Adams HP. The International Cooperative Study on the Timing of Aneurysm Surgery. Part 2: surgical results. *J Neurosurg* 1990;73:37–47.

96. Kato Y, Sano H, Dong PT, et al. The effect of clipping and coiling in acute severe subarachnoid hemorrhage after international subarachnoid aneurysmal trial (ISAT) results. *Minim Invasive Neurosurg* 2005;48:224–227.

97. Khurana VG, Wijdicks EFM, Parisi JE, Piepgras DG. Acute deterioration from thrombosis and rerupture of a giant intracranial aneurysm. *Neurology* 1999;52:1697–1699.

98. Kirkpatrick PJ, Turner CL, Smith C et al. Simvastatin in aneurysmal subarachnoid hemorrhage (STASH): a multicentre randomized phase 3 trial *Lancet Neurol* 2014;13:666–675.

99. Klimo P, Jr., Kestle JR, MacDonald JD, Schmidt RH. Marked reduction of cerebral vasospasm with lumbar drainage of cerebrospinal fluid after subarachnoid hemorrhage. *J Neurosurg* 2004;100:215–224.

100. Koivisto T, Vanninen R, Hurskainen H, et al. Outcomes of early endovascular versus surgical treatment of ruptured cerebral aneurysms: a prospective randomized study. *Stroke* 2000;31:2369–2377.

101. Komotar RJ, Schmidt JM, Starke RM, et al. Resuscitation and critical care of poor-grade subarachnoid hemorrhage. *Neurosurgery* 2009;64:397–410.

102. Konishi Y, Maemura E, Shiota M, et al. Treatment of vasospasm by balloon angioplasty: experimental studies and clinical experiences. *Neurol Res* 1992;14:273–281.

103. Kramer AH, Zygun DA, Bleck TP, et al. Relationship between hemoglobin concentrations and outcomes across subgroups of patients with aneurysmal subarachnoid hemorrhage. *Neurocrit Care* 2009;10:157–165.

104. Kumar R, Wijdicks EFM, Brown RD, Jr., Parisi JE, Hammond CA. Isolated angiitis of the CNS presenting as subarachnoid haemorrhage. *J Neurol Neurosurg Psychiatry* 1997;62:649–651

105. Kurre W, Berkefeld J. Materials and techniques for coiling of cerebral aneurysms: how much scientific evidence do we have? *Neuroradiology* 2008;50:909–927.

106. Lanzino G, Kanaan Y, Perrini P, Dayoub H, Fraser K. Emerging concepts in the treatment of intracranial aneurysms: stents, coated coils, and liquid embolic agents. *Neurosurgery* 2005;57:449–459.

107. Lanzino G, Murad MH, d'Urso PI, Rabinstein AA. Coil embolization versus clipping for ruptured intracranial aneurysms: a meta-analysis of prospective controlled published studies. *AJNR Am J Neuroradiol* 2013;34:1764–1768.

108. Le Roux PD, Newell DW, Eskridge J, Mayberg MR, Winn HR. Severe symptomatic vasospasm: the role of immediate postoperative angioplasty. *J Neurosurg* 1994;80:224–229.

109. Lee KH, Lukovits T, Friedman JA. "Triple-H" therapy for cerebral vasospasm following subarachnoid hemorrhage. *Neurocrit Care* 2006;4:68–76.

110. Lennihan L, Mayer SA, Fink ME, et al. Effect of hypervolemic therapy on cerebral blood flow after subarachnoid hemorrhage: a randomized controlled trial. *Stroke* 2000;31:383–391.

111. Levy ML, Rabb CH, Zelman V, Giannotta SL. Cardiac performance enhancement from dobutamine in patients refractory to hypervolemic therapy for cerebral vasospasm. *J Neurosurg* 1993;79:494–499.

112. Linn FH, Rinkel GJ, Algra A, van Gijn J. Incidence of subarachnoid hemorrhage: role of region, year, and rate of computed tomography: a meta-analysis. *Stroke* 1996;27:625–629.

113. Linn FH, Wijdicks EFM, van der Graaf Y, et al. Prospective study of sentinel headache in aneurysmal subarachnoid hemorrhage. *Lancet* 1994;344:590–593.

114. Linskey ME, Horton JA, Rao GR, Yonas H. Fatal rupture of the intracranial carotid artery during transluminal angioplasty for vasospasm induced by subarachnoid hemorrhage: case report. *J Neurosurg* 1991;74:985–990.

115. Liu JK, Couldwell WT. Intra-arterial papaverine infusions for the treatment of cerebral vasospasm induced by aneurysmal subarachnoid hemorrhage. *Neurocrit Care* 2005;2:124–132.

116. Lynch JR, Wang H, McGirt MJ, et al. Simvastatin reduces vasospasm after

aneurysmal subarachnoid hemorrhage: results of a pilot randomized clinical trial. *Stroke* 2005;36:2024–2026.

117. Macdonald RL. Lumbar drainage after subarachnoid hemorrhage: does it reduce vasospasm and delayed hydrocephalus? *Neurocrit Care* 2007;7:1–2.

118. Mayer SA, Fink ME, Homma S, et al. Cardiac injury associated with neurogenic pulmonary edema following subarachnoid hemorrhage. *Neurology* 1994;44:815–820.

119. Mayer SA, Solomon RA, Fink ME, et al. Effect of 5% albumin solution on sodium balance and blood volume after subarachnoid hemorrhage. *Neurosurgery* 1998;42:759–767.

120. McIver JI, Friedman JA, Wijdicks EFM, et al. Preoperative ventriculostomy and rebleeding after aneurysmal subarachnoid hemorrhage. *J Neurosurg* 2002;97:1042–1044.

121. Mitchell P, Kerr R, Mendelow AD, Molyneux A. Could late rebleeding overturn the superiority of cranial aneurysm coil embolization over clip ligation seen in the International Subarachnoid Aneurysm Trial? *J Neurosurg* 2008;108:437–442.

122. Molyneux A, Kerr R, Stratton I, et al. International Subarachnoid Aneurysm Trial (ISAT) of neurosurgical clipping versus endovascular coiling in 2143 patients with ruptured intracranial aneurysms: a randomised trial. *Lancet* 2002;360:1267–1274.

123. Molyneux AJ, Birks J, Clarke A, Sneade M, Kerr RS. The durability of endovascular coiling versus neurosurgical clipping of ruptured cerebral aneurysms: 18 year follow-up of the UK cohort of the International Subarachnoid Aneurysm Trial (ISAT). *Lancet* 2015;385:691–697.

124. Molyneux AJ, Kerr RS, Birks J, et al. Risk of recurrent subarachnoid haemorrhage, death, or dependence and standardised mortality ratios after clipping or coiling of an intracranial aneurysm in the International Subarachnoid Aneurysm Trial (ISAT): long-term follow-up. *Lancet Neurol* 2009;8:427–433.

125. Molyneux AJ, Kerr RS, Yu LM, et al. International subarachnoid aneurysm trial (ISAT) of neurosurgical clipping versus endovascular coiling in 2143 patients with ruptured intracranial aneurysms: a randomised comparison of effects on survival, dependency, seizures, rebleeding, subgroups, and aneurysm occlusion. *Lancet* 2005;366:809–817.

126. Morgenstern PF, Knopman J. Perimesencephalic hemorrhage with negative angiography: case illustration. *J Neurosurg* 2015:1–2.

127. O'Kelly CJ, Kulkarni AV, Austin PC, Wallace MC, Urbach D. The impact of therapeutic modality on outcomes following repair of ruptured intracranial aneurysms: an administrative data analysis: clinical article. *J Neurosurg* 2010;113:795–801.

128. Olson DM, Zomorodi M, Britz GW, et al. Continuous cerebral spinal fluid drainage associated with complications in patients admitted with subarachnoid hemorrhage. *J Neurosurg* 2013;119:974–980.

129. Pegoli M, Mandrekar J, Rabinstein AA, Lanzino G. Predictors of excellent functional outcome in aneurysmal subarachnoid hemorrhage. *J Neurosurg* 2015;122:414–418.

130. Petruk KC, West M, Mohr G, et al. Nimodipine treatment in poor-grade aneurysm patients: results of a multicenter double-blind placebo-controlled trial. *J Neurosurg* 1988;68:505–517.

131. Pfausler B, Belcl R, Metzler R, Mohsenipour I, Schmutzhard E. Terson's syndrome in spontaneous subarachnoid hemorrhage: a prospective study in 60 consecutive patients. *J Neurosurg* 1996;85:392–394.

132. Pickard JD, Murray GD, Illingworth R, et al. Effect of oral nimodipine on cerebral infarction and outcome after subarachnoid haemorrhage: British aneurysm nimodipine trial. *BMJ* 1989;298:636–642.

133. Rabinstein AA, Lanzino G, Wijdicks EFM. Multidisciplinary management and emerging therapeutic strategies in aneurysmal subarachnoid hemorrhage. *Lancet Neurol* 2010;9:504–519.

134. Rabinstein AA, Pichelmann MA, Friedman JA, et al. Symptomatic vasospasm and outcomes following aneurysmal subarachnoid hemorrhage: a comparison between surgical repair and endovascular coil occlusion. *J Neurosurg* 2003;98:319–325.

135. Rabinstein AA, Weigand S, Atkinson JL, Wijdicks EFM. Patterns of cerebral infarction in aneurysmal subarachnoid hemorrhage. *Stroke* 2005;36:992–997.

136. Rinkel GJ, van Gijn J, Wijdicks EFM. Subarachnoid hemorrhage without detectable aneurysm: a review of the causes. *Stroke* 1993;24:1403–1409.

137. Rinkel GJ, Wijdicks EFM, Hasan D, et al. Outcome in patients with subarachnoid haemorrhage and negative angiography according to pattern of haemorrhage on computed tomography. *Lancet* 1991;338:964–968.

138. Rinkel GJ, Wijdicks EFM, Vermeulen M, et al. The clinical course of perimesencephalic

nonaneurysmal subarachnoid hemorrhage. *Ann Neurol* 1991;29:463–468.

139. Rosen DS, Macdonald RL. Subarachnoid hemorrhage grading scales: a systematic review. *Neurocrit Care* 2005;2:110–118.

140. Salary M, Quigley MR, Wilberger JE, Jr. Relation among aneurysm size, amount of subarachnoid blood, and clinical outcome. *J Neurosurg* 2007;107:13–17.

141. Schievink WI, Wijdicks EFM. Origin of pretruncal nonaneurysmal subarachnoid hemorrhage: ruptured vein, perforating artery, or intramural hematoma? *Mayo Clinic Proc* 2000;75:1169–1173.

142. Schievink WI, Wijdicks EFM. Pretruncal subarachnoid hemorrhage: an anatomically correct description of the perimesencephalic subarachnoid hemorrhage. *Stroke* 1997;28:2572.

143. Schievink WI, Wijdicks EFM, Meyer FB, Sonntag VK. Spontaneous intracranial hypotension mimicking aneurysmal subarachnoid hemorrhage. *Neurosurgery* 2001;48:513–516.

144. Schievink WI, Wijdicks EFM, Parisi JE, Piepgras DG, Whisnant JP. Sudden death from aneurysmal subarachnoid hemorrhage. *Neurology* 1995;45:871–874.

145. Schievink WI, Wijdicks EFM, Piepgras DG, et al. The poor prognosis of ruptured intracranial aneurysms of the posterior circulation. *J Neurosurg* 1995;82:791–795.

146. Schievink WI, Wijdicks EFM, Piepgras DG, Nichols DA, Ebersold MJ. Perimesencephalic subarachnoid hemorrhage: additional perspectives from four cases. *Stroke* 1994;25:1507–1511.

147. Schmidt JM, Wartenberg KE, Fernandez A, et al. Frequency and clinical impact of asymptomatic cerebral infarction due to vasospasm after subarachnoid hemorrhage. *J Neurosurg* 2008;109:1052–1059.

148. Shojima M, Oshima M, Takagi K, et al. Magnitude and role of wall shear stress on cerebral aneurysm: computational fluid dynamic study of 20 middle cerebral artery aneurysms. *Stroke* 2004;35:2500–2505.

149. Sillberg VA, Wells GA, Perry JJ. Do statins improve outcomes and reduce the incidence of vasospasm after aneurysmal subarachnoid hemorrhage: a meta-analysis. *Stroke* 2008;39:2622–2626.

150. Tejada JG, Taylor RA, Ugurel MS, et al. Safety and feasibility of intra-arterial nicardipine for the treatment of subarachnoid hemorrhage-associated vasospasm: initial clinical experience with high-dose infusions. *AJNR Am J Neuroradiol* 2007;28:844–848.

151. Thomas AJ, Ogilvy CS. ISAT: equipoise in treatment of ruptured cerebral aneurysms? *Lancet* 2015;385:666–668.

152. Toussaint LG, 3rd, Friedman JA, Wijdicks EFM, et al. Survival of cardiac arrest after aneurysmal subarachnoid hemorrhage. *Neurosurgery* 2005;57:25–31.

153. Toyota BD. The efficacy of an abbreviated course of nimodipine in patients with good-grade aneurysmal subarachnoid hemorrhage. *J Neurosurg* 1999;90:203–206.

154. Treggiari-Venzi MM, Suter PM, Romand JA. Review of medical prevention of vasospasm after aneurysmal subarachnoid hemorrhage: a problem of neurointensive care. *Neurosurgery* 2001;48:249–261.

155. Tseng MY, Czosnyka M, Richards H, Pickard JD, Kirkpatrick PJ. Effects of acute treatment with pravastatin on cerebral vasospasm, autoregulation, and delayed ischemic deficits after aneurysmal subarachnoid hemorrhage: a phase II randomized placebo-controlled trial. *Stroke* 2005;36:1627–1632.

156. van Asch CJ, van der Schaaf IC, Rinkel GJ. Acute hydrocephalus and cerebral perfusion after aneurysmal subarachnoid hemorrhage. *AJNR Am J Neuroradiol* 2010;31:67–70.

157. van Donkelaar CE, Bakker NA, Veeger NJ. Predictive factors for rebleeding after aneurysmal subarachnoid hemorrhage: Rebleeding aneurysmal subarachnoid hemorrhage study. *Stroke* 2015 Aug;46(8):2100–2106.

158. van Gijn J, Hijdra A, Wijdicks EFM, Vermeulen M, van Crevel H. Acute hydrocephalus after aneurysmal subarachnoid hemorrhage. *J Neurosurg* 1985;63:355–362.

159. van Gijn J, van Dongen KJ, Vermeulen M, Hijdra A. Perimesencephalic hemorrhage: a nonaneurysmal and benign form of subarachnoid hemorrhage. *Neurology* 1985;35: 493–497.

160. Vanrossomme AE, Eker OF, Thiran JP, Courbebaisse GP, Zouaoui Boudjeltia K. Intracranial aneurysms: wall motion analysis for prediction of rupture. *Am J Neuroradiol* 2015;36(10):1796–1802.

161. Varelas P, Helms A, Sinson G, Spanaki M, Hacein-Bey L. Clipping or coiling of ruptured cerebral aneurysms and shunt-dependent hydrocephalus. *Neurocrit Care* 2006;4: 223–228.

162. Velthuis BK, Rinkel GJ, Ramos LM, Witkamp TD, van Leeuwen MS. Perimesencephalic hemorrhage: exclusion of vertebrobasilar aneurysms with CT angiography. *Stroke* 1999;30:1103–1109.

163. Vermeulen M, Lindsay KW, Murray GD, et al. Antifibrinolytic treatment in subarachnoid hemorrhage. *N Engl J Med* 1984;311:432–437.

164. Vermeulen M, van Gijn J, Hijdra A, van Crevel H. Causes of acute deterioration in patients with a ruptured intracranial aneurysm: a prospective study with serial CT scanning. *J Neurosurg* 1984;60:935–939.

165. Viñuela F, Duckwiler G, Mawad M. Guglielmi detachable coil embolization of acute intracranial aneurysm: perioperative anatomical and clinical outcome in 403 patients. *J Neurosurg* 1997;86:475–482.

166. White JB, Wijdicks EFM, Cloft HJ, Kallmes DF. Vanishing aneurysm in pretruncal nonaneurysmal subarachnoid hemorrhage. *Neurology* 2008;71:1375–1377.

167. White PM, Raymond J. Endovascular coiling of cerebral aneurysms using "bioactive" or coated-coil technologies: a systematic review of the literature. *AJNR Am J Neuroradiol* 2009;30:219–226.

168. Wijdicks EFM, Hasan D, Lindsay KW, et al. Short-term tranexamic acid treatment in aneurysmal subarachnoid hemorrhage. *Stroke* 1989;20:1674–1679.

169. Wijdicks EFM, Kallmes DF, Manno EM, Fulgham JR, Piepgras DG. Subarachnoid hemorrhage: neurointensive care and aneurysm repair. *Mayo Clinic Proc* 2005;80:550–559.

170. Wijdicks EFM, Schievink WI, Miller GM. MR imaging in pretruncal nonaneurysmal subarachnoid hemorrhage: is it worthwhile? *Stroke* 1998;29:2514–2516.

171. Wijdicks EFM, Schievink WI, Miller GM. Pretruncal nonaneurysmal subarachnoid hemorrhage. *Mayo Clinic Proc* 1998;73:745–752.

172. Wijdicks EFM, Vermeulen M, Murray GD, Hijdra A, van Gijn J. The effects of treating hypertension following aneurysmal subarachnoid hemorrhage. *Clin Neurol Neurosurg* 1990;92:111–117.

173. Wijdicks EF, Vermeulen M, ten Haaf JA, et al. Volume depletion and natriuresis in patients with a ruptured intracranial aneurysm. *Ann Neurol* 1985;18:211–216.

174. Wijdicks EFM, Vermeulen M, van Brummelen P, van Gijn J. The effect of fludrocortisone acetate on plasma volume and natriuresis in patients with aneurysmal subarachnoid hemorrhage. *Clin Neurol Neurosurg* 1988;90:209–214.

175. Wijdicks EFM. Worst-case scenario: management in poor-grade aneurysmal subarachnoid hemorrhage. *Cerebrovasc Dis* 1995;5:163–169.

176. Young N, Dorsch NW, Kingston RJ, Markson G, McMahon J. Intracranial aneurysms: evaluation in 200 patients with spiral CT angiography. *Eur Radiol* 2001;11:123–130.

177. Zoerle T, Lombardo A, Colombo A, et al. Intracranial pressure after subarachnoid hemorrhage. *Crit Care Med* 2015;43:168–176.

178. Zwienenberg-Lee M, Hartman J, Rudisill N, et al. Effect of prophylactic transluminal balloon angioplasty on cerebral vasospasm and outcome in patients with Fisher grade III subarachnoid hemorrhage: results of a phase II multicenter, randomized, clinical trial. *Stroke* 2008;39:1759–1765.

27

Ganglionic and Lobar Hemorrhages

By and large, intracerebral hematomas are caused by a ruptured penetrating arterial branch damaged by the effects of longstanding hypertension. This rupture may thus result in hemorrhages in the caudate nucleus, putamen, thalamus, cerebellum, or pons. Hematomas involving the subcortical white matter and cortex may have different causes, including vascular malformations. This fundamental distinction is clinically relevant because cerebral angiography may be urgently indicated in a lobar hematoma and may be of less importance in ganglionic hemorrhages in patients with known poorly controlled hypertension.

Ganglionic and lobar hemorrhages account for a considerable proportion of admissions to the neurosciences intensive care unit (NICU). Each type of cerebral hematoma has different characteristics, and they may be related to the risk of deterioration. Patients with expanding lobar hemorrhages with mass effect may be sent directly to the operating room. In most other patients, medical management is preferred and touches on nearly all aspects of critical care neurology.[28,66,100,105]

In the first hours, urgent treatment decisions may include management of uncontrolled hypertension and coagulopathy. These hemorrhages have the potential to enlarge in at least one-third of patients;[15] therefore, virtually every patient with a putaminal or lobar hemorrhage needs close clinical monitoring in the NICU.

CLINICAL RECOGNITION

Location of the hemorrhage typically is in the putamen or caudate nucleus. The cause is a ruptured lateral branch of the lenticulostriate artery. Equally common are hematomas in the thalamus from ruptured thalamoperforating arteries. Some of these hemorrhages are apoplectic, creating large, destructive volumes with extension into the ventricular system.[67]

The clinical hallmark of a spontaneous cerebral hemorrhage is rapid unfolding of a focal neurologic deficit and then fluctuating alertness. The neurologic manifestations of intra-cranial hematoma depend on the location of the hematoma.

Hemorrhages may be superficially in the subcortical white matter. Patients with frontal lobe hematoma are markedly disoriented in time and place, and many are abulic (from the Greek *abulia*, indecision).[34] Patients with abulia become diverted when asked to perform a simple task or to recall a recent major event in the world. They lack any initiative and truncate their conversation with a simple "yes," "no," or "I don't know," and even these answers require a disproportionately long time.

Patients with hematomas in the dominant (left for right-handed) parietal lobe display abnormalities in naming, reading, writing, calculations, finger identification, and left–right distinction. In contrast, patients with hematomas in the nondominant (right for right-handed) parietal lobe largely experience neglect of the opposite body half. Neglect of a hemiparesis may be associated with difficulty with writing, particularly omission of letters. Occipital hematomas may be manifested by visual hallucinations and bright colors, but homonymous hemianopia often remains the sole clinical finding on examination.

Seizures (mostly focal) have been reported, with an incidence of approximately 30% in lobar hemorrhages but a much lower incidence (5%) in ganglionic hemorrhages that spare the cortex.[122] Seizures occur close to the presentation of hemorrhage, and late-onset seizures are less common.[11,68]

Deep-seated hemorrhages involve the striatum—divided into the putamen and the caudate nucleus—or thalamus. The clinical syndromes in patients with hemorrhages in the putamen have been further divided on the basis of whether the lesion affects only the anterior part of the putamen close to the anterior limb of the internal capsule, the middle part, or the posterior part. Hemorrhage localized to the anterior part of the putamen may produce purely motor hemiparesis, eye deviation to the site of the lesion, and abulia. Extension into the middle part of the putamen may additionally result in spatial neglect and decreased sensation evidenced by diminished awareness of pinprick, touch, and position. Extension of the clot into the posterior putamen leads to a more prominent left-sided neglect in right-sided lesions and fluent aphasia in left-sided lesions. Large hemorrhages in the putamen may dissect along the white matter tracts into the temporal lobe, causing a Wernicke-type aphasia, but periclot edema may also impair the function of the temporal lobe.

The neurologic deficit in a putaminal hemorrhage is commonly stable when the patient is admitted to the NICU. However, neurologic deficits may become more pronounced, signaled by stupor instead of drowsiness or by development of a forced gaze.[19] Progression of neurologic symptoms, indicating enlargement of the hematoma with more mass effect, is commonly noted clinically within the first 6 hours after presentation.

Hemorrhages in the thalamus produce eye movement abnormalities, such as downward gaze, skew deviation, and limited abduction of both eyes, simulating a sixth-nerve palsy.[72] Hemiparesis occurs with paramedian extension. The pattern of anosognosia and visual spatial neglect in the nondominant thalamus and aphasia in the dominant thalamus holds. This type of aphasia is notable for mutism evolving into verbose jargon speech with relatively retained understanding and repetition. In patients who have extension of the thalamic hemorrhage into the striatum, verbal output may be less pronounced, and hypophonia and dysarthria may predominate.[70] Sentences offered for repetition are at times restated in a different manner.

Caudate hemorrhage is the least common of the classic hypertensive hemorrhages, and its clinical manifestations often can be inferred mainly from an extension to the ventricular system. Mostly patients are disoriented and confused, followed by a decline in consciousness from diffusely enlarged hemoventricles.[113,120] When the hematoma enlarges and extends from the caudate nucleus into the white matter, involving the internal capsule or putamen, level of consciousness decreases because of brain shift. Extension of the hemorrhage into the hypothalamus and diencephalon might produce complete Horner's syndrome on one side, a diagnostic clue to a large extending caudate hematoma.

As a rule, consciousness is impaired in lobar and putaminal hemorrhages when there is mass effect from the hematoma. Therefore, enlargement

of the hematoma must be suspected in patients who lapse into deeper stages of coma. In these situations, it is not uncommon to find a major discrepancy between clinical examination and initial computed tomography (CT) scan. Repeat CT scan often uncovers considerable enlargement commensurate with clinical findings.

Putaminal hemorrhages (more than 60 cm^3 on CT scan) may disconnect the diencephalon from the ascending reticular activating system by direct destruction, and this is the most common mechanism for coma. Any other large-volume hemorrhage may produce mass effect, displacing the thalamus and upper brainstem (Chapter 12) and may additionally compress the foramen of Monro.[123] This ventricular obstruction results in acute ventricular enlargement of the ventricles opposite to the hemorrhage. However, impaired consciousness in this clinical scenario is a clinical manifestation of tissue displacement[104] or destruction, and not acute hydrocephalus. An acutely placed ventriculostomy, therefore, does not improve the level of consciousness in this particular situation.

Primary intraventricular hemorrhage may be caused by arteriovenous malformations in the proximity of the ventricular system, intraventricular tumors, and use of thrombolytic agents. Uncommon causes are coagulopathy in patients with severe thrombocytopenia associated with a hematologic malignancy and moyamoya disease from rupture of the dilated periventricular arteries.[93] It may be difficult clinically and by CT scan criteria to differentiate spontaneous intraventricular hemorrhage from a small thalamic or caudate nucleus hemorrhage when there is overwhelming filling of the lateral portion of the ventricles. Intraventricular hemorrhage is also caused by a rupture of the anterior communicating aneurysm, which can dissect through the lamina terminalis to enter the third ventricle and connecting ventricles.

Primary intraventricular hemorrhage has a clinical presentation similar to that of aneurysmal subarachnoid hemorrhage. Although less severe presentations may occur, onset is acute, with immediate loss of consciousness and often spontaneous extensor posturing.[93] Many patients have rapid breathing with periods of apnea or barely audible air displacement and need to be immediately intubated and placed on a mechanical ventilator. Increased blood pressure most likely is a consequence of transmitted intracranial pressure affecting the brainstem, particularly at the rush of arterial blood through the ventricular system. Pupil reflexes may become sluggish and pupil size smaller if acute hydrocephalus develops rapidly. Any change in this direction should prompt a repeat CT scan to evaluate the progression of ventricular enlargement and need for ventriculostomy and thrombolytics.

NEUROIMAGING AND LABORATORY TESTS

CT scanning provides the opportunity for careful characterization of the parenchymal hemorrhage, and some measurements have clinical implication. The volume in cubic centimeters can be measured on CT scan by the ellipsoid ABC method:[14] [$A \times B \times C$]/2 (Figure 27.1). (A is the maximum diameter, B is the diameter perpendicular to A, and C is the number of slices in vertical plane with hematoma present multiplied by slice thickness in cm [usually 0.5 cm]). This approximation of hemorrhagic volume assumes that every hematoma is ellipsoidal. Overestimation (by as much as 30%) may occur when hematoma is irregularly shaped or separated in pieces.[121] However, mostly the value obtained correlates well with a direct CT scan measurement.

In 25% of patients, enlargement of the ganglionic hematoma may appear on CT scans when reimaged within the first hours of presentation. Patients with CT scans obtained more than 6 hours after the ictus and a volume of less than 25 cm³ are unlikely to have deterioration from further growth of the hematoma. However, anticoagulation with warfarin, despite rapid normalization of the international normalized ratio (INR), is a major factor in enlargement of the hematoma.

Putaminal hemorrhages are most prevalent and not infrequently massive. The volume on CT scan commonly approaches 60 cm³, but smaller hematomas may occur without further enlargement on serial CT scans. Types of putaminal hemorrhage with common pathway of extension are shown in Figure 27.2.

Thalamic hematomas are usually small (Figure 27.3), but because of close proximity to the ventricles, intraventricular hemorrhage may occur. Hydrocephalus may develop from obstruction of the cerebrospinal fluid (CSF) at the level of the foramen of Monro (Figure 27.4), more commonly with medially located thalamic hemorrhages. Enlargement of the hematoma has been observed in thalamic hemorrhages, typically in conjunction with progression to coma. The progression is destruction not only of the thalamus but also the mesencephalon, and this combination markedly reduces the chances of independent living. The CT scan and magnetic resonance imaging (MRI) features producing coma in patients with thalamic hematomas are shown in Figure 27.5.

Caudate hemorrhage (Figure 27.6) may be difficult to separate from intraventricular hemorrhage on CT scans, and often MRI is needed to locate the source in the caudate nucleus.

Lobar hematomas are peripheral and just under the cortex. Patients with lobar hematomas may have an underlying arteriovenous malformation or cavernous angioma. Simultaneous multiple hemorrhages should point to previous use of anticoagulants or thrombolytic agents, disseminated intravascular coagulation, metastatic disease, or as a result of infestation with aspergillus or toxoplasma.[80,124,126,128]

Several other CT scan characteristics of hematoma suggesting its origin should be recognized. Shift of midline structures on the initial CT scan in patients with lobar hematoma is highly predictive of further clinical deterioration.[39] The specific features are shift of the septum pellucidum, obliteration of the opposite ambient cistern, and early trapping of the temporal horn (Figure 27.7). Some

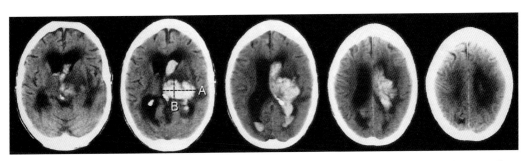

FIGURE 27.1: Volume of a thalamic hemorrhage as measured by the *ABC* method ($A \times B \times C$). In this example, *A* is 5 cm, *B* is 3 cm, and the number of slices (*C*) is four (hemorrhage is visible on four computed tomographic slices at 1 cm intervals). The total volume is calculated as 60 divided by 2, or 30 cm³.

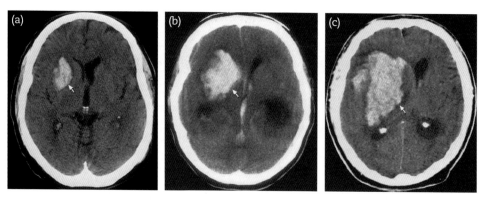

FIGURE 27.2: Putaminal hemorrhage. Computed tomographic scan examples of putaminal hemorrhage (*arrows*). (a) Localized. (b) Extensions to capsule and frontal lobe and ventricles. (c) Further extension into the thalamus.

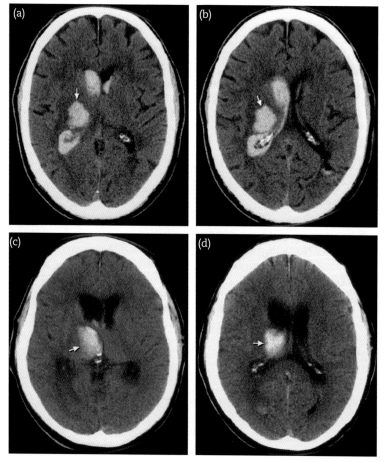

FIGURE 27.3: Thalamic hemorrhage. Computed tomographic scans of thalamic hemorrhage (*arrows*). (a, b) Lateral. (c, d) Medial.

of the CT scan changes may be subtle and involve effacement of the supracerebellar cistern from edema (Figure 27.8).

Lobar hematoma may indicate an underlying metastatic lesion or primary brain tumor, and it is evident by marked fingerlike white matter edema notably out of proportion to the size of the hematoma and seldom causing brain shift (Figure 27.9).

Superficially located hematomas commonly are a result of amyloid angiopathy (Capsule 27.1),

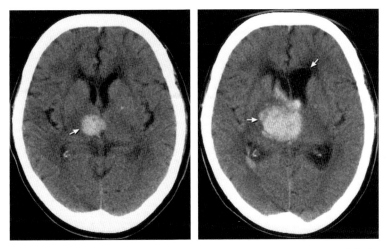

FIGURE 27.4: Thalamic hemorrhage. Computed tomographic images of enlargement of thalamic hemorrhage intraventricular extension and hydrocephalus.

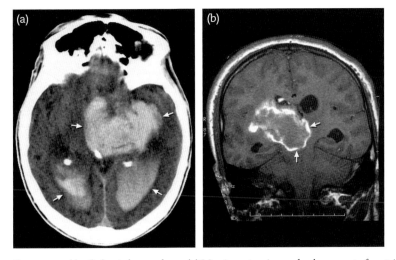

FIGURE 27.5: Coma caused by thalamic hemorrhage. (a) Massive extension and enlargement of ventricles (*arrows*). (b) Magnetic resonance image of the thalamic hemorrhage with extension into the midbrain.

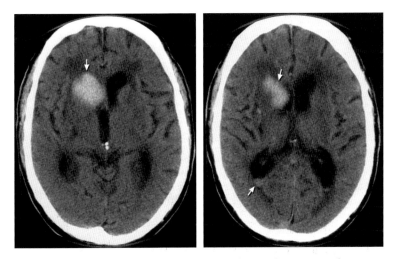

FIGURE 27.6: Computed tomographic images of caudate hemorrhage and intraventricular extension (*arrows*).

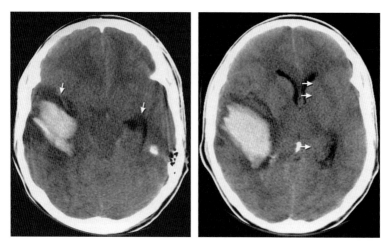

FIGURE 27.7: Computed tomographic scan signs predictive of deterioration in lobar hematoma (*arrow*). Note shift of septum pellucidum and pineal gland (*arrows*) and early temporal horn entrapment (*arrow*).

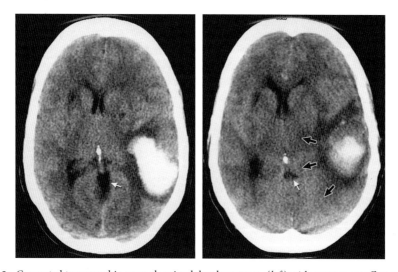

FIGURE 27.8: Computed tomographic scans showing lobar hematoma (*left*) with some mass effect and bowing of the midline structures. Several days later (*right*), the hematoma is resolving but edema is more pronounced, with progressive obliteration of the supracerebellar cistern without appreciable shift of the pineal gland from edema.

and MRI (preferably gradient-echo) may show earlier hemorrhages[59] (Figure 27.10).

Coagulation-associated hematomas are commonly multiple, involving multiple compartments. A blood–fluid interface inside the hematoma predicts an acquired (e.g., leukemia, idiopathic thrombocytopenic purpura, hemophilia) or drug-related (e.g., warfarin, heparin, thrombolytic agents) bleeding disorder[29,126] (Figure 27.11). Hematoma shape (regular, irregular, or separated) does not predict source of hemorrhage and is not more common in warfarin-associated cerebral hematomas. Intraventricular hemorrhage can be graded using the Graebe scale (Table 27.1).

Magnetic resonance imaging is a crucial study in lobar hematoma because it may identify an underlying structural lesion. In young adults, an arteriovenous malformation is common; in older adults, earlier amyloid hemorrhages may be found.

Magnetic resonance imaging with magnetic resonance angiography is a useful additional test that may demonstrate metastasis, occult vascular malformations, occasional previous hemorrhages associated with amyloid angiopathy, or cerebral venous thrombosis, all conditions beyond the detection of CT. Magnetic resonance imaging is able to estimate the age of the hematoma, and one of the earliest signs is peripheral deoxygenation,

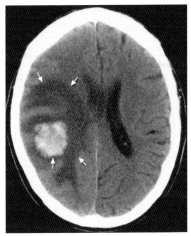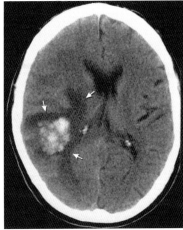

FIGURE 27.9: Hemorrhage in metastasis. Note the comparatively large, finger-like edema in the white matter out of proportion to the size of the hematoma. Computed tomographic scans mask underlying metastasis, which may be more clearly demonstrated by magnetic resonance imaging.

shown as a rim of hypodensity on T2-weighted spin echo images surrounding the hematoma. T1- and T2-weighted changes usually characterize the aging of the hematoma.[7,77] Gradient-echo MRI may demonstrate additional asymptomatic petechial or small-volume hemorrhages of different ages, suggesting cerebral amyloid angiopathy.[50] Finally, although uncommon, lobar hematomas may in fact be hemorrhagic cerebral infarcts associated with cerebral venous thrombosis (Chapter 32). Magnetic resonance imaging may also document a meningioma, which can easily be mistaken for a lobar hematoma on CT scan.[102]

Cerebral angiography is warranted in most patients with a lobar hematoma and may uncover an arteriovenous malformation (Figure 27.12). Its yield in a patient with normal findings on MRI and MRA is low.

The diagnostic value of cerebral angiography for underlying vascular abnormalities has been reviewed. Many of the studies are limited because selection criteria are unclear. The yield of arteriovenous malformations or aneurysms depends on the site of hemorrhage, a history of hypertension (or persistent hypertension 2 weeks after admission), and age.[133]

Normotensive patients with a hemorrhage in the putamen or thalamus who are younger than 45 years may have an underlying vascular lesion (50% occurrence). The detection rate drops to 7% in similar patients older than 45 years.[133] However, yield from cerebral angiography in chronically hypertensive patients with ganglionic hemorrhages is very low. The yield in patients with primary intraventricular hemorrhage varies from 30% to 75%.

Therefore, cerebral angiography is probably not warranted in patients with a typical putaminal or thalamic hemorrhage and long-standing hypertension. Putaminal hemorrhages are seldom associated with cerebral aneurysms, but when present are commonly visible on CT scans or the hematoma seems to originate from the middle cerebral artery implying an underlying aneurysm. Cerebral angiogram may lead to surprising results, and we found a P3 aneurysm in a patient with predominantly thalamic hematoma but also subarachnoid hemorrhage.[21] Repeat angiography may be needed as a follow-up study when cerebral angiography yields negative results in a patient with a lobar hematoma. (It is possible that the mass effect of a hematoma obscures a small arteriovenous malformation. Repeat angiography detected four

---

TABLE 27.1. GRAEBE SCALE: SYSTEM FOR GRADING SEVERITY OF IVH

Lateral Ventricles

1 = trace of blood or mild bleeding

2 = less than half of the ventricle filled with blood

3 = more than half of the ventricle filled with blood

4 = ventricle filled with blood and expanded

(Each lateral ventricle is scored separately)

Third and Fourth Ventricles

1 = blood present, ventricle size normal

2 = ventricle filled with blood and expanded

Total Score (maximum = 12)

CAPSULE 27.1 CEREBRAL AMYLOID ANGIOPATHY AND CEREBRAL HEMORRHAGE

Aging causes deposition of amyloid-β protein in blood vessels—mostly in the cortical and occipital regions—and compromises arterial wall integrity.[49,111] This process goes by the moniker of *cerebral amyloid angiopathy*.

It has been estimated that amyloid deposits are present in the vast majority of nonagenarians, but the lower cutoff age is unknown and may reach into the mid-40s. Their deposition may be due to reduced extracellular spaces that reduce drainage of these proteins and lead to deposition. (Familial forms have been described, most prominently in Dutch, Danish, and British families.)

Fibrinoid necrosis is seen, and may be a possible mechanism of rupture. The same mechanism of fibrinoid necrosis applies to hypertension-associated hemorrhages, and to make it more perplexing, long-standing hypertension may coexist with amyloid angiopathy. However, cerebral amyloid angiopathy typically spares the penetrating branches to the basal ganglia, thalamus, and brainstem. Amyloid may also impact on endothelial function and fail to inhibit plasmin and plasminogen activators, resulting in a hematoma with characteristics virtually similar to warfarin-associated hematomas (lobulated, fluid plasma levels). Cerebral hemorrhage after thrombolytic agents and anticoagulation may be linked to severe cerebral amyloid angiopathy, but the relationship is tentative.[112] Autopsy or careful evaluation of evacuated clot and brain tissue is needed to confirm the diagnosis. Neuropathologic studies require special staining methods (e.g., Congo red), but immunostaining of the protein is more specific (see accompanying illustration).

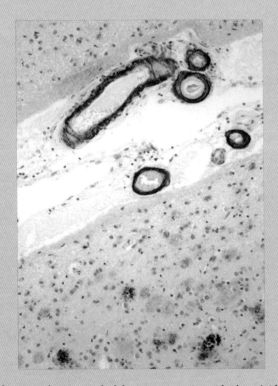

β-Amyloid staining showing marked deposits as seen in cerebral amyloid angiopathy.

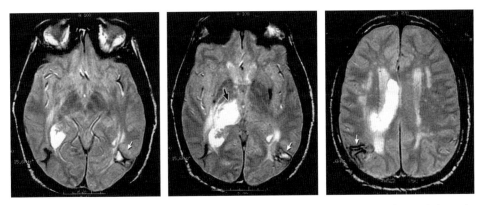

FIGURE 27.10: Amyloid angiopathy-associated hematoma. Magnetic resonance images show a thalamic hemorrhage (*black arrow*) and multiple areas of hemosiderin (*white arrows*), which are clues to earlier hemorrhages.

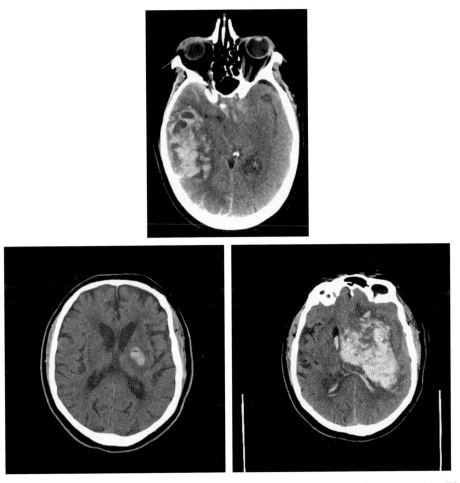

FIGURE 27.11. Upper row: Large lobar hematoma with multiple fluid levels ("footprints"). Lower row: Small hematoma at onset (hours after presentation) with massive enlargement.

arteriovenous malformations in 22 patients with initially negative cerebral angiograms.[58])

Laboratory evaluation should include, in addition to routine hematologic survey and chemistry group, other specific tests pertaining to possible causes (Table 27.2).

In patients with prior hypertension, chest radiography with measurement of cardiac ratio, electrocardiography, and urinalysis with quantification of proteinuria are required. They can be supplemented in younger patients by abdominal CT and vanillylmandelic acid analysis to screen for pheochromocytoma. Toxicologic screening for cocaine use should be considered in appropriate circumstances.

FIRST STEPS IN MANAGEMENT

Initial management in ganglionic and lobar cerebral hemorrhages is summarized in Table 27.3. If consciousness has decreased to a level at which protective laryngeal reflexes are lost, endotracheal intubation should follow. Mechanical ventilation with a combination of intermittent mandatory ventilation mode and pressure support is usually sufficient, because most patients retain the ability to trigger the ventilator. Prophylaxis for gastrointestinal bleeding and deep vein thrombosis is initiated. Early administration of low-molecular-weight heparin (LMWH) in patients at high risk is likely safe in patients with parenchymal hematoma but we prefer subcutaneous heparin starting 2 days after the ictus.[69]

TABLE 27.2. LABORATORY TESTS IN CEREBRAL HEMORRHAGE

Complete white cell count, platelet count, blood smear, sedimentation rate

Activated partial thromboplastin time, international normalized ratio

Aspartate transaminase, alkaline phosphatase

Fibrinogen and fibrinogen split products (optional)

Transthoracic echocardiography and serial blood cultures (optional)

Human immunodeficiency virus serology (optional)

Drug screen (optional)

Hemoglobin electrophoresis (optional)

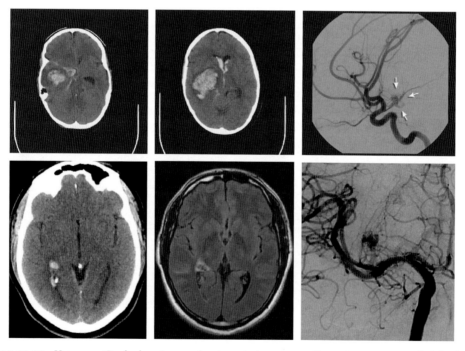

FIGURE 27.12: *Upper row:* Cerebral angiogram showing arteriovenous malformation as a cause of a lobar hematoma. *Lower row:* CT scan and MRI shows small deep posterior temporal lobe hematoma with extension into ventricle from a choroidal AVM.

TABLE 27.3. INITIAL MANAGEMENT OF GANGLIONIC AND LOBAR HEMORRHAGES

Airway management	Intubation if patient has hypoxemia despite facemask with 10 L of 60%–100% oxygen/minute, if abnormal respiratory drive or if abnormal protective reflexes (likely with motor response of withdrawal, or worse)
Mechanical ventilation	IMV/PS
	AC with aspiration pneumonitis
	Increase IMV to 15 when hyperventilation is indicated
Fluid management	2–3 L of 0.9% NaCl
	Mannitol, 1 g/kg, when shift appears on CT scan and patient deteriorates rapidly
Blood pressure management	Aim at systolic blood pressure between 130–140 mm Hg. IV labetalol, 10–15 mg every 15 min if needed. Hydralazine 10–20 mg IV if bradycardia. Consider nicardipine 5 mg/hr IV (maximum 15 mg/hr IV)
Nutrition	Enteral nutrition with continuous infusion (on day 2)
	Blood glucose control (goal 140–180 mg/dL)
Prophylaxis	DVT prophylaxis with pneumatic devices
	SC heparin 5,000 U t.i.d. after surgical evacuation or 2 days after ictus
	GI prophylaxis: pantoprazole 40 mg IV daily or lansoprazole 30 mg orally through nasogastric tube
	Levetiracetam 20 mg/kg IV over 60 minutes followed by 1,000 mg b.i.d. maintenance in lobar hematoma only
Other measures	Reverse anticoagulation (Table 27.4)
Surgical management	Evacuate hematoma if patient is deteriorating and has a lobar hematoma with shift
Access	Arterial catheter to monitor blood pressure (if IV antihypertensive drugs anticipated)
	Peripheral venous catheter or peripheral inserted central catheter

CT, computed tomography; DVT, deep vein thrombosis; GI, gastrointestinal; IMV, intermittent mandatory ventilation; IV, intravenously; MAP, mean arterial pressure; NaCl, sodium chloride; PS, pressure support; SC, subcutaneously.

Fluid management should focus on reduction of free water intake, and most patients are best managed with 2 L of isotonic saline. Patients with hematomas of large volume and evidence of rapid clinical deterioration can be additionally treated with 30 mL of hypertonic saline 3% (infused in 10 minutes) or mannitol, 1 g/kg in a bolus, to reduce intracranial pressure.

Many patients have greatly increased mean arterial pressure, and treatment may cause marked reduction of cerebral perfusion pressure. (One should be reminded here that chronic hypertension leads to a change in the autoregulation curve, with a shift to the right [Chapter 19]). Patients with significant and persistent increases in blood pressure may be treated cautiously. Patients with intracerebral hematoma from long-standing hypertension can be managed with an intravenous bolus of labetalol or angiotensin-converting enzyme inhibitors, which have the added advantage of dilating cerebral blood vessels in chronically hypertensive patients.

The control of hypertension may reduce rebleeding or continuing bleeding, but very few

data are available.[6,13,74] Conversely, aggressive lowering may change the cerebral blood flow, particularly in the tissue surrounding the clot. An important study using single-photon emission computed tomography (SPECT) in patients an average of 12 hours after onset did not show any reduction in cerebral blood flow with blood pressure reduction, but because the data were obtained in a small series of patients with small hematomas, hours after onset, the findings were inconclusive.[97]

The Intensive Blood Pressure Reduction in Acute Cerebral Hemorrhage Trial (INTERACT) was a randomized, open-labeled study in China targeting systolic blood pressure to less than 140 mm Hg within 6 hours after onset with blood pressures of less than 180 mm Hg in the control group. Initial results found no substantial clinical difference in outcome with only a minimal decrease in hematoma volume.[5] The best practice in managing blood pressure in cerebral hematoma is not clearly defined. The most recent American Heart Association/American Stroke Association (AHA/ASA) guidelines recommended a target systolic blood pressure of <130/80 mmHg (Part XIV, guidelines).

The management of comatose patients with deep-seated hematomas not eligible for evacuation could benefit from the monitoring of intracranial pressure using fiberoptic devices.[105] This monitoring could substantially facilitate management of blood pressure. With intracranial pressure and mean arterial pressure values, cerebral perfusion pressure can be calculated and titrated. Intracranial pressure should remain less than 20 mm Hg, and cerebral perfusion pressure ideally must remain in the range of 60–80 mm Hg to provide adequate cerebral blood flow. Nonetheless, this aggressive approach of ICP monitoring has not been well studied, and these practices are unknown (and likely uncommon). Combining reversal of INR to < 1.3 and keeping blood pressure < 160 reduced enlargement, but mortality and unfavorable outcome were still very high in this data set.[73]

The use of corticosteroids is discouraged. A randomized study of dexamethasone administered for 2 weeks in intracranial hemorrhage found no reduction in mortality.[96] In this study, many patients died from systemic complications tentatively linked to unnecessarily prolonged (up to 3 weeks) treatment with corticosteroids. In an elderly population, corticosteroids may also rapidly induce nonketotic hyperglycemia, certainly when osmotic agents, which may contribute to dehydration, are used. It is possible that high doses of corticosteroids (e.g., methylprednisolone) for only a brief period can be effective in these patients, but current data are not available.

Using antiepileptic medication is balancing risks. A generalized tonic-clonic seizure can result in marked hypoxemia from a direct effect on respiratory drive and from aspiration, and is a risk of cardiac arrhythmias. The adverse effects of antiepileptics are uncommon with a hypersensitivity syndrome (fever, rash, and a morbilliform [measles-like] eruption) occurring in 1 of 5,000 patients.

Thus, antiepileptic medication probably can be used selectively. In lobar hematomas, with a 30% prevalence of generalized seizures, one can argue that prophylaxis (e.g., 7–10 days) is justified.[30] The incidence of seizures in putaminal hemorrhage is so low that exposure to antiepileptic drugs is probably an added risk and expense. In patients with clearly documented generalized tonic-clonic seizures, phenytoin is indicated for an arbitrary period of 1 month. In patients with a likely poorly compliant brain tissue and expected increases in intracranial pressure with any type of stimulation, intravenous loading with (fos)phenytoin or intravenous levetiracetam is justified.

One approach to the treatment of cerebral hematoma is to minimize expansion (or even rebleeding). Acceleration of coagulation can be achieved with the hemostatic drug recombinant activated factor VIIa. The first promising trial[82] was followed by a second.[81] The Factor VIIa for Acute Hemorrhagic Stroke (FAST) trial found intracerebral hemorrhage volume reduction from 28% to 18% (20 mcg/kg) or 11% (80 mcg/kg), but outcome as measured by modified Rankin scale was not different. Myocardial ischemia increased significantly, with 15% in placebo to 22% in the 80 mcg/kg dose, but was similar to the 20 mcg/kg dose.[81] A subgroup that may benefit has been identified with age less than 70 years, intracerebral hemorrhage volume less than 60 mL, intraventricular volume less than 5 mL, and time to treatment less than 2.5 hours, but this would require a third trial with uncertain prospects for a benefit.[83] It is unlikely that Factor VIIa may become an established treatment for spontaneous cerebral hematoma.[36]

It is imperative to immediately reverse any anticoagulation. It is usually determined by INR. The INR measures the extrinsic pathway but depends mostly on factor VII levels. Correcting with fresh frozen plasma contains 1–2 units of each clotting factor and has an INR of 1.3. Recombinant factor VIIa instantaneously corrects INR, but factors II, IX, and X remain deficient. Prothrombin complex concentrate (PCC) will add more clotting factors. PCC contain all vitamin K-dependent factors—Factor II, VII, IX, and X. It has 25 times less volume than fresh frozen plasma and reduces the chance of TACO (transfusion-associated circulation overload). In one large prospective trial with PCC, 93% of patients had goal INR (< 1.3) at 30 minutes.[91] In another large study, PCC and vitamin K resulted in the best outcome.[92]

A wide variation of opinions exists among experts regarding the treatment of anticoagulation-associated hematomas.[3,17,43,44] Anticoagulation-related ganglionic or lobar hematoma may quickly expand and should be immediately reversed with two units of fresh frozen plasma and vitamin K.[65] The prolonged effect of oral anticoagulation often requires frequent repeated infusions. A difficult situation arises if a cerebral hematoma appears in a patient anticoagulated for a prosthetic valve, a patient who has atrial fibrillation with prior systemic embolization, or any other "high-risk" patient. However, in these clinical dilemmas, it appears that discontinuation of warfarin for a week in a patient with an intracranial hematoma seldom leads to systemic embolization. In a study of 26 patients with intracerebral hematomas and anticoagulation for metallic valves, discontinuation of 2 days to 3 months (median, 8 days) was safe.[127] Brief interruption of anticoagulation was also without complications in nine high-risk patients (defined as having the following criteria: cage-ball valve, atrial fibrillation, mitral valve position, and enlarged chambers on echocardiogram).[127] Resumption of anticoagulation using orally administered warfarin only was without rebleeding. An extension of this study in 141 patients showed that the risk of recurrent transient ischemic attack or stroke was small but not unsubstantial at 2.9% (95% confidence limit of 0–8%) in patients with prosthetic valves, 2.6% (0–7.6%) in patients with atrial fibrillation and stroke, and 4.8% (0–13.6%) in patients with prior recurrent transient ischemic attacks.[95]

Reversal of anticoagulation with fresh frozen plasma (mL/kg) has disadvantages.[56] Although fresh frozen plasma is readily available, there is serious concern about the length of time to complete reversal of INR.[1] This delay is caused by time required for thawing and the slow infusion rate (3–6 hours) of large volumes of plasma.[75]

Factor VIIa is more effective in rapidly correcting INR. The concern with factor VIIa—particularly in high doses—relates to the number of thromboembolic events in treated patients. Thromboembolic events are mostly arterial and involve acute myocardial infarction but also emboli to femoral, hepatic, pulmonary, renal, splenic, and iliac arteries. Deep vein thrombosis and pulmonary emboli have also been noted.[81,82] Nonetheless, factor VIIa or other drugs (e.g., prothrombin complex) might be a far more effective approach than fresh frozen plasma and vitamin K to correct a markedly abnormal INR.[25] It should be pointed out that factor VIIa usually is combined with fresh frozen plasma and vitamin K, but the number of units of fresh frozen plasma used can be markedly reduced.

In the United States, PCC has been made available in hospital formularies.[12,18,93,107] In addition to factor IX, PCC contains factors II, X and VII. (In 4 factor PCC factor VII is high) PCC is usually administered in 2,000 units (weight less than 90 kg) and 3,000 units (weight more than 90 kg) and combined with intravenous or subcutaneous vitamin K (5–10 mg). The cost of PCC is considerably less than Factor VIIa, works much longer, and there is no fresh frozen plasma requirement. Moreover, PCC consists of inactivated factors II, VII, IX, and X, "replacing" the missing factors, and thus may theoretically reduce the risk for thrombosis. It is not clear whether PCC complex is effective for limiting cerebral hematoma progression and may do nothing. One recent study found no major impact of reversal on expansion but timing of administration may remain critical.[99]

Albeit uncommon, intracranial hematomas in patients associated with recent use of thrombolytic agents requires immediate administration of tranexamic acid, reversal of heparin (often similarly given to reduce the risk of reocclusion of coronary or pulmonary arteries) with protamine sulfate (1 mg for every 100 U of heparin), 10 units of cryoprecipitate, and approximately 2 units of fresh frozen plasma.

A current unresolved issue is whether prior antiplatelet agent use increases hematoma volume and warrants platelet infusion. We consider platelet infusions in patients on dual antiplatelet agents and often if surgical evacuation is anticipated.[88]

A summary of options for correction of coagulopathies is shown Table 27.4.

Primary surgical intervention in ganglionic hemorrhages is practiced rarely in the United States but is widely used in Japan despite insufficient evidence of effect.[28,31,32,46,53,54,61,63,64,98] Stereotactic aspiration of the clot with the use of fibrinolytic drugs[8,57,62] has been proposed, but comparative

TABLE 27.4. ANTICOAGULATION REVERSAL

Warfarin
Fresh frozen plasma (2 Units), vitamin K, 10 mg IV
Factor VIIa 10–20 mcg/kg in one infusion
PCC 30–50 IU/kg.

Heparin
Stop infusion
Protamine sulfate, 1 mg per 100 U of heparin (maximal dose 50 mg)

Low molecular weight heparin
If within 12 hours, 1 mg protamine for each 1 mg of enoxaparin
Protamine not useful in LMWH when administered after 12 hours
Protamine does not reverse fondaparinux

IV tPA
Stop infusion
Tranexamic acid 1 gram in 20 minutes
Cryoprecipitate (0.15 U/kg) if fibrinogen is < 150 mg/dL
Platelet transfusion if platelets < 100 × 109/L

Thrombin inhibitors
Oral activated charcoal (if within 2 hours ingestion)
PCC 50 IU/kg
Hemodialysis (dabigatran only)
Monoclonal antibodies

Antiplatelets
Consider 2 units of platelets when prior use of dual antiplatelet therapy and surgery is anticipated.

TABLE 27.5. SPETZLER-MARTIN GRADING SYSTEM FOR ARTERIOVENOUS MALFORMATIONS

Variable	Score*
Size of arteriovenous malformation†	
Small (< 3 cm)	1
Medium (3–6 cm)	2
Large (> 6 cm)	3
Eloquence of adjacent brain‡	
No	0
Yes	1
Patterns of venous drainage§	
Superficial only	0
Deep	1

* Score of 1 equals grade I, score of 2 equals grade II, etc.
† Greatest diameter on magnetic resonance imaging, cerebral angiography, or computed tomography scan.
‡ Eloquent or functionally important areas are sensory-motor, language, visual cortex, diencephalon, internal capsule, brainstem, and peduncles or deep nuclei of the cerebellum.
§ Deep venous drainage and deep perforating arterial feeders.
From Martin NA, Vinters HV. Arteriovenous malformations. In Carter LP, Spetzler RF, eds., *Neurovascular Surgery.* New York: McGraw-Hill, 1995:875–903. With permission of the publisher.

studies are not available. Minimal invasive surgery (placement of 4 mm catheter under stereotactic guidance, followed by 1 mg recombinant tissue plasminogen activator infusion and draining the clot every 8 hours for several days) has been piloted and is currently being tested in a prospective trial (the MISTIE trial). Patients with a large lobar hematoma (e.g., volume of 30–60 cm³) and temporal lobe hematoma in particular may benefit from early surgery, possibly because of the increased risk of secondary deterioration from enlargement. This treatment should ideally be compared with the best medical management, including monitoring and control of intracranial pressure.

The international Surgical Treatment of Intracerebral Hemorrhage (STICH) trial randomized 1,033 patients to surgical evacuation within 96 hours of presentation or medical management, and outcome was similar.[85] The STICH II trial tested craniotomy in lobar hematoma (10–100 mL) but with no associated intraventricular clot but again found no significant differences in outcome.[86] We need to keep in mind that both these STICH trials did not enroll rapidly deteriorating patients.

Lobar hematomas associated with arteriovenous malformations require neurosurgical evaluation. The risk of fatal recurrent hemorrhage during the same admission is very low (≤ 1%), and surgical repair or other interventions (intravascular occlusion, stereotactic radiosurgery) often can be carefully planned. Untreated, the annual rebleeding risk is 15%–20% in some studies. Deep venous drainage emerged as a strong risk factor for recurrent hemorrhage. Arteriovenous malformations are usually graded (I to V) (Table 27.5), and the grade predicts postoperative morbidity and mortality. In the Barrow Neurological Institute experience, permanent major neurologic deficit was absent in grades I–III, but 22% in grade IV, and 17% in grade V arteriovenous malformation.[52] Surgical excision is preferred in grade I arteriovenous malformation, and perioperative mortality is low. Radiosurgery or combined therapies are reserved for other grades. More recently Spetzler and Ponce[110] suggested a 3 tier classification. Class A combines Grades I and II AVMs and they would recommend resection. Class B includes grade III and multimodality treatment is suggested, Class Combines Grades IV and V AVMs and management would be only considered with recurrent hemorrhages, progressive neurologic deficits, "steal-related symptoms" and AVM related aneurysms (twice more likely in posterior fossa AVM).[90] Effective treatment of a nidal aneurysm could potentially revert a symptomatic AVM into an asymptomatic AVM. Which approach is most satisfactory is decided by the neurosurgeon and is not further discussed here. Scholarly reviews of the management of arteriovenous malformations can be consulted.[4,37,79,89]

DETERIORATION: CAUSES AND MANAGEMENT

The condition of approximately 30% of patients with lobar and ganglionic hemorrhages deteriorates to a more significant neurologic deficit. In our series, one of four patients with a lobar hemorrhage had deterioration, which was more common in those with certain CT characteristics, such as a hematoma larger than 60 cm³, any shift of the septum pellucidum, effacement of the contralateral ambient cistern, and widening of the temporal horn.[39] Worsening in the degree of hemiparesis and decrease in the level of alertness are most common, and in others, a new neurologic deficit, such as speech and language difficulties, may become apparent. Pupil dilatation on the side of the hematoma indicates lateral brainstem displacement with damage to the third nerve in a temporal lobe hematoma, but may also indicate extension of the thalamic hemorrhage to the midbrain.

In the first 12–24 hours, enlargement of the hematoma is the cause of deterioration.[84,135] Patients with superficially located lobar hematomas from amyloid angiopathy are at comparatively low risk of deterioration, as are patients with a hematoma of small CT volume (< 30 cm³). Further growth of the hematoma is typically associated with a 50%–75% risk of mortality within 1 month.[47] Mortality in patients whose condition is deteriorating is the sum of systemic complications, progression to brain death, and, increasingly, withdrawal of support. Most commonly, withdrawal of support is instigated by advance directives or family requests in elderly patients with catastrophic hypertensive hemorrhage.

The volume of a hematoma may increase from continued bleeding, edema formation, and rebleeding.[9,15,24,48,125,129,130] The role of hemodynamic variables in expansion is minimal.[60] Continued bleeding occurs from a cascade effect. The mass exerts pressure and stretch on surrounding arteries, which subsequently rupture and build a mass in consecutive layers of fibrin. Edema in intra-cerebral hematoma is due to both cytotoxic and vasogenic mechanisms. It is maximal 1–3 days after the initial hemorrhage and resolves by day 5. The perilesional edematous regions contain significant clot-derived protein and expand the extracellular space, increasing the distance of white matter axons and cells from their blood supply. Thrombin is important in perilesional edema, because it causes inflammation, reactive gliosis, and retraction of axons and dendrites. In one experimental study, the effects of thrombin could be blocked by hirudin, which is a specific thrombin inhibitor, and edema could not be produced by other blood products. Edema is a form of reperfusion injury due to early ischemia after the hematoma, with flow improving significantly over time.[129] Influx of iron or prothrombin has also been implicated.[76] There may be a region of perihematoma tissue at risk, and glucose metabolism is disturbed. Ongoing damage may impact an outcome, but avenues for intervention are not yet known.[118,132]

The most comprehensive study on enlargement of intracerebral hematoma (from Niigata University in Japan) included 627 patients with serial CT scans (30 minutes after arrival and follow-up within 24 hours). Major risk factors for enlargement of hematoma (> 50% or an increase of 20 cm³) included daily heavy alcohol consumption, large hematoma, impaired consciousness on

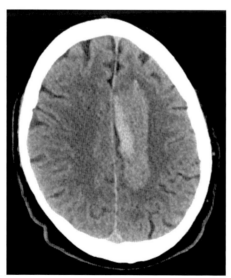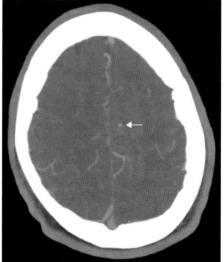

FIGURE 27.13: Computerized tomographic angiography in lobar hematoma, note contrast extravasation (spot sign).

TABLE 27.6. CT SCAN FINDINGS
SUGGESTING POTENTIAL FOR
ENLARGEMENT OF CEREBRAL
HEMATOMA

UHG > 10 ml/h
Baseline ICH volume > 60 ml
CTA spot sign
Fluid levels due to anticoagulation

admission, low level of fibrinogen, and a short time between onset and admission.[45]

The initial CT scan in ganglionic and lobar hematoma may provide early clues to clinical deterioration. Considerable CT volume of the clot (> 60 cm³) is one of the most important predictors of clinical neurologic deterioration, and the risk of further deterioration from enlargement of the hematoma is increased[19,24] (Figure 27.13). More recently, a CT angiogram "spot" sign has been identified as a predictor.[22,119] This sign can be found only on a CT angiogram and is defined as a 1–2 mm focus of enhancement within the hematoma, and it may represent active hemorrhage from ruptured perforators. The sign may have mimickers (notably AVM) and its predictive value for enlargement requires more prospective study. Patients with an irregularly shaped hematoma (possibly from active bleeding at multiple sites within the parenchyma) may be also at risk for further enlargement.[10] Another method of estimating enlargement is using the ultra early hematoma growth (UHG) formula determined by baseline ICH ABC/2 volume divided by time (in hours) between onset and first CT scan.[103] Speed of growth of more than 10 ml/h determines high risk of enlargement and outcome is already worse with ≥ 5 ml/h,[103,108] (Table 27.6).

Anticoagulation-related hemorrhages are significantly larger, often progress in size, and have a worse outcome.[35] Outcome in thrombolysis-associated hemorrhages is particularly poor. Expansion of the hematoma associated with thrombolysis may be dramatic, with virtually no time to successfully intervene medically or surgically.

Deterioration can be explained not only by enlargement of the hematoma but also by development of edema surrounding the hematoma, obstructive hydrocephalus, and systemic metabolic factors.

Acute hydrocephalus is a possible cause for deterioration, and when it is documented by serial CT scan, ventriculostomy can be considered as a diagnostic procedure. Patients who present in coma from intracranial hemorrhage with ventricular hemorrhage and dilatation seldom benefit from ventriculostomy, although it often seems the only rational option.[2,26] Ventriculostomy may be beneficial in patients with documented deterioration and enlarging hydrocephalus who have a comparatively small obstructing thalamic or caudate hemorrhage.

Treatment of patients with massive intraventricular hemorrhage and cast formation, particularly in caudate or thalamic hemorrhages, is difficult but a cause of neurologic deterioration.[78] We have used intraventricular tissue plasminogen activator (tPA) in patients with substantial intraventricular blood but, despite improved washout in ventricles, have not seen dramatic clinical improvement. Accurate predictions of clinical deterioration remain elusive and even in combination of findings would still marginally increase prediction.[16]

Surgical evacuation is pursued after deterioration, particularly if no effect is seen after osmotic diuretics. Ultra early removal of ganglionic hemorrhage may be associated with increased incidence of early rebleeding.[87] However, the literature consists of a heterogeneous mix of different techniques in different hemorrhages in patients with different prior states of health, and therefore comparison is quite difficult. Most clinical trials have only included stable patients.

Surgical evacuation in putaminal hemorrhage is often the only option to prevent further progression to brain death, but the procedure should be considered life-saving only, with often a dismal quality of life.

The options in lobar hematomas are clearly different. A particularly difficult clinical situation is a fluctuating level of consciousness in a patient with a moderate-sized hematoma and some shift but superficial localization in the frontal or temporal lobe. The threshold for evacuation should probably be low. Indeed, these hematomas are comparatively easy to evacuate, and it may be too intimidating to wait for the patient's condition to deteriorate.[38] Nonetheless, in some instances, we have been able to manage patients medically and have asked neurosurgeons to evacuate these hematomas after deterioration or when increasing brain shift on CT scans is present.

Emergency craniotomy in patients with hematomas was to no avail when comatose patients presented with absent pontomesencephalic reflexes (pupil, cornea, oculocephalic) and extensor posturing. In our series with predominantly younger patients and hematomas in the right hemisphere, functional independence was a possible outcome in approximately 20% of patients who had these

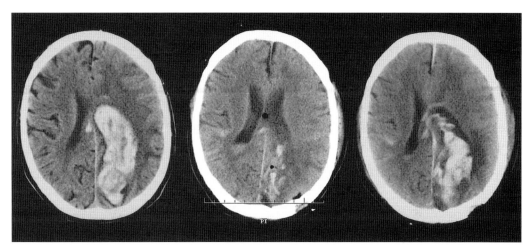

FIGURE 27.14: Rebleeding after evacuation of lobar hematoma. (*Left*) Large lobar hematoma (*Middle*) Immediate computed tomography (CT) scan hours after return from operating room showed near-total evacuation. (*Right*) CT scan on second postoperative day after failure to fully awaken showed rebleeding in operative bed.

brainstem reflexes preserved before surgery.[101] Therefore, massive hematomas producing brain tissue shift and features of herniation on CT scans were not incompatible with functional recovery. Patients should improve quickly after evacuation, and some in a very dramatic fashion, with reappearance of pupil reflexes. Failure to improve could represent rebleeding in the operating bed (Figure 27.14).

OUTCOME

Spontaneous intracerebral hematomas may constitute a diverse group in terms of prognosis.[23,27,33,115] Nonetheless, simple rules may apply. Mortality has been significantly increased in patients with a hematoma volume of 40–60 cm³, displacement of the pineal gland, stupor, and hyperglycemia.[27] Others found that patients with

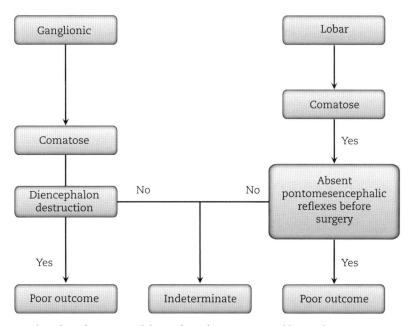

FIGURE 27.15: Algorithm of outcome in lobar and ganglionic intracranial hemorrhages.

Poor outcome: Severe disability or death, vegetative state. Indeterminate: Any statement would be a premature conclusion.

large intra-ventricular volumes[117] (fourth ventricle),[109] fever of any cause, hydrocephalus, warfarin use, increased systolic blood pressure, gaze palsy, neurologic deterioration after admission, and need for mechanical ventilation had a poor outcome.[40–42,51,106,109,114,116,131,134] Acute hydrocephalus in putaminal hemorrhage predicts 30-day mortality.[94] The FAST trial found baseline characteristics predictive of outcome (age, ganglionic location, severe neurologic deficit) but also early worsening.[20] Anemia (hemoglobin < 12 g/dL for women and < 13 g/dL for men) has been associated with larger hematoma volumes and thus worse outcome may be a marker for an underlying coagulopathy, particularly prior to undiagnosed malignancy. Whether erythropoietin has a role in reducing size is not known.[71]

Early mortality from intracranial hemorrhage in hospital-based series is approximately 20%, mortality 1 month from onset adds 10%, and mortality figures after 2 years may add an additional 20%, for a total mortality of 50% from neurologic causes and systemic complications from a persistent neurologic deficit.[55]

Survivors do relatively well, and independent survival has been reported in 50% of patients after 1 year. Early predictive factors for a significant handicap are virtually unknown. In many patients, marked improvement in motor function can be expected within 1 month. Patients who leave the NICU comatose but weaned from the ventilator and who show no clinical signs of improvement probably have no chance of independent recovery, although improvement to severe disability may be observed in the following month. An algorithm of outcome is shown in Figure 27.15. Resumption of anticoagulation in patients with warfarin associated hemorrhages and high embolic risk (prior prosthetic valve) or starting anticoagulation due to recent pulmonary embolism and deep venous thrombosis is reasonable 7–14 days after the ictus. When earlier initiation of anticoagulation is needed, initial use of IV heparin is preferred because it can be more rapidly reversed than oral anticoagulants.

CONCLUSION

- Medical management includes correction of possible coagulopathy (preferred prothrombin complex concentrate and vitamin K, but can consider factor VIIa and fresh frozen plasma), control of mass effect and shift (3% hypertonic saline or mannitol, 1 g/kg), early control of blood pressure to systolic blood pressure of less than 130 mm Hg with IV antihypertensives and antiepileptic drugs for 2–3 weeks in lobar hematoma only.
- Neurosurgical intervention is considered for marked clinical deterioration, but outcome in treated patients with ganglionic hemorrhages is not much better. Early surgical intervention is indicated in superficially located hematoma and brain tissue shift.

REFERENCES

1. Abdel-Wahab OI, Healy B, Dzik WH. Effect of fresh-frozen plasma transfusion on prothrombin time and bleeding in patients with mild coagulation abnormalities. *Transfusion* 2006;46:1279–1285.
2. Adams RE, Diringer MN. Response to external ventricular drainage in spontaneous intracerebral hemorrhage with hydrocephalus. *Neurology* 1998;50:519–523.
3. Aguilar MI, Hart RG, Kase CS, et al. Treatment of warfarin-associated intracerebral hemorrhage: literature review and expert opinion. *Mayo Clinic Proc* 2007;82:82–92.
4. Al-Shahi R, Warlow C. A systematic review of the frequency and prognosis of arteriovenous malformations of the brain in adults. *Brain* 2001;124:1900–1926.
5. Anderson CS, Huang Y, Wang JG, et al. Intensive blood pressure reduction in acute cerebral haemorrhage trial (INTERACT): a randomised pilot trial. *Lancet Neurol* 2008;7:391–399.
6. Arakawa S, Saku Y, Ibayashi S, Nagao T, Fujishima M. Blood pressure control and recurrence of hypertensive brain hemorrhage. *Stroke* 1998;29:1806–1809.
7. Atlas SW, Thulborn KR. MR detection of hyperacute parenchymal hemorrhage of the brain. *AJNR Am J Neuroradiol* 1998;19:1471–1477.
8. Auer LM, Deinsberger W, Niederkorn K, et al. Endoscopic surgery versus medical treatment for spontaneous intracerebral hematoma: a randomized study. *J Neurosurg* 1989;70:530–535.
9. Bae H, Jeong D, Doh J, et al. Recurrence of bleeding in patients with hypertensive intracerebral hemorrhage. *Cerebrovasc Dis* 1999;9:102–108.
10. Barras CD, Tress BM, Christensen S, et al. Density and shape as CT predictors of intracerebral hemorrhage growth. *Stroke* 2009;40:1325–1331.
11. Berger AR, Lipton RB, Lesser ML, Lantos G, Portenoy RK. Early seizures following intracerebral hemorrhage: implications for therapy. *Neurology* 1988;38:1363–1365.
12. Boulis NM, Bobek MP, Schmaier A, Hoff JT. Use of factor IX complex in warfarin-related intracranial hemorrhage. *Neurosurgery* 1999;45:1113–1118.

13. Broderick J, Connolly S, Feldmann E, et al. Guidelines for the management of spontaneous intracerebral hemorrhage in adults: 2007 update: a guideline from the American Heart Association/American Stroke Association Stroke Council, High Blood Pressure Research Council, and the Quality of Care and Outcomes in Research Interdisciplinary Working Group. *Circulation* 2007;116:e391–e413.

14. Broderick JP, Brott TG, Duldner JE, Tomsick T, Huster G. Volume of intracerebral hemorrhage: a powerful and easy-to-use predictor of 30-day mortality. *Stroke* 1993;24:987–993.

15. Brott T, Broderick J, Kothari R, et al. Early hemorrhage growth in patients with intracerebral hemorrhage. *Stroke* 1997;28:1–5.

16. Brouwers HB, Chang Y, Falcone GJ, et al. Predicting hematoma expansion after primary intracerebral hemorrhage. *JAMA Neurology* 2014;71:158–164.

17. Butler AC, Tait RC. Management of oral anticoagulant-induced intracranial haemorrhage. *Blood Rev* 1998;12:35–44.

18. Cartmill M, Dolan G, Byrne JL, Byrne PO. Prothrombin complex concentrate for oral anticoagulant reversal in neurosurgical emergencies. *Br J Neurosurg* 2000;14:458–461.

19. Chen ST, Chen SD, Hsu CY, Hogan EL. Progression of hypertensive intracerebral hemorrhage. *Neurology* 1989;39:1509–1514.

20. Christensen MC, Mayer SA, Ferran JM. Quality of life after intracerebral hemorrhage: results of the Factor Seven for Acute Hemorrhagic Stroke (FAST) trial. *Stroke* 2009;40:1677–1682.

21. Crum BA, Wijdicks EFM. Thalamic hematoma from a ruptured posterior cerebral artery aneurysm. *Cerebrovasc Dis* 2000;10:475–477.

22. d'Esterre CD, Chia TL, Jairath A, et al. Early rate of contrast extravasation in patients with intracerebral hemorrhage. *AJNR Am J Neuroradiol* 2011;32:1879–1884.

23. Daverat P, Castel JP, Dartigues JF, Orgogozo JM. Death and functional outcome after spontaneous intracerebral hemorrhage: a prospective study of 166 cases using multivariate analysis. *Stroke* 1991;22:1–6.

24. Davis SM, Broderick J, Hennerici M, et al. Hematoma growth is a determinant of mortality and poor outcome after intracerebral hemorrhage. *Neurology* 2006;66:1175–1181.

25. Deveras RA, Kessler CM. Reversal of warfarin-induced excessive anticoagulation with recombinant human factor VIIa concentrate. *Ann Intern Med* 2002;137:884–888.

26. Diringer MN, Edwards DF, Zazulia AR. Hydrocephalus: a previously unrecognized predictor of poor outcome from supratentorial intracerebral hemorrhage. *Stroke* 1998;29:1352–1357.

27. Dixon AA, Holness RO, Howes WJ, Garner JB. Spontaneous intracerebral hemorrhage: an analysis of factors affecting prognosis. *Can J Neurol Sci* 1985;12:267–271.

28. Duff TA, Ayeni S, Levin AB, Javid M. Nonsurgical management of spontaneous intracerebral hematoma. *Neurosurgery* 1981;9:387–393.

29. Ecker RD, Wijdicks EFM. Footprints of coagulopathy. *J Neurol Neurosurg Psychiatry* 2002;73:534.

30. Faught E, Peters D, Bartolucci A, Moore L, Miller PC. Seizures after primary intracerebral hemorrhage. *Neurology* 1989;39:1089–1093.

31. Fayad PB, Awad IA. Surgery for intracerebral hemorrhage. *Neurology* 1998;51:S69–S73.

32. Fernandes HM, Mendelow AD. Spontaneous intracerebral haemorrhage: a surgical dilemma. *Br J Neurosurg* 1999;13:389–394.

33. Fieschi C, Carolei A, Fiorelli M, et al. Changing prognosis of primary intracerebral hemorrhage: results of a clinical and computed tomographic follow-up study of 104 patients. *Stroke* 1988;19:192–195.

34. Fisher CM. Clinical syndromes in cerebral hemorrhage. In: Fields WS, ed. *Pathogenesis and Treatment of Cerebrovascular Disease*. Springfield, IL: Charles C. Thomas; 1961:318–342.

35. Flaherty ML, Tao H, Haverbusch M, et al. Warfarin use leads to larger intracerebral hematomas. *Neurology* 2008;71:1084–1089.

36. Flaherty ML, Woo D, Haverbusch M, et al. Potential applicability of recombinant factor VIIa for intracerebral hemorrhage. *Stroke* 2005;36:2660–2664.

37. Fleetwood IG, Steinberg GK. Arteriovenous malformations. *Lancet* 2002;359:863–873.

38. Flemming KD, Wijdicks EFM, Li H. Can we predict poor outcome at presentation in patients with lobar hemorrhage? *Cerebrovasc Dis* 2001;11:183–189.

39. Flemming KD, Wijdicks EFM, St Louis EK, Li H. Predicting deterioration in patients with lobar hemorrhages. *J Neurol Neurosurg Psychiatry* 1999;66:600–605.

40. Fogelholm R, Avikainen S, Murros K. Prognostic value and determinants of first-day mean arterial pressure in spontaneous supratentorial intracerebral hemorrhage. *Stroke* 1997;28:1396–1400.

41. Fogelholm R, Nuutila M, Vuorela AL. Primary intracerebral haemorrhage in the Jyvaskyla region, central Finland, 1985–89: incidence, case fatality rate, and functional outcome. *J Neurol Neurosurg Psychiatry* 1992;55:546–552.

42. Franke CL, van Swieten JC, Algra A, van Gijn J. Prognostic factors in patients with intracerebral haematoma. *J Neurol Neurosurg Psychiatry* 1992;55:653–657.

43. Fredriksson K, Norrving B, Stromblad LG. Emergency reversal of anticoagulation after intracerebral hemorrhage. *Stroke* 1992;23:972–977.

44. Freeman WD, Brott TG, Barrett KM, et al. Recombinant factor VIIa for rapid reversal of warfarin anticoagulation in acute intracranial hemorrhage. *Mayo Clinic Proc* 2004;79:1495–1500.

45. Fujii Y, Takeuchi S, Sasaki O, Minakawa T, Tanaka R. Multivariate analysis of predictors of hematoma enlargement in spontaneous intracerebral hemorrhage. *Stroke* 1998;29:1160–1166.

46. Fujitsu K, Muramoto M, Ikeda Y, et al. Indications for surgical treatment of putaminal hemorrhage: comparative study based on serial CT and time-course analysis. *J Neurosurg* 1990;73:518–525.

47. Gebel JM, Jr., Jauch EC, Brott TG, et al. Relative edema volume is a predictor of outcome in patients with hyperacute spontaneous intracerebral hemorrhage. *Stroke* 2002;33:2636–2641.

48. Gonzalez-Duarte A, Cantu C, Ruiz-Sandoval JL, Barinagarrementeria F. Recurrent primary cerebral hemorrhage: frequency, mechanisms, and prognosis. *Stroke* 1998;29:1802–1805.

49. Greenberg SM. Cerebral amyloid angiopathy and vessel dysfunction. *Cerebrovasc Dis* 2002;13 Suppl 2:42–47.

50. Greenberg SM, O'Donnell HC, Schaefer PW, Kraft E. MRI detection of new hemorrhages: potential marker of progression in cerebral amyloid angiopathy. *Neurology* 1999;53:1135–1138.

51. Gujjar AR, Deibert E, Manno EM, Duff S, Diringer MN. Mechanical ventilation for ischemic stroke and intracerebral hemorrhage: indications, timing, and outcome. *Neurology* 1998;51:447–451.

52. Hamilton MG, Spetzler RF. The prospective application of a grading system for arteriovenous malformations. *Neurosurgery* 1994;34:2–6.

53. Hankey GJ, Hon C. Surgery for primary intracerebral hemorrhage: is it safe and effective? A systematic review of case series and randomized trials. *Stroke* 1997;28:2126–2132.

54. Heiskanen O. Treatment of spontaneous intracerebral and intracerebellar hemorrhages. *Stroke* 1993;24:I94–95.

55. Helweg-Larsen S, Sommer W, Strange P, Lester J, Boysen G. Prognosis for patients treated conservatively for spontaneous intracerebral hematomas. *Stroke* 1984;15:1045–1048.

56. Hemphill JC, 3rd. Treating warfarin-related intracerebral hemorrhage: is fresh frozen plasma enough? *Stroke* 2006;37:6–7.

57. Higgins AC, Nashold BS, Jr. Stereotactic evacuation of large intracerebral hematoma. *Appl Neurophysiol* 1980;43:96–103.

58. Hino A, Fujimoto M, Yamaki T, Iwamoto Y, Katsumori T. Value of repeat angiography in patients with spontaneous subcortical hemorrhage. *Stroke* 1998;29:2517–2521.

59. Ishihara T, Takahashi M, Yokota T, et al. The significance of cerebrovascular amyloid in the aetiology of superficial (lobar) cerebral haemorrhage and its incidence in the elderly population. *J Pathol* 1991;165:229–234.

60. Jauch EC, Lindsell CJ, Adeoye O, et al. Lack of evidence for an association between hemodynamic variables and hematoma growth in spontaneous intracerebral hemorrhage. *Stroke* 2006;37:2061–2065.

61. Juvela S, Heiskanen O, Poranen A, et al. The treatment of spontaneous intracerebral hemorrhage: a prospective randomized trial of surgical and conservative treatment. *J Neurosurg* 1989;70:755–758.

62. Kandel EI, Peresedov VV. Stereotaxic evacuation of spontaneous intracerebral hematomas. *J Neurosurg* 1985;62:206–213.

63. Kaneko M, Tanaka K, Shimada T, Sato K, Uemura K. Long-term evaluation of ultra-early operation for hypertensive intracerebral hemorrhage in 100 cases. *J Neurosurg* 1983;58:838–842.

64. Kanno T, Nagata J, Nonomura K, et al. New approaches in the treatment of hypertensive intracerebral hemorrhage. *Stroke* 1993;24:96–100.

65. Kase CS, Robinson RK, Stein RW, et al. Anticoagulant-related intracerebral hemorrhage. *Neurology* 1985;35:943–948.

66. Kaufman HH. Treatment of deep spontaneous intracerebral hematomas: a review. *Stroke* 1993;24:101–106.

67. Kelley RE, Berger JR, Scheinberg P, Stokes N. Active bleeding in hypertensive intracerebral hemorrhage: computed tomography. *Neurology* 1982;32:852–856.

68. Kilpatrick CJ, Davis SM, Tress BM, et al. Epileptic seizures in acute stroke. *Arch Neurol* 1990;47:157–160.

69. Kiphuth IC, Staykov D, Kohrmann M, et al. Early administration of low molecular weight heparin after spontaneous intracerebral hemorrhage: a safety analysis. *Cerebrovasc Dis* 2009;27:146–150.

70. Kreisler A, Godefroy O, Delmaire C, et al. The anatomy of aphasia revisited. *Neurology* 2000;54:1117–1123.

71. Kumar MA, Rost NS, Snider RW, et al. Anemia and hematoma volume in acute intracerebral hemorrhage. *Crit Care Med* 2009;37:1442–1447.

72. Kumral E, Kocaer T, Ertubey NO, Kumral K. Thalamic hemorrhage: a prospective study of 100 patients. *Stroke* 1995;26:964–970.

73. Kuramatsu JB, Gerner ST, Schellinger PD, et al. Anticoagulant reversal, blood pressure levels, and anticoagulant resumption in patients with anticoagulation-related intracerebral hemorrhage. *JAMA* 2015;313:824–836.

74. Lee KS, Bae HG, Yun IG. Recurrent intracerebral hemorrhage due to hypertension. *Neurosurgery* 1990;26:586–590.

75. Lee SB, Manno EM, Layton KF, Wijdicks EFM. Progression of warfarin-associated intracerebral hemorrhage after INR normalization with FFP. *Neurology* 2006;67:1272–1274.

76. Levine JM, Snider R, Finkelstein D, et al. Early edema in warfarin-related intracerebral hemorrhage. *Neurocrit Care* 2007;7:58–63.

77. Linfante I, Llinas RH, Caplan LR, Warach S. MRI features of intracerebral hemorrhage within 2 hours from symptom onset. *Stroke* 1999;30:2263–2267.

78. Lord AS, Gilmore E, Choi HA, Mayer SA. Time course and predictors of neurological deterioration after intracerebral hemorrhage. *Stroke* 2015;46:647–652.

79. Mattle HP, Schroth G, Seiler RW. Dilemmas in the management of patients with arteriovenous malformations. *J Neurol* 2000;247:917–928.

80. Maurino J, Saposnik G, Lepera S, Rey RC, Sica RE. Multiple simultaneous intracerebral hemorrhages: clinical features and outcome. *Arch Neurol* 2001;58:629–632.

81. Mayer SA, Brun NC, Begtrup K, et al. Efficacy and safety of recombinant activated factor VII for acute intracerebral hemorrhage. *N Engl J Med* 2008;358:2127–2137.

82. Mayer SA, Brun NC, Begtrup K, et al. Recombinant activated factor VII for acute intracerebral hemorrhage. *N Engl J Med* 2005;352:777–785.

83. Mayer SA, Davis SM, Skolnick BE, et al. Can a subset of intracerebral hemorrhage patients benefit from hemostatic therapy with recombinant activated factor VII? *Stroke* 2009;40:833–840.

84. Mayer SA, Sacco RL, Shi T, Mohr JP. Neurologic deterioration in noncomatose patients with supratentorial intracerebral hemorrhage. *Neurology* 1994;44:1379–1384.

85. Mendelow AD, Gregson BA, Fernandes HM, et al. Early surgery versus initial conservative treatment in patients with spontaneous supratentorial intracerebral hematomas in the International Surgical Trial in Intracerebral Hemorrhage (STICH): a randomized trial. *Lancet* 2005;365:387–397.

86. Mendelow AD, Gregson BA, Rowan EN, et al. Early surgery versus initial conservative treatment in patients with spontaneous supratentorial lobar intracerebral hematomas (STICH II): a randomized trial. *Lancet* 2013;382:397–408.

87. Morgenstern LB, Demchuk AM, Kim DH, Frankowski RF, Grotta JC. Rebleeding leads to poor outcome in ultra-early craniotomy for intracerebral hemorrhage. *Neurology* 2001;56:1294–1299.

88. Naidech AM, Jovanovic B, Liebling S, et al. Reduced platelet activity is associated with early clot growth and worse 3-month outcome after intracerebral hemorrhage. *Stroke* 2009;40:2398–2401.

89. Ogilvy CS, Stieg PE, Awad I, et al. AHA Scientific Statement: Recommendations for the management of intracranial arteriovenous malformations: a statement for healthcare professionals from a special writing group of the Stroke Council, American Stroke Association. *Stroke* 2001;32:1458–1471.

90. Orning J, Amin-Hanjani S, Hamade Y, et al. Increased prevalence and rupture status of feeder vessel aneurysms in posterior fossa arteriovenous malformations. *J Neurointerv Surg.* 2016 in press.

91. Pabinger I, Brenner B, Kalina U, et al. Prothrombin complex concentrate (Beriplex P/N) for emergency anticoagulation reversal: a prospective multinational clinical trial. *J Thromb Haemost* 2008;6:622–631.

92. Parry-Jones AR, Di Napoli M, Goldstein JN, et al. Reversal strategies for vitamin K antagonists in acute intracerebral hemorrhage. *Ann Neurol* 2015 Jul;78(1):54–62.

93. Passero S, Ulivelli M, Reale F. Primary intraventricular hemorrhage in adults. *Acta Neurol Scand* 2002;105:115–119.

94. Phan TG, Koh M, Vierkant RA, Wijdicks EFM. Hydrocephalus is a determinant of early mortality in putaminal hemorrhage. *Stroke* 2000;31:2157–2162.

95. Phan TG, Koh M, Wijdicks EFM. Safety of discontinuation of anticoagulation in patients with intracranial hemorrhage at high thromboembolic risk. *Arch Neurol* 2000;57:1710–1713.

96. Poungvarin N, Bhoopat W, Viriyavejakul A, et al. Effects of dexamethasone in primary supratentorial intracerebral hemorrhage. *N Engl J Med* 1987;316:1229–1233.

97. Powers WJ, Zazulia AR, Videen TO, et al. Autoregulation of cerebral blood flow surrounding acute (6 to 22 hours) intracerebral hemorrhage. *Neurology* 2001;57:18–24.

98. Prasad K, Mendelow AD, Gregson B. Surgery for primary supratentorial intracerebral hemorrhage. *Cochrane Database Syst Rev* 2008:CD000200.

99. Purrucker JC, Haas K, Rizos T, et al. Early clinical and radiological course, management, and outcome of intracerebral hemorrhage related to new oral anticoagulants. *JAMA Neurol* 2016, 2016;73:169–177.

100. Qureshi AI, Tuhrim S, Broderick JP, et al. Spontaneous intracerebral hemorrhage. *N Engl J Med* 2001;344:1450–1460.

101. Rabinstein AA, Atkinson JL, Wijdicks EFM. Emergency craniotomy in patients worsening due to expanded cerebral hematoma: to what purpose? *Neurology* 2002;58:1367–1372.

102. Rabinstein AA, Wijdicks EFM, Fulgham JR. Meningioma disguised as cerebral hematoma. *Neurology* 2002;58:146.

103. Rodriguez-Luna D, Rubiera M, Ribo M, et al. Ultraearly hematoma growth predicts poor outcome after acute intracerebral hemorrhage. *Neurology* 2011;77:1599–1604.

104. Ropper AH, Gress DR. Computerized tomography and clinical features of large cerebral hemorrhages. *Cerebrovasc Dis* 1991;1:38–42.

105. Ropper AH, King RB. Intracranial pressure monitoring in comatose patients with cerebral hemorrhage. *Arch Neurol* 1984;41:725–728.

106. Rosenow F, Hojer C, Meyer-Lohmann C, et al. Spontaneous intracerebral hemorrhage: prognostic factors in 896 cases. *Acta Neurol Scand* 1997;96:174–182.

107. Safaoui MN, Aazami R, Hotz H, Wilson MT, Margulies DR. A promising new alternative for the rapid reversal of warfarin coagulopathy in traumatic intracranial hemorrhage. *Am J Surg* 2009;197:785–790.

108. Sato S, Arima H, Hirakawa Y, et al. The speed of ultraearly hematoma growth in acute intracerebral hemorrhage. *Neurology* 2014;83: 2232–2238.

109. Shapiro SA, Campbell RL, Scully T. Hemorrhagic dilation of the fourth ventricle: an ominous predictor. *J Neurosurg* 1994;80:805–809.

110. Spetzler RF, Ponce FA. 3-tier classification of cerebral arteriovenous malformations. *J Neurosurg* 2011;114: 842–849.

111. Smith EE, Greenberg SM. Beta-amyloid, blood vessels, and brain function. *Stroke* 2009;40:2601–2606.

112. Smith EE, Rosand J, Knudsen KA, Hylek EM, Greenberg SM. Leukoaraiosis is associated with warfarin-related hemorrhage following ischemic stroke. *Neurology* 2002;59:193–197.

113. Stein RW, Kase CS, Hier DB, et al. Caudate hemorrhage. *Neurology* 1984;34:1549–1554.

114. Toyoda K, Yasaka M, Nagata K, et al. Antithrombotic therapy influences location, enlargement, and mortality from intracerebral hemorrhage: the Bleeding with Antithrombotic Therapy (BAT) Retrospective Study. *Cerebrovasc Dis* 2009;27:151–159.

115. Tuhrim S, Dambrosia JM, Price TR, et al. Prediction of intracerebral hemorrhage survival. *Ann Neurol* 1988;24:258–263.

116. Tuhrim S, Horowitz DR, Sacher M, Godbold JH. Validation and comparison of models predicting survival following intracerebral hemorrhage. *Crit Care Med* 1995;23:950–954.

117. Tuhrim S, Horowitz DR, Sacher M, Godbold JH. Volume of ventricular blood is an important determinant of outcome in supratentorial intracerebral hemorrhage. *Crit Care Med* 1999;27:617–621.

118. Vespa PM. Metabolic penumbra in intracerebral hemorrhage. *Stroke* 2009;40:1547–1548.

119. Wada R, Aviv RI, Fox AJ, et al. CT angiography "spot sign" predicts hematoma expansion in acute intracerebral hemorrhage. *Stroke* 2007;38:1257–1262.

120. Waga S, Fujimoto K, Okada M, Miyazaki M, Tanaka Y. Caudate hemorrhage. *Neurosurgery* 1986;18:445–450.

121. Wang CW, Juan CJ, Liu YJ, et al. Volume-dependent overestimation of spontaneous intracerebral hematoma volume by the ABC/2 formula. *Acta Radiol* 2009;50:306–311.

122. Weisberg LA, Shamsnia M, Elliott D. Seizures caused by nontraumatic parenchymal brain hemorrhages. *Neurology* 1991;41:1197–1199.

123. Weisberg LA, Stazio A, Elliott D, Shamsnia M. Putaminal hemorrhage: clinical-computed tomographic correlations. *Neuroradiology* 1990;32:200–206.

124. Wijdicks EFM, Borleffs JC, Hoepelman AI, Jansen GH. Fatal disseminated hemorrhagic toxoplasmic encephalitis as the initial manifestation of AIDS. *Ann Neurol* 1991;29:683–686.

125. Wijdicks EFM, Fulgham JR. Acute fatal deterioration in putaminal hemorrhage. *Stroke* 1995;26:1953–1955.

126. Wijdicks EFM, Jack CR, Jr. Intracerebral hemorrhage after fibrinolytic therapy for acute myocardial infarction. *Stroke* 1993;24:554–557.

127. Wijdicks EFM, Schievink WI, Brown RD, Mullany CJ. The dilemma of discontinuation of anticoagulation therapy for patients with intracranial hemorrhage and mechanical heart valves. *Neurosurgery* 1998;42:769–773.

128. Wijdicks EFM, Silbert PL, Jack CR, Parisi JE. Subcortical hemorrhage in disseminated intravascular coagulation associated with sepsis. *AJNR Am J Neuroradiol* 1994;15:763–765.

129. Xi G, Hua Y, Bhasin RR, et al. Mechanisms of edema formation after intracerebral hemorrhage: effects of extravasated red blood cells on

blood flow and blood-brain barrier integrity. *Stroke* 2001;32:2932–2938.

130. Xi G, Wagner KR, Keep RF, et al. Role of blood clot formation on early edema development after experimental intracerebral hemorrhage. *Stroke* 1998;29:2580–2586.

131. Young WB, Lee KP, Pessin MS, et al. Prognostic significance of ventricular blood in supratentorial hemorrhage: a volumetric study. *Neurology* 1990;40:616–619.

132. Zazulia AR, Videen TO, Powers WJ. Transient focal increase in perihematomal glucose metabolism after acute human intracerebral hemorrhage. *Stroke* 2009;40:1638–1643.

133. Zhu XL, Chan MS, Poon WS. Spontaneous intracranial hemorrhage: which patients need diagnostic cerebral angiography? A prospective study of 206 cases and review of the literature. *Stroke* 1997;28:1406–1409.

134. Zubkov AY, Mandrekar JN, Claassen DO, et al. Predictors of outcome in warfarin-related intracerebral hemorrhage. *Arch Neurol* 2008;65:1320–1325.

135. Zurasky JA, Aiyagari V, Zazulia AR, Shackelford A, Diringer MN. Early mortality following spontaneous intracerebral hemorrhage. *Neurology* 2005;64:725–727.

28

Cerebellum and Brainstem Hemorrhages

Parenchymal hemorrhages in brain structures that make up the posterior fossa are unusual and uniquely different. The small confines of this compartment surrounded by a taut tentorium border leave little room for a cerebellar hemorrhage. Interruption of cerebrospinal fluid (CSF) circulation from compression of the fourth ventricle quickly follows.

Hemorrhage into the cerebellum is unquestionably a critical neurologic disorder that requires immediate neurosurgical attention. In fact, any sizable hemorrhage into the cerebellum is a neurosurgical emergency also because deterioration can be rapid in many of these seemingly stable patients. The decision is often either to evacuate the clot or, alternatively, to place a ventricular drain to manage acute obstructive hydrocephalus. There is immediacy when these patients are seen for the first time.

Hemorrhages in the brainstem are always more problematic, primarily because the therapeutic options are limited, if any. Pontine hemorrhages, which are uncommon, are highly destructive if due to hypertension, but patients have considerably better prospects if the hematoma is smaller and due to underlying vascular malformations such as leaking cavernomas.

This chapter focuses on the neurocritical care of patients with cerebellar hemorrhages, indications for suboccipital craniotomy, and a brief discussion of specific management problems with hemorrhages in the pons and medulla oblongata.

CLINICAL RECOGNITION

Cerebellar hemorrhages are difficult to diagnose. The delay in diagnosis may be due to lack of familiarity or atypical manifestations. The most consistent signs in cerebellar hemorrhage are an acute sense of vertigo, sudden onset of gait ataxia, dysarthria, and vomiting.[12,17,23,33] The imbalance can be striking; commonly, patients struggle to stand and need the assistance of two persons. Headache may have the characteristics of a thunderclap

headache or may rapidly build up to a profound occipital or holocephalic headache. Orthostatic headache may be prominent and may conceal other signs.[6] Impaired consciousness is common, and 10%–20% of these patients are stuporous at onset.[12,17,32] Cranial nerve deficits are invariably present. Nystagmus is typically horizontal rotary, but may additionally change in direction or become vertical. Gaze palsy to the side of the lesion is often found, but in patients with marked obstructive hydrocephalus, vertical gaze palsy may become more apparent. Many types of eye movement disorders have been reported, including ocular bobbing and skew deviation. Ipsilateral facial palsy is fairly common when compression of the brainstem occurs. However, the presenting triad of ipsilateral facial palsy, gaze preference, and limb ataxia is uncommon.[39,50] Patients with pontine compression have marked impairment of consciousness, bilateral miosis, and sluggish or absent oculocephalic responses. Fairly typical are breathing abnormalities, varying from hyperventilation to episodes of shallow breathing or apnea. Most patients in this stage of brainstem compression also have brief runs of bradycardia. Compression of the brainstem may result in increased vagal sensitivity and bradycardia, which may be observed during tracheal suctioning but may also be elicited with gentle pressure on the orbit. Surges of systolic hypertension (> 200 mm Hg) due to brainstem compression are associated with dysfunction of the sympathic projections but are not necessarily coupled with bradycardia.[49] When present, these signs indicate significant brainstem distortion, and evacuation of the hematoma becomes critical for survival. Loss of brainstem reflexes may be imminent, although patients with rapid deterioration often still have preserved gag reflex on tracheal suctioning. Despite extensor posturing, outcome can be surprisingly good after rapid evacuation of the hematoma.

Spontaneous hemorrhage into the pons justifies admission to the neurosciences intensive care unit (NICU) for mechanical ventilation and supportive therapy. The destruction is often more catastrophic than that in patients with cerebellar hematoma. Pontine hemorrhages are likely to be massive, from rupture of the distal midpontine perforating branches of the basilar artery, and occupy the entire pons or force their way into the ventricles. Patients are instantly comatose, have pinpoint but light-responsive pupils and no oculocephalic responses, and display vigorous extensor responses.[18,27] Ocular bobbing (fast downward disconjugate jerks with much slower return to midposition) is virtually diagnostic.[36] Oculovestibular testing using ice water injection may bring on bilateral internuclear ophthalmoplegia or loss of horizontal gaze in comatose patients. Irregular breathing, such as brief gasping marked hypoventilation or more often apneic spells, often necessitates intubation and support with mechanical ventilation. In addition, there is almost immediate significant pharyngeal and tongue weakness, causing obstructive pooling of secretions. Many patients with large pontine hemorrhages may become hyperthermic, and more than one-third have temperatures exceeding 40°C with profuse sweating.[36,61] Massive shivering may occur, which may mistakenly suggests seizures.

Coma from pons destruction should be differentiated from a locked-in syndrome if the hemorrhage remains confined to the basis pontis, but this is not common. Localization in the unilateral pons or tegmentum alone causes lesser degrees of impairment of consciousness, dysarthria, ataxic hemiparesis, crossed sensory loss, internuclear ophthalmoplegia, oculomotor palsy, and ipsilateral facial weakness.[10] One-and-a-half syndrome may occur in a unilateral tegmental lesion involving the paramedian pontine reticular formation or the abducens nucleus. There is a conjugate horizontal gaze palsy in one direction and an internuclear ophthalmoplegia in the other direction.[56] Oculopalatal tremor is often a later feature (the generator of the tremor is the inferior olive as part of the dentate nucleus and contralateral red nucleus connection or Guillain Mollaret triangle).[1] Visual hallucinations have been described, and the content of these hallucinations may include very graphic descriptions of landscapes and objects, as if the patient were in a dream. These hallucinations have not been satisfactorily explained—and are exceedingly rare—but could be due to a lesion in the reticular formation localized in the tegmentum of the pons.[36]

Hemorrhages in other parts of the brainstem are less common and more often are due to extension from a primary pontine hemorrhage. Primary midbrain hemorrhages have distinct clinical features, often from significant mass effect. As expected, third- and fourth nerve palsies are common,[30] but when the hemorrhage is situated in the rostral midbrain tegmentum, Parinaud syndrome (upgaze palsy, lid retraction, large pupils with absent pupil response to light but preservation of convergence) may be seen.[45] Drowsiness is noted in 50% of the patients but soon resolves. Outcome is invariably good, and stay in the NICU is usually overnight. In two-thirds of cases, the cause is unknown or is tentatively linked to long-standing hypertension.

Another very uncommon type of brainstem hemorrhage is primary medullary hemorrhage.[4] Vertigo and headache are often followed by progressive hemiparesis. Hiccups may occur. Recognized presenting signs are nystagmus, palatal weakness, hypoglossal palsy, cerebellar ataxia, and limb weakness—combinations of the classic descriptions of lateral and medial medullary syndromes (Chapter 30).

NEUROIMAGING AND LABORATORY TESTS

Cerebellar hematoma can be localized in the hemisphere or vermis (Figure 28.1). The overwhelming majority of cerebellar hemorrhages are due to a ruptured superior cerebellar artery branch from hypertension-induced lipohyalinosis, but not all cerebellar hematomas are a consequence of many years of poorly controlled hypertension. If there is no prior history of hypertension, or in a young patient with no comorbidity or prior drug use, an early MRI and MRA are warranted to look for an alternate cause. An MRI may show a cavernous malformation (Figure 28.2). A dural arteriovenous fistula can be considered if the hematoma is comparatively small and near the fourth ventricle, and this justifies cerebral angiography.[46] The simultaneous presence of subarachnoid hemorrhage and parenchymal hemorrhage may lead to a suspicion of a tentorial AVM[51] (Figure 28.3). It is important to consider hemorrhage into a metastasis, a not infrequently defining manifestation of widespread cancer—most probably breast and lung cancer and melanoma. Remote hemorrhages in the cerebellum following craniotomy are discussed in Chapter 44.

Neuroimaging in posterior fossa hemorrhages is important because it can classify patients at

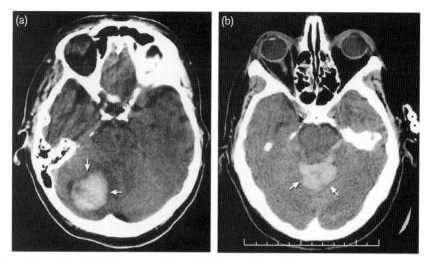

FIGURE 28.1: Types of cerebellar hematoma (*arrows*). (a) Hemisphere. (b) Vermis.

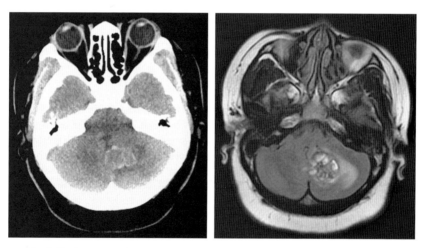

FIGURE 28.2: Cerebellar hematoma from cavernous angioma.

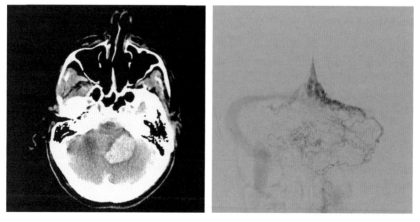

FIGURE 28.3: Cerebellar hematoma from dural AV fistula.

potential risk for further deterioration. In major textbooks, the size of the hematoma has traditionally been measured by using the axial cross-section diameter in centimeters and converting to true measurements. A diameter of 3 cm or more has been noted as a critical value to decide on evacuation. Cerebellar hematomas, well visualized on computed tomography (CT) scans, typically compress and distort surrounding structures. The fourth ventricle is partly or completely effaced, and there is early evidence of obstructive hydrocephalus, with enlargement of the temporal horns, dilatation of the third ventricle, and subependymal effusions surrounding the lateral ventricles and frontal horns. Less commonly, a cerebellar hematoma is small and only mildly displaces or distorts the fourth ventricle without obstructive hydrocephalus.

Important neuroradiologic signs of upward herniation are compression of the ambient cisterns and upward displacement of the vermis into the tentorial opening, and the posterior portion of the cistern surrounding the pineal gland changes from a diamond shape into a more blunted triangular shape[38] (Figure 28.4). These abnormalities have become known as signs of a *tight posterior fossa*[57] and, rightly so, have influenced clinical management. Complete obliteration of the quadrigeminal cistern predicts poor outcome despite surgical evacuation, whereas in partial obliteration, the predictive value is less clear.[52] Primary vermian hemorrhage or extension to the vermis is less common, but, due to its proximity with the brainstem, indicates a high probability of further deterioration.[49] On CT scans, therefore, the features of cerebellar hematoma that should be assessed are size, hydrocephalus, and, particularly, mass effect and degree of upward displacement.

In patients with a pontine hemorrhage, CT scans often show massive destruction. Four types of pontine hemorrhage have been described on CT scan. They can be classified as massive pontine, basal tegmental, bilateral tegmental, and small unilateral pontine hemorrhages (Figure 28.5).[7,31,58] Massive hemorrhages with complete destruction of the basis and tegmentum pontis are most frequent, almost invariably with intraventricular blood and prominent early hydrocephalus. Bilateral segmental hematoma with sparing of the basis pontis is less common. The basal tegmental type is an elliptical hematoma at the junction between the basis pontis and the tegmentum, along with some extension to the cerebellar peduncle and rupture into the fourth ventricle. A unilateral tegmental hemorrhage, with exclusive localization in one part of the tegmentum, often with a very small volume, has virtually no extension to the basis pontis or intraventricular rupture (Figure 28.5).

It is important to recognize whether the hematoma crosses over the midline, because this signifies a much worse prognosis than that in patients with unilateral tegmental hemorrhage.[7,11,13] Intraventricular blood or extension into the cerebellum has less prognostic value than the actual length of the hematoma.

Magnetic resonance imaging becomes an important study in survivors of pontine and cerebellar hemorrhages. The sensitivity for detection of underlying primary tumor, metastasis, and vascular malformations is good. It may detect the presence of cavernous malformations.[40]

Laboratory studies in patients with cerebellar hematoma should include complete blood cell count and smear, platelet count, and international normalized ratio (INR). In our hospital-based series, 25% of the patients with cerebellar hematomas were on warfarin, 75% of them beyond therapeutic range.[49] Involvement of other target organs from long-standing hypertension may be present and should be evaluated. The following should be done: renal function tests, full urinalysis, including measurement of total protein, if present; electrocardiography or echocardiography; and grading of atherosclerotic changes of the fundus. Results of liver function tests, which may indicate early evidence for a coagulopathy, must be known at admission; if they are abnormal, abdominal ultrasonography or CT of the liver is indicated. Optional tests include toxicology screen (for amphetamine and cocaine), human immunodeficiency virus testing, coagulation profile (fibrin degradation products, deficiency in factors VIII and IX), and hemoglobin electrophoresis if sickle cell disease is suspected.

FIRST STEPS IN MANAGEMENT

Immediately after arrival, a consultation with a neurosurgeon will lead to a decision and, in most cases, cerebellar hematoma must be evacuated immediately.[16,24,32] Evacuation may have to be postponed a few hours if platelet infusions or prothrombin complex are still pending. Neurosurgeons will proceed with an INR of 1.4 or less and a platelet count of at least 70,000. Platelets are usually administered if the patient

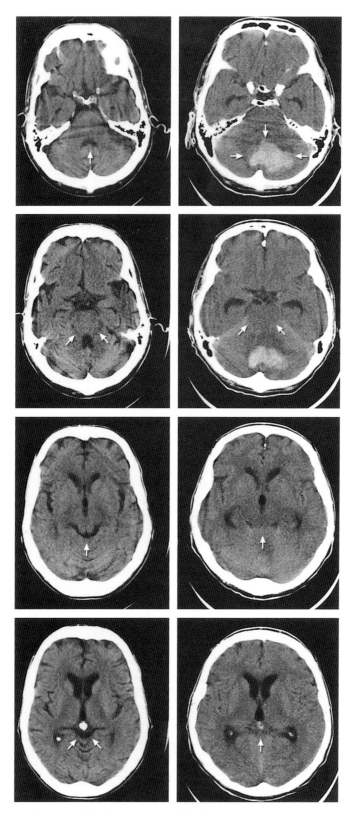

FIGURE 28.4: Computed tomographic changes with cerebellar hematoma.

Left column: Normal appearance for comparison. *Right column*: Typical features of a tight posterior fossa showing upward herniation (*arrow*): "toothy smile" appearance becomes "toothless frown" (from compression of the quadrigeminal cistern), diamond-shaped peritectal fluid space becomes squared off and more triangular, fourth ventricle and prepontine cisterns disappear, and temporal horns are enlarged.

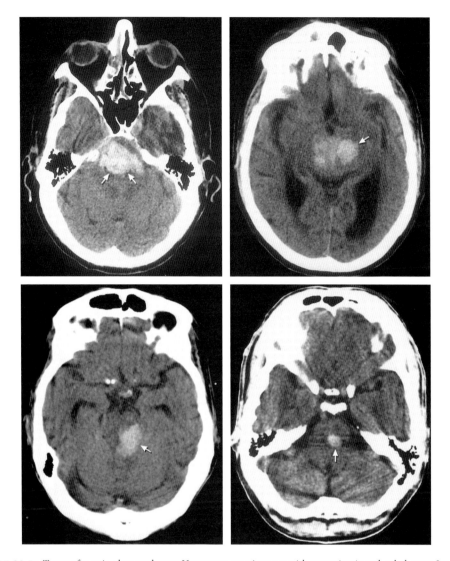

FIGURE 28.5: Types of pontine hemorrhages: *Upper row*: massive type with extension into the thalamus; *Lower row*: unilateral tegmental type; Bilateral tegmental type.

had antiplatelets, but this practice has not been tested. It remains crucially important to optimize hemostasis before surgery is attempted.

Monitoring in the NICU is imperative in patients who appear stable, because deterioration can occur in hours and sometimes abruptly. The initial steps in management are shown in Table 28.1. Airway management and endotracheal intubation in patients with progressive impairment of consciousness have a high priority because some patients may have unsuspected apnea. In others, marked hypoxemia occurs from aspiration during the ictus. Most intubated patients can breathe spontaneously with continuous positive airway pressure support of 5 cm H_2O, which is equivalent to a T-piece. Intermittent mandatory ventilation mode can be added if gas exchange remains insufficient or apnea spells continue.

Fluid management is important, and dehydration, if present, should be corrected. Swelling of the cerebellar hematoma is inevitable; it is not certain whether the amount of swelling can be reduced by marked free water restriction. A bolus of mannitol, 1 g/kg over 30 minutes, can be given en route to the operating room and can be repeated.

Anticoagulation should be reversed with fresh frozen plasma (2 units) and vitamin K (5–10 mg) given intravenously, or, much more preferably,

TABLE 28.1. INITIAL MANAGEMENT OF CEREBELLAR HEMATOMA

Airway management	Intubation if patient has hypoxemia despite facemask with 10 L of 60%–100% oxygen/minute, if abnormal respiratory drive or if abnormal protective reflexes (likely with motor response of withdrawal, or worse)
Mechanical ventilation	IMV/PS or CPAP mode
Fluid management	2–3 L of 0.9% NaCl
	Mannitol, 1 g/kg bolus, in patients with tight posterior fossa on CT scans. May consider 3%–23% hypertonic saline if a central access is available or pushing it through a femoral vein.
Blood pressure management	Labetalol, 10–20 mg IV every 15 min if needed for persistent hypertension (MAP > 130 mm Hg); hydralazine 10–20 mg IV if bradycardia
Cardiac arrhythmias	Sinus bradycardia: atropine, 0.5–2.0 mg IV
	Sinus tachycardia: fluid bolus, 500 mL of 0.9% NaCl or 250 mL of albumin 5%; metoprolol 5 mg IV
Nutrition	Enteral nutrition with continuous infusion (on day 2)
	Blood glucose control (goal 140–180 mg/dL)
Prophylaxis	DVT prophylaxis with pneumatic compression devices
	SC heparin 5000 U t.i.d. 2 days after craniotomy
	GI prophylaxis: pantoprazole 40 mg IV daily or lansoprazole 30 mg orally through nasogastric tube.
Surgical management	Surgical evacuation: hematoma size > 3 cm, obliterated 4th ventricle, or collapsed quadrigeminal cistern on CT scan
	Ventriculostomy for acute hydrocephalus
Access	Arterial catheter to monitor blood pressure (if IV antihypertensive drugs anticipated)
	Peripheral venous catheter or peripheral inserted central catheter

CPAP, continuous positive airway pressure; CT, computed tomography; DVT, deep vein thrombosis; GI, gastrointestinal; IMV, intermittent mandatory ventilation; IV, intravenously; MAP, mean arterial pressure; NaCl, sodium chloride; PS, pressure support; SC, subcutaneously.

prothrombin complex concentrate (PCC) should be administered (dosing is dependent on how high the INR is from a normal value, and dosing is dependent on brand used, but most patients need 20–30 IU/kg). Some neurosurgeons administer dexamethasone IV in a loading dose of 10 mg followed by 4 mg every 4 hours when craniotomy is anticipated, and this may potentially further reduce edema in the tight compartment of the posterior fossa.

Increases in blood pressure are treated only when persistently high. In most patients, however, hypertension is a manifestation of the Cushing response, a compensatory mechanism that probably should not tampered with. Bradycardia is also often a sign of brainstem compression. When it is associated with a decrease in blood pressure and when bradycardia occurs in runs, atropine (0.5–2 mg IV) should be considered. Tachycardia, however, may be related to dehydration, and fluid challenge should be considered first.

Decompressive suboccipital craniotomy is indicated in any patient with signs of compression on CT images, frequent episodes of bradycardia, less than localization to pain as a best motor response, or significant cranial nerve dysfunction. It is unclear whether size alone should prompt surgical evacuation. Most neurosurgeons favor craniotomy for cerebellar hemispheric hematomas and vermian hematomas larger than 3 cm, but mass effect (for example, obliteration of the fourth ventricle) and decreased level of alertness are probably more meaningful indicators than is absolute size of the hematoma.[44] One study of 50 consecutively treated patients with cerebellar hematoma found that 43% of patients with a completely effaced fourth ventricle deteriorated before transfer to the NICU.[23] In patients with small hematomas (clot diameter < 3 cm on CT scan) who have open ambient and quadrigeminal cisterns but hydrocephalus, ventriculostomy alone can be considered. In our series, this occurred in only 10% of patients, and suboccipital craniotomy followed soon after.[49] Medical management is probably the most reasonable choice in patients with maximal or nearly maximal

TABLE 28.2. INITIAL MANAGEMENT OF BRAINSTEM HEMORRHAGE

Airway management	Intubation if patient has hypoxemia despite facemask with 10 L of 100% oxygen/minute, if abnormal respiratory drive or if abnormal protective reflexes (likely with motor response of withdrawal, or worse)
Mechanical ventilation	IMV/PS or CPAP mode
Fluid management	2–3 L of 0.9% NaCl; increase amount in hyperthermia to 1 L per 1°C increase in temperature
Blood pressure management	Labetalol, 10–20 mg IV every 15 min if needed, for persistent hypertension (MAP > 120 mm Hg); hydralazine 10–20 mg IV if bradycardia.
Nutrition	Enteral nutrition with continuous infusion (on day 2)
	Blood glucose control (goal 140–180 mg/dL)
Prophylaxis	DVT prophylaxis with pneumatic compression devices
	GI prophylaxis: pantoprazole 40 mg IV daily or lansoprazole 30 mg orally through nasogastric tube
Access	Arterial catheter to monitor blood pressure (if IV antihypertensive drugs anticipated);
	Peripheral venous catheter or peripheral inserted central catheter

CPAP, continuous positive airway pressure; DVT, deep vein thrombosis; GI, gastrointestinal; IMV, intermittent mandatory ventilation; IV, intravenously; MAP, mean arterial pressure; NaCl, sodium chloride; PS, pressure support.

level of consciousness, no cranial nerve deficits, and a small hematoma without any major mass effect on CT scan. (For example, patients with marked cerebellar atrophy—as seen in chronic alcoholics—may tolerate hematomas of limited size.) Partial embolization and surgical resection are the best approach.

The management of patients with spontaneous brainstem hemorrhages is largely supportive (Table 28.2). Surgical management (Capsule 28.1) is considered in patients with an underlying cavernous angioma.

The almost universally large size of the brainstem hemorrhage destroys respiratory control and mandates mechanical ventilation. It is important to set the ventilator on intermittent-mandatory ventilation mode, because patients with markedly impaired ventilatory drive cannot breathe spontaneously. Patients with a pontine hemorrhage may have aspirated during the catastrophic ictus, and a large alveolar–arterial oxygen ratio may necessitate increasing positive end-expiratory pressure ventilation and high FIO_2. Hyperthermia has been noted in patients with pontine hemorrhages, and fluid intake could become insufficient. Cooling is indicated in patients with increased temperatures often exceeding 40°C. Blood pressures are markedly increased in patients with pontine hemorrhages. It is reasonable to mute marked elevations in mean arterial pressure, but in many patients, the increases are brief, disappearing within 24 hours. Extension of the lesion from edema may produce

complete loss of brainstem function. A change from hypertension to hypotension in patients with a large pontine hemorrhage and a sudden decrease in temperature to a subnormal level are ominous signs. As expected, diabetes insipidus is absent in patients with primary brainstem lesions.

Protection of the gastric mucosa in pontine hemorrhage with a proton-pump inhibitor is important. In a series of fatal cases of pontine hemorrhage, gastrointestinal bleeding was found within 1 week in one-third of the patients.[36] Enteral feeding can be started on the second or third day after admission, and in less severely affected cases, possible recovery of swallowing can be awaited during the first week. Percutaneous endoscopic gastrostomy is mandatory in patients with pontine hemorrhage who have an impaired swallowing mechanism and who are expected to require long-term care (Chapter 18).

For recovery to occur, a change for the better must be signaled by improvement in motor responses or in brainstem reflexes in the first week after the ictus. In patients with no change, the rationale (or lack thereof) for continuing supportive care, which includes tracheostomy and percutaneous endoscopic gastrostomy, must be discussed with the family.

DETERIORATION: CAUSES AND MANAGEMENT

Further deterioration in patients with cerebellar hematoma can be predicted with certainty. The odds are higher when systolic blood pressure

CAPSULE 28.1   SURGICAL OPTIONS IN PONTINE HEMORRHAGE

Stereotactic suction has been advocated in the treatment of pontine hemorrhage, and impressive results have been reported.[5,8,26] The architecture of the pons is quite delicate, but with stereotactic aspiration, good-to-fair recovery has been claimed in 65% of 20 patients with limited pontine hemorrhages (5–10 mL in volume). Outcome in patients with larger hematomas (> 10 mL) was poor and no better than that in a matched medically treated group.[47] Surgical intervention becomes a very important issue in patients with limited hematomas, particularly if additional MRIs demonstrate a cavernous angioma or cryptic arteriovenous malformation.[15,29,66] In patients with subependymal or tegmental localization of the hematoma, surgical removal through the vermis has resulted in good outcomes.[26] Recurrent hemorrhage is a major concern, up to 3% per patient year.[2,19,41] Although timing is uncertain, surgery is elective in most patients and most likely eliminates further risk of hemorrhage.[29] In reported cases, surgical excision may result in improvement or similar neurologic findings in 85% of the cases. Outcome may be worse in patients approached through the fourth ventricle as opposed to anterolateral pontine lesions.[19] Deep-seated lesions may be treated with stereotactic radiosurgery, but no proof exists that it reduces the rate of hemorrhage.[25,43]

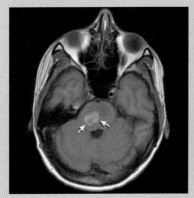 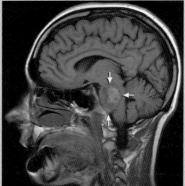

Sizable brainstem hemorrhage associated with cavernous hemangioma (arrows).

at admission is uncontrolled and higher than 200 mm Hg, corneal reflexes are abnormal, and oculocephalic reflexes are impaired. These signs reflect brainstem displacement. Neurologic deterioration also is likely in patients with vermian hemorrhage or hemispheric hemorrhage tracking into the vermis and in patients with early hydrocephalus on the initial CT scan. Risk of further clinical deterioration is low in patients without brainstem displacement, upward herniation, or, particularly, compression of the fourth ventricle.[49]

Most patients with a cerebellar hematoma have deterioration from direct brainstem compression rather than hydrocephalus.[2,23,55] The clinical features are progressive limitation

and loss of upward gaze and deepening coma. Pupils become asymmetrical in size and, soon after, pinpoint. Spontaneous hyperventilation with considerable respiratory alkalosis often occurs at the same time as marked deterioration in consciousness. Often, blood pressure increases with widening of the pulse pressure, and we have found this a helpful clinical sign of early deterioration. Bradycardia may be absent when vagal traffic, as a compensatory response, is interrupted by medullary compression and ischemia. Similar to cerebellar infarction with swelling (Chapter 31), the clinicopathologic correlate of upward herniation is subject to criticism. Whether a consistently recognizable pattern exists has been questioned after a careful autopsy report.[9] In addition, the relation of upward brain tissue displacement caused by ventriculostomy remains of doubtful causality. Of 52 patients with upward herniation noted in the literature, only 25% had ventriculostomy, but not all patients deteriorated minutes after ventriculostomy placement.[9]

Deterioration from hydrocephalus alone may occur in patients with cerebellar hematoma, usually in those with only marginal compression of the fourth ventricle, and presents with a much more gradual clinical course.[34] Computed tomography scanning confirms further enlargement of the lateral horns, shows bulging of the third ventricle, and, on lower CT scan slices, clearly visualizes the temporal horns. These patients gradually become more drowsy, new neurologic signs or symptoms seldom develop, and they are unable to protect the airway. The opening pressure is increased at the time of insertion of the ventricular drain, and several days of CSF drainage are required. A permanent ventriculoperitoneal drain is considered after 7–10 days, but rarely is necessary. Ventricular drains should be removed when the CSF is clear and there is no obstructive clot in the third or fourth ventricle, but also when the production of CSF is minimal and clamping has not resulted in an upsurge of intracranial pressure.

Placement of a ventricular catheter in patients with a pontine hemorrhage and an enlarged ventricular system but without a clinical history of deterioration is not only illogical but also unhelpful. Most patients with a massive pontine hemorrhage with an acute enlargement of the ventricular system present with clinical symptoms related to the pontine damage itself, not to hydrocephalus.

Patients with massive pontine hemorrhages may have progression to loss of all brainstem function on the day of admission.[37] Many patients, however, continue to trigger the ventilator and do not meet the clinical criteria for brain death. Ancillary tests are not helpful in this situation because blood flow to the brain may be preserved, certainly initially. In addition, electroencephalographic findings are expected to be abnormal but not isoelectric. In these patients, θ or δ activity may occur with sporadic α activity, but without reactivity to light or pain stimuli. Primary brainstem death is very uncommon. In these situations, we have extended our observation time to 24 hours. It can be expected that loss of all brain function occurs from progressive obstructive hydrocephalus.

OUTCOME

Mortality in hemorrhages of posterior fossa structures is considerable.[22,63] In addition, because most published data are from large medical centers with the most experience in treatment and probably also the best outcomes, the risk of fatal outcome most likely is underreported. Nonetheless, patients with cerebellar hematomas—particularly after decompressive surgery—may end up in a very acceptable functional state.

Predictive factors for poor outcome in cerebellar hemorrhage have not been studied prospectively. Patients of any age with loss of many brainstem functions may do surprisingly well after evacuation of the hematoma. In patients with less dramatic presentations, the prospects of independent recovery with preservation of gait are good.[32]

However, suboccipital craniotomy may be a futile surgical intervention. It is not known whether a dividing line exists between the potential for functional outcome and remaining in a crippled state. Absent corneal reflexes, acute hydrocephalus, and absent oculocephalic responses predict a poor outcome, but reversal of this poor clinical state has been documented in some cases.[50] In addition, neurosurgeons may favor toward younger patients and may be reluctant to consider surgical intervention in patients older than 70 years with clots of more than 3 cm in diameter on CT scans.[62] The degree of brainstem damage is important, and one study documented that T2 changes in the brainstem on postoperative MRI were correlated with poor outcome.[65] The timing of surgery in relation to the clinical signs of brainstem compression remains unknown but surgery consistently improved outcome.[20] A study of 16 comatose patients with abnormal pupils, compression of perimesencephalic cisterns, and hydrocephalus who were operated on within hours of admission found that all had poor outcomes.[64] In another study, comatose patients with a cerebellar hematoma and compressed quadrigeminal cistern on CT scan did not fare well, but the number of patients was small.[52]

Upward displacement of cerebellar tissue on CT scan (often also directly related to the total volume of the clot in cerebellar parenchyma) is a poor prognostic sign, but evacuation of the hematoma should nevertheless still be seriously considered. Coma alone should not be considered a reason to withdraw support or reduce the level of support, but some disagree.[32,54] Outcome in cerebellar hematoma, based on our series of 94 patients with cerebellar hematoma, is shown in Figure 28.6.[50] The decision whether to surgically

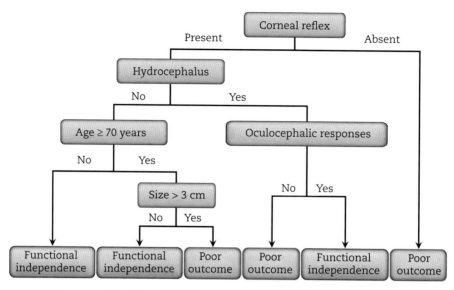

FIGURE 28.6: Outcome predictors in cerebellar hematoma.

Poor outcome: Severe disability or death, vegetative state. Functional independence: No assistance needed, minor handicap may remain.

intervene could be guided by these clinical and neuroimaging variables. Recurrence of a cerebellar hematoma is a possibility, but usually in patients with poorly controlled hypertension.[60]

The outcome in patients with pontine hemorrhage, coma within hours of onset, and horizontal vertical extension (> 2 cm on CT), and need for mechanical ventilation is invariably poor.[3,13,59] In our study, there were no survivors when patients presented with hyperthermia, extension to the thalamus, intraventricular hemorrhage, and acute hydrocephalus on the admission CT scan.[53] Surgically treated patients with large pontine hematomas have a better chance of survival, but very likely at the expense of devastating disability due to diplopia and ataxia.[53] A more recent scoring system from Japan predicted outcome on the presence of coma, hyperglycemia, and absent pupil reflexes, but such assessment lacks neurologic finesse and thus lacks prognostic finesse.[31]

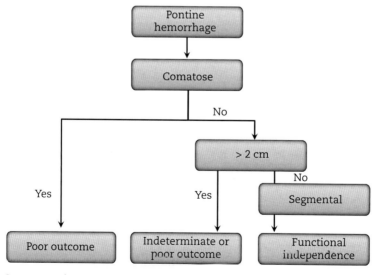

FIGURE 28.7: Outcome predictors in primary pontine hemorrhage.

Poor outcome: Severe disability or death, vegetative state. Indeterminate: Any statement would be a premature conclusion. Functional independence: No assistance needed, minor handicap may remain.

Lack of the N20 component on somatosensory evoked potentials has predicted poor outcome in pontine hemorrhage. In an unconfirmed study, preservation of one or both cortical somatosensory evoked potentials signified a chance for good recovery, even in a patient with a hemorrhage that crossed the midline of the pons.[14]

Patients with small lateral tegmental pontine hemorrhages do very well with medical management.[21,28,35,42,48] The first episode of hemorrhage in patients with brainstem vascular malformations is usually benign. Rebleeding of a brainstem cavernous malformation can be fatal. Neurosurgeons generally have no qualms about removing these lesions or to advise stereotactic therapy. Outcome predictors in pontine hemorrhage are shown in Figure 28.7.

CONCLUSIONS

- The CT scan signs in cerebellar hemorrhages are disappearance of the fourth ventricle, compression of ambient and quadrigeminal cisterns, and squaring off of the peritectal cistern, features most often seen in hematomas larger than 3 cm.
- Suboccipital decompressive craniotomy is the mainstay of management for large cerebellar hematomas.
- Management of cerebellar hematoma includes elective intubation in patients with rapid impairment of consciousness, mannitol in patients with CT evidence of tight posterior fossa, and labetalol intravenously for blood pressure control. Runs of bradycardia can be treated with atropine.
- Suboccipital craniotomy in comatose patients with cerebellar hemorrhage and loss of some brainstem reflexes may still result in independent recovery, but this is less likely when corneal reflexes are absent.
- Primary pontine hemorrhages carry a high mortality, often in patients with hyperthermia at presentation, intraventricular hematoma, and extension to midbrain and thalamus.
- In patients with a small localized hemorrhage, MRI studies are needed to demonstrate a possible arteriovenous malformation that can be successfully removed surgically.

REFERENCES

1. Aladdin Y, Scozzafava J, Muayqil T, Saqqur M. Pearls & oy-sters: oculopalatal tremor with one-and-a-half syndrome after pontine hemorrhage. *Neurology* 2008;71:e39–e41.
2. Aoki N, Mizuguchi K. Expanding intracerebellar hematoma: a possible clinicopathological entity. *Neurosurgery* 1986;18:94–96.
3. Balci K, Asil T, Kerimoglu M, Celik Y, Utku U. Clinical and neuroradiological predictors of mortality in patients with primary pontine hemorrhage. *Clin Neurol Neurosurg* 2005;108:36–39.
4. Barinagarrementeria F, Cantu C. Primary medullary hemorrhage: report of four cases and review of the literature. *Stroke* 1994;25:1684–1687.
5. Beatty RM, Zervas NT. Stereotactic aspiration of a brain stem hematoma. *Neurosurgery* 1983;13:204–207.
6. Chen WT, Fuh JL, Lu SR, Wang SJ. Cerebellar hemorrhage presenting as orthostatic headache: two case reports. *Neurology* 1999;53:1887–1888.
7. Chung CS, Park CH. Primary pontine hemorrhage: a new CT classification. *Neurology* 1992;42:830–834.
8. Colak A, Bertan V, Benli K, Ozek M, Gurcay O. Pontine hematoma: a report of three surgically treated cases. *Zentralbl Neurochir* 1991;52:33–36.
9. Cuneo RA, Caronna JJ, Pitts L, Townsend J, Winestock DP. Upward transtentorial herniation: seven cases and a literature review. *Arch Neurol* 1979;36:618–623.
10. Del-Brutto OH, Noboa CA, Barinagarrementeria F. Lateral pontine hemorrhage: reappraisal of benign cases. *Stroke* 1987;18:954–956.
11. Del Brutto OH, Campos X. Validation of intracerebral hemorrhage scores for patients with pontine hemorrhage. *Neurology* 2004;62:515–516.
12. Dunne JW, Chakera T, Kermode S. Cerebellar haemorrhage—diagnosis and treatment: a study of 75 consecutive cases. *Q J Med* 1987;64:739–754.
13. Dziewas R, Kremer M, Ludemann P, et al. The prognostic impact of clinical and CT parameters in patients with pontine hemorrhage. *Cerebrovasc Dis* 2003;16:224–229.
14. Ferbert A, Buchner H, Bruckmann H. Brainstem auditory evoked potentials and somatosensory evoked potentials in pontine hemorrhage: correlations with clinical and CT findings. *Brain* 1990;113 (Pt 1):49–63.
15. Ferroli P, Sinisi M, Franzini A, et al. Brainstem cavernomas: long-term results of microsurgical resection in 52 patients. *Neurosurgery* 2005;56:1203–1212.
16. Firsching R, Huber M, Frowein RA. Cerebellar haemorrhage: management and prognosis. *Neurosurg Rev* 1991;14:191–194.
17. Freeman RE, Onofrio BM, Okazaki H, Dinapoli RP. Spontaneous intracerebellar hemorrhage: diagnosis and surgical treatment. *Neurology* 1973;23:84–90.

18. Goto N, Kaneko M, Hosaka Y, Koga H. Primary pontine hemorrhage: clinicopathological correlations. *Stroke* 1980;11:84–90.
19. Gross BA, Batjer HH, Awad IA, Bendok BR. Brainstem cavernous malformations. *Neurosurgery* 2009;64:E805–818.
20. Han J, Lee HK, Cho TG, et al. Management and outcome of spontaneous cerebellar hemorrhage. *J Cerebrovasc Endovasc Neurosurg* 2015;17:185–193.
21. Iwasaki Y, Kinoshita M. Lateral pontine hemorrhage: atypical clinical manifestations and good outcome. *Comput Med Imaging Graph* 1988;12:371–373.
22. Jang JH, Song YG, Kim YZ. Predictors of 30-day mortality and 90-day functional recovery after primary pontine hemorrhage. *J Korean Med Sci* 2011;26:100–107.
23. Kirollos RW, Tyagi AK, Ross SA, van Hille PT, Marks PV. Management of spontaneous cerebellar hematomas: a prospective treatment protocol. *Neurosurgery* 2001;49:1378–1386.
24. Kobayashi S, Sato A, Kageyama Y, et al. Treatment of hypertensive cerebellar hemorrhage: surgical or conservative management? *Neurosurgery* 1994;34:246–250.
25. Kondziolka D, Lunsford LD, Flickinger JC, Kestle JR. Reduction of hemorrhage risk after stereotactic radiosurgery for cavernous malformations. *J Neurosurg* 1995;83:825–831.
26. Konovalov AN, Spallone A, Makhmudov UB, Kukhlajeva JA, Ozerova VI. Surgical management of hematomas of the brain stem. *J Neurosurg* 1990;73:181–186.
27. Kushner MJ, Bressman SB. The clinical manifestations of pontine hemorrhage. *Neurology* 1985;35:637–643.
28. Lancman M, Norscini J, Mesropian H, et al. Tegmental pontine hemorrhages: clinical features and prognostic factors. *Can J Neurol Sci* 1992;19:236–238.
29. Lanzino G, Spetzler RE. *Cavernous Malformations of the Brain and Spinal Cord.* New York: Thieme; 2007.
30. Link MJ, Bartleson JD, Forbes G, Meyer FB. Spontaneous midbrain hemorrhage: report of seven new cases. *Surg Neurol* 1993;39:58–65.
31. Meguro T.Kuwahara K,Tomita Y et al.Primary pontine hemorrhage in the acute stage: clinical features and a proposed new simple scoring system. *J Stroke Cerebrovasc Dis* 2015;24:860–865.
32. Mathew P, Teasdale G, Bannan A, Oluoch-Olunya D. Neurosurgical management of cerebellar haematoma and infarct. *J Neurol Neurosurg Psychiatry* 1995;59:287–292.
33. Melamed N, Satya-Murti S. Cerebellar hemorrhage: a review and reappraisal of benign cases. *Arch Neurol* 1984;41:425–428.
34. Mezzadri JJ, Otero JM, Ottino CA. Management of 50 spontaneous cerebellar haemorrhages: importance of obstructive hydrocephalus. *Acta Neurochir (Wien)* 1993;122:39–44.
35. Murata Y, Yamaguchi S, Kajikawa H, et al. Relationship between the clinical manifestations, computed tomographic findings and the outcome in 80 patients with primary pontine hemorrhage. *J Neurol Sci* 1999;167:107–111.
36. Nakajima K. Clinicopathological study of pontine hemorrhage. *Stroke* 1983;14:485–493.
37. Ogata J, Imakita M, Yutani C, Miyamoto S, Kikuchi H. Primary brainstem death: a clinicopathological study. *J Neurol Neurosurg Psychiatry* 1988;51:646–650.
38. Osborn AG, Heaston DK, Wing SD. Diagnosis of ascending transtentorial herniation by cranial computed tomography. *AJR Am J Roentgenol* 1978;130:755–760.
39. Ott KH, Kase CS, Ojemann RG, Mohr JP. Cerebellar hemorrhage: diagnosis and treatment: a review of 56 cases. *Arch Neurol* 1974;31:160–167.
40. Pandey P, Westbroek EM, Gooderham PA, Steinberg GK. Cavernous malformation of brainstem, thalamus, and basal ganglia: a series of 176 patients. *Neurosurgery* 2013;72:573–589.
41. Porter RW, Detwiler PW, Spetzler RF, et al. Cavernous malformations of the brainstem: experience with 100 patients. *J Neurosurg* 1999;90:50–58.
42. Rabinstein AA, Tisch SH, McClelland RL, Wijdicks EFM. Cause is the main predictor of outcome in patients with pontine hemorrhage. *Cerebrovasc Dis* 2004;17:66–71.
43. Rohde V, Berns E, Rohde I, Gilsbach JM, Ryang YM. Experiences in the management of brainstem hematomas. *Neurosurg Rev* 2007;30:219–223.
44. Salvati M, Cervoni L, Raco A, Delfini R. Spontaneous cerebellar hemorrhage: clinical remarks on 50 cases. *Surg Neurol* 2001;55:156–161.
45. Sand JJ, Biller J, Corbett JJ, Adams HP, Jr., Dunn V. Partial dorsal mesencephalic hemorrhages: report of three cases. *Neurology* 1986;36:529–533.
46. Satoh K, Satomi J, Nakajima N, Matsubara S, Nagahiro S. Cerebellar hemorrhage caused by dural arteriovenous fistula: a review of five cases. *J Neurosurg* 2001;94:422–426.
47. Shitamichi M, Nakamura J, Sasaki T, Suematsu K, Tokuda S. Computed tomography guided

stereotactic aspiration of pontine hemorrhages. *Stereotact Funct Neurosurg* 1990;54–55: 453–456.

48. Shuaib A. Benign brainstem hemorrhage. *Can J Neurol Sci* 1991;18:356–357.

49. St Louis EK, Wijdicks EFM, Li H. Predicting neurologic deterioration in patients with cerebellar hematomas. *Neurology* 1998;51:1364–1369.

50. St Louis EK, Wijdicks EFM, Li H, Atkinson JD. Predictors of poor outcome in patients with a spontaneous cerebellar hematoma. *Can J Neurol Sci* 2000;27:32–36.

51. Stein KP, Wanke I, Schlamann M, et al. Posterior fossa arterio-venous malformations: current multimodal treatment strategies and results. *Neurosurg Rev* 2014;37:619–628.

52. Taneda M, Hayakawa T, Mogami H. Primary cerebellar hemorrhage: quadrigeminal cistern obliteration on CT scans as a predictor of outcome. *J Neurosurg* 1987;67:545–552.

53. Teasell R, Foley N, Doherty T, Finestone H. Clinical characteristics of patients with brainstem strokes admitted to a rehabilitation unit. *Arch Phys Med Rehabil* 2002;83:1013–1016.

54. van der Hoop RG, Vermeulen M, van Gijn J. Cerebellar hemorrhage: diagnosis and treatment. *Surg Neurol* 1988;29:6–10.

55. van Loon J, Van Calenbergh F, Goffin J, Plets C. Controversies in the management of spontaneous cerebellar haemorrhage: a consecutive series of 49 cases and review of the literature. *Acta Neurochir (Wien)* 1993;122:187–193.

56. Wall M, Wray SH. The one-and-a-half syndrome—a unilateral disorder of the pontine tegmentum: a study of 20 cases and review of the literature. *Neurology* 1983;33:971–980.

57. Weisberg LA. Acute cerebellar hemorrhage and CT evidence of tight posterior fossa. *Neurology* 1986;36:858–860.

58. Weisberg LA. Primary pontine hemorrhage: clinical and computed tomographic correlations. *J Neurol Neurosurg Psychiatry* 1986;49:346–352.

59. Wessels T, Moller-Hartmann W, Noth J, Klotzsch C. CT findings and clinical features as markers for patient outcome in primary pontine hemorrhage. *AJNR Am J Neuroradiol* 2004;25:257–260.

60. Wijdicks EFM. Recurrent cerebellar hematomas. *Stroke* 1995;26:2198.

61. Wijdicks EFM, St Louis E. Clinical profiles predictive of outcome in pontine hemorrhage. *Neurology* 1997;49:1342–1346.

62. Wijdicks EFM, St Louis EK, Atkinson JD, Li H. Clinician's biases toward surgery in cerebellar hematomas: an analysis of decision-making in 94 patients. *Cerebrovasc Dis* 2000;10:93–96.

63. Witsch J, Neugebauer H, Zweckberger K, Juttler E. Primary cerebellar hemorrhage: complications, treatment and outcome. *Clin Neurol Neurosurg* 2013;115:863–869.

64. Yanaka K, Meguro K, Fujita K, Narushima K, Nose T. Immediate surgery reduces mortality in deeply comatose patients with spontaneous cerebellar hemorrhage. *Neurol Med Chir (Tokyo)* 2000;40:295–299.

65. Yanaka K, Meguro K, Fujita K, Narushima K, Nose T. Postoperative brainstem high intensity is correlated with poor outcomes for patients with spontaneous cerebellar hemorrhage. *Neurosurgery* 1999;45:1323–1327.

66. Zimmerman RS, Spetzler RF, Lee KS, Zabramski JM, Hargraves RW. Cavernous malformations of the brain stem. *J Neurosurg* 1991;75:32–39.

29

Major Hemispheric Ischemic Stroke Syndromes

Ischemic stroke embodies a diverse group of patients with different modes of presentation, progression, and outcome.[28] The diagnostic approach to these disorders is by the arterial system. In terms of severity, a large hemispheric stroke due to occlusion of the main arterial tributary is generally recognized as one of the major neurologic critical illnesses. Most seriously, the arterial occlusion may involve the carotid artery, stem, or one of the larger branches of the middle cerebral artery (MCA).

Although many neurologists are appreciably complacent about therapeutic interventions in patients with a massive stroke in whom expectations for functional recovery seem low, aggressive management in selected, often young, patients may result in a very reasonable outcome.[118] This may include use of thrombolytic agents in patients with hypoperfused but viable tissue. In others, decompressive craniectomy or induction of moderate hypothermia in massive cerebral swelling may be considered under appropriate circumstances.

This chapter discusses the most commonly encountered clinical presentations and the difficulties in management of major hemispheric ischemic stroke syndromes. Occlusion of the basilar artery is discussed in Chapter 30. Less frequently encountered disorders are mentioned when different therapies are recommended. Admission to the neurosciences intensive care unit (NICU) is largely determined by the proclivity for clinical deterioration or coexisting cardiopulmonary instability.

CLINICAL RECOGNITION

Recognition of clinical patterns of large artery occlusions is important because it allows an assessment of the severity of involvement and may predict the chance of further deterioration. Many of these clinical findings are captured by the National Institute of Health Stroke Scale (NIHSS,

Part XIII, Formulas and Scales),[13] and this scale has been widely used as a benchmark to delineate severity and to initiate thrombolysis or other interventional therapies.[23,56]

Middle Cerebral Artery Occlusion

Cerebral infarction often is catastrophic when caused by an occlusion of the MCA. Its arterial system can be occluded at the M1 segment (proximal MCA), proximal to the lateral lenticulostriatal arteries, and at the M2 segment. The M2 segment is further divided by the superior and inferior trunks, which supply the perisylvian area of the frontal and temporal lobes, respectively. The M2 MCA segment then is divided into the M3, or operculum, segment and the M4, or cortical, branches.

The most serious type of MCA occlusion is at M1 or the stem, with a thrombus possibly extending into the carotid artery. Occlusion at the origin of the MCA may lead to preferential direction of the gaze and head toward the side of the involved hemisphere.[128] Other major findings are hemianopsia, and flaccid hemiplegia of the arm, with some sparing of movement in the leg. Hemisensory loss with no grimacing or withdrawal to pinprick is typical. The patient has eyes open and may look about, but is unable to follow any command or does so in an inappropriate manner. There is an inability to move the lips and tongue and to blow out the cheeks. Speech may be characterized by repetitive stopping and starting and fumbling words. Other patients are mute. Occlusion of the superior trunk of the left MCA produces exactly the same characteristics and therefore cannot be differentiated clinically. However, occlusion of the inferior trunk of the left MCA produces a Wernicke-type aphasia and a superior homonymous quadrantanopsia ("pie in the sky").

An infarct may preferentially involve the perforating arteries of the MCA (lenticulostriate arteries) when the collateral supply from the anterior circulation and posterior cerebral artery (PCA) is sufficient to protect the remainder of the hemisphere from infarction. A comma-shaped infarct, or so-called *striatocapsular infarct*, occurs with hemiplegia equally severe in the arm and leg and with fairly mild sensory symptoms.

As mentioned, involvement of the upper division of the MCA produces aphasia when the infarction is located in the dominant hemisphere and results in unilateral neglect when it is located in the nondominant hemisphere.[2,28] Patients with a dominant MCA territory stroke usually have profound aphasia and may vocalize only single, distorted words. Comprehension is significantly impaired. Improvement to a less profound aphasia with some recovery of comprehension and grammatical order is possible in the first week.

In a nondominant large hemispheric stroke, spatial neglect is the major clinical feature. Denial of hemiplegia (anosognosia), flat affect, speech without much modulation in intonation (aprosody), and motor impersistence may be observed. Failure of the patient to recognize the paralyzed left body parts may result in a long delay before the stroke is discovered. Occasionally, patients fall and are not able to stand up from the floor. In others, a compartment syndrome with rhabdomyolysis from prolonged muscle compression may appear. Bilateral ptosis is typical in large nondominant hemispheric infarcts. This is an underrecognized sign, mistaken for drowsiness.[2] We and others have noted bilateral complete ptosis as the first sign of swelling preceding pupillary dilation in some patients (Figure 29.1). In others, ptosis improved with resolving edema on computed tomography (CT) scan.

Patients may appear indifferent and inert from frontal lobe or caudate nucleus involvement. Lack of concern (anosodiaphoria) is more common in nondominant lesions. However, the level of consciousness is normal unless swelling supervenes. Elderly patients can become less alert from dehydration alone, which can easily occur if they are unable to signal thirst. Other triggers for dehydration—a fairly constant observation during the initial encounter—are diuretics and poor oral fluid intake. Seizures are infrequent in patients with a large ischemic stroke; if they occur, they are usually observed within days of presentation and are focal. Complex partial seizures and progression of a single generalized tonic-clonic seizure to status epilepticus are not common. Brief loss of consciousness is very unusual but may implicate a cardiac source for stroke (e.g., transient atrial fibrillation with marked hypotension). Delirium or agitated confusion can decrease the level of consciousness and seems more frequent in patients with right hemispheric lesions. However, a patient with newly developing agitation soon after admission may, in fact, have a drug- or alcohol-withdrawal syndrome.

Forced eye deviation indicates involvement of a large territory, is more frequent in patients with right-sided infarcts of the brain, and possibly is also related to neglect of the left side of the body. However, the volume of infarcted tissue is larger in patients with a conjugate eye deviation associated with an infarct in the left hemisphere.[136] Homonymous hemianopia is invariably present, and an asymmetrical blink response is usually elicited by a rapidly approaching hand. Pupils are usually equal in size. New pupillary asymmetry and a blunted pupillary light response, when observed together with drowsiness, must be considered important early signs of brain swelling. Unilateral miosis from Horner's syndrome due to damage to the sympathetic terminals in the carotid

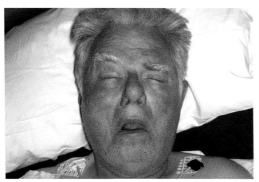 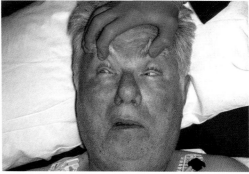

FIGURE 29.1: Patient with cerebral ptosis (apraxia of eyelid opening) associated with large hemispheric infarct. Note asymmetric eyelid closure, facial asymmetry, and eye deviation.

sheath may be evident and could indicate an acute carotid occlusion or dissection. Additional involvement of lower cranial nerves (IX, X, XII) in patients with an acute ischemic stroke should also point to possible carotid dissection.[135] Carotid dissection is almost certain when Horner's syndrome and tongue paresis with deviation to the involved side on protrusion are found. Displacement of the parapharyngeal space close to the internal carotid artery may compress these cranial nerves.

Asymmetrical facial grimacing spontaneously or to pain can involve all facial muscles and is responsible for a muted corneal reflex. The gag reflex is diminished. The tongue can be markedly involved as well and may rest virtually frozen in the mouth. This could place these patients at considerable risk of aspiration.

Hemiplegia of the upper limb involves complete hypotonic paralysis with some preservation of shoulder shrug. The lower limb is relatively preserved but usually is equally affected with large territorial infarction and, when ischemia involves the perforating arteries, to the internal capsule.

In many patients, the defect may further evolve or fluctuate and, in some, surprisingly, may disappear. Decrease in deficit may occur in patients with large territorial MCA occlusions ("spectacular shrinking deficit").[81] This is explained by fragmentation of the obstructing clot but could also be collateral artery compensation. In approximately one in 10 patients, deterioration occurs after initial dramatic improvement and is attributed to reocclusion or persistence of clot with failing collateral supply.[19,39]

Anterior Cerebral Artery Occlusion

Most anterior cerebral artery (ACA) distribution infarctions are caused by a cardioembolic source or by artery-to-artery embolization from internal carotid artery stenosis with a diameter reduction of more than 70%.[8] The clinical symptoms of acute ACA occlusion are complex and may not be obvious. Usually, occlusion involves severe weakness of the leg in combination with other frontal lobe symptoms, such as abulia and incontinence. Transcortical motor and sensory aphasia, characterized by lack of spontaneous speech and comprehension but the ability to repeat phrases, has been reported in an infarction involving the ACA territory. Apraxia of the left arm with normal use of the right arm is typical, and this dissociation can be explained by corpus callosum infarction interrupting connecting fibers and can occur irrespective of occlusion of the right or left ACA.

The disorder is revealed when patients can name objects placed in the right hand but are unable to recognize or name objects in the left hand.

An important artery that may become occluded is the recurrent artery of Heubner. Infarction of this territory (the head of caudate nucleus and the anterior portion of the lentiform nucleus and internal capsule) produces weakness in the contralateral arm and side of the face, with dysarthria and hemichorea. With bilateral occlusions, a minimally conscious state may appear.

Carotid Artery Occlusion

Acute carotid occlusion is usually due to gradual atherosclerotic narrowing, invading neck tumor, or direct trauma. Acutely occluded, it may result in a large territorial infarct with often massive swelling of both MCA and ACA territories. The occluded thrombus usually starts at the bifurcation and propagates to the skull base.[58,134] Organization of the thrombus is rapid, and restoration of flow is rare. A sudden carotid occlusion may be asymptomatic, with limited signs, or may result in a devastating stroke. Some patients may have sufficient collaterals that may limit the territory of infarction to the MCA only.

Arterial dissection leading to acute carotid occlusion or near occlusion is a more common mechanism in younger patients. A tear in the intima permits blood to dissect its way more distally into the muscular arterial wall and to create a double lumen into the artery. It occurs most commonly in the supraclinoid segment of the internal carotid artery. The clot may dissect under the intima (subintimal) or throughout the media (subadventitial), causing distention of the vessel wall inward (producing occlusion) or outward (creating a pseudoaneurysm). A false luminal channel can be created when intramural hemorrhage exits at a more distal site, but this is uncommon.

Dissection of the internal carotid artery is mostly spontaneous and may represent 10%–25% of ischemic strokes in adults aged 35–50.[73,124] The dissection can be the result of a direct force to the artery, possibly triggered by strenuous activity, head turning, or chiropractic maneuvers, but also by seemingly trivial insults, such as a brief Valsalva maneuver. There is a seasonal predilection for the fall.[116] An increased incidence of upper respiratory infection during this period may suggest an inflammatory cause or insults from repeated coughing. Dissections have been associated with congenital abnormalities of the wall of the artery, such as cystic medial necrosis, fibromuscular dysplasia, Marfan syndrome, Ehlers-Danlos syndrome type IV, α_1-anti-trypsin deficiency, autosomal-dominant polycystic kidney disease, and familial lentiginosis.[49,112,114,117] In a prospective study of dissections at Mayo Clinic, joint and skin laxity and facial stigmata of an underlying vasculopathy were found but could not be characterized as typical arteriopathy.[117]

Headache or neck pain is present in approximately 60% of patients. Headache may precede an ischemic stroke by several days and may not be clearly remembered or vocalized by the patient.[7] The character of the headache is dull and seldom throbbing. Retro-orbital headache of sudden onset should point to carotid artery dissection. Carotid artery dissection might be associated with a new presentation of Horner's syndrome, pulsatile tinnitus, and lower cranial nerve involvement, particularly the twelfth cranial nerve, causing weakness of the tongue. Other lower cranial nerves can become compressed in the cervical parapharyngeal space. The ninth to twelfth cranial nerves are in close proximity to the internal carotid artery and, alone or in combination, can become involved, producing dysarthria, dysphasia, dysphonia, and dysgeusia (metallic or bad taste).[135] Less common are a decreased sensation of the frontal division of the trigeminal nerve, oculomotor palsy, and abducens palsy.[62,83,84,115]

The interval between dissection and cerebral infarction varies widely, from minutes to 1 month, but is less than a week in most patients. Low-flow ("misery") infarction involving watershed areas is an uncommon mechanism.

Multiple Arterial Involvement

Acute multiple hemispheric infarctions may result in admission to the NICU, often because abnormal consciousness may lead to difficulty to protect the airway. Acute multiple territorial infarctions may also indicate a newly developing major medical illness, and this may include inflammatory or acute hematologic disorders. Both causes are discussed in more detail later.

Granulomatous vasculitis or isolated angiitis of the central nervous system (CNS) is an emergency and may rapidly lead to permanent devastating ischemic strokes or, less commonly, to intracranial hematomas or subarachnoid hemorrhage.[67,107,108] Progressive or recurrent neurologic symptoms are common, but because of the infrequent occurrence of this disorder, they may not be recognized as typical features of CNS vasculitis until the destruction is permanent. Delay in diagnosis has been established as an unfortunate fact.

Two-thirds of patients present with severe, persistent headache, overriding any other symptom. Profound aphasia, apraxia, or hemiparesis may occur, but acute confusion and, most typically, emotional lability, with crying or bizarre hysterical or childish behavior, are more common. Vasculitis may initially present as posterior reversible encephalopathy syndrome (PRES) on magnetic resonance imaging (MRI) only to worsen considerably, showing multiple territorial involvements.[156] Some patients become dull and abulic, particularly with preferential involvement of the anterior cerebral circulation. Multifocal neurologic findings can be expected because the pattern involves scattered inflammation of the medium- and small-sized arteries.

Central nervous system vasculitis may be secondary to a systemic illness or drug abuse. Skin lesions, joint swelling, or additional evidence of mononeuritis multiplex or progressive polyneuropathy may point to a connective tissue disorder or systemic vasculitis. The use of an amphetamine often can be inferred only from a careful history of drug use, which is not volunteered by most patients.

Infectious causes can produce CNS vasculitis, but other localizations should be evident (e.g., retina for cytomegalovirus, painful crusty skin lesions for herpes zoster, pulmonary manifestations associated with *Histoplasma* or *Coccidioides immitis*, or systemic manifestations of human immunodeficiency virus infection). Finally, lymphoproliferative disorders (Hodgkin's lymphoma) may be associated with vasculitis.

Moore's criteria for the diagnosis of isolated angiitis of the CNS are (1) recent severe onset of headaches, confusion, or multifocal neurologic deficits that are recurrent or progressive; (2) typical angiographic findings; (3) exclusion of systemic disease or infection; and (4) leptomeningeal and parenchymal biopsy findings that confirm vascular inflammation and exclude infection, neoplasia, and noninflammatory vascular disease.

Another major cause for multiple cerebral infarcts is hematologic disorders. Hematologic disorders may become complicated by ischemic strokes, and the attending neurologist has to contend with two simultaneous medical problems. Sickle-cell syndromes are rather prevalent, in most instances are caused by a single amino acid substitution in the globin β chains (valine instead of glutamic acid). Sickle-cell disease or sickle-cell trait (heterozygotic state) is more prevalent in African American patients, often manifested after a hypoxemic trigger, cold, or excessive alcohol consumption. Sickled masses of red blood cells occlude the arterial and venous systems, but other mechanisms, such as vasculopathy or fat embolization from infarcted bone marrow, may be operative. Stroke as a first presentation of sickle-cell disease has rarely been documented, but earlier ischemic strokes, predominantly those localized in the subcortical white matter, may be silent. One should inquire about previous episodes of *Streptococcus pneumoniae* infections, osteomyelitis by *Salmonella* species, painless hematuria, painful priapism, retinal–vitreous hemorrhage, or crises resulting in chest and abdominal pain.[44]

Polycythemia vera, a more complex disorder of increased erythrocytes and platelets, causes increased viscosity. It should be considered in patients with generalized pruritus, splenomegaly, headaches, and paresthesias. With a prevalence of five cases per 1 million persons, it is very uncommon.

Polycythemia may occur as a consequence of hypoxemia with cyanotic heart disease or obstructive pulmonary disease, but its association with ischemic stroke is less evident, because precise understanding of the mechanism is lacking.

Thrombotic thrombocytopenic purpura should be considered in multiple strokes of undetermined cause when patients present with a documented gradual decrease in platelet count. Middle-aged women are predominantly affected. Characteristic additional clinical signs are hematuria, myalgia, bloody diarrhea, fever, and, in some patients, rapidly developing renal failure. These symptoms, caused by platelet microthrombi, may not appear in 25% of cases, and ischemic stroke may be the defining illness. Seizures are comparatively frequent, and nonconvulsive status epilepticus may be a presenting feature. Headache, acute confusional episodes, and hemiparesis may progress to coma if not aggressively treated with plasma exchange.

Thrombocytosis may occur in many underlying disorders, often chronic myeloid leukemia and myelofibrosis, or as a myeloproliferative disorder itself. Cerebrovascular manifestations, although recognized as a complication of myeloproliferative disorders, are not well characterized.

Another increasingly recognized syndrome is associated with antiphospholipid antibodies, and it is a common manifestation in younger patients.[17,71] Both anticardiolipin antibodies and lupus anticoagulants can be demonstrated, but they may not be linked to each other. Evidence of arterial occlusions (ocular, peripheral artery, pulmonary, or mesenteric artery) or venous

occlusions (deep vein thrombosis or jugular venous thrombosis), miscarriages, and prior unexplained pulmonary hypertension are clues to the diagnosis. In 20% of patients, ischemic stroke is part of this syndrome. Inappropriate treatment results in a high rate of recurrence of cerebral infarction. Clinical features may include cardiac bruit (from associated mitral valve lesions or, possibly, Libman-Sacks endocarditis) and livedo reticularis. Blotchy hands and feet should point to the diagnosis. Multiorgan failure may be a presenting feature.

NEUROIMAGING AND LABORATORY TESTS

The vascular territories should be familiar when one views CT scans and are depicted in Figure 29.2. The signs of early ischemia can be recognized on CT scan of the brain even if no obvious hypodensity is present. The CT scan should be carefully scrutinized for early signs of cerebral infarction, such as sulci effacement and an obscured outline of the lentiform nucleus or decrease in tissue attenuation.[147–150] The subtle differences between gray and white matter are more easily detected when several CT window settings are used. Obscuration of the lentiform nucleus is the most frequent earliest sign and may appear within the first hour of infarction[139] (Figure 29.3). In a small study of 25 patients, it appeared in one of two patients within an hour of the ictus, in seven of eight patients in the second hour, in all three patients in the third hour, in seven of eight patients in the fourth hour, and in all four patients scanned thereafter. Early abnormalities on the CT scan also involve the parenchyma, with loss of the precise delineation between gray and white matter and, particularly, loss of the insular ribbon. The insular segment of the MCA supplies the insular ribbon, and with complete occlusion of the MCA, the insular region becomes a watershed arterial zone. In addition, the insular cortex is the region most distant from the collateral flow from the ACA and PCA.

In some patients, the extent of the ischemic territory is noted by eye deviation on CT (Figure 29.4a). A hyperdense MCA sign (Figure 29.4b) actually indicates the clot in the MCA and has been recognized as a prognostic feature.[63,137,138] In our studies, a hyperdense MCA, together with early swelling (sulci effacement), predicted deterioration from further brain swelling.[75] In other reports, hemorrhagic transformation was deemed more likely in patients who had a hyperdense MCA sign.[140] When the clot fragments

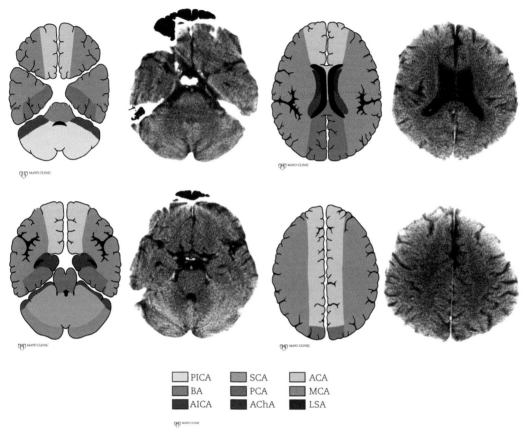

FIGURE 29.2: Vascular territories of the brain (computed tomographic scans and corresponding arterial territories).
ACA, anterior cerebral artery; AChA, anterior choroidal artery; AICA, anterior inferior cerebellar artery; BA, basilar artery; LSA, lenticulostriate artery; MCA, middle cerebral artery; PCA, posterior cerebral artery; PICA, posterior inferior cerebellar artery; SCA, superior cerebellar artery.

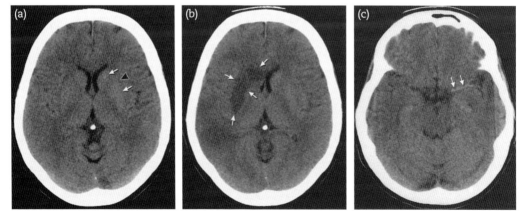

FIGURE 29.3. (a) Normal definition of the caudate nucleus, lentiform nucleus (*arrows*), and insular ribbon (*arrowhead*) in the left hemisphere has disappeared in the right hemisphere. (b) One day later, a computed tomography (CT) scan shows a hypodensity in that area (c) Hyperdense middle cerebral artery sign (*arrows*).

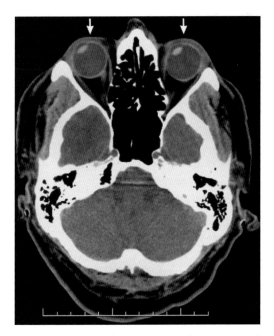

FIGURE 29.4. Eye deviation (*arrows*) on computed tomographic (CT) exam in MCA stem occlusion.

and breaks up, the hyperdense MCA sign disappears, often spontaneously or, at times, soon after intravenous administration of tissue plasminogen activator (tPA).

Hypodensity may involve the entire MCA territory (Figure 29.5a), but is usually evident days after onset. Hypodensity on CT scans may involve only the M2 territory (Figure 29.5b) or the lenticulostriate arteries (Figure 29.5c). A hypodensity can be seen within hours after MCA trunk occlusion. Transferred patients seen several hours after onset who had CT scanning during previous

hospitalization at the time of the ictus should have a repeat CT scan, which may show a developing hypodensity.

Computed tomography scanning remains the most important initial study and, in most institutions without immediate 24-hour MRI services, is not likely to be replaced soon by more sensitive tests for the diagnosis of ischemic stroke.[86] Until then, it is therefore of utmost importance that physicians treating ischemic stroke be familiar with the early signs on high-definition CT scans.

The CT scan in patients with acute MCA territory infarct can be further categorized by determining the size of the infarct, degree of swelling, and hemorrhagic conversion.[105] An early sizable hypodensity on CT scan predicts the further development of cerebral edema.[106] Different intervals of ictus to CT scan may define different CT predictors for swelling. The likelihood of progressive cerebral edema is 85% if a CT scan performed within 5 hours after onset shows a hypodensity that involves more than 50% of the MCA territory. The probability of deterioration is more than 70% when a CT scan done within 24 hours shows at least a combination of hyperdense MCA sign and sulcal effacement. In addition, a significantly higher incidence of hemorrhagic conversion (approximately 70%) is expected in patients with early hypodensity.[11]

Follow-up CT scanning within 3 days shows the characteristic triangular shape of the hypodensity, and mass effect may become more apparent with ventricular compression. Patients with a large infarct in the MCA territory may have some scattered petechial hemorrhages, indicating hemorrhagic conversion. The clinical significance

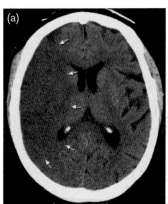 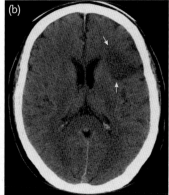 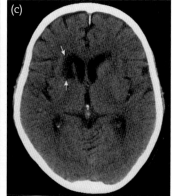

FIGURE 29.5: Computed tomographic scans (arrows point at hypodensities). (a) Middle cerebral artery stem occlusion. (b) Superior division occlusion. (c) Striatocapsular infarct.

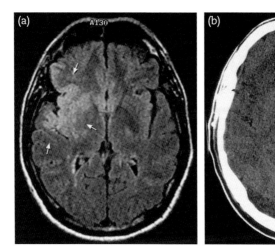

FIGURE 29.6: FLAIR. Fluid-attenuated inversion recovery (FLAIR) image of evolving right middle cerebral artery stroke (a) compared with virtually normal computed tomographic scan (b).

of hemorrhagic infarction is uncertain, and MRI studies have found that the phenomenon is more common and often underrecognized by CT scans.

Computed tomography angiography is often used initially to immediately provide the site of arterial occlusion and an estimate of the capacity of the collaterals.[127]

Cerebral infarction is better visualized on MRI than on CT scanning. Additional findings on MRI include lack of normal flow voids, representing the occluded vessel. Arterial enhancement of the T1-weighted images in the ischemic zone after administration of gadolinium contrast material is caused by slow flow in an otherwise high-flow arterial system distal to the obstructing lesion. This finding is seen in approximately 50% of patients with acute cortical infarcts.

Magnetic resonance imaging techniques using diffusion-weighted imaging (DWI) or fluid-attenuated inversion recovery (FLAIR) (Figure 29.6) are extremely sensitive for early infarction. Diffusion-weighted imaging may be very useful in determining the extent of ischemic injury.[3,129,143] In DWI, areas of hyperintensity (bright areas) indicate decreased movement of water, and reduction in the apparent diffusion coefficient of water is a marker of tissue loss. Diffusion-weighted imaging is superior within 6 hours of presentation when compared with CT or MRI alone. Several studies have shown that early infarction underlies the high signal intensity. It most likely reflects the failure of water movement in tissue in this zone of infarction. When these areas of restricted diffusion are quantified using the apparent diffusion coefficient, they are seen as a hypodense area (Figure 29.7). The size of the lesion with this abnormality

predicts future outcome; however, the critical size for possible improvement is not known, and DWI cannot distinguish which lesions may be reversible after specific treatment (particularly thrombolytic therapy). Practical use of DWI in acute situations remains undefined, and most currently published studies on these MR sequences represent a fraction of the admitted patients with acute stroke. Fluid-attenuated inversion recovery sequences are also superior to routine MR sequences, and one recent study comparing multimodality MR techniques found a sensitivity of 98% for DWI and 91% for FLAIR for detecting ischemic brain lesions within hours of the ictus.

A recent study compared FLAIR with DWI in the first 3 hours of stroke. A negative FLAIR study and positive DWI was commonly seen in patients with stroke onset of 3 hours or less. This FLAIR–DWI discrepancy had a 90% specificity and positive predictive value for early stroke recognition, and there was little change in predictive power with extension to the 4.5-hour window. This finding may have some value in determining the indication of thrombolytics in patients with uncertain stroke onset.[120]

Perfusion CT and other modalities have rapidly become established in acute stroke care.[27] Selection on the basis of penumbra or established infarction is commonly used in major institutions but this modality may not be predictive of outcome. We and others do not proceed with thrombolysis or endovascular treatment when a large territorial mismatch is found ("purple and black won't come back") and most certainly when it involves the entire middle cerebral artery (Figure 29.7).[15,37,74,132]

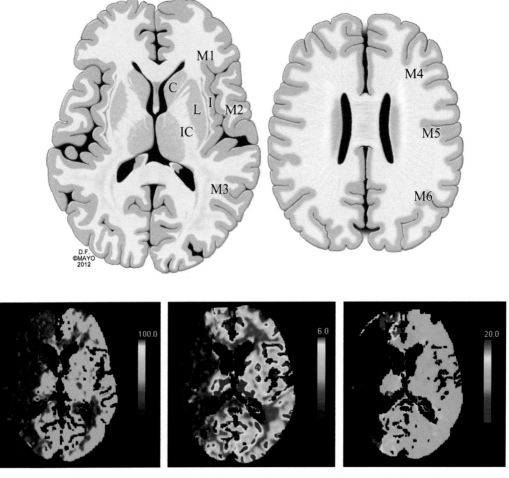

FIGURE 29.7: CT scan showing ASPECTS (0–10) one point subtracted for ischemic change in each region. Reconsideration thrombolytic or endovascular treatment with ASPECT of 6 or less. Perfusion CT scans in acute MCA stroke. From left to right note match between the cerebral blood flow, cerebral blood volume and time to peak.

With MRI, it seems from studies that a mismatch between DWI and PWI (hypoperfusion lesion more than diffusion lesion) may be present in a considerable proportion of patients and could suggest the presence of a reversible penumbra after thrombolysis.[94,145,146] These evolving techniques could be used to assess patients who may be eligible outside the accepted clinical windows, assuming that DWI abnormalities would indicate cell injury.[129]

Magnetic resonance imaging may show small, scattered infarcts within the MCA territory, a sign of early recanalization. The clinical correlate frequently is rapid improvement, often to only a fraction of the initial deficit (Figure 29.8).

Magnetic resonance angiography (MRA) is helpful in more precisely documenting not only the site of obstruction but also its configuration. When carotid dissection is considered, MRA can be helpful. If carotid dissection has resulted in an occlusion, typical flame-like tapering is seen (Figure 29.9). Ultrasound may detect carotid dissection, but the sensitivity for detection of dissection in the carotid system by MRI is approximately 80%.[22] Magnetic resonance angiography is highly sensitive and specific in the diagnosis of internal carotid artery dissection.[90] Magnetic resonance imaging also may show the typical dense "crescent" or "double-lumen" sign, which reflects an intramural thrombus, often found at lower slices (Figure 29.9).

Cerebral angiography may even better define arterial dissection. The most typical angiographic finding is relatively smooth, irregularly tapered luminal narrowing, often producing a very high stenosis (string sign) (Figure 29.10). Dissections may occur in both carotid arteries, in the carotid and vertebral arteries, or in all four arteries at the

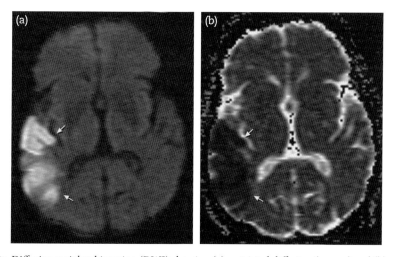

FIGURE 29.8: Diffusion-weighted imaging (DWI) showing (a) restricted diffusion (*arrows*) and (b) reduced ADC (*arrows*).

ADC, apparent diffusion coefficient.

same time. Fibromuscular dysplasia may be an additional finding.[49] A pseudoaneurysm might be found later, with typical fusiform appearance. The process of dissection and possible outcomes are shown in Figure 29.10.

The sensitivity of cerebral angiography in CNS vasculitis is high, approximately 95%–99%. However, a cerebral angiogram with negative findings has been described in biopsy-proven CNS vasculitis.[80] Suggestive findings are changed vessel caliber, with constriction, occlusion ("cutoffs"), irregularities, and dilatation showing a characteristic beading pattern (Figure 29.11). Alternative explanations for the angiographic findings include cerebral vasoconstriction syndrome (a mostly but not always benign angiopathy), advanced atherosclerosis (proximal carotid artery abnormalities or irregularities in the proximal vertebrobasilar system may be suggestive of atheromatous disease), and radiation-induced occlusive vasculopathy (abnormalities inside the radiation field). The inflammatory changes in the wall eventually lead to fibrosis and may lead to fixed angiographic narrowing.

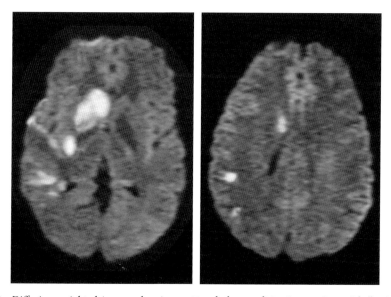

FIGURE 29.9: Diffusion-weighted images showing scattered abnormalities in a patient with "rapidly shrinking deficit."

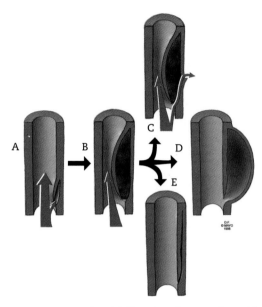

FIGURE 29.10: Arterial dissection. Process of arterial dissection (A) leading to near occlusion (B), rupture (C), pseudoaneurysm (D), or healing (E).

Other laboratory tests in acute ischemic stroke are potentially important in particular in hematologic disorders. Hemoglobin electrophoresis yields the diagnosis in sickle cell disease. Associated findings are increased leukocyte count, recent decrease in hemoglobin concentration (hemolytic anemia), and hyperbilirubinemia.

Polycythemia vera is diagnosed by increases in hematocrit and white cell count and, at later stages, bone marrow metaplasia. Laboratory criteria (minor criteria) are platelet level of less than 400,000/µL, leukocytes less than 12,000/µL, leukocyte alkaline phosphatase score greater than 100, and vitamin B_{12} level of more than 900 pg/mL.

Thrombotic thrombocytopenic purpura is considered when the following laboratory findings are present: fragmented red blood cells (schistocytes, or helmet cells), increased reticulocytes, unconjugated bilirubinemia with normal prothrombin time and partial thromboplastin time (PTT), and normal fibrin degradation products (differentiating it from disseminated intravascular coagulation and antiphospholipid antibody syndrome). Lactate dehydrogenase is greatly increased. Haptoglobin should be low or even unmeasurable.

Magnetic resonance imaging may show multiple infarcts in antiphospholipid syndrome (Figure 29.12). Anticardiolipin antibodies can be determined, but only a high titer of immunoglobulin G (IgG) is diagnostic (many laboratories define high titer as 20–100 IgG phospholipid units or more). IgM titers may vary significantly and can be increased by nonspecific stimuli, such as fever, infection, and pharmaceutical agents. Activated PTT is a good screening test and is prolonged in one-third of patients with antiphospholipid antibody syndrome.

FIRST STEPS IN MANAGEMENT

The management of acute ischemic stroke has been summarized in an American Heart Association guideline (Part XIV, Guidelines).

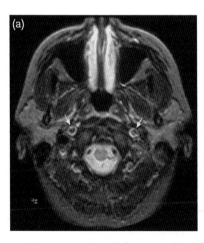
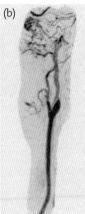
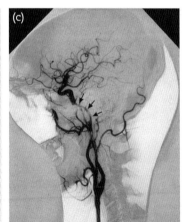

FIGURE 29.11: Carotid dissection. (a) MRI showing double lumen sign (*arrows*) in bilateral carotid dissection. (b) Magnetic resonance angiogram showing typical flame-like tapering in carotid dissection. (c) Distal carotid dissection (*arrows*). (d) Double lumen sign on cerebral angiogram.

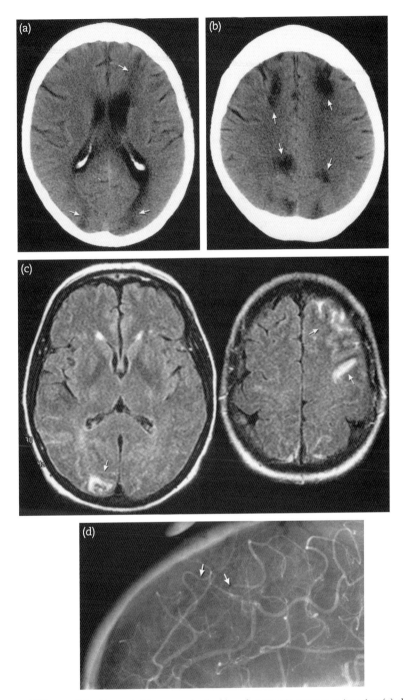

FIGURE 29.12: CNS vasculitis. Computed tomography (a, b) and magnetic resonance imaging (c) show multiple infarcts associated with central nervous system vasculitis. (d) Cerebral angiographic findings of segmental stenosis and beading are typical.

General Approach and Intervention

Patients seen within 4.5 hours after the ictus are potentially eligible to receive intravenous tPA.[1,4,13,40,42,72,79,85,110,151] Intravenous tPA (0.9 mg/ kg, 90 mg maximum, 10% bolus over 1 min and 90% in 1-hour infusion) is considered when less than 4.5 hours from ictus; intra-arterial tPA is considered when 4.5–6 hours from ictus (Figure 29.14).[125]

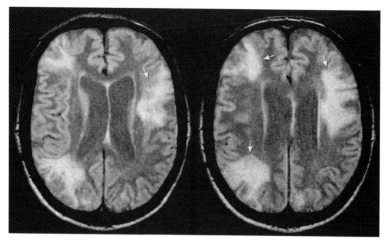

FIGURE 29.13: Magnetic resonance images showing multiple ischemic infarcts (*arrows*) in antiphospholipid antibody syndrome.

Intravenous thrombolysis may also be considered in patients with carotid artery dissection and a large distal embolus.[1,26] Initial concerns of extension of intramural hematoma or arterial rupture have not been substantiated in treated patients with a carotid dissection.

Endovascular intervention is now standard of care is in MCA stem occlusion, and can be very successful,[23,100] In referral hospitals it takes little time to set up a fully staffed neuroradiology suite.

There has been a rapid technical development and experience in the use of mechanical clot retrieval devices and stenting.[70,133] Initially referral centers began endovascular therapy with intra-arterial prourokinase since 1999.[33] The major first study, Mechanical Embolus Removal in Cerebral Ischemia (MERCI), albeit inconclusive, increased the use of these devices, and this option is available in selected patients in referral centers. This device originally consists of a corkscrew device, which has now been replaced with other devices.

A commonly used device is the Penumbra System (PS: Penumbra, Alameda, California). This device not only fragments thrombus but also aspirates. A prospective phase 1 single-arm trial employing this device resulted in an even higher recanalization rate than with the MERCI device.[9]

Use of self-expanding stents has been an alternative option when there was failure to open the artery. The success rate was variable, and clinical improvement was disappointing if flow restoration is achieved after a considerable time period has passed. These expanding stents

(e.g., Enterprise vascular reconstruction device-Codman Neurovascular/Cordis Corp.) are currently considered rescue interventions and off-label use.[82]

Endovascular treatment in proximal cerebral artery occlusions over the last few years is now stent assisted clot retrievers or clot extraction using aspiration after debulking of the thrombus. Clinical trials on endovascular therapy in large territorial stroke came in two waves. In 2013, three trials IMS III,[12] MR RESCUE,[59] and Synthesis[20] showed no benefit of endovascular treatment with embolectomy or intraarterial thrombolysis. These very disappointing (but questioned) results were followed by a second wave in 2015 with five randomized trials (Table 29.1) and significant benefit using stent-retriever devices, but also better selection of patients based on neuroimaging criteria.[34] The practice and the sequence of using thrombolytics and mechanical devices may not be uniform. Neurointerventionalists will try mechanical disruption, IA thrombolysis, an aspiration device, or stent retrievers. Early recanalization remains key whatever it takes.[78,126]

The management of carotid dissections is more complex.[30] Carotid dissections might resolve within 6 weeks, but reconstitution to a normal lumen after 6 months is uncommon. Many physicians favor anticoagulation with intravenous heparin, followed by warfarin (aiming at an international normalized ratio [INR] between 2 and 3) until MRA shows recanalization, but this is deferred if the dissection involves the intra-cranial portion because of the risk—albeit low—of causing subarachnoid hemorrhage. Antithrombotic

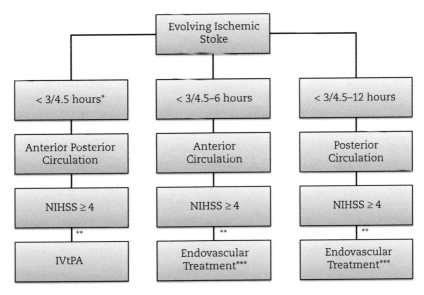

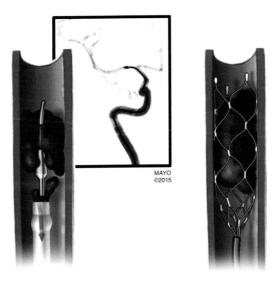

FIGURE 29.14: Decisions in acute evolving ischemic stroke. Endovascular treatment is now with stent retrievers or suction/aspiration devices.

therapy with aspirin 325 mg/day or clopidogrel 75 mg/day can be continued for another 3 months, but this period is arbitrary. A recent study found no difference in outcome between antiplatelet agents and warfarin.[35] Aneurysmal dilatation also may disappear spontaneously. However, it might become a source of recurrent transient ischemic attacks. If embolization occurs despite antiplatelet therapy, aneurysmal dilatation warrants surgical therapy or coil embolization of the artery with stenting of the occluded artery. Endovascular

treatment may be considered in patients with intracranial vertebral artery dissections, and possibly may be tailored to those with large or growing aneurysmal dilations, and certainly patients with subarachnoid hemorrhage.

Administration of corticosteroids in patients with presumed clinical CNS vasculitis is advised, and it should begin if no other causes are evident. (Brain biopsy within days in corticosteroid-treated patients should not mask inflammation and certainly not necrosis.) Methylprednisolone

TABLE 29.1. STENT RETRIEVAL STUDIES IN ACUTE STROKE

STUDY	MR CLEAN[6]	ESCAPE[38]	EXTEND-IA[16]	SWIFT PRIME[111]	REVAS CAT[52]
Size	500	316	70	196	206
Imaging selection	CTA	CTA	CTA/CTP	CTA	ASPECT > 7
	Any ASPECT	ASPECT 6–10 with good collaterals > 50% of MCA	(core < 70 ml)	ASPECT 6–10 No cervical ICA occlusion	
NIHSS* median	17/18	16/17	17/13	17/17*	17/17
Onset to puncture (median, min)	260	185	210	224	269
Onset to reperfusion (median, min)		241	248	250	355
% M1 occlusion	66.1 vs. 62	68.1 vs. 71.4	57 vs. 51	67 vs. 77	65 vs. 64
TICI 2b-3	58.7	72.4	86	88	65.7
% mRS -0–2 at 90 days	32.6 vs. 19.1	53 vs. 29.3	71 vs. 40	60.2 vs. 35.5	43.7 vs. 28.2
sICH*	6 vs. 5.2	3.6 vs. 2.7	0 vs. 6	1 vs. 3	2 vs. 2

* Treated vs. control
S = symptomatic.
Modified from Brinjikji W, Rabinstein AA, Cloft HJ et al. Radiology. 2015;276:8–11.

1 g IV per day for 3 days and cyclophosphamide 15 mg/kg IV (max 1 gram) using slow infusion should be started with active disease, and there is a reasonable consensus among experts that only such an aggressive treatment can reverse CNS vasculitis. It is followed by corticosteroids 1.5 mg/kg/day and cyclophosphamide 2 mg/kg/day orally. Corticosteroid administration can be tapered to a lower dose after 4 weeks, but cyclophosphamide, which has very low side effects with this dose, should be given for 1 year. The patient should be familiar with a 20% risk of infertility from cyclophosphamide, and egg or sperm harvesting should be offered. Proton-pump inhibitors should be added for stomach ulcer protection and Cotrimoxazole for *Pneumocystis carinii* pneumonia prophylaxis. Adequate hydration with intravenous fluids and frequent monitoring of the white blood cell count are needed to reduce the risk of hemorrhagic cystitis, and one should change the dose in case of neutropenia.

Acute Approach in Hemispheric Infarction

Guidelines have been recently published (Part XIV, Guidelines).[141,159] The management of patients with large hemispheric infarction first focuses on adequate stabilization (Table 29.2). Airway management is important, but many patients do not need endotracheal intubation for airway control. Oxygenation can be secured by 3 L of oxygen through nasal prongs. Elective intubation must be performed in patients who are unable to cough forcefully, are barely localizing to pain, or are stuporous. Early intubation, followed by mechanical ventilation, is certainly indicated in patients with poor oxygenation and chest radiographic evidence of aspiration, and at times is indicated in patients with a series of seizures treated with repeated doses of benzodiazepines.

There is reasonable evidence that increased core body temperature increases ischemia-induced lactate accumulation and has a deleterious effect. Body temperature has been associated with initial stroke severity and mortality, suggesting a causal relationship. Although the benefit of fever reduction in any patient with any type of stroke is clinically unproven, core temperature probably should initially be maintained at a point between 36°C and 37°C.

Patients with a major hemispheric stroke tend to be in a hypovolemic state and display marginal blood pressure readings when seen in the NICU.[152] Hypotension from hypovolemia is often manifested by low systolic blood pressure for age and mild sinus tachycardia, but also by an orthostatic pulse increase of 10 to 20 beats/min. Hypovolemia is almost always incurred during transport if adequate amounts of fluid—beyond an intravenous drip to keep an open venous access—are not

TABLE 29.2. INITIAL MANAGEMENT OF ACUTE HEMISPHERIC INFARCTION

Airway management	Intubation if patient has hypoxemia despite facemask with 10 L of 100% oxygen/minute, if abnormal respiratory drive or if abnormal protective reflexes (likely with motor response of withdrawal, or worse)
Mechanical ventilation	IMV/PS or CPAP mode
Fluid management	2–3 L of 0.9% NaCl per 24 hours
	Rehydrate with 500 mL of normal saline or albumin 5%
Blood pressure management	No antihypertensive agents unless MAP > 120 mm Hg
Nutrition	Enteral nutrition with continuous infusion (on day 2)
	Blood glucose control (goal 140–180 mg/dL)
Prophylaxis	DVT prophylaxis with pneumatic compression devices
	SC heparin 5,000 U t.i.d.
	GI prophylaxis: pantoprazole 40 mg IV daily or lansoprazole 30 mg orally through nasogastric tube
Other measures	Maintain normothermia with cooling blankets
Access	Arterial catheter to monitor blood pressure (if IV antihypertensive drugs anticipated)
	Peripheral venous catheter or peripheral inserted central catheter

CPAP, continuous positive airway pressure; DVT, deep vein thrombosis; GI, gastrointestinal; IMV, intermittent mandatory ventilation; IV, intravenously; MAP, mean arterial pressure; NaCl, sodium chloride; PS, pressure support; SC, subcutaneously.

provided. A bolus of fluid with 500 mL of saline or albumin is important to correct this volume deficit.

Maintenance fluid management in patients with acute hemispheric stroke includes 3 L of crystalloids such as isotonic saline. One may consider discontinuing administration of any diuretic agent for 24 hours. Glucose-containing fluids should be avoided, and blood glucose should be closely monitored in the first 2 days of admission and lowered (glucose 140–180 mg/dL). Hyperglycemia is very often stress-related and may require insulin protocol (Chapter 57). Progression to nonketotic hyperglycemic coma (values up to 1,000 mg/dL) is rare and, if present, is associated with marked dehydration.

Hypertension must be left alone in the first 24 hours after hemispheric stroke. Patients may have a marked hypertensive response after stroke, but it is seldom sustained, and aggressive blood pressure decrease may compromise compensatory collateral circulation.

Nutrition should not be deferred in patients with a large hemispheric stroke. Pantoprazole is indicated in patients with a history of gastric ulcers or prior use of nonsteroidal anti-inflammatory drugs, and in any patient on a mechanical ventilator.

Anticoagulation with heparin in patients with a large hemispheric stroke is problematic because of a true risk of significant hemorrhagic conversion of infarct. However, in one study of massive cerebral infarcts and swelling, hemorrhagic conversion developed in only four of 32 fully anticoagulated patients without significant deterioration.[18] Absolute indications are atrial fibrillation, clinical suspicion of myocardial infarction, and a large akinetic segment revealed by echocardiography. In this category of patients, the risk of re-embolization has been reported to be up to 21% in the first 3 weeks in patients with any type of acute cardioembolic infarction when anticoagulation is deferred. In patients treated with anticoagulation, recurrences are reduced to less than 3%. This reduction probably is more significant in patients with acute myocardial infarction or with atrial fibrillation and rapid ventricular response. Overcoagulation should be avoided, and the goal should be an aPTT of 1.5–2 times control. If no embolic source is evident, it may be prudent to defer intravenous heparin for several days to reduce hemorrhagic conversion, a complication that commonly evolves into a massive hematoma with displacement of the thalamus and upper brainstem.

DETERIORATION: CAUSES AND MANAGEMENT

Deterioration in patients with a large hemispheric stroke most often is caused by brain swelling. Brain swelling occurs invariably to some degree in patients with complete MCA territory occlusion, usually after a 2–7-day interval (median, 4 days).[10,103,125]

The pathophysiology of brain edema is complex and may have different explanations. The least common explanation probably is reperfusion of already irreversibly damaged brain and could be more common after thrombolytic therapy.[25,104] The formation of brain edema due to flooding of the infarcted territory may also be facilitated by the generation of reactive oxidants triggered after oxygen is provided to these ischemic parts. The delayed cerebral swelling is more difficult to explain. Cellular edema occurs from influx of water and sodium into the cells (cytotoxic edema phase), and osmotically active particles in the brain (e.g., *myo*-inositol) may contribute. Impairment of the blood–brain barrier follows later, adding more edema (vasogenic edema phase).[29]

As mentioned earlier, an important initial clinical sign of brain swelling is the development of anisocoria (≥ 2 mm) and bilateral ptosis. Very often, a Cheyne-Stokes breathing pattern changes into sustained hyperventilation, but periodic breathing may follow when coma deepens, and must prompt endotracheal intubation and mechanical ventilation.[161] A unilateral fixed, dilated pupil may be observed early, but small and constricted but reactive pupils from downward diencephalic displacement are more common.

The clinical course usually gradually worsens in most patients over days. However, drowsiness from brain swelling can be transient, and the level of consciousness can improve. Magnetic resonance imaging may show a massive expanding, swollen infarct (Figure 29.15).[43] Clinical course can worsen quickly, with relentless swelling and no improvement despite intervention. This type of rapidly developing edema is termed *malignant MCA territory infarction*.

Clinical and radiologic predictors of deterioration beyond drowsiness have been identified and have included an NIHSS score of greater than 25, additional territorial infarcts, and age.[45,57,65,66,76,77]

In many patients with early deterioration to stupor, intracranial pressure is normal or mildly increased.[32,119] Clinical deterioration is caused by progressive brainstem displacement both horizontally and vertically, but subtle pressure differences may not be measured by a peripherally located parenchymal monitor. More likely, the swollen hemisphere grows like a tumor mass, with some increase in intracranial pressure but much more displacement of the upper brainstem.[75,89]

Management of cerebral edema in patients with unilateral swelling in a large portion of the hemisphere is very difficult and often fails. However, considerable cerebral edema may resolve spontaneously if it remains in the MCA territory[153] (Figure 29.16). Corticosteroids have been ineffective in controlling cerebral edema.[98,131] This result is expected, because their membrane-stabilizing effect would not influence the cytotoxic edema phase. Osmotic agents (mannitol or hypertonic saline) are the first line of treatment, and the effect of mannitol should be observed first.[123] Mannitol is administered as a bolus of 1 g/kg IV over 30 minutes, and if no measurable effect is seen, a second intravenous dose of 2 g/kg is tried to reduce intracranial pressure. We have seen dramatic reversal of the clinical deterioration with mannitol and hyperventilation in brain edema associated with acute hemispheric infarction.[161] Lack of response to mannitol, as measured by MRI,[75] is often noted in more advanced stages of herniation.[109]

If deterioration continues and CT scans document further mass effect, the patient's next of kin is offered the choice of decompressive hemicraniectomy[24,50,51,54,109,120,122] (Figure 29.17). The timing of hemicraniectomy with duraplasty is unresolved, but it is reasonable to proceed when the patient's condition deteriorates to withdrawal to pain or new pupil abnormalities emerge.

Decompressive surgery has been mostly successful in patients with ischemic stroke in the nondominant hemisphere, including those with progression to coma and a fixed, dilated pupil (Figure 29.18). There is presumptive evidence that salvaged patients do well despite a fixed hemiparesis, and many return to their previous intellectual level.[14] (Capsule 29.1) The initial experience, largely from Germany, in more than 60 surgically treated patients suggests that mortality is substantially decreased, but one of four patients has severe disability. Early decompressive hemicraniectomy (arbitrarily defined as surgery before the first signs of herniation) has been advocated by some, but good results can also be explained by a favorable natural history. Reperfusion improved after decompression.[130] Concerns about major morbidity in survivors have been voiced,[154] and the functional outcome in elderly patients is marginal.[53,144,155] One study found severe disability even in patients older than 55 years.[99] (An insightful description of the burdens of surviving a craniotomy has been published by an anesthesiologist.[69])

Alternative therapies include a preemptive approach with repeated mannitol infusions in patients at very high risk (hypodensity involving more than 50% of the MCA territory on CT, hyperdense MCA sign, and sulcal effacement). Hypertonic saline may be effective when mannitol fails. One important study in Sprague-Dawley rats

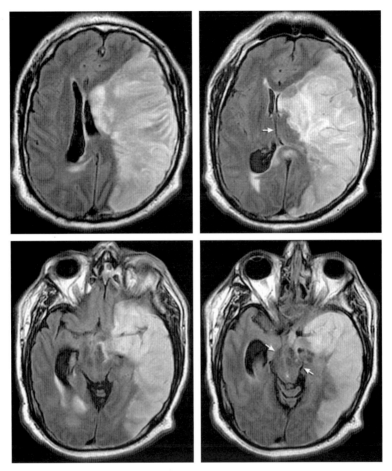

FIGURE 29.15: FLAIR MRI shows large MCA infarct with mass effect and tissue shift. Note bowing of the third ventricle and brainstem compression (*arrows*).

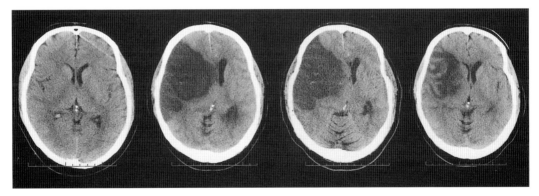

FIGURE 29.16: Serial computed tomography scans showing the evolution and resolution of a middle cerebral artery infarct with brain swelling. The patient had only brief periods of decreased level of consciousness but continued to localize to pain, occasionally followed commands, and protected his airway. At his last scan, he was alert but had major neglect and flaccid hemiplegia.

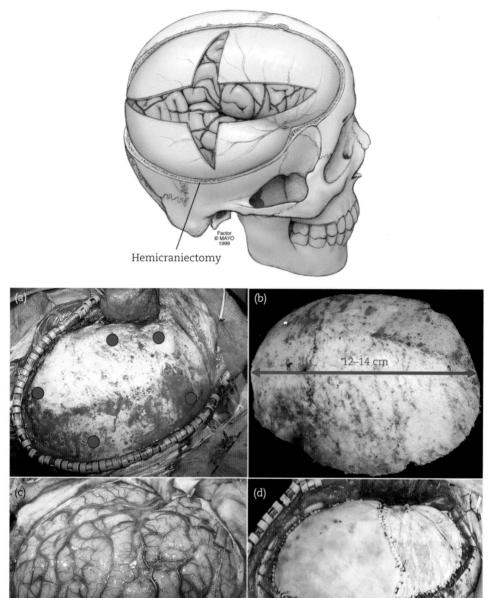

FIGURE 29.17: Hemicraniectomy.

Upper row left: Illustration showing the size of craniotomy of the skull with ample room left for the infarcted brain to swell.

Upper row right (actual surgery): (a) A curvilinear incision is used to raise a large scalp flap and mobilize the temporalis muscle and fascia, thereby gaining a wide fronto-parieto-temporal exposure; the positions of planned burr holes are indicated by *blue dots*. (b) The bone flap that is removed should measure 12–14 cm. (c) After opening the dura, the swollen brain herniates outward, relieving compression on medial structures and on the brainstem. (d) An augmentation duroplasty is performed to accommodate and protect the swollen brain (kindly provided by Dr. Simard).[68]

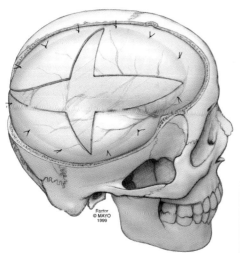
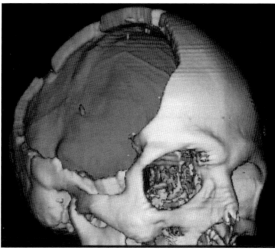

FIGURE 29.17: (Continued)

Lower row left (illustration): Duraplasty expands the intracranial vault.

Lower row right: Bone window of 3D reconstructed computed tomogram showing the extent of the skull removal.

suggested that albumin therapy virtually eliminated brain swelling. Albumin (2 g/kg) may reduce cerebral swelling by increasing the oncotic pressure of plasma without affecting osmolality because of the high molecular weight of plasma. There is little clinical experience with this approach.[5]

If family members refuse decompressive craniotomy, a regimen of moderate hypothermia (33°–34°C) can be instituted.[121]

Moderate hypothermia has received considerable interest as a treatment modality.[64,118] However, the evidence for reducing infarct size is much more compelling than that for treatment of cerebral swelling. Hypothermia could possibly suppress a glutamate flux and intraneuronal calcium mobilization, elements of excitotoxic neuronal damage. It may also decrease metabolic rate and the development of lactic acidosis. Experimental studies have consistently shown not only reduction in infarct volume but also continued neuroprotection after discontinuation of hypothermia even several hours after surgical occlusion of the MCA. Clinical trials of moderate hypothermia in massive hemispheric infarcts are in progress. Moderate hypothermia can be achieved by surface cooling or invasive devices. A simple way is to position the patient between two cooling blankets. The cooling blankets are set

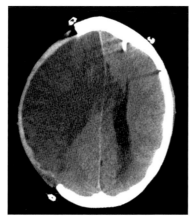
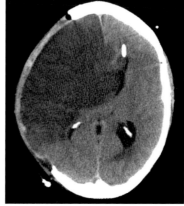

FIGURE 29.18: Serial computed tomography scans showing the marginal effect of decompressive hemicraniectomy with ventriculostomy.

CAPSULE 29.1   DECOMPRESSIVE HEMICRANIECTOMY AND OUTCOME

A large craniectomy with duraplasty to allow swelling outside the skull may be considered. Decompressive craniectomy involves removal of a large bone flap and duraplasty, but some have suggested that removal of the temporal muscle should be included.[93] Generally, the swollen infarct is left intact, and removal of necrotic tissue may cause major difficulty with hemostasis. The timing of surgery is unresolved. It is possible that decompressive craniectomy may result in good outcome in patients who may not necessarily need a decompressive craniectomy and may recover without any further clinical intervention. Some evidence suggests that this procedure has increased survival and resulted in 30%–50% functional outcome.[47,97,101,102] The surgical procedure should be offered to patients irrespective of the involved hemisphere. Hemicraniectomy has now been tested in three European trials, and pooled results show a benefit among patients treated

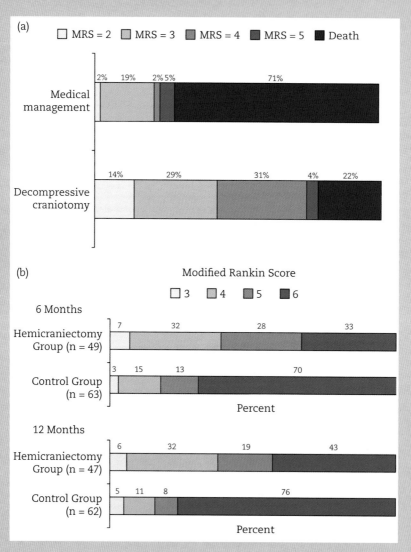

(a) Outcome in pooled analysis of hemicraniectomy trials. Outcomes are assessed with modified Rankin Scale (mRS). Poor outcome is generally considered mRS 3 or more. (b) Outcome of decompressive surgery in elderly.

with decompression[46] (see Capsule Figure). Mortality was reduced, but the number of severely disabled patients remains substantial, and there is a high prevalence of depression. In a more recent study in elderly patients[53] (see Capsule figure), mortality substantially decreased from 70% to 33%. There were no patients in mild disability category (mRS 2) and in the moderate category there was a decrease from 7% to 3% (mRS 3). Both worse categories increased. These results discourage hemicraniotomy in patients over 60 years old. The treatment may have been different between groups. In the group with worse outcome and receiving medical treatment alone, patients were often not admitted to ICUs, there was a higher incidence of multiterritorial infarcts, and less intubation and shorter time on the ventilator was noted.[21,41,46,145]

at 4.0°C initially and then adjusted to a core temperature of 33°–34°C. It may take up to 6 hours to reach this goal.[55] The process can be supplemented by alcohol rubbing and ice water gastric lavage and by intravenous infusion of cold fluids (Chapter 17).

Many NICUs in the United States use noninvasive means of cooling, by covering the patient with pads. Within these pads circulates cooled fluid that is kept at a certain set temperature. The ease of use and reliable cooling have made cooling pads a preferred method. An invasive option is the placement of a closed saline infusion loop after insertion of a probe into the vena cava or subclavian vein. Invasive cooling devices that have been introduced to the market all use the similar principle of core cooling. Maximal cooling rates of 5°–8°C/hr have been claimed. These devices greatly facilitate the management of hypothermia.

Shivering can be treated with meperidine, alfentanil, or propofol. A neuromuscular blocking agent is usually not needed. Intercurrent infections, particularly pneumonia, and hemorrhagic conversion of the infarct increase temperature significantly, and maintaining hypothermia becomes much more difficult.

Other complications have included reduced platelet count and cold-induced pancreatic failure, evidenced by increased serum amylase concentration. Drug metabolism is markedly affected (a major review has been recently published[142]).

A protocol for management in cerebral swelling is shown in Table 29.3.

Another neurologic cause for deterioration in patients with hemispheric stroke is hemorrhagic conversion of the infarct. The mechanism of development of an intracerebral hematoma in a large territory infarct is unresolved, but development of a large intracranial hematoma has tentatively been linked to excessive prolongation of activated partial thromboplastin time and surges in blood pressure. Early arterial recanalization would appear more likely as a possible explanation, but it was not confirmed in a study of four patients.[91]

It has been clearly established that most patients do not have clinical deterioration.[61] This can be explained by either petechial hemorrhage or small hematomas without significant mass effect. Patients with hemorrhagic conversion of infarcts are best managed by reduction of the intensity of anticoagulation to borderline anticoagulation. Certainly, in patients with excessive aPTT values, it is more prudent to hold heparin for 1 or 2 days. Studies of hemorrhagic infarction during heparinization, although retrospective, convincingly showed that this approach could be safe.[95,96]

Clinical worsening is much more prevalent and is often devastating in patients with large hematomas.[48,92] This uncommon cause of deterioration occurs in patients irrespective of anticoagulation.[48,91,92] In a large study of hemorrhagic transformation of ischemic stroke, a massive hematoma developed in 1 of 65 patients. Clinical deterioration may be gradual at first and usually during the day after admission. Often, large hemorrhagic infarcts are centrally located and may produce a downward compression of the thalamus and brainstem. The progression may be gradual and involves development of small midposition pupils, Cheyne-Stokes breathing, and hypertonia in previously flaccid limbs, evolving to pathologic flexion responses. Progression in many patients halts at this midbrain stage of central herniation, and they do not recover. Surgical removal of the clot is often a last resort, but many patients do poorly.

Seizures and status epilepticus are uncommon causes for deterioration.[36,60] Periodic lateralized epileptiform discharges are more commonly seen on electroencephalograms in patients with large ischemic strokes but are seldom accompanied by clinical manifestations.[131] These findings should

TABLE 29.3. TREATMENT OPTIONS
FOR CEREBRAL SWELLING
IN HEMISPHERIC INFARCTION

Maintain adequate hydration but restrict free water

Assess the effect of mannitol 20%, 1 g/kg

If mannitol is unsuccessful, place central catheter
and administer repeated doses of 30 mL of 23%
saline

If hypertonic saline therapy is unsuccessful, consider
decompressive hemicraniectomy

If decompressive hemicraniectomy is refused or
unsuccessful, consider hypothermia therapy,
reducing core body temperature to 33°–34°C by
using cooling blankets or cooling devices, gastric
lavage with ice water, and alcohol rubbing

Treat shivering with propofol (up to 3–5 mcg/kg/hr)
and alfentanil (0.5–3 µg/kg/min) if needed

Monitor serum amylase, activated partial
thromboplastin time, platelet count, and troponin
daily during hypothermia

Continue hypothermia for 3 days and rewarm,
ideally increasing temperature 1°C every 6 hours

not be interpreted as signs of subclinical seizures or nonconvulsive status epilepticus or lead to aggressive treatment with antiepileptic medication. These discharges, however, may predict later seizures, and in a patient with a single seizure, intravenous loading with fosphenytoin should be considered. Focal seizures can become notoriously difficult to treat and may need repeated use of benzodiazepines or valproate.

Because of comorbidity and poor general health, some patients with large hemispheric infarcts may have deterioration from systemic causes. Congestive heart failure may worsen rapidly with pulmonary edema, sometimes because of iatrogenic fluid loading or inadequate diuretic therapy. Almost half the patients who need mechanical ventilation have poor gas exchange from significant pulmonary edema associated with poor diastolic cardiac function, rather than from "neurogenic" pulmonary edema.

Similarly, cardiac arrhythmias emerge in patients with a large hemispheric stroke, and this may be the only reason for monitoring in the NICU. Rapid atrial fibrillation is more common in elderly patients but not exclusively in patients with coexisting cardiac disease. Significant arrhythmias, including ventricular tachycardia and series of ventricular ectopic beats, can be observed after hemispheric infarcts.[87] Recognition and treatment of the most common cardiac arrhythmias are discussed in Chapter 56.

Sudden death after a large territory hemispheric stroke may have its origin in a saddle pulmonary embolus. In our series of 30 patients with pulmonary emboli after stroke, pulmonary embolism defied ante-mortem detection in half the cases, and in one of three patients, it was associated with deep vein thrombosis in the paralyzed leg (Chapter 55).

OUTCOME

Although less appreciated in the NICU because of a bias toward the more severe cases, the clinical course in patients with a large hemispheric infarct is commonly a very gradual improvement. Mortality is high in patients with a large ischemic stroke. When acute stroke occurs in patients with acute myocardial infarction, cardiac arrhythmias may contribute to early mortality. Treatment of neurologic complications can be expected to substantially decrease mortality. Unrelenting cerebral swelling is a common cause of early death. Brain swelling may halt, and improvement may follow. These two entirely different clinical courses cannot be predicted at onset.

Mortality is high in patients who need mechanical ventilation.[127,158] In a study of 24 patients with acute MCA territory stroke who eventually needed ventilatory support, only five patients survived. We and others found that outcome is particularly poor (80%–100% mortality) in patients with CT scan evidence of swelling and a need for mechanical ventilation. Independent outcome is possible in surviving patients who needed prolonged ventilatory assistance and tracheostomy.

Whether patients reach an independent functional level depends on location, size, and comorbid condition. Intensive rehabilitation to improve walking, to optimize independence in daily living by significant adjustments in the home and at work, and to support psychological stress and depression is imperative for any survivor of a large hemispheric stroke.[31] Patients who remain in a coma for at least 1 week after a large ischemic stroke generally remain severely disabled and are often in need of nursing home placement.[157,160] There is little consensus among physicians concerning what constitutes "acceptable" outcome.[88]

Outcome in large hemispheric infarcts is also determined by its cause. Carotid dissection may recur in 1% per year (2% in the first month). Permanent stenosis of the carotid artery remains associated with a low incidence of recurrent stroke (0.7%), and ischemic strokes have occurred

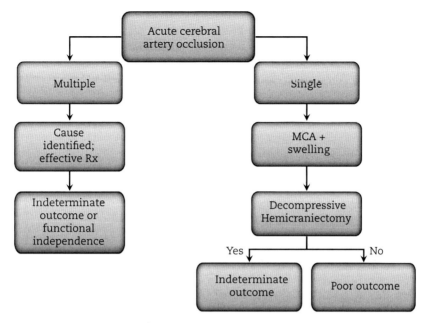

FIGURE 29.19: Outcome algorithm in hemispheric strokes. Poor outcome: Severe disability or death, vegetative state. Indeterminate: Any statement would be a premature conclusion. Functional independence or good outcome: No assistance needed, minor handicap may remain.

despite aspirin or warfarin.[113] Patients with associated hereditary disorders do not have a higher incidence of recurrence of dissection, and a history of dissection in a family member does not increase the incidence of recurrence. Outcome from infarction due to dissection appears more favorable in younger patients than in older patients with similar infarcts; the explanation is not known. Massive swelling may occur because of involvement of the anterior circulation; mortality is high without decompressive craniectomy.

Recurrence in CNS vasculitis is more common when patients are treated with corticosteroids alone. Outcome can be very good after aggressive combination therapy with administration of cyclophosphamide for at least 1 year (the estimated relapse rate then is < 10%). Corticosteroid doses can be tapered after 6 months. Mortality is uncommon, but functional outcome can be quite severely impacted when cerebral infarcts are widespread or located in both frontal lobes. An outcome algorithm in different types of hemispheric strokes is shown in Figure 29.19.

CONCLUSIONS
- The anatomy of vascular occlusion may indicate certain cause and direction of intervention.

- Acute occlusive disease can be treated with IV and IA thrombolytics, mechanical disruption, or stenting, and all three options can be considered.
- Deterioration in patients with MCA occlusion consists of brain swelling, cerebral hematoma from hemorrhagic conversion, or pulmonary edema due to aspiration or fluid overload.
- Primary control of brain swelling may initially be accomplished with scheduled mannitol or hypertonic saline. Decompressive surgery is a common occurrence and often best option in patients less than 60 years of age should be considered.

REFERENCES
1. Arnold M, Nedeltchev K, Sturzenegger M, et al. Thrombolysis in patients with acute stroke caused by cervical artery dissection: analysis of 9 patients and review of the literature. *Arch Neurol* 2002;59:549–553.
2. Averbuch-Heller L, Leigh RJ, Mermelstein V, Zagalsky L, Streifler JY. Ptosis in patients with hemispheric strokes. *Neurology* 2002;58: 620–624.
3. Barber PA, Darby DG, Desmond PM, et al. Identification of major ischemic change.

Diffusion-weighted imaging versus computed tomography. *Stroke* 1999;30:2059–2065.

4. Barber PA, Zhang J, Demchuk AM, Hill MD, Buchan AM. Why are stroke patients excluded from TPA therapy? An analysis of patient eligibility. *Neurology* 2001;56:1015–1020.

5. Belayev L, Liu Y, Zhao W, Busto R, Ginsberg MD. Human albumin therapy of acute ischemic stroke: marked neuroprotective efficacy at moderate doses and with a broad therapeutic window. *Stroke* 2001;32:553–560.

6. Berkhemer OA, Fransen PS, Beumer D, et al. A randomized trial of intraarterial treatment for acute ischemic stroke. *N Engl J Med* 2015;372:11–20.

7. Biousse V, D'Anglejan-Chatillon J, Touboul PJ, Amarenco P, Bousser MG. Time course of symptoms in extracranial carotid artery dissections: a series of 80 patients. *Stroke* 1995;26:235–239.

8. Bogousslavsky J, Regli F. Anterior cerebral artery territory infarction in the Lausanne Stroke Registry: clinical and etiologic patterns. *Arch Neurol* 1990;47:144–150.

9. Bose A, Henkes H, Alfke K, et al. The Penumbra System: a mechanical device for the treatment of acute stroke due to thromboembolism. *AJNR Am J Neuroradiol* 2008;29:1409–1413.

10. Bounds JV, Wiebers DO, Whisnant JP, Okazaki H. Mechanisms and timing of deaths from cerebral infarction. *Stroke* 1981;12:474–477.

11. Bozzao L, Angeloni U, Bastianello S, et al. Early angiographic and CT findings in patients with hemorrhagic infarction in the distribution of the middle cerebral artery. *AJNR Am J Neuroradiol* 1991;12:1115–1121.

12. Broderick JP, Palesch YY, Demchuk AM, et al. Endovascular therapy after intravenous t-PA versus t-PA alone for stroke. *N Engl J Med* 2013;368:893–903.

13. Brott T, Adams HP, Jr., Olinger CP, et al. Measurements of acute cerebral infarction: a clinical examination scale. *Stroke* 1989;20:864–870.

14. Brown MM. Surgical decompression of patients with large middle cerebral artery infarcts is effective: not proven. *Stroke* 2003;34:2305–2306.

15. Burton KR, Dhanoa D, Aviv RI, et al. Perfusion CT for selecting patients with acute ischemic stroke for intravenous thrombolytic therapy. *Radiology* 2015;274:103–114.

16. Campbell BC, Mitchell PJ, Kleinig TJ, et al. Endovascular therapy for ischemic stroke with perfusion-imaging selection. *N Engl J Med* 2015;372:1009–1018.

17. Cervera R, Piette JC, Font J, et al. Antiphospholipid syndrome: clinical and immunologic manifestations and patterns of disease expression in a cohort of 1,000 patients. *Arthritis Rheum* 2002;46:1019–1027.

18. Chamorro A, Vila N, Saiz A, Alday M, Tolosa E. Early anticoagulation after large cerebral embolic infarction: a safety study. *Neurology* 1995;45:861–865.

19. Cho KH, Kang DW, Kwon SU, Kim JS. Lesion volume increase is related to neurologic progression in patients with subcortical infarction. *J Neurol Sci* 2009;284:163–167.

20. Ciccone A, Valvassori L, Nichelatti M, et al. Endovascular treatment for acute ischemic stroke. *N Engl J Med* 2013;368:904–913.

21. Curry WT, Jr., Sethi MK, Ogilvy CS, Carter BS. Factors associated with outcome after hemicraniectomy for large middle cerebral artery territory infarction. *Neurosurgery* 2005;56:681–692.

22. de Bray JM, Lhoste P, Dubas F, Emile J, Saumet JL. Ultrasonic features of extracranial carotid dissections: 47 cases studied by angiography. *J Ultrasound Med* 1994;13:659–664.

23. del Zoppo GJ, Higashida RT, Furlan AJ, et al. PROACT: a phase II randomized trial of recombinant pro-urokinase by direct arterial delivery in acute middle cerebral artery stroke. PROACT Investigators. Prolyse in Acute Cerebral Thromboembolism. *Stroke* 1998;29:4–11.

24. Delashaw JB, Broaddus WC, Kassell NF, et al. Treatment of right hemispheric cerebral infarction by hemicraniectomy. *Stroke* 1990;21:874–881.

25. Delgado P, Sahuquillo J, Poca MA, Alvarez-Sabin J. Neuroprotection in malignant MCA infarction. *Cerebrovasc Dis* 2006;21 Suppl 2:99–105.

26. Derex L, Nighoghossian N, Turjman F, et al. Intravenous tPA in acute ischemic stroke related to internal carotid artery dissection. *Neurology* 2000;54:2159–2161.

27. Donahue J, Wintermark M. Perfusion CT and acute stroke imaging: foundations, applications, and literature review. *J Neuroradiol* 2015;42:21–29.

28. Donnan GA, Fisher M, Macleod M, Davis SM. Stroke. *Lancet* 2008;371:1612–1623.

29. Firlik AD, Yonas H, Kaufmann AM, et al. Relationship between cerebral blood flow and the development of swelling and life-threatening herniation in acute ischemic stroke. *J Neurosurg* 1998;89:243–249.

30. Fisher CM, Ojemann RG, Roberson GH. Spontaneous dissection of cervico-cerebral arteries. *Can J Neurol Sci* 1978;5:9–19.

31. Foerch C, Lang JM, Krause J, et al. Functional impairment, disability, and quality of life outcome after decompressive hemicraniectomy in malignant middle cerebral artery infarction. *J Neurosurg* 2004;101:248–254.

32. Frank JI. Large hemispheric infarction, deterioration, and intracranial pressure. *Neurology* 1995;45:1286–1290.

33. Furlan A, Higashida R, Wechsler L, et al. Intra-arterial prourokinase for acute ischemic stroke. The PROACT II study: a randomized controlled trial. Prolyse in Acute Cerebral Thromboembolism. *JAMA* 1999;282:2003–2011.

34. Furlan AJ. Endovascular therapy for stroke—it's about time. *N Engl J Med* 2015;372:2347–2349.

35. Georgiadis D, Arnold M, von Buedingen HC, et al. Aspirin vs anticoagulation in carotid artery dissection: a study of 298 patients. *Neurology* 2009;72:1810–1815.

36. Giroud M, Gras P, Fayolle H, et al. Early seizures after acute stroke: a study of 1,640 cases. *Epilepsia* 1994;35:959–964.

37. Gonzalez RG, Copen WA, Schaefer PW, et al. The Massachusetts General Hospital acute stroke imaging algorithm: an experience and evidence based approach. *J Neurointerv Surg* 2013;5 Suppl 1:i7–12.

38. Goyal M, Demchuk AM, Menon BK, et al. Randomized assessment of rapid endovascular treatment of ischemic stroke. *N Engl J Med* 2015;372:1019–1030.

39. Grotta JC, Welch KM, Fagan SC, et al. Clinical deterioration following improvement in the NINDS rt-PA Stroke Trial. *Stroke* 2001;32:661–668.

40. Group TNIoNDaSr-PSS. Tissue plasminogen activator for acute ischemic stroke. *N Engl J Med* 1995;333:1581–1587.

41. Gupta R, Connolly ES, Mayer S, Elkind MS. Hemicraniectomy for massive middle cerebral artery territory infarction: a systematic review. *Stroke* 2004;35:539–543.

42. Hacke W, Kaste M, Fieschi C, et al. Randomised double-blind placebo-controlled trial of thrombolytic therapy with intravenous alteplase in acute ischemic stroke (ECASS II). Second European-Australasian Acute Stroke Study Investigators. *Lancet* 1998;352:1245–1251.

43. Hacke W, Schwab S, Horn M, et al. 'Malignant' middle cerebral artery territory infarction: clinical course and prognostic signs. *Arch Neurol* 1996;53:309–315.

44. Hart RG, Kanter MC. Hematologic disorders and ischemic stroke: a selective review. *Stroke* 1990;21:1111–1121.

45. Hofmeijer J, Algra A, Kappelle LJ, van der Worp HB. Predictors of life-threatening brain edema in middle cerebral artery infarction. *Cerebrovasc Dis* 2008;25:176–184.

46. Hofmeijer J, Kappelle LJ, Algra A, et al. Surgical decompression for space-occupying cerebral infarction (the Hemicraniectomy After Middle Cerebral Artery infarction with Life-threatening Edema Trial [HAMLET]): a multicentre, open, randomised trial. *Lancet Neurol* 2009;8:326–333.

47. Holtkamp M, Buchheim K, Unterberg A, et al. Hemicraniectomy in elderly patients with space occupying media infarction: improved survival but poor functional outcome. *J Neurol Neurosurg Psychiatry* 2001;70:226–228.

48. Hornig CR, Dorndorf W, Agnoli AL. Hemorrhagic cerebral infarction: a prospective study. *Stroke* 1986;17:179–185.

49. Houser OW, Baker HL, Jr. Fibromuscular dysplasia and other uncommon diseases of the cervical carotid artery: angiographic aspects. *Am J Roentgenol Radium Ther Nucl Med* 1968;104:201–212.

50. Huttner HB, Juttler E, Schwab S. Hemicraniectomy for middle cerebral artery infarction. *Curr Neurol Neurosci Rep* 2008;8:526–533.

51. Ivamoto HS, Numoto M, Donaghy RM. Surgical decompression for cerebral and cerebellar infarcts. *Stroke* 1974;5:365–370.

52. Jovin TG, Chamorro A, Cobo E, et al. Thrombectomy within 8 hours after symptom onset in ischemic stroke. *N Eng J Med* 2015;372:2296–2306.

53. Juttler E, Unterberg A, Woitzik J, et al. Hemicraniectomy in older patients with extensive middle-cerebral-artery stroke. *N Engl J Med* 2014;370:1091–1100.

54. Kalia KK, Yonas H. An aggressive approach to massive middle cerebral artery infarction. *Arch Neurol* 1993;50:1293–1297.

55. Kammersgaard LP, Rasmussen BH, Jorgensen HS, et al. Feasibility and safety of inducing modest hypothermia in awake patients with acute stroke through surface cooling: a case-control study: the Copenhagen Stroke Study. *Stroke* 2000;31:2251–2256.

56. Kasner SE. Clinical interpretation and use of stroke scales. *Lancet Neurol* 2006;5:603–612.

57. Kasner SE, Demchuk AM, Berrouschot J, et al. Predictors of fatal brain edema in massive hemispheric ischemic stroke. *Stroke* 2001;32:2117–2123.

58. Katz BH, Quencer RM, Kaplan JO, Hinks RS, Post MJ. MR imaging of intracranial carotid occlusion. *AJR Am J Roentgenol* 1989;152:1271–1276.

59. Kidwell CS, Jahan R, Gornbein J, et al. A trial of imaging selection and endovascular treatment for ischemic stroke. *N Engl J Med* 2013;368:914–923.

60. Kilpatrick CJ, Davis SM, Hopper JL, Rossiter SC. Early seizures after acute stroke: risk of late seizures. *Arch Neurol* 1992;49:509–511.

61. Kimura K, Iguchi Y, Shibazaki K, Aoki J, Terasawa Y. Hemorrhagic transformation of ischemic brain tissue after t-PA thrombolysis as detected by MRI may be asymptomatic, but impair neurological recovery. *J Neurol Sci* 2008;272:136–142.

62. Klossek JM, Neau JP, Vandenmarq P, Fontanel JP. Unilateral lower cranial nerve palsies due to spontaneous internal carotid artery dissection. *Ann Otol Rhinol Laryngol* 1994;103:413–415.

63. Koo CK, Teasdale E, Muir KW. What constitutes a true hyperdense middle cerebral artery sign? *Cerebrovasc Dis* 2000;10:419–423.

64. Krieger DW, De Georgia MA, Abou-Chebl A, et al. Cooling for acute ischemic brain damage (cool aid): an open pilot study of induced hypothermia in acute ischemic stroke. *Stroke* 2001;32:1847–1854.

65. Krieger DW, Demchuk AM, Kasner SE, Jauss M, Hantson L. Early clinical and radiological predictors of fatal brain swelling in ischemic stroke. *Stroke* 1999;30:287–292.

66. Kucinski T, Koch C, Grzyska U, et al. The predictive value of early CT and angiography for fatal hemispheric swelling in acute stroke. *AJNR Am J Neuroradiol* 1998;19:839–846.

67. Kumar R, Wijdicks EFM, Brown RD, Jr, Parisi JE, Hammond CA. Isolated angiitis of the CNS presenting as subarachnoid haemorrhage. *J Neurol Neurosurg Psychiatry* 1997;62:649–651.

68. Kurland DB, Khaladj-Ghom A, Stokum JA, et al. Complications associated with decompressive craniectomy: a systematic review. *Neurocrit Care* 2015;23:292–304.

69. Larach DR, Larach DB, Larach MG. A life worth living: seven years after craniectomy. *Neurocrit Care* 2009;11:106–111.

70. Leary MC, Saver JL, Gobin YP, et al. Beyond tissue plasminogen activator: mechanical intervention in acute stroke. *Ann Emerg Med* 2003;41:838–846.

71. Levine SR, Brey RL, Sawaya KL, et al. Recurrent stroke and thrombo-occlusive events in the antiphospholipid syndrome. *Ann Neurol* 1995;38:119–124.

72. Lewandowski CA, Frankel M, Tomsick TA, et al. Combined intravenous and intra-arterial r-TPA versus intra-arterial therapy of acute ischemic stroke: Emergency Management of Stroke (EMS) Bridging Trial. *Stroke* 1999;30:2598–2605.

73. Lucas C, Moulin T, Deplanque D, Tatu L, Chavot D. Stroke patterns of internal carotid artery dissection in 40 patients. *Stroke* 1998;29:2646–2648.

74. Mair G, Wardlaw JM. Imaging of acute stroke prior to treatment: current practice and evolving techniques. *Br J Radiol* 2014;87:20140216.

75. Manno EM, Adams RE, Derdeyn CP, Powers WJ, Diringer MN. The effects of mannitol on cerebral edema after large hemispheric cerebral infarct. *Neurology* 1999;52:583–587.

76. Manno EM, Nichols DA, Fulgham JR, Wijdicks EFM. Computed tomographic determinants of neurologic deterioration in patients with large middle cerebral artery infarctions. *Mayo Clinic Proc* 2003;78:156–160.

77. Maramattom BV, Bahn MM, Wijdicks EFM. Which patient fares worse after early deterioration due to swelling from hemispheric stroke? *Neurology* 2004;63:2142–2145.

78. Menon BK, Saver JL, Goyal M, et al. Trends in endovascular therapy and clinical outcomes within the nationwide get with the guidelines: stroke registry. *Stroke* 2015;46:989–995.

79. Meschia JF, Miller DA, Brott TG. Thrombolytic treatment of acute ischemic stroke. *Mayo Clinic Proc* 2002;77:542–551.

80. Miller DV, Salvarani C, Hunder GG, et al. Biopsy findings in primary angiitis of the central nervous system. *Am J Surg Pathol* 2009;33:35–43.

81. Minematsu K, Yamaguchi T, Omae T. 'Spectacular shrinking deficit': rapid recovery from a major hemispheric syndrome by migration of an embolus. *Neurology* 1992;42:157–162.

82. Mocco J, Hanel RA, Sharma J, et al. Use of a vascular reconstruction device to salvage acute ischemic occlusions refractory to traditional endovascular recanalization methods. *J Neurosurg* 2010;112:557–562.

83. Mokri B, Schievink WI, Olsen KD, Piepgras DG. Spontaneous dissection of the cervical internal carotid artery. Presentation with lower cranial nerve palsies. *Arch Otolaryngol Head Neck Surg* 1992;118:431–435.

84. Mokri B, Sundt TM, Jr., Houser OW, Piepgras DG. Spontaneous dissection of the cervical internal carotid artery. *Ann Neurol* 1986;19:126–138.

85. Morris DL, Rosamond W, Madden K, Schultz C, Hamilton S. Prehospital and emergency department delays after acute stroke: the Genentech Stroke Presentation Survey. *Stroke* 2000;31:2585–2590.

86. Mullins ME, Schaefer PW, Sorensen AG, et al. CT and conventional and diffusion-weighted MR imaging in acute stroke: study in 691 patients at presentation to the emergency department. *Radiology* 2002;224:353–360.

87. Myers MG, Norris JW, Hachinski VC, Weingert ME, Sole MJ. Cardiac sequelae of acute stroke. *Stroke* 1982;13:838–842.

88. Neugebauer H, Creutzfeldt CJ, Hemphill JC, 3rd, Heuschmann PU, Juttler E. DESTINY-S: attitudes of physicians toward disability and treatment in malignant MCA infarction. *Neurocrit Care* 2014;21:27–34.

89. Ng LK, Nimmannitya J. Massive cerebral infarction with severe brain swelling: a clinicopathological study. *Stroke* 1970;1:158–163.

90. Nguyen Bui L, Brant-Zawadzki M, Verghese P, Gillan G. Magnetic resonance angiography of cervicocranial dissection. *Stroke* 1993;24:126–131.

91. Ogata J, Yutani C, Imakita M, et al. Hemorrhagic infarct of the brain without a reopening of the occluded arteries in cardioembolic stroke. *Stroke* 1989;20:876–883.

92. Okada Y, Yamaguchi T, Minematsu K, et al. Hemorrhagic transformation in cerebral embolism. *Stroke* 1989;20:598–603.

93. Park J, Kim E, Kim GJ, Hur YK, Guthikonda M. External decompressive craniectomy including resection of temporal muscle and fascia in malignant hemispheric infarction. *J Neurosurg* 2009;110:101–105.

94. Parsons MW, Barber PA, Chalk J, et al. Diffusion- and perfusion-weighted MRI response to thrombolysis in stroke. *Ann Neurol* 2002;51:28–37.

95. Pessin MS, Estol CJ, Lafranchise F, Caplan LR. Safety of anticoagulation after hemorrhagic infarction. *Neurology* 1993;43:1298–1303.

96. Pessin MS, Teal PA, Caplan LR. Hemorrhagic infarction: guilt by association? *AJNR Am J Neuroradiol* 1991;12:1123–1126.

97. Pillai A, Menon SK, Kumar S, et al. Decompressive hemicraniectomy in malignant middle cerebral artery infarction: an analysis of long-term outcome and factors in patient selection. *J Neurosurg* 2007;106:59–65.

98. Qizilbash N, Lewington SL, Lopez-Arrieta JM. Corticosteroids for acute ischaemic stroke. *Cochrane Database Syst Rev* 2002:CD000064.

99. Rabinstein AA, Mueller-Kronast N, Maramattom BV, et al. Factors predicting prognosis after decompressive hemicraniectomy for hemispheric infarction. *Neurology* 2006;67:891–893.

100. Rabinstein AA, Wijdicks EFM, Nichols DA. Complete recovery after early intraarterial recombinant tissue plasminogen activator thrombolysis of carotid T occlusion. *AJNR Am J Neuroradiol* 2002;23:1596–1599.

101. Rengachary SS, Batnitzky S, Morantz RA, Arjunan K, Jeffries B. Hemicraniectomy for acute massive cerebral infarction. *Neurosurgery* 1981;8:321–328.

102. Rieke K, Schwab S, Krieger D, et al. Decompressive surgery in space-occupying hemispheric infarction: results of an open, prospective trial. *Crit Care Med* 1995;23:1576–1587.

103. Ropper AH, Shafran B. Brain edema after stroke: clinical syndrome and intracranial pressure. *Arch Neurol* 1984;41:26–29.

104. Rudol J, Grond M, Stenzel C, Neveling M, Heiss WD. Incidence of space-occupying brain edema following systemic thrombolysis of acute supratentorial ischemia. *Cerebrovasc Dis* 1998;8:166–171.

105. Russell EJ. Diagnosis of hyperacute ischemic infarct with CT: key to improved clinical outcome after intravenous thrombolysis? *Radiology* 1997;205:315–318.

106. Saito I, Segawa H, Shiokawa Y, Taniguchi M, Tsutsumi K. Middle cerebral artery occlusion: correlation of computed tomography and angiography with clinical outcome. *Stroke* 1987;18:863–868.

107. Salvarani C, Brown RD, Jr., Calamia KT, et al. Angiography-negative primary central nervous system vasculitis: a syndrome involving small cerebral vessels. *Medicine (Baltimore)* 2008;87:264–271.

108. Salvarani C, Brown RD, Jr., Calamia KT, et al. Primary central nervous system vasculitis: analysis of 101 patients. *Ann Neurol* 2007;62:442–451.

109. Sandalcioglu IE, Schoch B, Rauhut F. Hemicraniectomy for large middle cerebral artery territory infarction: do these patients really benefit from this procedure? *J Neurol Neurosurg Psychiatry* 2003;74:1600.

110. Sandercock P, Berge E, Dennis M, et al. A systematic review of the effectiveness, cost-effectiveness and barriers to implementation of thrombolytic and neuroprotective therapy for acute ischemic stroke in the NHS. *Health Technol Assess* 2002;6:1–112.

111. Saver JL, Jahan R, Levy EI, et al. Solitaire flow restoration device versus the Merci Retriever in patients with acute ischemic stroke (SWIFT): a randomised, parallel-group, non-inferiority trial. *Lancet* 2012;380:1241–1249.

112. Schievink WI. Spontaneous dissection of the carotid and vertebral arteries. *N Engl J Med* 2001;344:898–906.

113. Schievink WI, Michels VV, Mokri B, Piepgras DG, Perry HO. Brief report: a familial syndrome of arterial dissections with lentiginosis. *N Engl J Med* 1995;332:576–579.

114. Schievink WI, Mokri B, Garrity JA, Nichols DA, Piepgras DG. Ocular motor nerve palsies in spontaneous dissections of the cervical internal carotid artery. *Neurology* 1993;43:1938–1941.

115. Schievink WI, Mokri B, O'Fallon WM. Recurrent spontaneous cervical-artery dissection. *N Engl J Med* 1994;330:393–397.

116. Schievink WI, Wijdicks EFM, Kuiper JD. Seasonal pattern of spontaneous cervical artery dissection. *J Neurosurg* 1998;89:101–103.

117. Schievink WI, Wijdicks EFM, Michels VV, Vockley J, Godfrey M. Heritable connective tissue disorders in cervical artery dissections: a prospective study. *Neurology* 1998;50:1166–1169.

118. Schwab S. Therapy of severe ischemic stroke: breaking the conventional thinking. *Cerebrovasc Dis* 2005;20 Suppl 2:169–178.

119. Schwab S, Aschoff A, Spranger M, Albert F, Hacke W. The value of intracranial pressure monitoring in acute hemispheric stroke. *Neurology* 1996;47:393–398.

120. Schwab S, Hacke W. Surgical decompression of patients with large middle cerebral artery infarcts is effective. *Stroke* 2003;34:2304–2305.

121. Schwab S, Schwarz S, Spranger M, et al. Moderate hypothermia in the treatment of patients with severe middle cerebral artery infarction. *Stroke* 1998;29:2461–2466.

122. Schwab S, Steiner T, Aschoff A, et al. Early hemicraniectomy in patients with complete middle cerebral artery infarction. *Stroke* 1998;29:1888–1893.

123. Schwarz S, Georgiadis D, Aschoff A, Schwab S. Effects of hypertonic (10%) saline in patients with raised intracranial pressure after stroke. *Stroke* 2002;33:136–140.

124. Shaw CM, Alvord EC, Jr, Berry RG. Swelling of the brain following ischemic infarction with arterial occlusion. *Arch Neurol* 1959;1:161–177.

125. Shaw GJ, Meunier JM, Lindsell CJ, Holland CK. Tissue plasminogen activator concentration dependence of 120 kHz ultrasound-enhanced thrombolysis. *Ultrasound Med Biol* 2008;34:1783–1792.

126. Sheth SA, Jahan R, Gralla J, et al. Time to endovascular reperfusion and degree of disability in acute stroke. *Ann Neurol* 2015;78:584–593.

127. Silver FL, Norris JW, Lewis AJ, Hachinski VC. Early mortality following stroke: a prospective review. *Stroke* 1984;15:492–496.

128. Simon JE, Morgan SC, Pexman JH, Hill MD, Buchan AM. CT assessment of conjugate eye deviation in acute stroke. *Neurology* 2003;60:135–137.

129. Singer MB, Chong J, Lu D, et al. Diffusion-weighted MRI in acute subcortical infarction. *Stroke* 1998;29:133–136.

130. Slotty PJ, Kamp MA, Beez T, et al. The influence of decompressive craniectomy for major stroke on early cerebral perfusion. *J Neurosurg* 2015:1–6.

131. So EL, Annegers JF, Hauser WA, O'Brien PC, Whisnant JP. Population-based study of seizure disorders after cerebral infarction. *Neurology* 1996;46:350–355.

132. Song SS. Advanced imaging in acute ischemic stroke. *Semin Neurol* 2013;33:436–440.

133. Stead LG, Gilmore RM, Bellolio MF, Rabinstein AA, Decker WW. Percutaneous clot removal devices in acute ischemic stroke: a systematic review and meta-analysis. *Arch Neurol* 2008;65:1024–1030.

134. Steinke W, Schwartz A, Hennerici M. Topography of cerebral infarction associated with carotid artery dissection. *J Neurol* 1996;243:323–328.

135. Sturzenegger M, Huber P. Cranial nerve palsies in spontaneous carotid artery dissection. *J Neurol Neurosurg Psychiatry* 1993;56:1191–1199.

136. Tijssen CC, van Gisbergen JA, Schulte BP. Conjugate eye deviation: side, site, and size of the hemispheric lesion. *Neurology* 1991;41:846–850.

137. Tomsick T, Brott T, Barsan W, et al. Prognostic value of the hyperdense middle cerebral artery sign and stroke scale score before ultraearly thrombolytic therapy. *AJNR Am J Neuroradiol* 1996;17:79–85.

138. Tomsick TA, Brott TG, Chambers AA, et al. Hyperdense middle cerebral artery sign on CT: efficacy in detecting middle cerebral artery thrombosis. *AJNR Am J Neuroradiol* 1990;11:473–477.

139. Tomura N, Uemura K, Inugami A, et al. Early CT finding in cerebral infarction: obscuration of the lentiform nucleus. *Radiology* 1988;168:463–467.

140. Toni D, Fiorelli M, Bastianello S, et al. Hemorrhagic transformation of brain infarct: predictability in the first 5 hours from stroke onset and influence on clinical outcome. *Neurology* 1996;46:341–345.

141. Torbey MT, Bosel J, Rhoney DH, et al. Evidence-based guidelines for the management of large hemispheric infarction: a statement for health care professionals from the Neurocritical Care Society and the German Society for Neuro-Intensive Care and Emergency Medicine. *Neurocrit Care* 2015;22:146–164.

142. Tortorici MA, Kochanek PM, Poloyac SM. Effects of hypothermia on drug disposition, metabolism, and response: a focus on hypothermia-mediated alterations on the cytochrome P450 enzyme system. *Crit Care Med* 2007;35:2196–2204.

143. Uno M, Harada M, Yoneda K, et al. Can diffusion- and perfusion-weighted magnetic resonance imaging evaluate the efficacy of acute thrombolysis in patients with internal carotid artery or middle cerebral artery occlusion? *Neurosurgery* 2002;50:28–34.

144. Vahedi K, Benoist L, Kurtz A, et al. Quality of life after decompressive craniectomy for malignant middle cerebral artery infarction. *J Neurol Neurosurg Psychiatry* 2005;76: 1181–1182.

145. Vahedi K, Hofmeijer J, Juettler E, et al. Early decompressive surgery in malignant infarction of the middle cerebral artery: a pooled analysis of three randomized controlled trials. *Lancet Neurol* 2007;6:215–222.

146. van Everdingen KJ, van der Grond J, Kappelle LJ, Ramos LM, Mali WP. Diffusion-weighted magnetic resonance imaging in acute stroke. *Stroke* 1998;29:1783–1790.

147. von Kummer R, Allen KL, Holle R, et al. Acute stroke: usefulness of early CT findings before thrombolytic therapy. *Radiology* 1997;205:327–333.

148. von Kummer R, Meyding-Lamade U, Forsting M, et al. Sensitivity and prognostic value of early CT in occlusion of the middle cerebral artery trunk. *AJNR Am J Neuroradiol* 1994;15:9–15.

149. von Kummer R, Nolte PN, Schnittger H, Thron A, Ringelstein EB. Detectability of cerebral hemisphere ischaemic infarcts by CT within 6 h of stroke. *Neuroradiology* 1996;38:31–33.

150. Warach S. Stroke neuroimaging. *Stroke* 2003;34:345–347.

151. Wardlaw JM, Warlow CP, Counsell C. Systematic review of evidence on thrombolytic therapy for acute ischaemic stroke. *Lancet* 1997;350:607–614.

152. Weinberg AD, Minaker KL. Dehydration. Evaluation and management in older adults. Council on Scientific Affairs, American Medical Association. *JAMA* 1995;274:1552–1556.

153. Wijdicks EFM. Hemicraniotomy in massive hemispheric stroke: a stark perspective on a radical procedure. *Can J Neurol Sci* 2000;27:271–273.

154. Wijdicks EFM. Management of massive hemispheric cerebral infarct: is there a ray of hope? *Mayo Clinic Proc* 2000;75:945–952.

155. Wijdicks EFM, Diringer MN. Middle cerebral artery territory infarction and early brain swelling: progression and effect of age on outcome. *Mayo Clinic Proc* 1998;73:829–836.

156. Wijdicks EFM, Manno EM, Fulgham JR, Giannini C. Cerebral angiitis mimicking posterior leukoencephalopathy. *J Neurol* 2003;250:444–448.

157. Wijdicks EFM, Rabinstein AA. Absolutely no hope? Some ambiguity of futility of care in devastating acute stroke. *Crit Care Med* 2004;32:2332–2342.

158. Wijdicks EFM, Scott JP. Causes and outcome of mechanical ventilation in patients with hemispheric ischemic stroke. *Mayo Clinic Proc* 1997;72:210–213.

159. Wijdicks EFM, Sheth KN, Carter BS, et al. Recommendations for the management of cerebral and cerebellar infarction with swelling: a statement for healthcare professionals from the American Heart Association/American Stroke Association. *Stroke* 2014;45:1222–1238.

160. Wijdicks EFM. *The Comatose Patient.* 2nd ed. New York: Oxford University Press; 2014.

161. Wijdicks EFM, Schievink WI, McGough PF. Dramatic reversal of the uncal syndrome and brain edema from infarction in the middle cerebral artery territory. *Cerebrovasc Dis* 1997;7:349–352.

30

Acute Basilar Artery Occlusion

Acute occlusion of the basilar artery can be such a devastating neurologic event that any therapeutic intervention with the potential to reverse outcome—even with a remote chance—is justified.[76] If recognized in time, endovascular clot retrieval but also IV and IA thrombolysis may improve outcome, even if patients are seen 12–24 hours after the first signs and symptoms.[2,33,37,46,55,57,92]

An acute embolus to the basilar artery and a terminal occlusion of a narrowed basilar artery have different time courses of presentation, but may not be easily distinguished clinically. Any acute occlusion of a basilar artery may progress rapidly, even after several hours of waxing and waning of brainstem signs, but when the medial pontine tegmentum is ischemic, patients become comatose and need to be intubated. In other patients, progression of brainstem dysfunction has not yet occurred or the neurologic deficit is limited. Patients in both categories are admitted with some frequency to the neurosciences intensive care unit (NICU). Endovascular intervention is often needed, but management may include blood pressure augmentation in a poorly perfused posterior circulation with little collateral rescue.

CLINICAL RECOGNITION

Acute vertebrobasilar occlusive disease leads to several major clinical presentations, each of which can progress to loss of virtually all brainstem function. Several syndromes have become known in the neurologic lexicon, such as locked-in syndrome[29] and top-of-the-basilar syndrome,[12] but there are also a host of other syndromes, known by mostly French eponyms (Capsule 30.1). These syndromes are characterized by partial involvement of the brainstem.[11,14,73]

Artery-to-artery embolus from atheromatous disease of the vertebral artery or ascending aortic arch, or an embolus from a cardiac source or a vertebral artery dissection can be implicated.[3,5,11,13,32] The sites of occlusion are shown in Figure 30.1.

Acute basilar artery occlusion results in median and paramedian pontine infarction. The most consistent signs and symptoms are altered consciousness from involvement of reticular formation in the tegmentum, ataxic or pseudobulbar speech, horizontal gaze palsy, ocular bobbing, facial diplegia, dysphagia, and profound tetraplegia that is notably asymmetrical in degree of motor weakness.[24]

The eye findings in acute basilar artery occlusion are often diagnostic. The following neuro-ophthalmologic signs are often seen: (a) a lesion of the medial longitudinal fasciculus that produces an internuclear ophthalmoplegia consisting of abnormal ipsilateral adduction and more profound nystagmus in the abducting eye; (b) one-and-a-half syndrome, consisting of one immobile eye in the horizontal plane and preservation of abduction alone in the other eye; (c) ocular bobbing, a type of vertical nystagmus that is a frequent finding in patients with extensive pontine infarction and is recognized by brisk conjugate downward eye movement, followed by slow correction to baseline midposition; (d) bilateral ptosis due to involvement of the sympathetic fibers in the pontine tegmentum, or unilateral ptosis due to infarction of the third-nerve nucleus; and (e) skew deviation, with eyes positioned out of their normal vertical axis. Pupils are abnormal and often anisocoric. Pinpoint pupils indicate a lesion in the pons and mid-position pupils in the mesencephalon. The simultaneous appearance of pontine and mesencephalic type pupil in a comatose patient is diagnostic (Figure 30.2).[8]

When hemiparesis occurs, the most affected side may alternate from left to right in the first hours. In the extreme form, patients may have hemiparesis for a few hours, resolution, and then newly appearing hemiparesis on the opposite side, return of the initial hemiparesis,[87,88] and eventually quite rapid progression to significant paresis of all four limbs. The fluctuation of signs and symptoms may be related to position change, and the virtual disappearance of symptoms in the

---

CAPSULE 30.1   THE CLASSIC BRAINSTEM SYNDROMES

Eponym	Lesion	Features
Midbrain		
Weber	Cerebral peduncle	Ipsilateral III nerve palsy
		Contralateral hemiparesis
Benedikt	Tegmentum, red nucleus	Ipsilateral III nerve palsy
		Contralateral tremor, chorea
Parinaud	Quadrigeminal plate	Paralysis of upward gaze
Chiray-Foix-Nicolesco	Lateral mesencephalon	Hemiataxia
		Hemichorea
		Decreased vibration and proprioception
		Arm and leg weakness with or without facial weakness
Pons		
Raymond	Paramedian area	Ipsilateral lateral rectus muscle paresis, contralateral hemiplegia
Millard-Gubler	Medial lower	Ipsilateral facial palsy with contralateral hemiplegia (often also VI)
Foville	Medial lower	Ipsilateral VII
		Ipsilateral paralysis of lateral gaze
		Contralateral hemiparesis
Raymond-Céstan	Medial	Quadriplegia
		Anesthesia
		Nystagmus
Brissaud	Ventral	Ipsilateral facial spasm
		Contralateral hemiparesis
Medulla Oblongata		
Wallenberg	Lateral	Horner's syndrome (ipsilateral), IX, X
		Crossed hemianesthesia
Avellis	Nucleus ambiguus	X, XI palsy (ipsilateral face, contralateral body)
		Tractus solitarius
	Spinothalamic tract	Contralateral dissociated hemianesthesia
Schmidt	Vagal nuclei	X, XI
	Bulbar and spinal nuclei of accessory fibers	
Jackson	Nuclear vagus, accessory, Hypoglossus nerve	X, XI, XII
Tapia	Motor nuclei vagus and Hypoglossus	X, XII

---

supine or Trendelenburg position has been tentatively linked to an improvement in perfusion pressure in a slow-flow system. Hemiplegia falsely suggesting hemispheric involvement can be present in 40% of patients seen early in the course of the disorder. Initial occlusion of the paramedian penetrating arteries may produce hemiparesis and horizontal gaze palsy in association with normal speech, swallowing, and level of consciousness (Foville syndrome).

The course of basilar artery occlusion is often rapidly progressive. In a large series of patients seen early for consideration of IV thrombolysis only a few had a deficit at maximal onset.[28]

Breathing becomes clearly irregular in many patients, coughing is very weak, and when the

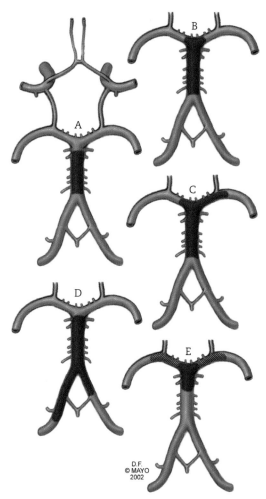

FIGURE 30.1: Sites of basilar artery occlusion.

Most likely as deduced from clinicopathologic correlation, (A) a thrombus occludes the paramedian or short circumferential branch, with possible further extension into the basilar artery (B), posterior cerebral artery (C), or vertebral artery (D). An embolus or thrombus may also lodge at the tip of the basilar artery (E), occluding supply to the thalamus, cerebral peduncle, and temporal and occipital lobes.

Modified from Kubik CS, Adams RD. Occlusion of the basilar artery: a clinical and pathological study. *Brain* 1946;69:73–121. With permission of Oxford University Press.

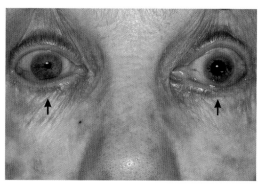

FIGURE 30.2: Patient with acute basilar artery occlusion and typical pontine and mesencephalic pupils.

From Burns et al.,[8] used with permission.

prompt immediate intubation and often further assistance with mechanical ventilation. Untreated, many patients become comatose, with bilateral unequal fixed pupils and extensor posturing. Terminal hyperthermia with temperatures reaching 40°C may occur.[43]

In complete occlusion of the basilar artery, the basis pontis may be destroyed, but the rostral tegmentum can be spared and level of consciousness is intact. In this so-called *locked-in syndrome*, patients are stuck in a motionless state, can feel and hear, and communication is possible only by vertical eye movements and blinking (Chapter 12).

Upon arrival in the NICU of any patient "comatose" due to acute basilar artery occlusion, one must eliminate the possibility of locked-in syndrome immediately by asking the patient to look up and blink on command. Failure of the examiner to recognize this condition may obviously cause unimaginable stress to the patient. Patients may hear any conversation and have to bear repetitive pain stimuli but cannot respond. In many patients, locked-in syndrome is not complete, and some motor function is preserved, including jaw opening and hand signaling. In other patients, consciousness is impaired from involvement of both thalami and extension to the tegmentum, and responses are not consistent.

Top-of-the-basilar artery syndrome is a constellation of signs and symptoms caused by an obstructing distal embolus. The strategic location of the clot at the juncture of the basilar artery with the posterior cerebral arteries and thalamic perforations produces, in addition to infarction in the mesencephalon, a fairly extensive area of infarction in thalamic nuclei, medial temporal lobes, and occipital lobes. At presentation, patients have

tegmentum is infarcted, sustained hyperventilation may occur. In patients with more extensive infarction of the pons, episodes with low respiratory rates, occasionally with superimposed gasps, may occur, all causing marginal gas exchange. Frequent episodes of apnea[44] or labored breathing from inability to protect the upper airway develop in most patients, and either condition should

an impaired, fluctuating level of consciousness from infarction of the bilateral paramedian rostral brainstem or the bithalamic nuclei. Typically, patients prefer to sleep most of the day, and response to questions is sluggish.

Visual hallucinations, which may include vivid colors, could be due to occipital lobe ischemia or brainstem involvement (peduncular hallucinations). Cortical blindness is unusual, but in some patients, brief episodes of sudden blindness have forewarned of basilar artery occlusion in this syndrome. As noted earlier, in addition to initial quadriplegia and dysarthria, findings often involve neuro-ophthalmologic signs, including pupillary abnormalities (pupils are poorly reactive and small), ptosis, third-nerve palsy, vertical or horizontal gaze abnormalities, skew deviation, and convergence nystagmus.

Brief extensor spasms—tonic fits[43,68]—are occasionally mistaken for seizures. These movements may be bizarre, including flapping, repetitive twitching, rhythmic shaking as in a chill, and head jerking with opisthotonos.[68] More often, they are myorhythmias involving facial musculature.

Acute basilar artery occlusion may have its origin in vertebral artery dissection.[32] This implies that not only the pons is affected but also the medulla oblongata and cerebellar hemispheres. The general physical examination of patients with a vertebral dissection should focus on predisposing conditions, although most dissections are spontaneous. Stigmata of Marfan disease[69] (dilated aortic root, joint laxity, and floppy mitral valve) and Ehlers-Danlos syndrome (easily bruising skin, hypermobile joints, and prolapse of mitral and tricuspid valves) should be recognized. Patients with vertebral artery dissection may present with severe neck pain and almost instantaneous brainstem findings. Although usually severe and intense, headache can be mild and may not even be present, further clouding recognition.[38] Most patients with vertebral artery dissection present with cerebellar symptoms (appendicular ataxia) or symptoms involving the lateral medulla oblongata (Horner's syndrome, horizontal-rotatory nystagmus directed away from the site of the lesion, ataxia, and crossed hemianesthesia).[32] Sensory involvement may include ipsilateral lower face, contralateral leg, and trunk hypalgesia or spinothalamic sensory loss (pinprick and temperature) at a midthoracic level. (This sensory level may falsely suggest a thoracic hemicord lesion.) The explanation is involvement of the far lateral spinothalamic fibers, sparing face and arm.[58,63] Dissection may be due to trauma, and other signs of traumatic brain injury may

be absent.[7] Sudden deterioration in level of consciousness may occur on the same day, quickly followed by brainstem signs.

Vertebral artery dissection may be associated with cerebellar infarction in young patients.[3,15,49,74,95] Neck manipulation from chiropractic therapy,[54,71] neck extension due to shampooing (beauty parlor stroke syndrome),[54,91] drinking ("bottoms up"), and polytrauma[7] have been particularly noted in young persons. Neck pain may be the only sign.[42] Although the relationship between chiropractic manipulation and vertebral artery dissection has been reported, the risk has not been appropriately defined in prospective studies.[71] Some patients may have sought a chiropractor for neck pain due to dissection. "Bone setters" in certain ethnic populations may apply vigorous neck manipulation.[66]

Dissection of the basilar artery is very uncommon, is more likely to occur in young patients, and is manifested by clinical symptoms of pontine infarction.[70,94] Dissection through the wall in the intradural, intracranial portion of the vertebral artery may lead to subarachnoid hemorrhage.[36]

NEUROIMAGING AND LABORATORY TESTS

Computed tomography (CT) scanning is the initial study, but in any lesion in the posterior fossa, it is significantly limited by degradation associated with bony artifacts. Computed tomography scanning may only demonstrate scattered hypodensities in cerebellar vascular territories in patients with massive pontine infarcts. In others, hypodensities on CT scan may be noted in the occipital lobe and thalamus, indicating a more distal basilar artery occlusion.

A fairly subtle early sign is a hyperdense basilar artery indicative of a clot and is virtually diagnostic if no intra-arterial density changes are seen in the supraclinoid portions of the carotid arteries.[31,77,89] This CT sign can be demonstrated at least 6 hours after onset,[31] with 71% sensitivity and 98% specificity (Figure 30.3). One study found attenuation measurement with a cut-off value of 46.5 HU is a reliable approach with high sensitivity.[22] The predictive value of the hyperdense basilar artery sign for outcome is not certain. Full recovery has been reported in patients with this sign, although it is often a predictor of long-term disability.[27,31] A CT scan may also show subarachnoid hemorrhage in some patients with dissection through the entire wall, predominantly in the basal cisterns but often with significant blood casts in the ventricles.[72]

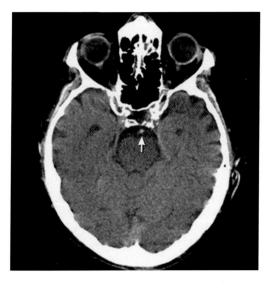

FIGURE 30.3: Computed tomography image showing characteristic hyperdense basilar artery sign (*arrow*).

Magnetic resonance imaging (MRI) confirms the diagnosis of acute basilar artery occlusion.[4,6,21,78] Magnetic resonance imaging not only delineates the area of pontine infarction but also may demonstrate absent flow in the basilar artery or a double lumen diagnostic of a dissection.[40] Magnetic resonance imaging can demonstrate abnormalities at the base of the pons, usually increased signal intensities on T2-weighted images, but findings can be normal as early as 12 hours after the episode, thus limiting its use in the early stage.[7,50] Magnetic resonance imaging fluid-attenuated inversion recovery (FLAIR) or diffusion-weighted sequences may be more useful to demonstrate early ischemic changes (Figure 30.4). Magnetic resonance angiography (MRA) may not be a perfect study in the detection of vertebral dissection,[45] tends to overestimate vertebrobasilar occlusive disease, and may falsely show lack of flow in a patent but severely narrowed lumen. Two-dimensional time-of-flight MRA is

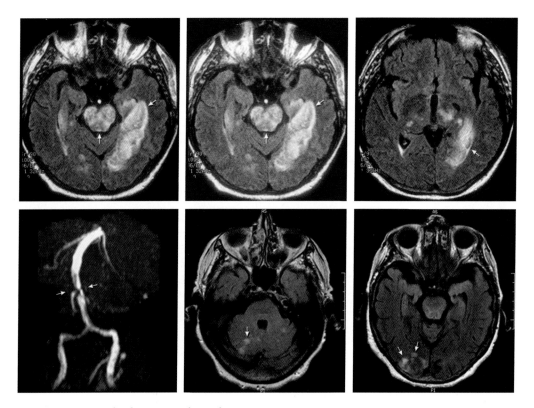

FIGURE 30.4: Acute basilar artery occlusive disease.

Upper row: Magnetic resonance imaging with fluid-attenuated inversion recovery sequence showing involvement of the pons, mesencephalon, mesial temporal lobe, thalamus, and occipital lobes typical of top-of the-basilar syndrome.
Lower row: Less severe involvement with mid-basilar stenosis and scattered cerebellar and occipital infarctions.

reasonably accurate (sensitivity, 100%; specificity, 75%–90%) in documenting occlusive disease in the basilar artery but less so in the vertebral artery.[6]

Transcranial Doppler ultrasonography may complement MRA, but the suboccipital probe usually cannot insonate the far distal portion of the basilar artery.

Computed tomography angiography has been used more frequently and is a useful first diagnostic test in many institutions throughout the world.[83] Although quite helpful to exclude major occlusive disease, it makes better sense to proceed with a selective cerebral angiogram when patients present early and have a limited deficit or deficit in flux.[9] With the arrival of intra-arterial thrombolytic therapy, cerebral angiography is performed more often and earlier.[92]

Cerebral angiography may demonstrate partial or complete occlusion of the basilar artery.[60] Most clots in the basilar artery are located in the middle or distal segments and often at the branching points. A proximal clot usually implies a trajectory from the confluence of the vertebral arteries to the branching of the anterior inferior cerebellar artery. A midbasilar clot is located between the anterior inferior and superior cerebellar arteries, and the remaining clots are designated distal clots. The distributions—proximal, middle, and distal—are, respectively, 45%, 35%, and 20%.[62] A typical pearl or string sign, double-contrast appearance, or sausage-like swelling strongly suggests vertebral dissection.

Assessment of collateral flow on cerebral angiography is important. One study suggested that lack of contralateral flow contributes to poor outcome despite recanalization of the basilar artery by thrombolysis.[61] Conversely, good collateral circulation (e.g., retrograde carotid artery to basilar artery, channeled through prominent posterior communicating arteries) may increase the chances of good functional survival with basilar artery occlusion.

Laboratory evaluation should include transesophageal echocardiography and studies of coagulation in young patients to exclude coagulopathy. Tests are needed to detect deficiency of antithrombin III and proteins C and S, as well as specific tests for the antiphospholipid syndrome, such as immunoglobulin (Ig)G or (less important and nonspecific) IgM antiphospholipid antibodies, Coombs test, antinuclear antibodies, activated partial thromboplastin time (aPTT) and partial prothrombin time (PTT), lupus anticoagulant, plasma homocysteine, and a blood smear.

FIRST STEPS IN MANAGEMENT

Management in acute basilar artery occlusion depends on clinical presentation—good or bad—and the availability of endovascular interventions (Table 30.1). Comparative studies of different modes of therapy are not available, and although therapeutic results remain anecdotal, most neurointensivists have no qualms about aggressive

TABLE 30.1. INITIAL MANAGEMENT OF ACUTE BASILAR ARTERY OCCLUSION

Airway management	Intubation if patient has hypoxemia despite facemask with 10 L of 60%–100% oxygen/minute, if abnormal respiratory drive or if abnormal protective reflexes (likely with motor response of withdrawal, or worse)
Mechanical ventilation	IMV/PS or CPAP mode; AC with aspiration pneumonitis
Fluid management	Maintenance with 3 L of 0.9% NaCl: Flat body position
Blood pressure management	Blood pressure augmentation with IV phenylephrine to mean arterial pressure of 100–120 mm Hg can be considered
Nutrition	Enteral nutrition with continuous infusion (on day 2)
	Blood glucose control (goal 140–180 mg/dL)
Prophylaxis	DVT prophylaxis with pneumatic compression devices
	SC heparin 5000 U t.i.d.
	GI prophylaxis: pantoprazole 40 mg IV daily or lansoprazole 30 mg orally through nasogastric tube.
Endovascular therapy	Mechanical retrieval of clot and possibly angioplasty
	Intraarterial tissue plasminogen activator
Access	Arterial catheter to monitor blood pressure (if vasopressors are anticipated)
	Peripheral venous catheter or Peripheral inserted central catheter

AC, Assist control; CPAP, continuous positive airway pressure; DVT, deep vein thrombosis; GI, gastrointestinal; IMV, intermittent mandatory ventilation; IV, intravenously; NaCl, sodium chloride; PS, pressure support; SC, subcutaneously.

endovascular intervention. Within the wide spectrum of presentations, we generally do not consider cerebral angiography and thrombolytic therapy in apneic patients who have lost virtually all brainstem reflexes and have early infarction in pons and cerebellum, but fortunately such a presentation is not common. Only a few case reports have noted dramatic awakening from coma with angiographically proven recanalization,[33,34,57] and in a larger experience in treated comatose patients with acute basilar artery occlusion, mortality was high (of 12 patients, 10 died, 6 of whom had basilar artery recanalization).[37] Little experience is reported in patients with locked-in syndrome who had successful opening of the basilar artery after thrombolytic treatment. In our experience, recanalization of the basilar artery resulted in no measurable neurologic deficit in two patients with locked-in syndrome.[92]

The approach is more or less as in a stroke in the anterior circulation. The main objective is to obtain recanalization of a proximal clot—in this situation, it is mostly mid-basilar. Earlier case series in management of basilar artery occlusion have clearly defined the potential of thrombolytic therapy, including the now suspended urokinase.[1,17,28,34,62,92] Thrombolysis may increase the risk of intracranial hematoma; in a series of 66 patients, fatal pontine hemorrhage developed in two patients after successful recanalization, but large doses were required to achieve clot lysis.[28] Mechanical clot fragmentation and suctioning or stent assisted clot retrieval is the most used endovascular technique, and it may include angioplasty. First, cerebral angiography maps out the extent of occlusion and collateral anatomy. Second, in some patients, mechanical fragmentation and retrieval alone may be successful with no need for additional IA thrombolysis.

IV thrombolytic therapy should remain standard also in the posterior circulation, but there is still an inability to reopen the occlusion in approximately 40%, and poor results are expected in patients who are comatose. Thrombolytic therapy may be withheld in patients who have marked fluctuation in clinical signs and are improving considerably. We have considered thrombolysis in a patient with fluctuating signs but sudden worsening of symptoms. Absence of tetraparesis and no alterations in consciousness probably also justify a more conservative approach.[62] In the Finnish IV thrombolysis experience, recanalization up to 48 hours resulted in 50% improvement in the absence of baseline ischemia and no increase in intracerebral hematoma.[82]

Limited areas of cerebral infarction noted on CT or We and others have been successful in reversing neurologic deficit in patients with limited MRI abnormalities, but whether to intervene with large infarctions is simply not known.[18,59,92] MRI should not be interpreted as low probability of success with thrombolytic agents, nor is the time beyond 12 hours considered a strict contraindication.

In contrast to clot occlusion in the anterior circulation, an embolus to the basilar artery may propagate, grow, knock out perforators one by one[48]. We have not hesitated to proceed with a cerebral angiogram to subsequently retrieve a clot more or less independent of the time of onset. Suction or stent retrieval of the clot is attempted and may be supplemented with intra-arterial thrombolysis with tissue plasminogen activator (tPA).[17,55] If after successful recanalization there is a remaining midbasilar occlusion, an angioplasty or expandable stent can be considered[84,85] (Figures 30.5 and 30.6). Dilatation of the basilar artery may reduce the risk of future occlusion of that artery, and clots may pass into the smaller branches with less damage. The potential for artery-to-artery embolization is not likely to be reduced with these procedures, and the potential for damage to the multiple perforations also remains considerable. Endovascular stenting after thrombolysis of an acutely thrombosed basilar artery resulted in good patency, but the risks of placement and choice of stent are unclear.[64]

Approaches to the management of acute basilar occlusion may vary substantially. For example, in one study, 32 patients with acute basilar artery occlusion were treated with intra-arterial tPA alone, and in 43 patients, intra-arterial tPA was preceded by intravenous abciximab. In addition, in this study, mechanical disruption was attempted in both groups. This approach resulted in better recanalization rates in the combination therapy (from 62% to 84%) without increase in symptomatic cerebral hemorrhage.[55] Studies with multiple drugs and use of a mechanical device in a single patient remain difficult to interpret, but there has been a tendency to use all available measures to improve outcome in these patients.[23,25,55,90,96]

Over the last few years, the experience with stent-assisted clot retrieval has rapidly increased. Most reported series start with IV thrombolysis first, and subsequently use a stent-retriever and this approach has significantly increased recanalization.[52,80] Recanalization (defined as TICI 2b + 3) occurred in three of four patients, but neurologic improvement (defined as ≥ 10 in NIHSS) in only one in two patients.[52]

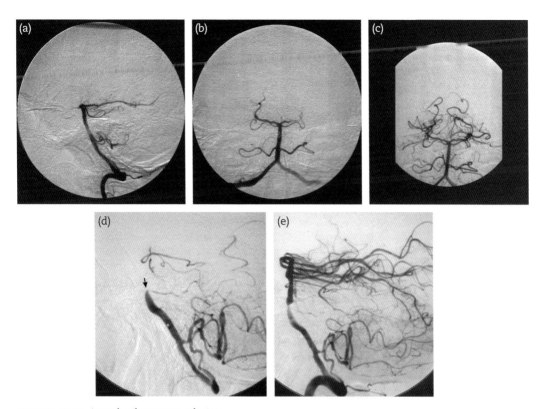

FIGURE 30.5: Acute basilar artery occlusion.

Thrombi in the mid-basilar artery distal to the origins of the anterior inferior cerebellar arteries and in the left posterior cerebral artery. (a, b, c) Dissolution of the thrombus in the basilar artery and restoration of flow of the distal left posterior cerebral artery after thrombolysis. The patient remained dysarthric, but left hemiparesis and an internuclear ophthalmoplegia resolved completely. (d) In another patient, occlusive thrombus in the proximal basilar artery was accompanied by some collateral reconstitution. (e) Complete opening was achieved, but a significant basilar artery stenosis remained. The patient made a complete recovery.

On the other hand, failure to recanalize doubles mortality and virtually leads to a poor outcome if there are also poor collaterals. Comparable results (but still 30% mortality) were found in other recent studies.[53,80] Time to intervention does not seem to impact outcome and is determined largely by the presence or absence of collateral circulation.[80]

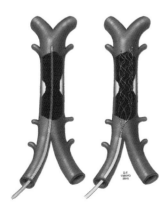

FIGURE 30.6: Stent retrieval of clot and balloon dilatation of remaining basilar artery stenosis.

If feasible, follow-up MRI can be performed. Scattered infarcts in the cerebellum or pons may account for any remaining clinical symptoms in patients with recanalization, but may also appear in clinically asymptomatic patients.

Patients who return to the NICU after thrombolysis need further supportive measures. Mechanical ventilation is continued if apneic episodes exist or if progressive drowsiness results in an inability to protect the airway. Death from sudden apnea has been reported, including in patients with a unilateral brainstem infarct.[39] Marked swallowing difficulties and difficulty in clearing secretions can be managed with glycopyrrolate to reduce secretions. In patients with a massive pontine infarct and no clinical change in 1–2 weeks, one should proceed with a tracheostomy if the patient or family members support further management despite expectations of poor outcome. Blood pressure needs to be carefully controlled and may be abnormal in both directions. Acute basilar artery occlusion is often associated with longstanding hypertension and cardiovascular disease, and hypertension may become difficult to control soon after the ictus. In other patients, blood pressure may border on hypotension. Fluctuations in motor weakness can be linked to hypotension, and may disappear with increasing blood pressure with low doses of vasopressors. One may find marginal ventricular function in some of these patients with acute basilar artery occlusion, with a decreased ejection fraction on echocardiography.

These patients are probably best treated flat or in a Trendelenburg position in the first 24 hours. Administration of diuretic and antihypertensive agents is discontinued. Blood pressure may be increased by use of vasopressors or inotropes. The use of vasopressors, however, is at the expense of ventricular irritability (predominantly premature ventricular contractions) and an increase in heart rate. Hemodynamic augmentation can be continued for a few days, and then the dose should be tapered. At that time, the clinical outcome should become clear, and further management decisions should be based on the severity of the clinical deficit.

The management of blood pressure may be different and more prudent, however, in patients with acute vertebral artery dissection. In patients with a typical history of vertebral dissection or angiographic confirmation, control of blood pressure should possibly be more aggressive. Whether normalization of blood pressure reduces the risk of extension of the dissection to a larger segment or dissection through the entire wall is not known. In fact, progression of the dissection when monitored by repeated angiography is seldom seen.[41] The ideal blood pressure in patients with vertebral artery dissection has not been established, but it may be prudent to attempt to attain normal mean arterial pressure values of 90–100 mm Hg. One should be particularly alert to vertebral artery dissection associated with a lateral medullary infarct (Wallenberg syndrome), which may be associated with dysautonomia, supine hypotension, and significant bradycardia.[39]

Normal maintenance fluids with 0.9% sodium chloride should suffice. In stable patients, swallowing should be assessed before liquid foods are given orally. In patients with massive pontine infarction and mechanical ventilation, it is reasonable to proceed with percutaneous endoscopic gastrostomy.

Intravenous heparin has been a common treatment in acute basilar occlusion (aPTT of 1.5–2 times control). However, whether heparin is effective in patients with acute basilar artery occlusion and major neurologic deficits is very doubtful, and often deterioration continues in most patients despite adequate anticoagulation.[93] It is important that a therapeutic level be achieved promptly, and a weight-based nomogram should be used to calculate the dose. The weight-based nomogram has a tendency to exceed the PTT value, but in a patient with a deteriorating basilar artery occlusion, it is probably less troublesome than inadequate anticoagulation. Survivors with a mild neurologic deficit and high-grade stenosis of the basilar trunk of the artery can be treated with warfarin, but management should be readdressed if marked ataxia is observed at the first attempts of mobilization from bed rest.

DETERIORATION: CAUSES AND MANAGEMENT

Fluctuating deficits, some of which are profound, are typical in basilar artery occlusion, but pathophysiologically are not fully explained. Failing collaterals with hypotension and recovery with blood pressure augmentation may be considered; but in others, a propagating clot knocks off a series of penetrations leading to clinical progressions with fits and starts.

A maximal deficit is present on the first day of admission in approximately one-third of the patients.[24] In another third, deterioration from further outgrowth of the clot results in successive occlusion of perforating arteries originating from the basilar artery. Many patients devastated by occlusion of the basilar artery remain in coma, with retention of some brainstem reflexes. Acute basilar artery occlusion rarely results in complete loss of brainstem reflexes, and some function of the medulla oblongata often remains.

An unfortunate cause of secondary deterioration is reocclusion after recanalization by thrombolysis. Patients with significant remaining stenosis of the basilar artery and possibly patients with small or absent posterior communicating arteries are at risk. We and others have been administering the intravenous antiplatelet drug abciximab in such instances. Successful improvement after reocclusion in at least one patient has been reported,[25,90] but with our very limited experience, we have not yet noted substantial clinical improvement.

Pontine hemorrhage may occur and is immediately devastating. As expected, it is most common after use of intra-arterial thrombolytic agents. Only survival in a disabled state has been reported, and most patients die.

Patients with vertebral artery dissection rarely have deterioration, and in most the event is monophasic. Patients with dissection and recurrent transient ischemic attacks in the posterior circulation can be successfully treated with balloon occlusion of the vertebral artery if sufficient collateral circulation is present. This usually implies retrograde flow from the contralateral vertebral artery to the ipsilateral posterior inferior cerebellar artery.[30,51]

OUTCOME

Persistent coma after the onset of acute basilar artery occlusion strongly predicts poor outcome.[20] Outcome is particularly poor in patients with acute basilar occlusion who remain comatose and are supported by mechanical ventilation. Of 25 comatose patients with acute basilar occlusion and mechanical ventilation, none had any improvement in neurologic function in the next 2–3 weeks.[93] Weaning from the ventilator and spontaneous breathing through a T-tube circuit were possible in patients intubated for airway protection. In eight patients, apneic episodes prompted intubation, and all had progression within 24–48 hours to locked-in syndrome or lost most brainstem reflexes. Most comatose patients with basilar artery occlusion and the need for mechanical ventilation died after withdrawal of support at the request of family members; in others, fatal aspiration pneumonitis or cardiac arrest in association with acute myocardial infarction occurred.[93]

Mortality remains high in patients with acute basilar artery occlusion, but a favorable outcome is possible in some patients with limited neurologic deficits.[10,26] Patients with limited infarcts in the pons may have a reasonable functional outcome, although diplopia may be a major handicap. If infarction remains limited to the lateral medulla, long-term outcome is good, and recurrent strokes in the posterior circulation are uncommon.[47,49,58] Patients with top-of-the-basilar syndrome may be severely disabled from a memory deficit caused by bilateral thalamic involvement.

Patients with locked-in syndrome from brainstem infarction have a high mortality. A review of the literature noted 67% mortality in 117 patients.[29] Long-term survival from locked-in syndrome is possible, even beyond a decade after the onset, but only with continuously dedicated nursing care. Recovery from complete locked-in syndrome is not expected but, recovery to a more functional state has been reported. It is impossible to predict which patients with locked-in syndrome will improve. They may have gradual improvement, over a period of months, regaining some muscle strength, but the ultimate result is marked pseudobulbar palsy with spastic tetraparesis. In addition, many patients die of intercurrent pulmonary infection. It should be pointed out that patients with incomplete locked-in syndrome (spared oropharyngeal function and some element of motor function) may improve considerably despite MRI documentation of pontine infarction. On multiple occasions, we have observed this pattern—poor outcome when complete, possible functional recovery when incomplete. MRI shows significant neuronal loss but despite all that clinical and functional improvement is still possible in patients with incomplete locked-in syndrome (Figure 30.7).[35]

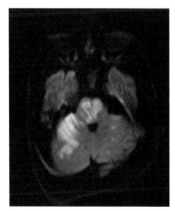 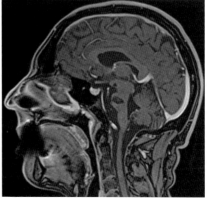

FIGURE 30.7: Serial MRI showing extensive pontine infarction in a patient with incomplete locked-in syndrome and good clinical improvement.[35]

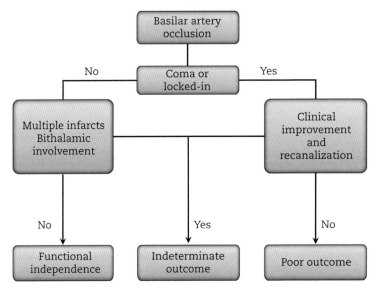

FIGURE 30.8: Outcome algorithm in acute basilar artery occlusion.

Functional independence: No assistance needed, minor handicap may remain. Indeterminate: Any statement would be a premature conclusion. Poor outcome: Severe disability, prolonged comatose state, or death.

There is no incentive to maintain a high level of critical care in comatose, ventilated patients with MRI-demonstrated massive pontine infarction. When diffusion-weighted MRI shows signal changes in multi-territorial areas it strongly correlates with poor clinical condition and poor outcome.[16,67] Life-prolonging procedures, such as cardiac resuscitation, tracheostomy, and percutaneous endoscopic gastrostomy, may not be warranted.

Long-term outcome in vertebral dissection has not been studied, but in patients with cervical artery dissection, the risk of recurrence is 1% and is greater in younger patients.[75] In most patients, brainstem stroke is a single event, and follow-up by MRA shows complete resolution of the dissection within 3 months.[65,75]

In summary, good outcome from acute basilar artery occlusion is possible in patients with limited clinical deficits and certain cerebral angiographic criteria, such as short segmental occlusions, distal clot, and good collateral supply.[10,18,19,60,79] Outcome does not seem to be measurably influenced by time between onset and recanalization.[81] In these fortunate patients the clinical course is usually recognized by slowly progressive deficits and often by marked fluctuation, whereas in patients with poor outcome, the maximal neurologic deficit often

arrives early. An outcome algorithm is shown in Figure 30.8.

CONCLUSIONS

- Tissue plasminogen activator, 90 mg intravenous dose in 1 hour (10% in bolus, 90% by infusion), should be considered standard before endovascular intervention.
- Endovascular treatment should be considered in patients with acute basilar artery occlusion seen within 12–24 hours. Intervention is determined by the appearance of a fixed deficit and not when fluctuation of signs started.
- Standard management includes IV heparin (aPTT 1.5–2 times the control value). In patients with hypotension, consider further blood pressure support with flat body position and vasopressors to achieve a mean arterial pressure of 100–120 mm Hg.
- Mechanical ventilation for apneic episodes, persistent coma for 1 week, and MRI showing entire pontine infarction carry a very poor prognosis.
- Good outcome can be expected in patients with a slowly progressive clinical course, limited neurologic deficits, short segmental abnormalities, and good collateral flow on cerebral angiography.

REFERENCES

1. US Food and Drug Administration. Letter to healthcare providers In: Food and Drug Administration, ed. Washington, DC, January 25, 1999.
2. Baird TA, Muir KW, Bone I. Basilar artery occlusion. *Neurocrit Care* 2004;1:319–329.
3. Barinagarrementeria F, Amaya LE, Cantu C. Causes and mechanisms of cerebellar infarction in young patients. *Stroke* 1997;28:2400 2404.
4. Bhadelia RA, Bengoa F, Gesner L, et al. Efficacy of MR angiography in the detection and characterization of occlusive disease in the vertebrobasilar system. *J Comput Assist Tomogr* 2001;25:458–465.
5. Biemond A. Thrombosis of the basilar artery and the vascularization of the brain stem. *Brain* 1951;74:300–317.
6. Biller J, Yuh WT, Mitchell GW, Bruno A, Adams HP, Jr. Early diagnosis of basilar artery occlusion using magnetic resonance imaging. *Stroke* 1988;19:297–306.
7. Blacker DJ, Wijdicks EFM. Clinical characteristics and mechanisms of stroke after polytrauma. *Mayo Clinic Proc* 2004;79:630–635.
8. Burns JD, Schiefer TK, Wijdicks EFM. Large and small: a telltale sign of acute pontomesencephalic injury. *Neurology* 2009;72:1707.
9. Caplan LR. Dissections of brain-supplying arteries. *Nat Clin Pract Neurol* 2008;4:34–42.
10. Caplan LR. Occlusion of the vertebral or basilar artery: follow up analysis of some patients with benign outcome. *Stroke* 1979;10:277–282.
11. Caplan LR. *Posterior Circulation Disease: Clinical Findings, Diagnosis, and Management.* Cambridge, MA: Blackwell Science; 1996.
12. Caplan LR. "Top of the basilar" syndrome. *Neurology* 1980;30:72–79.
13. Caplan LR. Vertebrobasilar embolism. *Clin Exp Neurol* 1991;28:1–22.
14. Caplan LR, Rosenbaum AE. Role of cerebral angiography in vertebrobasilar occlusive disease. *J Neurol Neurosurg Psychiatry* 1975;38:601–612.
15. Caplan LR, Wityk RJ, Glass TA, et al. New England Medical Center Posterior Circulation registry. *Ann Neurol* 2004;56:389–398.
16. Cho TH, Nighoghossian N, Tahon F, et al. Brain stem diffusion-weighted imaging lesion score: a potential marker of outcome in acute basilar artery occlusion. *AJNR Am J Neuroradiol* 2009;30:194–198.
17. Cross DT, 3rd, Derdeyn CP, Moran CJ. Bleeding complications after basilar artery fibrinolysis with tissue plasminogen activator. *AJNR Am J Neuroradiol* 2001;22:521–525.
18. Cross DT, 3rd, Moran CJ, Akins PT, et al. Collateral circulation and outcome after basilar artery thrombolysis. *AJNR Am J Neuroradiol* 1998;19:1557–1563.
19. Cross DT, 3rd, Moran CJ, Akins PT, Angtuaco EE, Diringer MN. Relationship between clot location and outcome after basilar artery thrombolysis. *AJNR Am J Neuroradiol* 1997;18:1221–1228.
20. Devuyst G, Bogousslavsky J, Meuli R, et al. Stroke or transient ischemic attacks with basilar artery stenosis or occlusion: clinical patterns and outcome. *Arch Neurol* 2002;59:567–573.
21. Du Mesnil de Rochemont R, Neumann-Haefelin T, Berkefeld J, Sitzer M, Lanfermann H. Magnetic resonance imaging in basilar artery occlusion. *Arch Neurol* 2002;59:398–402.
22. Ernst M, Romero JM, Buhk JH, et al. Sensitivity of hyperdense basilar artery sign on non-enhanced computed tomography. *PLoS One.* 2015 Oct 19;10(10):e0141096.
23. Favrole P, Saint-Maurice JP, Bousser MG, Houdart E. Use of mechanical extraction devices in basilar artery occlusion. *J Neurol Neurosurg Psychiatry* 2005;76:1462–1464.
24. Ferbert A, Bruckmann H, Drummen R. Clinical features of proven basilar artery occlusion. *Stroke* 1990;21:1135–1142.
25. Gaikwad SB, Padma MV, Moses EJ, et al. Intra-arterial thrombolysis in basilar artery occlusions combination of intra-arterial thrombolytics and Gp IIb/IIIa inhibitors in basilar artery thrombosis. *Neurol India* 2009;57:313–319.
26. Glass TA, Hennessey PM, Pazdera L, et al. Outcome at 30 days in the New England Medical Center Posterior Circulation Registry. *Arch Neurol* 2002;59:369–376.
27. Goldmakher GV, Camargo EC, Furie KL, et al. Hyperdense basilar artery sign on unenhanced CT predicts thrombus and outcome in acute posterior circulation stroke. *Stroke* 2009;40:134–139.
28. Hacke W, Zeumer H, Ferbert A, Bruckmann H, del Zoppo GJ. Intra-arterial thrombolytic therapy improves outcome in patients with acute vertebrobasilar occlusive disease. *Stroke* 1988;19:1216–1222.
29. Haig AJ, Katz RT, Sahgal V. Mortality and complications of the locked-in syndrome. *Arch Phys Med Rehabil* 1987;68:24–27.
30. Halbach VV, Higashida RT, Dowd CF, et al. Endovascular treatment of vertebral artery dissections and pseudoaneurysms. *J Neurosurg* 1993;79:183–191.
31. Harrington T, Roche J. The dense basilar artery as a sign of basilar territory infarction. *Australas Radiol* 1993;37:375–378.
32. Hart RG. Vertebral artery dissection. *Neurology* 1988;38:987–989.

33. Hayashi J, Oguma F, Miyamura H, Eguchi S, Koike T. Direct thrombolytic revascularization of the occluded basilar artery. *Cardiovasc Surg* 1993;1:547–549.

34. Herderschee D, Limburg M, Hijdra A, Koster PA. Recombinant tissue plasminogen activator in two patients with basilar artery occlusion. *J Neurol Neurosurg Psychiatry* 1991;54:71–73.

35. Hocker S, Wijdicks EFM. Recovery from locked-in syndrome. *JAMA Neurol* 2015;72:832–833.

36. Hosoda K, Fujita S, Kawaguchi T, et al. Spontaneous dissecting aneurysms of the basilar artery presenting with a subarachnoid hemorrhage: report of two cases. *J Neurosurg* 1991;75:628–633.

37. Huemer M, Niederwieser V, Ladurner G. Thrombolytic treatment for acute occlusion of the basilar artery. *J Neurol Neurosurg Psychiatry* 1995;58:227–228.

38. Iwase H, Kobayashi M, Kurata A, Inoue S. Clinically unidentified dissection of vertebral artery as a cause of cerebellar infarction. *Stroke* 2001;32:1422–1424.

39. Khurana RK. Autonomic dysfunction in pontomedullary stroke. [Abstract]. *Ann Neurol* 1982;12:86.

40. Kitanaka C, Tanaka J, Kuwahara M, Teraoka A. Magnetic resonance imaging study of intracranial vertebrobasilar artery dissections. *Stroke* 1994;25:571–575.

41. Kitanaka C, Tanaka J, Kuwahara M, et al. Nonsurgical treatment of unruptured intracranial vertebral artery dissection with serial follow-up angiography. *J Neurosurg* 1994;80:667–674.

42. Krespi Y, Gurol ME, Coban O, Tuncay R, Bahar S. Vertebral artery dissection presenting with isolated neck pain. *J Neuroimaging* 2002;12:179–182.

43. Kubik CS, Adams RD. Occlusion of the basilar artery; a clinical and pathological study. *Brain* 1946;69:73–121.

44. Levin BE, Margolis G. Acute failure of automatic respirations secondary to a unilateral brainstem infarct. *Ann Neurol* 1977;1:583–586.

45. Levy C, Laissy JP, Raveau V, et al. Carotid and vertebral artery dissections: three-dimensional time-of-flight MR angiography and MR imaging versus conventional angiography. *Radiology* 1994;190:97–103.

46. Lindsberg PJ, Mattle HP. Therapy of basilar artery occlusion: a systematic analysis comparing intra-arterial and intravenous thrombolysis. *Stroke* 2006;37:922–928.

47. Lindsberg PJ, Soinne L, Tatlisumak T, et al. Long-term outcome after intravenous thrombolysis of basilar artery occlusion. *JAMA* 2004;292:1862–1866.

48. Lindsberg PJ, Pekkola J, Strbian D, et al. Time window for recanalization in basilar artery occlusion: Speculative synthesis. *Neurology* 2015;85:1806–1815.

49. Malm J, Kristensen B, Carlberg B, Fagerlund M, Olsson T. Clinical features and prognosis in young adults with infratentorial infarcts. *Cerebrovasc Dis* 1999;9:282–289.

50. Martinez HR, Elizondo G, Herrera J, et al. Basilar artery thrombosis diagnosed by MR imaging. *AJNR Am J Neuroradiol* 1989;10:S81.

51. McCormick GF, Halbach VV. Recurrent ischemic events in two patients with painless vertebral artery dissection. *Stroke* 1993;24:598–602.

52. Mohlenbruch M, Stampfl S, Behrens L, et al. Mechanical thrombectomy with stent retrievers in acute basilar artery occlusion. *AJNR Am J Neuroradiol* 2014;35:959–964.

53. Mourand I, Machi P, Nogue E, et al. Diffusion-weighted imaging score of the brain stem: a predictor of outcome in acute basilar artery occlusion treated with the Solitaire FR device. *AJNR Am J Neuroradiol* 2014;35:1117–1123.

54. Mueller S, Sahs AL. Brain stem dysfunction related to cervical manipulation: report of three cases. *Neurology* 1976;26:547–550.

55. Nagel S, Schellinger PD, Hartmann M, et al. Therapy of acute basilar artery occlusion: intra-arterial thrombolysis alone vs bridging therapy. *Stroke* 2009;40:140–146.

56. Nakayama T, Tanaka K, Kaneko M, Yokoyama T, Uemura K. Thrombolysis and angioplasty for acute occlusion of intracranial vertebrobasilar arteries: report of three cases. *J Neurosurg* 1998;88:919–922.

57. Nenci GG, Gresele P, Taramelli M, Agnelli G, Signorini E. Thrombolytic therapy for thromboembolism of vertebrobasilar artery. *Angiology* 1983;34:561–571.

58. Norrving B, Cronqvist S. Lateral medullary infarction: prognosis in an unselected series. *Neurology* 1991;41:244–248.

59. Ostrem JL, Saver JL, Alger JR, et al. Acute basilar artery occlusion: diffusion-perfusion MRI characterization of tissue salvage in patients receiving intra-arterial stroke therapies. *Stroke* 2004;35:e30–e34.

60. Pessin MS, Gorelick PB, Kwan ES, Caplan LR. Basilar artery stenosis: middle and distal segments. *Neurology* 1987;37:1742–1746.

61. Pfeiffer G, Thayssen G, Arlt A, et al. Vertebrobasilar occlusion: outcome with and without local intra-arterial fibrinolysis. In: Hacke W, del Zoppo GJ, Hirschberg M, eds. *Thrombolytic Therapy in Acute Ischemic Stroke*. New York: Springer-Verlag; 1991:216–220.

62. Phan TG, Wijdicks EFM. Intra-arterial thrombolysis for vertebrobasilar circulation ischemia. *Crit Care Clin* 1999;15;719–742, vi

63. Phan TG, Wijdicks EFM. A sensory level on the trunk and sparing the face from vertebral artery dissection: how much more subtle can we get? *J Neurol Neurosurg Psychiatry* 1999;66:691–692.

64. Phatouros CC, Higashida RT, Malek AM, et al. Endovascular stenting of an acutely thrombosed basilar artery: technical case report and review of the literature. *Neurosurgery* 1999;44:667–673.

65. Pozzati E, Padovani R, Fabrizi A, Sabattini L, Gaist G. Benign arterial dissections of the posterior circulation. *J Neurosurg* 1991;75:69–72.

66. Quintana JG, Drew EC, Richtsmeier TE, Davis LE. Vertebral artery dissection and stroke following neck manipulation by Native American healer. *Neurology* 2002;58:1434–1435.

67. Renard D, Landragin N, Robinson A, et al. MRI-based score for acute basilar artery thrombosis. *Cerebrovasc Dis* 2008;25:511–516.

68. Ropper AH. 'Convulsions' in basilar artery occlusion. *Neurology* 1988;38:1500–1501.

69. Rose BS, Pretorius DL. Dissecting basilar artery aneurysm in Marfan syndrome: case report. *AJNR Am J Neuroradiol* 1991;12:503–504.

70. Ross GJ, Ferraro F, DeRiggi L, Scotti LN. Spontaneous healing of basilar artery dissection: MR findings. *J Comput Assist Tomogr* 1994;18:292–294.

71. Rothwell DM, Bondy SJ, Williams JI. Chiropractic manipulation and stroke: a population-based case-control study. *Stroke* 2001;32:1054–1060.

72. Sasaki O, Ogawa H, Koike T, Koizumi T, Tanaka R. A clinicopathological study of dissecting aneurysms of the intracranial vertebral artery. *J Neurosurg* 1991;75:874–882.

73. Savitz SI, Caplan LR. Vertebrobasilar disease. *N Engl J Med* 2005;352:2618–2626.

74. Schievink WI. Spontaneous dissection of the carotid and vertebral arteries. *N Engl J Med* 2001;344:898–906.

75. Schievink WI, Mokri B, O'Fallon WM. Recurrent spontaneous cervical-artery dissection. *N Engl J Med* 1994;330:393–397.

76. Schonewille WJ, Wijman CA, Michel P, et al. Treatment and outcomes of acute basilar artery occlusion in the Basilar Artery International Cooperation Study (BASICS): a prospective registry study. *Lancet Neurol* 2009;8:724–730.

77. Schuknecht B, Ratzka M, Hofmann E. The "dense artery sign": major cerebral artery thromboembolism demonstrated by computed tomography. *Neuroradiology* 1990;32:98–103.

78. Schwaighofer BW, Klein MV, Lyden PD, Hesselink JR. MR imaging of vertebrobasilar vascular disease. *J Comput Assist Tomogr* 1990;14:895–904.

79. Schwarz S, Egelhof T, Schwab S, Hacke W. Basilar artery embolism: clinical syndrome and neuroradiologic patterns in patients without permanent occlusion of the basilar artery. *Neurology* 1997;49:1346–1352.

80. Singer OC, Berkefeld J, Nolte CH, et al. Mechanical recanalization in basilar artery occlusion: the ENDOSTROKE study. *Ann Neurol* 2015;77:415–424.

81. Sliwka U, Mull M, Stelzer A, Diehl R, Noth J. Long-term follow-up of patients after intra-arterial thrombolytic therapy of acute vertebrobasilar artery occlusion. *Cerebrovasc Dis* 2001;12:214–219.

82. Strbian D, Sairanen T, Silvennoinen H, et al. Thrombolysis of basilar artery occlusion: impact of baseline ischemia and time. *Ann Neurol* 2013;73:688–694.

83. Sylaja PN, Puetz V, Dzialowski I, et al. Prognostic value of CT angiography in patients with suspected vertebrobasilar ischemia. *J Neuroimaging* 2008;18:46–49.

84. Terada T, Higashida RT, Halbach VV, et al. Transluminal angioplasty for arteriosclerotic disease of the distal vertebral and basilar arteries. *J Neurol Neurosurg Psychiatry* 1996;60:377–381.

85. Terada T, Yokote H, Tsuura M, et al. Tissue plasminogen activator thrombolysis and transluminal angioplasty in the treatment of basilar artery thrombosis: case report. *Surg Neurol* 1994;41:358–361.

86. Veltkamp R, Jacobi C, Kress B, Hacke W. Prolonged low-dose intravenous thrombolysis in a stroke patient with distal basilar thrombus. *Stroke* 2006;37:e9–e11.

87. Voetsch B, DeWitt LD, Pessin MS, Caplan LR. Basilar artery occlusive disease in the New England Medical Center Posterior Circulation Registry. *Arch Neurol* 2004;61:496–504.

88. von Campe G, Regli F, Bogousslavsky J. Heralding manifestations of basilar artery occlusion with lethal or severe stroke. *J Neurol Neurosurg Psychiatry* 2003;74:1621–1626.

89. Vonofakos D, Marcu H, Hacker H. CT diagnosis of basilar artery occlusion. *AJNR Am J Neuroradiol* 1983;4:525–528.

90. Wallace RC, Furlan AJ, Moliterno DJ, et al. Basilar artery rethrombosis: successful treatment with platelet glycoprotein IIB/IIIA receptor inhibitor. *AJNR Am J Neuroradiol* 1997;18:1257–1260.

91. Weintraub MI. Beauty parlor stroke syndrome: report of five cases. *JAMA* 1993;269:2085–2086.

92. Wijdicks EFM, Nichols DA, Thielen KR, et al. Intra-arterial thrombolysis in acute basilar artery thromboembolism: the initial Mayo Clinic experience. *Mayo Clinic Proc* 1997;72:1005–1013.

93. Wijdicks EFM, Scott JP. Outcome in patients with acute basilar artery occlusion requiring mechanical ventilation. *Stroke* 1996;27:1301–1303.

94. Yoshimoto Y, Hoya K, Tanaka Y, Uchida T. Basilar artery dissection. *J Neurosurg* 2005;102:476–481.

95. Youl BD, Coutellier A, Dubois B, Leger JM, Bousser MG. Three cases of spontaneous extracranial vertebral artery dissection. *Stroke* 1990;21:618–625.

96. Yu W, Binder D, Foster-Barber A, et al. Endovascular embolectomy of acute basilar artery occlusion. *Neurology* 2003;61:1421–1423.

31

Cerebellar Infarct

Sizable cerebellar infarcts may require monitoring in the neurosciences intensive care unit (NICU). Cerebellar infarction can be isolated or can coexist with other regions such as the brainstem, thalamus, or cortical infarcts. Cerebellar infarcts may become of greater relevance when swollen tissue produces a mass effect and usually within 3 days, signs of swelling could overshadow vertigo and ataxia. Mass effect develops more frequently in patients with full territorial cerebellar infarcts, although only half deteriorate.[21] Clinical deterioration may be particularly more frequent in patients with a posterior inferior cerebellar artery (PICA) occlusion or superior cerebellar artery (SCA) occlusion and in those with infarcts confined to the medial vermian hemispheric branches of these arteries.[11,17,20] Involvement of the anterior inferior cerebellar artery (AICA) is much less associated with mass effect.[21]

The initial phase of cerebellar infarction is punctuated by clinical signs from cerebellar dysfunction, and physicians need to recognize the subsequent stage of brainstem compression or ventricular obstruction. Deterioration could prompt neurosurgical intervention to remove the necrotic tissue or to place a ventriculostomy tube.

There are some similarities in clinical course with cerebellar hemorrhage (Chapter 28), but swelling after infarction of a cerebellar hemisphere is more protracted. Nonetheless, one must implicitly assume that early recognition of deterioration in cerebellar stroke cannot be guaranteed in a neurologic ward, and not much should stand in the way to admit these patients to the NICU for observation.

CLINICAL RECOGNITION

The clinical spectrum of cerebellar infarction has been investigated in much detail.[1-4] (Capsule 31.1). Patients with a cerebellar infarct in the PICA territory (approximately 30% of cases) complain of severe vertigo, headache, nausea, vomiting, and unsteadiness of gait with dysarthria.[5,7,10,16,17]

Hiccups may emerge and can be extremely invalidating. Patients with a PICA infarct may present with a lateral medullary (Wallenberg) syndrome, consisting of Horner's syndrome, weakness of the vocal cords or tongue, ataxia, unilateral facial analgesia, and contralateral analgesia in the trunk and limbs.

In patients with an AICA infarct, acute vertigo may develop and can be followed by acute deafness, tinnitus, peripheral facial palsy, hemiataxia, and thermoanalgesia. However, AICA infarcts can also produce more isolated cerebellar signs.

Infarction of the SCA predominantly produces dysarthria and ataxia, and although it may superficially mimic a lacunar syndrome, it is typically recognized by ipsilateral dysmetria, choreiform movements, Horner's syndrome, and crossed thermoanalgesia with palsy of the trochlear nerve. Bilateral infarcts in the SCA territory may appear, pointing to the presence of an embolus in the distal basilar artery. Only complete involvement of these territories can lead to brainstem compression, which is uncommon.[31] The clinical syndromes of infarction in the distribution of the cerebellar arteries are summarized in Table 31.1.

NEUROIMAGING AND LABORATORY TESTS

The typical occurrence of a cerebellar infarct may not be recognized clinically. In addition, hypodensity indicating infarction may not be visible on the initial computed tomography (CT) scan, and the appearance of distinctive hypodensity in the cerebellar hemisphere on CT scans may be delayed up to a few days ("stroke somewhere, stroke nowhere, stroke in the cerebellum").[21] Moreover, the specificity of a single CT scan is poor, and space-occupying lesions, including metastasis or abscess, may underlie the hypodensity. When cerebellar infarction appears, it is an ill-defined area of decreased density and can obliterate or distort the fourth ventricle. Disappearance of the quadrigeminal and ambient cisterns is a prominent CT

CAPSULE 31.1   VASCULARIZATION OF THE CEREBELLUM

The arterial topography is depicted in the accompanying illustration. Three main arteries supply the cerebellum: the posterior-inferior cerebellar artery (PICA), which arises from the vertebral artery and supplies the caudal part of the cerebellar hemisphere and vermis; the anterior-inferior cerebellar artery (AICA), originating from the basilar artery and supplying a small area of the anterior and medial cerebellum, including the middle cerebellar peduncle and flocculus on the lower posterior border of the cerebellum; and the superior cerebellar artery (SCA), which originates from the distal basilar artery close to the posterior cerebral artery and supplies the rostral half of the cerebellar hemisphere and vermis as well as the dentate nucleus.[1,28] Cerebellar infarcts involve occlusion of these major branches, but other infarcts may involve territories between two major arterial territories (junctional infarcts).[6] Multiple cerebellar infarcts may occur.[30] Most likely, a single large PICA providing branches to both cerebellar hemispheres is occluded in these situations.[30]

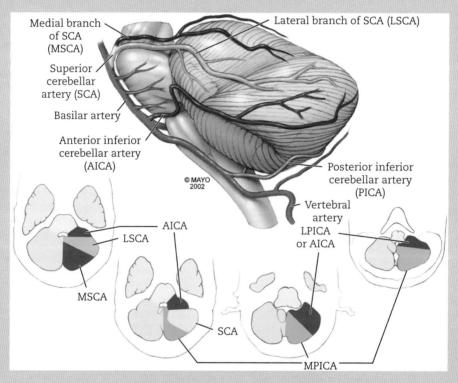

Vascular bed of cerebellum. Serial horizontal cuts identify single territories.

LPICA, lateral branch of posterior inferior cerebellar artery; MPICA, medial branch of posterior inferior cerebellar artery.

Modified from Amarenco P. The spectrum of cerebellar infarctions. *Neurology* 1991;41:973–979. With permission of the American Academy of Neurology.

scan indicator of cerebellar infarction but also of swelling and tissue displacement. Another important feature of CT scanning is obstructive hydrocephalus. Hydrocephalus is evidenced on CT scans by enlargement of the temporal horns, followed by enlargement of the lateral and third ventricles. Obstructive hydrocephalus sometimes becomes more apparent on serial CT scans; therefore, it is useful to repeat CT scanning with specific attention to deformity or disappearance of the fourth ventricle

TABLE 31.1. CLINICAL SYNDROMES OF INFARCTION IN THE DISTRIBUTION OF THE CEREBELLAR ARTERIES

Arterial Territory	Structures Affected	Clinical Manifestations
Posterior inferior cerebellar artery	Restiform body, inferior surface of cerebellar hemisphere Descending tract and nucleus of fifth nerve Nucleus ambiguus Descending sympathetic tract Spinothalamic tract Vestibular nuclei	Limb ataxia, gait ataxia Facial hypesthesia to pain and temperature Palatal weakness, decreased gag reflex, dystonia (vocal cord paresis) Horner's syndrome Hypesthesia to pain and temperature of limbs and trunk Vertigo, nystagmus
Anterior inferior cerebellar artery	Brachium pontis, inferior surface of cerebellar hemisphere Descending sympathetic tract Cochlear nucleus Intrapontine course of seventh nerve Trigeminal nuclei (descending tract and main sensory tract) Spinothalamic tract Vestibular nuclei	Limb ataxia, gait ataxia Horner syndrome Deafness Facial paralysis Facial hypesthesia Hypesthesia to pain and temperature of limbs and trunk Vertigo, nystagmus
Superior cerebellar artery	Brachium pontis, superior surface of cerebellar hemisphere (including vermis), dentate nucleus Brachium conjunctivum Descending sympathetic tract Spinothalamic tract Pontine tectum	Limb ataxia, gait ataxia Choreiform dyskinesia Horner's syndrome Hypesthesia to pain and temperature of limbs and trunk Trochlear nerve palsy

Modified from Kase CS. Cerebellar infarction. *Heart Dis Stroke* 1994;3:38–45. With permission of the American Heart Association.

and further enlargement of the third and lateral ventricles. Hemorrhagic conversion is more common in larger infarcts and anticoagulated patients and may be associated with later deterioration.[21]

When a CT scan is obtained, thin slices of the posterior fossa can be considered, but magnetic resonance imaging (MRI) and magnetic resonance angiography (MRA) have the major advantages of localizing the lesion, delineating the extent of infarction and the presence of swelling (Figure 31.1), and documenting occlusion in the posterior circulation. In younger patients, cerebellar infarcts can be a result of vertebral artery dissection.[24] This dissection can be found in any type of cerebellar infarct but, as expected, due to its branching off the vertebral artery, more frequently in the PICA territory. Magnetic resonance angiography can be diagnostic and should be the initial test.

Radiologic landmarks are helpful to determine brainstem displacement and tonsillar descent. Swelling outside these demarcations may influence the neurosurgeon's decision to proceed with decompression. Examination of the cerebrospinal fluid is contraindicated. However, in a hectic emergency department, lumbar puncture may already have been performed. Typically, this occurs in patients with prominent initial severe headache that masks the cerebellar findings and with "normal" CT findings. Lumbar puncture could cause marked compartmental shifts and compression of the medulla oblongata, resulting in sudden death from apnea, but there is little documentation to support this commonly stated assertion. A recent study found that 25–30 cc volume of cerebellar stroke on diffusion-weighted imaging (DWI) MRI predicted secondary deterioration and need for surgical decompression.[33]

Further laboratory tests are tailored toward possible causes of cerebellar infarction. In a series of 115 patients with cerebellar infarcts, one study found that 35% had a cardiac source of emboli.[3] Therefore, transesophageal echocardiography should be performed to document an important cardioembolic source, as evidenced by markedly akinetic segments or intramural clots, or to find complex atherosclerotic aortic arch disease.

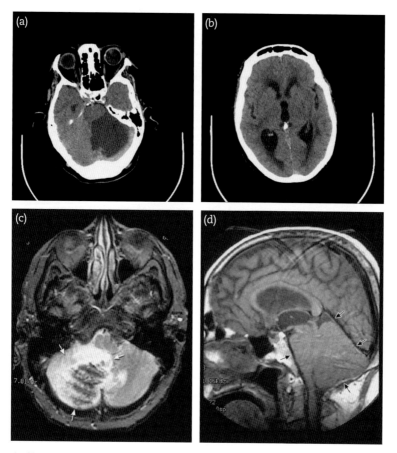

FIGURE 31.1. (a, b) Posterior inferior cerebellar artery distribution infarct on computed tomography scan with acute hydrocephalus from fourth ventricle obstruction. (c, d) Example of how axial and sagittal magnetic resonance images can show marked brainstem compression with upward and downward tissue displacement.

FIRST STEPS
IN MANAGEMENT

The decision to admit patients to the NICU depends occasionally on the degree of arousal, but more often on evidence of a mass effect on the initial CT scan. Airway management is important, and many patients require intubation for airway protection because of inability to maintain an open airway from drowsiness or from reduced oropharyngeal function.

Intravenous administration of heparin must be started immediately, because cerebellar infarcts can be the first manifestation of a propagating clot in the basilar artery. Heparin may also reduce recurrence of embolization from a cardioembolic source. Heparin is particularly germane in patients who have atrial fibrillation and in patients with a recent myocardial infarct or ventricular failure. Generally, the risk of clinically relevant hemorrhagic conversion in the cerebellar infarct is low,

and, if present, often only petechial hemorrhages appear on CT scans.[8] Follow-up CT scan may also discover hemorrhagic conversion without much evidence of clinical worsening. Even if deterioration occurs, it may be due to larger volumes of infarction and swelling, rather than to expanding hematoma. Cerebellar hemorrhagic infarction most commonly occurs in infarcts involving the SCA territory.[21]

Patients with concomitant brainstem infarction may have hiccups that can be difficult to manage. These hiccups not only are tiresome to the patient but also can increase the risk of aspiration. Baclofen in a starting dose of 5 mg orally three times a day may substantially relieve hiccups and should be the drug of choice.[23] Alternative choices are chlorpromazine 25–50 mg intravenously over 30 minutes, and then 50–60 mg/day orally in 3 divided doses; metoclopramide 10 mg intravenously, and then 10–40 mg orally; haloperidol, 2 mg intramuscularly every 4–8 hours; and valproic acid, 5 mg/kg orally four times a day.

Progressive swelling in patients with cerebellar infarcts can be associated with brief episodes of asymptomatic sinus bradycardia. If these episodes of bradycardia are associated with marked hypotension (systolic blood pressure of < 90 mm Hg), atropine (0.5–2.0 mg IV) should be administered. Patients who have marked hypertension as part of a Cushing response possibly should not be treated unless hypertension persists at high values (mean arterial pressure > 130 mm Hg).

Nutrition can be started only after swallowing mechanisms have been assessed. Typically, a nasogastric tube must be placed (also when patients are vomiting profusely).

The initial management of cerebellar infarct is summarized in Table 31.2. The criteria for "conservative treatment" or "watchful waiting" remain difficult to define, knowing that patients can deteriorate suddenly, that respiratory and cardiac arrest can occur, and also that ventriculostomy alone does prevent further brainstem compression. Some neurosurgeons place a ventriculostomy and only decompress after clinical deterioration.[27] Others feel that the risk of decompressive craniotomy is small and proceed.[22]

DETERIORATION: CAUSES AND MANAGEMENT

The clinical course in patients admitted to the NICU may evolve along three possible clinical scenarios. The mechanism of deterioration in a patient with a cerebellar infarct is direct compression of the brainstem, development of obstructive hydrocephalus, or progression of concurrent brainstem infarction. First, patients may be alert at presentation with cerebellar symptoms and signs that seem to stabilize in the first days but then change, often with rapid deterioration in level of consciousness. Progressive compression of the brainstem from swelling of the infarcted tissue is the most probable explanation in these patients. Second, patients may develop fluctuating responsiveness without progressive brainstem symptoms. Most often, CT scans show early enlargement of the ventricular system from obstruction at the level of the fourth ventricle. Third, in an almost invariably hopeless situation, patients become comatose within hours of the first initial symptoms. It is likely that this clinical course is most often observed in patients with additional extensive brainstem infarction. Pinpoint pupils, loss of oculocephalic reflexes, and ocular bobbing are present. Clearly

TABLE 31.2. INITIAL MANAGEMENT OF CEREBELLAR INFARCT

Airway management	Intubation if patient has hypoxemia despite face mask of 10% oxygen/min, if abnormal respiratory drive or if abnormal protective reflexes, likely with motor response of withdrawal or worse
Mechanical ventilation	IMV/PS or CPAP mode
Fluid management	2 L of 0.9% NaCl
Blood pressure management	No treatment of hypertension unless persistently MAP > 130 mm Hg
Nutrition	Assess swallowing mechanism and place nasogastric tube
	Enteral nutrition with continuous infusion (on day 2)
	Blood glucose control (goal 140–180 mg/dL)
Prophylaxis	DVT prophylaxis with pneumatic compression devices
	Consider SC heparin 5000 U t.i.d.
	GI prophylaxis: pantoprazole 40 mg IV daily or lansoprazole 30 mg orally through nasogastric tube
Other measures	Heparin IV (activated partial thromboplastin time twice control value)
	Baclofen for hiccups (15 mg qid orally)
Surgical Management	Ventriculostomy if progressive hydrocephalus but no compression of the brainstem
	Suboccipital decompressive craniotomy if further neurologic deterioration from brainstem compression
Access	Arterial catheter to monitor blood pressure (if IV antihypertensive drugs anticipated)
	Peripheral venous catheter or peripheral inserted central catheter

CPAP, continuous positive airway pressure; DVT, deep vein thrombosis; GI, gastrointestinal; IMV, intermittent mandatory ventilation; IV, intravenously; MAP, mean arterial pressure; NaCl, sodium chloride; PS, pressure support; SC, subcutaneously.

distinguishing these mechanisms on clinical grounds alone remains difficult. Autopsy may not be revealing either. In a postmortem study of 16 patients with space-occupying cerebellar infarcts, tetraplegia correlated strongly with massive paramedian pontine infarction rather than with compression.[1] In another autopsy study, however, only a few structural changes in the brainstem were found in patients who died of space-occupying cerebellar infarcts.[29]

Compression of the brainstem can be at the midbrain level in patients who have cerebellar tissue expanding upward and at the medullary level in patients with cerebellar tissue expanding downward and descending tonsils.

Upward cerebellar tissue expansion from swelling has some distinguishing features. These patients have signs of progressive drowsiness, paralysis of upward gaze from pretectal compression, and development of unreactive pinpoint pupils. The distinction between brainstem compression and rapid development of acute hydrocephalus, however, can be very difficult, and both can be present at the same time. These clinical features can be accompanied by radiologic progression that begins with fourth ventricle deformity and continues to fourth ventricle shift, obstructive hydrocephalus, brainstem deformity, and effacement of the basal cisterns. Upward cerebellar displacement has been attributed to ventriculostomy,[18] but this dramatic development—similar to that in cerebellar hematoma—is not commonly seen, if at all.

Earlier clinical observations have linked descending swollen cerebellar tonsils with increasing neck stiffness (occasionally with a tendency toward opisthotonos), development of cardiac arrhythmias (usually bradycardia), and irregular respiration (leading to frequent apneic episodes), but the reliability of these signs can be questioned. More certain symptoms of brainstem compression are gaze deviation in the horizontal plane, ipsilateral hemiparesis (from compression of the contralateral pyramid against the clivus),[15] and development of bilateral Babinski signs.[11] Other clinical signs that particularly localize brainstem compression are peripheral facial nerve palsy and loss of corneal reflexes. Eventually, further brain-stem displacement produces extensor motor responses, oculocephalic responses disappear, and apnea occurs.

The management of a swollen cerebellar infarct remains suboccipital craniotomy with resection of necrotic material[9] (Figure 31.2). Ventriculostomy alone has been proposed as a temporary measure, but many neurosurgeons agree that suboccipital craniotomy should be offered in deteriorating patients to relieve brainstem compression. Ventriculostomy is reasonable if deterioration can be clearly attributed only to obstructive hydrocephalus.[12,32] The typical development in these patients is marked impairment of consciousness associated with substantial enlargement of the ventricles, and disappearance of the fourth ventricle but with retained visualization of the ambient cisterns.

Compression of the brainstem and simultaneously developing hydrocephalus in patients

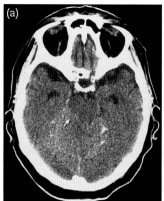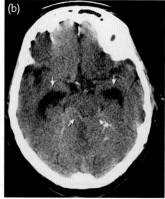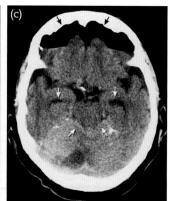

FIGURE 31.2: Progressive clinical deterioration in a patient with cerebellar infarct and swelling. (a) Brainstem compression and disappearance of fourth ventricle (note indentation of brainstem) (*arrow*). (b) Brainstem compression with developing hydrocephalus (*arrows*). (c) After decompressive surgery, ambient cistern is partially open and bifrontal air appears associated with surgery in the sitting position (*arrows*).

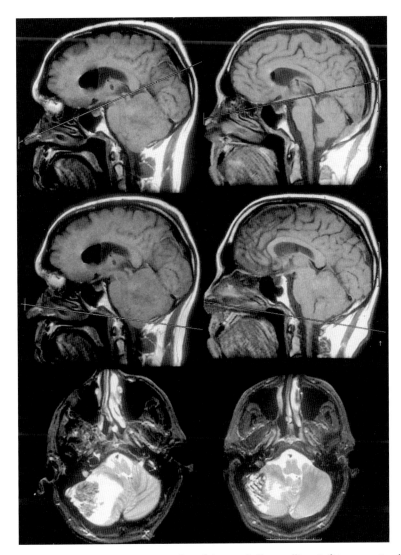

FIGURE 31.3: Serial magnetic resonance images of resolving cerebellar swelling. Left image series shows massive cerebellar infarct with obstruction of the fourth ventricle and upward and downward herniation. The incisural line (*top line*) connects the anterior tuberculum sellae to the confluence of the straight sinus, great cerebral vein, and inferior sagittal sinus. The iter (tip of the aqueduct) is exactly on this line. The foramen magnum line (*bottom line*) extends from the inferior tip of the clivus to the posterior tip of the foramen magnum. In this image, the radiographic landmarks show upward displacement of the iter and tonsillar descent with spontaneous resolution. Right image series shows resolution without suboccipital decompressive craniotomy.

From Wijdicks et al.[35]

with cerebellar softening can rarely be managed conservatively. If acute hydrocephalus progresses on CT images, clinical deterioration soon follows, and improvement is commonly dramatic after decompression and ventriculostomy. The decision to proceed with suboccipital craniotomy to decompress the posterior fossa should probably not be made solely on the basis of CT or MRI findings.[9] We have documented significant compression on MRI but virtually no impairment of consciousness after ventriculostomy (Figure 31.3), and later, spontaneous resolution.[35] In addition, vertical displacement on MRI did not correlate with clinical presentation[21] or deterioration. Again, some patients with cerebellar infarcts can improve with conservative treatment alone. In a series of 11 patients with large cerebellar infarcts (eight with

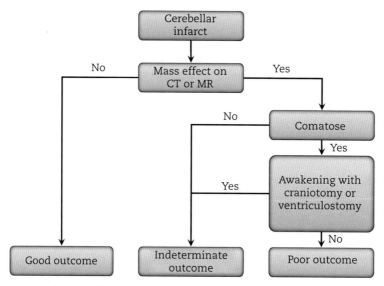

FIGURE 31.4: Outcome algorithm for cerebellar infarction. Good outcome: No assistance needed, minor handicap may remain. Indeterminate outcome: Any statement would be a premature conclusion. Poor outcome: Severe disability or death, vegetative state.

CT, computed tomography; MR, magnetic resonance imaging.

CT scan evidence of hydrocephalus), five were treated with ventriculostomy and six with supportive care alone. One patient died of progressive brainstem infarction, and the others had a good to fair outcome.[20]

OUTCOME

Poor surgical outcome after craniotomy for cerebellar swelling can be expected in patients older than 60 years, patients with brainstem signs at presentation, and patients in a late clinical stage, defined as coma with extensor posturing at the time of admission.[13,14] Mortality in a recent series was 18% and poor outcome in 32%.[26] Some have suggested BAEP studies may predict outcome, but this practice is highly unusual and not established. Outcome is determined by early recognition, and every year patients succumbed because of late recognized swelling.[25]

Patients with acute bilateral cerebellar infarcts (AICA or PICA) also can make a good recovery. Two studies using more comprehensive measures of functional independence found a less favorable outcome in patients with SCA occlusion.[19,34] Involvement of the dentate nucleus or superior cerebellar peduncle has been implicated.

The long-term outcome in patients with surgical treatment of expanding cerebellar infarcts has been studied only sparingly.[36] Dysphagia and ataxia may remain significant handicaps. Patients with persistent dysphagia may benefit from cricopharyngeal myotomy, but recovery may not occur until after 3 years.[27] Many patients are able to function independently at home with only mild, nondisabling instability of gait, although some have transient ischemic attacks in the posterior circulation in the following years.[21] An outcome prediction algorithm is shown in Figure 31.4.

CONCLUSIONS

- Important CT scan criteria for the diagnosis of cerebellar swelling are hypodensity with obliteration of the fourth ventricle, brainstem deformity, obstructive hydrocephalus, and obliteration of the ambient cistern. Magnetic resonance imaging findings of brainstem displacement do not predict deterioration.
- Patients with PICA infarcts have a 30% risk of further deterioration from swelling.
- Symptoms of brainstem compression are gaze deviation in the horizontal plane, disappearing corneal reflexes, paralysis of upward gaze, and pinpoint pupils.
- Definitive management of cerebellar infarcts remains suboccipital craniotomy in patients with deterioration or who fail to improve. Ventriculostomy is considered only if deterioration is from obstructive hydrocephalus alone.

REFERENCES

1. Amarenco P. The spectrum of cerebellar infarctions. *Neurology* 1991;41:973–979.
2. Amarenco P, Hauw JJ, Gautier JC. Arterial pathology in cerebellar infarction. *Stroke* 1990;21:1299–1305.
3. Amarenco P, Levy C, Cohen A, et al. Causes and mechanisms of territorial and nonterritorial cerebellar infarcts in 115 consecutive patients. *Stroke* 1994;25:105–112.
4. Amarenco P, Roullet E, Hommel M, Chaine P, Marteau R. Infarction in the territory of the medial branch of the posterior inferior cerebellar artery. *J Neurol Neurosurg Psychiatry* 1990;53: 731–735.
5. Barth A, Bogousslavsky J, Regli F. The clinical and topographic spectrum of cerebellar infarcts: a clinical-magnetic resonance imaging correlation study. *Ann Neurol* 1993;33:451–456.
6. Canaple S, Bogousslavsky J. Multiple large and small cerebellar infarcts. *J Neurol Neurosurg Psychiatry* 1999;66:739–745.
7. Chaves CJ, Caplan LR, Chung CS, et al. Cerebellar infarcts in the New England Medical Center Posterior Circulation Stroke Registry. *Neurology* 1994;44:1385–1390.
8. Chaves CJ, Pessin MS, Caplan LR, et al. Cerebellar hemorrhagic infarction. *Neurology* 1996;46:346–349.
9. Chen HJ, Lee TC, Wei CP. Treatment of cerebellar infarction by decompressive suboccipital craniectomy. *Stroke* 1992;23:957–961.
10. Edlow JA, Newman-Toker DE, Savitz SI. Diagnosis and initial management of cerebellar infarction. *Lancet Neurol* 2008;7:951–964.
11. Hornig CR, Rust DS, Busse O, Jauss M, Laun A. Space-occupying cerebellar infarction: clinical course and prognosis. *Stroke* 1994;25:372–374.
12. Horwitz NH, Ludolph C. Acute obstructive hydrocephalus caused by cerebellar infarction: treatment alternatives. *Surg Neurol* 1983;20:13–19.
13. Jauss M, Krieger D, Hornig C, Schramm J, Busse O. Surgical and medical management of patients with massive cerebellar infarctions: results of the German-Austrian Cerebellar Infarction Study. *J Neurol* 1999;246:257–264.
14. Juttler E, Schweickert S, Ringleb PA, et al. Long-term outcome after surgical treatment for space-occupying cerebellar infarction: experience in 56 patients. *Stroke* 2009;40:3060–3066.
15. Kanis KB, Ropper AH, Adelman LS. Homolateral hemiparesis as an early sign of cerebellar mass effect. *Neurology* 1994;44:2194–2197.
16. Kase CS. Cerebellar infarction. *Heart Dis Stroke* 1994;3:38–45.
17. Kase CS, Norrving B, Levine SR, et al. Cerebellar infarction. Clinical and anatomic observations in 66 cases. *Stroke* 1993;24:76–83.
18. Kase CS, Wolf PA. Cerebellar infarction: upward transtentorial herniation after ventriculostomy. *Stroke* 1993;24:1096–1098.
19. Kelly PJ, Stein J, Shafqat S, et al. Functional recovery after rehabilitation for cerebellar stroke. *Stroke* 2001;32:530–534.
20. Khan M, Polyzoidis KS, Adegbite AB, McQueen JD. Massive cerebellar infarction: "conservative" management. *Stroke* 1983;14:745–751.
21. Koh MG, Phan TG, Atkinson JL, Wijdicks EFM. Neuroimaging in deteriorating patients with cerebellar infarcts and mass effect. *Stroke* 2000;31:2062–2067.
22. Kudo H, Kawaguchi T, Minami H, et al. Controversy of surgical treatment for severe cerebellar infarction. *J Stroke Cerebrovasc Dis* 2007;16:259–262.
23. Launois S, Bizec JL, Whitelaw WA, Cabane J, Derenne JP. Hiccup in adults: an overview. *Eur Respir J* 1993;6:563–575.
24. Malm J, Kristensen B, Carlberg B, Fagerlund M, Olsson T. Clinical features and prognosis in young adults with infratentorial infarcts. *Cerebrovasc Dis* 1999;9:282–289.
25. Neugebauer H, Witsch J, Zweckberger K, Juttler E. Space-occupying cerebellar infarction: complications, treatment, and outcome. *Neurosurg Focus* 2013;34:E8.
26. Ng ZX, Yang WR, Seet E, et al. Cerebellar strokes: a clinical outcome review of 79 cases. *Singapore Med J* 2015;56:145–149.
27. Raco A, Caroli E, Isidori A, Salvati M. Management of acute cerebellar infarction: one institution's experience. *Neurosurgery* 2003;53:1061–1065.
28. Savoiardo M, Bracchi M, Passerini A, Visciani A. The vascular territories in the cerebellum and brainstem: CT and MR study. *AJNR Am J Neuroradiol* 1987;8:199–209.
29. Scotti G, Spinnler H, Sterzi R, Vallar G. Cerebellar softening. *Ann Neurol* 1980;8:133–140.
30. Sorenson EJ, Wijdicks EFM, Thielen KR, Cheng TM. Acute bilateral infarcts of the posterior inferior cerebellar artery. *J Neuroimaging* 1997;7:250–251.
31. Stangel M, Stapf C, Marx P. Presentation and prognosis of bilateral infarcts in the territory of the superior cerebellar artery. *Cerebrovasc Dis* 1999;9:328–333.
32. Taneda M, Ozaki K, Wakayama A, et al. Cerebellar infarction with obstructive hydrocephalus. *J Neurosurg* 1982;57:83–91.
33. Tchopev Z, Hiller M, Zhuo J, et al. Prediction of poor outcome in cerebellar infarction by diffusion MRI. *Neurocrit Care* 2013;19:276–282.
34. Tohgi H, Takahashi S, Chiba K, Hirata Y. Cerebellar infarction: clinical and neuroimaging analysis in 293 patients. The Tohoku

Cerebellar Infarction Study Group. *Stroke* 1993;24:1697–1701.

35. Wijdicks EFM, Maus TP, Piepgras DG. Cerebellar swelling and massive brain stem distortion: spontaneous resolution documented by MRI. *J Neurol Neurosurg Psychiatry* 1998;65:400–401.

36. Wijdicks EFM, Sheth KN, Carter BS, et al. Recommendations for the management of cerebral and cerebellar infarction with swelling: a statement for healthcare professionals from the American Heart Association/American Stroke Association. *Stroke* 2014;45:1222–1238.

32

Cerebral Venous Thrombosis

Precisely because its presentation commonly confuses clinicians, cerebral venous thrombosis remains a disorder that is difficult to diagnose. Certainly, the diagnosis of cerebral venous thrombosis has been greatly aided by magnetic resonance venography (MRV), but the test is neither uniformly available, nor ordered in the evaluation of some cases. Reasons for admission to the neurosciences intensive care unit (NICU) include the development of hemorrhagic infarction, seizures, and other less common life-threatening complications in patients with a hypercoagulable state, such as pulmonary embolus or peripheral arterial occlusion. Less commonly, patients are admitted to the NICU with obstruction at the cavernous sinus, which results in painful ophthalmoplegia, which involves the third, fourth, fifth (first two divisions), and sixth cranial nerves.

Most challenging are management difficulties in association with increased intracranial pressure due to a culmination of bilateral cerebral infarctions and edema. Thrombus formation in the cerebral venous system may result in a cascade of clinical problems, and early aggressive treatment—anticoagulation, endovascular clot retraction or intravenous thrombolysis—may prevent serious disability and death. However, fortunately, it can be estimated that fewer than 10% of patients with cerebral venous thrombosis will need neurologic intensive care during the course of the disease.

CLINICAL RECOGNITION

Knowledge of the anatomic ramifications of the larger veins is needed to understand the propagation of clot. Most of the cortical veins drain into the superior sagittal sinus, which follows the falx cerebri. The inferior sagittal sinus follows the ventral side of the falx and drains into the straight sinus. Both transverse sinuses are located at the tentorium cerebelli. The superior sagittal sinus, straight sinus, and both transverse sinuses form a confluence called the *torcular Herophili*. The anatomy of the cerebral venous system, including important anastomoses (Trolard and Labbé), is shown in Figure 32.1.

The defining characteristics of cerebral venous thrombosis include profound headache, papilledema, and, in more severe cases, seizures, weakness, and speech abnormalities.[3,13,18,31,77] Patients with cerebral venous thrombosis (most often, the superior sagittal sinus) invariably complain of a persistent headache of new onset. The headache is dull but intense and bilateral. Movements of the head, sneezing, and coughing may be aggravating, but the headache can also be instantaneous in onset, mimicking a thunderclap-type headache (Chapter 4). If the headache becomes worse when the patient bends forward and suddenly exacerbates with a sharp throb of pain after sneezing, an underlying sinusitis must be suspected, although septic sagittal sinus thrombosis is very uncommon.

Papilledema is an important early clinical finding and may be manifested by obscurations.[80] These typical blackouts last only seconds, are often in one eye, and may be either spontaneous or elicited by change in posture. In a few instances, pressure on the globe by the examiner may bring them on. When papilledema is subtle, it is detected only by disappearance of the venous pulsation. Disk elevation, blurring of disk margins, and dilated and tortuous veins occur in fewer than half of patients with the diagnosis of sagittal sinus thrombosis.[12] Visual loss may ensue in longstanding papilledema, but visual blurring may occur early when retinal exudate extends to the macula. Diplopia in a horizontal plane may occur as a result of an associated sixth-nerve palsy. In patients with unilateral transverse sinus thrombosis alone, compression of the contralateral jugular vein may cause unilateral facial venous engorgement (Crowe's test), but the diagnostic value of this test is uncertain.

Patients with sagittal sinus thrombosis may become confused and may exhibit bizarre behavior,

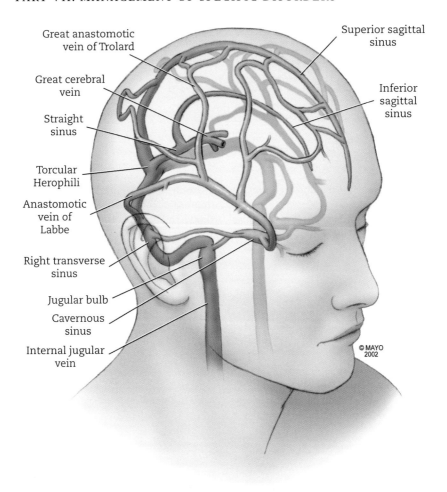

FIGURE 32.1: Anatomy of the cerebral venous system. The superficial and deep draining veins are depicted with anastomoses.

as well as nonspecific signs such as progressive anorexia and forgetfulness.[42,82] However, localizing deficits, such as hemiparesis, aphasia, abnormal visual fields, and anosognosia, likely denote the development of venous cerebral infarction.

Because initially small cortical areas are involved, seizures are focal, and presenting generalized tonic-clonic seizures are less common. Seizures are often isolated events and may not herald further progression into status epilepticus. A focal seizure may result in hemiparesis of several hours' duration (Todd's paresis) and may not indicate permanent infarction of the brain.

Progression to coma may be caused by diffuse cerebral edema or bilateral cerebral, often hemorrhagic, infarctions. The volume of one hemorrhagic infarct, however, may predominate over the other and may cause mass effect with marked brain shift. Diffuse massive brain edema occurs

rarely, and the outcome is often poor despite aggressive measures to reduce edema.

Venous infarction in both thalami may produce marked fluctuations in arousal and substantial memory deficits later. Other clinical signs of bilateral hemorrhagic thalamic infarcts are delirium, abulia, dyscalculia, confabulation, and atypical transcortical sensory aphasia with impaired naming and comprehension but preserved fluency and repetition.[8,42] Unusual presenting symptoms are acute micrographia and hypophonia from venous infarction in both thalami, the putamen, and the caudate nucleus.[57]

Isolated multiple cranial nerve palsy (III, VII, VIII) has been reported in patients with unilateral occlusion of the transverse-sigmoid sinus. This atypical presentation has been explained by venous congestion of the ventral pontine and lateral medullary veins.[50]

NEUROIMAGING AND LABORATORY TESTS

Cerebral venous sinus thrombosis is often without an identifiable precipitating trigger, and the results of a battery of diagnostic tests may be unremarkable. A comprehensive investigation of potential causes is negative in 20% of the patients, including those with 2-year follow-up, in whom an underlying disorder, if present, should have become apparent.[12]

Major causes for cerebral sinus thrombosis are all stages of pregnancy (but more likely the puerperium) and the use of oral contraceptives.[56,77] Other causes are coagulation disorders, connective tissue disorders, cancer[65] chemotherapeutic treatment,[46] nephrotic syndrome, bacteremia or disseminated intravascular coagulation, and conditions of extreme dehydration. Hematologic cancers such as adult acute lymphoblastic leukemia treated with asparaginase or intrathecal methotrexate were associated with cerebral venous thrombosis.[97] Occlusion of the transverse sinus may occur in patients with mastoiditis (Chapter 33). Local invasion of the sagittal sinus by metastatic disease should be considered in patients with metastatic carcinoma. Behçet's disease, Crohn's disease, ulcerative colitis, and acquired immunodeficiency syndrome may appear with cerebral venous thrombosis and should all be considered.[24,47] One group of investigators reported that approximately 40% of a large series of patients had an underlying systemic disease.[64] Damage to the jugular vein from trauma or surgical procedures involving the neck is a well-recognized cause. In rare occasions, cerebral venous thrombosis has been associated with placement of a jugular vein catheter for parenteral nutrition[69] or perioperative monitoring or after placement of pacemaker wires.[33,38,52] Other rare causes for cerebral venous thrombosis are dural arteriovenous fistula[29] and antifibrinolytic agents.[1]

Superior sagittal sinus thrombosis has been reported in at least 12 patients after nonpenetrating head injury.[44] The mechanism in head injury remains unresolved. No studies are available to prove the theory that thromboplastin, which is present in large quantities in the brain after injury, alters blood coagulation. In fact, clot in the transverse sinus may occur after a far more trivial trauma to the head.

Table 32.1 summarizes a complete evaluation schedule. Cerebral venous thrombosis may be the first defining disorder in patients with a hypercoagulable state. The therapeutic consequences of a once-detected thrombophilia are quite important. Recurrent spontaneous abortions, recurrent deep vein thrombosis, pulmonary embolism at a young age, and arterial occlusions at uncommon sites may have been earlier indicators of a coagulation abnormality.[3,29,48,72,87] Congenital thrombophilias, such as protein S deficiency,[37] anticardiolipin antibodies,[14] activated protein C resistance, hyperhomocysteinemia, and increased levels of factors VIII and XI, should be investigated. Both a heterozygous and a homozygous state for factor V Leiden and a 20210A sequence variation of the prothrombin gene have been associated with cerebral venous thrombosis in sporadic cases and in up to 9% of patients in larger series.[10,11,67,72] Inherited coagulopathy associated with cerebral venous thrombosis may be more common than is generally appreciated, and a study from Germany found that the incidence approached 40%.[79] Simultaneous occurrence of factor V Leiden mutation and the 20210A genotype of the prothrombin gene has also been reported in one patient,[54] and in another patient with a lateral and sagittal sinus thrombosis, protein C deficiency and mastoiditis.[66]

TABLE 32.1. LABORATORY STUDIES IN PATIENTS WITH CEREBRAL VENOUS THROMBOSIS

Blood smear, platelet count, differential count
Antithrombin III, protein C, and protein S
Heparin cofactor II
Plasma fibrinogen
Lupus anticoagulant
Anticardiolipin antibodies
MTHFR mutation
Plasma homocysteine
Hemoglobin electrophoresis
Urinalysis with quantification of protein and determination of hemosiderin
Coombs test, rheumatoid factor, antineutrophil cytoplasmic autoantibody, antinuclear antibody
Drug screen
Computed tomography scan of chest or abdomen, or both
Optional
  Human immunodeficiency virus
  Colonoscopy
  Skin and conjunctiva biopsy
  Blood cultures
  Bone marrow
  Hematology consultation
  Rheumatology consultation
  Otorhinolaryngology consultation

MTHFR, methylenetetrahydrofolate reductase.

In one study of 163 patients with cerebral venous thrombosis at Mayo Clinic with comprehensive testing for thrombophilia, abnormalities were found in 29% of the cases. (Anticardiolipin antibodies were present in the majority of patients.[91])

Computed tomography scanning is the first test in patients with suspicious signs of cerebral venous thrombosis, but the radiologic features are mostly subtle and findings are normal in 50% of patients.[4,40,60] Computed tomography (CT) may nevertheless show hemorrhagic cerebral infarction, decreased ventricular size as a consequence of diffuse edema, or compression of the ventricles from swelling in the thalamus. Diffuse cerebral edema may be difficult to appreciate in young patients, whose sulci often are poorly visualized on CT scans. The "empty triangle sign" (thrombosis in the sagittal or straight sinus) after contrast administration is not often present, but remains a classic CT imaging sign.[84] The cord sign (hyperdense superficial lesion that represents a thrombosed vein) may be seen as well, usually close to the bone structures (Figure 32.2). Computed tomography scan may show multiple hemorrhages with early swelling (Figure 32.3). Trapping of the third ventricle may occur as a result of thalamic edema or hemorrhagic infarction.[96]

Magnetic resonance imaging (MRI) has become the standard imaging test.[62,73,92] The combination of spin-echo T2-weighted sequences[81] and two-dimensional time-of-flight (2DTOF) probably is the most sensitive technique. The 2DTOF images may better visualize the deeper venous structures; spin-echo sequences clearly image the parenchymal lesions but also differentiate a thrombus from an artifact. The T1 images may demonstrate the lack of flow void in the sinuses, and the T2 images may show abnormal periventricular and thalamic signals that most likely represent increased interstitial edema or may show an intracerebral hematoma with surrounding edema. The thrombus is initially isointense on T1-weighted and hypointense on T2-weighted images but 1–2 weeks after onset becomes hyperintense in both images. Examples of cerebral venous thrombosis on magnetic resonance cerebral venography (MRV) are shown in Figure 32.4.

Magnetic resonance venography (2DTOF) is useful in the diagnosis and assessment of the propagation of cerebral sinus thrombosis. However, hypoplastic nondominant transverse sinuses (commonly left) may appear as an artifactual flow gap, a finding that should not be interpreted as thrombosis without clear clinical features (Figure 32.5).[3] In addition, not all veins are identified on 2DTOF sequences. Using 2DTOF technology, one study in 100 normal controls found the inferior sagittal sinus in only 52%, occipital sinus in 10%, vein of Rosenthal in 91%, vein of Trolard in 37%, and vein of Labbé in 91% on the right and 96% on the left.[6] Gadolinium-enhanced 3-dimensional MRV is currently used and is most sensitive (Figure 32.4a).

Diffusion-weighted imaging with echo-planar imaging has been studied in cerebral venous thrombus.[92] Diffusion-weighted MRI may discriminate between vasogenic and cytotoxic edema, but it is not clear whether this distinction contributes to prognosis.[17,61] Cytotoxic edema is a

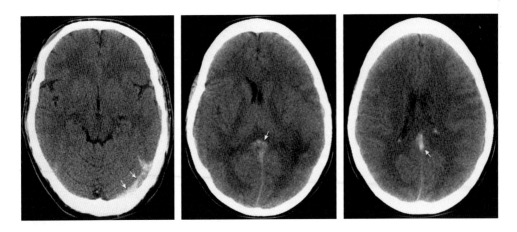

FIGURE 32.2: Computed tomographic scan with "cord sign" (transverse sinus) and vein of Galen and straight sinus (*arrows*).

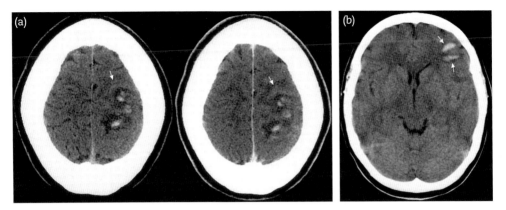

FIGURE 32.3: CT scans showing hemorrhagic infarct from sagittal sinus thrombosis (a) and cortical venous thrombosis (b).

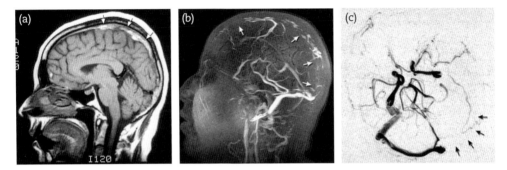

FIGURE 32.4: Variations in severity of cerebral venous thrombosis. MRI showing extensive clot in sagittal sinus and magnetic resonance venography demonstrating extensive sagittal sinus (a, b) and in left transverse sinus (c) thrombosis.

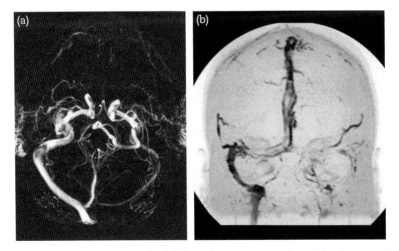

FIGURE 32.5: Magnetic resonance venography. (a) Hypoplastic transverse sinus with a flow gap mimicking transverse sinus thrombosis (often the length of the flow gap is one-third the length of the ipsilateral sinus). (b) Extensive clot in the superior sagittal sinus and both transverse sinuses but with partial recanalization. No flow in the left transverse sinus.

common radiologic finding early in the course of cerebral venous thrombosis.[34,53] Decreased apparent diffusion coefficient values suggest cellular edema, and increased values suggest vasogenic edema. However, in a small study, reduced apparent diffusion coefficient values did not correlate with later development of infarction.[26]

Generally, the abnormalities on neuroimaging correspond to the site of occlusion (e.g., transverse or sigmoid sinus occlusion leading to posterior temporal lesions, deep cerebral venous occlusion leading to bithalamic lesions), but the degree of brain lesions is variable. Some patients may have extensive clots in multiple venous systems but with only minimal parenchymal involvement. Bilateral lesions, however, were more often seen if the superior sagittal sinus occlusion was accompanied by occlusion of the vein of Galen or internal cerebral veins.[95] Cerebral angiography is not necessary if MRI and MRV have demonstrated cerebral venous sinus thrombosis, and the procedure has become more important in patients for whom endovascular treatment is considered.

Examination of the cerebrospinal fluid (CSF) could exclude an inflammatory disorder, but must be deferred in patients with progression to hemorrhagic infarction and brain shift. The CSF pressure is typically abnormal and often increased, with values of more than 200 mm H$_2$O.

Transcranial Doppler ultrasonography (TCD) has shown a fairly typical pattern of a prominent venous signal with a high amplitude bilaterally. Insonation uses the transtemporal and transorbital approaches, and the basal vein of Rosenthal is insonated posteriorly.[85,88] Normal mean venous values are 11 ± 2 cm/sec in the deep middle cerebral vein, 10 ± 2 cm/sec in the basal vein of Rosenthal, and 27 ± 17 cm/sec in the anterior cavernous sinus, but they are highly variable.[85] It may also show increased drainage to cavernous sinus and deep cerebral veins, flow reversal in basal veins, and reversed flow in transverse sinus. Its diagnostic usefulness in clinical practice is not well defined.

FIRST STEPS IN MANAGEMENT

Besides prompt anticoagulation, initial management in patients with cerebral venous thrombosis is largely supportive (Table 32.2).

Most patients can adequately protect the airway, and endotracheal intubation is indicated only for those with developing cerebral edema. Patients with cerebral venous thrombosis are at risk for pulmonary embolism, and a spiral CT of the chest

may be indicated if an increased alveolar–arterial gradient and hypoxemia intervene.

Fluid intake is standard while avoiding further dehydration. Certainly, patients with an infectious trigger for cerebral venous thrombosis should receive a fluid bolus with albumin 5% or increased intake of crystalloids to ensure adequate fluid status. The danger of fluid overload is of much less concern in these patients, who are often young and previously healthy.

Anticoagulation is the standard therapy in any patient with cerebral venous thrombosis, albeit based on the findings in a few trials of small groups of patients.[9,27,28,76,89] Intravenous heparin remains indicated in patients with CT evidence of either cerebral ischemia or hemorrhagic conversion of the infarcts. In a randomized trial of anticoagulation in cerebral venous thrombosis, outcome also improved in patients with hemorrhagic infarcts or hematomas.[28] Overall outcome in anticoagulated patients was significantly better than that in the placebo group. In two retrospective studies of patients with moderate-sized hematomas, anticoagulation was not associated with increased hemorrhage volume, neurologic deterioration, or worse outcome. Both studies suggested that deterioration from intracerebral hematoma was related more to untreated progression of the disease than to worsening by anticoagulation.[32,90]

Heparin administration begins with an infusion of 10,000 units, and the dose is adjusted to achieve an activated partial thromboplastin time that is two times the control value. A weight-based nomogram can also be considered to rapidly achieve full anticoagulation (Chapter 20). Warfarin administration can begin after approximately 5 days of observation. One trial concluded that low-molecular-weight heparin (LMWH) followed by warfarin for 3 months did not result in a statistically significant improvement or worsening from placebo results. In this study, 50% of 59 patients had CT- or MRI-documented cerebral hemorrhage.[22]

Prophylactic administration of antiepileptic medication is hardly justified in adults because of the low incidence of seizures (10%–15%), most of which are focal. Treatment is usually only initiated when focal or generalized seizures occur.

Corticosteroids are administered only to patients in whom cerebral venous thrombosis is a first manifestation of a collagen vascular disease, Behçet's disease, Crohn's disease, or sarcoidosis. In others, corticosteroids are of no demonstrated benefit in reducing cerebral edema.

Patients with marked papilledema are best treated with repeat lumbar punctures, but

TABLE 32.2. INITIAL MANAGEMENT OF CEREBRAL VENOUS THROMBOSIS

Airway management	Intubation if patient has hypoxemia despite face mask with 10 L of 100% oxygen/minute, if abnormal respiratory drive or presence of abnormal protective reflexes (likely with motor response of withdrawal, or worse)
Mechanical ventilation	IMV/PS or CPAP in most patients
Fluid management	Rapid hydration with normal saline
	Maintenance fluid intake, 3 L of 0.9% NaCl
Nutrition	Enteral nutrition with continuous infusion (on day 2)
	Blood glucose control (goal 140–180 mg/dL)
Prophylaxis	DVT prophylaxis with pneumatic compression devices
	GI prophylaxis: pantoprazole 40 mg IV daily or lansoprazole 30 mg orally through nasogastric tube.
Other measures	Heparin infusion, per weight based nomogram, activated partial thromboplastin time two times control
	Endovascular thrombolysis
	Fenestration can be considered if papilledema is present
Access	Peripheral venous catheter or peripheral inserted central catheter

CPAP, continuous positive airway pressure; DVT, deep vein thrombosis; GI, gastrointestinal; IMV, intermittent mandatory ventilation; IV, intravenously; NaCl, sodium chloride; PS, pressure support.

fenestration of the optic nerve may be needed to reduce the risk of visual loss.[7] Serial perimetry may reveal an enlarging blind spot that may guide the decision to proceed.

DETERIORATION: CAUSES AND MANAGEMENT

Patients can be expected to remain relatively stable despite development of cerebral infarction and impressive occlusion on MRV. In addition, hemorrhagic cerebral infarcts may be located in the occipital lobes and may not produce a significant mass effect. Monitoring of these patients with serial CT scans is necessary.

Clinical neurologic deterioration is probably a consequence of further thrombosis in the venous system. Impaired consciousness may indicate extension of the thrombosis into the tributary cortical veins. An increase in sagittal sinus pressure may result in the formation of hemorrhagic infarction, often bilaterally in the parietal lobes, and an increase in capillary filtration, causing cerebral edema (Capsule 32.1).

Deterioration from an enlarging hematoma with progressive brainstem compression may have to be treated with a craniotomy or decompressive craniotomy to evacuate the hematoma.[51] In our experience, we have seen patients rapidly deteriorating with the diagnosis first established at surgery. Examples of intracranial hematoma associated with cerebral venous thrombosis are shown in Figure 32.6.

When deterioration occurs despite aggressive use of intravenous heparin, an attempt to lyse the clot with thrombolytic agents is warranted. This practice with an invasive technique may not be more beneficial than anticoagulation alone. The bulk of the evidence is drawn from small case studies with different endpoints (recanalization or clinical improvement). To complicate matters further, patients have recovered from coma with medical management alone.

Endovascular intervention with lysis of the clot has been successful in a large proportion of patients, including comatose patients with pretreatment hemorrhagic infarcts resulting in significant neurologic improvement.[78] A catheter is inserted via puncture of the jugular vein or through the transfemoral route, advanced to the transverse sinus, and, if possible, advanced to the superior sagittal sinus or placed at the torcular Herophili.[30,45,83] Tissue plasminogen activator is usually infused at 1 mg/hour and may take 12–20 hours. One may start a 2-mg bolus tPA with suction thrombectomy with penumbra. Reimaging is considered after 12 hours.

The timing of endovascular thrombolysis is unresolved.[58,74] There is some consensus that endovascular treatment should be considered in a patient with deterioration from clot propagation despite adequate intravenous heparinization or use of LMWH. However, the often impressive recanalization with local administered intravenous tPA (Figure 32.7) will undoubtedly prompt a discussion on why it is that endovascular

---

CAPSULE 32.1   PATHOLOGY OF CEREBRAL VENOUS OCCLUSION

The typical sequence of events in cerebral venous thrombosis is dilatation of the venous and capillary bed, gradual progression of interstitial edema, disruption of veins, and formation of hematomas (see accompanying illustration). Cytotoxic edema may occur early; some animal studies, in fact, suggest that cytotoxic edema is followed by vasogenic edema, and that treatment with tissue plasminogen activator may partially resolve cytotoxic edema.[68] Generally, the venous system is most commonly obstructed at the superior sagittal sinus, with a possible extension to the cortical veins, leading to hemorrhagic cerebral infarction. Obstruction at the level of the deep internal cerebral veins may result in hemorrhagic infarction of the thalami or caudate heads.[93] Clot can be identified easily at autopsy (see Capsule Figure).

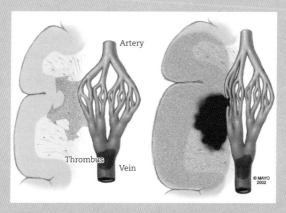

Mechanism of cerebral edema and hemorrhagic infarction.

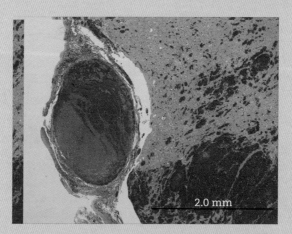

Neuropathology specimen showing clot in sagittal sinus.

---

treatment should be postponed until heparinization fails. We can expect increase in early endovascular intervention now that this option is available in many centers. Another option is mechanical disruption of the clot by use of a microsnare or high-pressure saline jets.[2,15,63,94] Saline jets macerate the thrombus, which is then aspirated into the catheter. Major limitations for use in cerebral venous thrombosis are difficult navigation and inability to advance beyond vein of Galen.[16,25,70]

Several major concerns remain, including treatment in patients with hemorrhagic infarcts, the exact time window, and whether tPA infusion needs to be repeated after a failed or partially

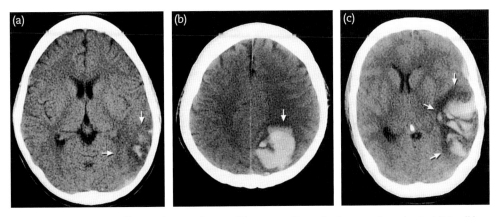

FIGURE 32.6: Three types of hemorrhagic infarcts and hematoma in cerebral venous thrombosis. (a) Small hemorrhages (*arrows*). (b) Occipital-parietal lobe hematoma without significant mass effect (*arrows*). (c) Large parietal lobe hematoma with swelling and significant shift of midline structures (*arrows*).

failed first attempt. Thrombolysis is less successful if the disorder has been present for days and pupils are fixed,[78] but recanalization can be achieved in patients who have had symptoms for weeks.[45]

Current data on endovascular thrombolysis may also be biased toward less severe cases, and in some reports, it is unclear whether the effects of intravenous heparin have been properly evaluated.[59] Worsening intracerebral hematoma in patients treated endovascularly or administered thrombolytics has been reported in some series but not in others.[36,45,49,75] Management remains complex and time-consuming, and complete lysis of an extensive clot often cannot be expected.

Patients with progressive cerebral edema become progressively drowsy, fail to localize pain, and cannot protect the airway. After endotracheal intubation and mechanical ventilation, hyperventilation (PCO_2 of approximately 30 mm Hg) can be tried. Patients with multiple hemorrhagic infarcts or progressive cerebral edema may not be successfully treated with osmotic agents. The blood–brain barrier may be defective at several locations, and an osmotic agent may be drawn into the brain with the theoretical potential for further worsening. Treatment of increased intracranial pressure cannot be guided by values obtained by fiberoptic monitoring, because patients are on heparin infusion. Propofol (1–5 mcg/kg/hr) may be a useful alternative way to treat intracranial pressure, but experience is limited.

As a last resort, cerebral blood flow can be reduced by barbiturates. Barbiturate coma can effectively reduce intracranial pressure in this situation. A report of successful management in two patients by the administration of high doses of pentobarbital has been published,[43] but there is very little recent experience. Barbiturate coma can be continued for at least 1 week, and improvement on CT scans or MRI may guide timing of tapering the barbiturate dose.

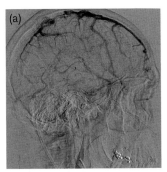
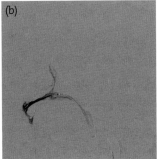
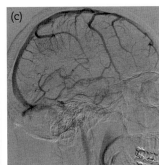

FIGURE 32.7: Extensive cerebral venous thrombus. (a) Pre tPA image. (b) microcatheter is placed. (c) recanalization after infusion of 0.5 mg/hr of tPA for 8 hours.

Patients with cerebral venous thrombosis may have sudden deterioration from pulmonary emboli. This was noted in 11% of 203 patients reported in the literature, with a 95% mortality.[23] Emboli may originate from the thrombosed jugular veins rather than, for example, from deep vein thrombosis associated with immobilization. Spiral CT of the chest is needed in any patients with a sudden increase in alveolar–arterial gradient.

OUTCOME

Because the disorder is infrequent, series of patients with cerebral venous thrombosis have been small, and the prognosis may be determined by underlying disease.[21,39] Cerebral sinus thrombosis is caused by direct destruction and invasion of malignant cells in some patients; in others, cerebral venous thrombosis is related to coagulopathy from hematologic malignant disease or infection. However, a review from Memorial Sloan-Kettering Cancer Center documented a 0.3% incidence of cerebral sinus thrombosis in cancer patients seen in consultation.[65] Notable features were involvement of multiple veins and more than one contributing factor, such as dural metastasis and antiestrogen therapy, but good clinical neurologic recovery with anticoagulation.

In a review of 103 cases reported in the literature before anticoagulation was recommended, only 14 of 66 patients (21%) with complete sagittal sinus thrombosis survived. Outcome was significantly better in patients with only partial occlusion. Early diagnosis (and thus treatment) appears to influence outcome, and mortality decreases when the diagnosis is made within 1 week of symptoms.[71]

In a series of patients after the introduction of anticoagulation who were usually treated with heparin, outcome was considerably better, with a mortality of 10% but persistent neurologic deficits in approximately 20% of the patients.[3] Coma at presentation or its development during hospitalization, seizures, or underlying disease has no effect on short-term outcome, and thus these features should not preclude any type of therapeutic intervention. Morbidity in cerebral venous thrombosis can be devastating and may include akinetic mutism, blindness from optic atrophy, and ataxia.[64]

Bilateral thalamic infarcts may cause marked memory impairment and hypersomnia, but improvement has been reported.[35] Long-term cognitive impairment seems prevalent, with nearly half the patients not returning to the workforce.[20]

Generally, parenchymal lesions on MRI correlate with outcome, but there are exceptions.[5]

A recent large series found that women have a much better outcome than men, which may be related to seeking earlier physician consultation and to pregnancy-related cerebral venous thrombosis.[19]

Long-term outcome is most likely worse in patients in coma and involvement of superior sagittal and straight sinuses on MRV, but recovery can be observed.[10,16] Another follow-up study (77 patients) emphasized good recovery in 86% and a very low (4%) incidence of epilepsy, but in that study altered consciousness was an infrequent presentation.[64] Recurrent seizures usually appeared within 1 year and expectedly more often in patients who presented with seizures. Long-term antiepileptic therapy (> 1 year) is not indicated.

When evaluation for possible causes of cerebral venous thrombosis has been repeatedly negative, the cerebral venous system has recanalized, and no other systemic clotting sites have appeared on MRV, administration of warfarin may be discontinued. Some investigators have continued anticoagulation for 12 months when venous occlusion was still detectable on MRV at follow-up. Recurrence is unusual, affecting fewer than 10% of patients without underlying systemic illness.[41,64] Long-term follow-up in patients with specific congenital thrombophilia is not available, but one study of cerebral venous thrombosis and factor V Leiden mutation suggested an increased risk of pulmonary emboli and deep vein thrombosis but not cerebral venous thrombosis.[55] Recurrence of puerperal cerebral venous thrombosis has not been reported, most likely because patients have been advised against future pregnancies. However, pregnancies in 12 patients with a history of cerebral venous thrombosis not related to pregnancy were without complications.[64] One patient with prior puerperal thrombosis treated with heparin for 3 weeks before delivery and anticoagulation for 3 months postpartum did not have a relapse.[86] Coverage with LMWH around the time of delivery seems an appropriate measure.

Generally, outcome remains difficult to accurately predict in young patients, and we have personally observed excellent recoveries in patients with extensive clot burden, but all these patients remained alert and did not progress beyond drowsiness. An outcome algorithm is shown in Figure 32.8.

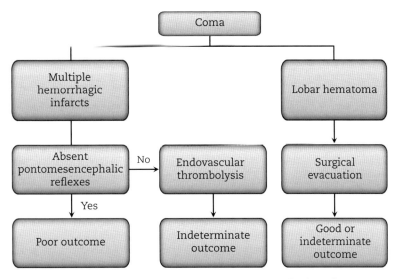

FIGURE 32.8: Outcome algorithm for cerebral venous thrombosis. Functional independence: No assistance needed, minor handicap may remain. Poor outcome: Severe disability or death, vegetative state. Indeterminate: Any statement would be a premature conclusion.

CONCLUSIONS

- Magnetic resonance imaging and gadolinium bolus MRV remain the preferred diagnostic tests. Cerebral angiography should be performed if thrombolysis is considered.
- Management consists of rehydration, rapid anticoagulation with heparin to an activated partial thromboplastin time of two times the control value, and control of intracranial pressure in comatose patients.
- Intravenous administration of heparin should be continued in patients with hemorrhagic infarcts or hematomas without mass effect.
- Increased intracranial pressure can be controlled by hyperventilation (diffuse edema or bilateral cerebral infarcts) or barbiturates.
- Evacuation of a hemorrhagic infarct may be needed in deteriorating patients from mass effect.

REFERENCES

1. Achiron A, Gornish M, Melamed E. Cerebral sinus thrombosis as a potential hazard of anti-fibrinolytic treatment in menorrhagia. *Stroke* 1990;21:817–819.
2. Agner C, Deshaies EM, Bernardini GL, Popp AJ, Boulos AS. Coronary angiojet catheterization for the management of dural venous sinus thrombosis: technical note. *J Neurosurg* 2005;103:368–371.
3. Ameri A, Bousser MG. Cerebral venous thrombosis. *Neurol Clin* 1992;10:87–111.
4. Anxionnat R, Blanchet B, Dormont D, et al. Present status of computerized tomography and angiography in the diagnosis of cerebral thrombophlebitis cavernous sinus thrombosis excluded. *J Neuroradiol* 1994;21:59–71.
5. Appenzeller S, Zeller CB, Annichino-Bizzachi JM, et al. Cerebral venous thrombosis: influence of risk factors and imaging findings on prognosis. *Clin Neurol Neurosurg* 2005;107:371–378.
6. Ayanzen RH, Bird CR, Keller PJ, et al. Cerebral MR venography: normal anatomy and potential diagnostic pitfalls. *AJNR Am J Neuroradiol* 2000;21:74–78.
7. Banta JT, Farris BK. Pseudotumor cerebri and optic nerve sheath decompression. *Ophthalmology* 2000;107:1907–1912.
8. Baumgartner RW, Landis T. Venous thalamic infarction. *Cerebrovasc Dis* 1992;2:353–358.
9. Benamer HT, Bone I. Cerebral venous thrombosis: anticoagulants or thrombolytic therapy? *J Neurol Neurosurg Psychiatry* 2000;69:427–430.
10. Biousse V, Conard J, Brouzes C, et al. Frequency of the 20210 G-->A mutation in the 3'-untranslated region of the prothrombin gene in 35 cases of cerebral venous thrombosis. *Stroke* 1998;29:1398–1400.
11. Bloem BR, van Putten MJ, van der Meer FJ, van Hilten JJ, Bertina RM. Superior sagittal sinus

thrombosis in a patient heterozygous for the novel 20210 A allele of the prothrombin gene. *Thromb Haemost* 1998;79:235.

12. Bousser MG. Cerebral venous thrombosis: diagnosis and management. *J Neurol* 2000;247:252–258.

13. Bousser MG, Chiras J, Bories J, Castaigne P. Cerebral venous thrombosis: a review of 38 cases. *Stroke* 1985;16:199–213.

14. Carhuapoma JR, Mitsias P, Levine SR. Cerebral venous thrombosis and anticardiolipin antibodies. *Stroke* 1997;28:2363–2369.

15. Chahlavi A, Steinmetz MP, Masaryk TJ, Rasmussen PA. A transcranial approach for direct mechanical thrombectomy of dural sinus thrombosis: report of two cases. *J Neurosurg* 2004;101:347–351.

16. Chow K, Gobin YP, Saver J, et al. Endovascular treatment of dural sinus thrombosis with rheolytic thrombectomy and intra-arterial thrombolysis. *Stroke* 2000;31:1420–1425.

17. Chu K, Kang DW, Yoon BW, Roh JK. Diffusion-weighted magnetic resonance in cerebral venous thrombosis. *Arch Neurol* 2001;58:1569–1576.

18. Coutinho JM, Gerritsma JJ, Zuurbier SM, Stam J. Isolated cortical vein thrombosis: systematic review of case reports and case series. *Stroke* 2014;45:1836–1838.

19. Coutinho JM, Majoie CB, Coert BA, Stam J. Decompressive hemicraniectomy in cerebral sinus thrombosis: consecutive case series and review of the literature. *Stroke* 2009;40:2233–2235.

20. de Bruijn SF, Budde M, Teunisse S, de Haan RJ, Stam J. Long-term outcome of cognition and functional health after cerebral venous sinus thrombosis. *Neurology* 2000;54:1687–1689.

21. de Bruijn SF, de Haan RJ, Stam J. Clinical features and prognostic factors of cerebral venous sinus thrombosis in a prospective series of 59 patients. For The Cerebral Venous Sinus Thrombosis Study Group. *J Neurol Neurosurg Psychiatry* 2001;70:105–108.

22. de Bruijn SF, Stam J. Randomized, placebo-controlled trial of anticoagulant treatment with low-molecular-weight heparin for cerebral sinus thrombosis. *Stroke* 1999;30:484–488.

23. Diaz JM, Schiffman JS, Urban ES, Maccario M. Superior sagittal sinus thrombosis and pulmonary embolism: a syndrome rediscovered. *Acta Neurol Scand* 1992;86:390–396.

24. Doberson MJ, Kleinschmidt-DeMasters BK. Superior sagittal sinus thrombosis in a patient with acquired immunodeficiency syndrome. *Arch Pathol Lab Med* 1994;118:844–846.

25. Dowd CF, Malek AM, Phatouros CC, Hemphill JC, 3rd. Application of a rheolytic thrombectomy device in the treatment of dural sinus

thrombosis: a new technique. *AJNR Am J Neuroradiol* 1999;20:568–570.

26. Ducreux D, Oppenheim C, Vandamme X, et al. Diffusion-weighted imaging patterns of brain damage associated with cerebral venous thrombosis. *AJNR Am J Neuroradiol* 2001;22:261–268.

27. Einhaupl K, Bousser MG, de Bruijn SF, et al. EFNS guideline on the treatment of cerebral venous and sinus thrombosis. *Eur J Neurol* 2006;13:553–559.

28. Einhaupl KM, Villringer A, Meister W, et al. Heparin treatment in sinus venous thrombosis. *Lancet* 1991;338:597–600.

29. Enevoldson TP, Russell RW. Cerebral venous thrombosis: new causes for an old syndrome? *Q J Med* 1990;77:1255–1275.

30. Eskridge JM, Wessbecher FW. Thrombolysis for superior sagittal sinus thrombosis. *J Vasc Interv Radiol* 1991;2:89–93; discussion 93–84.

31. Ferro JM, Canhao P. Cerebral venous sinus thrombosis: update on diagnosis and management. *Curr Cardiol Rep* 2014;16:523.

32. Fink JN, McAuley DL. Safety of anticoagulation for cerebral venous thrombosis associated with intracerebral hematoma. *Neurology* 2001;57:1138–1139.

33. Floyd WL, Mahaley MS. Cerebral dural venous sinus thrombosis following cardiac pacemaker implantation. *Arch Intern Med* 1969;124:368–372.

34. Forbes KP, Pipe JG, Heiserman JE. Evidence for cytotoxic edema in the pathogenesis of cerebral venous infarction. *AJNR Am J Neuroradiol* 2001;22:450–455.

35. Forsting M, Krieger D, Seier U, Hacke W. Reversible bilateral thalamic lesions caused by primary internal cerebral vein thrombosis: a case report. *J Neurol* 1989;236:484–486.

36. Frey JL, Muro GJ, McDougall CG, Dean BL, Jahnke HK. Cerebral venous thrombosis: combined intrathrombus rtPA and intravenous heparin. *Stroke* 1999;30:489–494.

37. Galan HL, McDowell AB, Johnson PR, Kuehl TJ, Knight AB. Puerperal cerebral venous thrombosis associated with decreased free protein S: a case report. *J Reprod Med* 1995;40:859–862.

38. Girard DE, Reuler JB, Mayer BS, Nardone DA, Jendrzejewski J. Cerebral venous sinus thrombosis due to indwelling transvenous pacemaker catheter. *Arch Neurol* 1980;37:113–114.

39. Girot M, Ferro JM, Canhao P, et al. Predictors of outcome in patients with cerebral venous thrombosis and intracerebral hemorrhage. *Stroke* 2007;38:337–342.

40. Goldberg AL, Rosenbaum AE, Wang H, et al. Computed tomography of dural sinus thrombosis. *J Comput Assist Tomogr* 1986;10:16–20.

41. Gosk-Bierska I, Wysokinski W, Brown RD, Jr., et al. Cerebral venous sinus thrombosis: incidence of venous thrombosis recurrence and survival. *Neurology* 2006;67:814–819.

42. Haley EC, Jr, Brashear HR, Barth JT, Cail WS, Kassell NF. Deep cerebral venous thrombosis. Clinical, neuroradiological, and neuropsychological correlates. *Arch Neurol* 1989;46:337–340.

43. Hanley DF, Feldman E, Borel CO, Rosenbaum AE, Goldberg AL. Treatment of sagittal sinus thrombosis associated with cerebral hemorrhage and intracranial hypertension. *Stroke* 1988;19:903–909.

44. Hesselbrock R, Sawaya R, Tomsick T, Wadhwa S. Superior sagittal sinus thrombosis after closed head injury. *Neurosurgery* 1985;16:825–828.

45. Horowitz M, Purdy P, Unwin H, et al. Treatment of dural sinus thrombosis using selective catheterization and urokinase. *Ann Neurol* 1995;38: 58–67.

46. Hotton KM, Khorsand M, Hank JA, et al. A phase Ib/II trial of granulocyte-macrophage-colony stimulating factor and interleukin-2 for renal cell carcinoma patients with pulmonary metastases: a case of fatal central nervous system thrombosis. *Cancer* 2000;88:1892–1901.

47. Imai WK, Everhart FR, Jr., Sanders JM, Jr. Cerebral venous sinus thrombosis: report of a case and review of the literature. *Pediatrics* 1982;70:965–970.

48. Kalbag RM, Woolf AL. Thrombosis and thrombophlebitis of cerebral veins and dural sinuses. In: Vinken PJ, Bruyn GW, eds. *Handbook of Clinical Neurology.* Vol 12. Amsterdam: North-Holland; 1972:422–446.

49. Kim SY, Suh JH. Direct endovascular thrombolytic therapy for dural sinus thrombosis: infusion of alteplase. *AJNR Am J Neuroradiol* 1997;18:639–645.

50. Kuehnen J, Schwartz A, Neff W, Hennerici M. Cranial nerve syndrome in thrombosis of the transverse/sigmoid sinuses. *Brain* 1998;121 (Pt 2):381–388.

51. Lanterna LA, Gritti P, Manara O, et al. Decompressive surgery in malignant dural sinus thrombosis: report of 3 cases and review of the literature. *Neurosurg Focus* 2009;26:E5.

52. Larkey D, Williams CR, Fanning J, et al. Fatal superior sagittal sinus thrombosis associated with internal jugular vein catheterization. *Am J Obstet Gynecol* 1993;169:1612–1614.

53. Leach JL, Fortuna RB, Jones BV, Gaskill-Shipley MF. Imaging of cerebral venous thrombosis: current techniques, spectrum of findings, and diagnostic pitfalls. *Radiographics* 2006;26 Suppl 1:S19–S41.

54. Liu XY, Gabig TG, Bang NU. Combined heterozygosity of factor V leiden and the G20210A prothrombin gene mutation in a patient with cerebral cortical vein thrombosis. *Am J Hematol* 2000;64:226–228.

55. Ludemann P, Nabavi DG, Junker R, et al. Factor V Leiden mutation is a risk factor for cerebral venous thrombosis: a case-control study of 55 patients. *Stroke* 1998;29:2507–2510.

56. Martinelli I, Sacchi E, Landi G, et al. High risk of cerebral-vein thrombosis in carriers of a prothrombin-gene mutation and in users of oral contraceptives. *N Engl J Med* 1998;338:1793–1797.

57. Murray BJ, Llinas R, Caplan LR, Scammell T, Pascual-Leone A. Cerebral deep venous thrombosis presenting as acute micrographia and hypophonia. *Neurology* 2000;54:751–753.

58. Nimjee SM, Powers CJ, Kolls BJ, et al. Endovascular treatment of venous sinus thrombosis: a case report and review of the literature. *J Neurointerv Surg* 2011;3:30–33.

59. Novak Z, Coldwell DM, Brega KE. Selective infusion of urokinase and thrombectomy in the treatment of acute cerebral sinus thrombosis. *AJNR Am J Neuroradiol* 2000;21:143–145.

60. Nussel F, Huber P. High resolution computed tomography of superior sagittal sinus-thrombosis and -abnormalities. *Neuroradiology* 1989;31:307–311.

61. Peeters E, Stadnik T, Bissay F, Schmedding E, Osteaux M. Diffusion-weighted MR imaging of an acute venous stroke: case report. *AJNR Am J Neuroradiol* 2001;22:1949–1952.

62. Perkin GD. Cerebral venous thrombosis: developments in imaging and treatment. *J Neurol Neurosurg Psychiatry* 1995;59:1–3.

63. Philips MF, Bagley LJ, Sinson GP, et al. Endovascular thrombolysis for symptomatic cerebral venous thrombosis. *J Neurosurg* 1999;90:65–71.

64. Preter M, Tzourio C, Ameri A, Bousser MG. Long-term prognosis in cerebral venous thrombosis: follow-up of 77 patients. *Stroke* 1996;27:243–246.

65. Raizer JJ, DeAngelis LM. Cerebral sinus thrombosis diagnosed by MRI and MR venography in cancer patients. *Neurology* 2000;54:1222–1226.

66. Ram B, Meiklejohn DJ, Nunez DA, Murray A, Watson HG. Combined risk factors contributing to cerebral venous thrombosis in a young woman. *J Laryngol Otol* 2001;115:307–310.

67. Reuner KH, Ruf A, Grau A, et al. Prothrombin gene G20210-->A transition is a risk factor for cerebral venous thrombosis. *Stroke* 1998;29:1765–1769.

68. Rother J, Waggie K, van Bruggen N, de Crespigny AJ, Moseley ME. Experimental cerebral venous thrombosis: evaluation using magnetic resonance imaging. *J Cereb Blood Flow Metab* 1996;16:1353–1361.

69. Saxena VK, Heilpern J, Murphy SF. Pseudotumor cerebri: a complication of parenteral hyperalimentation. *JAMA* 1976;235:2124.

70. Scarrow AM, Williams RL, Jungreis CA, Yonas H, Scarrow MR. Removal of a thrombus from the sigmoid and transverse sinuses with a rheolytic thrombectomy catheter. *AJNR Am J Neuroradiol* 1999;20:1467–1469.

71. Schell CL, Rathe RJ. Superior sagittal sinus thrombosis: still a killer. *West J Med* 1988;149:304–307.

72. Seligsohn U, Lubetsky A. Genetic susceptibility to venous thrombosis. *N Engl J Med* 2001;344:1222–1231.

73. Selim M, Fink J, Linfante I, et al. Diagnosis of cerebral venous thrombosis with echo-planar T2*-weighted magnetic resonance imaging. *Arch Neurol* 2002;59:1021–1026.

74. Siddiqui FM, Banerjee C, Zuurbier SM, et al. Mechanical thrombectomy versus intrasinus thrombolysis for cerebral venous sinus thrombosis: a non-randomized comparison. *Interv Neuroradiol* 2014;20:336–344.

75. Spearman MP, Jungreis CA, Wehner JJ, Gerszten PC, Welch WC. Endovascular thrombolysis in deep cerebral venous thrombosis. *AJNR Am J Neuroradiol* 1997;18:502–506.

76. Stam J. Sinus thrombosis should be treated with anticoagulation. *Arch Neurol* 2008;65:984–985.

77. Stam J. Thrombosis of the cerebral veins and sinuses. *N Engl J Med* 2005;352:1791–1798.

78. Stam J, Majoie CB, van Delden OM, van Lienden KP, Reekers JA. Endovascular thrombectomy and thrombolysis for severe cerebral sinus thrombosis: a prospective study. *Stroke* 2008;39:1487–1490.

79. Stolz E, Kemkes-Matthes B, Potzsch B, et al. Screening for thrombophilic risk factors among 25 German patients with cerebral venous thrombosis. *Acta Neurol Scand* 2000;102:31–36.

80. Subash M, Parmar DN. Papilloedema as the sole presenting feature of postpartum cerebral venous sinus thrombosis. *Can J Ophthalmol* 2009;44:e1–2.

81. Sze G, Simmons B, Krol G, et al. Dural sinus thrombosis: verification with spin-echo techniques. *AJNR Am J Neuroradiol* 1988;9:679–686.

82. Thaler DE, Frosch MP. Case records of the Massachusetts General Hospital. Weekly clinicopathological exercises. Case 16–2002: a 41-year-old woman with global headache and an intracranial mass. *N Engl J Med* 2002;346:1651–1658.

83. Tsai FY, Higashida RT, Matovich V, Alfieri K. Acute thrombosis of the intracranial dural sinus: direct thrombolytic treatment. *AJNR Am J Neuroradiol* 1992;13:1137–1141.

84. Ulmer JL, Elster AD. Physiologic mechanisms underlying the delayed delta sign. *AJNR Am J Neuroradiol* 1991;12:647–650.

85. Valdueza JM, Hoffmann O, Weih M, Mehraein S, Einhaupl KM. Monitoring of venous hemodynamics in patients with cerebral venous thrombosis by transcranial Doppler ultrasound. *Arch Neurol* 1999;56:229–234.

86. van der Stege JG, Engelen MJ, van Eyck J. Uncomplicated pregnancy and puerperium after puerperal cerebral venous thrombosis. *Eur J Obstet Gynecol Reprod Biol* 1997;71:99–100.

87. Villringer A, Bousser MG, Einhäupl KM. Cerebral sinus venous thrombosis. In: Hacke W, Hanley DF, Einhäupl KM, et al., eds. *Neurocritical Care*. Berlin: Springer-Verlag; 1994:654–660.

88. Wardlaw JM, Vaughan GT, Steers AJ, Sellar RJ. Transcranial Doppler ultrasound findings in cerebral venous sinus thrombosis: case report. *J Neurosurg* 1994;80:332–335.

89. Wasay M, Kamal AK. Anticoagulation in cerebral venous sinus thrombosis: are we treating ourselves? *Arch Neurol* 2008;65:985–987.

90. Wingerchuk DM, Wijdicks EFM, Fulgham JR. Cerebral venous thrombosis complicated by hemorrhagic infarction: factors affecting the initiation and safety of anticoagulation. *Cerebrovasc Dis* 1998;8:25–30.

91. Wysokinska EM, Wysokinski WE, Brown RD, et al. Thrombophilia differences in cerebral venous sinus and lower extremity deep venous thrombosis. *Neurology* 2008;70:627–633.

92. Yoshikawa T, Abe O, Tsuchiya K, et al. Diffusion-weighted magnetic resonance imaging of dural sinus thrombosis. *Neuroradiology* 2002;44:481–488.

93. Yuh WT, Simonson TM, Wang AM, et al. Venous sinus occlusive disease: MR findings. *AJNR Am J Neuroradiol* 1994;15:309–316.

94. Zhang A, Collinson RL, Hurst RW, Weigele JB. Rheolytic thrombectomy for cerebral sinus thrombosis. *Neurocrit Care* 2008;9:17–26.

95. Zubkov AY, McBane RD, Brown RD, Rabinstein AA. Brain lesions in cerebral venous sinus thrombosis. *Stroke* 2009;40:1509–1511.

96. Zuurbier SM, van den Berg R, Troost D, et al. Hydrocephalus in cerebral venous thrombosis. *J Neurol* 2015;262:931–937.

97. Zuurbier SM, Lauw MN, Coutinho JM, et al. Clinical course of cerebral venous thrombosis in adult acute lymphoblastic leukemia. *J Stroke Cerebrovasc Dis* 2015;24:1679–1684.

33

Acute Bacterial Meningitis

Community-acquired acute bacterial meningitis remains a potentially devastating neurologic disorder, prone to fatal outcome. Not only is meningitis at times difficult to control, but, in some patients, pathogens (*Neisseria meningitidis*) continue to pose a threat to close contacts. Overall survival has improved, but major risks for persistent neurologic sequelae remain, predominantly from late recognition, delayed initiation of antibiotic therapy, or complications.[55,65,69] Sepsis and septic shock are major outcome determinants.

Some introductory remarks on epidemiology are appropriate. Acute bacterial meningitis can be community-acquired or nosocomial, and the circumstances are different. Many patients have otogenic meningitis and may have had chronic otitis.[5] In neurosurgical patients, penetrating injury, foreign bodies, placement of ventricular catheters, and instrumentation of the spine are the main potential triggers. The risk of acute bacterial meningitis is considerable in patients with wounds inflicted by high-velocity missiles. A cerebrospinal fluid (CSF) leak followed by bacterial meningitis is uncommon (3%) and is not always prevented by antibiotic prophylaxis.

In 30%–50% of adults, bacterial meningitis is caused by *Streptococcus pneumoniae*. In another 10%–15% each, *Escherichia coli, N. meningitidis*, and *Staphylococcus* species can be implicated.[21,29,36,53,59,65,69] Less common organisms, including *Listeria monocytogenes* and *Pseudomonas aeruginosa*, are found in the remaining patients with acute bacterial meningitis.[7,23] *L. monocytogenes* has been a major cause of bacterial meningitis in transplant recipients, but also is seen in debilitated patients with alcohol abuse and diabetes.[7,40,42] *L. monocytogenes* may be on the rise as a cause of bacterial meningitis because of increased life expectancy.[6] Human immunodeficiency virus (HIV) infection is a major risk factor for *Listeria* infection, increasing the odds substantially.[32,37] The distribution of organisms causing acute bacterial meningitis in adults is summarized in Figure 33.1. Gram-negative bacilli include *E. coli, P. aeruginosa, Klebsiella pneumoniae*, and *Acinetobacter*. Streptococci include groups A, B, and G, *viridans, bovis*, and other species. Vaccines have greatly reduced *Haemophilus influenzae* type B in children to 5 years of age, at least in the United States, and it has not been replaced by other types. *H. influenzae* is now most commonly detected in adults, although its prevalence is low.

The pathologic inflammatory cascade induced by bacterial meningitis is complicated and mostly unresolved[60] (Capsule 33.1). Operative factors that may be avenues for new therapies include reactive oxygen (e.g., superoxide),[39] nitrogen (e.g., nitric oxide and peroxynitrite), and matrix metalloproteinases.

In the emergency department, once evaluation of the patient leads to diagnosis, initial treatment is with broad-spectrum antibiotics together with corticosteroids (Chapter 3). Some patients are directly admitted from another hospital with an uncertain clinical diagnosis. Bacterial meningitis in the emergency department is often not recognized in a timely manner.[57] When data are acquired in the modern era, the time toward recognition and diagnostic tests remains markedly delayed. A recent study showed that the average time from entry to the emergency department to performance of radiologic examination was on average 2½ hours, and a time of diagnosis of meningitis resulting in antibiotics was over 2 hours after entry.[45,57] On average, the time to lumbar puncture was nearly 5 hours. Only 64% of the patients with suspected meningitis who had a normal CT scan were treated with antibiotics before CT scan and lumbar puncture. All these delays must be considered significant. Moreover, because of the complexity of acute bacterial meningitis and possible systemic involvement, very few patients with the disease are properly managed and monitored on wards. Those admitted to the neurosciences intensive care unit (NICU) often are patients lapsing into coma or patients with early complications (such as seizure, pulmonary infection, or sepsis).

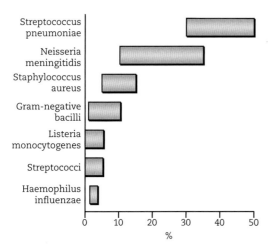

FIGURE 33.1: Distribution of causes of bacterial meningitis.

CLINICAL RECOGNITION

In most adults, a normal state of health is first interrupted by an upper respiratory tract infection or ear infection, against which antibiotic therapy does not make any major progress. These potential sources for acute bacterial meningitis, such as pneumonia, paranasal sinusitis, and middle ear infection,[5] should be sought. These causes are more prevalent in patients with profound comorbidity, such as diabetes mellitus, prior transplantation, long-term dialysis, splenectomy, alcoholism, and certain malignancies such as Hodgkin's disease.

The clinical features of acute bacterial meningitis have a very recognizable pattern. A history of myalgias, ear pain, sore throat, joint stiffness, and fatigue occurring several days before major clinical deterioration is often obtained. Fever and vomiting are the most constant early signs, present in more than three-fourths of the patients, without much variation between age groups. Headache, often described as bursting and splitting, is severe enough to overcome most commonly prescribed medications. Altered consciousness is characteristic, but may vary from delirium to drowsiness and stupor. Therefore, an acute confusional state in a febrile elderly patient should always raise the possibility of acute bacterial meningitis, and symptoms should not be assumed to have resulted from a trivial pneumonia or urinary tract infection (Chapter 3). In contrast, diagnosing acute bacterial meningitis in a fully alert patient is unusual. More than 75% of patients with bacterial meningitis are confused, irritable, or stuporous. Most patients can be roused with a forcible command or painful stimulus. Elderly patients may simply

have a blank expression and may be motionless and withdrawn.

The degree of fever in bacterial meningitis may vary, but temperature is usually constantly elevated. Most patients have so-called hectic temperature, with a surge to 39°C or 40°C, but low-grade fever (or none at all) may be present in the elderly, immunosuppressed patients, or patients who have been taking oral antibiotics or antipyretic drugs, all of whom may have greatly reduced mechanisms to mount this febrile response. Marked temperature oscillations may suggest a localized collection of pus (e.g., tonsillar, mastoid, or middle ear abscess).

Nuchal rigidity, an important sign, is common in bacterial meningitis. Neck stiffness is obscured in patients who are comatose. In patients who are drowsy and stuporous, testing of neck stiffness by neck flexion or passive extension of the knees with the hips flexed at 90° (Kernig sign) results in pain, opening of the eyes, a verbal response, and occasional combative behavior. A Brudzinski sign may be useful as well: neck flexion results in flexion of the knees and hips (one hand prevents patient from rising). The sensitivity of these classic diagnostic tests is not great, and they may not identify patients with meningitis[63] (Figure 33.2).

Papilledema in the early stages is unusual but may point to an evolving sagittal sinus thrombosis or progressive brain edema. Papilledema is most likely to be observed in a comatose patient with a fulminant clinical course.

Cranial nerves are generally not affected in patients with acute bacterial meningitis, but if they are (most commonly oculomotor nerves III, IV, and VI), tuberculosis, syphilis, or carcinomatous meningitis should be considered. Cranial nerve involvement may include abducens nerve palsy as a false localizing sign of increased intracranial pressure, facial nerve palsy associated with mastoiditis and, most worrisome, inflammation of the cochlear nerve leading to hearing loss, and reducing the patient's response to voice.

Seizures are more prevalent in children and young adults but may occur in up to 10% of adults or the elderly.[74] Seizures, particularly focal, can be attributed to focal edema, early cortical venous thrombosis, and cerebral infarction from occlusion of penetrating branches encased by the basal purulent exudate.

Focal or generalized tonic-clonic seizures should also raise the suspicion of extension of bacterial meningitis to the parenchyma. Persistent generalized or focal seizures may also be seen in patients with subdural empyema, a disorder

CAPSULE 33.1   PATHOGENESIS OF ACUTE BACTERIAL MENINGITIS

A common sequence in the development of bacterial meningitis is as follows: Nasopharyngeal colonization occurs and is dependent on fimbriae and specific surface cell receptors. Attachment may be facilitated by previous viral infection. This stage is followed by the development of bacteremia. The polysaccharide capsule should counter the classic complement pathway or alternative complement pathway (common in patients with underlying sickle cell disease and splenectomy) and defy phagocytosis. Next is meningeal invasion and entrance into the CSF through the choroid plexus, again facilitated by receptors. The bactericidal activity in the subarachnoid space is poor because the complement activity needed to initiate phagocytosis is low. Then, an inflammatory response is mounted by components of the lysed bacterial cell mass (teichoic acid endotoxin),[22,39] which induces production of inflammatory cytokines (tumor necrosis factor, interleukin-1, and macrophage inhibitory protein). Matrix metalloproteinases are endopeptidases induced by tumor necrosis factor; they degrade extracellular matrix and open the blood–brain barrier.[48] Eventually, this leads to disruption of the blood–brain barrier, brain edema, and neuronal damage due to vasculitis. Neutrophils invade, and blood–brain barrier permeability increases, finally causing vasogenic brain edema. The toxic oxygen metabolites cause cytotoxic edema, and CSF outflow resistance from protein-rich exudate in the subarachnoid space produces interstitial edema and hydrocephalus.

Cerebral infarcts from vasculitis,[70] vasospasm of basal arteries, or thrombosis of the major venous sinuses may occur, possibly only in the most fulminant cases with virulent pathogens.[58]

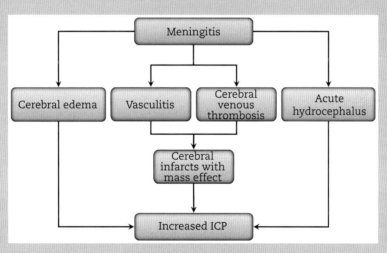

Complications of meningitis leading to increased intracranial pressure (ICP).

associated with sinusitis or mastoiditis that not only strongly resembles acute bacterial meningitis but also may be documented only by magnetic resonance imaging (MRI).

Generalized myoclonus may be noted several days into the illness and may indicate toxic levels of cephalosporins. It is occasionally noted in patients with coexistent renal disease, which reduces excretion and allows penicillin or cephalosporins to accumulate to high levels.

Rapidly developing coma with pathologic motor responses is uncommon in adults, but when present, it signals a fulminant variant with diffuse cerebral edema or multiple cerebral infarcts from secondary inflammatory vasculitis. Increased intracranial pressure occurs in approximately 10% of patients. Rarely, meningeal veins become necrotic or thrombosed, a condition leading to extensive hemorrhagic cortical infarction and bihemispheric swelling. Transverse sinus

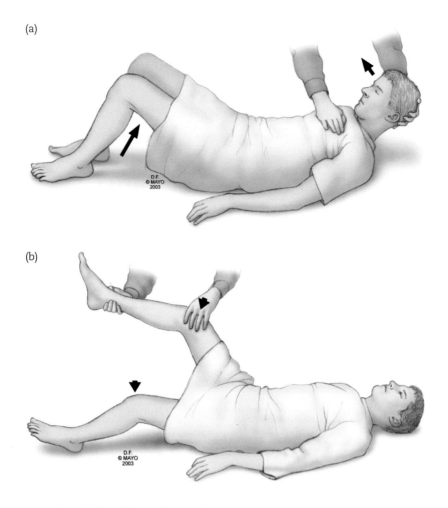

FIGURE 33.2: Brudzinski (a) and Kernig (b) signs of meningismus.

thrombosis is a possible consequence of bacterial meningitis in patients with mastoiditis, and the clot may propagate to the sagittal sinus. The true prevalence of transverse sinus thrombosis in mastoiditis is unknown and likely under investigated.

Meningococcal meningitis may progress to shock from adrenal hemorrhages.[56] Petechiae, widespread purpuric rash with patches of necrotic skin, conjunctival hemorrhage, and punctate lesions inside the mouth and on the lips are seen in conjunction with shock, profound hyponatremia and hyperkalemia (Addison's disease), and laboratory evidence of intravascular coagulation (Chapter 12).

Systemic manifestations of acute bacterial meningitis may occur but do not predict a specific cause. Shock arises more frequently in meningitis from *N. meningitidis* or *S. aureus*. However, any fulminant acute bacterial meningitis may result in hypovolemic shock from dehydration, sometimes provoked by rigorous fluid restriction in an erroneous attempt to treat brain edema.

Rashes are not specific for any cause, nor is there any characteristic distribution. Petechiae and erythematous rashes may be seen in Rocky Mountain spotted fever, West Nile fever, and echovirus 9 infection. A maculopapular rash, however, may suggest acute bacterial meningitis caused by *S. pneumoniae* or *S. aureus*. A limited petechial rash may occur in *S. aureus* meningitis or *N. meningitidis* meningitis and in any type of viral meningitis.

Septic arthritis has been reported in over 100 patients with streptococcus pneumonia with the knee commonly involved. Multiple joint involvement should be anticipated.[52] Debridement with needle aspiration or arrhoscopic lavage is needed.

Finally, the differentiation of post-neurosurgical chemical meningitis from bacterial meningitis on the basis of clinical and CSF data is very difficult. A review of 70 patients suggested a very low probability when wound infection, new focal findings, coma, new-onset seizures, temperature exceeding 39.4°C, rhinorrhea, and otorrhea were all absent. Whether antibiotic therapy can be withheld in these patients is debatable.[10,24]

Certain organisms are expected to be more frequent in particular circumstances (Table 33.1). Gram-negative bacilli meningitis (*Pseudomonas* and *E. coli*) should be considered in neutropenic patients after treatment with neoplastic agents and in patients with hematologic malignant disease. Bacterial meningitis in immunocompromised patients is often a more severe manifestation of *S. pneumoniae* or could be caused by *L. monocytogenes*. With the re-emergence of *Mycobacterium tuberculosis*, extrapulmonary manifestations may become prevalent in HIV-infected patients and intravenous drug abusers.[13]

Tuberculous meningitis should be suspected in patients with HIV infection, malnutrition, drug abuse, homelessness, or any immunosuppressed state. Prodromal symptoms of coughing, weight loss, and night sweats, followed by confusion and rapidly developing coma with cranial nerve deficits, are frequent but nonspecific. Choroidal tubercles at ophthalmoscopy, hilar adenopathy on chest radiographs, and hydrocephalus on computed

TABLE 33.1. CAUSES OF BACTERIAL MENINGITIS

Clinical Situation	Highly Probable Organism
Otitis media, mastoiditis, sinusitis	*Streptococcus pneumoniae, Haemophilus influenzae*
Pneumonia	*S. pneumoniae, Neisseria meningitidis*
Endocarditis	*Staphylococcus aureus, S. pneumoniae*
Asplenism	*S. pneumoniae, H. influenzae, N. meningitidis*
Alcoholism	*S. pneumoniae, Listeria monocytogenes*
Cerebrospinal fluid shunt	*Staphylococcus epidermidis*
Penetrating trauma	*S. aureus*
Intravenous drug abuse	*S. aureus*
Immunosuppression, acquired immunodeficiency syndrome, and transplantation	*L. monocytogenes, Pseudomonas aeruginosa, Escherichia coli*

tomography (CT) scan are additional indicators of tuberculous meningitis. In one series, 32 of 48 patients with adult tuberculous meningitis had an extrameningeal tuberculous location.[46] When younger patients are seen on admission, white cell counts of less than $10,000 \times 10^3$ per mL and protracted history of illness are more common features seen with tuberculous meningitis than with other causes of meningitis. Clear CSF with moderate number of lymphocytes and monocytes and a reduced ratio of cerebral fluid–blood glucose are important differentiating factors.

Chest radiography may be helpful, and miliary lesions have been found in 25%–50% of patients.

NEUROIMAGING AND LABORATORY TESTS

Turbid CSF often confirms the initial diagnosis of acute bacterial meningitis.[33] Conversely, crystal-clear CSF decreases the probability of acute bacterial meningitis, since only a few hundred leukocytes are necessary to reduce CSF clarity. Cerebrospinal fluid with a high viscosity or early clotting indicates very high protein content. Increasing CSF protein levels is a reflection of damage to the blood–brain barrier by the inflammatory process. Cerebrospinal fluid opening pressures are often increased (200–500 mm H_2O) in acute bacterial meningitis. The characteristic CSF profile in bacterial meningitis is a markedly increased cell count (10 to 10,000 leukocytes/mm^3, with more than 80% neutrophils), but may be much less very early in the illness or in immunocompromised patients. Typical CSF findings in tuberculous meningitis are pleocytosis with a lymphocytic predominance, a greatly increased protein level (about 200 mg/dL), and a markedly reduced glucose value. Smears are often negative, and only cultures identify the organism.

A traumatic lumbar puncture—inevitable in some agitated patients—may increase the leukocyte count. The true leukocyte count can be estimated by subtracting 1 leukocyte for every 700 erythrocytes. In patients with a marginal increase in the total number of cells, differentiation from viral meningitis becomes virtually impossible, and a second sample of CSF is needed 24 hours later.[14]

The CSF glucose concentration is normally 70% of the serum glucose value, and in acute bacterial meningitis may be normal or decreased. Any ratio of CSF to serum that is less than 0.50 indicates a decrease in glucose concentration. (A decreased glucose ratio may be less reliable in patients who have had a recent infusion of glucose-containing fluids, and 2 hours are required for equilibration.) Protein values are usually more than 100 mg/dL and may be less discriminating between viral and bacterial meningitides. An unconfirmed study in children suggested that urine reagent strips may be helpful in the initial assessment of bacterial meningitis. Normal CSF was differentiated from infected CSF by use of semiquantitative measurements of glucose, protein, and leukocytes; specificity was 100% and sensitivity 97%.[44] The test, if results are replicated, may indeed be useful during the wait for laboratory results, which can easily require 45–60 minutes.

An essential diagnostic procedure is a Gram stain of the first uncentrifuged CSF sample. The sample and positive staining may suggest specific organisms (lancet-shaped indicate *S. pneumoniae*, rods indicate *L. monocytogenes*, and cocci in clusters indicate *Staphylococcus*). Gram-negative bacilli often point to *Klebsiella*, *P. aeruginosa*, or *E. coli*. Gram-negative diplococci indicate *N. meningitidis*. One must be certain, however, that there is no technical error, possibly caused by delayed processing of the CSF or by faulty use of the dye material, that falsely suggests *Neisseria* species in patients with streptococcal meningitis. This error may unnecessarily cause an upsetting alert and distribution of chemoprophylaxis to all individuals in close contact with the patient. The availability of a polymerase chain reaction has facilitated recognition of *Neisseria*.[49]

Cultures of CSF coupled with blood cultures remain the standard for evaluation of suspected acute bacterial meningitis (Chapter 3). However, 2 days may be required for classification of the responsible species. In one study of bacterial meningitis, positive identification in blood cultures was 79% for *H. influenzae*, 56% for *S. pneumoniae*, 33% for *N. meningitidis*, 29% for β-hemolytic streptococcus meningitis, and only 17% for *S. aureus* meningitis.

Other diagnostic tests are readily available. Latex particle agglutination, which may rapidly test for bacterial antigens, has a specificity in CSF of 95% in *H. influenzae* and 50% in *S. pneumoniae* but only 30% in *N. meningitidis*. Measurement of C-reactive protein for differentiation between viral and bacterial meningitides, particularly in patients partially treated with oral antibiotics, is not very reliable in adults. The Limulus amebocyte lysate assay detects gram-negative endotoxin with a sensitivity of almost 100% but a specificity of about 90%.

At the time of admission to the NICU, a baseline CT scan has been performed in most patients in the emergency department.[34] A CT scan may unexpectedly demonstrate a subdural empyema or epidural abscess, either of which can clinically mimic acute bacterial meningitis. An otherwise normal CT scan of the brain should be additionally scrutinized for sinusitis or mastoiditis (associated with free air), which requires additional bone windows (Figure 33.3).

CT scanning is definitely indicated in patients without improvement after appropriate antibiotic treatment. Cerebral edema, an indication of poor prognosis, is occasionally seen. Resistance to antibiotic therapy seems a probable explanation in some of these unfortunate patients. CT scan is also indicated in patients with marked decrease in level of consciousness, papilledema, or neurologic findings, indicating a parenchymal lesion. A prospective study of 301 adults with "suspected" meningitis suggested that very few patients (2%) had a mass effect on CT.[34] Computed tomography

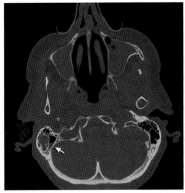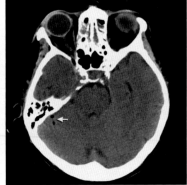

FIGURE 33.3: Acute bacterial meningitis. Computed tomography scan showing fluid pockets in mastoid and intracranial air in patient with acute bacterial meningitis (*arrows*).

scanning had a higher yield of abnormal findings in patients who were older than 60 years, were in an immunocompromised state, had a history of seizures, had focal signs and a prior central nervous system lesion, and had reduction in level of consciousness.[34]

Magnetic resonance imaging is more sensitive in diagnosing possible complications of bacterial meningitis, such as subdural effusions, cerebritis or abscess, cerebral venous thrombosis, early hydrocephalus (most commonly in patients with tuberculous meningitis), and cerebral infarcts (Figure 33.4.). Pus can be documented by MRI.[26] The magnetic resonance characteristics include irregularly contoured sedimentary material in the posterior horns and a bright signal on diffusion-weighted sequences (Figure 33.5).

Endocarditis may be more commonly associated with staphylococcus meningitis, and echocardiogram as well as a more systemic source control may be needed and could include MRI of the entire neuraxis to look for a possible epidural spinal abscess.[43]

FIRST STEPS IN MANAGEMENT

The initial management of patients with acute bacterial meningitis is shown in Table 33.2.

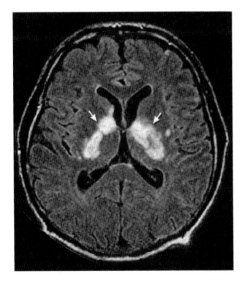

FIGURE 33.4: Magnetic resonance image with fluid-attenuated inversion recovery (FLAIR) sequences in patient with fulminant pneumococcal meningitis. Bilateral thalamic infarcts (*arrows*) from penetrating branch occlusions produce coma.

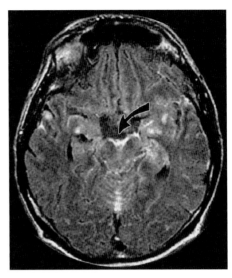

FIGURE 33.5: Magnetic resonance image with fluid-attenuated inversion recovery (FLAIR) sequences in patient with meningitis. Hyperintensity represents pus.

Respiratory isolation precaution is indicated only for patients in whom the possibility of *N. meningitidis* infection is high, and is continued for the first 24 hours of treatment. For all other patients, no specific measures other than handwashing are necessary.

Patients with acute bacterial meningitis are almost invariably dehydrated from vomiting and fever. Adequate fluid replacement should be established with at least 3 L of isotonic saline. Hyponatremia is frequently seen and has traditionally been attributed to the syndrome of inappropriate antidiuretic hormone, although this mechanism has recently been questioned (Chapter 57). The clinical manifestations of hyponatremia are mild in most cases and seldom affect the level of consciousness. Free water administration should be avoided because it aggravates hyponatremia in some patients.[66] A rapid decrease in plasma sodium may, however, decrease the threshold of seizures. Mild free water restriction is mostly sufficient for the treatment of hyponatremia associated with bacterial meningitis, but the electrolyte abnormality often is self-limiting.

Patients with acute severe bacterial meningitis could benefit from cannulation of the radial artery for monitoring of intra-arterial blood pressure but need a large-bore, peripherally placed intravenous catheter for administration of fluids and antibiotics.

Hemodynamic management in patients who develop endotoxic septic shock is complex. Septic

TABLE 33.2. INITIAL MANAGEMENT OF PATIENTS WITH ACUTE BACTERIAL MENINGITIS

Airway management	Intubation if patient has hypoxemia despite face mask with 10 L of 100% oxygen/minute, if abnormal respiratory drive or if abnormal protective reflexes (likely with motor response of withdrawal, or worse)
Mechanical ventilation	IMV/PS or CPAP mode
Blood pressure management	Maintain MAP 70–100 mm Hg
Fluid management	3 L of NaCl
	Evidence of septic shock: fluid challenges of 1L of crystalloids
	Add norepinephrine or dopamine. Vasopressin may be subsequently added to norepinephrine.
Nutrition	Enteral nutrition with continuous infusion (on day 2)
	Blood glucose control (goal 140–180 mg/dL)
Prophylaxis	DVT prophylaxis with pneumatic compression devices and SC heparin 5000 U t.i.d.
	GI prophylaxis: pantoprazole 40 mg IV daily or lansoprazole 30 mg orally through nasogastric tube.
Antibiotic treatment	Cefotaxime, 2–4 g/day IV in divided doses every 12 hours, or ceftriaxone 4 g/day in divided doses every 12 hours
	Vancomycin, 20 mg/kg IV every 12 hours (trough goal 15–20 mcg/ml).
	Ampicillin, 12 g/day in divided doses every 4 hours, in immunosuppressed patients and those older than 50 years
Other measures	Dexamethasone, 10 mg IV every 6 hours for 4 days
Access	Peripheral inserted central catheter or subclavian catheter

CPAP, continuous positive airway pressure; DVT, deep vein thrombosis; GI, gastrointestinal; IMV, intermittent mandatory ventilation; IV, intravenously; MAP, mean arterial pressure; NaCl, sodium chloride; PS, pressure support; SC, subcutaneously.

shock is recognized by hypotension, clammy skin, and poor perfusion of the kidneys, evidenced by oliguria. Aggressive fluid resuscitation and vasopressors are needed for a prolonged period of time (Chapter 51).

As alluded to in Chapter 3, antibiotics must be administered intravenously before transport to the CT scanner. Antibiotic treatment affects CSF cultures, but not significantly if the specimen is obtained within 2 hours after antibiotic administration. When samples were obtained 4–12 hours after administration of antibiotics, CSF cultures were positive in approximately 50% of the patients.[64] In addition, the latex particle agglutination test can be helpful when a significant delay between antibiotic administration and lumbar puncture has occurred.

Empirical antibiotic coverage generally includes a cephalosporin (cefotaxime or ceftriaxone), and definitive treatment should be adjusted when cultures and sensitivities become known. The minimal inhibitory concentration for each of the antibiotics is shown in Table 33.3. The addition of vancomycin is strongly recommended for coverage of penicillin-resistant pneumococci strains, particularly in geographic areas where it is more prevalent. The recommended antibiotic

dosages for each of the pathogens is shown in Table 33.4.[64,69] Chemoprophylaxis is given to household contacts of patients admitted with N. meningitidis meningitis and to healthcare workers who have intimate contact with respiratory secretions (Table 33.5). The prophylactic effect may be minimal if the drug is given 14 days after onset.[56]

Corticosteroids (dexamethasone) in acute bacterial meningitis are now considered standard therapy.[3,68] On a cellular level, corticosteroids may mute the inflammatory response by reducing cytokines (e.g., interleukin-1β), reducing expression of adhesion molecules, and lessening alteration of the blood–brain barrier by reducing matrix metalloproteinases.[17,48,62] Dexamethasone in randomized studies has reduced mortality and hearing loss in children with meningitis from H. influenzae.[20,28,31,35,41] Its effect in adults with bacterial meningitis due to totally different pathogens has been established, but it appears most effective in S. pneumoniae.[18] Initially, one prospective controlled trial found significantly fewer neurologic complications and reduced hearing loss in adults using dexamethasone 0.6 mg/kg/day in four divided doses for the first 4 days of antibiotic therapy.[30] A large

TABLE 33.3. MINIMAL INHIBITORY CONCENTRATION BREAKPOINTS FOR ANTIMICROBIAL AGENTS USED TO TREAT *STREPTOCOCCUS PNEUMONIAE* INFECTIONS (MG/ML)

Antimicrobial Agent	Susceptible	Non-Susceptible	
		Intermediate	Resistant
Penicillin	≤ 0.06	0.1–1.0	≥ 2.0
Ceftriaxone	≤ 0.5	1.0	≥ 2.0
Cefotaxime	≤ 0.5	1.0	≥ 2.0
Cefepime	≤ 0.5	1.0	≥ 2.0
Vancomycin	≤ 1.0	—	—
Rifampin	≤ 1.0	2.0	≥ 4.0
Chloramphenicol	≤ 4.0	—	≥ 8.0
Imipenem	≤ 0.12	0.25–0.5	≥ 1.0
Meropenem	≤ 0.12	≥ 0.25	—

Data from National Committee for Clinical Laboratory Standards: *Methods for Dilution Antimicrobial Susceptibility Tests for Bacteria That Grow Aerobically: Approved Standard*, 4th ed., NCCLS Document M7-A4. Wayne, PA, National Committee for Clinical Laboratory Standards, 1997.

trial found significant reduction in mortality and improved outcome in survivors. However, most patients had *S. pneumoniae* meningitis without resistance to antibiotics.[18] Therefore, a concern in areas with high prevalence of ceftriaxone or cefotaxime resistance is that vancomycin penetration into the CSF could be reduced by dexamethasone. It remains unknown if these hydrophilic antibiotics may not penetrate well as a result of corticosteroid-diminished inflammation. Some studies claimed reductions in concentration of vancomycin up to 77%.[11,47] One recent study found adequate penetration of vancomycin. However, in this prospective trial in a small group of patients, a high dose

TABLE 33.4. RECOMMENDED ANTIMICROBIAL THERAPY FOR BACTERIAL MENINGITIS

Organism	Antibiotic, Total Daily Dose (Dosing Interval)
Neisseria meningitidis	Penicillin G 24 million U/day in divided doses q4h
	or
	Aztreonam 6–8g/day IV in divided doses every 6 hours
Streptococcus pneumoniae	Cefotaxime 8–12 g/day (q4h) and vancomycin 20 mg/kg IV (q12h)
Gram-negative bacilli (except *Pseudomonas aeruginosa)*	Ceftriaxone 4 g/day IV (q12h)
	or
	Cefotaxime 8–12 g/day IV (q4h)
Pseudomonas aeruginosa	Ceftazidime 6–12 g/day IV (q8h)
Haemophilus influenzae type b	Ceftriaxone 4 g/day (q12h)
	or
	Cefepime 29 IV (q8h)
Staphylococcus aureus	
Methicillin-sensitive	Oxacillin 9–12 g/day IV (q4h)
Methicillin-resistant	Vancomycin 20 mg/kg IV (q12h) or nafcillin 8–12 g/day IV (q4h)
Listeria monocytogenes	Ampicillin 12 g/day IV (q4h)
Enterobacteriaceae	Cefotaxime 8–12 g/day (q4h)
	or
	Ceftriaxone 4 g/day (q12h)

TABLE 33.5. CHEMOPROPHYLAXIS OPTIONS FOR MENINGOCOCCAL MENINGITIS

Antibiotic	Dose
Rifampin (oral)	Adults: 600 mg q12h for 2 days
	Children > 1 month of age: 10 mg/kg q12h for 2 days
	Infant < 1 month of age: 5 mg/kg q12h for 2 days
Ciprofloxacin (oral)	Adults: 500 mg single dose; children: 125 mg
Ceftriaxone (IM)	Adults: 250 mg; children: 125 mg

IM: intramuscular.

of vancomycin was administered in a continuous infusion and after a loading dose, which may have influenced the results.[54] Addition of rifampin could enhance absorption, or a larger dose of vancomycin could be used.[71] Our practice is to give dexamethasone (10 mg IV every 6 hours for 4 days), starting just before the first dose of an antibiotic, to all patients with a bacterial meningitis, and to patients with a high likelihood of tuberculous meningitis.[50] We consider the addition of rifampin to vancomycin—until susceptibility is known—in patients with low CSF proteins levels that may be indicative of a relatively intact blood–brain barrier.

Recommendations for the duration of antibiotic therapy vary, but the following duration has been proposed: *H. influenzae* and *N. meningitidis*, 7 days; *S. pneumoniae*, 10–14 days; *L. monocytogenes* and group B streptococci, more than 21 days; and other gram-negative bacilli, at least 21 days[51,64] (see Part XIV, Guidelines). Multidrug-resistant gram-negative bacilli may prompt use of fluoroquinolones, but the toxicity of these agents may be concerning. There are insufficient data to support its use.[16]

DETERIORATION: CAUSES AND MANAGEMENT

Many patients quickly do well after intravenous antibiotic therapy, but in a few, further deterioration is marked by progression to persistent coma. The course of this progression is rapid, usually beginning soon after admission. In the advanced stage of cerebral edema, pupils become sluggish and dilated and papilledema appears. Computed tomography scanning may show signs of cortical effacement, but this may be very difficult to appreciate in young patients with less prominent sulci. Progressive effacement of the sylvian fissure

and compression of ventricles and the basal cisterns are more diagnostic for cerebral edema on CT scans. Patients with acute brain edema require intubation and mechanical ventilation to a respiratory alkalosis with $PaCO_2$ in the low 30s. Administration of a bolus of mannitol (1 g/kg) is guided using standard criteria (Chapter 21). A parenchymal intracranial pressure monitor is placed to determine the effect of treatment, but the development of brain edema is an ominous sign.

In a rapidly worsening patient, subdural empyema should be considered for what at first seems to be acute bacterial meningitis.[67] The clinical presentation of headache and worsening coma can be analogous to acute bacterial meningitis. Important clues are prior paranasal sinusitis and recent sinus surgery, both of which are associated with subdural empyema in a considerable number of patients. To complicate matters further, noncontrast CT scanning can yield normal results or may not have been performed initially. Magnetic resonance imaging may demonstrate multilocular collections that cannot be seen with CT scanning, particularly those localized at the convexity.[72] In most patients, however, CT scanning with contrast demonstrates the subdural pus pocket (Figures 33.6 and 33.7). A large craniotomy is needed to salvage the patient.[4] Treatment is shown in Table 33.6. Outcome is poor if patients are comatose.

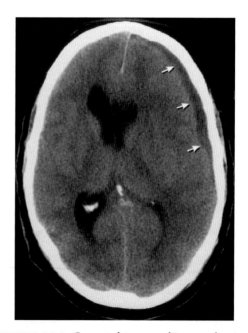

FIGURE 33.6: Computed tomographic scan showing subdural empyema with mass effect (*arrows*).

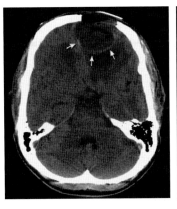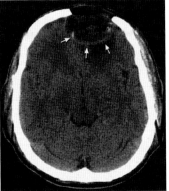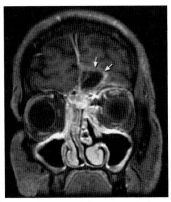

FIGURE 33.7: Computed tomographic scans and magnetic resonance image after frontal craniotomy show new epidural pus collections (*arrows*).

Another important cause for clinical deterioration is therapeutic failure. In recent years, penicillin-resistant *S. pneumoniae* strains have increased in frequency.[3,12,25] Any patient with bacterial meningitis, rapid clinical deterioration, persistent high fever despite antibiotic treatment, and diplococci in a repeated CSF culture after several days of treatment may have a penicillin-resistant strain of *S. pneumoniae*. As mentioned earlier, the addition of vancomycin to the initial empirical antibiotic treatment should reduce therapeutic failures. Rarely, intrathecal vancomycin with monitoring of CSF levels is needed in addition to systemic therapy.

The patient's condition may deteriorate from seizures, but the low incidence of 10% does not justify prophylactic treatment. Nonconvulsive status epilepticus is a rare cause of deterioration in patients with meningitis, but we monitor patients with video electroencephalogram when seizures have occurred, if they fail to awaken promptly or their level of consciousness waxes and wanes.

OUTCOME

Prognostic factors in acute bacterial meningitis depend on the organism.[8,22] The odds of unfavorable outcome are six times higher in patients infected with *Streptococcus pneumoniae* when compared with patients infected with *Neisseria meningitidis*. Acute obstructive hydrocephalus requiring a ventriculostomy is a poor prognosticator, and the same applies to diffuse brain edema.[39] Most studies have found that delay in onset of treatment is associated with adverse clinical outcome. Other well-recognized risk factors are age and duration of illness before effective antibiotic therapy begins, hypotension, and seizures.[2,15,68] Splenectomy or functional hyposplenia is a major risk factor for bacterial meningitis particularly if patients are not systematicallt vaccinated against *Streptococcus pneumoniae* and results in a high rate of mortality and unfavorable outcome.[1] Delay to diagnosis, delay to antibiotic treatment, delay to treatment of associated critical illness, and delay of treatment of increased

TABLE 33.6. EMPIRICAL ANTIBIOTIC THERAPY IN SUBDURAL EMPYEMA AND EPIDURAL ABSCESS

Likely Source	Covers	Antimicrobial Therapy
Otitis media or mastoiditis	Streptococci Anaerobes Enterobacteria	Cefotaxime 8–12 g/day IV (q4h divided doses) Metronidazole 15 mg/kg loading, 7.5 mg/kg IV (q4h)
Sinusitis	Streptococci Anaerobes	*or*
	Enterobacteria	Piperacillin sodium and tazobactam sodium 3.375 g (q6h) IV
	Staphylococcus aureus *Haemophilus* species	

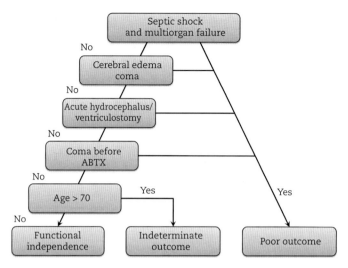

FIGURE 33.8: Outcome algorithm for bacterial meningitis. Functional independence: No assistance needed, minor handicap may remain. Indeterminate: Any statement would be a premature conclusion. Poor outcome: Severe disability or death, vegetative state.

ABTX, antibiotic therapy.

intracranial pressure remain major concerns in management of acute bacterial meningitis. Deescalation of care may be the most common reason of death in patients who remain comatose after fulminant meningitis. Early withdrawal may be inappropriate because even patients who are nearly moribund may actually survive and some of them may fully recover.

In one recent study, the time to treat with antibiotics in the emergency department was on average 3 hours (1–5 hours range), and the time to treat with dexamethasone in the ED was on average 6 hours (2–9 hours range).[45] The study had an unfavorable outcome in 73% of controls and with a large proportion of patients in severe sepsis. Therefore, delay to diagnosis, delay to antibiotic treatment, delay to treatment of critical illness, and delay of treatment of increased intracranial pressure remain major concerns in the management of acute bacterial meningitis.[9] Expertise of care can only be found in tertiary centers. The mortality remains high in the fulminant bacterial meningitis group (40%–50%, and in some studies 70%), but this is related to the development of sepsis and time to treatment. The case fatality rate is 19% for *S. pneumoniae* and 13% for *N. meningitidis*, and even in the current era, one in five adults with bacterial meningitis dies.[69] Mortality is higher in *N. meningitidis* meningitis when septicemia is present.[27] *Klebsiella*, a rare cause of acute bacterial meningitis, has a much higher reported mortality of 43%.[61]

Long-term neurologic deficits remain uncommon and are less than 10%.[2,42] Outcome in meningitis-associated traumatic CSF leak is good when the cause is *S. pneumoniae* and treatment with a third-generation cephalosporin is begun early. Nonetheless, the major disabling sequelae of acute bacterial meningitis are hearing loss and a seizure disorder. The risk of significant hearing impairment is approximately 15% in patients with *N. meningitidis* meningitis. Gadolinium-enhanced, high-resolution MRI documented abnormalities in the cochlear nerve, but because many patients in the study received brief courses of gentamicin in addition to standard therapy, the relationship between meningitis and cochlear damage was uncertain.[19] One study identified multiple laboratory and clinical features that predict poor outcome as early as several hours after onset. These variables are abnormal consciousness, cranial nerve palsy, decreased white cell count, and the presence of gram-positive cocci.[73] However, the most important variable is initial management and appropriate treatment with antibiotics within an hour in the emergency department and before neuroimaging.[16] An outcome algorithm for acute bacterial meningitis is shown in Figure 33.8.

CONCLUSION

- *S. pneumoniae* is the cause of most cases of adult bacterial meningitis. *S. aureus* can be implicated in penetrating trauma and intravenous drug abuse. In immunosuppressed patients, alcoholics, and debilitated patients with diabetes, *L. monocytogenes* or *P. aeruginosa* should be considered.

- Empirical therapy for adult bacterial meningitis consists of cefotaxime or ceftriaxone. Ampicillin is added in immunosuppressed patients and in patients older than 50 years.
- Vancomycin is currently recommended in the empirical regimen to treat penicillin-resistant pneumococci.
- Rapid deterioration in patients with presumed acute bacterial meningitis has three major causes: fulminant meningitis or penicillin-resistant *S. pneumoniae* not properly covered with vancomycin, cerebral edema, and failure to diagnose empyema.

REFERENCES

1. Adriani KS, Brouwer MC, van der Ende A, van de Beek D. Bacterial meningitis in adults after splenectomy and hyposplenic states. *Mayo Clin Proc* 2013;88:571–578.
2. Aronin SI, Peduzzi P, Quagliarello VJ. Community-acquired bacterial meningitis: risk stratification for adverse clinical outcome and effect of antibiotic timing. *Ann Intern Med* 1998;129:862–869.
3. Assiri AM, Alasmari FA, Zimmerman VA, et al. Corticosteroid administration and outcome of adolescents and adults with acute bacterial meningitis: a meta-analysis. *Mayo Clinic Proc* 2009;84:403–409.
4. Bannister G, Williams B, Smith S. Treatment of subdural empyema. *J Neurosurg* 1981;55:82–88.
5. Barry B, Delattre J, Vie F, Bedos JP, Gehanno P. Otogenic intracranial infections in adults. *Laryngoscope* 1999;109:483–487.
6. Behrman RE, Meyers BR, Mendelson MH, Sacks HS, Hirschman SZ. Central nervous system infections in the elderly. *Arch Intern Med* 1989;149:1596–1599.
7. Beninger PR, Savoia MC, Davis CE. Listeria monocytogenes meningitis in a patient with AIDS-related complex. *J Infect Dis* 1988;158:1396–1397.
8. Bohr V, Rasmussen N, Hansen B, et al. Pneumococcal meningitis: an evaluation of prognostic factors in 164 cases based on mortality and on a study of lasting sequelae. *J Infect* 1985;10:143–157.
9. Brouwer MC, Van de Beek D, Wijdicks EFM. Update in bacterial meningitis. *Intensive Care Med* 2016 42;415–417.
10. Brown EM, de Louvois J, Bayston R, Lees PD, Pople IK. Distinguishing between chemical and bacterial meningitis in patients who have undergone neurosurgery. *Clin Infect Dis* 2002;34:556–558.
11. Cabellos C, Martinez-Lacasa J, Martos A, et al. Influence of dexamethasone on efficacy of ceftriaxone and vancomycin therapy in experimental pneumococcal meningitis. *Antimicrob Agents Chemother* 1995;39:2158–2160.
12. Catalan MJ, Fernandez JM, Vazquez A, et al. Failure of cefotaxime in the treatment of meningitis due to relatively resistant Streptococcus pneumoniae. *Clin Infect Dis* 1994;18:766–769.
13. Clark WC, Metcalf JC, Jr, Muhlbauer MS, Dohan FC, Jr, Robertson JH. Mycobacterium tuberculosis meningitis: a report of twelve cases and a literature review. *Neurosurgery* 1986;18:604–610.
14. Connolly KJ, Hammer SM. The acute aseptic meningitis syndrome. *Infect Dis Clin N Am* 1990;4:599–622.
15. Conte HA, Chen YT, Mehal W, Scinto JD, Quagliarello VJ. A prognostic rule for elderly patients admitted with community-acquired pneumonia. *Am J Med* 1999;106:20–28.
16. Cottagnoud P, Tauber MG. Fluoroquinolones in the treatment of meningitis. *Curr Infect Dis Rep* 2003;5:329–336.
17. Coyle PK. Glucocorticoids in central nervous system bacterial infection. *Arch Neurol* 1999;56:796–801.
18. de Gans J, van de Beek D. Dexamethasone in adults with bacterial meningitis. *N Engl J Med* 2002;347:1549–1556.
19. Dichgans M, Jager L, Mayer T, Schorn K, Pfister HW. Bacterial meningitis in adults: demonstration of inner ear involvement using high-resolution MRI. *Neurology* 1999;52:1003–1009.
20. Diseases AAoPCoI. Dexamethasone therapy for bacterial meningitis in infants and children. *Pediatrics* 1990;86:130–133.
21. Durand ML, Calderwood SB, Weber DJ, et al. Acute bacterial meningitis in adults: a review of 493 episodes. *N Engl J Med* 1993;328:21–28.
22. Fiore AE, Moroney JF, Farley MM, et al. Clinical outcomes of meningitis caused by Streptococcus pneumoniae in the era of antibiotic resistance. *Clin Infect Dis* 2000;30:71–77.
23. Fong IW, Tomkins KB. Review of *Pseudomonas aeruginosa* meningitis with special emphasis on treatment with ceftazidime. *Rev Infect Dis* 1985;7:604–612.
24. Forgacs P, Geyer CA, Freidberg SR. Characterization of chemical meningitis after neurological surgery. *Clin Infect Dis* 2001;32:179–185.

25. Friedland IR, Klugman KP. Failure of chloramphenicol therapy in penicillin-resistant pneumococcal meningitis. *Lancet* 1992;339:405–408.

26. Fukui MB, Williams RL, Mudigonda S. CT and MR imaging features of pyogenic ventriculitis. *AJNR Am J Neuroradiol* 2001;22:1510–1516.

27. Gedde-Dahl TW, Bjark P, Hoiby EA, Host JH, Bruun JN. Severity of meningococcal disease: assessment by factors and scores and implications for patient management. *Rev Infect Dis* 1990;12:973–992.

28. Geiman BJ, Smith AL. Dexamethasone and bacterial meningitis: a meta-analysis of randomized controlled trials. *West J Med* 1992;157:27–31.

29. Geiseler PJ, Nelson KE, Levin S, Reddi KT, Moses VK. Community-acquired purulent meningitis: a review of 1,316 cases during the antibiotic era, 1954–1976. *Rev Infect Dis* 1980;2:725–745.

30. Gijwani D, Kumhar MR, Singh VB, et al. Dexamethasone therapy for bacterial meningitis in adults: a double blind placebo control study. *Neurol India* 2002;50:63–67.

31. Girgis NI, Farid Z, Mikhail IA, et al. Dexamethasone treatment for bacterial meningitis in children and adults. *Pediatr Infect Dis J* 1989;8:848–851.

32. Gould IA, Belok LC, Handwerger S. Listeria monocytogenes: a rare cause of opportunistic infection in the acquired immunodeficiency syndrome (AIDS) and a new cause of meningitis in AIDS: a case report. *AIDS Res* 1986;2:231–234.

33. Gray LD, Fedorko DP. Laboratory diagnosis of bacterial meningitis. *Clin Microbiol Rev* 1992;5:130–145.

34. Hasbun R, Abrahams J, Jekel J, Quagliarello VJ. Computed tomography of the head before lumbar puncture in adults with suspected meningitis. *N Engl J Med* 2001;345:1727–1733.

35. Havens PL, Wendelberger KJ, Hoffman GM, Lee MB, Chusid MJ. Corticosteroids as adjunctive therapy in bacterial meningitis: a meta-analysis of clinical trials. *Am J Dis Child* 1989;143:1051–1055.

36. Jensen AG, Espersen F, Skinhoj P, Rosdahl VT, Frimodt-Moller N. Staphylococcus aureus meningitis: a review of 104 nationwide, consecutive cases. *Arch Intern Med* 1993;153:1902–1908.

37. Jurado RL, Farley MM, Pereira E, et al. Increased risk of meningitis and bacteremia due to Listeria monocytogenes in patients with human immunodeficiency virus infection. *Clin Infect Dis* 1993;17:224–227.

38. Kasanmoentalib ES, Brouwer MC, van der Ende A, van de Beek D. Hydrocephalus in adults with community-acquired bacterial meningitis. *Neurology* 2010;75:918–923.

39. Kastenbauer S, Koedel U, Becker BF, Pfister HW. Oxidative stress in bacterial meningitis in humans. *Neurology* 2002;58:186–191.

40. Koziol K, Rielly KS, Bonin RA, Salcedo JR. Listeria monocytogenes meningitis in AIDS. *CMAJ* 1986;135:43–44.

41. Lebel MH, Freij BJ, Syrogiannopoulos GA, et al. Dexamethasone therapy for bacterial meningitis: results of two double-blind, placebo-controlled trials. *N Engl J Med* 1988;319:964–971.

42. Lorber B. Listeriosis. *Clin Infect Dis* 1997;24:1–9; quiz 10–11.

43. Lucas MJ, Brouwer MC, van der Ende A, van de Beek D. Endocarditis in adults with bacterial meningitis. *Circulation* 2013;127:2056–2062.

44. Moosa AA, Quortum HA, Ibrahim MD. Rapid diagnosis of bacterial meningitis with reagent strips. *Lancet* 1995;345:1290–1291.

45. Mourvillier B, Tubach F, van de Beek D, et al. Induced hypothermia in severe bacterial meningitis: a randomized clinical trial. *JAMA* 2013;310:2174–2183.

46. Ogawa SK, Smith MA, Brennessel DJ, Lowy FD. Tuberculous meningitis in an urban medical center. *Medicine (Baltimore)* 1987;66:317–326.

47. Paris MM, Hickey SM, Uscher MI, et al. Effect of dexamethasone on therapy of experimental penicillin- and cephalosporin-resistant pneumococcal meningitis. *Antimicrob Agents Chemother* 1994;38:1320–1324.

48. Paul R, Lorenzl S, Koedel U, et al. Matrix metalloproteinases contribute to the blood-brain barrier disruption during bacterial meningitis. *Ann Neurol* 1998;44:592–600.

49. Porritt RJ, Mercer JL, Munro R. Detection and serogroup determination of Neisseria meningitidis in CSF by polymerase chain reaction (PCR). *Pathology* 2000;32:42–45.

50. Prasad K, Volmink J, Menon GR. Steroids for treating tuberculous meningitis. *Cochrane Database Syst Rev* 2000:CD002244.

51. Quagliarello VJ, Scheld WM. Treatment of bacterial meningitis. *N Engl J Med* 1997;336:708–716.

52. Raad J, Peacock JE Jr. Septic arthritis in the adult caused by Streptococcus pneumoniae: a report of 4 cases and review of the literature. *Semin Arthritis Rheum* 2004 Oct;34(2):559–569.

53. Ragunathan L, Ramsay M, Borrow R, et al. Clinical features, laboratory findings and management of meningococcal meningitis in England and Wales: report of a 1997 survey. Meningococcal meningitis: 1997 survey report. *J Infect* 2000;40:74–79.

54. Ricard JD, Wolff M, Lacherade JC, et al. Levels of vancomycin in cerebrospinal fluid of adult

patients receiving adjunctive corticosteroids to treat pneumococcal meningitis: a prospective multicenter observational study. *Clin Infect Dis* 2007;44:250–255.

55. Roos KL. Acute bacterial meningitis. *Semin Neurol* 2000;20:293–306.

56. Rosenstein NE, Perkins BA, Stephens DS, Popovic T, Hughes JM. Meningococcal disease. *N Engl J Med* 2001;344:1378–1388.

57. Schuh S, Lindner G, Exadaktylos AK, Muhlemann K, Tauber MG. Determinants of timely management of acute bacterial meningitis in the ED. *Am J Emerg Med* 2013;31:1056–1061.

58. Schut ES, Brouwer MC, de Gans J, et al. Delayed cerebral thrombosis after initial good recovery from pneumococcal meningitis. *Neurology* 2009;73:1988–1995.

59. Sigurdardottir B, Bjornsson OM, Jonsdottir KE, Erlendsdottir H, Gudmundsson S. Acute bacterial meningitis in adults: a 20-year overview. *Arch Intern Med* 1997;157:425–430.

60. Simon RP, Beckman JS. Why pus is bad for the brain. *Neurology* 2002;58:167–168.

61. Tang LM, Chen ST. Klebsiella pneumoniae meningitis: prognostic factors. *Scand J Infect Dis* 1994;26:95–102.

62. Tauber MG, Moser B. Cytokines and chemokines in meningeal inflammation: biology and clinical implications. *Clin Infect Dis* 1999;28:1–11; quiz 12.

63. Thomas KE, Hasbun R, Jekel J, Quagliarello VJ. The diagnostic accuracy of Kernig's sign, Brudzinski's sign, and nuchal rigidity in adults with suspected meningitis. *Clin Infect Dis* 2002;35:46–52.

64. Tunkel AR, Hartman BJ, Kaplan SL, et al. Practice guidelines for the management of bacterial meningitis. *Clin Infect Dis* 2004;39.1267–1284.

65. Tunkel AR, Scheld WM. Acute bacterial meningitis. *Lancet* 1995;346:1675–1680.

66. van de Beek D, Brouwer MC, de Gans J. Hypernatremia in bacterial meningitis. *J Infect* 2007;55:381–382.

67. van de Beek D, Campeau NG, Wijdicks EFM. The clinical challenge of recognizing infratentorial empyema. *Neurology* 2007;69:477–481.

68. van de Beek D, de Gans J, Spanjaard L, et al. Clinical features and prognostic factors in adults with bacterial meningitis. *N Engl J Med* 2004;351:1849–1859.

69. van de Beek D, de Gans J, Tunkel AR, Wijdicks EFM. Community-acquired bacterial meningitis in adults. *N Engl J Med* 2006;354:44–53.

70. van de Beek D, Patel R, Wijdicks EFM. Meningococcal meningitis with brainstem infarction. *Arch Neurol* 2007;64:1350–1351.

71. Viladrich PF, Gudiol F, Linares J, et al. Evaluation of vancomycin for therapy of adult pneumococcal meningitis. *Antimicrob Agents Chemother* 1991;35:2467–2472.

72. Weingarten K, Zimmerman RD, Becker RD, et al. Subdural and epidural empyemas: MR imaging. *AJR Am J Roentgenol* 1989;152:615–621.

73. Weisfelt M, van de Beek D, Spanjaard L, Reitsma JB, de Gans J. A risk score for unfavorable outcome in adults with bacterial meningitis. *Ann Neurol* 2008;63:90–97.

74. Zoons E, Weisfelt M, de Gans J, et al. Seizures in adults with bacterial meningitis. *Neurology* 2008;70:2109–2115.

34

Brain Abscess

Several traditional causes of brain abscess, such as otitis media and sinusitis, have decreased in prevalence because of improved diagnosis and management and have been displaced by other causes, such as infections of molar teeth, staphylococcal endocarditis, and hematogenous dissemination from pulmonary infections.[36] The clinical spectrum of pathogens causing brain abscess has also most likely changed with the arrival of human immunodeficiency virus (HIV) infections and, to a lesser degree, with the increase in the number of immunocompromised transplant patients.

Admission to the neurosciences intensive care unit (NICU) is mostly dictated by the complexity of management, such as neurosurgical management of the abscess, or by a complication, such as ventriculitis or cerebral edema. When a brain abscess is located in the brainstem,[20] it may cause impaired swallowing, difficulty with clearing of secretions, and respiratory problems. Merely the anticipation of clinical deterioration in a patient with a sizable brain abscess and mass effect or an abscess situated in close proximity to the ventricular system qualifies for admission to the NICU. The number of patients with brain abscess in the NICU is small, and sometimes even the diagnosis becomes apparent after elective biopsy for a solitary mass thought to be a glioma.

Definitive treatment of brain abscess is often neurosurgical, although several successful attempts have been reported using antibiotic therapy alone, particularly in patients with lesions that were not easily accessible. The management of brain abscess often requires expertise from specialists in infectious diseases, otolaryngologists, pulmonologists, and dental surgeons. This chapter focuses on the diagnostic evaluation and options for medical treatment in brain abscess. It also proposes neurosurgical indications.

CLINICAL RECOGNITION

A careful history and physical examination may provide additional clues in the evaluation of patients with a brain abscess. The potential source of infection may lie in dental abscess or periodontal disease, otitis media or suppurative sinusitis, congenital heart disease,[5,25,26,28,36,61] acquired valvular disease, pulmonary disease, skin infections, or recent travel or occupational exposure. Pulmonary arteriovenous malformations have been associated with brain abscesses, most frequently in patients with hereditary hemorrhagic telangiectasia (Osler disease).[6,16,47] In any single mass suspicious for a bacterial abscess other causes should be considered and immune status is important (Table 34.1).

Brain abscess is usually diagnosed on the basis of three important clinical signs: headache, focal neurologic deficit, and, perhaps less commonly, change in level of consciousness.[2,8,62,66] In a review from the University of California at San Francisco, 56% of the patients with a brain abscess were drowsy to stuporous at presentation.[41] In another report, full alertness was noted in approximately 70% of 140 patients, a discrepancy that may reflect recognition of cerebral abscess by early timing of neuroimaging studies.[66]

Pronounced neck stiffness is present in only 40% of patients with a brain abscess, but may be more apparent in patients with ventriculitis. Fever and focal neurologic signs remain more

TABLE 34.1. DIFFERENTIAL DIAGNOSIS OF A SINGLE MASS SUSPICIOUS FOR BACTERIAL ABSCESS

Noncompromised Host	Compromised Host
Cysticercosis	*Cryptococcus neoformans*
Glioma	Kaposi sarcoma
Herpes simplex	*Listeria monocytogenes*
Metastasis	Lymphoma
Multiple sclerosis	*Mycobacterium*
Sarcoidosis	*Nocardia*
	Progressive multifocal leukoencephalopathy
	Toxoplasma

distinctive signs, but both may also be absent.[64,66] Fever occurs in only 50% of patients in most series. Most patients have hemiparesis, which may be subtle; in others, a single cerebral abscess produces behavioral changes alone. Brain abscess frequently lodges in the frontal (or frontoparietal) lobe (Capsule 34.1), and this location may explain the lack of obvious clinical signs. Many patient with frontal abscesses are delirious with no fever. In patients with an abscess in the dominant hemisphere, symptoms may become more evident during reading, spelling out loud, or writing, although many patients have clearly recognizable Broca aphasia. Otogenic brain abscesses are most frequent in the temporal lobe or cerebellum.[31,55] An abscess in the brainstem can be associated with impaired consciousness if it abuts the reticular formation, and involvement of major

CAPSULE 34.1   NEUROPATHOLOGY OF ABSCESS

Five neuropathologic stages in brain abscess development have been recognized. The first stage is a presuppurative stage (1–3 days) and inoculation causing a cerebritis. During this stage, injury occurs to the microvasculature, and bacteria enter the white matter, where they replicate in these ischemic and necrotic areas. The microscopic hallmark at this stage is vascular congestion, perivascular exudates, petechial hemorrhages, microthrombi, and nests of polymorphonuclear cells. The second stage (days 4–9) is characterized by the emergence of a purulent center surrounded by granulation tissue, neutrophils, lymphocytes, and sporadic macrophages. Perivascular cuffing of neutrophils is characteristic. The formation of an abscess capsule is the third stage and takes up to 2 weeks (see accompanying illustration). The capsule is thin at this stage and can easily rupture into the ventricles.

The fourth stage is the development of a well-organized capsule (see accompanying figure) with surrounding edema and can be found more than 14 days into the infection. At this stage, multiple capsular layers are found. In the final stage, the abscess becomes a mass of collagen.[37]

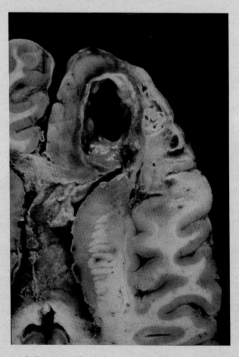

Frontal abscess with perforation into ventricular system.

nuclei produces cranial nerve deficits. Depending on localization in the brainstem, patients have involvement of cranial nerves VI and VII and, less commonly, III, and these findings are almost always associated with marked horizontal nystagmus, ataxia, or hemiparesis. Localization in the medulla mostly produces impaired swallowing.

The clinical characteristics in patients with multiple brain abscesses are fairly similar, and most have headache, impaired consciousness, and focal neurologic deficits.[40] Seizures are common in patients with multiple brain abscesses, and the incidence in several studies approached 30%. Symptoms depend on size and tissue shift, and one lesion may be responsible for the clinical presentation.

NEUROIMAGING AND LABORATORY TESTS

Advances in neuroimaging leading to early recognition may have improved the outcome in brain abscess. Currently, magnetic resonance imaging (MRI) is the preferred neuroimaging technique, but computed tomography (CT) scanning remains important in the initial diagnosis, during stereotactic biopsy, and in serial monitoring after antibiotic therapy and surgical drainage[43] (Figure 34.1). Typically, an abscess is manifested as a round, thick capsule with a central low density, representing pus. Surrounding edema in the white matter usually is found and often is the only clearly visible determinant of the lesion in a noncontrast CT scan. In cerebritis, these CT features are less developed. Contrast enhancement is seen in most cases but can be insignificant in patients treated with corticosteroids. The inner wall layer becomes smooth when the abscess is firm, which occurs almost invariably 2 weeks after the first symptoms. Multiloculation within the abscess is also an important CT feature, because it indicates that surgical intervention is a less favorable

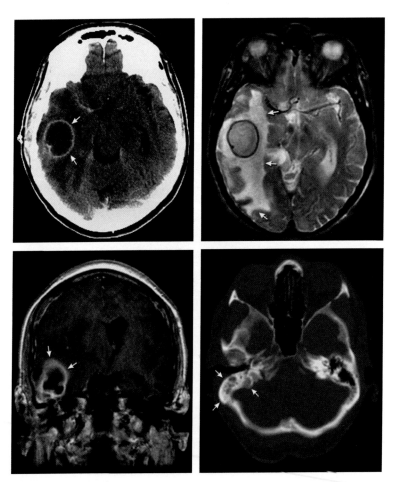

FIGURE 34.1: Brain Abscesses. Upper row: Computed tomographic scans showing abscess in the temporal lobe with perilesional edema on MRI (*arrows*). Lower row: MRI showing temporal lobe abscess associated with otitis media. Aeration is absent in the mastoid cells on CT (*arrows*).

option. Features that require attention are shift of midline structures and release of pus into the ventricular system. Contrast enhancement in the ventricular wall is seen in ventriculitis or ependymitis. Bone windows on CT scans are necessary to carefully evaluate the sinuses and mastoids for loss of air pockets and presence of fluid collection, which may be a source of the infection.[44]

The advantage of MRI is a greater sensitivity in detection of cerebritis and abscesses that are either not detected or uncertain by CT.[12] Diffusion-weighted MRI may also be helpful in differentiating cerebral abscess from necrotic tumor and ventricular extension of pus.[14,41] In brain abscess the typical finding is high signal intensity on DWI and a low ADC value, findings that are not noted in gliomas or metastasis.[50]

Magnetic resonance imaging may be helpful in further differentiating between a pyogenic or fungal abscess. Apart from differences in morphology (pyogenic smooth and lobulated; fungal irregular and with intracavitary projections), MR in a fungal abscess may more often show no enhancement and no restricted diffusion in the core of the abscess.[39]

Lumbar puncture may not be helpful, and rapid deterioration after the procedure has been demonstrated, not necessarily only in patients with massive shift on CT scans. However, one study reported no complications after lumbar puncture in 17 patients, including three with papilledema.[56] The yield of cerebrospinal fluid (CSF) cultures in patients with brain abscess is low. The frequency varies from 0 to 7%,[11] although the number of reported patients who have had CSF examination is small. As expected, identification of the organism is more common in surgical specimens[41] (only 4% of the patients had sterile cultures)

Findings on peripheral blood examination can be supportive, with increased sedimentation rate and increased leukocyte count in most patients. Blood cultures should be part of the evaluation in any patient with brain abscess. Three consecutive blood samples should be taken; they may demonstrate, for example, *Staphylococcus aureus* or *Aspergillus* in highly susceptible patients, such as intravenous drug abusers and transplant recipients. (Aspergillemia in a single sample is often spurious.) The bacteriologic cause of pyogenic brain abscess depends on its source, (Table 34.2) but cultures may yield a polymicrobial flora, and results are inconclusive in more than half of the cases. Ribosomal DNA sequencing techniques may become important future tests in identifying the causative organism.[1] *Streptococcus milleri* is most common in abscesses associated with paranasal sinusitis.[17] Otogenic abscesses

TABLE 34.2. BRAIN ABSCESS: PREDISPOSING CONDITION, SITE OF ABSCESS, AND MICROBIOLOGY

Predisposing Condition	Site of Abscess	Usual Microbial Isolates
Contiguous Focus or Primary Infection		
Otitis media or mastoiditis	Temporal lobe or cerebellum	Streptococci (anaerobic or aerobic), *Bacteroides fragilis*, Enterobacteriaceae
Frontoethmoidal sinusitis	Frontal lobe	Predominantly streptococci (anaerobic or aerobic), *Bacteroides* spp., Enterobacteriaceae, *Staphylococcus aureus*, *Haemophilus* spp.
Sphenoidal sinusitis	Frontal or temporal lobe	Same as frontoethmoidal sinusitis
Periodontal abscess	Frontal lobe	Mixed *Fusobacterium, Bacteroides*, and *Streptococcus* spp.
Penetrating head injury or postsurgical infection	Near the laceration	*S. aureus*, streptococci, Enterobacteriaceae, *Clostridium* spp.
Hematogenous Spread or Distant Site of Infection		
Congenital heart disease	Multiple sites	Streptococci (aerobic, anaerobic, or microaerophilic), *Haemophilus* spp.
Lung abscess, empyema, bronchiectasis	Multiple sites	*Fusobacterium* spp., *Actinomyces* spp., *Bacteroides* spp., *Streptococcus* spp., *Nocardia asteroides*
Bacterial endocarditis	Multiple sites	*S. aureus*, *Streptococcus* spp.

are commonly caused by *Proteus* anaerobes, *Streptococcus* species, Enterobacteriaceae, or *Pseudomonas aeruginosa*.[55] Unusual species are *Klebsiella* bacteria,[37] *Streptococcus pneumoniae*,[24] and *Streptococcus bovis*.[42] The right to left shunt in cyanotic heart disease reduces filtering of bacteria in the lungs, and *Streptococcus milleri* or *Staphylococcus spp* are common microorganisms in these patients. Intratumoral abscess, facilitated by breakdown of the blood–brain barrier through tumor and prior surgery, is rare but has been described in more than 25 cases.[33] Diagnostic criteria for neurocysticercosis have been published and should be considered in individuals from an endemic area.[8] In brief, they include cystic lesions showing the scolex on neuroimaging and funduscopic demonstration of subretinal parasites, positive serum enzyme-linked immunoelectrotransfer blot assay, and response to albendazole and praziquantel.[13] Paracoccidiomycosis is a common (potentially fatal) fungal infection with up to 35% CNS involvement in areas in Central and South America.[7,46,53] The essential laboratory tests in evaluation of brain abscess are summarized in Table 34.3.

FIRST STEPS IN MANAGEMENT

The argument in favor of medical management of cerebral abscess is compelling. Early antibiotic therapy alone in patients with an abscess is indicated for a small solitary abscess (< 3 cm), an abscess in a surgically inaccessible area, multilocular or multiple localizations, brainstem localization,[9,21,22,54] early abscess formation without clear capsule formation (cerebritis stage), and a paucity of clinical

---

TABLE 34.3. LABORATORY STUDIES IN THE INITIAL EVALUATION OF BRAIN ABSCESS

Cultures	Blood, urine, sputum, cerebrospinal fluid
	Selected cases: gastric washings, bronchial brushing, pleural or ascitic fluid, aspirate or biopsy
Serologic studies	Viral, fungal, *Toxoplasma gondii*
Imaging studies	Chest radiograph, sinus radiograph and Panorex, electrocardiogram, echocardiography, computed tomography images of chest or abdomen

---

signs. In other patients, surgical aspiration, not necessarily with reduction of the mass itself, should be considered to obtain pus for cytologic examination and cultures. Obviously, antibiotic coverage is of utmost importance, but if surgery is performed within hours and the diagnosis of cerebral abscess is very uncertain, administration probably should be postponed to reduce the risk of sterile cultures.

Surgical management includes freehand or stereotactic aspiration, endoscopic aspiration, or craniotomy with excision. Neurosurgeons may use intraoperative guidance with MRI or intraoperative ultrasound.[26] Location and multiplicity of brain abscesses are important factors in surgical decision-making. When surgical aspiration is considered, the stereotactic approach is preferred. The risk of further morbidity from the stereotactic procedure remains low. A study from the University of Lille, France, comparing medical management, surgical aspiration, and excision in brain abscess found no differences in survival, but seizures and focal deficits occurred more often in the surgically approached group.[38] In general, for lesions that are very superficially located and are not over the motor strip of the cortex, catheter drainage can be tried by placing a burr hole and puncturing the parenchyma with a small soft catheter. Catheter drainage is continued for at least 1 week, with alternative aspiration and saline irrigation. In deep-seated lesions, stereotactic aspiration can be considered, but most argue that antibiotic therapy is the first therapeutic choice.[58,59] Excision of the abscess by open craniotomy with additional damage to the surrounding white matter is not an attractive first option, even in large, encapsulated abscesses. On the other hand, cerebellar abscesses are preferably healed surgically, and the outcome is much better than that with supratentorial abscess.

Multiple abscesses occur in 1%–15% of the patients.[3,35] Surgical treatment is controversial,[4,51] and antimicrobial therapy seems more appropriate in patients with superficially located abscesses and in immunosuppressed patients with a high likelihood of toxoplasmosis or aspergillosis.[15] Stereotactic aspiration by CT-guided techniques should be considered in patients with deep lesions larger than 3 cm.

It is difficult to marshal all the different options for the management of cerebral abscess, but some guidance is shown in Figure 34.2. The surgical technique usually consists of stereotactic aspiration, aspiration after craniotomy, or excision.[27,29,45] Surgical management is clearly indicated for superficial abscesses, lesions with a well-defined wall

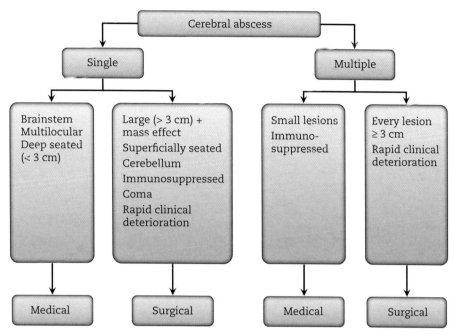

FIGURE 34.2: Guideline for management of brain abscess.

on imaging studies, and abscesses abutting the ventricles at risk of rupture, causing ventriculitis. Abscesses located in the parietooccipital region are more commonly associated with ventricular rupture than are those in other locations.[60] Abscesses originating from the sinus or middle ear may rupture into the subarachnoid space.[48] Abscesses in the posterior fossa should be surgically removed if the fourth ventricle is effaced and, as in cerebellar infarcts and hematomas, if CT features of a tight posterior fossa are present. Aspiration is clearly indicated if the lesion causes significant mass effect or produces coma or rapid clinical deterioration.[32]

Conversely, medical management is more reasonable in patients with deep-seated lesions that are surgically inaccessible, multiple small abscesses, or multilocular abscesses. A primary lesion in the brainstem probably should be managed medically and may not need stereotactic aspiration. However, in a survey of 71 patients with brainstem masses who had stereotactic surgery, there was no procedure-related mortality and only one patient had permanent morbidity.[49]

Surgical intervention by stereotactic aspiration must be strongly considered in immunosuppressed patients with acquired immunodeficiency syndrome (AIDS) or HIV infection. A 2-week trial with therapy directed against *Toxoplasma gondii* is recommended, but tissue must be obtained for culture and histologic examination

if failure to improve is apparent clinically or by CT scan. On the other hand, an abscess caused by *Nocardia* is difficult to cure with aspiration and antibiotics and probably must be excised.[19] Local instillation of amphotericin B, next to systemic treatment, was entertained in a patient with cerebellar aspergillosis.[15]

Another approach favors surgically aggressive treatment of multiple cerebral abscesses, albeit based on a review of only 16 patients.[40] In this protocol, every abscess greater than 2.5 cm in diameter was treated surgically (excision or aspiration). Antibiotic therapy followed, CT scan or MRI was repeated in 2 weeks, and stereotactic drainage or craniotomy was repeated if new large lesions emerged. Abscesses with more than two aspirations were surgically excised. This management protocol resulted in low mortality and reflects a low threshold for aspiration in large lesions (> 2.5 cm) and the investigators' willingness to repeat aspiration if a good response was not observed by clinical and neuroimaging criteria.

The initial medical management in patients with a brain abscess is summarized in Table 34.4. Brain abscess is treated empirically by cephalosporins in combination with metronidazole and vancomycin.[23,30,52,57,65] Vancomycin should be administered to patients with penicillin allergy. Parenteral treatment should be continued for 3–4 weeks after excision and for 4–6 weeks after aspiration.[10] Empirical

TABLE 34.4. INITIAL MANAGEMENT OF PATIENTS WITH BRAIN ABSCESS

Airway management	Intubation if patient has hypoxemia despite facemask with 10 L of 100% oxygen/minute, if abnormal respiratory drive or presence of abnormal protective reflexes (likely with motor response of withdrawal, or worse)
Mechanical ventilation	IMV/PS or CPAP mode
Fluid management	2 L of 0.9% NaCl (adjust with fever)
Nutrition	Enteral nutrition with continuous infusion (on day 2)
	Blood glucose control (goal 140–180 mg/dL)
Prophylaxis	DVT prophylaxis with pneumatic compression devices
	Consider SC heparin 5,000 U t.i.d.
	GI prophylaxis: pantoprazole 40 mg IV daily or lansoprazole 30 mg orally through nasogastric tube
	Consider seizure prophylaxis when surgery anticipated (levetiracetam 20 mg/kg IV over 60 minutes) maintenance 1,000 mg b.i.d. orally
Medical management	Third-generation cephalosporin and metronidazole
Surgical management	Aspiration with rapid deterioration, coma, mass effect, and > 3 cm
Access	Peripheral inserted central catheter

CPAP, continuous positive airway pressure; DVT, deep vein thrombosis; GI, gastrointestinal; IMV, intermittent mandatory ventilation; IV, intravenously; NaCl, sodium chloride; PS, pressure support; SC, subcutaneously.

treatment in immunocompromised patients or in patients who most likely have an unusual infection is complex (Table 34.5). Rifampin, isoniazid, pyrazinamide, and ethambutol (RIPE) therapy is instituted for patients with tertiary TB meningoencephalitis (Figure 34.3) (combination therapy with

ethambutol 1,600 mg/day, pyrazinamide to 2,000 mg/day, rifampin 600 mg/day, isoniazid 300 mg/day, and pyridoxine 50 mg/day).

Listeria is more commonly seen in immunocompromised patients and post transplantation and present with an abscess (Figure 34.4).

TABLE 34.5. EMPIRICAL ANTIBIOTIC TREATMENT FOR PATIENTS WITH BRAIN ABSCESS

Nonimmunocompromised Patients	
Cefotaxime	8–12 g/day IV in divided doses q4h
Metronidazole	15 mg/kg IV load; 7.5 mg/kg IV q6h
Vancomycin (with penicillin allergy)	20 mg/kg IV in divided doses q12h
Immunocompromised Patients or Those with Possible Unusual Bacterial Infection, Atypical Bacteria, or Nonbacterial Infection	
Antituberculous therapy	Rifampin, 10 mg/kg/day orally
	Isoniazid, 5 mg/kg/day orally
	Pyrazinamide, 2,000 mg/day/orally
	Ethambutol, 15 mg/kg/day orally
Antifungal therapy	Amphotericin B, 0.25–1.0 mg/kg/day IV to total dose of 1.5 mg/kg/day infused over 2–6 hours
Antiparasitic therapy	
Toxoplasma gondii	Pyrimethamine, initially 200 mg po and then 50–75 mg/day orally
	Sulfadiazine, 1–1.5 g q6h/day (leucovorin [folinic acid], 10 mg orally)
Taenia solium	Praziquantel, 60 mg/kg/day (in divided doses tid) or albendazole, 15 mg/kg/day (in divided doses tid)
Atypical bacteria	
Nocardia asteroides	Trimethoprim, sulfamethoxazole, 15 mg TMP/kg/day in 2 divided doses IV or orally qid per day or sulfisoxazole, 4–8 g/day (in 4 divided doses)

IV, intravenous.

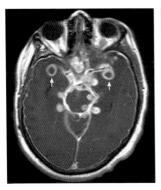
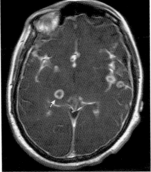
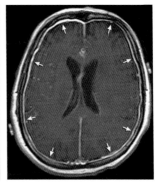

FIGURE 34.3: Multiple abscesses associated with tuberculosis.

Treatment is surgical extirpation, if accessible, and ampicillin 12 grams daily plus gentamycine 5mg/kg/day every 8 hour.

Central access should be obtained in expectation of several weeks of antibiotic administration. Preferably, a Hickman-Broviac catheter is inserted. This catheter is tunneled under the skin and brought out several inches from the site of insertion. The catheter should be placed in the superior vena cava or the proximal right atrium, because malpositioning in smaller veins may produce phlebitis and thrombosis. The complications of long-term placement of a central venous catheter are few, and most are related to insertion. Nonetheless, we observed pulmonary emboli in one patient at the end of an 8-week course of intravenously administered antibiotics.[19] Daily flushing with heparin is advised.

Fluid intake should not exceed maintenance amounts but must be adjusted if fever occurs. (Fos)phenytoin or levetiracetam is given when surgical treatment is planned but can be deferred in patients receiving medical management alone. Antiepileptic coverage is reasonable, however, when considerable edema and shift are seen on CT scans. Furthermore, the risk of late seizures is considerable in patients with abscess. Although extremely rare, if the level of consciousness waxes and wanes, one should also consider cephalosporin toxicity causing nonconvulsive status epilepticus.[34]

DETERIORATION: CAUSES AND MANAGEMENT

Most patients with a solitary abscess remain neurologically stable and begin to improve soon after antibiotic treatment. Deterioration in level of consciousness is more common in patients with multiple abscesses and in patients with multilocular abscesses; as expected, mortality is very high. In two series of patients who died before surgical procedures could be performed, multiple abscesses and rupture of abscesses into the ventricular system were prevalent.[54,66]

Enlargement of the abscess with clinical deterioration is an absolute indication for stereotactic aspiration or extirpation (Figure 34.5). Brain edema surrounding the abscess may be the cause of significant displacement and can be determined

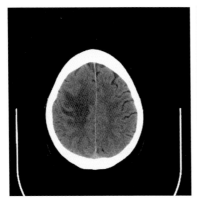
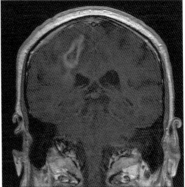

FIGURE 34.4: Listeria abscess (CT nondistinctive, MRI more delineated abscess).

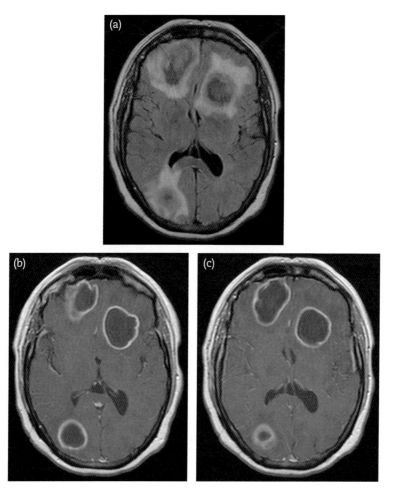

FIGURE 34.5: Multiple large ring enhancing cerebral abscesses in a patient with declining consciousness from bifrontal mass effect.

only by comparison of recent and previous CT images. Corticosteroids to reduce edema may not have the disadvantage of spreading the infection, as commonly thought, and should be administered promptly in deteriorating patients (dexamethasone: loading dose of 10 mg IV, then 4 mg IV q 6h). Waiting for the effect of dexamethasone, which may take hours, is ill-advised, and one should proceed with aspiration. A bolus of mannitol (1 g/kg IV) should be used additionally to reduce intracranial pressure in anticipation of surgery. Surgical intervention is the only lifesaving measure if deterioration is rapid. Aspiration through a burr hole may involve 15–30 cc of pus and may be repeated if needed (in about 20% of cases).

In unfortunate circumstances, the abscess ruptures into the ventricular system and the outcome is often fatal.[18,60] Magnetic resonance imaging often shows enhancement of the ventricular

wall adjacent to the abscess (Figure 34.6), which may precede rupture.

Deterioration from hydrocephalus associated with abscess located in the posterior fossa has been reported. Extirpation of the compressing abscess alone with antibiotic therapy is sufficient. Ventriculostomy alone probably should be avoided to reduce the risk of upward tissue displacement.

OUTCOME

Intravenous antibiotic therapy may cure a solitary brain abscess with or without aspiration. Use of a Hickman-Broviac catheter allows the administration of antibiotics on an outpatient basis, greatly reducing hospital costs. Outcome in patients with medically treated brainstem abscesses is quite good; most neurologic function returns, and ataxia and diplopia diminish significantly (Figure 34.7). Outcome seems correlated with location of lesion

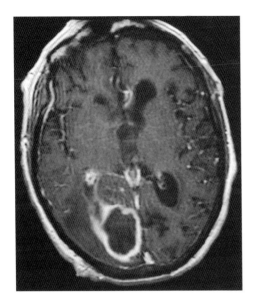

FIGURE 34.6: Brain abscess suspicious for early rupture to the ventricles. Note dumbbell shape and enhancement, suggesting ventriculitis.

(deep-seated), progression to coma before intervention, and, particularly, ventricular rupture.[60,63] However, outcome in patients with brain abscess also depends on the clinical features on admission, the type of infectious agent, or whether abscess is single or multiple. Salvage therapy with relatively new agents (such as linezolid or daptomycin) should be used in patients with brain abscesses caused by MRSA strains who do not have a response or who have an elevated minimum inhibitory concentration of vancomycin.[5]

Multiple staphylococcal abscesses associated with endocarditis are often fatal. Cerebral abscesses in immunocompromised patients have a less favorable outcome because of fungal origin in most patients. In contrast, brain abscesses caused by *Toxoplasma* may virtually disappear after appropriate therapy, although the underlying illness may shorten the long-term outcome. Mortality varies considerably in most series and currently probably approaches 20%. One study found that a shorter duration of symptoms before

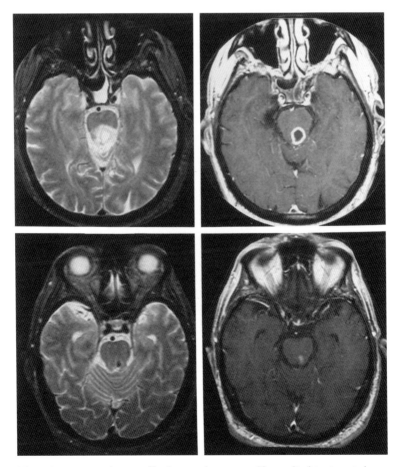

FIGURE 34.7: Magnetic resonance images of brainstem abscess cured by medical treatment alone.

From Fulgham JR, Wijdicks EFM, Wright AJ. Cure of a solitary brainstem abscess with antibiotic therapy: case report. *Neurology* 1996;46:1451–1454. With permission of the American Academy of Neurology.

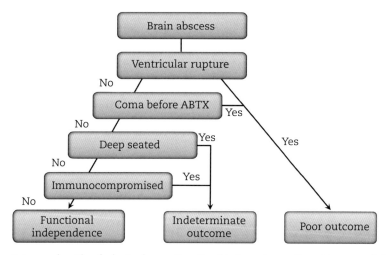

FIGURE 34.8: Outcome algorithm for brain abscess. Functional independence: No assistance needed, minor handicap may remain. Indeterminate: Any statement would be a premature conclusion. Poor outcome: Severe disability or death, vegetative state.

ABTX, antibiotic therapy.

admission predicted death or severe sequelae, reflecting a fulminant course and its consequences.[56] Outcome prediction is shown as an algorithm in Figure 34.8.

CONCLUSIONS

- Medical treatment is indicated for brainstem abscess, multilocular abscesses, and surgically inaccessible deep-seated lesions.
- Surgical treatment is indicated (craniotomy or stereotactic aspiration) if abscesses are causing mass effect and rapid clinical deterioration. The threshold for a surgical approach should also be low if the abscess is superficially placed or in the cerebellum.
- Empirical therapy in nonimmunocompromised patients is vancomycin, cefotaxime with metronidazole.
- Empirical therapy in immunocompromised patients (particularly those infected with HIV) is indicated if multiple abscesses suggestive of toxoplasmosis are found. Therapy is guided by repeat CT scan or MRI.

REFERENCES

1. Al Masalma M, Armougom F, Scheld WM, et al. The expansion of the microbiological spectrum of brain abscesses with use of multiple 16S ribosomal DNA sequencing. *Clin Infect Dis* 2009;48:1169–1178.

2. Bagdatoglu H, Ildan F, Cetinalp E, et al. The clinical presentation of intracranial abscesses: a study of seventy-eight cases. *J Neurosurg Sci* 1992;36:139–143.

3. Basit AS, Ravi B, Banerji AK, Tandon PN. Multiple pyogenic brain abscesses: an analysis of 21 patients. *J Neurol Neurosurg Psychiatry* 1989;52:591–594.

4. Boom WH, Tuazon CU. Successful treatment of multiple brain abscesses with antibiotics alone. *Rev Infect Dis* 1985;7:189–199.

5. Brouwer MC, Tunkel AR, van de Beek D. Brain abscess. *N Engl J Med* 2014;371:1758.

6. Brydon HL, Akinwunmi J, Selway R, Ul-Haq I. Brain abscesses associated with pulmonary arteriovenous malformations. *Br J Neurosurg* 1999;13:265–269.

7. Buitrago MJ, Bernal-Martinez L, Castelli MV, Rodriguez-Tudela JL, Cuenca-Estrella M. Histoplasmosis and paracoccidioidomycosis in a non-endemic area: a review of cases and diagnosis. *J Travel Med* 2011;18:26–33.

8. Carpenter J, Stapleton S, Holliman R. Retrospective analysis of 49 cases of brain abscess and review of the literature. *Eur J Clin Microbiol Infect Dis* 2007;26:1–11.

9. Carpenter JL. Brain stem abscesses: cure with medical therapy, case report, and review. *Clin Infect Dis* 1994;18:219–226.

10. Infection in Neurosurgery Working Party of the British Society for Antimicrobial Chemotherapy. The rational use of antibiotics in the treatment of brain abscess. *Br J Neurosurg* 2000;14:525–530.

11. Chun CH, Johnson JD, Hofstetter M, Raff MJ. Brain abscess: a study of 45 consecutive cases. *Medicine (Baltimore)* 1986;65:415–431.

12. Davidson HD, Steiner RE. Magnetic resonance imaging in infections of the central nervous system. *AJNR Am J Neuroradiol* 1985;6:499–504.

13. Del Brutto OH, Rajshekhar V, White AC, Jr., et al. Proposed diagnostic criteria for neurocysticercosis. *Neurology* 2001;57:177–183.

14. Desprechins B, Stadnik T, Koerts G, et al. Use of diffusion-weighted MR imaging in differential diagnosis between intracerebral necrotic tumors and cerebral abscesses. *AJNR Am J Neuroradiol* 1999;20:1252–1257.

15. Erdogan E, Beyzadeoglu M, Arpaci F, Celasun B. Cerebellar aspergillosis: case report and literature review. *Neurosurgery* 2002;50:874–876.

16. Faughnan ME, Lui YW, Wirth JA, et al. Diffuse pulmonary arteriovenous malformations: characteristics and prognosis. *Chest* 2000;117:31–38.

17. Fenton JE, Smyth DA, Viani LG, Walsh MA. Sinogenic brain abscess. *Am J Rhinol* 1999;13:299–302.

18. Ferre C, Ariza J, Viladrich PF, et al. Brain abscess rupturing into the ventricles or subarachnoid space. *Am J Med* 1999;106:254–257.

19. Fried J, Hinthorn D, Ralstin J, Gerjarusak P, Liu C. Cure of brain abscess caused by Nocardia asteroides resistant to multiple antibiotics. *South Med J* 1988;81:412–413.

20. Fuentes S, Bouillot P, Regis J, Lena G, Choux M. Management of brain stem abscess. *Br J Neurosurg* 2001;15:57–62.

21. Fujino H, Kobayashi T, Goto I, Nagata E, Shima F. Cure of a man with solitary abscess of the brainstem. *J Neurol* 1990;237:265–266.

22. Fulgham JR, Wijdicks EFM, Wright AJ. Cure of a solitary brainstem abscess with antibiotic therapy: case report. *Neurology* 1996;46:1451–1454.

23. Green HT, O'Donoghue MA, Shaw MD, Dowling C. Penetration of ceftazidime into intracranial abscess. *J Antimicrob Chemother* 1989;24:431–436.

24. Grigoriadis E, Gold WL. Pyogenic brain abscess caused by Streptococcus pneumoniae: case report and review. *Clin Infect Dis* 1997;25:1108–1112.

25. Hakan T. Management of bacterial brain abscesses. *Neurosurg Focus* 2008;24:E4.

26. Hall WA, Truwit CL. The surgical management of infections involving the cerebrum. *Neurosurgery* 2008;62 Suppl 2:519–530.

27. Hasdemir MG, Ebeling U. CT-guided stereotactic aspiration and treatment of brain abscesses: an experience with 24 cases. *Acta Neurochir (Wien)* 1993;125:58–63.

28. Helweg-Larsen J, Astradsson A, Richhall H, et al. Pyogenic brain abscess, a 15 year survey. *BMC Infect Dis* 2012;12:332.

29. Itakura T, Yokote H, Ozaki F, et al. Stereotactic operation for brain abscess. *Surg Neurol* 1987;28:196–200.

30. Jansson AK, Enblad P, Sjolin J. Efficacy and safety of cefotaxime in combination with metronidazole for empirical treatment of brain abscess in clinical practice: a retrospective study of 66 consecutive cases. *Eur J Clin Microbiol Infect Dis* 2004;23:7–14.

31. Jim KK, Brouwer MC, van der Ende A, van de Beek D. Cerebral abscesses in patients with bacterial meningitis. *J Infect* 2012;64:236–238.

32. Kala M. Aspiration or extirpation in cerebral abscess surgery? *Neurosurg Rev* 1993;16:121–124.

33. Kalita O, Kala M, Svebisova H, et al. Glioblastoma multiforme with an abscess: case report and literature review. *J Neurooncol* 2008;88:221–225.

34. Klion AD, Kallsen J, Cowl CT, Nauseef WM. Ceftazidime-related nonconvulsive status epilepticus. *Arch Intern Med* 1994;154:586–589.

35. Kratimenos G, Crockard HA. Multiple brain abscess: a review of fourteen cases. *Br J Neurosurg* 1991;5:153–161.

36. Kulai A, Ozatik N, Topcu I. Otogenic intracranial abscesses. *Acta Neurochir (Wien)* 1990;107:140–146.

37. Liliang PC, Lin YC, Su TM, et al. Klebsiella brain abscess in adults. *Infection* 2001;29:81–86.

38. Love S, Louis D, Ellison DW. *Greenfield's Neuropathology.* 8th ed. London: Hodder Arnold; 2008.

39. Luthra G, Parihar A, Nath K, et al. Comparative evaluation of fungal, tubercular, and pyogenic brain abscesses with conventional and diffusion MR imaging and proton MR spectroscopy. *AJNR Am J Neuroradiol* 2007;28:1332–1338.

40. Mamelak AN, Mampalam TJ, Obana WG, Rosenblum ML. Improved management of multiple brain abscesses: a combined surgical and medical approach. *Neurosurgery* 1995;36:76–85.

41. Mampalam TJ, Rosenblum ML. Trends in the management of bacterial brain abscesses: a review of 102 cases over 17 years. *Neurosurgery* 1988;23:451–458.

42. Maniglia RJ, Roth T, Blumberg EA. Polymicrobial brain abscess in a patient infected with human immunodeficiency virus. *Clin Infect Dis* 1997;24:449–451.

43. Miller ES, Dias PS, Uttley D. CT scanning in the management of intracranial abscess: a review of 100 cases. *Br J Neurosurg* 1988;2:439–446.

44. Nalbone VP, Kuruvilla A, Gacek RR. Otogenic brain abscess: the Syracuse experience. *Ear Nose Throat J* 1992;71:238–242.

45. Nauta HJ, Contreras FL, Weiner RL, Crofford MJ. Brain stem abscess managed with computed tomography-guided stereotactic aspiration. *Neurosurgery* 1987;20:476–480.

46. Pedroso VS, Vilela Mde C, Pedroso ER, Teixeira AL. [Paracoccidioidomycosis compromising the central nervous system: a systematic review of the literature]. *Rev Soc Bras Med Trop* 2009;42:691–697.

47. Preston DC, Shapiro BE. Pulmonary arteriovenous fistula and brain abscess. *Neurology* 2001;56:418.

48. Quijano M, Schuknecht HF, Otte J. Temporal bone pathology associated with intracranial abscess. *ORL J Otorhinolaryngol Relat Spec* 1988;50:2–31.

49. Rajshekhar V, Chandy MJ. Computerized tomography-guided stereotactic surgery for brainstem masses: a risk-benefit analysis in 71 patients. *J Neurosurg* 1995;82:976–981.

50. Rana S, Albayram S, Lin DD, Yousem DM. Diffusion-weighted imaging and apparent diffusion coefficient maps in a case of intracerebral abscess with ventricular extension. *AJNR Am J Neuroradiol* 2002;23:109–112.

51. Rousseaux M, Lesoin F, Destee A, Jomin M, Petit H. Developments in the treatment and prognosis of multiple cerebral abscesses. *Neurosurgery* 1985;16:304–308.

52. Ruelle A, Zerbi D, Zuccarello M, Andrioli G. Brain stem abscess treated successfully by medical therapy. *Neurosurgery* 1991;28:742–745.

53. Salaki JS, Louria DB, Chmel H. Fungal and yeast infections of the central nervous system: a clinical review. *Medicine (Baltimore)* 1984;63:108–132.

54. Schliamser SE, Backman K, Norrby SR. Intracranial abscesses in adults: an analysis of 54 consecutive cases. *Scand J Infect Dis* 1988;20:1–9.

55. Sennaroglu L, Sozeri B. Otogenic brain abscess: review of 41 cases. *Otolaryngol Head Neck Surg* 2000;123:751–755.

56. Seydoux C, Francioli P. Bacterial brain abscesses: factors influencing mortality and sequelae. *Clin Infect Dis* 1992;15:394–401.

57. Sjolin J, Lilja A, Eriksson N, Arneborn P, Cars O. Treatment of brain abscess with cefotaxime and metronidazole: prospective study on 15 consecutive patients. *Clin Infect Dis* 1993;17:857–863.

58. Stapleton SR, Bell BA, Uttley D. Stereotactic aspiration of brain abscesses: is this the treatment of choice? *Acta Neurochir (Wien)* 1993;121:15–19.

59. Stroobandt G, Zech F, Thauvoy C, et al. Treatment by aspiration of brain abscesses. *Acta Neurochir (Wien)* 1987;85:138–147.

60. Takeshita M, Kagawa M, Izawa M, Takakura K. Current treatment strategies and factors influencing outcome in patients with bacterial brain abscess. *Acta Neurochir (Wien)* 1998;140:1263–1270.

61. Takeshita M, Kagawa M, Yato S, et al. Current treatment of brain abscess in patients with congenital cyanotic heart disease. *Neurosurgery* 1997;41:1270–1278.

62. Takeshita M, Kawamata T, Izawa M, Hori T. Prodromal signs and clinical factors influencing outcome in patients with intraventricular rupture of purulent brain abscess. *Neurosurgery* 2001;48:310–316.

63. Tseng JH, Tseng MY. Brain abscess in 142 patients: factors influencing outcome and mortality. *Surg Neurol* 2006;65:557–562.

64. Wispelwey B, Scheld WM. Brain abscess. *Semin Neurol* 1992;12:273–278.

65. Yamamoto M, Jimbo M, Ide M, et al. Penetration of intravenous antibiotics into brain abscesses. *Neurosurgery* 1993;33:44–49.

66. Yang SY, Zhao CS. Review of 140 patients with brain abscess. *Surg Neurol* 1993;39:290–296.

35

Acute Encephalitis

All of us, in a way, see a fair number of patients with acute encephalitis—at least often we think that's what it is. Patients with acute encephalitis are admitted to the NICU when they become stuporous and have an urgent need for airway protection. Not infrequently, admission to the NICU is also justified if seizures have developed and in some situations have progressed to status epilepticus. Other patients in earlier stages are agitated and combative, difficult to restrain effectively, and in need of sedation and respiratory monitoring.

Neurologists are adept at recognizing the emerging clinical picture, but a critically important part in the care of these patients is to sort out a cause, which may in some situations radically change therapy.

Acute encephalitis is not an uncommon critical neurologic illness, and when of viral origin, herpes simplex encephalitis is statistically most common.[11,78] On the other hand, the ability to recognize the beginning of an outbreak of arboviral encephalitis is difficult, and it may take time for the outbreak to become fully established. The season is important in epidemic forms of encephalitis, with peak occurrence from June to September. In addition, an immunosuppressed state (including human immunodeficiency virus [HIV] infection) requires specific attention, because it places the patient in a different category of differential diagnosis and outcome.

This chapter discusses the most pertinent therapeutic targets in the management of acute encephalitis. The treatment of acute viral encephalitis is the major focus.

CLINICAL RECOGNITION

Any acutely progressive encephalitis will present with confusion, followed by a decline in consciousness, often punctuated by seizures. No clinical feature is characteristic of encephalitis, but clues in the history may help in sorting out possible causes. Essential inquiries in the evaluation of any encephalitis are recent vaccination, travel, animal contact (pets, bats, or wild animals),

deaths in horse populations, tick exposure, long-term immunosuppression or possible exposure to HIV, or recent diagnosis of acquired immunodeficiency syndrome (AIDS). Immunosuppressed patients are also at risk for herpes zoster encephalitis when disseminated cutaneous zoster is present. Prodromal pharyngitis may suggest cytomegalovirus (CMV) or Epstein-Barr virus (EBV) as a potential pathogen.

The typical clinical characteristics of acute viral encephalitis are the rapid development of fever (which may begin cyclically and reach 40°C), headache, acute confusional state, and new neurologic signs. Several human herpes types can produce neurologic complications after reactivation from peripheral sensory ganglia. Herpes simplex virus (HSV)-1 causes herpes simplex encephalitis; HSV-2 is sexually transmitted, causing recurrent meningitis, and presents with cranial nerve deficit and confusion; in certain recurrent cases, it has been misdiagnosed as Mollaret meningitis (a relapsing meningitis with no identifiable infectious source[15]).

In herpes simplex encephalitis, the clinical features are altered consciousness, and fever (> 39°C).[46,47,73] Initial neurologic signs, such as seizures, visual field defects, aphasia, and bizarre behavior, including hypomania, have been reported.[31] Seizures, often focal and transient, are present in one-third of patients.[6] As the disorder progresses, epilepsia partialis continua and temporal lobe seizures may reflect frontal or temporal lobe involvement. Auras of temporal lobe seizures may consist of hallucinations and dysgeusia. Memory impairment with abnormal recall alone and complete absence of fever and other accompanying signs have been noted as a presentation of herpes simplex encephalitis.[87] A proclivity for brainstem involvement with diplopia, dysarthria, and ataxia exists in immunosuppressed patients with herpes simplex encephalitis.[7]

An anterior operculum syndrome has been reported, and failure to recognize its distinguishing features may potentially delay therapy.[54]

Involvement of the anterior operculum (the operculum is the cortex and white matter tissue overlying the insula) results in difficulty chewing, a tendency for the mouth to be half open, bifacial palsy, dysphagia, drooling, anarthria, and trismus. Automatic facial movements, such as yawning, are preserved.[54] Cerebellitis with profound swelling, a location more preferentially affected in children, has been reported in an adult.[23] All these complex presentations should alert the physician to herpes simplex encephalitis, but such an untraditional presentation may not be recognized.

Progression may take days but can be rapid, and even the interval between the development of febrile illness and coma may be surprisingly short. Some patients may be healthy in the morning and meet the criteria for brain death at night. Autonomic dysfunction with profound instability in blood pressure, tachypnea, and sweating may occur and, in exceptional cases, may further deteriorate into a sympathetic overdrive with catatonia and extensive rigidity.[46,47]

Epstein-Barr virus-related encephalitis is rare, but the outcome is quite good. Epstein-Barr virus encephalitis usually occurs in systemic infections, and the classic findings are lymphadenopathy, pharyngitis, and splenomegaly.

Encephalitis may occur during the yearly influenza season, and both influenza A and influenza B have been implicated. The damage may be quite impressive, including patients remaining in a minimally conscious state.

Varicella zoster virus (VZV) encephalitis should be the first consideration in immunosuppressed (e.g., HIV-infected) patients with recent shingles.[1] In most reported cases, however, a rash developed days to weeks before the onset but was not always remembered by the patients. In several reports, VZV encephalitis actually occurred without a skin eruption.

Varicella zoster virus (VZV) encephalitis also occurs more often in the elderly, and in patients with malignant disease.[35] Varicella zoster virus encephalitis has been associated with hematologic–oncologic malignant disease, sarcoidosis, rheumatoid arthritis, tuberculosis, transplantation, and AIDS. Cutaneous localization of herpes zoster invariably may have to be confirmed by skin biopsy. Herpes zoster encephalitis is not common in patients with herpes zoster infection involving several dermatomes alone but is more often present in patients with a disseminated form.[3] Reduced state of arousal may be accompanied by borderline fever, acute hemiparesis, language abnormalities, or apraxia, which can be

due to ischemic stroke from vasculitis. Seizures are less common. Cranial nerve involvement in herpes zoster encephalitis may be more prevalent than in other types of encephalitis.[46]

The patterns of VZV encephalitis have been classified into three major categories:[3,43] (1) large- or medium-vessel vasculopathy, involving arteries at the base of the brain or convexity, which may affect large territories and cause hemorrhagic infarctions; (2) small-vessel vasculopathy, producing demyelinating ischemic lesions with a more subacute clinical course; and (3) ventriculitis.

Progressive multifocal neurologic deficits occur, and more specific neurocognitive syndromes, such as Gerstmann syndrome (acalculia, finger agnosia, right–left confusion, and agraphia) and Anton syndrome (cortical blindness). Mental impairment with frontal release signs and spastic paraparesis has been observed in patients with a type of small-vessel vasculopathy causing widespread white matter demyelination without cortical involvement.

Cytomegalovirus encephalitis occurs predominantly in patients with a severely impaired cellular immune system.[40] It occurs often in patients with therapy for another manifestation of CMV infection (e.g., CMV retinitis). Cytomegalovirus is an opportunistic infectious agent. CMV ventriculoencephalitis is the hallmark of the infection and the cause of death.

Confusion and lethargy in a patient with a history of CMV retinitis or pneumonitis should suggest the diagnosis. The clinical features include confusion, coma, cranial nerve palsy, and seizures. Patients with CMV encephalitis may manifest apathy and social withdrawal that closely mimic AIDS dementia. Ventriculitis and hydrocephalus may be the cause of reduced consciousness. Hyponatremia from CMV adrenalitis is common and an important laboratory indicator in patients with AIDS and rapidly developing encephalitis.

One of the most dramatic types of encephalitis in the United States is the arbovirus encephalitides.[66] Arboviral encephalitis is caused by a mosquito or tick vector. Outbreaks are seasonal, usually occurring in the summer. In encephalitides transmitted by ticks, outbreaks occur in high-risk areas during the tick feeding season (late spring and early summer).

The mosquito-borne eastern equine encephalomyelitis (EEE) is prevalent along the eastern seaboard and on the Gulf Coast; mortality from this disease is 40% (the virus causes acute encephalitis in horses and can be isolated from brain tissue specimen).[29] The agent is a single-stranded RNA α-virus. The onset is rather sudden, with a high incidence of seizures and dysautonomia, manifested by sympathetic hyperactivity. A short prodrome of several days is common, with headache and abdominal distress. Focal weakness occurs in half the patients. Cranial nerve palsies (III, VII, XII) have been noted in one-third of the patients. Virtually all patients have a progression to coma. In contrast, western equine encephalomyelitis (WEE) is less often characterized by a devastating clinical course and mostly peaks in August and September.

St. Louis encephalitis occurs commonly in the United States. Its manifestations appear to be milder in children than in adults. The susceptible populations are persons living in public housing projects and, possibly, patients infected with HIV.

In the tropics, Venezuelan equine encephalitis is most common, particularly in Central and South America, and is very comparable to WEE in prevalence, clinical presentation, morbidity, and mortality. Japanese encephalitis is endemic in Southeast Asia and India. Vaccination of children has markedly decreased its prevalence in Japan, and vaccination for travelers to endemic areas is recommended. Most cases occur in China, India, and Thailand.

Japanese encephalitis peaks during the rainy season, and there has been a change in genotype. The culex mosquitoes have transmitted the virus mostly from pigs.[88] It may occur during only brief stays, such as a vacation, although the risk of exposure increases with a longer stay. The clinical features of Japanese encephalitis are nonspecific, but seizures are very common, with elements of diffuse involvement of both hemispheres.[36,39,56] Spinal cord involvement (often leading to the incorrect diagnosis of fulminant multiple sclerosis) has been noted.

Tick-borne encephalitis is caused by flaviviruses and is transmitted by tick bites. Encephalitis develops in only 1 of 10 infected persons, usually after a flu-like illness. Tick-borne encephalitis has been a serious health problem in forested areas of Europe and Russia, but vaccination has reduced manifestation.[30]

Headache and fever may be the only signs of tick-borne encephalitides, and the disorder may remain limited as aseptic meningitis. The most severe form is a meningoencephalomyelitis occurring up to 2 weeks after resolution of the febrile prodrome. Flaccid paralysis and involvement of the cranial nerve nuclei, particularly the bulbar nuclei, lead to poor outcome and often death.

West Nile encephalitis is commonly found on all continents, with prior outbreaks in Africa, Romania, Russia, and Israel. West Nile encephalitis swept the western and midwestern United States in the summer of 2002, and later moved to western states and the east coast.[9,38,61] The outbreaks are severe, and the ravages in survivors are not yet entirely known. The flavivirus is amplified in mosquitoes in the characteristic spring to fall season and is spread through birds. The risk of developing encephalitis is estimated to be 1 in 150 infected persons and increases with age and prior poor immunologic state. Fatalities have been common. The combination of neck stiffness, pleocytosis in the cerebrospinal fluid (CSF), hyponatremia (30%), and clinical or electrophysiologic signs of asymmetric flaccid paralysis should suggest the diagnosis.[60] Polio-like syndromes (marked asymmetry and pure motor involvement involving facial, cervical, and limb muscles) have been described.[32,52,68,79]

In general, the clinical manifestations of other viral encephalitides are similar. However, several features are noticeable, such as involvement of facial, glossopharyngeal, and oculomotor nerves (St. Louis encephalitis);[80] marked abulia (Colorado tick fever); high incidence of focal and generalized seizures with propensity toward development of status epilepticus (La Crosse encephalitis[55]); and fear of water, vigorous muscle spasms in swallowing muscles, and violent behavior (rabies encephalitis).[10] La Crosse (California) encephalitis is most commonly reported to the Centers for Disease Control and Prevention and predominates in children younger than 15 years.[55] The adult epidemic viral encephalitides are summarized in Table 35.1.

Rickettsial diseases are transmitted through ticks, mites, lice, and fleas. The stings are often not remembered because they are painless and may not be followed by a rash at the injection site. The most important and potentially fatal disorder is Rocky Mountain spotted fever, which causes a generalized vasculitis and meningoencephalitis. It emerges in late spring and summer, predominantly in the Southeast region of the United States (regardless of its name, which suggests the West).[49]

Other rickettsial infections that may involve the central nervous system (CNS) are encephalitides from the typhus group. The typhus group includes Q fever, epidemic typhus, murine typhus, and scrub typhus. Epidemics can be worldwide and produce similar neurologic manifestations, with typical maculopapular rash and multifocal CNS manifestations.[69]

TABLE 35.1. ADULT EPIDEMIC VIRAL ENCEPHALITIS

Type	Virus	Severity	Mortality (%)
Eastern equine encephalomyelitis	Alphavirus	+++	50–70
Western equine encephalomyelitis	Alphavirus	++	5–10
Venezuelan equine encephalomyelitis	Alphavirus	+	< 1
Japanese encephalitis	Flavivirus	+++	25–50
St. Louis encephalitis	Flavivirus	++	70*
Murray Valley encephalitis	Flavivirus	++	10–20
Colorado tick fever	Orbivirus	+	< 1
La Crosse encephalitis	Bunyavirus	++	< 5
Lymphocytic choriomeningitis	Arenavirus	++	< 1
Argentine hemorrhagic fever	Arenavirus	++	< 10
Lassa fever	Arenavirus	++	< 15
Rabies	Rabies virus	+++	~100[†]
West Nile	Flavivirus	++	~70[‡]

* In elderly patients only
† Occasional survivors in a mildly disabled state have been reported.
‡ Experience too limited for findings to be entirely accurate
+++ Often progressing to coma
++ Variable presentation, but may be severe deficit
+ Often mild.

Rocky Mountain spotted fever is evident in patients with fever who have a marked purpuric rash involving the palms and soles. The flexor surfaces of the hands and feet are involved first before the rash spreads over the body. The purpuric lesions are a consequence of rickettsiae invading small blood vessels and causing occlusion and necrosis (Chapter 12).

The findings in Rocky Mountain spotted fever are multiple, small subcortical infarcts (often in the basal ganglia), development of cerebral edema with loss of gray–white matter differentiation, and sulci effacement.

Neurologic manifestations are protean, but severe headache, profound neck stiffness, and clouding of consciousness are common, with progression to stupor in more than one-fourth of affected patients.[48]

Q fever occurs as a result of exposure to farm animals, rabbits, or deer and may result in fever, pneumonia, myocarditis, endocarditis, and meningoencephalitis. The involvement of the CNS is less common in Q fever, but may mimic herpes simplex encephalitis.[21] Neurologic involvement from the responsible agent, *Coxiella burnetii*, can be dramatic. Severe headache and myalgias are common. Neurologic manifestations that may precede stupor are cranial nerve involvement and cerebellar signs. Epidemic, murine, and scrub types, which occur widely in Southeast Asia, the Pacific Islands, India, and Nepal, are not further considered here.

Parasitic or fungal infections may cause encephalitis. Toxoplasmic encephalitis is a leading cause of acute encephalitis in patients with AIDS or in immunosuppressed patients.[58] *Toxoplasma* infestation can be a defining illness in previously HIV-positive patients.[84] It is much less common in transplant recipients, patients with Hodgkin's disease, or patients with systemic lupus erythematosus.

Toxoplasma infection may result in a single mass effect, multiple abscesses, or multiple hemorrhages in abscesses mimicking coagulopathy-associated hemorrhages. The total parasite burden to the brain determines the clinical manifestations, but many of these abscesses do not produce clinical signs other than headache and lethargy. Progression may be in days or protracted over months. Decreasing alertness, onset of seizures, and persisting headache should alert one to the diagnosis. *Toxoplasma* has a predilection for the basal ganglia and cerebellum, but hemichorea, hemiballismus, and ataxia are uncommon manifestations.

Fungal encephalitis should always be considered in endemic regions. One should be especially alert if an acute presentation is followed by an insidious course.

The lung is the port of entry of the fungus and generally the primary site of infection. Evidence of infection in organ systems outside the CNS, such as skin, bone, and prostate, is commonly needed to implicate fungal infection. Typical clinical features are headaches, myalgia, fever, intermittent nausea, and photophobia. Cognition may rapidly become impaired, and patients may have marked abulia and lethargy due to irreversible, severe brain damage. The presentation often is nonspecific and atypical, making the diagnosis very difficult.

Coccidioides immitis is endemic to the southwestern United States and the central valley of California. Dissemination is usually seen only in immunosuppressed patients but occurs in 1% of infected patients. Central nervous system involvement is typically severe and fatal if untreated.

Other fungal causes must be considered in the differential diagnosis. Organisms include *Cryptococcus neoformans, Blastomyces dermatitidis, Histoplasma capsulatum, Aspergillus* species, and a number of uncommon pathogens, all with possibly similar presentations and CSF formulae. Meningitis is the most common manifestation of infection by *C. neoformans* and is generally found in immunocompromised patients. It is ubiquitous and protean in its presentation, ranging from indolent changes in cognitive function to florid meningoencephalitis. *H. capsulatum* is found in the Ohio and Mississippi River valleys, and most persons in endemic areas have positive skin tests for previous infection. Active disease is rare and, again, is seen most commonly in immunocompromised hosts. *Aspergillus* is a common fungal pathogen with a predilection for the brain parenchyma over the meninges. Abscess formation is common, as is CNS vasculitis.

Case reports of blastomycotic meningitis are noteworthy for the frequent misdiagnosis of tuberculous meningitis. The similar clinical characteristics and the nodular appearance of meningeal enhancement on magnetic resonance imaging (MRI) in both diseases make distinction between the two difficult.[33] Not infrequently, patients have been treated with antituberculous agents before the accurate diagnosis of blastomycotic meningitis. This can further confuse the diagnosis, because rifampin has some therapeutic benefit in treating blastomycosis, and incomplete treatment with that drug may lead to the reactivation of disease.

Paraneoplastic limbic encephalitis should be considered when infectious agents seem highly unlikely. The pathologic changes can be extensive, with neuronal loss, perivascular monocytic infiltrates, and microglial nodules, predominantly in the limbic and insular cortices but also located in the brain stem, spinal cord, and dorsal root ganglia.[4,14,27,77,85] The condition can be the first manifestation or can appear in a patient with a previous diagnosis of small-cell (oat cell) carcinoma, Hodgkin's disease, or testicular seminoma. Certain antibodies may point to certain cancers (Capsule 35.1).

The rapid onset of mood changes, usually sadness, detachment, and prominent decline in memory domains, is the characteristic presentation, but more fulminant forms are manifested by agitation, hallucinations, and bizarre behavior, preceding a decrease in alertness.[4,14] The diagnosis is often suggested when the psychiatric symptoms progress despite psychotropic drugs.

CAPSULE 35.1   PARANEOPLASTIC NEURONAL ANTINEURAL ANTIBODIES AND ENCEPHALITIS

Antibody	Associated Cancer
Ma 1	Various causes
Ma 2 (Ta)	Testicular cancer
Hu (ANNA-1)	Small-cell lung cancer
Ri (ANNA-2)	Breast cancer
CV2/CRMP5	Small-cell lung cancer (thymoma)
ANNA-3	Small-cell lung cancer
PCA-2	Small-cell lung cancer
TR	Hodgkin lymphoma
NMDA	Ovarium teratoma

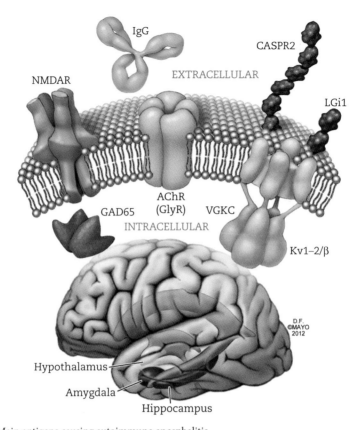

FIGURE 35.1: Main antigens causing autoimmune encephalitis.

From Wijdicks. Handling Difficult Situations. Core Principles of Acute Neurology: Oxford University Press, 2014.

There has been increased recognition and understanding of autoimmune encephalitis, a condition that had been categorized as "cryptic" before. A severe form of this type of encephalitis is anti-*N*-methyl-D-aspartate (NMDA) receptor encephalitis.[25] Seen most often in young female patients (median age of 23 years), the disease rapidly progresses to coma and status epilepticus. This disorder has now been better characterized, and several subsets of antineural antibodies are now known. These antibodies can be against NMDA receptors, GABA (B) receptors, CASPR2, and against LGI1 and contactin-2 (Figure 35.1). Antibodies are best measured in CSF.

Clinical syndromes have been linked to specific antibodies. Antibodies to LGI1 result in worsening memory loss, seizures, agitation, and a new psychotic break in men older than 40 years.[26,45,51,53] Movement disorders are more common in patients with voltage-gated potassium channel antibodies (VGCK); and this may involve dystonia of face and arm, often named facial-brachial dystonia. Neuropsychiatric features always precede movement disorders, and autonomic dysfunction and abnormal consciousness follow about 2 weeks after onset. Limbic encephalitis associated with GABA$_B$R and AMPAR antibodies do present with amnesia, as seen in limbic encephalitis, but with no clearly identifiable other clinical features. Limbic encephalitis associated with GAD antibodies may present itself with stiff-man syndrome, cerebellar ataxia, or recurrent seizures.

In summary, numerous clinical neurologic conditions can closely mimic viral encephalitis. Obviously, each of these rapidly progressive disorders will lead to a totally different therapeutic approach and thus should be considered when evaluation of the patient is not supportive of the clinical impression.[11] The most commonly considered alternative diagnoses for viral encephalitis are cerebral venous thrombosis, isolated granulomatous angiitis, CNS intravascular lymphoma, acute hemorrhagic leukoencephalitis, acute disseminated encephalomyelitis, progressive multifocal leukoencephalopathy, subdural empyema, fulminant bacterial meningitis, and even neurosyphilis.[13,74] Infectious diseases that can mimick viral encephalitis are shown in Table 35.2.

TABLE 35.2. INFECTIOUS DISEASES
THAT CAN MASQUERADE AS VIRAL
CENTRAL NERVOUS SYSTEM
INFECTIONS

Bacteria
    Spirochetes
        Syphilis (secondary or meningovascular)
        Leptospirosis
Borrelia burgdorferi infection (Lyme disease)
Mycoplasma pneumoniae infection
Cat-scratch fever
Listeriosis
Brucellosis (particularly due to *Brucella melitensis*)
Tuberculosis
Typhoid fever
Parameningeal infections (epidural infection,
    petrositis)
Partially treated bacterial meningitis
Brain abscesses
Whipple disease
Fungi
    Cryptococcosis
    Coccidioidomycosis
    Histoplasmosis
    North American blastomycosis
    Candidiasis
Parasites
    Toxoplasmosis
    Cysticercosis
    Echinococcosis
    Trichinosis
    Trypanosomiasis
    Plasmodium falciparum infection
    Amebiasis (due to *Naegleria* and *Acanthamoeba*)

Modified from Johnson RT. Acute encephalitis. *Clin Infect Dis*
1996;23:219. With permission of the University of Chicago.

NEUROIMAGING AND LABORATORY TESTS

The evaluation of a patient with suspected encephalitis has been carefully summarized in a recent publication (Part XIV, Guidelines) and in Chapter 3. The diagnostic value of computed tomography (CT) or MRI in patients early in the disease is low. The CT scan findings become abnormal in 60% of patients with biopsy proven herpes simplex encephalitis (Figure 35.2), but are often initially normal in other encephalitides.

Magnetic resonance imaging is much more sensitive than CT scan in patients with herpes simplex encephalitis.[59] Magnetic resonance imaging demonstrates lesions that are hypointense on T1-weighted and hyperintense on T2-weighted images, with occasional mass effect and additional petechial hemorrhages in at least 50% of the patients. A very suggestive finding for herpes simplex encephalitis on MRI is a density change in the inferomedial temporal lobe, including the limbic system and extending into the insular cortex, with typical sparing of the putamen (Figure 35.3) The internal capsule, cingulate gyrus, and frontal lobe can be involved.[28,34] However, involvement of the medial and temporal lobes has also been described in a patient with limbic encephalitis associated with carcinoma of the lung and in a patient with Q fever and neurosyphilis, again emphasizing the need for proper diagnosis with polymerase chain reaction (PCR) or brain biopsy. Strictly unilateral lesions are uncommon in herpes simplex encephalitis and should raise suspicion of other causes (e.g., brain abscess, multiple sclerosis, malignant glioma, CNS lymphoma, brain metastasis). Diffusion-weighted imaging in patients with herpes simplex encephalitis may be more sensitive than conventional MRI and may point to the development of cytotoxic edema. Generally, in our experience, the MRI findings in patients with herpes simplex encephalitis are virtually always present, but may further evolve over time. Conversely, a normal MRI likely excludes a herpes simplex infection.

In patients with CMV encephalitis, MRI findings may be normal or later may show nonspecific atrophy. MRI in CMV encephalitis may show nonspecific brain atrophy and enlarged ventricles with typical ependymal signal enhancement. Brainstem and cerebellar abnormalities detected only after gadolinium administration have been reported.[40]

In patients with VZV encephalitis, both neuroimaging studies show multiple T1-weighted hypointensity and T2-weighted hyperintensity involving the white and gray matter. Subcortical enhancing, coalescing lesions, followed by gray matter involvement, are characteristic. Involvement of multiple territories is compatible with intracranial vasculitides representing infarction (Figure 35.4).

Magnetic resonance imaging findings in EEE and rabies are predominantly in the basal ganglia and thalamus and are nearly always abnormal in comatose patients. Magnetic resonance imaging findings in a review of St. Louis encephalitis were mostly nonspecific, but edema in the substantia nigra was noted in two patients. The MRI findings in different types of viral encephalitis are summarized in Table 35.3.

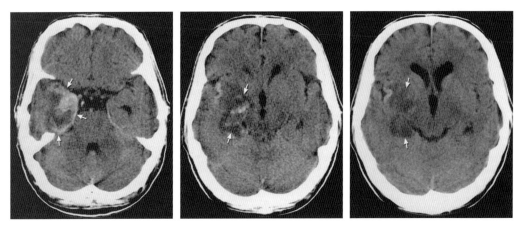

FIGURE 35.2: Herpes simplex encephalitis. Computed tomographic scans showing unilateral swollen, hypodense, and partly hemorrhagic temporal lobe lesion from herpes simplex encephalitis (*arrows*).

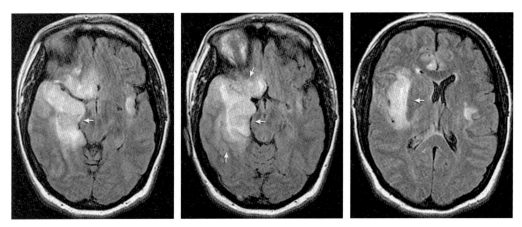

FIGURE 35.3: Herpes simplex encephalitis. Magnetic resonance images with typical hyperintensities in temporal, frontal lobe, and insular regions (*arrows*).

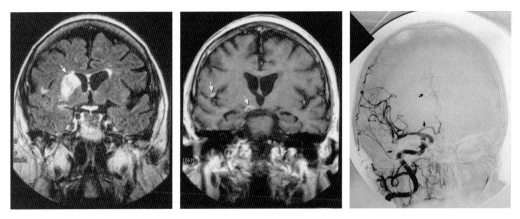

FIGURE 35.4: Varicella-zoster virus encephalitis. Multiple cerebral infarcts (*white arrows*) and marked arterial narrowing consistent with vasculitis (*black arrows*) on cerebral angiogram.

TABLE 35.3. MAGNETIC RESONANCE IMAGING FINDINGS IN VIRAL ENCEPHALITIS

Site	HSE	EEE	CMV	La Crosse	St. Louis	Rabies
Frontal	X			X		
Temporal	X			X		
Basal ganglia		X				X
Thalamus		X				X
White matter			X			
Substantia nigra					X	
Meningeal enhancement			X			

CMV cytomegalovirus; EEE, eastern equine encephalomyelitis; HSE, herpes simplex encephalitis.
X = Abnormal signal.

In toxoplasma encephalitis, CT scanning underestimates the number of abscesses (Figure 35.5). Acute hydrocephalus without defined abscesses may point to the diagnosis in the proper clinical situation. Multiple intracerebral hemorrhages in patients with AIDS often indicate *Toxoplasma* (or *Aspergillus*) rather than a coagulopathy.[84]

Magnetic resonance imaging of toxoplasmic encephalitis (Figure 35.6), which displays multiple abscesses, is nonspecific because very similar signal abnormalities and ring enhancement can be seen with lymphoma, tuberculous abscesses, nocardiosis, and cryptococcosis.

Hyperintensity on T2-weighted images is common, but after treatment, it evolves into T2-weighted isointensity comparable with that of necrotizing abscesses.[17] Marked perilesional edema is typical. Prominent enhancement of the meninges can be found. In fungal meningoencephalitis, a nodular appearance is common on MR imaging. Scattered hyperintensities in the basal ganglia may represent extension of infection along penetrating arteries (Figure 35.6).

The findings in Rocky Mountain spotted fever are multiple small subcortical infarcts (often in the basal ganglia), development of cerebral edema with loss of gray–white matter differentiation, and sulci effacement. A survivor in one report had multiple punctate areas of increased intensity throughout the white matter in the distribution of the perivascular (Virchow-Robin) spaces, possibly representing a perivascular inflammatory response.[16] Meningeal enhancement after gadolinium is typical.

In limbic encephalitis, normal CT findings are common, and MRI often suggests the diagnosis in the proper situation. T2-weighted hyperintensity changes in the medial temporal lobes may appear with contrast enhancement in the temporal lobes, amygdala, and hippocampus (Figure 35.7). Magnetic resonance abnormalities may improve with successful treatment of underlying cancer.

Cerebrospinal fluid examination is the preferred diagnostic test after the initial CT scan with contrast has excluded some of the most obvious mimicking disorders. Cerebrospinal fluid examination probably should be deferred in patients with mass effect, particularly those with swollen temporal lobes from herpes simplex encephalitis. When CSF is analyzed, pleocytosis with predominant lymphocytes is common at the first presentation, but exceptions exist. A five- to tenfold increase in protein concentration can be expected, although protein values may be normal. Lactate in CSF is increased, particularly in patients with a viral encephalitis that carries a poor prognosis. Red blood cells may be present in CSF, but this finding is not specific for any type of encephalitis. Cerebrospinal fluid glucose concentration tends to be in the normal range, but may be decreased in herpes simplex encephalitis and EEE. In patients with EEE, the CSF formula may strongly suggest acute bacterial meningitis.

Serologic testing may identify the cause of encephalitis, and acute and convalescent serum samples separated by 6 weeks should be obtained. Cerebrospinal fluid samples must be obtained for identification of the most common epidemic encephalitides, such as EEE, WEE, La Crosse, and St. Louis, which may demonstrate at least a fourfold increase in immunoglobulin M antibody responses.[19,20,57] A guideline for serologic testing of CSF is presented in Table 35.4. Other samples for virus identification may include throat swab (influenza, enterovirus), rectal swab (enterovirus), urine (adenovirus, CMV), saliva (rabies), and skin exudate (herpes).

The detection of virus by PCR may markedly facilitate the diagnosis of viral encephalitis from

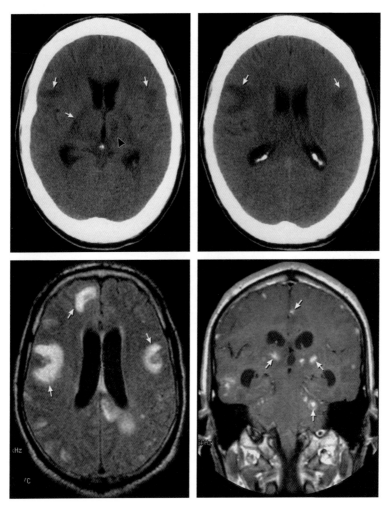

FIGURE 35.5: Toxoplasmic encephalitis with multiple abscesses (*arrows and arrowhead*). The abscesses are poorly defined by computed tomographic scan and more evident by magnetic resonance imaging fluid-attenuated inversion recovery and postcontrast T1-weighted scan.

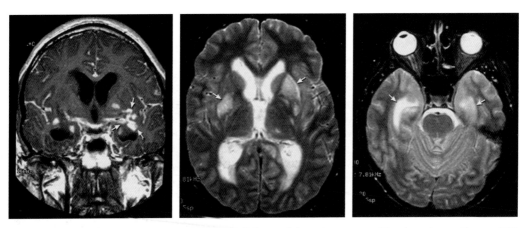

FIGURE 35.6: Magnetic resonance images showing diffuse nodular enhancement of basal meninges. Abnormal T2 signal in the basal ganglia bilaterally and bitemporal lesions represent encephalitis (*arrows*). The fungus isolated from brain biopsy culture was *Blastomyces*.

From Friedman J, Wijdicks EFM, Fulgham J, et al. Meningoencephalitis due to blastomycosis dermatitis: a case report and literature review. *Mayo Clin Proc* 2000;75:403–408. With permission of the publisher.

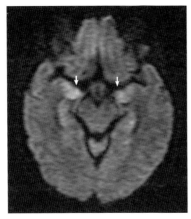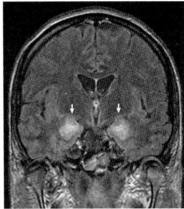

FIGURE 35.7: Limbic paraneoplastic encephalitis. Magnetic resonance images of limbic paraneoplastic encephalitis, showing symmetric T2 signal in mesial temporal lobes (*arrows*).

herpes simplex,[5,67] CMV, EBV, enteroviruses, and, recently, influenza. The laboratory procedure can be completed within 10 hours. The sensitivity and specificity of PCR in the CSF in herpes simplex are very high, but false-negative samples very occasionally exist when collection is early.[8,42,44] Possible reasons for a negative PCR finding are the absence of DNA in the CSF sample from early clearing of the viral genome (as early as 5 days after symptoms), variation in the amplification of HSV strains, and, less likely, institution of antiviral therapy. Nested PCR includes a second amplification and increases detection. In a study of 28 patients, 30% still had a positive herpes simplex virus PCR up to 6 weeks months after acyclovir treatment. The PCR result can be positive as early as the first day into the illness, and only very rarely is herpes simplex virus DNA genome detected in patients without encephalitis.

One report by the National Institute of Allergy and Infectious Diseases Collaborative Antiviral Study Group[50] found a sensitivity of 98% and a specificity of 94% when CSF PCR was compared with brain biopsy. Of 54 patients with biopsy-proven herpes simplex encephalitis, 53 had a positive PCR result. Of 47 patients with a negative biopsy result, 44 had a negative PCR finding. The three positive PCR test results in biopsy-negative patients were considered to represent herpes simplex encephalitis and a "missed" biopsy. In virtually all patients, PCR could detect herpes simplex encephalitis DNA within 1 week of therapy.[50] Most laboratories have reached excellent predictive value.

Electroencephalography (EEG) is an important test in patients with herpes simplex

encephalitis in whom neuroimaging findings are normal. Electroencephalography demonstrates diffuse arrhythmic δ activity or diffuse polymorphic slowing of the background but more typically shows periodic lateralized epileptiform discharges in the temporal lobe as early as the second day, although it lacks specificity.[41,72]

Although many authoritative reviews emphasize brain biopsy, in clinical practice open brain biopsy is currently indicated only in patients with atypical clinical presentation and unusual MRI findings, in patients with clinical deterioration despite antiviral treatment, and in patients with nondiagnostic PCR test findings. In addition, the threshold for brain biopsy in immunosuppressed patients should be lower, particularly because opportunistic infection (CMV, *Toxoplasma*, fungi)

TABLE 35.4. MANDATORY SEROLOGIC TESTS OF CEREBROSPINAL FLUID IN ENCEPHALITIS OF UNKNOWN CAUSE

Herpes simplex
Cytomegalovirus
Human immunodeficiency virus
Varicella-zoster virus
Epstein-Barr virus
Toxoplasma gondii
Borrelia burgdorferi
Mycoplasma pneumoniae
Leptospira species
Legionella pneumophila
Brucella species
Syphilis
Aspergillus

may mimic herpes simplex encephalitis and may result in a different therapeutic approach. Brain biopsy in patients with acute encephalitis without any CT or MRI abnormalities most likely has a very low yield.

Brain biopsy has a low complication rate in patients with encephalitis, with approximately 1% morbidity in the National Institute of Allergy and Infectious Diseases collaborative study, and virtually no mortality. Higher complication rates from intracranial hemorrhage and edema have been reported. However, brain biopsies may have been performed in moribund patients, and further progressive temporal lobe edema in these cases may simply have represented the natural history of herpes simplex encephalitis. Intracranial hematoma at the biopsy site may be devastating, and this risk may indeed be increased in patients with herpes simplex encephalitis and a hemorrhagic necrotic lesion.

Brain tissue should be targeted at the lesion; and if no lesion can be identified or if neurosurgeons are reluctant to biopsy the temporal lobe of the dominant hemisphere, tissue in the form of a large sample of white matter should be obtained from the right frontal cortex. Handling of specimens from patients with HIV-associated encephalitis requires efficiency and care.

Tissue should be processed unfixed in a special medium for subsequent viral culture and routine bacterial, fungal, and mycobacterial studies. (Usually, brain tissue is fixed in formaldehyde not only for routine hematoxylin-eosin examination but also for studies of lymphoma surface markers.) In patients with undiagnosed encephalitis, a major portion of the tissue should remain unfixed for cultures, and a portion should be fixed in glutaraldehyde for electron microscopic examination, which may identify certain viral particles. The specimen should be kept cool, but freezing destroys many viruses. The time to isolation of herpes simplex virus from brain tissue is 1–7 days. Immunohistochemical staining can diagnose the virus after microscopic examination.

Rabies encephalitis requires pathologic confirmation of hemorrhages and necrosis in the basal ganglia and brainstem, which can be documented on MRI if time allows.[10] Intraneuronal, round eosinophilic intracytoplasmic bodies (Negri bodies) emerge in the hippocampal cortex and Purkinje cells. Corneal impression smears and biopsy of oral mucosa or skin can be diagnostic.[37] However, antemortem diagnosis can be achieved in only a few cases, because the centrifugal spread of the virus takes time.

FIRST STEPS IN MANAGEMENT

Treatment of patients with acute encephalitis is largely by supportive measures (Table 35.5).

Airway management has the highest priority, especially in patients who are becoming progressively drowsier and in patients who have had a flurry of seizures. The adequacy of ventilation must be immediately assessed. Endotracheal intubation must be performed in patients with hypoxemia. Most patients have normal respiratory drive and mechanics and breathe spontaneously on a T-piece only, but continuous positive airway pressure (5–10 cm H_2O) can be added. In addition, patients may become progressively agitated, and aspiration becomes a great risk in patients who are thrashing around. Particularly vexing are patients who are wildly delirious. In these patients, the combination of sedation (e.g., intravenous midazolam) and ventilatory support is more appropriate than trying to combat these episodes with antipsychotic drugs or a variety of benzodiazepines.

Normal maintenance fluids consist of 2 L of isotonic saline and incremental increases in intake in patients with fever (500 mL for every 1°C increase). Daily fluid balance must be estimated by measuring fluid intake and output, with insensible losses of 500–1,000 mL per day. Renal function should be evaluated daily. Certain viral encephalitides may coincide with acute renal involvement (St. Louis encephalitis, rabies); but renal failure may be caused by direct nephrotoxicity associated with acyclovir or, less commonly, by dehydration associated with fever.

It is important to supply proper nutrition, because protein catabolism begins early and continues throughout the period of relative starvation that follows. Protein wasting should be avoided, and adequate calories must be provided to counteract the effects of infection.

In patients with a strong likelihood of viral encephalitis, treatment is begun with acyclovir.[81-83] Specific antiviral therapy is limited in viral encephalitides other than herpes simplex encephalitis, but acyclovir therapy is typically started while awaiting PCR results. Interestingly, in a recent study from France, "late" administration of acyclovir (> 1 day of admission) was noted in 37% of patients. Cerebrospinal fluid with leukocytes counts of less than 10/mm³, prior alcohol abuse, or atypical presentations hindered recognition and thus early administration of acyclovir.[63] Randomized clinical studies in patients treated with acyclovir have found that mortality is reduced to 25% (predominantly in patients with

TABLE 35.5. INITIAL MANAGEMENT OF ACUTE VIRAL ENCEPHALITIS

Airway management	Intubate early if deterioration is rapid. Intubation if patient has hypoxemia despite facemask with 10 L of 100% oxygen/minute, if abnormal respiratory drive or presence of abnormal protective reflexes (likely with motor response of withdrawal, or worse)
Mechanical ventilation	IMV/ PS or CPAP mode
Fluid management	Maintenance, 3 L of 0.9% NaCl (500 mL increase/°C); in patients with hyponatremia, consider dilution (treat with free-water restriction) or Addison's disease (treat with corticosteroids)
Nutrition	Enteral nutrition with continuous infusion (on day 2)
	Blood glucose control (goal 140–180 mg/dL)
Prophylaxis	DVT prophylaxis with pneumatic compression devices
	SC heparin 5,000 U t.i.d.
	GI prophylaxis: pantoprazole 40 mg IV daily or lansoprazole 30 mg orally through nasogastric tube.
Specific treatment	Antiviral: HSE: acyclovir, 10 mg/kg q8h
	CMV: ganciclovir, 5 mg/kg q12 h
	Autoimmune: PLEX/IVIG/Methylprednisolone
Other measures	Seizures: Fosphenytoin, 20 mg PE/kg followed by 300 mg IV or Levetiracetam 20 mg/kg IV over 60 minutes. Maintenance 1,000 mg bid IV or orally
	Agitation: Midazolam (0.02 mg/kg/hr) or lorazepam (0.025 mg/kg/hr) infusion
Surgical management	Consider brain biopsy for diagnostic purposes
	Removal of necrotic temporal mass
Access	Peripheral venous catheter or Peripheral inserted central catheter

CMV, cytomegalovirus; CPAP, continuous positive airway pressure; DVT, deep vein thrombosis; GI, gastrointestinal; HSE, herpes simplex encephalitis; IMV, intermittent mandatory ventilation; IV, intravenously; IVIG: intravenous immunoglobulin; NaCl, sodium chloride; PLEX, plasma exchange; PS, pressure support; SC, subcutaneously.

impaired consciousness) and that almost 40% of the treated patients have good recovery or only minimal deficits.[81] Acyclovir is administered at a dose of 10 mg/kg every 8 hours and is continued for 10–14 days. If recognized, the side effects of acyclovir are reversible; they include renal failure with increases in creatinine and blood urea nitrogen in 10% of patients. An adjusting schedule based on calculated creatinine clearance is shown in Table 35.6. Other side effects are thrombocytopenia (6%), aspartate transaminase elevation (3%), fever, and, less commonly (< 1%), leukopenia and tremors.

The usefulness of corticosteroids is very uncertain. A reported trial of dexamethasone in Japanese encephalitis did not show any effect on outcome, a result that may discourage its use in other types of encephalitis.[39] However, corticosteroids are advised in patients scheduled for diagnostic brain biopsy.

In patients with CMV encephalitis, ganciclovir is the preferred drug (5 mg/kg every 12 hours). Ganciclovir is much more toxic and is associated with bone marrow depression, nausea, and vomiting. Not infrequently, patients with CMV encephalitis have already been treated for CMV retinitis with a maintenance dose of ganciclovir. In these patients, foscarnet is indicated as additional therapy (60 mg/kg infused over 1 hour, every 8 hours), along with restarting of the intravenous dose of ganciclovir. Toxicity, including electrolyte abnormalities and renal failure, is common with foscarnet.

TABLE 35.6. ACYCLOVIR DOSES IN RENAL IMPAIRMENT

CRCL, mL/min*	mg/kg	Frequency
> 50	10	q8h
30–50	10	q12h
10–30	10	q24h
< 10	5	q24h

*Calculation of creatinine clearance (CRCL).

$$\text{Male: CRCL}(\text{mL / min}) = \frac{(140 - \text{age}) \times (\text{ideal body weight}[\text{kg}])}{\text{serum creatine}(\text{mg / dL}) \times 72}$$

Female: 0.85 × CRCL for men
Ideal body weight: males, 50 kg + 2.3 kg for each inch over 5 feet; females, 45.5 kg + 2.3 kg for each inch over 5 feet.

The standard therapeutic agents for toxoplasmic encephalitis are pyrimethamine (50–75 mg/day) and sulfadiazine (4–8 g/day), combined with folinic acid (10 mg/day) to reduce bone marrow depression.

Adverse reactions are a rash and anemia, leukopenia, or thrombocytopenia, occurring in 20% of patients. Any allergic reaction should result in replacement of sulfadiazine by clindamycin (600–900 mg PO or IV every 6 hours). When *Toxoplasma* is the culprit, within 3 weeks radiologic improvement (defined as less edema and isointense signals rather than hyperintense signals on MRI) or complete resolution should be expected in 70% of patients.

Ketoconazole, or more recently itraconazole, is the first-line agent for pulmonary blastomycosis. Amphotericin B is usually reserved for more serious clinical situations or refractory disease, but many experts believe that it is the drug of choice in patients with meningeal involvement. Most authorities recommend a total dose of amphotericin B of 0.25 mg–1 mg/kg/day IV infusion over 6 hours. One should also consider intrathecal amphotericin B (intrathecal test dose of amphotericin B 0.01 and 0.05 mg have been given prior to doses of 0.2–0.5 mg intrathecally 3–5 times per week). Hydrocephalus may become considerable, and ventriculostomy is needed. This provides the opportunity to culture CSF, but brain biopsy may be needed to find the fungus.

Treatment of paraneoplastic encephalitis is supportive care, treatment of seizures, and surgical removal of the underlying neoplasm. The immune response can be attained by using not only intravenous immunoglobulins and plasma exchange, but also corticosteroids, cyclophosphamide, and rituximab.

Treatment in autoimmune encephalitis is often initially 5–10 infusions of IV immunoglobulin, 5–10 sessions of plasma exchange, and 1 gram of methylprednisolone for 5–10 days. Treatment of severe agitation may include intubation and IV midazolam as only option. This treatment may be needed for weeks. In many patients, seizures can only be controlled when the disease is treated more aggressively using a combination of rituximab and cyclophosphamide.[62,76] Rituximab is usually used in a dose of 375 mg/m² every week for 4 weeks and in severe cases combined with cyclophosphamide 750 mg/m² given with the first dose of rituximab, which is then followed by monthly cycles of cyclophosphamide. Oral cyclophosphamide or intravenous cyclophosphamide will lead to hair loss and bone marrow suppression (marked neutropenia days after administration, as expected in most chemotherapeutic agents). Both rituximab and cyclophosphamide are effective many weeks after administration and, thus, an early effect is not expected. Aggressive and prolonged treatment of status epilepticus might be necessary, and there have been full recoveries in patients who have been treated for several months. However, outcome in others are less favorable, with refractory status epilepticus in several patients despite ovariectomy and combinations of rituximab and cyclophosphamide.

DETERIORATION: CAUSES AND MANAGEMENT

Deterioration is common in patients with an acute encephalitis and is a very discouraging experience when there are no specific options for treatment.

In some encephalitides the worsening is relentless (e.g., fungal encephalitis and paraneoplastic encephalitis). Deterioration in a patient with viral encephalitis is most often the result of an overwhelming infection and may be associated with the development of cerebral edema. Deterioration can be expected in patients with a more virulent encephalitis. In the collaborative antiviral study, two-thirds of the patients had progression after the diagnosis was confirmed by brain biopsy, and one-third of the patients lapsed into coma. Occasionally, sudden deterioration occurs in a patient who has recently had a diagnostic brain biopsy and may be caused by hemorrhage into a necrotic biopsy site.

Intracranial pressure (ICP) monitoring should be considered if the level of consciousness deteriorates to coma. Placement of a ventricular catheter is very difficult, because slit-like ventricles may have appeared on CT scans. Whether or not aggressive management of increased ICP changes outcome is not known. The most extensive experience (albeit observations in only eight comatose patients), predominantly in patients with herpes simplex encephalitis, was reported from Massachusetts General Hospital.[12] Placement of an ICP monitor in comatose patients with encephalitis revealed that ICP was initially abnormal, but continuous ICP monitoring showed a progressive increase in ICP approximately 2 weeks after onset. Patients in whom increased ICP was controlled had a better outcome than those in whom no change in ICP was observed. The latter patients often had progression to brain death or died from sepsis while remaining in a severely disabled or vegetative state. Elevation of the head position and osmotic diuretics may control ICP.

There is virtually no clinical experience with the use of barbiturates in this situation, but it may be the last resort.

Patients whose condition deteriorates despite optimal treatment of increased ICP and who have unilateral swelling of a nondominant temporal lobe can be salvaged with craniotomy and decompression by careful removal of the necrotic tissue of the anterior temporal lobe.[2,86] The options in patients with bilateral swelling or brainstem compression from a swollen dominant temporal lobe are very limited. Decompressive craniotomy increases the probability of survival in patients with bilateral involvement, but unlike patients with unilateral swelling, they are virtually certain to have a major handicap.[2,75,86]

Seizures occur more often in certain viral encephalitides, and repeated EEG is important at least to exclude the possibility that deterioration or fluctuation in consciousness is associated with nonconvulsive status epilepticus.[6]

In any patient with acute encephalitis who has rapid deterioration in level of consciousness and a marked febrile response, the possibility of early sepsis must be considered. Patients with acute encephalitis are at considerable risk of urosepsis and aspiration pneumonia that may evolve into bilateral pneumonitis.

Hyponatremia is another potential problem in patients with encephalitis, because in some cases it becomes severe (serum sodium concentration < 120 mmol/L). Fluid restriction corrects dilutional hyponatremia and possibly its incumbent risks of seizures. In many patients, fluid restriction with replacement of insensible loss and urine output alone corrects hyponatremia. Hyponatremia in CMV encephalitis may be due to adrenalitis. Adrenalitis may cause a characteristic addisonian syndrome with hyponatremia, hyperkalemia, and shock, and corticosteroids are urgently indicated.

OUTCOME

Outcome varies and depends on the type of encephalitis. Poor outcome in any type of viral encephalitis is determined by a multiplicity of factors. These include the virulence of the virus, age greater than 60 years, absent or late initiation (later than 4 days) of antiviral treatment, altered consciousness or status epilepticus at presentation, and whether secondary complications, such as brain edema, have occurred. A recent study from Mayo Clinic reported a high percentage of patients with poor recovery potential if all of the following clinical characteristics were present: age > 65 years, mechanical ventilation, coma,

acute thrombocythemia, and when patients were immunocompromised. CSF polymorphonuclear cell count was more often associated with poor outcome in viral encephalitis.[71] Mortality in La Crosse and California encephalitides is fortunately low, but neurologic sequelae with hemiparesis or aphasia are possible in 15% of patients. Eastern equine encephalitis may cause numerous deaths, and up to 70% of patients have severe neurologic disability.[64] In WEE, in contrast, full recovery occurs, although elderly patients are at higher risk of major complications. The mortality in St. Louis encephalitis is approximately one in four for elderly patients. Neuropsychologic sequelae seem more common than overt localizing neurologic signs in tick-borne encephalitis. Fatality is high in West Nile encephalitis, but it appears that several patients awaken from coma without residual symptoms.[22] Abnormal neuroimaging could predict outcome in Rocky Mountain spotted fever. One study of 34 patients' abnormalities on MRI (diffuse enhancement, infarctions, and edema) were uncommon but were correlated with poor outcome.[16]

Coma from brain edema in herpes simplex encephalitis implies a poor prognosis and increases the likelihood of fatal outcome.[18] Early EEG findings, such as diffuse slowing, spikes, and sharp waves, do not predict poor outcome or future seizure disorder. However, later diffuse slowing of the background pattern on EEG correlates with poor outcome.

In patients with treated herpes simplex encephalitis, mortality is 15%, and 60% of the patients survive without any appreciable functional deficit. Marked cognitive deficits as well as seizures (up to 20%) are well-recognized sequelae. The cognitive deficits can frankly be devastating, with loss of memory, significant intellectual decline, and behavioral and personality changes. Restricted DWI on MRI is strongly correlated with poor outcome.[70] Young age, early administration of acyclovir, and smaller areas of involvement increase the probability of a successful outcome.[24,65] Early treatment with acyclovir may not prevent cognitive sequelae. Patients treated as early as 5 days into the illness have shown marked neurologic deficits and the inability to function at a similar intellectual level. Average survival with CMV encephalitis in AIDS is 2 months after diagnosis despite therapy, and successful outcome is exceptional. The outcome in VZV encephalitis is entirely determined by associated vasculitis; without it, full recovery is possible. These disorders are rare, but morbidity is substantial.

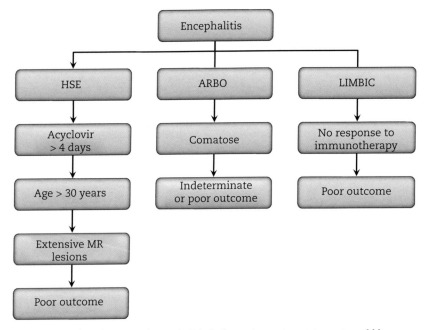

FIGURE 35.8: Outcome algorithm in viral encephalitis. Indeterminate: Any statement would be a premature conclusion. Functional independence: No assistance needed, minor handicap may remain. Poor outcome: Severe disability or death, vegetative state.

HSE, herpes simplex encephalitis.

Brain death is a possible outcome in patients with viral encephalitis. Patients with rabies encephalitis (or strong suspicion) cannot become organ donors because of the potential risk of transmission by organs or cornea. As expected, outcome in patients with severe manifestations of limbic encephalitis is poor if seizures cannot be controlled and no response to immunotherapy is seen. In autoimmune encephalitis–so common in young previously healthy persons–all efforts to treat the immunoresponse pay off. Many experts feel it is important to continue aggressive and sustained immunotherapy for several months to allow improvement.

An outcome algorithm for acute encephalitis is shown in Figure 35.8.

CONCLUSIONS

- Treatment of acute encephalitis is largely supportive, including seizure control and management of agitation.
- Polymerase chain reaction can reliably detect herpes simplex DNA in CSF and has largely replaced the need for brain biopsy; PCR is also available for CMV, EBV, and enteroviruses.
- Brain edema in acute viral encephalitis warrants ICP monitoring. Aggressive management, including decompressive craniectomy, may increase the chance of survival.

REFERENCES

1. Case records of the Massachusetts General Hospital. Weekly clinicopathological exercises. Case 36–1996. A 37-year-old man with AIDS, neurologic deterioration, and multiple hemorrhagic cerebral lesions. *N Engl J Med* 1996;335:1587–1595.
2. Adamo MA, Deshaies EM. Emergency decompressive craniectomy for fulminating infectious encephalitis. *J Neurosurg* 2008;108:174–176.
3. Amlie-Lefond C, Kleinschmidt-DeMasters BK, Mahalingam R, Davis LE, Gilden DH. The vasculopathy of varicella-zoster virus encephalitis. *Ann Neurol* 1995;37:784–790.
4. Anderson NE, Barber PA. Limbic encephalitis: a review. *J Clin Neurosci* 2008;15:961–971.
5. Anderson NE, Powell KF, Croxson MC. A polymerase chain reaction assay of cerebrospinal fluid in patients with suspected herpes simplex encephalitis. *J Neurol Neurosurg Psychiatry* 1993;56:520–525.

6. Annegers JF, Hauser WA, Beghi E, Nicolosi A, Kurland LT. The risk of unprovoked seizures after encephalitis and meningitis. *Neurology* 1988;38:1407–1410.

7. Armstrong RW, Fung PC. Brainstem encephalitis (rhombencephalitis) due to Listeria monocytogenes. case report and review. *Clin Infect Dis* 1993;16:689–702.

8. Aslanzadeh J, Skiest DJ. Polymerase chain reaction for detection of herpes simplex virus encephalitis. *J Clin Pathol* 1994;47:554–555.

9. Asnis DS, Conetta R, Waldman G, Teixeira AA. The West Nile virus encephalitis outbreak in the United States (1999–2000): from Flushing, New York, to beyond its borders. *Ann N Y Acad Sci* 2001;951:161–171.

10. Awasthi M, Parmar H, Patankar T, Castillo M. Imaging findings in rabies encephalitis. *AJNR Am J Neuroradiol* 2001;22:677–680.

11. Bale JF, Jr. Viral encephalitis. *Med Clin North Am* 1993;77:25–42.

12. Barnett GH, Ropper AH, Romeo J. Intracranial pressure and outcome in adult encephalitis. *J Neurosurg* 1988;68:585–588.

13. Bash S, Hathout GM, Cohen S. Mesiotemporal T2-weighted hyperintensity: neurosyphilis mimicking herpes encephalitis. *AJNR Am J Neuroradiol* 2001;22:314–316.

14. Bataller L, Kleopa KA, Wu GF, et al. Autoimmune limbic encephalitis in 39 patients: immunophenotypes and outcomes. *J Neurol Neurosurg Psychiatry* 2007;78:381–385.

15. Berger JR, Houff S. Neurological complications of herpes simplex virus type 2 infection. *Arch Neurol* 2008;65:596–600.

16. Bonawitz C, Castillo M, Mukherji SK. Comparison of CT and MR features with clinical outcome in patients with Rocky Mountain spotted fever. *AJNR Am J Neuroradiol* 1997;18:459–464.

17. Brightbill TC, Post MJ, Hensley GT, Ruiz A. MR of Toxoplasma encephalitis: signal characteristics on T2-weighted images and pathologic correlation. *J Comput Assist Tomogr* 1996;20:417–422.

18. Buttner T, Dorndorf W. Prognostic value of computed tomography and cerebrospinal fluid analysis in viral encephalitis. *J Neuroimmunol* 1988;20:163–164.

19. Calisher CH, Berardi VP, Muth DJ, Buff EE. Specificity of immunoglobulin M and G antibody responses in humans infected with eastern and western equine encephalitis viruses: application to rapid serodiagnosis. *J Clin Microbiol* 1986;23:369–372.

20. Calisher CH, Pretzman CI, Muth DJ, Parsons MA, Peterson ED. Serodiagnosis of La Crosse virus infections in humans by detection of immunoglobulin M class antibodies. *J Clin Microbiol* 1986;23:667–671.

21. Cameron DA, Freedman AR, Wansbrough-Jones MH. Q fever encephalitis. *J Infect* 1990;20:159–162.

22. Campbell GL, Marfin AA, Lanciotti RS, Gubler DJ. West Nile virus. *Lancet Infect Dis* 2002;2:519–529.

23. Ciardi M, Giacchetti G, Fedele CG, et al. Acute cerebellitis caused by herpes simplex virus type 1. *Clin Infect Dis* 2003;36:e50–e54.

24. Counsell CE, Taylor R, Whittle IR. Focal necrotising herpes simplex encephalitis: a report of two cases with good clinical and neuropsychological outcomes. *J Neurol Neurosurg Psychiatry* 1994;57:1115–1117.

25. Dalmau J, Gleichman AJ, Hughes EG, et al. Anti-NMDA-receptor encephalitis: case series and analysis of the effects of antibodies. *Lancet Neurol* 2008;7:1091–1098.

26. Dalmau J, Lancaster E, Martinez-Hernandez E, Rosenfeld MR, Balice-Gordon R. Clinical experience and laboratory investigations in patients with anti-NMDAR encephalitis. *Lancet Neurol* 2011;10:63–74.

27. Darnell RB, Posner JB. Paraneoplastic syndromes involving the nervous system. *N Engl J Med* 2003;349:1543–1554.

28. Demaerel P, Wilms G, Robberecht W, et al. MRI of herpes simplex encephalitis. *Neuroradiology* 1992;34:490–493.

29. Deresiewicz RL, Thaler SJ, Hsu L, Zamani AA. Clinical and neuroradiographic manifestations of eastern equine encephalitis. *N Engl J Med* 1997;336:1867–1874.

30. Dumpis U, Crook D, Oksi J. Tick-borne encephalitis. *Clin Infect Dis* 1999;28:882–890.

31. Fisher CM. Hypomanic symptoms caused by herpes simplex encephalitis. *Neurology* 1996;47:1374–1378.

32. Flaherty ML, Wijdicks EFM, Stevens JC, et al. Clinical and electrophysiologic patterns of flaccid paralysis due to West Nile virus. *Mayo Clinic Proc* 2003;78:1245–1248.

33. Friedman JA, Wijdicks EFM, Fulgham JR, Wright AJ. Meningoencephalitis due to Blastomyces dermatitidis: case report and literature review. *Mayo Clinic Proc* 2000;75:403–408.

34. Gasecki AP, Steg RE. Correlation of early MRI with CT scan, EEG, and CSF: analyses in a case of biopsy-proven herpes simplex encephalitis. *Eur Neurol* 1991;31:372–375.

35. Gilden D. Varicella zoster virus and central nervous system syndromes. *Herpes* 2004;11 Suppl 2:89A–94A.

36. Hanna JN, Ritchie SA, Phillips DA, et al. Japanese encephalitis in north Queensland, Australia, 1998. *Med J Aust* 1999;170:533–536.

37. Hantson P, Guerit JM, de Tourtchaninoff M, et al. Rabies encephalitis mimicking the electrophysiological pattern of brain death: a case report. *Eur Neurol* 1993;33:212–217.

38. Hochberg LR, Sims JR, Davis BT. West Nile encephalitis in Massachusetts. *N Engl J Med* 2002;346:1030–1031.

39. Hoke CH, Jr., Vaughn DW, Nisalak A, et al. Effect of high-dose dexamethasone on the outcome of acute encephalitis due to Japanese encephalitis virus. *J Infect Dis* 1992;165:631–637.

40. Holland NR, Power C, Mathews VP, et al. Cytomegalovirus encephalitis in acquired immunodeficiency syndrome (AIDS). *Neurology* 1994;44:507–514.

41. Illis LS, Taylor FM. The electroencephalogram in herpes-simplex encephalitis. *Lancet* 1972;1:718–721.

42. Jeffery KJ, Read SJ, Peto TE, Mayon-White RT, Bangham CR. Diagnosis of viral infections of the central nervous system: clinical interpretation of PCR results. *Lancet* 1997;349:313–317.

43. Jemsek J, Greenberg SB, Taber L, et al. Herpes zoster-associated encephalitis: clinicopathologic report of 12 cases and review of the literature. *Medicine (Baltimore)* 1983;62:81–97.

44. Kamei S, Takasu T, Morishima T, Yoshihara T, Tetsuka T. Comparative study between chemiluminescence assay and two different sensitive polymerase chain reactions on the diagnosis of serial herpes simplex virus encephalitis. *J Neurol Neurosurg Psychiatry* 1999;67:596–601.

45. Kayser MS, Dalmau J. Anti-NMDA receptor encephalitis, autoimmunity, and psychosis. *Schizophr Res* 2014;pii: S0920–9964.

46. Kennedy PG. Viral encephalitis. *J Neurol* 2005;252:268–272.

47. Kennedy PG, Chaudhuri A. Herpes simplex encephalitis. *J Neurol Neurosurg Psychiatry* 2002;73:237–238.

48. Kirk JL, Fine DP, Sexton DJ, Muchmore HG. Rocky Mountain spotted fever: a clinical review based on 48 confirmed cases, 1943–1986. *Medicine (Baltimore)* 1990;69:35–45.

49. Koskiniemi M, Piiparinen H, Mannonen L, Rantalaiho T, Vaheri A. Herpes encephalitis is a disease of middle aged and elderly people: polymerase chain reaction for detection of herpes simplex virus in the CSF of 516 patients with encephalitis. The Study Group. *J Neurol Neurosurg Psychiatry* 1996;60:174–178.

50. Lakeman FD, Whitley RJ. Diagnosis of herpes simplex encephalitis: application of polymerase chain reaction to cerebrospinal fluid from brainbiopsied patients and correlation with disease. National Institute of Allergy and Infectious Diseases Collaborative Antiviral Study Group. *J Infect Dis* 1995;171:857–863.

51. Leypoldt F, Armangue T, Dalmau J. Autoimmune encephalopathies. *Ann N Y Acad Sci.* 2015 Mar;1338:94–114.

52. Li J, Loeb JA, Shy ME, et al. Asymmetric flaccid paralysis: a neuromuscular presentation of West Nile virus infection. *Ann Neurol* 2003;53:703–710.

53. Linnoila JJ, Rosenfeld MR, Dalmau J. Neuronal surface antibody-mediated autoimmune encephalitis. *Semin Neurol* 2014;34:458–466.

54. McGrath NM, Anderson NE, Hope JK, Croxson MC, Powell KF. Anterior opercular syndrome, caused by herpes simplex encephalitis. *Neurology* 1997;49:494–497.

55. McJunkin JE, de los Reyes EC, Irazuzta JE, et al. La Crosse encephalitis in children. *N Engl J Med* 2001;344:801–807.

56. Misra UK, Kalita J. Seizures in Japanese encephalitis. *J Neurol Sci* 2001;190:57–60.

57. Monath TP, Nystrom RR, Bailey RE, Calisher CH, Muth DJ. Immunoglobulin M antibody capture enzyme-linked immunosorbent assay for diagnosis of St. Louis encephalitis. *J Clin Microbiol* 1984;20:784–790.

58. Montoya JG, Liesenfeld O. Toxoplasmosis. *Lancet* 2004;363:1965–1976.

59. Mook-Kanamori B, van de Beek D, Wijdicks EFM. Herpes simplex encephalitis with normal initial cerebrospinal fluid examination. *J Am Geriatr Soc* 2009;57:1514–1515.

60. Nash D, Mostashari F, Fine A, et al. The outbreak of West Nile virus infection in the New York City area in 1999. *N Engl J Med* 2001;344:1807–1814.

61. Petersen LR, Marfin AA. West Nile virus: a primer for the clinician. *Ann Intern Med* 2002;137:173–179.

62. Pham HP, Daniel-Johnson JA, Stotler BA, Stephens H, Schwartz J. Therapeutic plasma exchange for the treatment of anti-NMDA receptor encephalitis. *J Clin Apher* 2011;26:320–325.

63. Poissy J, Wolff M, Dewilde A, et al. Factors associated with delay to acyclovir administration in 184 patients with herpes simplex virus encephalitis. *Clin Microbiol Infect* 2009;15:560–564.

64. Przelomski MM, O'Rourke E, Grady GF, Berardi VP, Markley HG. Eastern equine encephalitis in Massachusetts: a report of 16 cases, 1970–1984. *Neurology* 1988;38:736–739.

65. Raschilas F, Wolff M, Delatour F, et al. Outcome of and prognostic factors for herpes simplex encephalitis in adult patients: results of a multicenter study. *Clin Infect Dis* 2002;35:254–260.

66. Reimann CA, Hayes EB, DiGuiseppi C, et al. Epidemiology of neuroinvasive arboviral disease in the United States, 1999–2007. *Am J Trop Med Hyg* 2008;79:974–979.

67. Rowley AH, Whitley RJ, Lakeman FD, Wolinsky SM. Rapid detection of herpes-simplex-virus DNA in cerebrospinal fluid of patients with herpes simplex encephalitis. *Lancet* 1990;335:440–441.

68. Sejvar JJ. The long-term outcomes of human West Nile virus infection. *Clin Infect Dis* 2007;44:1617–1624.

69. Sempere AP, Elizaga J, Duarte J, et al. Q fever mimicking herpetic encephalitis. *Neurology* 1993;43:2713–2714.

70. Singh TD, Fugate JE, Hocker S, et al. Predictors of outcome in HSV encephalitis. *J Neurol* 2016 in press.

71. Singh TD, Fugate JE, Rabinstein AA. The spectrum of acute encephalitis: causes, management, and predictors of outcome. *Neurology* 2015;84:359–366.

72. Siren J, Seppalainen AM, Launes J. Is EEG useful in assessing patients with acute encephalitis treated with acyclovir? *Electroencephalogr Clin Neurophysiol* 1998;107:296–301.

73. Steiner I, Kennedy PG, Pachner AR. The neurotropic herpes viruses: herpes simplex and varicella-zoster. *Lancet Neurol* 2007;6:1015–1028.

74. Szilak I, Marty F, Helft J, Soeiro R. Neurosyphilis presenting as herpes simplex encephalitis. *Clin Infect Dis* 2001;32:1108–1109.

75. Taferner E, Pfausler B, Kofler A, et al. Craniectomy in severe, life-threatening encephalitis: a report on outcome and long-term prognosis of four cases. *Intensive Care Med* 2001;27:1426–1428.

76. Titulaer MJ, McCracken L, Gabilondo I, et al. Treatment and prognostic factors for long-term outcome in patients with anti-NMDA receptor encephalitis: an observational cohort study. *Lancet Neurol* 2013;12:157–165.

77. Toothaker TB, Rubin M. Paraneoplastic neurological syndromes: a review. *Neurologist* 2009;15:21–33.

78. Tyler KL. Emerging viral infections of the central nervous system: part 1. *Arch Neurol* 2009;66:939–948.

79. Tyler KL. Neurological infections: advances in therapy, outcome, and prediction. *Lancet Neurol* 2009;8:19–21.

80. Wasay M, Diaz-Arrastia R, Suss RA, et al. St Louis encephalitis: a review of 11 cases in a 1995 Dallas, Tex, epidemic. *Arch Neurol* 2000;57:114–118.

81. Whitley RJ. Herpes simplex encephalitis: adolescents and adults. *Antiviral Res* 2006;71:141–148.

82. Whitley RJ. Viral encephalitis. *N Engl J Med* 1990;323:242–250.

83. Whitley RJ, Alford CA, Hirsch MS, et al. Vidarabine versus acyclovir therapy in herpes simplex encephalitis. *N Engl J Med* 1986;314:144–149.

84. Wijdicks EFM, Borleffs JC, Hoepelman AI, Jansen GH. Fatal disseminated hemorrhagic toxoplasmic encephalitis as the initial manifestation of AIDS. *Ann Neurol* 1991;29:683–686.

85. Wingerchuk DM, Noseworthy JH, Kimmel DW. Paraneoplastic encephalomyelitis and seminoma: importance of testicular ultrasonography. *Neurology* 1998;51:1504–1507.

86. Yan HJ. Herpes simplex encephalitis: the role of surgical decompression. *Surg Neurol* 2002;57:20–24.

87. Young CA, Humphrey PR, Ghadiali EJ, Klapper PE, Cleator GM. Short-term memory impairment in an alert patient as a presentation of herpes simplex encephalitis. *Neurology* 1992;42:260–261.

88. Zhang JS, Zhao QM, Zhang PH, Jia N, Cao WC. Genomic sequence of a Japanese encephalitis virus isolate from southern China. *Arch Virol* 2009;154:1177–1180.

36

Acute Spinal Cord Disorders

Acute spinal cord injury (SCI) is caused by traffic accidents in more than 50% of patients arriving at emergency departments. The demographic profile consists of men in their 30s, admitted most often during weekends in the summer months. Complete cord lesions have decreased in prevalence, which is tentatively explained by improved care in the field, increased use of seat belts, and, possibly, surgical care of unstable spine trauma. It is prudent to assume that SCI may have occurred in patients who have had multiple trauma, motor vehicle or sports accidents, or a documented spine fracture.

The spectrum of causes in other acute spinal cord disorders is wide,[11] and there are regional differences in the cause of SCI in published series. In a study from France of 79 patients with acute myelopathy, the most common causes were multiple sclerosis, systemic disease such as cancer, and spinal cord infarction.[17] In contrast, tuberculosis of the spine, acute transverse myelitis, and primary cord tumor were common in a series of patients with paraplegia from India.[56]

This chapter is not intended to comprehensively discuss all traumatic spinal lesions and surgical management, which can be properly addressed only by experienced spine surgeons or neurosurgeons with special qualifications in the management of spine trauma. Spine trauma has evolved into a subspecialty in which the role of the neurointensivist or neurologist is important, but is limited to accurate clinical description of the damage, appropriate stabilization, early recognition of unstable spine fractures or dislocations, and, when necessary, specific medical management.[43,45]

The arrival of a patient with acute SCI to the neurosciences intensive care unit (NICU) is awaited with trepidation, and for good reason. Uncertainty about the etiology of an acute myelopathy justifies admission to the NICU not only to observe the clinical course but also to aggressively continue the search for a cause. Early clinical signs and symptoms of acute SCI have also been discussed in Chapter 9 and are repeated here for completeness.

The overarching theme of this chapter is the management of acute SCI, and the immediate priorities are stabilization of respiration, cardiac rhythm, and blood pressure, and the management of neurogenic bladder and bowel dysfunction.[3] Ischemic spinal cord infarction associated with aortic surgery is discussed in Chapter 48.

CLINICAL RECOGNITION

The course of development of symptoms (insidious, abrupt, or maximal at onset) could indicate a certain cause. Tumors in the spinal cord may have different and unpredictable courses of development. Even a remitting, relapsing course can occur, and some benign tumors can cause rapid progression to quadriplegia in days. Traumatic spinal cord lesions are often determined at the time of injury.

Sensory symptoms are the most frequent presenting symptoms in patients with multiple sclerosis, whereas motor and sphincter dysfunction appear to be more frequent in other causes.[17] The manifestations of acute transverse myelitis at onset may be paresthesias, interscapular pain followed by paraparesis, and urinary retention. Acute catastrophic onset has been reported.[4,15,51] Neuromyelitis optica (Devic disease) is possibly linked to multiple sclerosis, but its pathologic substrate of severe necrosis and axonal degeneration indicates that it could be a separate disorder. The absence of demyelinating lesions outside the optic nerve and spinal cord is required for the diagnosis. Respiratory failure due to cervical cord involvement in Devic disease is common in relapsing forms. The optic neuritis and myelitis may not coincide with each other and may occur several years apart.

The clinical course in necrotic myelopathy may be vacillating. Rapid decline is common, but gradual worsening, alternating with sudden progression and followed by slow progression, may be observed.[36,62] An ascending sensory level, pain, and urinary incontinence are common presenting symptoms, together with lower motor neuron signs (areflexia, atrophy, and flaccidity) on examination.

Spinal cord ischemia due to occlusion of the anterior spinal artery and tributaries results in acute maximal motor paralysis and sensory level. Causes are invariably dissecting aneurysm, shock, ruptured abdominal aneurysm, trauma, and, in young patients, fibrocartilaginous embolization.[13]

Pain is an important clinical feature that may point to a certain cause, but it may also result in a mistaken referral to a cardiologist (pain involving the T1–T5 roots), gastroenterologist (pain referred to the upper abdomen; T6–T10 roots), or urologist (pain involving the lower back and radiation to genitalia; T12– S4). The pain associated with spinal cord disease is sharp and stabbing and therefore can be differentiated from the duller, nagging pain associated with visceral disease. Percussion pain may be elicited over the spine, but this symptom is generally considered unreliable. Patients with extensive metastatic disease and collapsed vertebrae may not feel any pain with percussion. Pain that feels as if something were "ripped open" is fairly typical in a patient with an acute epidural hematoma. It commonly mimics a ruptured abdominal aorta or ureter obstruction due to a kidney stone. Failures to support one's weight and urinary retention within the first few hours after onset of an excruciating stab of back pain are fairly diagnostic.

Neurologic examination should determine the level and the extent of spinal cord involvement in the horizontal axis. The function of the spinal cord is graded to determine whether the lesion is complete or incomplete. It is complete when the absence of both motor and sensory function below the lesion level is documented. The degree of weakness can be assessed by grading muscle strength on the grading scale of the British Medical Research Council (Table 36.1). Although one may grade the weakness of all muscles for documentation and comparison over time, some muscles are localizing: arm abduction (C5), forearm extension (C5), forearm flexion (C5 and C6), knee extension (L3 and L4), foot and great toe dorsiflexion (L5), and plantar flexion (S1). Assessing muscle tone is also important, although many patients have a flaccid paralysis due to so-called spinal shock—a poorly understood pathophysiologic phenomenon. Muscle tone, or the resistance a muscle has against passive movement of the joint, may distinguish between upper motor neuron disease and lower motor neuron disease. Upper motor neuron disease typically causes spasticity in which

TABLE 36.1. BRITISH MEDICAL RESEARCH COUNCIL SCALE OF MUSCLE STRENGTH

0 No muscular contraction
1 A flicker of contraction either seen or palpated but insufficient to move a joint
2 Muscular contractions sufficient to move a joint but not against the force of gravity
3 Muscular contractions sufficient to maintain a position against the force of gravity
4 Muscular contractions sufficient to resist the force of gravity plus additional force
5 Normal motor power

Modified from *Aids to the Examination of the Peripheral Nervous System*, 4th ed. Edinburgh: W. B. Saunders, 2000. With permission of *The Guarantors of Brain*.

the flexors in the upper extremities and extensors of the lower extremities are more commonly involved. It is worthwhile to inspect the muscles for atrophy, which may indicate a long-standing process that has evolved into cord compression. Acute radiculopathy does not produce atrophy, but long-standing compression root lesions produce fasciculations and significant atrophy of the muscle bulk. Myoclonic twitching may occur and can be widespread in acute SCI.

All sensory modalities should be tested (pinprick, position, and vibration sense; light touch with a wisp of cotton; pressure touch; and temperature). Abnormal pinprick is usually interpreted as touch without identification of a sharp sting and is most valuable in localizing segments. When a tuning fork is unavailable to test vibration, at least position sense should be tested. Normally, movement of a few degrees in the position of the toe joints should be easily appreciated. In addition, tactile discrimination should be tested, and normally a 2- to 3-cm difference between two points should be appreciated. Normal function suggests intact posterior column tracts but also nerve root function.

Saddle anesthesia (S3–S5) is an indication of a conus medullaris lesion, which can be accurately delineated but may be missed with superficial examination in a supine patient. The sensory loss is often dissociated, with sparing of touch but loss of pinprick. Absence of dissociation suggests involvement of the cauda equina, not just the conus.

Sacral sparing of the sensory symptoms is an important sign because it implies a centrally located intramedullary lesion. (The representation of the sacral fibers is very peripheral in the cord;

thus, pinprick and temperature sensation may be spared in acute central cord lesions.)

The presence of dissociating sensory findings may further localize. Brown-Séquard syndrome is strongly indicative of extramedullary compression, but it may occur in patients with cancer and radiation myelopathy. Its clinical hallmark is loss of pain and temperature (involvement of the crossed spinothalamic tract), sensation opposite the lesion, with loss of position and vibration (involvement of the ascending posterior column tracts), and more prominent leg weakness (corticospinal tract) at the level of the lesion. (The patient may be puzzled by numbness in one leg and weakness in the other.) Brown-Séquard syndrome

is rarely uniform in presentation, but marked unilateral leg weakness with a Babinski sign and lack of position recognition of the toe should point to acute extramedullary compression.

The classic patterns of sensory loss in myelopathies are depicted in Figure 36.1. Again, important pointers are nipple at level T4; umbilicus at level T10; and thumb, middle finger, and fifth digit innervated by C6, C7, and C8. The C4 and T2 dermatomes are continuous. A notable finding, when present, is the preservation of sacral sensation, implying an intra-axial lesion due to ventrolateral localization of sacral spinothalamic tracts.

It is important to assess anal sphincter tone (S3–S4). The examining finger should be held

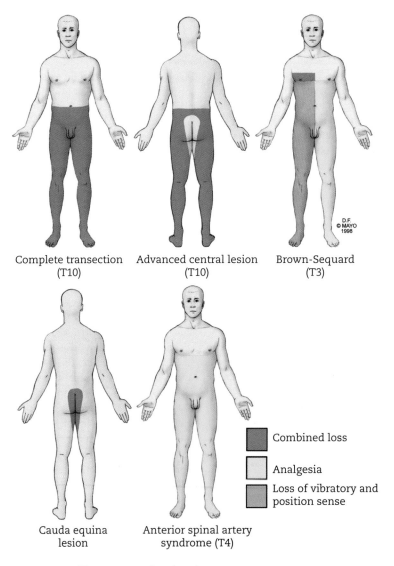

Complete transection (T10)   Advanced central lesion (T10)   Brown-Sequard (T3)

Cauda equina lesion   Anterior spinal artery syndrome (T4)

Combined loss

Analgesia

Loss of vibratory and position sense

FIGURE 36.1: The major spinal cord syndromes.

firmly against the anal verge to allow gradual passive relaxation. The strength of the external anal sphincter can be assessed by having the patient tighten the pelvic floor as if to prevent stool from escaping. The puborectalis should also be palpated a few inches inside the anal canal. Gentle pressure is applied toward the sacrum to assess the puborectalis for tone, strength, and spasticity. In addition, the bulbocavernous reflexes can be elicited by pinching the dorsal glans penis or by pressing the clitoris and palpating for bulbocavernosus and external anal sphincter contraction. If these rarely tested reflexes are intact, conus medullaris function is normal. Priapism is present in some cases but resolves.[27]

The SCI can be classified by the American Spinal Injury Association (ASIA) impairment scale specifically designed for traumatic injury (see Table 36.2 and Part XIV, Guidelines).

Clinical differentiation of an extramedullary tumor from an intramedullary tumor of the spinal cord can be difficult and may be unreliable. Nonetheless, an extramedullary tumor may appear as a Brown-Séquard type of lesion and then become more widespread. Extramedullary tumors often produce radicular and regional pain rather than the poorly localized burning pain of intramedullary tumors. Sphincter disturbances are also considered very unusual in patients with extramedullary and intramedullary tumors. (Magnetic resonance imaging [MRI] may eventually resolve this clinical uncertainty.)

TABLE 36.2. AMERICAN SPINAL INJURY ASSOCIATION (ASIA) IMPAIRMENT SCALE

Grade	Description
A	Complete; no sensory or motor function preserved in the sacral segments S4–S5
B	Incomplete; sensory but not motor function preserved below the neurologic level and extending through the sacral segment S4–S5
C	Incomplete; motor function preserved below the neurologic level; most key muscles have an MRC grade 3
D	Incomplete; motor function preserved below the neurologic level; most key muscles have an MRC grade 3
E	Normal motor and sensory function

MRC, Medical Research Council.
From McDonald JW, Sadowsky C. Spinal-cord injury. *Lancet* 2002; 359:417–425. With permission of Elsevier Science.

Two specific problems need to be addressed. First, respiration can be very seriously affected when the lesion involves the cervical cord C3 and C4 segments.[24] Patients often have shortness of breath with an increased work of breathing, but also may have a sensation of air hunger and chest tightness. When lesions reach C3, diaphragmatic expansion and abdominal muscle function are absent, so rapid intubation and full mechanical ventilation are needed. Later, tracheostomy is indicated with use of cannulas that allow for speech. Noninvasive assisted ventilation could be tried, but the criteria have not been well outlined in this condition. In SCI, weakness of the respiratory muscles, as in any type of impaired neuromuscular respiratory function, is determined by weakness of the diaphragm and the intercostal and abdominal muscles.[52,64] Innervation of these muscles is organized as follows: diaphragm (phrenic nerve, C3–C5), intercostal muscles (T1–T12), and abdominal muscles (T7–L1).[28] Therefore, effective coughing is determined by the level of injury. Lower levels of injury may spare intercostal muscles, resulting in better volume of respiratory function.[52] When myelitis or myelopathy involves levels in the lower cervical segments, breathing depends on posture. Vital capacity increases in the supine position (unlike diaphragmatic failure in Guillain-Barré syndrome and myasthenia gravis, which worsens breathing in this position). The abdominal contents produce a pressure effect, and this is the principle underlying the use of abdominal binders.

Second, the delicate autonomic balance of sympathetic and parasympathetic output is skewed toward vagal output in lesions involving the low cervical midthoracic cord (C1–T6).[38] This leads to hypotension (reduced sympathetic arteriolar tone) and bradycardia (vagal innervation unopposed). Tonic and reflex control of sympathetic and sacral parasympathetic function in cord lesions above T5 leads to hypotension with head-up tilt but also to frequent bradycardia.[20] Bradycardia can remain asymptomatic (Figure 36.2), but cardiac pauses are common reasons for "calling a code." Bradycardia usually resolves within several weeks to months,[41] but the patient may need a temporary pacemaker. Injury to the cervical cord completely disrupts sympathetic traffic, which explains the much higher frequency of bradycardia with a lesion in this location. Tracheal suctioning is perhaps the most noticeable trigger. These vagal discharges clearly respond to 1 mg of atropine or revert spontaneously.

Many patients are poikilothermic (temperature fluctuations from ambient temperature).

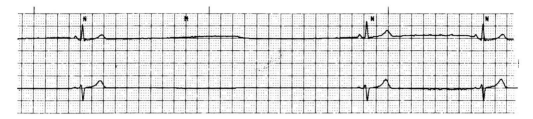

FIGURE 36.2: Spell of bradycardia with brief pause in a patient with cervical necrotic myopathy.

Hypothermia may occur from lack of shivering (loss of sympathetic tone) and profound vasodilatation, and some patients may not notice decreases in core temperature to 33°C. It may also lead to a prolonged QT interval on the electrocardiogram. Lack of sweating from loss of sympathetic control of the apocrine glands may produce hyperthermia. However, sweating above the lesion often prevents hyperthermia.

Gastric atony may be evident on a routine chest radiograph that reveals large air pockets. Atony also affects the bladder.[33] Catheterization and placement of an indwelling catheter are required to assess possible retention. Bladder retention of more than 1 L may not be noted by the patient. Retention may continue even when the patient is catheterized, particularly if urinary flow is minimal or obstructed. Bowel dysfunction significantly affects management, and most reflex activity below the level of SCI is lost.

NEUROIMAGING AND LABORATORY TESTS

Neuroimaging of the spine and spinal cord has a high priority after presumed trauma. The extent of imaging is determined by neurologic findings at presentation. Careful clinical delineation of level of involvement may tailor orientation and selection of the studies.

Neuroradiologists should have access to clinical information that may further determine certain MRI sequences. The first priority is to diagnose unstable cervical or thoracic spine fractures or spine compression.[12]

Screening cervical spine radiographs for alert patients with no neck tenderness and no neurologic abnormalities have a very low yield. Combined lateral, anteroposterior, and odontoid views have a high diagnostic yield and should recognize more than 90% of the lesions. The lateral cervical spine radiograph and odontoid views should be viewed systematically. A common pitfall is focusing on a single fracture or misalignment while overlooking other abnormalities. The essentials of spine film viewing are summarized in Table 36.3, and an overview of spinal fractures can be found in a companion textbook.[61] Only the trained eye of an experienced physician can identify fractures, but even then, a computed tomography (CT) scan is often needed for confirmation. The threshold for ordering a CT scan of the cervical spine must be very low, particularly when plain films of the cervical spine give dubious information or are of marginal quality.

First, the cervical vertebral bodies should be identified, and particular attention should be paid to the lower cervical spine. Hand traction should be used to pull both arms and shoulders of the patient down. Inadequate films should prompt CT scanning of the spine. When a lateral spine film is evaluated, four lordotic curves and alignments are assessed to look for displacement (Figure 36.3).

Common findings are compression of the vertebral bodies (vertebral body often several millimeters less anteriorly than posteriorly), displacement in the lateral view (> 3 mm between adjacent vertebral bodies), and displacement of the odontoid bone (odontoid tip should be aligned with tip of clivus).

TABLE 36.3. SPINE INSTABILITY

Cervical
- Widened interspinous space or facet joints
- Anterior listhesis > 3.5 mm
- Narrowed or widened disk space
- Focal angulation > 11 degrees
- Vertebral compression > 25%

Thoracic
- Fracture dislocation
- Posttraumatic kyphosis > 40 degrees
- Spine fractures associated with sternal fractures
- Concomitant rib fracture or costovertebral dislocation

Imhof H, Fuchsjäger M. Traumatic injuries: imaging of spinal injuries. *Eur Radiol* 2002;12:1262. With permission of Springer.

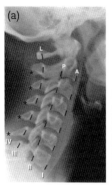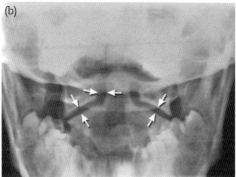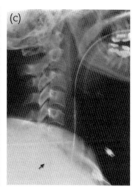

FIGURE 36.3: Plain spine radiographs with examination techniques to uncover fractures and dislocations. (a) Normal alignment lines: I, normal alignment along the anterior (*A*) vertebral margins; II, posterior (*P*) vertebral margin alignment line; III, spinal laminar (*L*) line; IV, relation of the dorsal spinous processes. (b) Indicators of normal odontoid interspace (*arrows*). (c) Incomplete cervical spine examination (C7 is missing, *arrow*).

Indications of instability are displacement of a vertebral body, widening of the interspinous or interlaminar distance, widening of the facet joints or spinal canal, disruption of the posterior spinal line, and anterolisthesis or retrolisthesis with flexion or extension. The odontoid bone typically lies within 13 mm of the posterior cortex of the anterior C1 arch.

Hyperflexion injuries of the cervical spine—direct trauma to the head, spine in the flexed position—can be seen in various degrees, from mild widening of the posterior intervertebral space to subluxation of the vertebra; and the inferior articular facet may become lodged on the superior facet of the vertebra below (so-called *perched facet*). A cord lesion is common or easily induced with further manipulation, making this a highly unstable condition. Unilateral facet distortion can be recognized by an alteration in the laminar space, namely, the distance between the spinolaminar line and the posterior margin of the articular mass.

Hyperextension injuries (sudden deceleration impact) produce fairly characteristic features, such as a hyperextension teardrop fracture (avulsion of the site of attachment of the anterior longitudinal ligament); hangman's fracture with bilateral fracture through the pars interarticularis of C2; Jefferson's fracture (fracture of the ring of C1); and odontoid fractures (tip is type I, base is type II, and extension into the body of C2 is type III). Figure 36.4 illustrates the most common unstable cervical fractures. Facial injury is more common as a result of direct impact.

Computed tomography scans added to a plain cervical spine film are unsurpassed in diagnostic value for the demonstration of fractures. Computed tomography scan reconstructions are very useful in imaging loose bone fragments and facet dislocation. Myelography combined with CT can more clearly demonstrate the cord and nerve roots and determine whether they are compressed by the misalignment or fracture. In most instances, specific areas are scanned with axial slices 1.5–3 mm thick for the cervical spine and 3–5 mm thick for the thoracic and lumbar spines.

Intrathecal administration of contrast medium (myelography, CT scanning) is usually reserved for patients who cannot undergo MRI (presence of a pacemaker, aneurysm clips, cochlear implants, bullet fragments, and morbid obesity). It has become the second-choice imaging modality in spine injury because it is time-consuming and requires patient movement.

Nontraumatic acute SCIs also require a set of neuroimaging tests. A plain radiograph of the spine may also identify bone destruction from metastatic disease and the consequences for stability of the spine. Plain radiographs can appear misleadingly normal in approximately 25% of patients with documented metastatic spinal cord compression; furthermore, plain radiographic abnormalities may not correspond to the location of the tumor, often showing cord compression at a much higher or lower thoracic level.

Bone scan with technetium 99m diphosphonate is occasionally used for screening and as a supplementary test,[58] but MRI of the spine, with specific attention to the level determined by clinical localization, should be considered the standard in acute spinal cord compression.

An adequate MRI study of the spine should have sagittal T1- and T2-weighted images with thin (4–5 mm) sections. Several important features can be identified on MRI of the spine. On

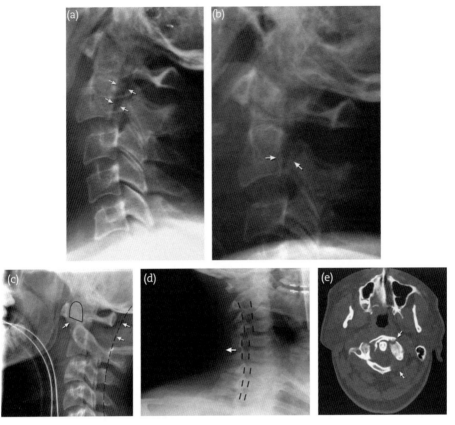

FIGURE 36.4. (a, b) Two examples of hangman fracture (*C2* bilateral fracture through pars articularis), common with windshield injuries (*arrows*). (c) Odontoid fracture. The spinal laminar line is disrupted (*arrows*). Dens is outlined. (d) Locked facet dislocation (hyperflexion injury). (e) Jefferson C1 fracture (*arrows*).

T1-weighted images, bone marrow in the vertebral bodies produces a high intensity but a low signal of the cortical bone. T1-weighted images may underestimate the width of the spinal canal, because CSF characteristics are of low signal as well. The nerve roots may emerge on axial slices against the high-intensity signal of epidural fat and the low intensity of CSF. Disks also have a low T1 signal. The spinal cord signal is intermediate, but higher than that of surrounding CSF. On T2-weighted images, the CSF is bright. The intravertebral disks are brighter. The nerve roots are much better appreciated on T2 images because of the distinctive bright signal of the CSF. Motion artifacts may produce hyperintense or hypointense bands (phantom images or harmonics), suggesting a cavity in the cord or neoplasm.

Magnetic resonance imaging in spine injury should first obtain sagittal T1-weighted images, with axial images through abnormal areas. A T1-weighted image is important to rule out major abnormalities and can be followed by T2 or gradient echo sequences (short time to acquire and sensitive for early hemorrhages in the spine). On T1-weighted images, subacute hemorrhage is bright and cerebrospinal fluid (CSF) is dark. On T2-weighted images, CSF is bright, cord edema is bright, and acute hemorrhage is dark.[65] An example of cord trauma and swelling is shown in Figure 36.5. Magnetic resonance imaging of the spine can classify abnormalities as intramedullary or extramedullary, in which the lesions are often intradural. Often more than one lesion is involved, supporting a policy of MRI of the whole spine in these patients.

Gadolinium does not penetrate the central nervous system; therefore, if the blood–brain barrier is intact, the spine should not become enhanced. T1-weighted images enhance the basivertebral veins, epidural venous plexus, and spinal ganglion. Necrosis in the spine appears as a high-intensity signal in T1-weighted images after gadolinium injection. Because tumor has a high signal enhancement, gadolinium is useful in further evaluation of intramedullary, intradural, and extramedullary lesions.

Nerve root enhancement with gadolinium ordinarily does not appear unless disease is

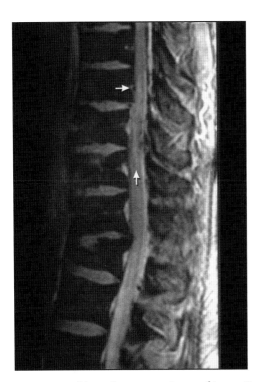

FIGURE 36.5: Magnetic resonance image of traumatic cord swelling (*arrows*).

present, but occasionally is observed when a dose of very high contrast is used (0.3 mmol/kg of body weight). Enhancement of the spinal nerve roots is an important finding, and several patterns have been described. Diffuse enhancement of the cauda can occur in leptomeningeal metastasis, most often associated with systemic malignant disease, such as breast, lung, or skin cancer. However, diffuse enhancement can be seen in inflammatory polyradiculopathy, such as cytomegalovirus radiculopathy in acquired immunodeficiency syndrome (AIDS). Tuberculosis should be considered in persons from endemic areas and, more recently, in patients with AIDS. Epidural compression may be caused by granuloma formation, which is apparent as thickening of the nerve roots. Virtually any leptomeningeal infection can cause enhancement, including *Mycobacterium tuberculosis* infection and cysticercosis. Sarcoidosis should be considered when enhancement is linear at the nerve roots.

In spinal cord compression from cancer, vertebral compression fractures may not coexist with an epidural mass. Malignant lesions on MRI most often have a low-intensity signal on T1-weighted images and a high-intensity signal on T2-weighted images. Contrast enhancement increases the sensitivity of detecting malignant lesions in further

defining epidural mass effect, which may not be evident on unenhanced images.[39]

The diagnosis of epidural hematoma has been greatly facilitated by MRI.[2,26,59] A high T2-weighted signal often identifies a hematoma that may be scattered throughout the spinal canal, with various degrees of compression at different levels. However, a hyper-acute hematoma (within an hour or so) may be isointense on T1-weighted images.[25,30]

Magnetic resonance imaging is the preferred test in epidural abscess, and sometimes after gadolinium enhancement, compartmentalization becomes evident.[37] Acute spinal cord syndromes may be caused by infarction or an arteriovenous malformation. An isolated increased centromedullary signal on MRI is diagnostic for a spinal cord infarct. Arteriovenous malformation may be located in the dura and may cause significant backlog of venous flow and a dramatic swelling of the cord.

Spinal cord swelling can also accompany multiple sclerosis and initially suggests a tumor. In multiple sclerosis, the lesions are frequently small and localized in the lateral or posterior regions.[55] In addition, MRI of the brain detects areas of demyelination, typically in the corpus callosum. Some patterns of abnormality on MRI encountered in acute spinal cord disorders are shown in Figure 36.6.

Visual evoked potentials are possibly helpful in documenting previous or simultaneous involvement of the optic nerves, pointing to Devic (optic neuromyelitis) disease.[63] Somatosensory evoked potentials or corticomotor evoked potentials are not helpful in diagnosis but may hold promise as an indicator of prognosis. Tibial and pudendal somatosensory evoked potentials seem to indicate recovery of ambulatory capacity,[16] but one study suggested that this finding applied only to ischemic spinal cord lesions.[35]

Cerebrospinal fluid analysis can be helpful because oligoclonal bands and a cell count higher than 30 cells are common in multiple sclerosis. Pleocytosis (> 30 cells without oligoclonal bands) suggests an infectious cause and may indicate a postinfectious myelopathy. In spinal cord infarction, the CSF should be normal, although a mild pleocytosis has been reported. The diagnostic tests are summarized in Table 36.4.

FIRST STEPS IN MANAGEMENT

Emergency stabilization of traumatic SCI includes immediate cervical spine immobilization and endotracheal intubation when needed.

Hypotension from unopposed parasympathetic tone is common, particularly with change

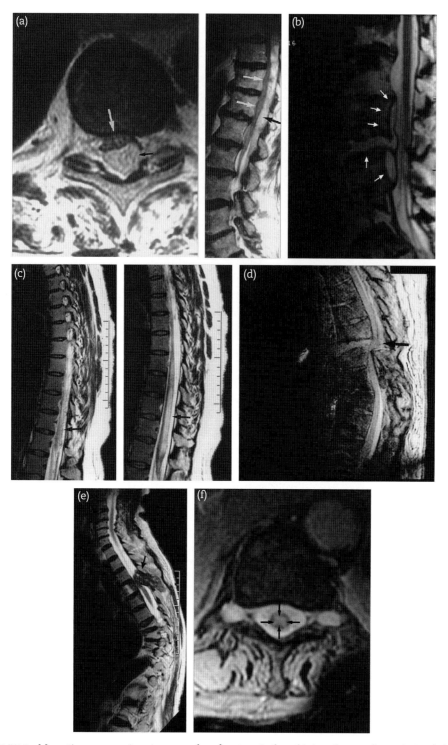

FIGURE 36.6: Magnetic resonance imaging examples of acute spinal cord injury (*arrows* denote lesions). (a) (left and right) Epidural hematoma (*black arrows*); *white arrows* show compressed cord. (b) Epidural abscess (*arrows*). (c) (left and right) Dural arteriovenous fistula with a typical dilated vein (*arrow*) and T2 hyperintensity in patient with progressive paraplegia (*arrow*). (d) Central cord lesion due to trauma. (e) Spinal cord compression due to a paraspinal mass. (f) Spinal cord infarction (*arrows*).

Image A is from Henderson RD, Pittock SJ, Piepgras DG, et al. Acute spontaneous spinal epidural hematoma. *Arch Neurol* 2001;58:1145–1146. With permission of the American Medical Association.

TABLE 36.4. COMMON DIAGNOSTIC CONSIDERATIONS IN ACUTE SPINAL CORD DISEASE

Disorder	Diagnostic Test
Myelopathy	
Compressive myelopathy	MRI of spine
Acute necrotic myelopathy	MRI of spine, biopsy
Vacuolar myelopathy	CSF (PMN), HIV-1
Anterior spinal artery occlusion	MRI of spine, RF, SLE, ANA
Foix-Alajouanine syndrome	MRI of spine, spinal angiogram
Radiation myelopathy	Radiation field, irradiation dose
Paraneoplastic myelopathy	CT scan of chest-abdomen, bone marrow, thyroid scan
Myelitis	
Acute disseminated encephalomyelitis	CSF (MN), MRI of brain
Postinfectious myelitis	Echovirus, coxsackievirus
Demyelinating myelitis	CSF (protein, IgG, oligoclonal bands)
Neuromyelitis optica	VEP, MRI of spine, CSF protein)
Viral myelitis	Herpes zoster, CSF (PCR), HTLV-1
Bacterial myelitis	VDRL, FTA-ABS, CSF (cells, protein)
Tropical myelitis	Circulating antigen, stools, ELISA (schistosomiasis, trichinosis)

ANA, antinuclear antibody; CSF, cerebrospinal fluid; CT, computed tomography; ELISA, enzyme-linked immunosorbent assay; FTA-ABS, fluorescent treponemal antibody absorption test; HIV, human immunodeficiency virus; MN, mononuclear leukocytes; MRI, magnetic resonance imaging; PCR, polymerase chain reaction; PMN, polymorphonuclear leukocytes; RF, rheumatoid factor; SLE, systemic lupus erythematosus; VEP, visual evoked potential.
From Berman M, Feldman S, Alter M, et al. Acute transverse myelitis: incidence and etiologic considerations. *Neurology* 1981;31:966–971; and Campi A, Filippi M, Comi G, et al. Acute transverse myelopathy: spinal and cranial MR study with clinical follow-up. *AJNR Am J Neuroradiol* 1995;16:115–123.

in position or in the first minutes after connection to the mechanical ventilator (decreased preload due to positive pressure effect). Three of four spinal cord trauma victims experience one or more episodes of hypotension.[32,60] Volume resuscitation or intravenous phenylephrine infusion is needed. In occasional patients, autonomic dysregulation is manifested as marked hypertensive surges, which should be treated with labetalol. Positional hypotension may also later be treated with midodrine or fludrocortisone.

Spinal cord experts state that a mean arterial pressure of $\geq$ 85 mm Hg or $\geq$ 120 mm Hg systolic for 7 days provides the best hemodynamic support. Another crucial decision in any patient with acute spinal cord symptoms is whether immediate neurosurgical intervention is needed. Many neurosurgical conditions of the spinal cord, particularly acute epidural hematoma and penetrating injury, are successfully treated only when decompression has been achieved early in the course. Acute epidural hematoma due to rupture of the epidural venous plexus is commonly associated with the use of warfarin. Immediate administration of fresh frozen plasma and evacuation within 12 hours result in good ambulatory function and bladder control.[22] A nonsurgical approach should be considered only in patients with stable or improving minimal neurologic deficits and a lesion not compressing the cord. It is not commonly an option. Above all, these conservatively managed patients belong in the NICU with a neurosurgeon in attendance.[18]

Other emergency neurosurgical indications are removal of foreign objects (e.g., bullet), obtaining tissue samples of an unknown tumor, and spinal instability from any cause in a patient whose condition is rapidly worsening. Patients with significant traumatic displacement, perching, and burst fracture need stabilization with instrumentation.[6] However, an uncertain neurosurgical indication is progression of paraplegia after or during radiotherapy.

The initial measures for patients with acute SCI are fairly standard for each of the disorders (Table 36.5). After admission to the NICU, the patient should be placed in a special rotating or air-fluidized bed to decrease decubitus ulcers. These turning beds and specialty care beds may also reduce the complication of pulmonary embolization, although no hard data are available. Every patient should receive heparin subcutaneously (5,000 U twice a day) or intermittent pneumonic devices.[1,9,34] Subcutaneous heparin is

TABLE 36.5. INITIAL MANAGEMENT OF ACUTE SPINAL CORD DISORDER

Airway management	Incentive spirometry and assisted cough
	Intubation if patient has hypoxemia despite facemask with 10 L of 100% oxygen/ minute or with abnormal respiratory drive
Mechanical ventilation	AC or IMV mode in high cervical lesions (C3–C5)
Blood pressure management	Maintain MAP 90–100 mm Hg (MAP of 85 mmHg or more for at least 7 days in traumatic spine injury) IV norepinephrine may be needed.
Fluid management	2 L of 0.9% NaCl
	Consider crystalloid infusions with shock
Nutrition	Enteral nutrition with continuous infusion (on day 2)
	Blood glucose control (goal 140–180 mg/dL)
Prophylaxis	DVT prophylaxis: Pneumatic compression devices
	SC heparin 5,000 U t.i.d.
	GI prophylaxis: Pantoprazole 40 mg daily IV or lansoprazole 30 mg orally through nasogastric tube
	Inspect skin with each turn and every 8 hours
	Bisacodyl supp and digital stimulation daily for bowel care
	Indwelling urinary catheter
Specific management	*In spinal cord compression and acute myelitis*: dexamethasone, 100 mg IV, followed by 4–25 mg/day q.i.d.
	In traumatic spine injury: Methylprednisolone < 3 hr (30 mg/kg bolus, followed by infusion of 5.4 mg/kg/hr for 23 hours); 3–8 hr (30 mg/kg bolus, followed by infusion of 5.4 mg/kg/hr for 48 hours)
Surgical management	Surgical stabilization and instrumentation in spinal cord compression from cancer
	Immediate evacuation in spinal epidural hematoma
Other measures	Consider temporary pacemaker
	Consider atropine, 0.5 mg, or isoproterenol infusion, 2–10 μg per minute
	Abdominal binders and elastic leg wraps with upright position
	Consider midodrine (2.5–10 mg orally t.i.d.) for orthostatic hypotension
	Aggressive postural drainage, rotating beds
Access	Arterial catheter to monitor blood pressures (particularly if labile blood pressures)
	Peripheral venous catheter or Peripheral inserted central catheter

AC, assist control; DVT, deep vein thrombosis; GI, gastrointestinal; IMV, intermittent mandatory ventilation; IV, intravenously; NaCl, sodium chloride; SC, subcutaneously.

not contraindicated in patients after surgery for an acute epidural hematoma, and the claim that heparin increases the risk of recurrence after the operation is somewhat baseless. Aggressive pulmonary techniques and prevention are important to reduce the development of pulmonary complications, which substantially increase the length of hospital stay and costs.[10,40] Early tracheostomy is important in these patients.[29] Abdominal binders and leg wraps are needed when patients are placed in an upright position (Figure 36.7). Bradycardia associated with hypotension can be treated with 0.5 mg of atropine intravenously, a low-dose infusion of isoproterenol (2–10 μg per minute titrating to response), or a temporary pacemaker.[41] Neurogenic bladder is prone to become associated with asymptomatic bacteriuria, and renal failure may occur.[48] Antimicrobial therapy reduces its frequency, but not the frequency of symptomatic

infections and therefore is not recommended for prophylaxis.[33,47]

Priapism may be treated with intracorporal phenylephrine.[27]

Corticosteroids are indicated if an acute spinal cord lesion is due to a tumor, trauma, or demyelination. In patients with acute cord compression, 100 mg of dexamethasone intravenously is given immediately and is followed by 4–25 mg four times a day. A tapering of the high doses of corticosteroid is started after 3 days. We routinely administer proton pump inhibitors to patients receiving corticosteroids. Corticosteroids or plasma exchange has also been useful in patients with acute SCI due to exacerbation of multiple sclerosis. We reversed ventilatory dependence in one patient after use of high-dose corticosteroid treatment.[49]

In patients with traumatic SCI seen within 3 hours of injury, methylprednisolone 30 mg/kg IV

cervical spine injury with average total length of cooling time of about 100 hours. Catheter insertion for cooling may be delayed in patients under evaluation for abdominal or chest injuries, and injury to initiation of hypothermia time was on average 9 hours (3–33 hours); target temperature was achieved another 2 hours later.[12]

DETERIORATION: CAUSES AND MANAGEMENT

Deterioration in the NICU after surgical intervention is not very common. A fixed deficit or improvement in function is more commonly observed. However, in patients with significant spinal cord trauma, secondary deterioration may occur associated with postoperative edema, likely as a result of vasogenic edema (Figure 36.8). Such a clinical picture may also become apparent when there has been vertebral artery injury but then the deficit is fixed. Studies have found no proof of dexamethasone or mannitol, but a short course of corticosteroids is often administered. In some specific disorders, further deterioration is possible despite early resolution of signs and symptoms that prompted a conservative wait-and-see approach. In epidural hematoma, outcome is clearly linked to prompt intervention, and any delay reduces chances of later ambulation, adequate pain control, and bladder and bowel control.[2] Postoperative deterioration due to recurrence is rarely observed, and usually an epidurally placed drain prevents further accumulation of a sizable hematoma.

Necrotic myelopathy may be rapidly ascending without response to corticosteroids. Immunomodulating therapy, such as plasma exchange or intravenous immunoglobulin, may not be helpful but is used in these patients without much success. In some of these patients, it may be difficult to clearly distinguish between multiple sclerosis and necrotic myelopathy (considered a separate entity), and these aggressive modes of therapy are then considered.

Spinal epidural abscess may worsen insidiously despite aggressive antibiotic therapy and surgical drainage, all of which hinder recovery. Delay in early recognition—understandable because of the mimicking of infectious disease—possibly is partly to blame.[31] Rapid progression of signs in patients with spinal metastasis may be due to vertebral collapse, and some patients continue to worsen after radiotherapy. Indications for surgical decompression remain uncertain in these patients.

OUTCOME

Rehabilitation with hope of restoration of function has been organized and established and

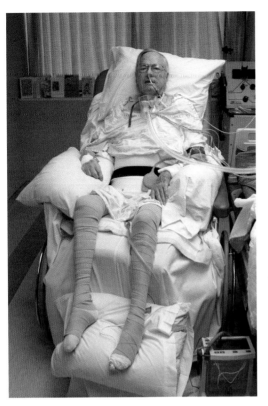

FIGURE 36.7: Patient with cervical cord lesion in a sitting position. Note abdominal binders and leg wraps.

over 30 minutes infusion is followed by infusion of 5.4 mg/kg/hr for 23 hours.[5,7,8] For patients seen between 3 and 8 hours, similar doses are given by intravenous bolus and infusion, but treatment is maintained for 48 hours. The design and results of the National Acute Spinal Cord Injury Study 2 and 3 trials have been criticized, and claims of success are not generally accepted.[8,55] One study found that gastrointestinal and pulmonary complications were higher with methylprednisolone (17% and 35%, respectively) compared with placebo (0% and 4%, respectively).[44]

Now many years later the evidence for methylprednisone use in traumatic spinal cord disorders remains questioned with variable practices throughout the world. Many spine surgeons and neurosurgeons do not feel these is enough benefit despite marked short-term motor score improvement if methylprednisolone is administered within eight hours of injury. Pooled evidence does not demonstrate a significant long-term benefit for methylprednisolone in patients with acute TSCIs and suggests it may be associated with increased gastrointestinal bleeding.[19]

Induced hypothermia (using invasive cooling device) has been used in 14 patients with acute

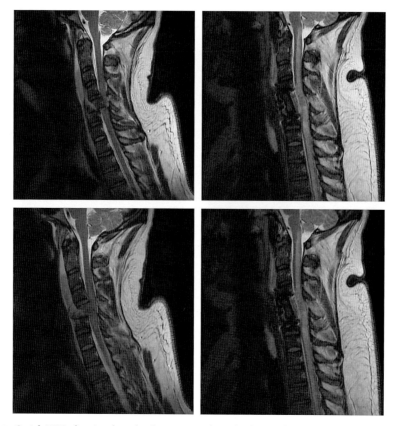

FIGURE 36.8: Serial MRI showing late developing spinal cord edema after instrumentation to treat cervical dislocation.

should start soon in the NICU.[57] Compelling data suggest that outcome (measured by paralysis) is better when patients with traumatic SCI are admitted to trauma centers. Regeneration of SCI is an active field of research (Capsule 36.1). The improved outcome can be attributed to the availability of early surgical decompression and is most evident in patients with American Spinal Injury Association (ASIA) scores of 4 or higher.[16] Acute complete loss of spinal cord function rarely results in significant improvement.[45,46] Impaired respiratory function in high cervical lesions is permanent, and long-term mechanical ventilation is needed. Ventilatory support may be needed in many patients with cervical or high-thoracic lesions, but improvement and weaning from the ventilator can be expected in lesions lower than C4 (estimated 50%–80% of patients).[14] Pulmonary function test results improve gradually and may increase to 60% of predicted values at 5 months. Weaning from the ventilator in patients with acute SCI may be predicted by needle electromyelogram of the diaphragm and pulmonary function tests but not fluoroscopic examination of the diaphragm

or phrenic nerve conduction studies. A PI_{max} of –40 cm H_2O and the presence of diaphragm motor recruitment predicted weaning in one small study.[14] Stiffening of the chest wall associated with spasticity of the abdominal and intercostal muscles reduces collapse with breathing, but also the diaphragm may condition itself to larger workloads of breathing.

Mortality in spinal cord infarction remains high (22%).[54] Some spinal cord disorders, such as epidural hematoma, have surprisingly good outcomes if surgical intervention is prompt. Relapse is uncommon after one bout of transverse myelitis, but studies found that 80% of patients with acute partial transverse myelitis had acquired definite multiple sclerosis within a 3-year follow-up period.[15,23] Our recent review of 115 patients with spinal cord infarcts found 23% mortality and 42% confined to a wheelchair. Worst outcome (no improvement and paraplegic) was found in patients who reached ASIA A or B. Most improvement was seen in 6 months, but gradual recovery over several years was noted in some. Presence of longitudinal extensive multilevel ischemic signal changes on MRI predicted poor outcome.[50] Pain

Within the first 2 hours of trauma to the spinal cord, swelling occurs with hemorrhages in the central gray matter. Surrounding white matter becomes injured due to vascular disruption. Microglial cells are activated with upregulation of proinflammatory cytokines and increase in excitotoxic glutamate. Secondary injury processes follow for up to 48 hours, with increased production of free radicals, ionic dysregulation (calcium), and receptors. There is marked increase in blood–brain barrier permeability. Neuronal inflammation may be the most important component of secondary injury. After 2 days, phagocytosis begins, and astrocytes proliferate and may restore some blood–brain barrier integrity. Therapies are directed to either replace oligodendrocytes or neurons or enhance axonal regeneration.[21,32,53] In mouse models, transplanted neural precursor cells may differentiate into oligodendrocytes and myelinate. Whether this translates to functional improvement is a crucial challenge. The mechanisms involved with regeneration are shown in the accompanying illustration.

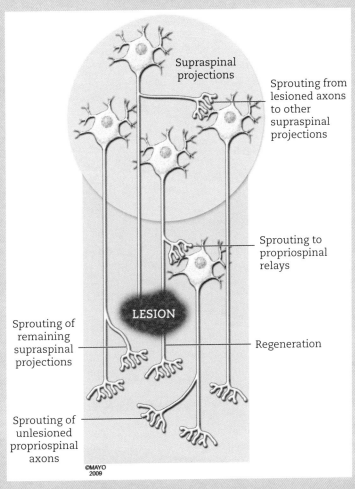

Several mechanisms can potentially contribute to spontaneous, or experimentally enhanced, plasticity after spinal cord injury. These include rapid responses (unmasking) in addition to delayed responses (sprouting). Delayed mechanisms include the following: (a) a lesioned supraspinal projection can sprout onto another unlesioned supraspinal projection and enhance descending activity; (b) a lesioned supraspinal axon can sprout onto a spinal interneuron, forming a novel intraspinal relay; (c) an unlesioned intraspinal neuron can undergo compensatory sprouting in response to loss of supraspinal inputs; (d) spared supraspinal axons can undergo compensatory collateral sprouting below a lesion; and (e) axons can be experimentally induced to undergo axonal regeneration through or around a lesion site.

Adapted from Blesh A, Tuszynski MH. Spinal cord injury: plasticity, regeneration and the challenge of translational drug development. *Trends Neurosci* 2009;32:41–47.

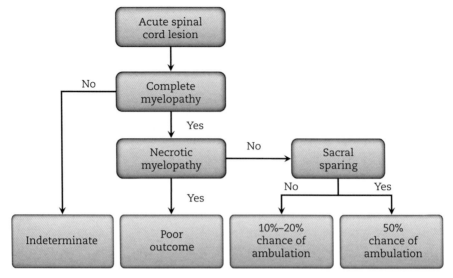

FIGURE 36.9: Algorithm of outcome in acute spinal cord disorder. Poor outcome: Severe disability or death; vegetative state. Indeterminate: Any statement would be a premature conclusion.

remained a major disabling sign that could disappear but also appear in the ensuing months.

Approximately 70% of patients with malignant spinal extradural compression remain or become mobile after surgical treatment. Radiotherapy is preferred in patients with known radiosensitive tumors. A short fractionated course, often with corticosteroids, is appropriate in most patients. Single-fraction therapy should be considered when the aim of treatment is palliation of pain only. Reirradiation in patients with recurrent spinal cord compression from cancer also preserves ambulation. In one study, ambulation was achieved in two-thirds of patients, but median survival was 4 months. Primary chemotherapy has been advocated for lymphoma, myeloma, and germ cell tumors, but in most patients is combined with radiotherapy.

Generally, outcome in acute SCI is difficult to judge, but sparing of pinprick sensation in the sacral area could predict improvement. It has been claimed that more than 50% of patients with sacral sensory sparing may have conversion from ASIA grade B to grade C–D.[45] Outcome in epidural abscess is much better than initially suspected with many patients improving to ASIA grade D.[37] An outcome algorithm is shown in Figure 36.9.

CONCLUSIONS

- Traumatic spine injury requires not only radiologic studies but also expert evaluation.
- Magnetic resonance imaging complements clinical localization and should be performed urgently.

- Respiratory compromise and severe bradycardia should be expected in patients with complete cervical lesions.
- Methylprednisolone may be effective in traumatic SCI if administration begins within 3 hours. An intravenous bolus of 30 mg/kg is followed by infusion of 5.4 mg/kg/hr for 23 hours.
- Plasma exchange should be considered in acute demyelinating disorders not responding to corticosteroids.
- Prompt neurosurgical intervention is generally indicated for acute epidural hematoma, spinal instability from trauma or cancer destruction, and removal of a foreign object.

REFERENCES

1. Agarwal NK, Mathur N. Deep vein thrombosis in acute spinal cord injury. *Spinal Cord* 2009;47:769–772.
2. Ananthababu PS, Anbuselvam M, Radhakrishnan MK. Spontaneous spinal epidural hematoma: report of two cases and review of the literature. *J Clin Neurosci* 2005;12:90–92.
3. Ball PA. Critical care of spinal cord injury. *Spine (Phila Pa 1976)* 2001;26:S27–30.
4. Berman M, Feldman S, Alter M, Zilber N, Kahana E. Acute transverse myelitis: incidence and etiologic considerations. *Neurology* 1981;31: 966–971.
5. Blight AR, Zimber MP. Acute spinal cord injury: pharmacotherapy and drug development perspectives. *Curr Opin Investig Drugs* 2001;2:801–808.

6. Botel U, Glaser E, Niedeggen A. The surgical treatment of acute spinal paralysed patients. *Spinal Cord* 1997;35:420–428.

7. Bracken MB. Methylprednisolone and spinal cord injury. *J Neurosurg* 2000;93:175–179.

8. Bracken MB, Shepard MJ, Holford TR, et al. Administration of methylprednisolone for 24 or 48 hours or tirilazad mesylate for 48 hours in the treatment of acute spinal cord injury: results of the Third National Acute Spinal Cord Injury Randomized Controlled Trial. National Acute Spinal Cord Injury Study. *JAMA* 1997;277:1597–1604.

9. Brambilla S, Ruosi C, La Maida GA, Caserta S. Prevention of venous thromboembolism in spinal surgery. *Eur Spine J* 2004;13:1–8.

10. Burns SP. Acute respiratory infections in persons with spinal cord injury. *Phys Med Rehabil Clin N Am* 2007;18:203–216, v–vi.

11. Byrne TN, Benzel EC, Waxman SG. *Diseases of the Spine and Spinal Cord.* New York: Oxford University Press; 2000.

12. Charles YP, Steib JP. Management of thoracolumbar spine fractures with neurologic disorder. *Orthop Traumatol Surg Res* 2015;101:S31–S40.

13. Cheshire WP, Santos CC, Massey EW, Howard JF, Jr. Spinal cord infarction: etiology and outcome. *Neurology* 1996;47:321–330.

14. Chiodo AE, Scelza W, Forchheimer M. Predictors of ventilator weaning in individuals with high cervical spinal cord injury. *J Spinal Cord Med* 2008;31:72–77.

15. Christensen PB, Wermuth L, Hinge HH, Bomers K. Clinical course and long-term prognosis of acute transverse myelopathy. *Acta Neurol Scand* 1990;81:431–435.

16. Curt A, Dietz V. Ambulatory capacity in spinal cord injury: significance of somatosensory evoked potentials and ASIA protocol in predicting outcome. *Arch Phys Med Rehabil* 1997;78:39–43.

17. de Seze J, Stojkovic T, Breteau G, et al. Acute myelopathies: clinical, laboratory and outcome profiles in 79 cases. *Brain* 2001;124:1509–1521.

18. Duffill J, Sparrow OC, Millar J, Barker CS. Can spontaneous spinal epidural haematoma be managed safely without operation? A report of four cases. *J Neurol Neurosurg Psychiatry* 2000;69:816–819.

19. Evaniew N, Belley-Côté EP, Fallah N, Noonan V, Rivers CS, Dvorak MF. Methylprednisolone for the treatment of patients with acute spinal cord injuries: A systematic review and meta-analysis. *J Neurotrauma* 2016, in press.

20. Fehlings MG, Tighe A. Spinal cord injury: the promise of translational research. *Neurosurg Focus* 2008;25:E1.

21. Fleming JC, Norenberg MD, Ramsay DA, et al. The cellular inflammatory response in human spinal cords after injury. *Brain* 2006;129:3249–3269.

22. Foo D. Operative treatment of spontaneous spinal epidural hematomas: a study of the factors determining postoperative outcome. *Neurosurgery* 1997;41:1218–1220.

23. Ford B, Tampieri D, Francis G. Long-term follow-up of acute partial transverse myelopathy. *Neurology* 1992;42:250–252.

24. Frisbie JH. Breathing and the support of blood pressure after spinal cord injury. *Spinal Cord* 2005;43:406–407.

25. Fukui MB, Swarnkar AS, Williams RL. Acute spontaneous spinal epidural hematomas. *AJNR Am J Neuroradiol* 1999;20:1365–1372.

26. Gallia GL, Sobotta MH. Images in clinical medicine: traumatic epidural hematoma. *N Engl J Med* 2009;360:615.

27. Gordon SA, Stage KH, Tansey KE, Lotan Y. Conservative management of priapism in acute spinal cord injury. *Urology* 2005;65:1195–1197.

28. Gotway MB, Mason RJ, Broaddus VC, Murray JF, Nadel JA. *Murray and Nadel's Textbook of Respiratory Medicine.* 4th ed. Philadelphia: W. B. Saunders; 2005.

29. Harrop JS, Sharan AD, Scheid EH, Jr., Vaccaro AR, Przybylski GJ. Tracheostomy placement in patients with complete cervical spinal cord injuries: American Spinal Injury Association Grade A. *J Neurosurg* 2004;100:20–23.

30. Henderson RD, Pittock SJ, Piepgras DG, Wijdicks EFM. Acute spontaneous spinal epidural hematoma. *Arch Neurol* 2001;58:1145–1146.

31. Holt T, Hoskin P, Maranzano E, et al. Malignant epidural spinal cord compression: the role of external beam radiotherapy. *Curr Opin Support Palliat Care* 2012;6:103–108.

32. Hurlbert RJ. Strategies of medical intervention in the management of acute spinal cord injury. *Spine (Phila Pa 1976)* 2006;31:S16–21.

33. Inatomi Y, Itoh Y, Fujii N, Nakanishi K. The spinal cord descending pathway for micturition: analysis in patients with spinal cord infarction. *J Neurol Sci* 1998;157:154–157.

34. Investigators SCIT. Prevention of venous thromboembolism in the acute treatment phase after spinal cord injury: a randomized, multicenter trial comparing low-dose heparin plus intermittent pneumatic compression with enoxaparin. *J Trauma* 2003;54:1116–1124.

35. Iseli E, Cavigelli A, Dietz V, Curt A. Prognosis and recovery in ischaemic and traumatic spinal cord injury: clinical and electrophysiological evaluation. *J Neurol Neurosurg Psychiatry* 1999;67:567–571.

36. Katz JD, Ropper AH. Progressive necrotic myelopathy: clinical course in 9 patients. *Arch Neurol* 2000;57:355–361.

37. Koo DW, Townson AF, Dvorak MF, Fisher CG. Spinal epidural abscess: a 5-year case-controlled review of neurologic outcomes after rehabilitation. *Arch Phys Med Rehabil* 2009;90:512–516.

38. Krassioukov A, Warburton DE, Teasell R, Eng JJ. A systematic review of the management of autonomic dysreflexia after spinal cord injury. *Arch Phys Med Rehabil* 2009;90:682–695.

39. Kwon BK, Tetzlaff W, Grauer JN, Beiner J, Vaccaro AR. Pathophysiology and pharmacologic treatment of acute spinal cord injury. *Spine J* 2004;4:451–464.

40. Ledsome JR, Sharp JM. Pulmonary function in acute cervical cord injury. *Am Rev Respir Dis* 1981;124:41–44.

41. Lehmann KG, Lane JG, Piepmeier JM, Batsford WP. Cardiovascular abnormalities accompanying acute spinal cord injury in humans: incidence, time course and severity. *J Am Coll Cardiol* 1987;10:46–52.

42. Levi AD, Green BA, Wang MY, et al. Clinical application of modest hypothermia after spinal cord injury. *J Neurotrauma* 2009;26:407–415.

43. Macias CA, Rosengart MR, Puyana JC, et al. The effects of trauma center care, admission volume, and surgical volume on paralysis after traumatic spinal cord injury. *Ann Surg* 2009;249:10–17.

44. Matsumoto T, Tamaki T, Kawakami M, et al. Early complications of high-dose methylprednisolone sodium succinate treatment in the follow-up of acute cervical spinal cord injury. *Spine (Phila Pa 1976)* 2001;26:426–430.

45. McDonald JW, Sadowsky C. Spinal-cord injury. *Lancet* 2002;359:417–425.

46. McKinley WO, Seel RT, Gadi RK, Tewksbury MA. Nontraumatic vs. traumatic spinal cord injury: a rehabilitation outcome comparison. *Am J Phys Med Rehabil* 2001;80:693–699.

47. Morton SC, Shekelle PG, Adams JL, et al. Antimicrobial prophylaxis for urinary tract infection in persons with spinal cord dysfunction. *Arch Phys Med Rehabil* 2002;83:129–138.

48. Pettersson-Hammerstad K, Jonsson O, Svennung IB, Karlsson AK. Impaired renal function in newly spinal cord injured patients improves in the chronic state: effect of clean intermittent catheterization? *J Urol* 2008;180:187–191.

49. Pittock SJ, Rodriguez M, Wijdicks EFM. Rapid weaning from mechanical ventilator in acute cervical cord multiple sclerosis lesion after steroids. *Anesth Analg* 2001;93:1550–1551, table of contents.

50. Robertson CE, Brown RD, Jr, Wijdicks EFM, Rabinstein AA. Recovery after spinal cord infarcts: long-term outcome in 115 patients. *Neurology* 2012;78:114–121.

51. Ropper AH, Poskanzer DC. The prognosis of acute and subacute transverse myelopathy based on early signs and symptoms. *Ann Neurol* 1978;4:51–59.

52. Roth EJ, Lu A, Primack S, et al. Ventilatory function in cervical and high thoracic spinal cord injury: relationship to level of injury and tone. *Am J Phys Med Rehabil* 1997;76:262–267.

53. Rowland JW, Hawryluk GW, Kwon B, Fehlings MG. Current status of acute spinal cord injury pathophysiology and emerging therapies: promise on the horizon. *Neurosurg Focus* 2008;25:E2.

54. Salvador de la Barrera S, Barca-Buyo A, Montoto-Marques A, et al. Spinal cord infarction: prognosis and recovery in a series of 36 patients. *Spinal Cord* 2001;39:520–525.

55. Simnad VI, Pisani DE, Rose JW. Multiple sclerosis presenting as transverse myelopathy: clinical and MRI features. *Neurology* 1997;48:65–73.

56. Srivastava S, Sanghavi NG. Non traumatic paraparesis: aetiological, clinical and radiological profile. *J Assoc Physicians India* 2000;48:988–990.

57. Stampas A, Tansey KE. Spinal cord injury medicine and rehabilitation. *Semin Neurol* 2014;34:524–533.

58. Taoka T, Mayr NA, Lee HJ, et al. Factors influencing visualization of vertebral metastases on MR imaging versus bone scintigraphy. *AJR Am J Roentgenol* 2001;176:1525–1530.

59. Thiele RH, Hage ZA, Surdell DL, et al. Spontaneous spinal epidural hematoma of unknown etiology: case report and literature review. *Neurocrit Care* 2008;9:242–246.

60. Vale FL, Burns J, Jackson AB, Hadley MN. Combined medical and surgical treatment after acute spinal cord injury: results of a prospective pilot study to assess the merits of aggressive medical resuscitation and blood pressure management. *J Neurosurg* 1997;87:239–246.

61. Wijdicks EFM. *Neurologic Complications of Critical Illness*. 3rd ed. Oxford: Oxford University Press; 2009.

62. Wiley CA, VanPatten PD, Carpenter PM, Powell HC, Thal LJ. Acute ascending necrotizing myelopathy caused by herpes simplex virus type 2. *Neurology* 1987;37:1791–1794.

63. Wingerchuk DM, Lennon VA, Lucchinetti CF, Pittock SJ, Weinshenker BG. The spectrum of neuromyelitis optica. *Lancet Neurol* 2007;6:805–815.

64. Winslow C, Rozovsky J. Effect of spinal cord injury on the respiratory system. *Am J Phys Med Rehabil* 2003;82:803–814.

65. Wittenberg RH, Boetel U, Beyer HK. Magnetic resonance imaging and computer tomography of acute spinal cord trauma. *Clin Orthop Relat Res* 1990:176–185.

37

Acute White Matter Disorders

Acute white matter disorders are fulmi-nant multiple sclerosis (MS), transverse myelitis, and disseminated encephalomyelitis. These disorders are sporadically seen, even in referral centers. A related disorder, often with an acute onset, is acute leukoencephalopathy, occur-ring in a diverse group of patients. In this entity, edema rather than demyelination is part of a more global involvement of white matter structures. Toxicity from immunosuppressive and chemo-therapeutic agents is commonly implicated, or a persistent surge in blood pressure may touch off damage to the blood brain barrier and seepage of plasma in the white matter. These disorders may resolve after elimination of the trigger alone.

Generally, the morbidity with acute white matter disorders is substantial. Aggressive immu-nosuppression or plasma exchange may, in cer-tain disorders, resolve most of the manifestations or shorten the relapse. In some situations, acute demyelination of the neuraxis may be ultimately catastrophic. This chapter discusses the more pro-gressive fulminant forms that will require close observation and management in the neurosci-ences intensive care unit (NICU).

CLINICAL RECOGNITION

One of the most recognizable disorders is acute disseminated encephalomyelitis (ADEM), and this dramatic monophasic illness results from an autoimmune response activated by a viral infec-tion or vaccination.[52,56,57,61] Pathologic features of ADEM include multifocal patchy perivenous demyelination.

ADEM occurs more often in children and young adults, and most infections are mundane viral respiratory episodes.[5] ADEM may also follow any well-defined illness (e.g., rubeola, varicella, mycoplasmal pneumonia, infectious mononucle-osis, and hepatitis C), or may occur without an identifiable antecedent event.[13,56] Even in the most severe fatal cases, use of polymerase chain reac-tion analysis to recover a virus (e.g., enterovirus, adenovirus, herpesvirus, and respiratory syncytial virus) from the cerebrospinal fluid or from the brain during autopsy has not been successful.

Neurologic manifestation may occur sev-eral weeks after the infection or vaccination but progresses rapidly to a maximum within days.[45] Widespread involvement of the central nervous system (CNS) may affect many eloquent areas of the brain and cord. White matter destruction involving the optic tract, brainstem, and spinal cord is a classic finding if the disorder progresses. ADEM may preferentially involve the brainstem.[60]

The clinical presentation is fairly charac-teristic, and consulted family members recall a flu-like illness with a variable combination of fever and complaints of aching joints and fatigue. Some of these constitutional symptoms may still be present at onset. Initially, head-aches with transient focal neurologic signs may be prominent and fluctuating. Neurologic find-ings further reflect acute myelin destruction and may consist of any degree of impairment of consciousness, with several prompts needed to alert patients to their surroundings. In others, ophthalmoplegia, cerebellar ataxia, and speech abnormality may evolve to muteness.

Spinal cord involvement may be the first pre-senting symptom, or may quickly merge into a more diffuse or multifocal neurologic symptom complex. Progressive quadriparesis may result in early inability to walk, but level of conscious-ness should also become involved at this time. Progression is within days, but a clinical course with up to 2 months of gradual, protracted change has been documented.

ADEM can be mistaken for CNS lymphoma, vasculitis, viral encephalitis, paraneoplastic encephalopathy,[40] and manifestations of flaring up of rheumatologic disorders, some of which were not previously known[19] (Table 37.1). Equally important we have diagnosed ADEM on repeat MRI in patients who were transferred to us with "worsening encephalitis".

Fulminant MS is another rare but occasion-ally encountered disorder. Patients with clinically

TABLE 37.1. DISORDERS MIMICKING ACUTE DISSEMINATED ENCEPHALOMYELITIS

Acute viral encephalitis (arboviruses)
Herpes simplex encephalitis
Central nervous system vasculitis
Gliomatosis cerebri
Intravascular lymphoma
Progressive multifocal leukoencephalopathy
Neurosarcoidosis
Systemic lupus erythematosus
Sjögren disease

TABLE 37.2. CAUSES OF ACUTE TRANSVERSE MYELITIS

Echovirus
Varicella
Herpes zoster
Herpes simplex virus (HSV1, HSV2)
Influenza
Epstein-Barr virus
Cytomegalovirus
Mycoplasma
Parasites (e.g., schistosomiasis)
Vaccination
Multiple sclerosis
Lupus erythematosus
Sjögren disease
Syphilis
Lyme disease

definitive or laboratory-supported MS may have very severe exacerbations, but progression to a devastating condition or death rarely is the first presentation. The designation "fulminant" in this condition is usually defined by symptoms and signs emerging in days, rather than weeks, and presupposes involvement of multiple areas in the cerebral white matter and often the brainstem.[24,29,36,44] A brain biopsy, usually performed to characterize the source of a new mass, shows fairly typical neuropathologic features of marked inflammatory perivascular infiltrates, extensive myelin breakdown that spares the nerve cell bodies and axis cylinders, and diffuse macrophage infiltration.[16,36]

Earlier descriptions of this fulminant variant emphasized an accelerated development of ataxia, hemiparesis, or paraparesis; blindness or progressive ophthalmoplegia. Brainstem involvement is a common feature in acute fulminant MS, with notable bulbar involvement leading to dysphagia and aspiration.[24,29,44] Quadriparesis and involvement of the lower cranial nerves with sparing of only the oculomotor nerves closely resemble a locked-in syndrome and often are linked to a fatal outcome.[7,15]

The most dramatic form of MS, one with high mortality, is the Marburg variant.[24] Within days, progressive ophthalmoplegia, dysarthria, dysphagia, and blindness may develop, and the patient becomes comatose. Rapid brainstem displacement may appear when a large inflammatory demyelinating tumefactive lesion shifts brain tissue.

Acute white matter disorders can preferentially involve the spinal cord.[48] Acute transverse myelitis is an uncommon, potentially devastating disorder associated with many illnesses[27] (Table 37.2). Diagnostic criteria for idiopathic transverse myelitis have been published.[14,19] It is not a likely consideration if there had been prior

radiation to the spine within the last 10 years, evidence of connective tissue disease, or a variety of infectious agents. Its pathogenesis is attributed to a vigorously mounted immune response. Demyelination and inflammation involve the spinal cord at any level, but often the effects are limited to a few segments. However, patients presenting with acute paraparesis and a distinct sensory level more commonly have extramedullary cord compression or another cause of myelitis[53,55] (Chapters 9 and 34).

Rapid ascending sensory deficit and difficulty walking within days are hallmarks of the disorder. Fever and nuchal rigidity may occur in 27% and 13% of patients, respectively.[9,14,19] Paresthesias may be widespread, but usually a sensory level below which sensation is abnormal is pointed out by the patient. Motor weakness may vary substantially, with a maximum deficit usually within 1–2 days, although subacute progression up to 2 months is known. However, maximal motor deficit may be reached within several hours. The neurologic findings are typical of a functional spinal cord transection at one segment, with loss of motor and sensory function and areflexia. All spinal cord levels can become involved. Partial variants have been described, with incomplete involvement, patchy and dissociated sensory symptoms, and sparing of the bladder.

Several acute leukoencephalopathies in adults have been described. Chronic, protracted leukoencephalopathies consist of a very wide array of disorders, including aminoacidopathy, organic acid disorders, and lysosomal storage disease. Selective white matter damage with acute forms has become more apparent with the introduction of immunosuppressive agents and chemotherapeutic agents. These lipophilic substances preferentially target myelin because of its high lipid content. Magnetic resonance imaging (MRI) predominance in the bilateral parieto-occipital hemispheric regions justifies the term posterior leukoencephalopathy.[6,21,22,31,43] The term posterior reversible encephalopathy syndrome (PRES) has been suggested, connoting a relationship with changes in blood pressure.

Decreases in level of consciousness and marked cognitive decline, but also behavioral changes alone, may be presenting symptoms of acute leukoencephalitis.[27,35] Headache is prominent. Seizures are prevalent, mostly generalized tonic-clonic, but focal onset has been noted. The disorder may progress rapidly to cortical blindness, marked ataxia, and speech or language abnormalities. Akinetic mutism may occur if the disorder is not recognized in the earlier stages of presentation. Akinetic mutism (summarized by neurosurgeon Cairns as "motionless, mindless wakefulness") can be explained by extensive involvement of the thalamofrontal fibers and, in particular, disconnection from the anterior cingulate cortex.

Immunosuppressive agents (cyclosporine and tacrolimus) in transplantation recipients have been used in many well-documented cases of acute leukoencephalopathy. Breakdown of the blood–brain barrier or facilitated transport is required for these immunosuppressive drugs to enter the brain.[6] Cyclosporine or tacrolimus may have a direct damaging effect on the vasculature, leading to microvascular damage and access to the brain.

Tremors, vivid visual hallucinations, and behavioral changes with paranoid behavior and wide mood swings are common and are associated with rambling, nonsensible speech. Commonly, the speech disorder is characterized by stuttering when words are spoken rapidly or even at a normal pace, but there is normal speech output when the patient is instructed to speak slowly. Speech may be distorted, with similarity to a foreign accent, and a single, generalized tonic-clonic seizure may be the only clue to toxicity. Less common presentations are blindness, cerebellar syndrome, orofacial dyskinesias, and mutism. Presentation is similar in tacrolimus and cyclosporine neurotoxicity: less severe signs and symptoms regress rapidly after discontinuation but may recur after substitution of another immunosuppressive agent is substituted. With the oral microemulsion of cyclosporine (Neoral), neurotoxicity is less severe, mostly tremor and headache only. There are no reports of neurotoxicity with sirolimus (the term suggests a pharmacologic similarity with tacrolimus; however, even though receptor linkage is similar, the two agents differ in their target).[38,63]

Another well identified leukoencephalopathy has been associated with chemotherapeutic agents, predominantly 5-fluorouracil and levamisole. The estimated incidence of this toxic leukoencephalopathy is low.[59]

The lesions are more confluent and multifocal when tissue is examined. Perivascular lymphocytic inflammation is found next to demyelination. A more delayed manifestation, often with seizures, has been reported with chemotherapeutic agents. In these patients, a history of insidious decline in intellectual function is obtained, together with clinical evidence of a progressive disorder characterized by spasticity and bulbar palsy. Its clinical presentation can be nothing more specific than depression and withdrawal, sometimes mistaken for a psychological response to the diagnosis of cancer. Ataxia, impaired thinking, slurring of speech, and memory impairment follow, and profound stupor or coma may ensue. The predominant trigger of neurotoxicity is 5-fluorouracil, but toxicity with levamisole alone has been reported.

Methotrexate is used intravenously, intrathecally, and orally. All of these modes of administration may be associated with toxic damage to the white matter. Methotrexate barely crosses the blood–brain barrier because it is an ionized and lipid-insoluble compound, but prior radiation-induced damage to the integrity of the blood–brain barrier may facilitate its transport. Intra-arterially administered nimustine (ACNU) has produced leukoencephalopathy in the treatment of glioma. However, combined use of radiation and chemotherapy may complicate finding a precise cause-and-effect relationship. It may occur without prior radiation.

In the management of leukemia, three recognized chemotherapy-associated leukoencephalopathy syndromes have been described: (1) an acute syndrome within 24 hours after intrathecal administration of methotrexate, cranial irradiation, or use of cytarabine, resulting in an acute confusional state, cerebellar symptoms, and seizures resolving in 2–3 days; (2) subacute leukoencephalopathy 1–2 weeks after intravenous administration of methotrexate, with focal motor neurologic signs, behavioral changes, and seizures; and (3) insidious leukoencephalopathy progressing over months, with personality changes, marked intellectual decline, and spasticity.[59]

TABLE 37.3. ACUTE
LEUKOENCEPHALOPATHY IN ADULTS

Immunosuppressive agents (cyclosporine,
  tacrolimus)

Hypertensive crisis

Eclampsia, HELLP syndrome

Chemotherapeutic agents (methotrexate, 5-
  fluorouracil, levamisole, intra-arterial nimustine
  [ACNU])

Fulminant multiple sclerosis

Postradiation

Human immunodeficiency virus

Erythropoietin

Interferon-α

Ecstasy

Bath salts

Heroin inhalation

Progressive multifocal leukoencephalopathy

ACNU, 1-(4-amino-2-methyl-5-pyrimidinyl)-methyl-(2-chloroethyl)-
3-nitrosourea; HELLP, hemolysis, elevated liver enzymes, and low
platelet count
Data extracted from Filley CM, Kleinschmidt-deMasters BK. Toxic
encephalopathy. *N Engl J Med* 2001;345:425–432. With permission
of the publisher.

Leukoencephalopathy may occur after heroin abuse, particularly after inhalation of heroin vapor ("chasing the dragon"). Progression from cerebellar symptoms to extrapyramidal involvement to spasticity to persistent coma is due to involvement of both cerebral hemispheres, the cerebellar peduncles, and the midbrain.[18,41] We have seen a fatal toxic leukoencephalopathy after bath salt inhalation, presenting with acute liver failure and massive rhabdomyolysis.[32]

Anecdotal reports of acute leukoencephalopathy with erythropoietin, amphotericin, and interferon have appeared. Eclampsia may cause headache, seizures, cortical blindness, and papilledema and may produce a similar reversible posterior leukoencephalopathy syndrome. It remains important to exclude multifocal leukoencephalopathy associated with human immunodeficiency virus (HIV) and progressive multifocal leukoencephalopathy associated with JC virus by examination of cerebrospinal fluid (CSF),[23,33] polymerase chain reaction, or brain biopsy. Causes are summarized in Table 37.3.

NEUROIMAGING AND LABORATORY TESTS

Computed tomographic (CT) and MRI findings are fairly typical but may be rather subtle in earlier stages.[4] The typical appearance in ADEM is multiple discrete lesions in the cerebral white matter and rarely in periventricular areas, a location much more typical of fulminant MS.[37] The lesions predominate in occipital-parietal white matter, but may involve the basal ganglia, thalamus, and brainstem[28] (Figure 37.1). Symmetrical cerebellar white matter and basal ganglia involvement may differentiate it from MS.[10,11] All of these abnormalities may hardly be detected by CT, and only some decreased attenuation in the white matter of the centrum semiovale is seen, even at the stage of prominent neurologic manifestations. Magnetic resonance imaging remains a crucial determinant for its diagnosis, and more advanced techniques are developed to follow pathologic changes.[2,3,58] Gadolinium enhancement is a reflection of the blood–brain barrier breakdown in the earlier stages of demyelination. Enhancement may appear in some lesions on MRI and not in others, suggesting different stages in demyelination. Enhancement may be marginal because of corticosteroid treatment, which reduces the blood–brain barrier permeability. If enhancement is found, abnormal signal intensity is more commonly found in the optic nerves (as opposed to unilateral optic neuritis in MS). Generally, these MRI features cannot be easily differentiated from those of MS, nor has a more distinct histologic feature been identified in brain tissue specimens.

Hemorrhagic changes suggest an acute hemorrhagic leukoencephalitis (Weston-Hurst disease); and this disorder, noted after similar triggering circumstances, may primarily be an aggressive variant of ADEM.[17,50] Not infrequently, it presents with massive brain edema. Hyperintense lesions on T2-weighted images, with ringlike solid enhancing lesions and perifocal edema, have been reported as well (Figure 37.1). Cortical involvement is compatible with the diagnosis, albeit less extensively distributed. A single bout in the brainstem has been reported,[1] and pathologic lesions may show predominant perivascular inflammation and hemorrhage without evidence of demyelination (Figure 37.2).

Magnetic resonance imaging assists in the diagnosis of fulminant MS, but findings are nonspecific.[8] Magnetic resonance imaging suggests demyelination when lesions are hypointense or isointense on T1-weighted images, occasionally display hyperintense edges, and are small, irregular, or confluent. White matter lesions are invariably located in the pons, medulla, additional hemispheric areas involving the junctions of gray and white matter, and corpus callosum (Figure 37.3). Larger confluent areas in periventricular white

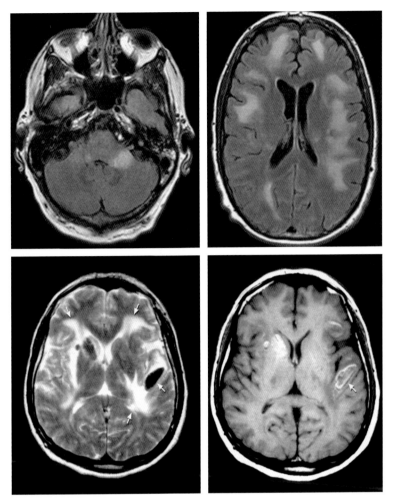

FIGURE 37.1: Different patterns of severity in acute disseminated encephalomyelitis. *Upper row*: Magnetic resonance imaging acute disseminated encephalomyelitis with cerebellar location. *Middle row*: Magnetic resonance imaging with coronal views showing severe involvement in acute disseminated encephalomyelitis (ADEM). *Lower row*: Hemorrhagic component (*arrows*) to severe acute disseminated encephalomyelitis (Weston-Hurst type).

matter can be seen as well. Ovoid lesions at right angles to the ventricular surface are characteristic. Unilateral mass effect with developing edema may occur. Mass effect may be the most prominent CT scan manifestation (Figure 37.4). Ring-like structures may appear, corresponding to layers of macrophages, which generate free radicals to produce this paramagnetic effect.

Magnetic resonance imaging is essential in acute transverse myelitis, to exclude potentially reversible causes. The rarity of the disorder implies that other causes of paraplegia are more frequent in clinical practice. Magnetic resonance imaging should be performed at once and, if necessary, patients should be referred to a tertiary center. Magnetic resonance imaging findings are

swelling of the cord, increased T2-weighted signal, and often abnormal enhancement throughout the cord.[8] More extensive involvement may be found on MRI than is clinically evident, and vice versa (Figure 37.5). Magnetic resonance imaging of the brain and visual evoked potentials are useful to demonstrate other demyelinating lesions that increase the probability of MS or Devic disease, with acute transverse myelitis as the first defining lesion.[64]

Routine MRI sequences, gadolinium enhancement, and, if available, diffusion-weighted imaging may further delineate the white matter lesion. Restricted diffusion on diffusion-weighted MRI may support cytotoxic edema, which indicates ischemia and is associated with reduced ADC

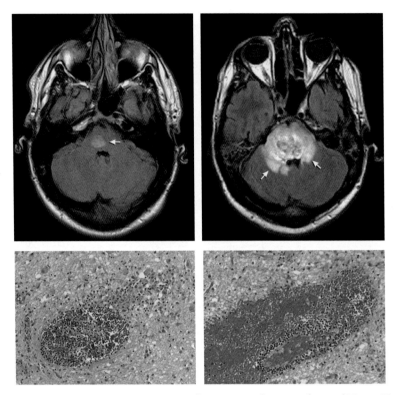

FIGURE 37.2: *Upper row*: Magnetic resonance imaging demonstrating brainstem lesions (Weston-Hurst) disease at presentation and at 2 weeks progression with early hemorrhage. Axial T2 without gadolinium shows extension of the lesion with marked edema and hemorrhage. *Lower row*: Pathology of brainstem shows hemorrhage and necrosis and on microscopy perivascular inflammation with hemorrhage.

From Abou Zeid NE, Burns JD, Wijdicks EFM, et al. Atypical acute hemorrhagic leukoencephalitis (Hurst's disease) presenting with focal hemorrhagic brainstem lesion. *Neurocrit Care* 2010;12:95–97. Used with permission.

values. The extensive lesions are nonspecific, but some MRI characteristics may point to a certain cause. These are sparing of the U fibers (cytomegalovirus and HIV encephalopathy); capping of the lateral ventricles, centrum semiovale, and corpus callosum (MS); additional gray matter involvement (CNS vasculitis, organic acidurias, postanoxic ischemic encephalopathies, including carbon monoxide and cyanide); enhancement with gadolinium (ADEM, MS, Alexander disease, Schilder diffuse sclerosis); and sparing of the basal ganglia (lysosomal disorders, including sphingolipidosis). Most patients with mild forms of cyclosporine or tacrolimus neurotoxicity do not have MRI abnormalities, which are typically seen in the most severe instances, often in patients with seizures at presentation. Progressive multifocal leukoencephalopathy may mimic these disorders. Little or no mass effect or gadolinium enhancement is noted. The lesions are in focal areas of the gray–white junction. Several examples of these acute leukoencephalopathies are shown in Figures 37.6–37.10.

Cerebrospinal fluid may show moderate pleocytosis (up to 200 cells/mm^3). In ADEM, the CSF contains lymphocytes; in Weston-Hurst disease, polymorphonuclear leukocytes are prominent. The pleocytosis is usually out of proportion to what is expected during a flare-up of MS. Oligoclonal bands can be found in up to 50% of cases and may disappear after treatment (oligoclonal bands commonly persist in MS).[42]

The diagnostic criteria of MS, including laboratory abnormalities, have been expertly outlined.[47] A modification of the Poser criteria is shown in Capsule 37.1.

In MS, evoked potential studies may detect asymptomatic lesions. Pattern reversal visual evoked potential is sensitive for lesions in the optic nerve and chiasm, and findings are abnormal in 40%–60% of patients with early MS.[34] The sensitivity in median nerve somatosensory evoked potentials is similar. Brainstem auditory evoked potentials are less sensitive and positive in only 20%–25% of patients with MS.

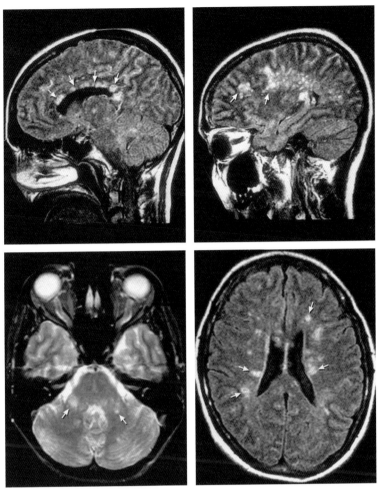

FIGURE 37.3: MRI of fulminant multiple sclerosis with multiple periventricular white matter lesions and characteristic scattered lesions in the corpus callosum and brainstem.

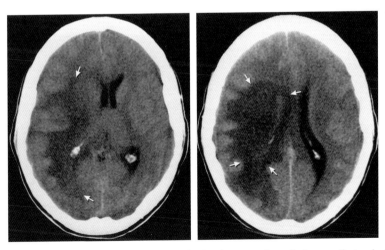

FIGURE 37.4: CT scan showing Marburg variant of multiple sclerosis with marked mass effect and edema (*arrows*).

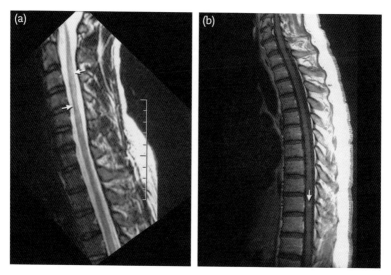

FIGURE 37.5: Acute transverse myelitis (magnetic resonance images, sagittal view). (a) Long segment of T2 signal in cervical cord. (b) Subtle enhancing thoracic cord abnormality. Both patients had complete spinal cord lesions on examination.

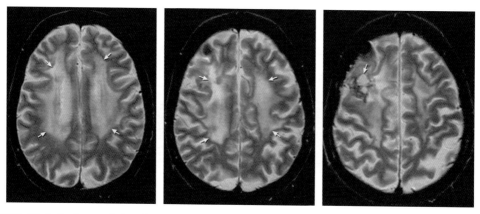

FIGURE 37.6: Leukoencephalopathy. Magnetic resonance images demonstrate radiation leukoencephalopathy (radiation for glioma) (*arrows*).

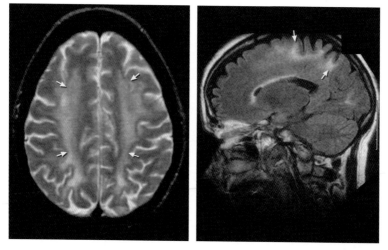

FIGURE 37.7: Methotrexate leukoencephalopathy as shown on axial T2-weighted and sagittal fluid-attenuated inversion recovery magnetic resonance imaging (similar findings are seen with 5-fluorouracil and levamisole).

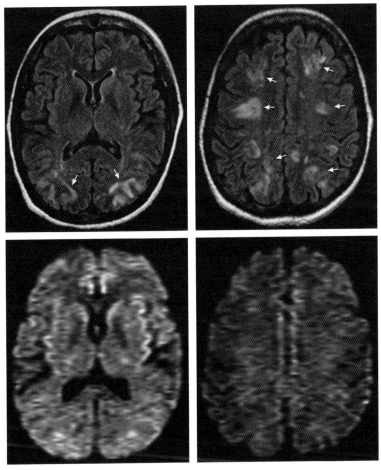

FIGURE 37.8: Cyclosporine-associated leukoencephalopathy. Multiple areas of involvement but normal diffusion-weighted imaging suggest edema.

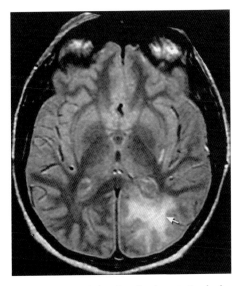

FIGURE 37.9: MRI showing focal posterior leukoencephalopathy due to progressive multifocal leukoencephalopathy (*arrow*).

Evoked potentials probably are most useful for providing supportive laboratory evidence of MS when additional diagnostic tests are abnormal.

Cell count can vary from 10–50 lymphocytes/mm³, with a mixture of monocytes, plasma cells, and macrophages. Total protein is mildly increased, and immunoglobulin G (IgG) is increased in 70% of clinically definite MS. Two or more oligoclonal bands in the gamma field may be detected in only 40% of patients with first presentation of MS. Intrathecal immunoglobulin in the CSF is a result of increased plasma cell synthesis and leakage from the brain through a defective blood–brain barrier. Oligoclonal bands in the CSF (at least two different and distinct bands) but not in the serum are typical for MS but can occur in 8% of patients with other neurologic diseases that may superficially mimic MS (viral meningoencephalitis, neurosyphilis, sarcoidosis, and fungal meningitis). The sensitivity of oligoclonal bands in CSF for MS is more than 90%.

In acute transverse myelitis, CSF examination may show pleocytosis of up to 10,000 cells

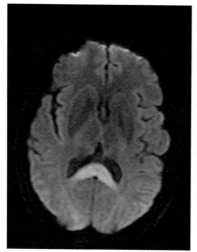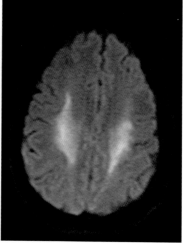

FIGURE 37.10: Bath salt inhalation causing restricted diffusion in splenium and corona radiata.

(both lymphocytes and polymorphonuclear leukocytes), but CSF cell count can be almost normal. Cerebrospinal fluid protein is commonly increased (in more than three-fourths of patients) and may reach values as high as 500 mg/dL.

Transverse myelitis needs to be differentiated from neuromyelitis optica—an autoimmune disorder—that may present with recurrent optic neuritis but also recurrent transverse myelitis as part of what is now recognized as NMO spectrum disorder. NMO lesions may involve hypothalamus, corpus callosum, brainstem, or periventricular, and may have antiaquaporin-4-IgG antibodies. This distinction is important because long-term immunosuppression is needed.[30,46] Viral serology may be useful because well-known viruses may cause acute transverse myelitis.

Cerebrospinal fluid examination is useful to obtain material for detecting the JC virus, and the test has 100% specificity in immunosuppressed patients after transplantation. Oligoclonal bands and IgG index are not diagnostic and can be seen in many demyelinating disorders.

Finally, in toxic leukoencephalopathies the correlation of cyclosporine and tacrolimus with blood or plasma levels is unreliable, and in some patients progression may occur despite declining blood levels. In only 30%–40% of reported cases, trough plasma levels are increased or show a significant upward trend. Plasma levels of these

---

CAPSULE 37.1   DIAGNOSTIC CLINICAL AND LABORATORY CRITERIA FOR MULTIPLE SCLEROSIS

Category	Subcategory	No. of Clinical Attacks	Clinically Evident Lesions	Paraclinical Evidence*	No. of CSF Oligoclonal Bands
CDMS	A1	2	2	N/A	N/A
	A2	2	1	and 1 (or more)	N/A
	A3	1	1	2†	N/A
LSDMS	B1	2	1	or 1 (or more)	+
	B2	1	2		+
	B3	1	1	and 1 (or more)	+

CDMS, clinically definite multiple sclerosis; CSF, cerebrospinal fluid; LSDMS, laboratory-supported definite multiple sclerosis; N/A, not applicable; +, present.
* Implies magnetic resonance imaging, evoked potentials, or CSF.
† A diagnosis of CDMS A3 requires paraclinical evidence for dissemination over time.
In DW Paty, GC Ebers, eds., *Multiple Sclerosis. Contemporary Neurology Series* Philadelphia: FA Davis, 1998, p. 48. With permission of Oxford University Press.

immunosuppressive agents are more likely to be increased when leukoencephalopathy is demonstrated on MRI, but correlation remains poor.

FIRST STEPS IN MANAGEMENT

A brief period of observation in the NICU and support with mechanical ventilation may be needed, but many patients are soon able to protect their airway and ventilate normally.

Brain biopsy should be deferred until the effect of immunosuppressive therapy or plasma exchange has been evaluated. High-dose methylprednisolone (1 g/day IV for 5 consecutive days) remains the first therapy of choice for many acute white matter disorders (Table 37.4).[62] Excellent recovery has also been observed with plasma exchange, and failure to improve rapidly (arbitrarily defined as 1–2 days) with corticosteroids should prompt its use. The exact number of plasma exchanges is unknown, although exchanges for up to 10 days (or until improvement) have been proposed.[26,39,49] Alternatively, intravenous immunoglobulin, 0.4 g/kg for 5 days, can be used,[20,51] again, typically in patients who have been worsening while receiving methylprednisolone.

Early aspiration pneumonia, fever, or major oropharyngeal involvement justifies admission to an NICU. Placement of an intracranial pressure device is warranted in the Marburg variant of MS,

to monitor clinical progression and treat increased intracranial pressure. Neurosurgical consultation for craniotomy or biopsy may be needed to pathologically confirm the diagnosis.

In fulminant MS, mechanical ventilation is often needed in patients whose condition deteriorates to coma and in patients with bulbar signs. Neurogenic pulmonary edema as a result of sympathetic disinhibition may accompany the fulminant form. In most patients, marked bulbar failure and an inability to swallow secretions lead to aspiration pneumonitis, and upper cervical or spinal cord involvement impairs pulmonary mechanics.

In any form of fulminant MS, intravenous administration of methylprednisolone 1 g/day for 3–5 days, is followed by 60 mg/day of prednisone. Tapering of oral prednisone should be completed in 14 days. Overall prognosis is not affected by corticosteroids.

Treatment of acute transverse myelitis with corticosteroids is controversial. No measurable effect has been reported, and with marked variability in recovery time, improvement cannot be attributed to this treatment without a formal clinical trial. Most physicians, however, still prefer a brief course with methylprednisolone. It is unknown whether specific antibiotic or antiviral therapy improves outcome. The AAN guideline advises that plasma exchange may be considered in patients with transverse myelitis

TABLE 37.4. INITIAL MANAGEMENT OF ACUTE WHITE MATTER DISORDERS

Airway management	Intubation if patient has hypoxemia despite facemask with 10 L of 100 oxygen/minute, if abnormal respiratory drive or presence of abnormal protective reflexes (likely with motor response of withdrawal, or worse)
Mechanical ventilation	IMV/PS or AC needed with high cervical cord lesions in acute transverse myelitis CPAP or PS mostly suffices for ADEM or acute leukoencephalopathies
Fluid management	2 L of 0.9% NaCl per 24 hours
Nutrition	Enteral nutrition with continuous infusion (on day 2) Blood glucose control (goal 140–180 mg/dL)
Prophylaxis	DVT prophylaxis with pneumatic compression devices SC heparin 5,000 U t.i.d. GI prophylaxis: Pantoprazole 40 mg IV daily or lansoprazole 30 mg orally through nasogastric tube
Other measures	IV methylprednisone 1 g/day for 3–5 days Series of plasma exchanges (7–10) or series of IV immunoglobulin 0.4 g/kg/day for 5 days Discontinue chemotherapy (if applicable) Substitute immunosuppression with sirolimus (if applicable)
Access	Peripheral venous catheter or peripheral inserted central catheter

AC, assist control; ADEM, acute disseminated encephalomyelitis; CPAP, continuous positive airway pressure; DVT, deep vein thrombosis; GI, gastrointestinal; IMV, intermittent mandatory ventilation; IV, intravenously; NaCl, sodium chloride; PS, pressure support; SC, subcutaneously.

who fail to improve after corticosteroid treatment. Rituximab may be considered in patients with transverse myelitis due to NMO antibodies to decrease the number of relapses. There is no evidence of effect using plasmapheresis and intravenous immunoglobulin.[54]

It is important to place an indwelling catheter in patients with minimal bladder reflex activity. Dysautonomia may occur alone from a distended bladder when the lesion is above the sympathetic outflow (T6), and any stimulus may produce severe hypertension. Prophylaxis for deep vein thrombosis (heparin 5,000 U subcutaneously t.i.d. or intermittent compression devices) should begin early.

In some forms of leukoencephalopathy, discontinuation of therapy with the causative drug may resolve most of the symptoms within 2 days. Cyclosporine or tacrolimus can be replaced by mycophenolate mofetil (CellCept) or sirolimus. Methylprednisolone (1 g/day for 3–5 days) has been administered intravenously in inflammatory leukoencephalopathies associated with chemotherapeutic agents, with a good result but no proof of its effect.

Suspicion of progressive multifocal leukoencephalopathy should be high in patients who have acquired immunodeficiency syndrome (AIDS) and in transplantation recipients. Treatment with cytarabine (2 mg/kg) should await biopsy determination. This drug may retard progression only for several months.

DETERIORATION: CAUSES AND MANAGEMENT

When acute treatment of multiple sclerosis with IV methylprednisolone fails, additional daily treatments can be considered, up to 7 days of 1,000 mg daily infusion (slow infusion over 90 minutes). Peak effect may take 15 days to achieve and, if not, should lead to plasma exchange (one exchange of 1.1 plasma volume units every other day over 14 days). IVIG has no role in acute treatment of MS.[25] If this approach fails after 2 weeks, alternative treatments are cyclophosphamide, alemtuzumab, and natalizumab. Current immunomodulatory treatments are shown in Table 37.5. Many immunosuppressive agents are unlikely to be started in the NICU and more often are considered in follow-up clinics.

OUTCOME

In ADEM, improved arousal can be rather rapid and is followed by improvement in diplopia, bulbar dysfunction, and, more gradually, ambulation. Residual symptoms may remain but are in

TABLE 37.5. THERAPY IN MULTIPLE SCLEROSIS

Tier 1 medication	interferon-B
	glatiramer acetate
	dimethyl fumarate
Tier 2 medication	fingolimod
	natalizumab
	cyclophosphamide
	mitoxantrone
Promising medication	daclizumab
	alemtuzumab
	rituximab

From Kantarci et al. Novel immunomodulatory approaches for the management of multiple sclerosis. *Clin Pharmacol Ther* 2014;95:32–44.

a minority disabling. Magnetic resonance image findings closely parallel clinical improvement. Full recovery after Weston-Hurst disease has been described in several cases. One study suggested that one of three patients with ADEM develops MS within 3 years; this included patients with well-established triggers such as infection or vaccination. This report also emphasized that the diagnosis of ADEM as a monophasic demyelinating disorder becomes likely only if the patient has remained asymptomatic for at least 1 year.[52]

Fulminant MS is associated with a high probability of permanent disability and with a somewhat shortened life span, strongly dependent on the degree of disability. Unfavorable prognostic factors are age over 40, male gender, and extensive MRI abnormalities (increased T2 lesion load and number of active enhancing lesions).[12] The relapse rate varies after a first major attack but decreases over time. After the first attack, approximately 25% of patients have a relapse within 1 year and 50% within 3 years. The extent of disability 5 years after the diagnosis strongly determines the future clinical course. Recovery may be protracted, lasting 3–4 weeks; and intercurrent infections may contribute to early mortality.

One-third of patients with acute transverse myelitis do not recover ambulation or bladder or bowel control. Partial recovery with a considerable handicap and good recovery each account for one-third of patients. Acute transverse myelitis has a much better prognosis if there is no progression to a complete cord syndrome and sensation remains preserved. Magnetic resonance image findings are not predictive of outcome. No correlation has been found with extent of the initial deficit, neurologic deficit and prognosis, and MRI findings.

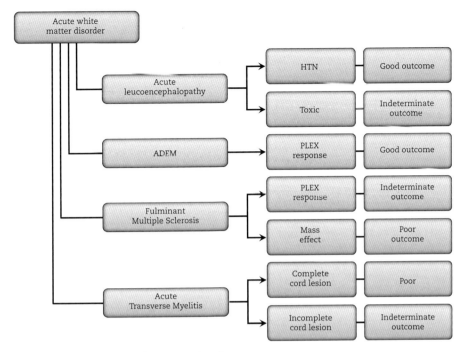

FIGURE 37.11: Outcome in acute white matter disorders.

ADEM, acute disseminated encephalomyelitis; HTN, hypertension; PLEX, plasma exchange.

The prognosis for recovery in drug-induced leukoencephalopathy is excellent, and both clinical resolution and MRI resolution are expected after cessation of the immunosuppressive and chemotherapeutic agents. Incomplete recovery, persistent vegetative state, or minimally conscious state has been noted, from illicit drug use. Outcome of white matter disorders is summarized in Figure 37.11.

CONCLUSIONS

- Progressive demyelinating disorders may need both plasma exchange and high-dose methylprednisolone to reduce morbidity.
- Acute transverse myelitis is likely not responsive to specific therapy.
- Mass effect from acute necrotic or demyelinating disease requires early ICP reduction and possible surgical evacuation.

REFERENCES

1. Abou Zeid NE, Burns JD, Wijdicks EFM, Giannini C, Keegan BM. Atypical acute hemorrhagic leukoencephalitis (Hurst's disease) presenting with focal hemorrhagic brainstem lesion. *Neurocrit Care* 2010;12:95–97.
2. Arnold DL. Evidence for neuroprotection and remyelination using imaging techniques. *Neurology* 2007;68:S83–90.
3. Arnold DL, Goodin DS. Magnetic resonance imaging as a surrogate for treatment effect on multiple sclerosis relapses. *Ann Neurol* 2009;65:237–238.
4. Atlas SW, Grossman RI, Goldberg HI, et al. MR diagnosis of acute disseminated encephalomyelitis. *J Comput Assist Tomogr* 1986;10:798–801.
5. Banwell B, Kennedy J, Sadovnick D, et al. Incidence of acquired demyelination of the CNS in Canadian children. *Neurology* 2009;72:232–239.
6. Bartynski WS. Posterior reversible encephalopathy syndrome, part 2: controversies surrounding pathophysiology of vasogenic edema. *AJNR Am J Neuroradiol* 2008;29:1043–1049.
7. Blunt SB, Boulton J, Wise R, Kennard C, Lewis PD. Locked-in syndrome in fulminant demyelinating disease. *J Neurol Neurosurg Psychiatry* 1994;57:504–505.
8. Bot JC, Barkhof F. Spinal-cord MRI in multiple sclerosis: conventional and nonconventional MR techniques. *Neuroimaging Clin N Am* 2009;19:81–99.
9. Bruna J, Martinez-Yelamos S, Martinez-Yelamos A, Rubio F, Arbizu T. Idiopathic acute transverse myelitis: a clinical study and prognostic markers in 45 cases. *Mult Scler* 2006;12:169–173.
10. Caldemeyer KS, Harris TM, Smith RR, Edwards MK. Gadolinium enhancement in acute

disseminated encephalomyelitis. *J Comput Assist Tomogr* 1991;15:673–675.

11. Caldemeyer KS, Smith RR, Harris TM, Edwards MK. MRI in acute disseminated encephalomyelitis. *Neuroradiology* 1994;36:216–220.

12. Daumer M, Neuhaus A, Morrissey S, Hintzen R, Ebers GC. MRI as an outcome in multiple sclerosis clinical trials. *Neurology* 2009;72:705–711.

13. de Seze J, Debouverie M, Zephir H, et al. Acute fulminant demyelinating disease: a descriptive study of 60 patients. *Arch Neurol* 2007;64:1426–1432.

14. de Seze J, Lanctin C, Lebrun C, et al. Idiopathic acute transverse myelitis: application of the recent diagnostic criteria. *Neurology* 2005;65:1950–1953.

15. Forti A, Ambrosetto G, Amore M, et al. Locked-in syndrome in multiple sclerosis with sparing of the ventral portion of the pons. *Ann Neurol* 1982;12:393–394.

16. Frohman EM, Racke MK, Raine CS. Multiple sclerosis: the plaque and its pathogenesis. *N Engl J Med* 2006;354:942–955.

17. Gibbs WN, Kreidie MA, Kim RC, Hasso AN. Acute hemorrhagic leukoencephalitis: neuroimaging features and neuropathologic diagnosis. *J Comput Assist Tomogr* 2005;29:689–693.

18. Ginat DT. MRI of toxic leukoencephalopathy syndrome associated with methylenedioxymethamphetamine. *Neurology* 2015;84:757.

19. Group TMCW. Proposed diagnostic criteria and nosology of acute transverse myelitis. *Neurology* 2002;59:499–505.

20. Hahn JS, Siegler DJ, Enzmann D. Intravenous gammaglobulin therapy in recurrent acute disseminated encephalomyelitis. *Neurology* 1996;46:1173–1174.

21. Hefzy HM, Bartynski WS, Boardman JF, Lacomis D. Hemorrhage in posterior reversible encephalopathy syndrome: imaging and clinical features. *AJNR Am J Neuroradiol* 2009;30:1371–1379.

22. Hinchey J, Chaves C, Appignani B, et al. A reversible posterior leukoencephalopathy syndrome. *N Engl J Med* 1996;334:494–500.

23. Jelcic I, Faigle W, Sospedra M, Martin R. Immunology of progressive multifocal leukoencephalopathy. *J Neurovirol* 2015;21: 614–622.

24. Johnson MD, Lavin P, Whetsell WO, Jr. Fulminant monophasic multiple sclerosis, Marburg's type. *J Neurol Neurosurg Psychiatry* 1990;53:918–921.

25. Kantarci OH, Pirko I, Rodriguez M. Novel immunomodulatory approaches for the management of multiple sclerosis. *Clin Pharmacol Ther* 2014;95:32–44.

26. Kanter DS, Horensky D, Sperling RA, et al. Plasmapheresis in fulminant acute disseminated encephalomyelitis. *Neurology* 1995;45:824–827.

27. Kelley CE, Mathews J, Noskin GA. Acute transverse myelitis in the emergency department: a case report and review of the literature. *J Emerg Med* 1991;9:417–420.

28. Kesselring J, Miller DH, Robb SA, et al. Acute disseminated encephalomyelitis: MRI findings and the distinction from multiple sclerosis. *Brain* 1990;113 (Pt 2):291–302.

29. Khoshyomn S, Braff SP, Penar PL. Tumefactive multiple sclerosis plaque. *J Neurol Neurosurg Psychiatry* 2002;73:85.

30. Kitley J, Leite MI, Kuker W, et al. Longitudinally extensive transverse myelitis with and without aquaporin 4 antibodies. *JAMA Neurology* 2013;70:1375–1381.

31. Kozak OS, Wijdicks EFM, Manno EM, Miley JT, Rabinstein AA. Status epilepticus as initial manifestation of posterior reversible encephalopathy syndrome. *Neurology* 2007;69:894–897.

32. Kramer CL, Wetzel DR, Wijdicks EFM. Devastating delayed leukoencephalopathy associated with bath salt inhalation. *Neurocrit Care.* 2016 in press.

33. Lee HC, Mulanovich V, Nieto Y. Progressive multifocal leukoencephalopathy after allogeneic bone marrow transplantation for acute myeloid leukemia. *J Natl Compr Canc Netw* 2014;12:1660–1664.

34. Lee KH, Hashimoto SA, Hooge JP, et al. Magnetic resonance imaging of the head in the diagnosis of multiple sclerosis: a prospective 2-year follow-up with comparison of clinical evaluation, evoked potentials, oligoclonal banding, and CT. *Neurology* 1991;41:657–660.

35. Lee VH, Wijdicks EFM, Manno EM, Rabinstein AA. Clinical spectrum of reversible posterior leukoencephalopathy syndrome. *Arch Neurol* 2008;65:205–210.

36. Lucchinetti CF, Gavrilova RH, Metz I, et al. Clinical and radiographic spectrum of pathologically confirmed tumefactive multiple sclerosis. *Brain* 2008;131:1759–1775.

37. Mader I, Stock KW, Ettlin T, Probst A. Acute disseminated encephalomyelitis: MR and CT features. *AJNR Am J Neuroradiol* 1996;17:104–109.

38. Maramattom BV, Wijdicks EFM. Sirolimus may not cause neurotoxicity in kidney and liver transplant recipients. *Neurology* 2004;63:1958–1959.

39. Markus R, Brew BJ, Turner J, Pell M. Successful outcome with aggressive treatment of acute haemorrhagic leukoencephalitis. *J Neurol Neurosurg Psychiatry* 1997;63:551.

40. McKeon A, Ahlskog JE, Britton JW, Lennon VA, Pittock SJ. Reversible extralimbic paraneoplastic encephalopathies with large abnormalities on magnetic resonance images. *Arch Neurol* 2009;66:268–271.

41. Metkees M, Meesa IR, Srinivasan A. Methadone-induced acute toxic leukoencephalopathy. *Pediatr Neurol* 2015;52:256–257.

42. Moulin D, Paty DW, Ebers GC. The predictive value of cerebrospinal fluid electrophoresis in 'possible' multiple sclerosis. *Brain* 1983;106 (Pt 4):809–816.

43. Mueller-Mang C, Mang T, Pirker A, et al. Posterior reversible encephalopathy syndrome: do predisposing risk factors make a difference in MRI appearance? *Neuroradiology* 2009;51:373–383.

44. Niebler G, Harris T, Davis T, Roos K. Fulminant multiple sclerosis. *AJNR Am J Neuroradiol* 1992;13:1547–1551.

45. Noorbakhsh F, Johnson RT, Emery D, Power C. Acute disseminated encephalomyelitis: clinical and pathogenesis features. *Neurol Clin* 2008;26:759–780, ix.

46. Pandit L, Asgari N, Apiwattanakul M, et al. Demographic and clinical features of neuromyelitis optica: a review. *Mult Scler* 2015;21:845–853.

47. Paty DW, Noseworthy JH, Ebers GC. Diagnosis of multiple sclerosis. In: Paty DW, Ebers GC, eds. *Multiple Sclerosis*. Philadelphia: FA Davis; 1998.

48. Pittock SJ, Lucchinetti CF. Inflammatory transverse myelitis: evolving concepts. *Curr Opin Neurol* 2006;19:362–368.

49. Rodriguez M, Karnes WE, Bartleson JD, Pineda AA. Plasmapheresis in acute episodes of fulminant CNS inflammatory demyelination. *Neurology* 1993;43:1100–1104.

50. Rossi A. Imaging of acute disseminated encephalomyelitis. *Neuroimaging Clin N Am* 2008;18:149–161; ix.

51. Sahlas DJ, Miller SP, Guerin M, Veilleux M, Francis G. Treatment of acute disseminated encephalomyelitis with intravenous immunoglobulin. *Neurology* 2000;54:1370–1372.

52. Schwarz S, Mohr A, Knauth M, Wildemann B, Storch-Hagenlocher B. Acute disseminated encephalomyelitis: a follow-up study of 40 adult patients. *Neurology* 2001;56:1313–1318.

53. Scott TF. Nosology of idiopathic transverse myelitis syndromes. *Acta Neurol Scand* 2007;115:371–376.

54. Scott TF, Frohman EM, De Seze J, Gronseth GS, Weinshenker BG. Evidence-based guideline: clinical evaluation and treatment of transverse myelitis: report of the Therapeutics and Technology Assessment Subcommittee of the American Academy of Neurology. *Neurology* 2011;77:2128–2134.

55. Scott TF, Kassab SL, Pittock SJ. Neuromyelitis optica IgG status in acute partial transverse myelitis. *Arch Neurol* 2006;63:1398–1400.

56. Sejvar JJ. Acute disseminated encephalomyelitis. *Curr Infect Dis Rep* 2008;10:307–314.

57. Sonneville R, Klein I, de Broucker T, Wolff M. Post-infectious encephalitis in adults: diagnosis and management. *J Infect* 2009;58:321–328.

58. Sormani MP, Bonzano L, Roccatagliata L, et al. Magnetic resonance imaging as a potential surrogate for relapses in multiple sclerosis: a meta-analytic approach. *Ann Neurol* 2009;65:268–275.

59. Soussain C, Ricard D, Fike JR, et al. CNS complications of radiotherapy and chemotherapy. *Lancet* 2009;374:1639–1651.

60. Tateishi K, Takeda K, Mannen T. Acute disseminated encephalomyelitis confined to brainstem. *J Neuroimaging* 2002;12:67–68.

61. Tenembaum S, Chitnis T, Ness J, Hahn JS. Acute disseminated encephalomyelitis. *Neurology* 2007;68:S23–36.

62. Tumani H. Corticosteroids and plasma exchange in multiple sclerosis. *J Neurol* 2008;255 Suppl 6:36–42.

63. van de Beek D, Kremers WK, Kushwaha SS, McGregor CG, Wijdicks EFM. No major neurologic complications with sirolimus use in heart transplant recipients. *Mayo Clinic Proc* 2009;84:330–332.

64. Wingerchuk DM, Lennon VA, Lucchinetti CF, Pittock SJ, Weinshenker BG. The spectrum of neuromyelitis optica. *Lancet Neurol* 2007;6:805–815.

38

Acute Obstructive Hydrocephalus

Acute hydrocephalus is a consequence of many acute critical neurologic disorders, but this chapter will focus on acute obstructive hydrocephalus as a presenting problem that attracts the most attention and dictates the course of action. Generally speaking, acute obstructive hydrocephalus indicates a much more complex clinical neurologic problem, with several diagnostic causes to consider. In a large proportion of patients, the cause of acute hydrocephalus in adults admitted to the NICU is ventricular dilatation associated with subarachnoid hemorrhage, lobar hematoma, cerebellar hematoma, primary intraventricular hemorrhage, or, less commonly, malfunctioning ventriculolumbar or peritoneal shunts for previous hydrocephalus. Once recognized, urgent ventriculostomy results in adequate diversion of flow and, in fact, may be life-saving.

This chapter describes the clinical presentation, causes, and shunt placement of acute hydrocephalus. Enlargement of the ventricular system may be acutely created by a mass obstructing cerebrospinal fluid (CSF) outflow, or may be a result of sudden ballooning out, such as may occur after introduction of a jet of arterial blood. Definitive management, carefully planned later, could include resection or debulking of the tumor or permanent placement of a ventriculoperitoneal shunt.[12]

CLINICAL RECOGNITION

Patients with acute obstructive hydrocephalus have diminished alertness at presentation. In retrospect, episodes of headache are common and are frequently intense. Papilledema may occur, implying long-standing increased CSF pressure, but this remains an uncommon clinical finding in most intraventricular, pineal, or choroid plexus tumors. Earlier periods of blurred vision and obscuration (sudden blackouts lasting seconds) are reported by the patient and are explained by pressure-induced ischemia of the optic nerve. Unfortunately, the diagnosis in some patients is made only after symptoms and signs referable to brainstem compression or brainstem shift have occurred.

Decreased consciousness from ventricular enlargement may have several mechanisms. First, hydrocephalus may impair the ascending reticular activating system (ARAS) at the level of the aqueduct, which pushes against relay nuclei and fibers of the ARAS when it expands. Second, displacement of the upper brainstem by a massively enlarged third ventricle may tilt it backward and kink its structure. Third, when intracranial pressure (ICP) from increased ventricular pressure rises above the cerebral perfusion pressure, and certainly when the increase in pressure occurs rapidly, global ischemic damage to both hemispheres or displacement of brain tissue bilaterally through the tentorium or foramen magnum produces a terminal stage of coma. Fourth, and by an indirect mechanism, decreased arousal may also be caused by tumor infiltration into paramedian thalamic nuclei or the mesencephalon, which at the same time obstructs normal CSF flow.

Tumors that obstruct the ventricles may produce clinical signs from compression of the brainstem (e.g., pinealoma). These signs may combine to form Parinaud's syndrome, consisting of upward gaze palsy (Figure 38.1) and impaired convergence, with a so-called light-near dissociation of the pupillary light reflex (pupil constriction to accommodation, if cooperation by the patient is possible, and not to light). The lesion for the classic finding of Parinaud's syndrome is in the dorsal midbrain (pretectum) and interrupts the supra-nuclear mechanisms for upward gaze.

Pineal gland tumors may directly compress the midbrain, and compression may persist despite CSF diversion methods. However, the dorsal midbrain can also be distorted by enlargement of the posterior third ventricle and periaqueductal structures.[3] Colloid cysts are incidentally found, but they obstruct the foramen of Monro only after reaching a critical size. Intermittent headaches may precede acute deterioration, which can lead to sudden death. The causes of acute hydrocephalus associated with masses in adults are shown in Table 38.1. The

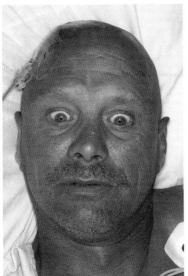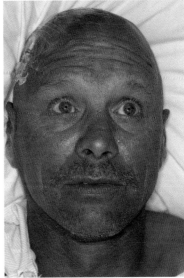

FIGURE 38.1: Lid retraction (*left*) and upward gaze limitation (*right*) in patient with aneurysmal subarachnoid hemorrhage and acute hydrocephalus. Symptoms persisted several days after placement of ventriculostomy.

pathophysiology of acute hydrocephalus is discussed in Capsule 38.1.

NEUROIMAGING AND LABORATORY TESTS

Different sites of obstruction in acute hydrocephalus are shown in Figures 38.2 through 38.5. Computed tomography (CT) scanning clearly delineates the degree of hydrocephalus and, in many instances, the obstructing tumor. Usually, the largest parts of the ventricular system (the anterior horns of the lateral ventricles) enlarge first, the temporal horns next, and then the third and fourth ventricles. When hydrocephalus has developed over weeks, subependymal effusions are clear evidence of increased CSF pressure. These periventricular hypodensities may occur in up to 40% of patients with acute obstructing hydrocephalus, but

TABLE 38.1. MASSES CAUSING ACUTE OBSTRUCTIVE HYDROCEPHALUS

Type	CT Scan Characteristics	Treatment
Intraventricular tumors		
Colloid cyst	Rounded, anterior 3V, widened SP, collapse of posterior 3V, ID, or HYP	Surgery or stereotactic aspiration
Plexus papilloma	Oval, 4V, LV, HYP	Total excision
Ependymoma	Lobulated, 4V, LV, ID	Excision and radiotherapy
Oligodendroglioma	Lobulated, LV, HYP, calcification	Resection
Ganglioglioma	3V, ID, HYP	Resection
Astrocytoma	LV, HD or HYP, irregular shape	Radiation, resection
Epidermoid cyst	4V, HYP, ID	Resection
Masses in pineal region		
Pineoblastoma	Lobulated, HD at peripheral rim, calcifications	Resection, radiation
Germinoma	ID, rounded	Radiation
Teratoma	HD or HYP, calcifications, lipid content	Resection
Vein of Galen aneurysm	HYP, rounded, triangular	Endovascular occlusion

CT, computed tomography; HD, hypodense; HYP, hyperdense; ID, isodense; LV, lateral ventricle; SP, septum pellucidum; 3V, third ventricle; 4V, fourth ventricle.
Data obtained from references 2, 17, 21, 22, 33, 35.

CAPSULE 38.1   PATHOPHYSIOLOGY OF ACUTE HYDROCEPHALUS

Cerebrospinal fluid is produced in the choroid plexus of the lateral ventricle; it is circulated throughout a system with critical passages at the foramen of Monro, third ventricle, and aqueduct of Sylvius; and it is absorbed through arachnoid villi (see accompanying illustration). Any obstruction of flow at these sites causes increased hydrostatic pressure in a matter of hours. Acute hydrocephalus occurs when normal physiologic equilibrium is disturbed. Cerebrospinal fluid (an ultrafiltrate from capillaries) is produced in the choroid plexus and may increase in the plexus papilloma. The circulation of CSF depends on several variables, such as rate of production (400–600 mL/day or 20 ml per hour), choroid plexus pulsations (filling of choroid plexus with each arterial pulse generates a pumping force), resistance (series of conduits, including foramina, aqueduct of Sylvius, and arachnoid villi), and sagittal sinus pressure (CSF pressure is greater, and flow depends on this pressure gradient). Absorption is linearly related to CSF pressure. Some of the CSF is merely recycled. Reduction in CSF volume therefore may be achieved by decreasing CSF production (carbonic anhydrate inhibitors; acetazolamide, which takes hours to achieve the effect), removing an obstructing tumor, and improving absorption (e.g., corticosteroids to reduce inflammatory response in arachnoid villi). Enlargement of the ventricles is incremental, with elevation of the corpus callosum after dilation of the lateral ventricles and eventual reduction of the convexity gray matter. CSF has a constant production rate and drains into the dural venous system, using a valvular system maintaining a one-direction flow outward. CSF reabsorption is dependent on CSF pressure and virtually nonexistent with CSF pressure < 5 mm Hg. CSF is very position dependent, and when upright, venous blood in cortical veins draws into jugular vein. CSF drains more easily into the spinal arachnoid space in an erect position and may even become negative; this is one of the reasons that valves are used in permanent ventriculoperitoneal CSF shunts.

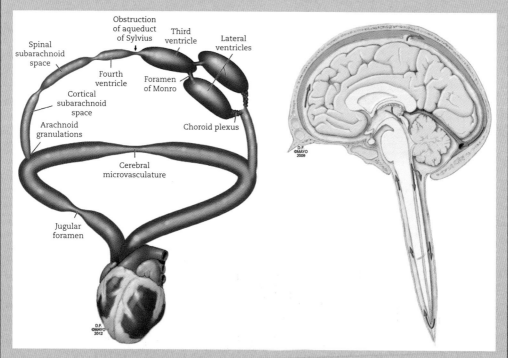

Circulation of cerebrospinal fluid.

Adapted from Sakka L, Coll G, Chazal J. Anatomy and physiology of cerebrospinal fluid. *Eur Ann Otorhinolaryngol Head Neck Dis* 2011;128:309–316.

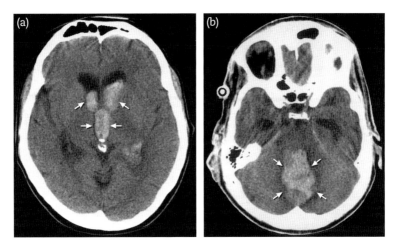

FIGURE 38.2. (a) Acute hydrocephalus in intraventricular hemorrhage due to sudden arterial jet of blood (*arrows*). (b) Acute hydrocephalus (note enlarged temporal horns) associated with cerebellar hematoma effacing the fourth ventricle (*arrows*).

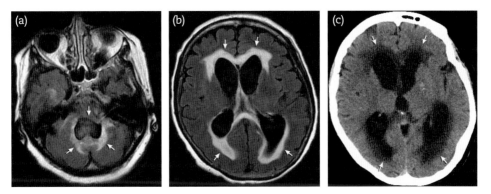

FIGURE 38.3. (a) Acute obstructive hydrocephalus associated with obstructive fourth ventricle tumor. (b, c) There are marked periventricular effusions on magnetic resonance imaging and computed tomography (*arrows*).

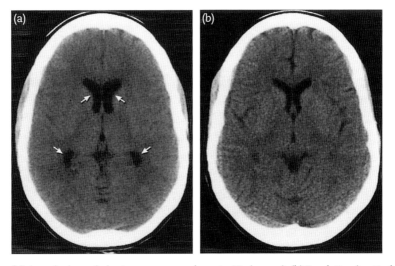

FIGURE 38.4. (a) Acute hydrocephalus in pneumococcal meningitis (*arrows*). (b) Resolution (particularly temporal horns) of the enlargement but also reappearance of sulci 4 days after antibiotic therapy.

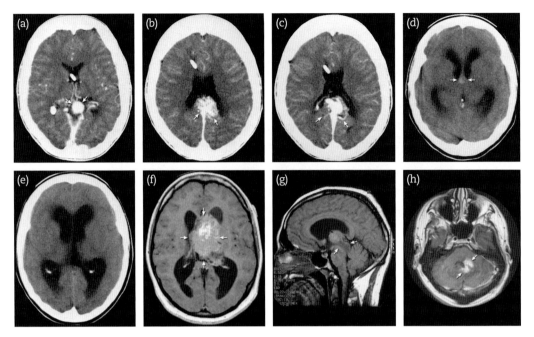

FIGURE 38.5: Examples of different sites of obstruction (*arrows*). *a–c:* Arteriovenous malformation with giant vein of Galen. *d, e:* Colloid cyst in third ventricle (note absence of third ventricle). *f:* Neurocytoma in third ventricle. *g:* Low-grade glioma in pineal region. *h:* Central nervous system lymphoma compressing fourth ventricle.

this capping surrounding the ventricle may also be evident in elderly patients with long-standing hypertension and diabetes but no hydrocephalus.

The degree of hydrocephalus can be carefully assessed by several measuring systems. These simple linear measurements not only determine the degree of hydrocephalus but also can be used to monitor change.[34] The ventricular size index measures the bifrontal diameter (transverse inner diameter) and divides it by the frontal horn diameter. The bicaudate index might be more reliable because normal values have been established. This index is determined by the width of the frontal horns at the level of the caudate nuclei divided by the maximum width of the brain at the same level (Figure 38.6). Alternatively, ventricular volume can be measured on CT or magnetic resonance imaging (MRI), outlining each slice and multiplying the area of outline by slice thickness.[34] The total volume is the sum of these volumes, including the calculated interslice gaps. In adults, there is little experience with this technique in acute neurologic disorders.

The temporal horns remain sensitive indicators for hydrocephalus on CT scans. Temporal horns, usually barely visible, become large, boomerang-shaped ventricles in acute hydrocephalus. This configuration often clearly differentiates obstruction from cortical cerebral atrophy. Other features compatible with atrophy rather than hydrocephalus

are widening sylvian and interhemispheric fissures, leaving marked hypodense fluid-filled spaces and prominent dilated cortical sulci.[28] It is important to identify tumors that may obstruct the ventricular system, particularly those located in the intraventricular compartment, which may be isodense to the brain tissue. Characteristically, colloid cysts of the third ventricle are very subtle and difficult to detect because they blend in with brain tissue. A mass should be strongly considered if the third ventricle cannot be identified or the septum pellucidum is widened, separating the posterior medial aspects of the frontal horns. It is important to scrutinize the posterior fossa for a mass lesion that may be evident only from distortion of the fourth ventricle.

However, MRI should disclose any obstructive mass lesion. Magnetic resonance imaging also is particularly important to demonstrate meningeal enhancement (e.g., in sarcoidosis or carcinomatous meningitis) and lesions typically not well recognized on CT scanning (e.g., smaller pineal region cysts).

Neoplastic growth of the epithelial lining on the ventricular surface is most commonly supratentorial in adults and more commonly intratentorial in children. Seeding throughout the CSF occurs in some instances. These malignant tumors grow slowly, and outcome is determined by grade, with 5-year survival of 80% in patients with

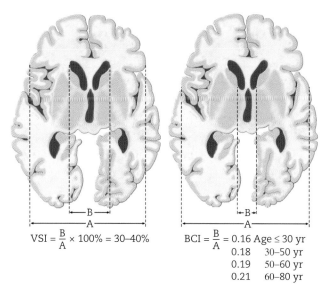

$$VSI = \frac{B}{A} \times 100\% = 30\text{–}40\%$$

$$BCI = \frac{B}{A} = 0.16 \quad \text{Age} \le 30 \text{ yr}$$
$$0.18 \quad 30\text{–}50 \text{ yr}$$
$$0.19 \quad 50\text{–}60 \text{ yr}$$
$$0.21 \quad 60\text{–}80 \text{ yr}$$

FIGURE 38.6: Measurement on computed tomographic scan of the ventricular system in acute hydrocephalus. Numbers indicate normal values. The ventricular size index (VSI) is not corrected for age.

BCI, bicaudate index.

low-grade tumors. Anaplastic or poorly differentiated ependymoma with typical histologic features of high mitotic activity, vascular proliferation, and necrosis reduces survival to 50%.

Tumors of the choroid plexus often are papillary and highly vascularized. Intratumoral hemorrhage is frequent. Localization is commonly in the fourth ventricle in adults. These tumors do not invade, and are comparatively easy to resect.

Epidermoid cysts are ectodermal elements displaced during embryogenesis that become symptomatic in adults. Rupture of the cyst may cause aseptic ventriculitis. Predilection is for the fourth ventricle; because of compression of the brainstem, cranial nerve palsy, ataxia, and hemiparesis may occur. Because of its slow growth and pliable nature, however, it may produce only intermittent headaches.

Pineal region tumors predominate in young adults (and children). Compression of the quadrigeminal plate depends on the size of the tumor, and compression of the cerebral aqueduct or tumor growth into the posterior third ventricle produces obstructive hydrocephalus.

Pineal parenchymal neoplasms can be divided into pineoblastoma (with histologic characteristics nearly identical to those of medulloblastoma) and pineocytoma (characteristic rosette formation).

Germinomas are very radiosensitive, and long-term survival or cure is expected after resection. Cerebrospinal fluid should be sampled at the time of ventricular shunting. Choriocarcinoma and pineal germinoma secrete human chorionic gonadotropin. α-fetoprotein is increased in endodermal sinus tumors, infiltrating teratoma, embryonal carcinoma, and choriocarcinoma. Cerebrospinal fluid markers may help in differentiation.

The incidence of colloid cyst of the third ventricle is about 0.5%–2% of all intracranial tumors. This developmental abnormality is filled with homogeneous viscous material containing cellular debris. Its location in the third ventricle causes intermittent marked enlargement of the ventricles or ventricular diverticula, and death may ensue if recurrent headaches are not sufficiently investigated. Colloid cysts are a cause of sudden death in pediatric and adult patients. Deterioration was observed in 32% of symptomatic patients, emphasizing its less than benign presence.[12,18]

In the Karolinska Hospital–based series of 37 consecutive patients with colloid cysts, five patients were admitted to the ED and two died despite emergency ventriculostomy. Full resection should be planned. Unfavorable long-term results were associated with aspiration and subtotal resection. However, transcallosal microsurgery produced excellent results.[24]

FIRST STEPS IN MANAGEMENT

Untreated obstructive hydrocephalus leads to altered arousal, coma, and in some cases brain death and, thus, urgent neurosurgical intervention is needed irrespective of its cause. The initial management is shown in Table 38.2. Unfortunately, the rarity and rapid progression of acute obstructive hydrocephalus often delay diagnosis and limit the ability to treat. The emphasis is therefore on early intervention with ventriculostomy and identification of the trigger. Acute CSF diversion with placement of a ventriculostomy drain into the largest ventricle has priority and, if feasible, should be performed in the NICU or even the ED. The ventriculostomy tube is connected to a manometric CSF drainage system draining at 10–15 cm H$_2$O. If the CSF is bloody, drainage at 0 cm H$_2$O or lower should be considered, to reduce clotting in the catheter, or tPA is considered (Chapter 26). Ventricular clearing of blood with ventriculostomy is not optimal and may lead to obstruction of the catheter. Use of intraventricular thrombolytic agents is currently under investigation.[11,16,26,33] Ventriculitis is uncommon, and probably has been reduced with antibiotic prophylaxis and subcutaneous tunneling or antibiotic-coated catheters.[6,7] In our series of 169 ventriculostomies, only four (2.4%) patients developed an infection.[29] Malplacement occurs in approximately 10% of patients.[19,29] Complications are rare and include epidural, subdural, or intraparenchymal hematoma (mostly in patients with severe coagulopathy); malfunctioning through blood clot obstruction; migration against the ventricular wall; and, rarely, creation of a dural arteriovenous fistula.[4,15] All are reasons to replace the catheter. Heparin can be safely used after placement of ventriculostomy, though not all neurosurgeons agree.[17]

Definitive treatment of the obstructing mass warrants endoscopic removal in most cases, and some patients need permanent ventriculoperitoneal shunts or fenestration of the third ventricle, accomplished by endoscopic techniques.[2,10,30,31] The lamina terminalis, septum pellucidum, and floor of the third ventricle can all be punctured and then dilated with catheters to divert CSF. Techniques such as fenestration of the septum pellucidum or third ventriculostomy are alternative approaches.[14,22] Ventriculoperitoneal shunts usually employ valve systems draining at CSF pressures of more than 10 mm Hg. Overdrainage may lead to subdural effusions or subdural hematomas, particularly in patients with low pressure or no pressure valves. However, some patients do not tolerate median value shunts and improve immediately with an external shunt at 0 cm H$_2$O, or even as low as –5 cm H$_2$O; in these cases, low-pressure valve shunts are needed.

DETERIORATION: CAUSES AND MANAGEMENT

Primary intraventricular hemorrhage commonly causes acute hydrocephalus, although a more

TABLE 38.2. INITIAL MANAGEMENT OF ACUTE HYDROCEPHALUS

Airway management	Protect airway with nasal trumpet or intubate if patient has hypoxemia despite facemask with 10 L of 100 oxygen/minute or if abnormal respiratory drive or if abnormal protective reflexes (likely with motor response of withdrawal, or worse)
Mechanical ventilation	CPAP mode IMV/PS may be needed in obstructing lesions in the posterior fossa
Fluid management	2 L of 0.9% NaCl
Nutrition	Enteral nutrition with continuous infusion (on day 2) Blood glucose control (goal 140–180 mg/dL)
Prophylaxis	DVT prophylaxis with pneumatic compression devices SC heparin 5,000 U t.i.d. GI prophylaxis: Pantoprazole 40 mg IV daily or lansoprazole 30 mg orally through nasogastric tube
Surgical management	Ventriculostomy at 5–10 cm H$_2$O Revision prior shunt Ventricular peritoneal shunt (pressure valve varies) Surgical extirpation of obstructing mass
Access	Peripheral venous catheter or peripheral inserted central catheter

CPAP, continuous positive airway pressure; DVT, deep vein thrombosis; GI, gastrointestinal; IMV, intermittent mandatory ventilation; IV, intravenously; NaCl, sodium chloride; PS, pressure support; SC, subcutaneously.

delayed course has been noted. Usually, the hemorrhage is massive. Intraventricular introduction of a thalamic, caudate, or large lobar hematoma also produces acute ventricular enlargement. Acute hemorrhage in the cerebellum, particularly when it extends to the vermis, may rapidly block the fourth ventricle, leading to obstructive hydrocephalus. Further deterioration from cerebellar hematoma and acute hydrocephalus can be treated by ventriculostomy when the fourth ventricle is blocked and no brainstem compression is evident on CT scans. Only in this particular clinical situation can ventriculostomy be beneficial; in all other instances, decompression of the pons by suboccipital craniotomy is more logical.

Computed tomography scan evidence of acute hydrocephalus is common in aneurysmal subarachnoid hemorrhage (Chapter 26). Acute hydrocephalus may be caused by obstruction of CSF outflow at the level of the ambient cisterns, by clogging of the arachnoid space with subarachnoid blood, or occasionally from the mass effect of a giant aneurysm obstructing the third ventricle. Commonly, the temporal horns are dilated early, typically before identifiable dilatation of the third and lateral ventricles. Ventriculostomy is certainly justified when clinical worsening in level of consciousness is clearly documented, when serial CT scans unmistakably demonstrate further enlargement, or when the third ventricle has changed into a balloon-shaped structure. One may argue that early ventriculostomy is a safeguard against rebleeding in the first hours; but conversely, it may be argued that reducing the CSF pressure may reduce the sealing pressures of the aneurysm and thus increase the risk of bleeding. We and others have found no such relationship and believe that ventriculostomy placement is indicated in patients with persistent stupor, vertical downgaze, pinpoint pupils, and documented enlarging size in CT.[25] Some endovascular radiologists prefer a ventriculostomy drain in place to safeguard the effects of rebleeding associated with placement of coils. (Its presence will allow the release of ventricular blood that otherwise would massively enlarge the ventricular system.)

In bacterial meningitis, obstruction of the ventricular communication with the subarachnoid space by inflammatory exudate is the most likely mechanism. Acute obstructive hydrocephalus can occur several weeks after bacterial meningitis begins and typically appears insidiously. The ventricular system, however, can be enlarged soon after the illness but usually to a minor degree and transiently. Rarely is there a need to proceed with a ventriculostomy when hydrocephalus occurs within the first days. Delayed hydrocephalus (10% in adult bacterial meningitis) may require placement of a drain. Once ventriculostomy is needed, outcome is much worse.

OUTCOME

Acute hydrocephalus in intracerebral hematoma is an independent predictor of poor outcome.[13,27] In addition, one study seriously questioned the use of ventriculostomy in parenchymal supratentorial hemorrhage.[1] Ventricular drainage controlled ICP but did not consistently improve level of consciousness, suggesting direct irreversible tissue damage from hydrocephalus.[23] Moreover, hemorrhagic dilatation of the fourth ventricle has been identified as an important indicator of poor outcome, confirming the impression that sudden massive enlargement causes damage to the periaqueductal area.[32]

Acute hydrocephalus in pontine hemorrhage is merely a consequence of its destructive hemorrhage, and ventriculostomy will not reverse coma. Extension to the mesencephalon and occasionally bilaterally to the thalamus precludes awakening.

As expected, outcome in tumor-related acute hydrocephalus is determined by the malignancy grade. The outcome of pineoblastoma is poor, with survival rarely extending beyond 2 years. Pineocytoma with neuronal differentiation, such as large rosette formation or ganglion cells, has a much better long-term outcome, up to three decades after diagnosis, resection, and radiotherapy.[5,8,9,20,21] Radiosurgery may be useful as adjuvant therapy. Germinomas may arise from this location, as may other germ cell tumors, such as teratomas, embryonal carcinoma, endodermal sinus tumor, and choriocarcinoma.

Generally the outcome of acute hydrocephalus is also determined by a response to interventions (Figure 38.7).

CONCLUSIONS

- Acute obstructive hydrocephalus may be life-threatening and in many circumstances requires an urgent ventriculostomy.
- Primary intraventricular hemorrhage and acute hydrocephalus may need additional treatment with thrombolytics.

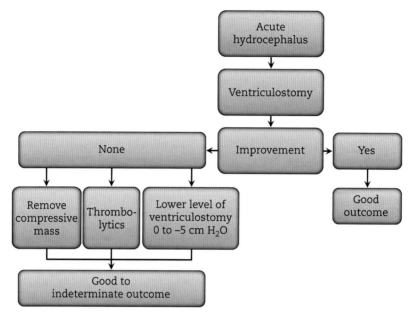

FIGURE 38.7: Outcome prediction in acute obstructive hydrocephalus. Good outcome: No assistance needed, minor handicap may remain. Indeterminate outcome: Any statement would be a premature conclusion.

- Treatment of acute hydrocephalus often comes first, followed by management of the obstructing tumor.
- Ventriculostomy may need to be internalized. Some patients require no valve or a low-pressure valve to maintain a normal ventricular size.

REFERENCES

1. Adams RE, Diringer MN. Response to external ventricular drainage in spontaneous intracerebral hemorrhage with hydrocephalus. *Neurology* 1998;50:519–523.
2. Ahmed AI, Zaben MJ, Mathad NV, Sparrow OC. Endoscopic biopsy and third ventriculostomy for the management of pineal region tumours. *World Neurosurg* 2015;83:543–547.
3. Baloh RW, Furman JM, Yee RD. Dorsal midbrain syndrome: clinical and oculographic findings. *Neurology* 1985;35:54–60.
4. Binz DD, Toussaint LG, 3rd, Friedman JA. Hemorrhagic complications of ventriculostomy placement: a meta-analysis. *Neurocrit Care* 2009;10:253–256.
5. Blakeley JO, Grossman SA. Management of pineal region tumors. *Curr Treat Options Oncol* 2006;7:505–516.
6. Brown EM, Edwards RJ, Pople IK. Conservative management of patients with cerebrospinal fluid shunt infections. *Neurosurgery* 2008;62(Suppl 2): 661–669.
7. Brown EM, Edwards RJ, Pople IK. Conservative management of patients with cerebrospinal fluid shunt infections. *Neurosurgery* 2006;58:657–665.
8. Bruce JN, Ogden AT. Surgical strategies for treating patients with pineal region tumors. *J Neurooncol* 2004;69:221–236.
9. Chang SM, Lillis-Hearne PK, Larson DA, et al. Pineoblastoma in adults. *Neurosurgery* 1995;37:383–390.
10. Cheng H, Hong W, Mei Z, Wang X. Surgical management of non-communicating hydrocephalus in patients: meta-analysis and comparison of endoscopic third ventriculostomy and ventriculoperitoneal shunt. *J Craniofac Surg* 2015;26:481–486.
11. Coplin WM, Vinas FC, Agris JM, et al. A cohort study of the safety and feasibility of intraventricular urokinase for nonaneurysmal spontaneous intraventricular hemorrhage. *Stroke* 1998;29:1573–1579.
12. de Witt Hamer PC, Verstegen MJ, De Haan RJ, et al. High risk of acute deterioration in patients harboring symptomatic colloid cysts of the third ventricle. *J Neurosurg* 2002;96:1041–1045.
13. Diringer MN, Edwards DF, Zazulia AR. Hydrocephalus: a previously unrecognized predictor of poor outcome from supratentorial intracerebral hemorrhage. *Stroke* 1998;29:1352–1357.
14. Feng H, Huang G, Liao X, et al. Endoscopic third ventriculostomy in the management of obstructive hydrocephalus: an outcome analysis. *J Neurosurg* 2004;100:626–633.

15. Gardner PA, Engh J, Atteberry D, Moossy JJ. Hemorrhage rates after external ventricular drain placement. *J Neurosurg* 2009;110:1021–1025.

16. Hall B, Parker D, Jr., Carhuapoma JR. Thrombolysis for intraventricular hemorrhage after endovascular aneurysmal coiling. *Neurocrit Care* 2005;3:153–156.

17. Hoh BL, Nogueira RG, Ledezma CJ, Pryor JC, Ogilvy CS. Safety of heparinization for cerebral aneurysm coiling soon after external ventriculostomy drain placement. *Neurosurgery* 2005;57:845–849.

18. Humphries RL, Stone CK, Bowers RC. Colloid cyst: a case report and literature review of a rare but deadly condition. *J Emerg Med* 2011;40:e5–e9.

19. Huyette DR, Turnbow BJ, Kaufman C, et al. Accuracy of the freehand pass technique for ventriculostomy catheter placement: retrospective assessment using computed tomography scans. *J Neurosurg* 2008;108:88–91.

20. Kano H, Niranjan A, Kondziolka D, Flickinger JC, Lunsford D. Role of stereotactic radiosurgery in the management of pineal parenchymal tumors. *Prog Neurol Surg* 2009;23:44–58.

21. Kano H, Niranjan A, Kondziolka D, Flickinger JC, Lunsford LD. Outcome predictors for intracranial ependymoma radiosurgery. *Neurosurgery* 2009;64:279–287.

22. Lehto H, Dashti R, Karatas A, Niemela M, Hernesniemi JA. Third ventriculostomy through the fenestrated lamina terminalis during microneurosurgical clipping of intracranial aneurysms: an alternative to conventional ventriculostomy. *Neurosurgery* 2009;64:430–434.

23. Liliang PC, Liang CL, Lu CH, et al. Hypertensive caudate hemorrhage prognostic predictor, outcome, and role of external ventricular drainage. *Stroke* 2001;32:1195–1200.

24. Mathiesen T, Grane P, Lindgren L, Lindquist C. Third ventricle colloid cysts: a consecutive 12-year series. *J Neurosurg* 1997;86:5–12.

25. McIver JI, Friedman JA, Wijdicks EFM, et al. Preoperative ventriculostomy and rebleeding after aneurysmal subarachnoid hemorrhage. *J Neurosurg* 2002;97:1042–1044.

26. Moradiya Y, Murthy SB, Newman-Toker DE, Hanley DF, Ziai WC. Intraventricular thrombolysis in intracerebral hemorrhage requiring ventriculostomy: a decade-long real-world experience. *Stroke* 2014;45:2629–2635.

27. Phan TG, Koh M, Vierkant RA, Wijdicks EFM. Hydrocephalus is a determinant of early mortality in putaminal hemorrhage. *Stroke* 2000;31:2157–2162.

28. Pople IK. Hydrocephalus and shunts: what the neurologist should know. *J Neurol Neurosurg Psychiatry* 2002;73 Suppl 1:i17–i22.

29. Saladino A, White JB, Wijdicks EFM, Lanzino G. Malplacement of ventricular catheters by neurosurgeons: a single institution experience. *Neurocrit Care* 2009;10:248–252.

30. Schroeder HW. Intraventricular tumors. *World Neurosurg* 2013;79:S17 e15–e19.

31. Shahinian H, Ra Y. Fully endoscopic resection of pineal region tumors. *J Neurol Surg B Skull Base* 2013;74:114–117.

32. Shapiro SA, Campbell RL, Scully T. Hemorrhagic dilation of the fourth ventricle: an ominous predictor. *J Neurosurg* 1994;80:805–809.

33. Varelas PN, Rickert KL, Cusick J, et al. Intraventricular hemorrhage after aneurysmal subarachnoid hemorrhage: pilot study of treatment with intraventricular tissue plasminogen activator. *Neurosurgery* 2005;56:205–213.

34. Xenos C, Sgouros S, Natarajan K. Ventricular volume change in childhood. *J Neurosurg* 2002;97:584–590.

39

Malignant Brain Tumors

Intracranial tumors are unusual in adults and are much less common than other systemic cancers. About 6 per 100,000 patients annually receive a diagnosis of primary malignant brain tumor, but this disease is ranked among the 10 most common causes of cancer death in the United States.[3] Infiltrating astrocytic tumors are found in the majority of all brain tumors, but histologically they can be further divided into malignant gliomas (70%), anaplastic astrocytomas (15%), and anaplastic oligodendrogliomas and oligoastrocytoma (10%), followed by such rare neoplasms as pleomorphic xanthoastrocytoma or other mixed gliomas (5%).[52]

Care of patients with a malignant brain tumor is directed by neurosurgeons and initially involves mostly surgical resection. Admission to the neurosciences intensive care unit (NICU) is usually reserved for patients after craniotomy, but their stay in the unit may be prolonged for several reasons. First, recurrent seizures may become a major management problem after debulking of the mass. Second, the tumor may involve precarious brainstem structures that could result in apneic spells, hypercapnia, or marked oropharyngeal weakness. Third—and most problematic—brain tumors may swell, and swell rapidly. This chapter discusses the care of patients with worsening symptoms of a recently diagnosed malignant brain tumor. Tumors located in the ventricular system causing acute hydrocephalus are discussed in Chapter 38. The managment of biopsy complications is discussed in Chapter 44.

CLINICAL RECOGNITION

The most common presenting feature is seizures for patients with astrocytomas, whether low- or high-grade astrocytoma. A new, unprovoked, and unexpected seizure leads to neuroimaging and discovery of a worrisome lesion. Partial seizures are less common and are seen more in the immediate postoperative debulking phase. Earlier studies have suggested that seizures are more common with slow-growing, low-grade astrocytomas.[1,2] Headache is uncommon, probably occurring in not more than 50% of patients and with no distinguishing features other than that it is a new symptom. Personality change is far more likely than headache, with patients having aggressive and accusatory behavior, with no insight of or ability to correct this behavior. In other patients, clinical suspicion arises when they become confused in familiar social settings.[1,2] Nausea and vomiting may occur, but they are rarely a presenting feature. With increased intracranial pressure, nausea and vomiting may develop, and blurred vision becomes more prominent.

The frontal lobe is most often involved in patients with a glioblastoma, followed in frequency by involvement of the temporal and parietal lobes. Therefore, clinical manifestations in most instances relate to the manifestations of a frontal syndrome. Tumors that arise in the right frontal lobe need to be a sizable growth to produce symptoms. Not infrequently, persons with such tumors become abulic and lack initiative, and brain tumor is identified only after persistent problematic conduct or work-related difficulties. Some persons become aloof and start simply napping through the day.

As expected, tumors that extend to the parietooccipital region result in visual agnosia. Tumors involving the temporal and frontal lobes may present with aphasia, dysphasia, and anosognosia.

Neurologic examination may document papilledema or oculomotor palsies, but they are an unusual clinical finding. Localizing the neurologic findings depends on the origin of the tumor spread and the development of secondary manifestations, such as cerebral infarcts from arterial encroachment and occlusion or development of obstructive hydrocephalus. Oculomotor abnormalities are expected when tumors originate in or extend to the base of the brain. Visual field cuts may be detected, but often abnormalities develop in the person's visual acuity. Invasion of the tumor into the basal ganglia may produce acute dystonic posturing. Tumors in the posterior fossa are most problematic because of displacement of the brainstem, which produces dysphagia, diplopia, and dysarthria—often with noticeable gait ataxia. Infiltrating brainstem glioma may also obstruct the fourth ventricle and become symptomatic from acute hydrocephalus (Chapter 38). These patients may have developed marked difficulty clearing secretions and may have changed their diet to more frequent thick liquids to avoid choking. Nocturnal apneas or desaturations may occur, and these patients may need a tracheostomy, particularly after surgery.

Some patients may present with a rapid-onset decline of consciousness, and a computed tomographic (CT) scan may show a ring-enhancing lesion with massive tumoral edema. Although clinical deterioration may occur within days, rarely is brain edema of such severity that it does not respond to an immediate dose of corticosteroids. Generally, patients with an anaplastic oligoastrocytoma present with a short clinical history.

NEUROIMAGING AND LABORATORY TESTS

After CT scanning documents a mass lesion, a contrast CT scan or, better, a magnetic resonance imaging (MRI) scan can characterize the mass.[4] Symmetric tumor infiltration through the corpus callosum may appear as a "butterfly." Generally, when compared with the subtle clinical presentation, the significant edema and tissue displacement indicate a long-standing process (Figure 39.1). Many patients who are alert or drowsy at best may have massive lesions with displacement that otherwise would not be tolerated in an acute process, and even small hemorrhages may be seen. An MRI with gadolinium enhancement can provide substantial new information and also determine whether a breakdown is present in the blood–brain barrier. Central areas of necrosis and peritumoral edema are more often seen in glioblastomas, and numerous areas may be present. Malignant brain tumors may be multifocal (Figure 39.2). Tumors of the posterior fossa (notably medulloblastoma) may be better defined with MRI (Figure 39.3). Proton magnetic resonance spectroscopy is occasionally used to

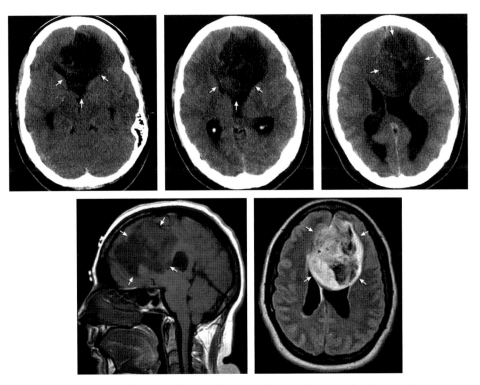

FIGURE 39.1: Examples of glioblastoma. Computed tomography scan (*upper row*) and magnetic resonance imaging (*lower row, sagittal and axial views*) of butterfly glioblastoma with significant mass effect and early hemorrhage (*arrows*).

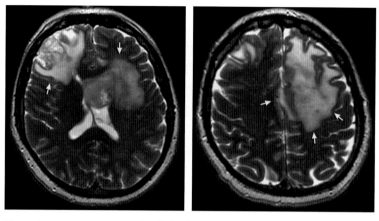

FIGURE 39.2: Magnetic resonance imaging of multifocal grade IV fibrillary astrocytoma (*arrows*).

document an increase in the choline concentration peak with a concomitant decrease in the acetylaspartate concentration peak, and these findings indicate necrosis.

Low-grade astrocytoma on CT scan ranges from appearing isodense to appearing hypodense to the adjacent brain and does not show enhancement with contrast medium on CT scan. On MRI scan, the tumor is homogeneously hyperintense on T2-weighted imaging, with little enhancement and peritumoral edema. In glioblastoma multiforme and anaplastic astrocytoma, the T2 signal clearly shows an irregular, enhanced rim. This finding is a consequence of increased cellularity but also of endothelial proliferation and necrosis. Positron emission tomographic scanning has been used occasionally, and tumors with increased metabolism show more intense uptake of fludeoxyglucose F18.[5] More recently, perfusion MRI scanning has been used, and has shown that the cerebral blood volume is markedly increased in glioblastomas compared with anaplastic gliomas.

Eventually, the patient requires a biopsy to confirm the diagnosis. Some centers use diffusion tensor imaging–based functional neuronavigation to identify and spare eloquent regions.[54]

The complexity of the World Health Organization (WHO) classification of central nervous system tumor is outside the scope of this book[28] (Capsule 39.1). Gemistocytic astrocytomas are more aggressive and more often progress to glioblastoma. An absence of miotic cells distinguishes WHO grade II astrocytoma from WHO grade III astrocytoma. Testing for Ki-67 protein is a recognized marker of proliferation and a useful additional analysis.

FIRST STEPS IN MANAGEMENT

The initial management steps for malignant brain tumor are shown in Table 39.1. The major treatment focus for a patient with a recently discovered brain tumor who is admitted to the NICU is the control of cerebral edema and its mass effect. Usually, the

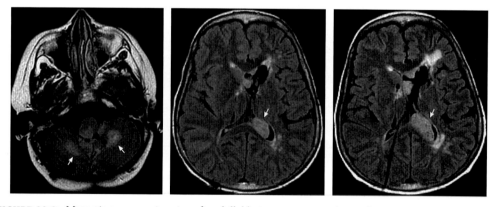

FIGURE 39.3: Magnetic resonance imaging of medulloblastoma recurrence (*arrows*).

CAPSULE 39.1   WHO GRADING OF TUMORS OF THE CENTRAL NERVOUS SYSTEM

Grade	Description
I	Low proliferative potential and potential for curative resection
II	Infiltrative, low-level proliferative potential but often reoccur
III	Histologic evidence of malignancy with nuclear atypia and mitotic activity
IV	Cytologically malignant with rapid evolution and fatal outcome

WHO, World Health Organization.
Adapted from Louis DN, Ohgaki H, Wiestler OD, et al. The 2007 WHO classification of tumors of the central nervous systems. *Acta Neuropathol* 2007;114:97–109. With permission of the publisher.

Astrocytic tumors	I	II	III	IV
Subependymal giant cell astrocytoma	✓			
Pilocytic astrocytoma	✓			
Pilomyxoid astrocytoma		✓		
Diffuse astrocytoma		✓		
Pleomorphic xanthoastrocytoma		✓		
Anaplastic astrocytoma			✓	
Glioblastoma				✓
Giant cell glioblastoma				✓
Gliosarcoma				✓
Oligodendroglial tumors				
Oligodendroglioma		✓		
Anaplastic oligodendroglioma			✓	
Oligoastrocytic tumors				
Oligoastrocytoma		✓		
Anaplastic oligoastrocytoma			✓	
Ependymal tumors				
Subependymoma	✓			
Myxopapillary ependymoma	✓			
Ependymoma		✓		
Anaplastic ependymoma			✓	
Choroid plexus tumors				
Choroid plexus papilloma	✓			
Atypical choroid plexus papilloma		✓		
Choroid plexus carcinoma			✓	
Other neuroepithelial tumors				
Angiocentric glioma	✓			
Chordoid glioma of the third ventricle		✓		
Neuronal and mixed neuronal-glial tumors				
Gangliocytoma	✓			
Ganglioglioma	✓			
Anaplastic ganglioglioma			✓	
Desmoplastic infantile astrocytoma and ganglioglioma	✓			
Dysembryoplastic neuroepithelial tumor	✓			

	I	II	III	IV
Central neurocytoma		✓		
Extraventricular neurocytoma		✓		
Cerebellar liponeurocytoma		✓		
Paraganglioma of the spinal cord	✓			
Papillary glioneuronal tumor	✓			
Rossette-forming glioneuronal tumor of the fourth ventricle	✓			
Pineal tumor				
Pineocytoma	✓			
Pineal parenchymal tumor of intermediate differentiation		✓	✓	
Pineoblastoma				✓
Papillary tumor of the pineal region		✓	✓	
Embryonal tumors				
Medulloblastoma				✓
CNS primitive neuroectodermal tumor (PNET)				✓
Atypical teratoid/rhabdoid tumor				✓
Tumors of the cranial and paraspinal nerves				
Schwannoma	✓			
Neurofibroma	✓			
Perineurioma	✓	✓	✓	
Malignant peripheral nerve sheath tumor (MPNST)		✓	✓	✓
Meningeal tumors				
Meningioma	✓			
Atypical meningioma		✓		
Anaplastic/malignant meningioma			✓	
Hemangiopericytoma		✓	✓	
Anaplastic haemangiopericytoma			✓	
Hemangioblastoma	✓			
Tumors of the sellar region				
Craniopharyngioma	✓			
Granular cell tumor of the neurohypophysis	✓			
Pituicytoma	✓			
Spindle cell oncocytoma of the adenohypophysis	✓			

WHO grading of tumors of the central nervous system.

patient is treated with a bolus of 10 mg of dexamethasone, followed by a daily dose of 16 mg (4 mg every 6 hours). In many patients, early improvement is seen within hours, and corticosteroid therapy can prevent further brain tissue shift. Dexamethasone reduces vascular permeability and cerebral blood flow and blood volume.[30] If long-term management of tumor is anticipated, the patient should receive trimethoprim-sulfamethoxazole to reduce the risk of pneumocystic pneumonitis. Adrenal suppression precluding sudden discontinuation of the drug is expected only after 2 weeks of usage. Whether a patient should receive prophylactic antiepileptic drugs is unclear, particularly because, in the later use of chemotherapy, the effect of the antiepileptic drugs may increase the metabolism of chemotherapeutic agents. Recently, the Quality Standards Subcommittee of the American Academy of Neurology found no evidence of benefit with routine use of antiepileptic drugs for brain tumors.[16] However, most neurosurgeons prefer to treat the patient with antiepileptic drugs after stereotactic biopsy or debulking of the mass. Levetiracetam is the drug that is probably best tolerated, and at Mayo Clinic, we start with 1,000 mg IV (over 15 min) as a loading dose.

TABLE 39.1. INITIAL MANAGEMENT OF MALIGNANT BRAIN TUMOR

Airway management	Intubation when patient's consciousness declines, and if abnormal protective reflexes (likely with motor response of withdrawal, or worse)
	Tracheostomy for brainstem tumors
Mechanical ventilation	Usually CPAP or IMV/PS
Fluids management	2L of 0.9% NaCl
Nutrition	Enteral nutrition with continuous infusion (on day 2)
	Blood glucose control (goal 140–180 mg/dL)
Prophylaxis	DVT prophylaxis with pneumatic compression devices
	Consider SC heparin 5000 U t.i.d.
	GI prophylaxis: Pantoprazole 40 mg IV daily or lansoprazole 30 mg orally through nasogastric tube
	Administration of trimethoprim-sulfamethoxazole DS (160 mg) in patients with dexamethasone
	Levetiracetam 1,000 mg IV over 15 minutes and 1,000 mg bid maintenance
Specific management	Bolus administration of dexamethasone (10 mg intravenously)
	Maintenance dexamethasone (8–16 mg/day)
Access	Peripheral venous catheter or peripheral inserted central catheter
Surgical treatment	Debulking procedure
	Stereotactic biopsy

CPAP, continuous positive airway pressure; DVT, deep vein thrombosis; GI, gastrointestinal; IMV, intermittent mandatory ventilation; IV, intravenous; LMWH, low-molecular-weight heparin; NaCl, sodium chloride; PS, pressure support; SC, subcutaneous.

Patients with tumors in the brainstem are at high risk for respiratory difficulties, and careful attention to nocturnal desaturation is required. Some of these patients are unable to protect their airway because of pooling secretions and need to be intubated or, more likely, to receive a transient tracheostomy until definitive treatment has been completed. Even for patients with retained mobility, aggressive treatment to prevent deep vein thrombosis is advised.[15] Some studies have claimed a 30% incidence of deep vein thrombosis in patients with a brain tumor, and suggested low-molecular-weight heparin (LMWH) is needed to prevent a pulmonary embolus.[26,27,37] Hemorrhage into the tumor mostly occurs in patients receiving complete anticoagulation therapy, and the risk is less than 1% in patients treated with LMWH or subcutaneous heparin. The risk of long term use of LMWH is indeterminate and the prematurely stopped PRODIGE study suggested reduced venous thrombosis and increased intracranial bleeding.[33]

Treatment of malignant glioma is determined by tumor classification, and several options may be offered to the patient.[6,7,9,17,39] Therapy is targeted to tumor-associated endothelial cells and glioma cells and involves signal transduction pathways and the regulation of tumor growth. Treatment is aimed at targets on multiple levels and at different pathways to increase its efficacy.[43,45,49,51,53] One target is to mute the tumor growth; another target is to attack angiogenesis and cell migration. No accepted standard treatment exists for the patient with a glioma after surgical debulking.[52] Most patients are treated with maximal surgical resection, radiotherapy, and chemotherapy[13,24,47,48] (Table 39.2). Sufficient evidence shows that therapy with temozolomide (75 mg/m^2/day) for 6 weeks, followed by adjuvant temozolomide therapy (150–200 mg/m^2/day) for 5 days every 28 days for 6 cycles, improves outcome, with a survival rate of about 50% at 2 years.

DETERIORATION: CAUSES AND MANAGEMENT

Management of malignant brain tumor for most deteriorating patients involves difficulty in the treatment of refractory seizures and the treatment of worsening cerebral edema.

Focal seizures are common major later manifestations. Seizures may be seen after initial treatment but also may be a sign of tumor progression. Persistent focal seizures are difficult to treat and may require high doses (30 mg/kg IV) of sodium phenobarbital (aiming at serum levels of 40–80 µg/mL) or large doses (30 mg/kg IV) of sodium valproate (aiming at serum levels of 40–100 µg/mL). Intervention with intravenous anesthetic drugs

TABLE 39.2. CURRENT TREATMENT OF MALIGNANT GLIOMAS

Type of Tumor	Treatment
Newly diagnosed tumors	
Glioblastomas (WHO grade IV)	Maximal surgical resection, plus radiotherapy plus concomitant and adjuvant TMZ or carmustine wafers
Angioplastic astrocytomas (WHO grade III)	Maximal surgical resection, TMZ alone, or radiotherapy plus concomitant and adjuvant TMZ
Anaplastic oligodendrogliomas and anaplastic oligoastrocytoma (WHO grade III)	Maximal surgical resection, radiotherapy alone, TMZ or PVC with or without radiotherapy afterward, radiotherapy plus concomitant and adjuvant TMZ, or radiotherapy plus adjuvant TMZ
Recurrent tumors	Reoperation in selected patients, carmustine wafers, conventional chemotherapy (e.g., lomustine, carmustine PCV, carboplatin, irinotecan hydrochloride, etoposide phosphate, bevacizumab plus irinotecan), experimental therapies

PCV, procarbazine; TMZ, temozolomide; WHO, World Health Organization.
Adapted from Wen PY, Kesari S. Malignant gliomas in adults. *N Engl J Med* 2008;359:492–507. Used with permission.

may be warranted, but such an aggressive intervention may be withheld if there is tumor recurrence and no neurosurgical option. Propofol may be an option, but high doses are often needed, thus substantially increasing the risk of propofol infusion syndrome (Chapter 16). Recurrence of focal seizures is high after weaning off these third-line drugs, but in some patients this intervention is successful in controlling focal status epilepticus.[18,40]

Worsening cerebral edema (Figure 39.4) is another management challenge. Investigators have suggested four processes related to the edema associated with primary brain tumors: (1) tumor angiogenesis of vessels with a defective blood–brain barrier, characterized by large interendothelial gaps;[11,14] (2) increased microvascular permeability from production of mediators, such as prostaglandin E_2 and thromboxane B_2, in the process;[8] (3) an immunologic mechanism (e.g., interleukin-2) that, when the substance is injected, has resulted in brain edema in experimental studies; and, finally, (4) an inflammatory mechanism activated through substances, such as platelet-activating factor, released from polynuclear leukocytes surrounding the tumor-associated edema.[21–23]

Other factors that may potentiate tumor-associated edema are seizures, use of chemotherapeutic agents, and therapeutic radiation.[10] Plasma osmolality may have an important role, and one experimental study found a direct relation between plasma osmolality and the formation of brain edema.[19] Brain edema is preferentially in the white matter, often sparing the gray matter, and generally involves a proteinaceous plasma infiltrate in the extracellular space, as opposed to a cytotoxic (i.e., gray matter) infiltration.[31] Brain edema caused by cellular swelling from the influx of water and sodium is seen in cerebral infarcts and may occur when tissue shift obliterates cerebral arteries (anterior cerebral artery against the falx) or venous occlusion develops (dural seeding).

Clearing of brain edema occurs predominantly through the cerebrospinal fluid (CSF). Clearance of extravasated proteins by the glial cells is also closely linked to the resolution of edema fluid; this clearance suggests a major role for colloid osmotic pressure generated by the proteins.[29,34]

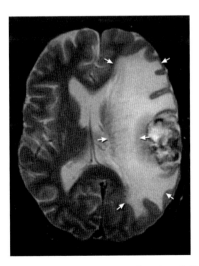

FIGURE 39.4: Magnetic resonance imaging of glioblastoma with peritumoral edema (*arrows*).

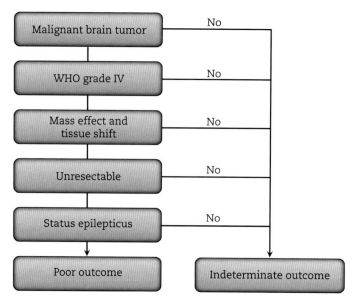

FIGURE 39.5: Outcome in malignant brain tumors. Poor outcome: Severe disability or death, negative state. Indeterminate outcome: Any statement would be a premature conclusion.

Edema spreads through bulk flow and a downhill pressure gradient between the white matter and the CSF compartment, a mechanism that may be further facilitated when CSF pressure is reduced. A centrally located arterial natriuretic factor has been found to moderate the brain water content, and it might decrease edema formation.[12,22,32,35,46] Another mechanism may be due to water channel proteins (aquaporin-4), which are widely expressed in the brain.[46]

Brain edema associated with recent tumor growth responds within hours of intravenous administration of 10 mg of dexamethasone. Osmotic diuretics—mannitol or hypertonic (23%) saline—are the best next options, and the dose can be titrated to a target serum sodium concentration of 145–155 mmol/L or a serum osmolality of 320 mOsmol/L.

Urgent craniotomy with duraplasty and debulking is considered when these measures are unsuccessful, when aggressive management continues to be warranted (e.g., when histological characteristics of the tumor are unknown), and when cerebral infarction appears to be the major component of swelling. However, such procedures are not commonly performed and lead to substantial morbidity.

OUTCOME

The prognosis is not only determined by the degree of neurologic deficit after tumor debulking (often reflected in a poor Karnofsky performance status), but also by the WHO grade (histologic features and, more recently, specific genetic alterations).[25,38,42,44,50] Certain gene deletions may be associated with improved chances of survival and improved response to chemotherapy.[20,36] Progression-free survival is determined by preoperative tumor diameter, histologic type, and residual tumor seen on MRI. However, even a residual tumor of less than 1 cm or more had a 26% recurrence rate at 5 years.[41] Status epilepticus in patients with a previously treated malignant brain tumor is a major complication, and in these cases, outcome is mostly poor. Outcome in malignant brain tumor is shown in (Figure 39.5).

CONCLUSIONS

- Patients in the NICU with a recent malignant brain tumor need close monitoring for seizures, post-debulking cerebral edema or hemorrhage, and control of airway.
- Dexamethasone may rapidly reduce clinical signs of mass effect.
- Status epilepticus (epilepsia partialis continua) does occur with recurrence and may need surgical resection or anesthetic drugs.

REFERENCES

1. Brandsma D, Stalpers L, Taal W, Sminia P, van den Bent MJ. Clinical features, mechanisms, and

management of pseudoprogression in malignant gliomas. *Lancet Oncol* 2008;9:453–461.

2. Buckner JC, Brown PD, O'Neill BP, et al. Central nervous system tumors. *Mayo Clinic Proc* 2007;82:1271–1286.

3. CBTRUS 2008 statistical report: primary brain tumors in the United States. Central Brain Tumor Registry of the United States, 2000–2004. http://www.cbtrus.org/reports/2007 2008/2007report.pdf.

4. Cha S. Update on brain tumor imaging: from anatomy to physiology. *AJNR Am J Neuroradiol* 2006;27:475–487.

5. Chen W. Clinical applications of PET in brain tumors. *J Nucl Med* 2007;48:1468–1481.

6. Citrin D, Menard C, Camphausen K. Combining radiotherapy and angiogenesis inhibitors: clinical trial design. *Int J Radiat Oncol Biol Phys* 2006;64:15–25.

7. Combs SE, Steck I, Schulz-Ertner D, et al. Long-term outcome of high-precision radiotherapy in patients with brain stem gliomas: results from a difficult-to-treat patient population using fractionated stereotactic radiotherapy. *Radiother Oncol* 2009;91:60–66.

8. Cooper C, Jones HG, Weller RO, Walker V. Production of prostaglandins and thromboxane by isolated cells from intracranial tumours. *J Neurol Neurosurg Psychiatry* 1984;47:579–584.

9. Dancey JE, Chen HX. Strategies for optimizing combinations of molecularly targeted anticancer agents. *Nat Rev Drug Discov* 2006;5:649–659.

10. DeAngelis LM, Posner JB. *Neurologic Complications of Cancer.* 2nd ed. New York: Oxford University Press; 2008.

11. Del Maestro RF, Megyesi JF, Farrell CL. Mechanisms of tumor-associated edema: a review. *Can J Neurol Sci* 1990;17:177–183.

12. Doczi T, Joo F, Szerdahelyi P, Bodosi M. Regulation of brain water and electrolyte contents: the possible involvement of central atrial natriuretic factor. *Neurosurgery* 1987;21:454–458.

13. Fine HA, Dear KB, Loeffler JS, Black PM, Canellos GP. Meta-analysis of radiation therapy with and without adjuvant chemotherapy for malignant gliomas in adults. *Cancer* 1993;71:2585–2597.

14. Fishman RA. *Cerebrospinal Fluid in Diseases of the Nervous System.* 2nd ed. Philadelphia: W. B. Saunders; 1992.

15. Gerber DE, Grossman SA, Streiff MB. Management of venous thromboembolism in patients with primary and metastatic brain tumors. *J Clin Oncol* 2006;24:1310–1318.

16. Glantz MJ, Cole BF, Forsyth PA, et al. Practice parameter: anticonvulsant prophylaxis in patients with newly diagnosed brain tumors. Report of the Quality Standards Subcommittee of the American Academy of Neurology. *Neurology* 2000;54:1886–1893.

17. Glas M, Happold C, Rieger J, et al. Long-term survival of patients with glioblastoma treated with radiotherapy and lomustine plus temozolomide. *J Clin Oncol* 2009;27:1257–1261.

18. Goonawardena J, Marshman LA, Drummond KJ. Brain tumor-associated status epilepticus. *J Clin Neurosci* 2015;22:29–34.

19. Hansen TD, Warner DS, Traynelis VC, Todd MM. Plasma osmolality and brain water content in a rat glioma model. *Neurosurgery* 1994;34:505–511.

20. Houillier C, Lejeune J, Benouaich-Amiel A, et al. Prognostic impact of molecular markers in a series of 220 primary glioblastomas. *Cancer* 2006;106:2218–2223.

21. Ito U, Baethmann A, Hossmann KA, et al. Brain edema XI. *Acta Neurochir (Wien)* 1993;60:1–11.

22. Kimelberg HK. Current concepts of brain edema: review of laboratory investigations. *J Neurosurg* 1995;83:1051–1059.

23. Klatzo I. Presidental address. Neuropathological aspects of brain edema. *J Neuropathol Exp Neurol* 1967;26:1–14.

24. Kondziolka D, Shin SM, Brunswick A, Kim I, Silverman JS. The biology of radiosurgery and its clinical applications for brain tumors. *Neuro Oncol* 2015;17:29–44.

25. Lamborn KR, Chang SM, Prados MD. Prognostic factors for survival of patients with glioblastoma: recursive partitioning analysis. *Neuro Oncol* 2004;6:227–235.

26. Lee AY, Levine MN, Baker RI, et al. Low-molecular-weight heparin versus a coumarin for the prevention of recurrent venous thromboembolism in patients with cancer. *N Engl J Med* 2003;349:146–153.

27. Levin JM, Schiff D, Loeffler JS, et al. Complications of therapy for venous thromboembolic disease in patients with brain tumors. *Neurology* 1993;43:1111–1114.

28. Louis DN, Ohgaki H, Wiestler OD, et al. The 2007 WHO classification of tumours of the central nervous system. *Acta Neuropathol* 2007;114:97–109.

29. Marmarou A, Hochwald G, Nakamura T, et al. Brain edema resolution by CSF pathways and brain vasculature in cats. *Am J Physiol* 1994;267:H514–520.

30. McClelland S, 3rd, Long DM. Genesis of the use of corticosteroids in the treatment and prevention of brain edema. *Neurosurgery* 2008;62:965–967.

31. Milhorat TH. *Cerebrospinal Fluid and the Brain Edemas.* New York: Neuroscience Society of New York; 1987.

32. Nakao N, Itakura T, Yokote H, Nakai K, Komai N. Effect of atrial natriuretic peptide on ischemic brain edema: changes in brain water and electrolytes. *Neurosurgery* 1990;27:39–43.

33. Perry JR, Julian JA, Laperriere NJ,et al. PRODIGE: a randomized placebo-controlled trial of dalteparin low-molecular-weight heparin thromboprophylaxis in patients with newly diagnosed malignant glioma. *J Thromb Haemost* 2010;8:1959–1965.

34. Reulen HJ, Graham R, Spatz M, Klatzo I. Role of pressure gradients and bulk flow in dynamics of vasogenic brain edema. *J Neurosurg* 1977;46:24–35.

35. Rosenberg GA, Estrada EY. Atrial natriuretic peptide blocks hemorrhagic brain edema after 4-hour delay in rats. *Stroke* 1995;26:874–877.

36. Ruano Y, Ribalta T, de Lope AR, et al. Worse outcome in primary glioblastoma multiforme with concurrent epidermal growth factor receptor and p53 alteration. *Am J Clin Pathol* 2009;131:257–263.

37. Ruff RL, Posner JB. Incidence and treatment of peripheral venous thrombosis in patients with glioma. *Ann Neurol* 1983;13:334–336.

38. Sanai N, Berger MS. Glioma extent of resection and its impact on patient outcome. *Neurosurgery* 2008;62:753–764.

39. Sathornsumetee S, Reardon DA, Desjardins A, et al. Molecularly targeted therapy for malignant glioma. *Cancer* 2007;110:13–24.

40. Sayegh ET, Fakurnejad S, Oh T, Bloch O, Parsa AT. Anticonvulsant prophylaxis for brain tumor surgery: determining the current best available evidence. *J Neurosurg* 2014;121:1139–1147.

41. Shaw EG, Berkey B, Coons SW, et al. Recurrence following neurosurgeon-determined gross-total resection of adult supratentorial low-grade glioma: results of a prospective clinical trial. *J Neurosurg* 2008;109:835–841.

42. Smith JS, Chang EF, Lamborn KR, et al. Role of extent of resection in the long-term outcome of low-grade hemispheric gliomas. *J Clin Oncol* 2008;26:1338–1345.

43. Stewart LA. Chemotherapy in adult high-grade glioma: a systematic review and meta-analysis of individual patient data from 12 randomized trials. *Lancet* 2002;359:1011–1018.

44. Stummer W, Reulen HJ, Meinel T, et al. Extent of resection and survival in glioblastoma multiforme: identification of and adjustment for bias. *Neurosurgery* 2008;62:564–576.

45. Stupp R, Roila F. Malignant glioma: ESMO clinical recommendations for diagnosis, treatment and follow-up. *Ann Oncol* 2009;20(Suppl 4):126–128.

46. Sun MC, Honey CR, Berk C, Wong NL, Tsui JK. Regulation of aquaporin-4 in a traumatic brain injury model in rats. *J Neurosurg* 2003;98:565–569.

47. Tentori L, Graziani G. Pharmacological strategies to increase the antitumor activity of methylating agents. *Curr Med Chem* 2002;9:1285–1301.

48. Tentori L, Graziani G. Recent approaches to improve the antitumor efficacy of temozolomide. *Curr Med Chem* 2009;16:245–257.

49. van den Bent MJ, Carpentier AF, Brandes AA, et al. Adjuvant procarbazine, lomustine, and vincristine improves progression-free survival but not overall survival in newly diagnosed anaplastic oligodendrogliomas and oligoastrocytomas: a randomized European Organisation for Research and Treatment of Cancer phase III trial. *J Clin Oncol* 2006;24:2715–2722.

50. van den Bent MJ, Dubbink HJ, Sanson M, et al. MGMT promoter methylation is prognostic but not predictive for outcome to adjuvant PCV chemotherapy in anaplastic oligodendroglial tumors: a report from EORTC Brain Tumor Group Study 26951. *J Clin Oncol* 2009;27:5881–5886.

51. van den Bent MJ, Taphoorn MJ, Brandes AA, et al. Phase II study of first-line chemotherapy with temozolomide in recurrent oligodendroglial tumors: the European Organization for Research and Treatment of Cancer Brain Tumor Group Study 26971. *J Clin Oncol* 2003;21:2525–2528.

52. Wen PY, Kesari S. Malignant gliomas in adults. *N Engl J Med* 2008;359:492–507.

53. Westphal M, Hilt DC, Bortey E, et al. A phase 3 trial of local chemotherapy with biodegradable carmustine (BCNU) wafers (Gliadel wafers) in patients with primary malignant glioma. *Neuro Oncol* 2003;5:79–88.

54. Wu JS, Zhou LF, Tang WJ, et al. Clinical evaluation and follow-up outcome of diffusion tensor imaging-based functional neuronavigation: a prospective, controlled study in patients with gliomas involving pyramidal tracts. *Neurosurgery* 2007;61:935–948.

40

Status Epilepticus

Status epilepticus is a neurologic emergency that not only needs rapid pharmacologic intervention but also is more properly treated when its cause is identified. Fortunately, about two-thirds of patients with status epilepticus become seizure-free in the emergency department (ED) from treatment with repeated boluses of lorazepam and intravenous loading with a sufficient amount of phenytoin (Chapter 11). Thus, persistent and therapy-refractory generalized tonic-clonic seizures after admission to the neurosciences intensive care unit (NICU) indicate a more severe form of status epilepticus with undoubtedly higher probability of permanent neurologic damage. Aggressive use of benzodiazepines and rapid escalation of a number of intravenous antiepileptic (anesthetic) drugs may lead to longer ICU stays and may increase infection complications.[72,95] A critical juncture is the time of successful administration of antiepileptic agents, and duration of status epilepticus less than 10 hours predicts a better outcome.[34]

The cause of tonic-clonic status epilepticus is diverse (Chapter 11). Withdrawal of antiepileptic medication or poor compliance has traditionally been implicated. Discontinuation of antiepileptic agents for seizure localization in the epilepsy monitoring unit may bring patients to the NICU with status epilepticus. One study noted that the vast majority of patients with status epilepticus and a seizure disorder had therapeutic or subtherapeutic antiepileptic drug levels at the time of presentation.[5] Clearly identified causes of status epilepticus in adults are alcohol withdrawal, primary brain tumors, traumatic brain injury, ischemic and hemorrhagic stroke, posterior reversible encephalopathy syndrome, encephalitis, meningitis, poisoning, illicit drug abuse, toxicity of immunosuppressive agents and, occasionally, metabolic derangements, such as marked shifts in plasma sodium and serum glucose.[6,7,20,21,59,78,113] In older adults without a history of epilepsy, half of all instances could be attributed to acute stroke.[30] Worldwide, neurocysticercosis is a common cause of seizures and status epilepticus.[18] Some drugs used in the NICU can lower the seizure threshold and trigger a single seizure, particularly in patients with a proclivity to seizures, but status epilepticus is unlikely (Table 40.1).

Status epilepticus in adults can be classified broadly into tonic-clonic status epilepticus, nonconvulsive status epilepticus, and complex partial status epilepticus (Chapter 11).[40,44] This chapter mainly concentrates on the management of refractory tonic-clonic status epilepticus.[33,35]

CLINICAL RECOGNITION

Tonic-clonic status epilepticus and its refractory stage are difficult to define. The definition "continuous seizures of more than 5-minute duration or two or more discrete seizures without full recovery of consciousness" is currently considered the most reasonable operational definition. The time limit of several minutes demands rapid intervention.[69]

Tonic-clonic status epilepticus may begin as a single seizure with initial full recovery of consciousness. In typical tonic-clonic status epilepticus, the fits begin to overlap one another. In the extreme case, some body parts may be in a resolving clonic stage and others in a new tonic spell as status epilepticus progresses.[4,9,17] The tonic phase seems to become progressively shorter or may even disappear. Additionally, the clonic phase may lose its characteristics and become brief and less intense, even dispersing into multiple twitches.

Most of the time, a tonic-clonic seizure starts with a tonic contraction lasting 15–30 seconds, and continues with several minutes of repeated muscle contractions, loss of pupillary light response and corneal reflexes, and emergence of bilateral Babinski signs. Very notable at this stage in some patients, as the result of a sympathetic outpouring, is profuse sweating, tachycardia, increased bronchial secretion, and marked hypertension. Before the next seizure begins, patients cannot be roused, and this interval is often marked by labored breathing with frothing at the mouth.

TABLE 40.1. PHARMACEUTICAL AGENTS USED IN THE NICU THAT CAN REDUCE SEIZURE THRESHOLD

Antibiotics	Imipenem
	Norfloxacin
	Ciprofloxacin
	Cefepime
	Penicillin derivatives
Antidepressants	Amitriptyline
	Doxepin
	Nortriptyline
	Fluoxetine, sertraline
Antipsychotics	Chlorpromazine
	Haloperidol
	Thioridazine
	Perphenazine
	Trifluoperazine

Tonic-clonic status epilepticus can lead to remote effects involving vital organs;[27,38,45,92,109] the most pertinent consequences are illustrated in Figure 40.1. These manifestations of status epilepticus can be brief and transient, but also are potentially concerning (e.g., pulmonary edema or aspiration).

NEUROIMAGING AND LABORATORY TESTS

Computed tomography (CT) scan may document a structural lesion and is mandatory in patients with tonic-clonic status epilepticus. It may not be sensitive enough to rule out an underlying new structural lesion and therefore at some point must be supplemented by magnetic resonance imaging (MRI). Changes in CT scan—effacement of sulci from edema or infarction in watershed territories—can be seen in patients who have had a major additional hypoxic–ischemic insult to the brain. Traumatic subarachnoid blood or small hemorrhagic contusions may be noted that could be a consequence of trauma from a fall, rather than a trigger for status epilepticus.

Magnetic resonance imaging may document evidence of encephalitis, evolution of an ischemic stroke, a low-grade astrocytoma, or cavernous malformations. Magnetic resonance imaging scanning may also show small areas of hyperintensity on T2-weighted images in the gray and white matter, often in the posterior vascular watershed

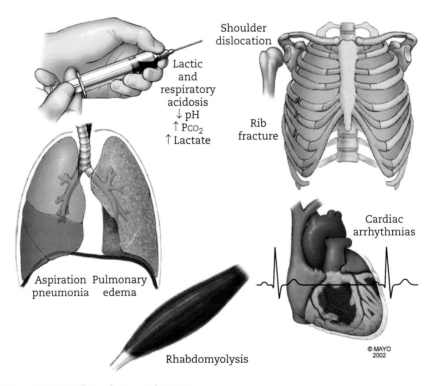

Shoulder dislocation

Lactic and respiratory acidosis
$\downarrow$ pH
$\uparrow$ P_{CO_2}
$\uparrow$ Lactate

Rib fracture

Cardiac arrhythmias

Aspiration Pulmonary
pneumonia   edema

Rhabdomyolysis

© MAYO 2002

FIGURE 40.1: Systemic effects of status epilepticus.

From Wijdicks EFM. The multifaceted care of status epilepticus. *Epilepsia* 2013;54 Suppl 6:61–63.

areas, abnormalities that resolve after seizures are under control. Cerebral edema is the most likely cause for these reversible MRI abnormalities.[119] Diffusion-weighted MRI may document transient increased diffusion in the subcortical white matter and decrease in the cortex, possibly from water flux toward the seizing cortical neurons.[111] Damage to the hippocampus with subsequent hippocampal sclerosis and amygdala kindling may occur as a direct result of status epilepticus and may appear as hyperintensity on T2-weighted images with fluid-attenuated inversion recovery[57,97] (Capsule 40.1). Single-photon emission CT in the interictal phase may show global reduced perfusion after sampling of both hemispheres, but has less value in localizing an epileptic focus. Single-photon emission CT co-registered with MRI may be a helpful test in the documentation of seizure focus after recovery from status epilepticus, particularly when epilepsy surgery is under consideration.[94]

We have noted in our patients with refractory status epilepticus with initially normal MR imaging a gradual development of generalized cerebral atrophy over several months. As expected, none of these patients recovered beyond severe disability, and many not beyond even a minimally conscious state (Figure 40.2). MRI may also show high signal densities in pulvinar structures and opposite cerebellum (crossed cerebellar diaschisis).[1]

Examination of the cerebrospinal fluid (CSF) is obligatory in patients with fever and increased white blood cell counts to exclude bacterial meningitis. Status epilepticus may transiently increase the cell count up to 65 total nucleated cells. Obviously, an increased cell count in the CSF in any patient with status epilepticus should prompt further cultures and empirical antibiotic and antiviral therapy.[90,91] Polymerase chain reaction should be performed for certain types of encephalitis (e.g., herpes simplex). Herpes simplex encephalitis should be considered if family

---

CAPSULE 40.1   NEURONAL DAMAGE ASSOCIATED WITH STATUS EPILEPTICUS

Neuropathologic studies in humans have unequivocally shown that status epilepticus or recurrent generalized seizures can seriously damage the brain.[48,75,77] The most striking abnormalities have been found in the hippocampus and reflect the clinically observed memory deficits in some patients. The hippocampus may swell and have complete cell loss in the CA1 region.[28] The major confounding factor in clinicopathologic correlation of hippocampal damage is hypoxemia, which may be particularly severe in patients with prolonged status epilepticus. Nonetheless, carefully controlled experimental studies have shown that despite adequate oxygenation, 2 hours of status epilepticus can produce neuronal changes, not only in the Sommer sector, but also in thalamic nuclei and pyramidal cortical layers.[75]

The mechanisms of self-sustaining status epilepticus are largely unknown. Maladaptive changes—increased expression of proconvulsive neuropeptides (substance P, neurokinin B) and reduced inhibitory neuropeptides (galanin, dynorphin)—may perpetuate excitability.[20,76]

Convulsive status epilepticus may greatly increase the excitatory amino acid glutamate, which in turn opens cation channels to calcium through N-methyl-D-aspartate receptors ("excitotoxic theory"). Whether this damage, with a proclivity for the hippocampus, thalamus, cerebellum, and neocortex, is also caused by additional hyperglycemia, anoxia, hyperpyrexia, or severe acidosis in humans remains unresolved. Neuronal dropout in the neocortex is predominantly apparent in inappropriately treated or unrecognized long-standing status epilepticus. It can take the form of dramatic MR changes.

With ongoing seizures, the GABA receptors reduce in numbers and are internalized into endocytic vessels and destroyed, which results in decreased GABAergic inhibition.[43] On the other hand, there is increased transport of the NMDA receptors to the synaptic membrane, resulting in an increased number of excitatory NMDA receptors per synapse. Therefore, lack of inhibition and increased excitation as a result of the interplay of these two receptors may perpetuate sustained seizures or status epilepticus.[110]

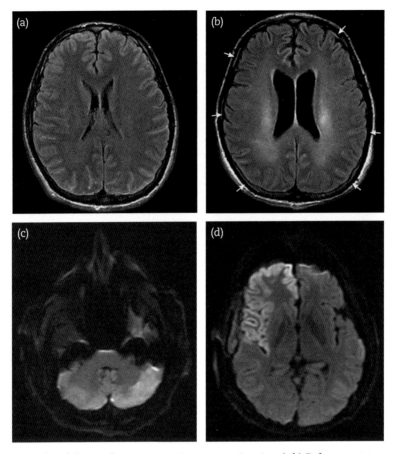

FIGURE 40.2: Examples of abnormalities in magnetic resonance imaging. (a,b) Refractory status epilepticus in a young woman showing emerging cerebral atrophy as evidenced by widening sulci (*arrows*) and ventricular system. (c,d) DWI demonstrates diffusion restriction in the right frontal cortex and insula and left cerebellum as a result of crossed cerebellar diaschisis.

members mention that acute confusion, aphasia, and abruptly high temperatures occurred before seizures began. *Aspergillus* and *Cryptococcus* antigens need to be determined in immunosuppressed patients (Chapter 33). Neuron-specific enolase may be found in increased titers in the CSF (a less robust association is present in serum) and indicate brain injury, but usefulness of this finding in determining outcome is not known.[25]

Results of arterial blood gas examination are often abnormal after status epilepticus. Respiratory acidosis (due to reduced respiratory drive) is common, occurring alone or in combination with metabolic acidosis (due to lactate from muscle injury). Most acid–base abnormalities disappear spontaneously within hours. There is no consistent relation of any of the acid–base abnormalities to cardiac arrhythmias occurring after status epilepticus.[114]

Chest radiography may give an early indication of gastric aspiration. Seldom are typical features of neurogenic pulmonary edema shown.[27] Fractures of the long bones and vertebral bodies may occur, more often, as expected, in elderly patients. Bilateral or unilateral posterior fracture-dislocation of the humeral head is a characteristic fracture (Figure 40.3), but rib fractures and vertebral body compression fractures should be considered when pain suggests those regions. Radiographs are indicated in patients with localized pain, and sometimes MRI of the shoulder is needed to document a major tear or fracture. Pain in the shoulder should not be attributed simply to muscle soreness following seizures.

Conventional electroencephalogram (EEG) documents status epilepticus, and it becomes even more important in patients who need second-line drugs for treatment.[55] Many EEG patterns are seen

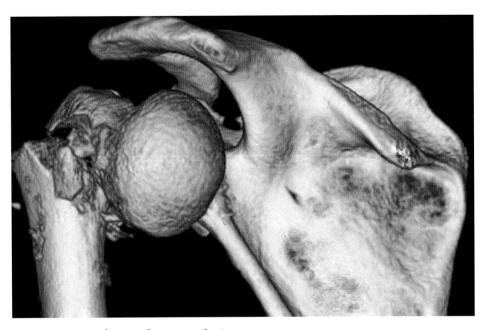

FIGURE 40.3: Humerus fracture after status epilepticus.

(Chapter 11), but in convulsive status epilepticus a five-phase evolution has been proposed.[100] The initial stage shows single epileptic activity followed by high-voltage slow activity. The EEG characteristically shows an episode of silence in the postictal phase. The next stages are characterized by merging of electrographic seizures, accompanied by fluctuating amplitude and frequency of EEG rhythms, continuous ictal activity, or continuous ictal activity punctuated by low-voltage flat periods that finally evolve into a burst-suppression pattern of periodic epileptiform discharges on a flat background. This classification has been criticized because the progressive temporal evolution observed in animal experiments does not appear in clinically encountered cases. A major controversy exists about whether the periodic epileptic discharges in the final stage represent continuing seizure activity, requiring more aggressive treatment, or reflect postictal recovery. Moreover, the claim that the response to treatment declines proportionally with each stage, with a response of almost 20% remaining in patients with periodic epileptic discharges, has not been substantiated in series of adults with status epilepticus.[100]

Mostly electroencephalographic recordings characteristically show a discrete seizure with intermittent flattening that may evolve into periodic lateralized epileptiform discharges (PLEDs). During the course of status epilepticus, EEG may continue to demonstrate outbursts of epileptic activity without any clinically observed motor accompaniment. Whether PLEDs represent potentially reversible continuing epileptic activity or severe cerebral damage is uncertain,[41] but many experts consider PLEDs (bilaterally independent or bilaterally synchronous-generalized) an interictal phenomenon if no motor manifestations occur.

A single EEG infrequently captures all elements of status epilepticus. An EEG should be obtained in a patient with prolonged (about 1 hour) postictal unresponsiveness, to differentiate coma due to continuing seizures from postictal sleep, but earlier in a patient who has received neuromuscular blocking agents and sedative agents with a prolonged anesthetic effect. Generally, to best monitor effect of treatment, video-EEG monitoring is required in any patient with status epilepticus.[62]

FIRST STEPS IN MANAGEMENT

Management of status epilepticus should begin in the emergency department and even ideally in the field[49] (Chapter 11). The first measure is airway control[62,108] (Table 40.2). Many patients have been aspirating, may have copious secretions, and, in fact, may already have an obstructed bronchial branch. Often, endotracheal intubation is necessary because large doses of benzodiazepines have caused drowsiness and upper airway collapse. Invariably, all benzodiazepines greatly depress respiratory drive, causing hypoventilation, transient apneic episodes, and, occasionally, tongue obstruction. However, not all patients in status epilepticus need endotracheal intubation, and a surprising number tolerate multiple doses of lorazepam. Endotracheal intubation is needed when a second-line agent midazolam or propofol is administered.

Mechanical ventilation is necessary after endotracheal intubation, and oxygen delivery is substantially improved by intermittent-mandatory ventilation and pressure support. If oxygenation does not noticeably improve, fiberoptic bronchoscopy may be indicated to investigate possible bronchial obstruction from a foreign body (e.g., tooth fragment) or mucus plug. In the rare situation of neurogenic pulmonary edema, mechanical ventilation with high settings of positive end-expiratory pressure is necessary, but pulmonary edema is short-lived. Aspiration occurred much more often than pulmonary edema in one series of patients with status epilepticus.[114] In none of a consecutive series of 35 patients with treatment-refractory status epilepticus could neurogenic pulmonary edema be implicated as a potential cause for hypoxemia and respiratory acidosis,[114] though others have reported well-documented instances.[27]

After the airway has been secured, two intravenous peripheral catheters must be placed in large arm veins for administration of antiepileptic drugs and possibly a peripherally inserted central catheter for vasopressors.

In patients with multiple seizures, hydration with 0.9% saline (200 mL/hr) is started immediately to reduce the risk of renal failure from rhabdomyolysis, particularly if the admission serum creatine kinase is considerably increased.

Excessive muscle activity depletes glycogen, promotes anaerobic glycolysis, and results in lactate production; thus, metabolic acidosis is frequently found but should not be corrected with bicarbonate until the pH has declined to 7.0.

Acute nonoliguric renal failure from rhabdomyolysis may become apparent with acutely rising serum creatinine, hyperkalemia, and hyperphosphatemia. Initial treatment is to change intravenous fluids from normal saline to D5W with 3

TABLE 40.2. INITIAL MANAGEMENT OF STATUS EPILEPTICUS

Airway management	Intubation if patient has hypoxemia despite facemask with 10 L of 100% oxygen/minute, if abnormal respiratory drive or if abnormal protective reflexes (likely with motor response of withdrawal, or worse)
	Elective endotracheal intubation if second-line treatment (propofol or midazolam) is anticipated
Mechanical ventilation	IMV/PS
	AC with use of anesthetic drugs
Fluid management	2–3 L of 0.9% NaCl; increase with fever or evidence of rhabdomyolysis
Nutrition	Enteral nutrition with continuous infusion (on day 2)
	Blood glucose control (goal 140–180 mg/dL)
Prophylaxis	DVT prophylaxis with pneumatic compression devices
	SC heparin 5,000 U t.i.d.
	GI prophylaxis: pantoprazole 40 mg IV daily or lansoprazole 30 mg orally through nasogastric tube.
	Consider β-blockade or diltiazem infusion in patients with persistent rapid ventricular rate
Specific management	Lorazepam, 4 mg (total dose, 8 mg)
	Phenytoin loading, 20 mg/kg (rate, 50 mg/min or, in elderly, 25 mg/min), or fosphenytoin, 20 mg PE/kg (rate 100–150 mg PE/min)
	If unsuccessful (recurrent clinical seizure or electrographic seizures) proceed with IV midazolam bolus 0.2 mg/kg, start 0.1 mg/kg/hr and increase until seizures stop
Access	Two large-bore intravenous catheters
	Peripheral inserted central catheter or internal jugular central venous line if vasopressors are needed or anticipated

AC, assist control; DVT, deep vein thrombosis; GI, gastrointestinal; IMV, intermittent mandatory ventilation; IV, intravenously; NaCl, sodium chloride; PE, phenytoin equivalents; PS, pressure support; SC, subcutaneously.

ampules of bicarbonate at 200 mL/hr to maintain urinary output of more than 100 mL/hr. Phosphate binders (calcium acetate) are needed until laboratory values normalize.

The effect of status epilepticus on heart muscle has been poorly studied in humans, but recent animal experiments suggest that myocardial hemorrhage, contraction bands, and cardiac pump failure occur within minutes after seizure induction[45,54,71] (Chapter 56). Cardiac arrhythmias are present in 50% of the patients.[98] Sinus tachycardia (ST) is most prevalent. In other patients, multifocal atrial tachycardia, ventricular tachycardia, or a brief asystole after bradycardia has been found. Although ST depressions can be transient in patients with electrocardiographic abnormalities, suggesting ventricular strain or myocardial ischemia, selective protective β-blockade (e.g., with metoprolol) should be considered.[98]

As discussed in Chapter 11, benzodiazepines are the first line of treatment and are virtually immediately followed by intravenous phenytoin loading. The choice of benzodiazepine is arbitrary. Diazepam has traditionally been one of the most successful agents, but it is associated with severe respiratory depression when used repeatedly and may lead to unnecessary intubation.[29] Lorazepam is the preferred benzodiazepine, and has the advantage of terminating seizures in almost 80% of patients.[63] It is effective for approximately 1–3 hours, and is administered in a dose of 4 mg at 1–2 mg/min to a maximum of 8 mg total. Lorazepam is not more effective than phenobarbital or a combination of diazepam and phenytoin for initial treatment, but a randomized trial found the highest response rate and fewest side effects in lorazepam-treated patients.[101] Lorazepam appeared to be more effective than diazepam in a clinical randomized trial investigating its safety when administered by paramedics.[2] Lorazepam should, therefore, be considered the most appropriate first-line agent to terminate status epilepticus.

In general, intravenous loading with phenytoin is standard after patients have been treated with benzodiazepines.[88] Oral administration of 300 mg of phenytoin after intravenous loading should begin 6 hours after infusion and produces steady serum levels of phenytoin after 4 days of treatment.[26] Phenytoin is infused in isotonic saline, the infusion rate must not exceed 50 mg/min, and the rate must be halved in elderly patients. Infusion in a typical patient of 80 kg takes 30 minutes, but seizures should stop after approximately 10 minutes. A more rapid infusion has the disadvantage of increasing the risk of hypotension and cardiac arrhythmias.[36] These side effects are more common in elderly patients and, in addition to a direct cardiotoxic effect, may be more common in poorly hydrated patients.[10]

Some of the major side effects have been overcome with the introduction of fosphenytoin. The drug, however, is not widely available outside the United States. Fosphenytoin (Cerebyx), a water-soluble disodium phosphate ester of phenytoin, does not require the propylene glycol vehicle that is often responsible for hypotension and cardiac arrhythmias.[87] We have been using fosphenytoin intravenously for status epilepticus; the dose is similar to that of phenytoin and is expressed in phenytoin equivalents, but the recommended rate for status epilepticus is 100–150 mg of phenytoin equivalents per minute three times (faster than that for intravenous phenytoin). Careful checking of labels is required, because rapid infusion of phenytoin mistaken for fosphenytoin may cause life-threatening cardiac arrhythmias.[115] If status epilepticus is not reversed with lorazepam, phenytoin, or fosphenytoin, several more options are available, but recommendations are not based on comparative studies, vary considerably, are guided by personal opinion, and follow trends. This approach is consistent with a recent recommendation from the Neurocritical Care Society (NCS). The NCS has published an approach based on a consensus statement (Part XIV, Guidelines). The major recommendations reflect current practices and include (1) rapid treatment of clinical and electrographic seizures; (2) IV lorazepam, intramuscular midazolam, or rectal diazepam as first-line drugs; (3) IV (fos)phenytoin, valproic acid, or levetiracetam as second-line drugs; (4) anesthetic drugs should be titrated to burst suppression or isoelectric EEG; (5) duration of treatment should be at least 24 hours before weaning from anesthetic drugs; and (6) maintenance drugs should be provided before weaning.[15]

DETERIORATION: CAUSES AND MANAGEMENT

Two major forms of clinical deterioration occur in status epilepticus: first, recurrence of seizures almost immediately after completion of phenytoin (or fosphenytoin) infusion, and second, breakthrough seizures every time the anesthetic agent is tapered. Both forms are considered therapy-refractory status epilepticus.

Failure to control seizures has several causes, and each should be explored.[8] The most common cause is an inadequate dose of phenytoin. Most often, a typical but highly insufficient 1,000 mg infusion of phenytoin has been ordered. This dose, originally from the landmark paper by Wallis et al.,[107] is most likely used because a dose of 1 g is easily remembered; however, it translates to a body weight of 50 kg. Other causes of failure to control seizures, besides an acute structural brain lesion, are persistence of a metabolic derangement (e.g., hyponatremia, recurrent hypoglycemia, or hyperglycemia), drug toxicity, and CNS infection. In some patients, the reason for the poor initial response remains unknown, and treatment with lorazepam and phenytoin is simply not sufficient to control seizures.

It is best to have a predetermined idea of which agent to use, rather than to frequently switch agents. Algorithms on status epilepticus have a short shelf life and drugs often change priority. A reasonable guideline is shown in Figure 40.4. The doses of antiepileptic drugs are summarized in Table 40.3. Drug interactions are found in the Part XIV, Guidelines.

Before a new antiepileptic agent is considered, an additional infusion of fosphenytoin at one-third or half of the original infusion dose (usually 5–10 mg/kg) is useful to maximize fosphenytoin loading. This probably should be given after an additional intravenous dose of 4 mg of lorazepam.

Many neurointensivists and epileptologists now directly proceed with midazolam, propofol, or pentobarbital anesthesia.[10,22,62,66,82,85,123] Midazolam has emerged as a preferred second-line antiepileptic drug for status epilepticus.[10-12,39,52,61,80,106] The recommended loading dose is 0.2 mg/kg intravenously in a bolus, and this is followed by an infusion of 0.1–0.6 mg/kg/hr until the EEG is free of seizure activity. However, midazolam is several times more expensive than barbiturates when used in an intravenous infusion. In addition, with increasing doses, blood pressure may decrease significantly, with a need for long-term vasopressors. A comparative study with pentobarbital is not available.

An alternative approach is to use high doses of propofol.[56,70,117] Propofol is administered in a bolus of 2 mg/kg, followed by an infusion of 5 mg/kg/hr, later tapered to 1–5 mg/kg/hr. Propofol acts through enhancement of γ-aminobutyric acid (GABA)-mediated transmission, possibly at the chloride ion channel, different from that with benzodiazepines and barbiturates.[16]

The enthusiasm for propofol has diminished after an early initially unexplained report of four-fold higher mortality.[82] As discussed in Chapter 16, there have been many reports of a propofol infusion syndrome (PRIS), an unexplained sudden cardiovascular collapse in patients treated with high doses (more than 10 mg/kg/hr) and for more than 3 days, although PRIS may occur hours after infusion of propofol and in much lower doses. Propofol is currently ill-advised in the treatment of status epilepticus when frequent high doses or prolonged treatment is anticipated.[118,121]

Pentobarbital can be strongly considered if prior drugs fail. Pentobarbital is administered intravenously as an initial bolus of 10–15 mg/kg over 1–2 hours, followed by infusion of 1–3 mg/kg/

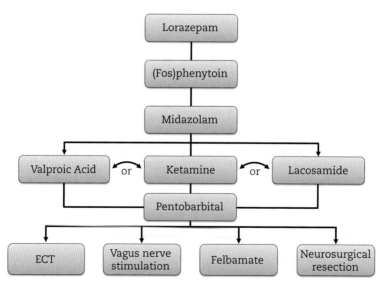

FIGURE 40.4: Algorithm for treatment-refractory status epilepticus.

ECT, electro-convulsive therapy.

TABLE 40.3. INTRAVENOUS ANTIEPILEPTIC AGENTS USED TO TREAT CONVULSIVE STATUS EPILEPTICUS

Drug	Initial Dose (Bolus)	Rate	Infusion (Maintenance)	Precautions
Midazolam	0.2 mg/kg	< 4 mg/min	0.1–0.6 mg/kg/hr	Mechanical ventilation invariably needed; vasopressors for hypotension
Lorazepam	4 mg	1–2 mg/min		Cardiac monitoring for cardiac arrhythmias (bradycardia)
Phenytoin	18–20 mg/kg	50 mg/min		Cardiac and blood pressure monitoring
Fosphenytoin	18–20 mg PE/kg	100–150 mg PE/min		Cardiac and blood pressure monitoring
Phenobarbital	10–20 mg/kg	30–50 mg/min	1–3 mg/kg/hr	Mechanical ventilation with high dose (> 40 mg/kg) may be needed
Pentobarbital	10–15 mg/kg	1–2 hours	1–3 mg/kg/hr	Vasopressors for hypotension
Lidocaine	1.5–2 mg/kg	< 50 mg/min	3 mg/kg/hr	Cardiac monitoring (bradycardia, heart block)
Isoflurane	Inhalation to MAC (0.8%–1.1%)			Full anesthetic system and anesthesia support
Propofol	2 mg/kg initially	Slow push	1–5 mg/kg/hr	Vasopressors for hypotension (monitoring for metabolic acidosis)
Ketamine	1 mg/kg	2 min	10–50 mg/kg/min	Tachyphylaxis (increasing dose needed)
Valproate	20–30 mg/kg	20 mg/min	1–4 mg/kg/hr	Monitoring of albumin

MAC, minimum alveolar concentration; PE, phenytoin equivalents.

hr until seizures stop clinically and on EEG.[68,81,83] Pentobarbital has a marked cardiodepressant effect, and many patients need vasopressors for blood pressure support. A burst-suppression pattern, up to 30 seconds, is preferable, but one may argue that an EEG without superimposed epileptic discharges is equally effective. In fact, burst suppression on EEG recording does not mean that intermittent brief seizures cannot occur. Pushing the pentobarbital dosage to a burst-suppression or flat EEG pattern may markedly increase the need for more vasopressors. Thus, aiming for an EEG without seizure activity may considerably reduce the side effects of pentobarbital. However, in daily practice, the EEG may fluctuate from burst

suppression to bilateral PLEDs without appreciable bursts of seizures. This EEG recording may be a satisfactory endpoint.

A major management problem arises when generalized tonic-clonic seizures are not controlled or continue to recur after discontinuation of barbiturate therapy. Failure to control seizures with barbiturate anesthesia seems very uncommon, but if it happens, the chance of effectively controlling seizures is low, and morbidity is high in these patients.

The third line of therapy in refractory status epilepticus is even more anecdotal.

Isoflurane is an attractive option and highly effective.[58,74,84,120] In a series of 11 patients with treatment-refractory status epilepticus, morbidity and mortality remained high despite seizure control. In our experience with several patients, control of seizures is achieved almost immediately. Isoflurane is used in concentrations of minimum alveolar concentration (MAC of 1.15%), but progressively higher concentrations are often needed to control seizures. Isoflurane is a great way to control status epilepticus, but whether it is successful long term is unknown.[122]

Lidocaine has shown efficacy in therapy-refractory status epilepticus, but we have little experience with the drug.[73,105] Lidocaine is injected in a bolus of 1.5–2 mg/kg in several minutes, followed by an infusion of 3 mg/kg/hr. The infusion should not be continued for more than 12 hours. Its use is limited in patients with a history of cardiac arrhythmias or electrocardiographic evidence of any type of heart block and poor ejection fraction on echocardiography. Use in patients with liver failure is also contraindicated due to decreased hepatic clearance, and a high level of lidocaine, which itself can lead to seizures, may result.

New alternative agents for the treatment of refractory status epilepticus include ketamine and valproate. Experience is limited, and undoubtedly only successful cases have been published, so the physician must exercise great caution in their use as a treatment for status epilepticus. A short-acting anticonvulsant, an N-methyl-D-aspartate receptor antagonist, ketamine, surprisingly controlled status epilepticus in one patient refractory to phenytoin, phenobarbital, midazolam, propofol, valproate, and lidocaine infusion. This unconfirmed experience is valuable. Ketamine was used in a bolus of 2 mg/kg over 2 minutes, followed by an infusion of 10–50 mg/kg/min, a dose that does not cause respiratory depression. The infusion dose is then tapered to 7.5 mg/kg/hr for 7–14 days.[13,89] We have gradually moved ketamine up in priority and use it as a second-line agent.[60]

Intravenous valproate has been recently introduced, but its efficacy is unknown, and control of seizures is only 30%. Its major advantage may be that it does not reduce blood pressure and thus may be a good alternative in patients who have become cardio-vascularly unstable with midazolam and propofol.[51] It also has virtually no respiratory depression. Intravenous loading doses of valproate can be 25–30 mg/kg, with infusion rate of 20 mg/min to attain a steady-state serum concentration of 75 mg/L. It is highly bound to albumin, and toxicity may rapidly arise in patients with poor nutritional intake; it has been implicated in abnormal hemostasis.[31,42,56,93]

When all else fails, it makes common sense to try to treat seizures with a radically different approach. Lacosamide,[53,79] levetiracetam,[3] nimodipine,[14] resection of an (identifiable) epileptic focus, vagus nerve stimulation, high-dose phenobarbital (100–300 mg/mL plasma levels), and electroconvulsive therapy[24,54,64] have all been considered with variable success.

Weaning from intravenous antiepileptic drugs has not been carefully studied. We prefer to treat patients aggressively (burst-suppression or mostly suppressed EEG pattern) for at least 24 hours, aiming for a seizure-free period of another 24 hours. Then we reduce the dose 10% every hour, while monitoring with video-EEG for recurrence, and then either stop weaning or increase the dose. An aggressive approach with prolonged use of anesthetic drugs for several months may be justified only in young patients with traumatic brain injury, in encephalitis, and in patients with MRI findings that do not suggest widespread cortical damage.

OUTCOME

The prognosis of status epilepticus depends on several factors.[37,47,50,86,96,104] The most important finding has been the association of the actual time that patients have remained in tonic-clonic status epilepticus and later morbidity. This finding, however, probably does not hold for patients in nonconvulsive status epilepticus. Nonconvulsive status epilepticus lasting many days may result in a favorable outcome, but data are sparse in this category of patients.[19,46,116]

Patients with tonic-clonic status epilepticus have a considerable risk of permanent morbidity. A duration of status epilepticus of less than 10 hours[34,35] seems an important cutoff point, and good outcome is possible within this time period. Considerable neurologic improvement can be expected in some patients. A neuropsychologic study in nine patients with previous epilepsy who were tested before and after status epilepticus found no substantial changes in cognitive ability.[32]

In most of our patients—some treated for 3–6 months—seizures stopped ("burned out") or became stimulus-induced myoclonic twitches, but often leading to long-term disability.[124] Status epilepticus in young patients with normal MRI warrants long-term management, and a satisfactory outcome is not an unrealistic possibility.

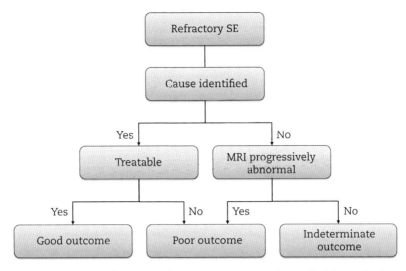

FIGURE 40.5: Outcome algorithm for status epilepticus. Poor outcome: Severe disability or death, vegetative state. Functional independence: No assistance needed, minor handicap may remain.

Mortality in status epilepticus is based on hospital series alone; therefore, considerable referral bias exists. A review of deaths related to status epilepticus found a mortality of 2% in adult status epilepticus.[90] In a study of 282 consecutive admissions, mortality from status epilepticus could be linked to an underlying disorder in all but two patients.[44] Mortality was higher in patients with stroke if status epilepticus occurred within 7 days of stroke.[103] Anoxic–ischemic insult to the brain and older age predicted mortality in status epilepticus and could be related to cardiac resuscitation in the first place.[23,65] The role of withdrawal of support in a patient failing to improve is difficult to abstract from those studies.

The risk of subsequent epilepsy in adult patients with de novo status epilepticus is 12% and includes a similar risk of recurrent status epilepticus of 13%.[90,102] Risks are higher in patients with known structural lesions, onset of seizure disorder during adolescence, and neurologic abnormalities.[17] In general, predictive factors for poor outcome include the lack of response to first treatment and the underlying cause of status epilepticus, particularly when these are associated with anoxic–ischemic encephalopathy, acute stroke, encephalitis, diffuse axonal head injury, or a primary malignant tumor.[67] Status epilepticus associated with anoxic–ischemic injury and older age significantly increase the odds of a higher incidence of severe, persistent disability.[99] An outcome algorithm is shown in Figure 40.5.

CONCLUSION

- One can expect that a large proportion of patients with status epilepticus can be controlled with benzodiazepines (lorazepam 4–8 mg) and an adequate loading dose of phenytoin (20 mg/kg, 50 mg/min).
- Recurrence of seizures after adequate phenytoin loading could be treated with midazolam or propofol infusion.
- If all else fails, intravenous administration of ketamine, pentobarbital, isoflurane, or electroconvulsive therapy should be considered.
- Outcome of status epilepticus is strongly related to the response to the first dose of antiepileptic agent and to the underlying trigger.

REFERENCES

1. Ahn HS, Kim KK. Two cases of crossed cerebellar diaschisis with or without thalamic lesion on brain MRI in status epilepticus. *J Epilepsy Res* 2014;4:74–77.
2. Alldredge BK, Gelb AM, Isaacs SM, et al. A comparison of lorazepam, diazepam, and placebo for the treatment of out-of-hospital status epilepticus. *N Engl J Med* 2001;345:631–637.
3. Altenmuller DM, Kuhn A, Surges R, Schulze-Bonhage A. Termination of absence status epilepticus by low-dose intravenous levetiracetam. *Epilepsia* 2008;49:1289–1290.

4. Aminoff MJ, Simon RP. Status epilepticus: causes, clinical features and consequences in 98 patients. *Am J Med* 1980;69:657–666.

5. Barry E, Hauser WA. Status epilepticus and antiepileptic medication levels. *Neurology* 1994;44:47–50.

6. Barry E, Hauser WA. Status epilepticus: the interaction of epilepsy and acute brain disease. *Neurology* 1993;43:1473–1478.

7. Bateman BT, Claassen J, Willey JZ, et al. Convulsive status epilepticus after ischemic stroke and intracerebral hemorrhage: frequency, predictors, and impact on outcome in a large administrative dataset. *Neurocrit Care* 2007;7:187–193.

8. Betjemann JP, Lowenstein DH. Status epilepticus in adults. *Lancet Neurol* 2015;14:615–624.

9. Bleck TP. Convulsive disorders: status epilepticus. *Clin Neuropharmacol* 1991;14:191–198.

10. Bleck TP. Intensive care unit management of patients with status epilepticus. *Epilepsia* 2007;48(Suppl 8):59–60.

11. Bleck TP. Management approaches to prolonged seizures and status epilepticus. *Epilepsia* 1999;40(Suppl 1):S59–S63.

12. Bleck TP. Transatlantic similarities and differences in the management of status epilepticus. *Epilepsia* 2008;49:1285–1287.

13. Borris DJ, Bertram EH, Kapur J. Ketamine controls prolonged status epilepticus. *Epilepsy Res* 2000;42:117–122.

14. Brandt L, Saveland H, Ljunggren B, Andersson KE. Control of epilepsy partialis continuans with intravenous nimodipine: report of two cases. *J Neurosurg* 1988;69:949–950.

15. Brophy GM, Bell R, Claassen J, et al. Guidelines for the evaluation and management of status epilepticus. *Neurocrit Care* 2012;17:3–23.

16. Brown LA, Levin GM. Role of propofol in refractory status epilepticus. *Ann Pharmacother* 1998;32:1053–1059.

17. Browne TR, Holmes GL. Epilepsy. *N Engl J Med* 2001;344:1145–1151.

18. Carpio A, Hauser WA. Epilepsy in the developing world. *Curr Neurol Neurosci Rep* 2009;9:319–326.

19. Cascino GD. Nonconvulsive status epilepticus in adults and children. *Epilepsia* 1993;34 Suppl 1:S21–S28.

20. Chen JW, Wasterlain CG. Status epilepticus: pathophysiology and management in adults. *Lancet Neurol* 2006;5:246–256.

21. Claassen J, Bateman BT, Willey JZ, et al. Generalized convulsive status epilepticus after nontraumatic subarachnoid hemorrhage: the nationwide inpatient sample. *Neurosurgery* 2007;61:60–64.

22. Claassen J, Hirsch LJ, Mayer SA. Treatment of status epilepticus: a survey of neurologists. *J Neurol Sci* 2003;211:37–41.

23. Claassen J, Lokin JK, Fitzsimmons BF, Mendelsohn FA, Mayer SA. Predictors of functional disability and mortality after status epilepticus. *Neurology* 2002;58:139–142.

24. Cline JS, Roos K. Treatment of status epilepticus with electroconvulsive therapy. *J Ect* 2007;23:30–32.

25. Correale J, Rabinowicz AL, Heck CN, et al. Status epilepticus increases CSF levels of neuron-specific enolase and alters the blood-brain barrier. *Neurology* 1998;50:1388–1391.

26. Cranford RE, Leppik IE, Patrick B, Anderson CB, Kostick B. Intravenous phenytoin: clinical and pharmacokinetic aspects. *Neurology* 1978;28:874–880.

27. Darnell JC, Jay SJ. Recurrent postictal pulmonary edema: a case report and review of the literature. *Epilepsia* 1982;23:71–83.

28. DeGiorgio CM, Tomiyasu U, Gott PS, Treiman DM. Hippocampal pyramidal cell loss in human status epilepticus. *Epilepsia* 1992;33:23–27.

29. Delgado-Escueta AV, Enrile-Bacsal F. Combination therapy for status epilepticus: intravenous diazepam and phenytoin. *Adv Neurol* 1983;34:477–485.

30. DeLorenzo RJ, Hauser WA, Towne AR, et al. A prospective, population-based epidemiologic study of status epilepticus in Richmond, Virginia. *Neurology* 1996;46:1029–1035.

31. Devinsky O, Leppik I, Willmore LJ, et al. Safety of intravenous valproate. *Ann Neurol* 1995;38:670–674.

32. Dodrill CB, Wilensky AJ. Intellectual impairment as an outcome of status epilepticus. *Neurology* 1990;40:23–27.

33. Drislane FW. Who's afraid of status epilepticus? *Epilepsia* 2006;47:7–9.

34. Drislane FW, Blum AS, Lopez MR, Gautam S, Schomer DL. Duration of refractory status epilepticus and outcome: loss of prognostic utility after several hours. *Epilepsia* 2009;50:1566–1571.

35. Drislane FW, Lopez MR, Blum AS, Schomer DL. Detection and treatment of refractory status epilepticus in the intensive care unit. *J Clin Neurophysiol* 2008;25:181–186.

36. Earnest MP, Marx JA, Drury LR. Complications of intravenous phenytoin for acute treatment of seizures: recommendations for usage. *JAMA* 1983;249:762–765.

37. Ferlisi M, Shorvon S. The outcome of therapies in refractory and super-refractory convulsive status epilepticus and recommendations for therapy. *Brain* 2012;135:2314–2328.

38. Finelli PF, Cardi JK. Seizure as a cause of fracture. *Neurology* 1989;39:858–860.

39. Fountain NB, Adams RE. Midazolam treatment of acute and refractory status epilepticus. *Clin Neuropharmacol* 1999;22:261–267.

40. Gaitanis JN, Drislane FW. Status epilepticus: a review of different syndromes, their current evaluation, and treatment. *Neurologist* 2003;9:61–76.

41. Garzon E, Fernandes RM, Sakamoto AC. Serial EEG during human status epilepticus: evidence for PLED as an ictal pattern. *Neurology* 2001;57:1175–1183.

42. Gidal B, Spencer N, Maly M, et al. Valproate-mediated disturbances of hemostasis: relationship to dose and plasma concentration. *Neurology* 1994;44:1418–1422.

43. Goodkin HP, Yeh JL, Kapur J. Status epilepticus increases the intracellular accumulation of GABAA receptors. *J Neurosci* 2005;25:5511–5520.

44. Goulon M, Levy-Alcover MA, Nouailhat F. [Status epilepticus in the adult. Epidemiologic and clinical study in an intensive care unit]. *Rev Electroencephalogr Neurophysiol Clin* 1985;14:277–285.

45. Gravenstein JS, Anton AH, Wiener SM, Tetlow AG. Catecholamine and cardiovascular response to electro-convulsion therapy in man. *Br J Anaesth* 1965;37:833–839.

46. Guberman A, Cantu-Reyna G, Stuss D, Broughton R. Nonconvulsive generalized status epilepticus: clinical features, neuropsychological testing, and long-term follow-up. *Neurology* 1986;36:1284–1291.

47. Hauser WA. Status epilepticus: epidemiologic considerations. *Neurology* 1990;40:9–13.

48. Hauser WA, Lee JR. Do seizures beget seizures? *Prog Brain Res* 2002;135:215–219.

49. Hirsch LJ. Intramuscular versus intravenous benzodiazepines for prehospital treatment of status epilepticus. *N Engl J Med* 2012;366:659–660.

50. Hocker SE, Britton JW, Mandrekar JN, Wijdicks EFM, Rabinstein AA. Predictors of outcome in refractory status epilepticus. *JAMA Neurol* 2013;70:72–77.

51. Hodges BM, Mazur JE. Intravenous valproate in status epilepticus. *Ann Pharmacother* 2001;35:1465–1470.

52. Jagoda A, Riggio S. Refractory status epilepticus in adults. *Ann Emerg Med* 1993;22:1337–1348.

53. Jain V, Harvey AS. Treatment of refractory tonic status epilepticus with intravenous lacosamide. *Epilepsia* 2012;53:761–762.

54. Kamel H, Cornes SB, Hegde M, Hall SE, Josephson SA. Electroconvulsive therapy for refractory status epilepticus: a case series. *Neurocrit Care* 2010;12:204–210.

55. Kaplan PW. EEG monitoring in the intensive care unit. *Am J Electroneurodiagnostic Technol* 2006;46:81–97.

56. Kaplan PW. Intravenous valproate treatment of generalized nonconvulsive status epilepticus. *Clin Electroencephalogr* 1999;30:1–4.

57. Kim JA, Chung JI, Yoon PH, et al. Transient MR signal changes in patients with generalized tonicoclonic seizure or status epilepticus: periictal diffusion-weighted imaging. *AJNR Am J Neuroradiol* 2001;22:1149–1160.

58. Kofke WA, Young RS, Davis P, et al. Isoflurane for refractory status epilepticus: a clinical series. *Anesthesiology* 1989;71:653–659.

59. Kozak OS, Wijdicks EFM, Manno EM, Miley JT, Rabinstein AA. Status epilepticus as initial manifestation of posterior reversible encephalopathy syndrome. *Neurology* 2007;69:894–897.

60. Kramer AH. Early ketamine to treat refractory status epilepticus. *Neurocrit Care* 2012;16:299–305.

61. Kumar A, Bleck TP. Intravenous midazolam for the treatment of refractory status epilepticus. *Crit Care Med* 1992;20:483–488.

62. Lawn ND, Wijdicks EFM. Progress in clinical neurosciences: status epilepticus: a critical review of management options. *Can J Neurol Sci* 2002;29:206–215.

63. Leppik IE, Derivan AT, Homan RW, et al. Double-blind study of lorazepam and diazepam in status epilepticus. *JAMA* 1983;249:1452–1454.

64. Lisanby SH, Bazil CW, Resor SR, et al. ECT in the treatment of status epilepticus. *J Ect* 2001;17:210–215.

65. Logroscino G, Hesdorffer DC, Cascino GD, et al. Long-term mortality after a first episode of status epilepticus. *Neurology* 2002;58:537–541.

66. Lowenstein DH. Treatment options for status epilepticus. *Curr Opin Pharmacol* 2005;5:334–339.

67. Lowenstein DH, Alldredge BK. Status epilepticus at an urban public hospital in the 1980s. *Neurology* 1993;43:483–488.

68. Lowenstein DH, Aminoff MJ, Simon RP. Barbiturate anesthesia in the treatment of status epilepticus: clinical experience with 14 patients. *Neurology* 1988;38:395–400.

69. Lowenstein DH, Bleck T, Macdonald RL. It's time to revise the definition of status epilepticus. *Epilepsia* 1999;40:120–122.

70. Mackenzie SJ, Kapadia F, Grant IS. Propofol infusion for control of status epilepticus. *Anaesthesia* 1990;45:1043–1045.

71. Manno EM, Pfeifer EA, Cascino GD, Noe KH, Wijdicks EFM. Cardiac pathology in status epilepticus. *Ann Neurol* 2005;58:954–957.

72. Marchi NA, Novy J, Faouzi M, et al. Status epilepticus: impact of therapeutic coma on outcome. *Crit Care Med* 2015 May;43(5):1003–1009.

73. Marik PE, Varon J. The management of status epilepticus. *Chest* 2004;126:582–591.

74. Meeke RI, Soifer BE, Gelb AW. Isoflurane for the management of status epilepticus. *Dicp* 1989;23:579–581.

75. Meldrum BS, Brierley JB. Prolonged epileptic seizures in primates: ischemic cell change and its relation to ictal physiological events. *Arch Neurol* 1973;28:10–17.

76. Murdoch D. Mechanisms of status epilepticus: an evidence-based review. *Curr Opin Neurol* 2007;20:213–216.

77. Nevander G, Ingvar M, Auer R, Siesjo BK. Status epilepticus in well-oxygenated rats causes neuronal necrosis. *Ann Neurol* 1985;18:281–290.

78. Oxbury JM, Whitty CW. Causes and consequences of status epilepticus in adults:a study of 86 cases. *Brain* 1971;94:733–744.

79. Paquette V, Culley C, Greanya ED, Ensom MH. Lacosamide as adjunctive therapy in refractory epilepsy in adults: a systematic review. *Seizure* 2015;25:1–17.

80. Parent JM, Lowenstein DH. Treatment of refractory generalized status epilepticus with continuous infusion of midazolam. *Neurology* 1994;44:1837–1840.

81. Parviainen I, Uusaro A, Kalviainen R, et al. High-dose thiopental in the treatment of refractory status epilepticus in intensive care unit. *Neurology* 2002;59:1249–1251.

82. Prasad A, Worrall BB, Bertram EH, Bleck TP. Propofol and midazolam in the treatment of refractory status epilepticus. *Epilepsia* 2001;42:380–386.

83. Rashkin MC, Youngs C, Penovich P. Pentobarbital treatment of refractory status epilepticus. *Neurology* 1987;37:500–503.

84. Ropper AH, Kofke WA, Bromfield EB, Kennedy SK. Comparison of isoflurane, halothane, and nitrous oxide in status epilepticus. *Ann Neurol* 1986;19:98–99.

85. Rossetti AO. Which anesthetic should be used in the treatment of refractory status epilepticus? *Epilepsia* 2007;48 Suppl 8:52–55.

86. Rossetti AO, Hurwitz S, Logroscino G, Bromfield EB. Prognosis of status epilepticus: role of etiology, age, and consciousness impairment at presentation. *J Neurol Neurosurg Psychiatry* 2006;77:611–615.

87. Runge JW, Allen FH. Emergency treatment of status epilepticus. *Neurology* 1996;46:S20–23.

88. Shaner DM, McCurdy SA, Herring MO, Gabor AJ. Treatment of status epilepticus: a prospective comparison of diazepam and phenytoin versus phenobarbital and optional phenytoin. *Neurology* 1988;38:202–207.

89. Sheth RD, Gidal BE. Refractory status epilepticus: response to ketamine. *Neurology* 1998;51:1765–1766.

90. Shorvon S. Tonic clonic status epilepticus. *J Neurol Neurosurg Psychiatry* 1993;56:125–134.

91. Shorvon S, Ferlisi M. The treatment of super-refractory status epilepticus: a critical review of available therapies and a clinical treatment protocol. *Brain* 2011;134:2802–2818.

92. Simon RP. Physiologic consequences of status epilepticus. *Epilepsia* 1985;26 Suppl 1:S58–66.

93. Sinha S, Naritoku DK. Intravenous valproate is well tolerated in unstable patients with status epilepticus. *Neurology* 2000;55:722–724.

94. So EL. Integration of EEG, MRI, and SPECT in localizing the seizure focus for epilepsy surgery. *Epilepsia* 2000;41 Suppl 3:S48–54.

95. Spatola M, Alvarez V, Rossetti AO. Benzodiazepine overtreatment in status epilepticus is related to higher need of intubation and longer hospitalization. *Epilepsia* 2013;54:e99–e102.

96. Tiamkao S, Pranboon S, Thepsuthammarat K, Sawanyawisuth K. Incidences and outcomes of status epilepticus: a 9-year longitudinal national study. *Epilepsy Behav* 2015;49:135–137.

97. Tien RD, Felsberg GJ. The hippocampus in status epilepticus: demonstration of signal intensity and morphologic changes with sequential fast spin-echo MR imaging. *Radiology* 1995;194:249–256.

98. Tigaran S, Rasmussen V, Dam M, et al. ECG changes in epilepsy patients. *Acta Neurol Scand* 1997;96:72–75.

99. Towne AR, Pellock JM, Ko D, DeLorenzo RJ. Determinants of mortality in status epilepticus. *Epilepsia* 1994;35:27–34.

100. Treiman DM. Generalized convulsive status epilepticus in the adult. *Epilepsia* 1993;34 Suppl 1:S2–11.

101. Treiman DM, Meyers PD, Walton NY, et al. A comparison of four treatments for generalized convulsive status epilepticus. Veterans Affairs Status Epilepticus Cooperative Study Group. *N Engl J Med* 1998;339:792–798.

102. Tsetsou S, Novy J, Rossetti AO. Recurrence of status epilepticus: prognostic role and outcome predictors. *Epilepsia* 2015;56:473–478.

103. Velioglu SK, Ozmenoglu M, Boz C, Alioglu Z. Status epilepticus after stroke. *Stroke* 2001;32:1169–1172.

104. Vignatelli L, Tonon C, D'Alessandro R. Incidence and short-term prognosis of status epilepticus in adults in Bologna, Italy. *Epilepsia* 2003;44:964–968.

105. Walker IA, Slovis CM. Lidocaine in the treatment of status epilepticus. *Acad Emerg Med* 1997;4:918–922.

106. Walker M. Status epilepticus: an evidence based guide. *BMJ* 2005;331:673–677.

107. Wallis W, Kutt H, McDowell F. Intravenous diphenylhydantoin in treatment of acute repetitive seizures. *Neurology* 1968;18:513–525.

108. Walls RM, Sagarin MJ. Status epilepticus. *N Engl J Med* 1998;339:409.

109. Walton NY. Systemic effects of generalized convulsive status epilepticus. *Epilepsia* 1993;34 Suppl 1:S54–S58.

110. Wasterlain C, Treiman D. *Status Epilepticus: Mechanisms and Management*. Cambridge, MA: MIT Press; 2006.

111. Wieshmann UC, Symms MR, Shorvon SD. Diffusion changes in status epilepticus. *Lancet* 1997;350:493–494.

112. Wijdicks EFM. The multifaceted care of status epilepticus. *Epilepsia* 2013;54 Suppl 6:61–63.

113. Wijdicks EFM. Neurologic complications in critically ill patients. *Anesth Analg* 1996;83:411–419.

114. Wijdicks EFM, Hubmayr RD. Acute acid-base disorders associated with status epilepticus. *Mayo Clinic Proc* 1994;69:1044–1046.

115. Wilder BJ. Use of parenteral antiepileptic drugs and the role for fosphenytoin. *Neurology* 1996;46:S1–S2.

116. Williamson PD, Spencer DD, Spencer SS, Novelly RA, Mattson RH. Complex partial status epilepticus: a depth-electrode study. *Ann Neurol* 1985;18:647–654.

117. Wood PR, Browne GP, Pugh S. Propofol infusion for the treatment of status epilepticus. *Lancet* 1988;1:480–481.

118. Wysowski DK, Pollock ML. Reports of death with use of propofol (Diprivan) for nonprocedural (long-term) sedation and literature review. *Anesthesiology* 2006;105:1047–1051.

119. Yaffe K, Ferriero D, Barkovich AJ, Rowley H. Reversible MRI abnormalities following seizures. *Neurology* 1995;45:104–108.

120. Young GB, Blume WT, Bolton CF, Warren KG. Anesthetic barbiturates in refractory status epilepticus. *Can J Neurol Sci* 1980;7:291–292.

121. Zarovnaya EL, Jobst BC, Harris BT. Propofol-associated fatal myocardial failure and rhabdomyolysis in an adult with status epilepticus. *Epilepsia* 2007;48:1002–1006.

122. Zeiler FA, Zeiler KJ, Teitelbaum J, Gillman LM, West M. Modern inhalational anesthetics for refractory status epilepticus. *Can J Neurol Sci* 2015:1–10.

123. Ziai WC, Kaplan PW. Seizures and status epilepticus in the intensive care unit. *Semin Neurol* 2008;28:668–681.

124. Zubkov AY, Rabinstein AA, Manno EM, Wijdicks EFM. Prolonged refractory status epilepticus related to thrombotic thrombocytopenic purpura. *Neurocrit Care* 2008;9:361–365.

41

Traumatic Brain Injury

Assault or accidental trauma to the brain merits stabilization in the emergency department (ED) and, as a matter of course, admission to the neurosciences intensive care unit (NICU) or trauma unit for expeditious management. Traumatic brain injury (TBI) is a major cause of disability in young persons, and leads to the expenditure of billions of dollars in health care. Epidemiologic surveys have estimated that the number of newly disabled survivors of TBI in the United States each year is nearly 80,000, thus amounting to a "silent epidemic."[27,33] The fact is that few options are available, other than primary prevention (seat belts, air bags, and helmets) of mechanical neuronal injury. Several drug options for secondary damage are currently tested. Most are promising, but a string of failures (nimodipine, tirilazad, dexamethasone, magnesium, eliprodil, and dexanabinol) has dampened enthusiasm for this line of treatment.

One of the most tragic, and often entirely avoidable, events is admission to the NICU of an inebriated young adult extracted from a motor vehicle accident and facing, as a result, either death or a life of severe disability. Equally as tragic, assault has been increasing as a cause of TBI in cohort studies of younger patients.[12,33] Even more serious is TBI in young troops returning from major conflicts, with its accompanying characteristics of penetrating blast injury.[77,107] The late consequences (morbidity and epilepsy) of these war injuries are not well known.

The management of patients with TBI requires a multidisciplinary approach.[106] There are also some indications that outcome in TBI is better if patients are managed in recognized trauma centers with extensive experience in managing deterioration.[33] In large hospitals, trauma to the central nervous system is primarily managed by neurosurgical services. Patients with multiple trauma are often cared for in surgical trauma units with a neurologic or neurosurgical consultative service. The contribution of the neurointensivist can be substantial during every step of the way.

A large proportion of patients with TBI are not considered candidates for neurosurgical intervention to remove contusional brain or extra-axial hematomas. Management is largely directed to reducing increased intracranial pressure (ICP) and maintaining cerebral perfusion pressure, closely observing patients at high risk of deterioration, and preventing systemic complications associated with coma. Early surgical removal and larger craniotomies may improve outcomes.[38,131] Neurologists or neurosurgeons involved in the management of head injury, whether seeing patients in the ED or in the NICU, recognize that outcome after head injury depends greatly on whether the injury is accompanied by hypoxemia, hypercapnia, and hypovolemia.[2,18,63] Moreover, these factors may obscure the neurologic examination and patients may improve after resuscitation.[105]

This chapter discusses the management of TBI and the neurosurgical options in a patient whose condition is deteriorating. Standardized trauma care protocols improve outcome.[47] Admission to the NICU is warranted in patients who have impaired consciousness or are at risk for further deterioration. The threshold for observation in the ICU should be low in patients with skull fracture, trauma by fall, blunt head trauma from fists, or a temporal or frontal lobe intracranial hematoma on computed tomography (CT) scan.[109]

CLINICAL RECOGNITION

The vast majority of patients with severe TBI have clinical symptoms of diffuse axonal brain injury. Depending on the impact and the damage to brain parenchyma, patients may be alert and able to follow commands, or they may be combative, agitated, or comatose with abnormal motor responses. In major head injury registries, the Glasgow Coma Scale (GCS) score is the most commonly used measure of the severity of TBI and is related to prognosis. The responses measured by the GCS may significantly improve after successful fluid replacement in patients in shock.

Thus, the GCS after any type of resuscitation may have changed greatly from that at first evaluation. In an analysis of 746 patients from the Traumatic Coma Data Bank, approximately 40% were comatose with a GCS sum score of 3 at presentation, whereas 20% had this score after resuscitation.[1]

Of all available brainstem reflexes, pupillary size and light reflex have been tested most often, and they are considered the most important indicators of brain damage. The diagnostic values of all other brainstem reflexes or certain combinations have not been tested. Although intuitively obvious, it is not known whether the absence of pontomesencephalic reflexes portends poor outcome. In the Traumatic Coma Data Bank analysis, 74% of patients with initial bilateral fixed pupils from all causes became vegetative.[1] In addition, 50% of patients with later abnormal pupils after admission died or became vegetative. However, good outcome is particularly possible in patients with an extradural hematoma and fixed pupils.[89] Unfortunately, lack of details in neurologic examination, such as those that can be captured by the FOUR score, predominates in most TBI databases. Recent studies confirmed the value of using the FOUR score in traumatic brain injury.[45,76]

In the absence of direct trauma to the globe, dilatation of one pupil and absent or sluggish light response usually suggest an intracranial contusional mass that produces brain tissue and brainstem shifts. Often, the ipsilateral pupil dilates and becomes fixed, and this reaction soon follows in the opposite pupil. The presenting signs of epidural and subdural hematomas are similar, with a decline in consciousness, focal signs, and unilateral pupil enlargement. The course in epidural hematoma is very rapid and is related to its growth under arterial pressure.

Trauma to the cervical spine should be clinically ruled out before eye movements are investigated with use of oculocephalic responses, and determination of oculovestibular responses by cold caloric testing is safer in comatose patients. Abnormal responses with failure to adduct or abduct may suggest a third or sixth cranial nerve palsy (Chapter 12).

Post-traumatic injury may involve cranial nerves I, II, VI, and VII. Post-traumatic anosmia due to shearing of olfactory fibers at the cribriform plate is usually permanent, with some return and regeneration, although rarely noticeable, in one-third of the patients.[46] Traumatic optic neuropathy may result in no light perception, and if it is associated with orbital fracture, visual loss is not likely to improve. (Visual acuities of at least 20/400 may improve with corticosteroids. In any patient with less visual acuity, optic decompression needs to be considered.[116])

Sixth-nerve palsy may be seen and, in extreme cases, is bilateral. The inability to abduct past the midline and bilateral involvement at presentation predict poor outcome, and incisional strabismus surgery is needed.[42] Traumatic facial palsy is predominantly in the geniculate ganglion area. Surgical decompression is indicated if facial palsy is total and noted immediately after trauma.[21] Many patients recover well within 6 months.

In the initial assessment, it is important to examine the patient for facial fractures. Midface fractures are more frequently associated with TBI than are mandibular fractures. Facial fractures increase the chance of severe intracranial injury and are more often present in patients with decreased consciousness.[39] As part of a routine trauma examination, one should specifically note if the patient has a Battle sign (named after the British surgeon William Henry Battle), who noted clearly visible bruising at the level of the mastoid, indicating fracture of the basal skull and mastoid. Another more common manifestation are "raccoon eyes" (periorbital ecchymosis, indicating soft tissue damage but also facial fractures or a frontobasal skull fracture; Figure 41.1). Periorbital hematomas from the use of blunt instruments or fist impact are common in spousal abuse. Left-sided facial injuries are more frequent than right-sided impacts, reflecting the simple logic that most assailants are right-handed.

Seizures are comparatively uncommon in patients with TBI (5%–10%).[94] The incidence of seizures in patients with mild head injury is probably very low (< 1%). In patients with severe head

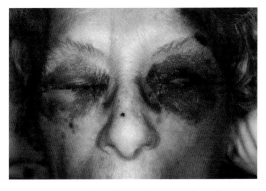

FIGURE 41.1: Periorbital edema and ecchymosis ("raccoon eyes").

injury, alcohol-related seizures should be considered, but only if there is a history of heavy drinking. The most significant risk factors associated with developing late post-traumatic seizures are decreased level of consciousness, cortical contusion, depressed skull fracture and dural tear, penetrating head wound, and a seizure within 24 hours of injury. The additional presence of an intra-cranial hematoma may markedly increase the risk of seizures, with incidences up to 35%.[22]

Patients with severe head injury and coma on admission may be affected by a significant and often dramatic sympathetic outburst. The exact pathophysiology is not known, but the sympathoexcitatory centers in the upper brainstem and diencephalon are likely intermittently stimulated. Besides agitation, clenching of fists, grinding of teeth, profuse sweating, sustained tachycardia, and marked hypertension are all part of the picture. These episodes can be associated with hyperthermia (to 40°C) and increased respiratory rate, often with inadequate gas exchange, and ICP often increases during these episodes (Figure 41.2). These sympathetic storms are inappropriately termed diencephalic seizures[4,11] (electroencephalographic recordings during these episodes have not shown epileptiform activity). The more appropriate term is *paroxysmal sympathetic hyperactivity*.

After an initial neurologic examination, the physical examination should be repeated to recognize possible additional systemic injuries, such as lung and heart contusion, splenic rupture, and any type of bony fracture. Hypotension usually signals hypovolemia from significant blood loss, and should not be considered a manifestation of severe head injury. Hypotension directly related to head injury occurs only in patients who fulfill the clinical criteria for brain death, patients with marked spinal cord injury, and children with large epidural hematomas. The head should be carefully examined for lacerations of the scalp. Blood loss from facial fractures or scalp lacerations can be profound and is never completely appreciated in the initial assessment. Hypotension is commonly associated with fractures of the pelvis or femur, and blood loss (> 1 L) can be life-threatening. However, even when long-bone fractures are found in a patient with hypotension, other sites need to be considered, including the chest, peritoneal cavity, and retroperitoneal space. Chest radiographs, thoracocentesis, and diagnostic peritoneal lavage are fairly reliable tests to demonstrate internal bleeding (Chapters 51 and 58).

In a patient with multitrauma, one must consider fat embolism syndrome from bone marrow of fractured long bones. This rare condition is signaled generally 12–72 hours after the traumatic impact, when the patient's condition suddenly deteriorates in parallel with laboratory changes. The common manifestations are acute confusional state, or sudden coma and generalized tonic-clonic seizures. A pathognomonic sign, present in 50% of patients, is a petechial rash appearing suddenly on the chest, axillary folds (Chapter 12) and, occasionally, conjunctiva. A typical fat embolization syndrome, however, appears in only 3%–4% of patients, and clinical signs may resolve within 24 hours.[10,54]

NEUROIMAGING AND LABORATORY TESTS

Computed tomography (CT) scan of the brain is imperative in any traumatic head injury. The current use for alert and stable patients with trauma is not very selective, but it is very difficult to identify a set of criteria that could result in a CT scan deferral.[102] Moreover, normal findings on CT do not preclude delayed traumatic hemorrhage. Five risk factors that could lead to a neurosurgical intervention have been identified. They are failure to become fully alert within the first hour, suspected open skull fracture, signs of basal skull fracture, vomiting more than twice, and age over 65 years.[102] In contrast, in a large series of consecutive fully alert patients, only 9% had CT scan abnormalities, and only two of these patients required neurosurgical intervention.[55] Nevertheless, because of possible medicolegal consequences, many patients, if not all, irrespective of any type of head injury, are likely to have a CT scan in the ED.

The types of abnormalities that can be seen on CT scans in TBI are summarized in Table 41.1.[53,62] A traumatic intracerebral hematoma may not appear on the first CT scan[26] (Figure 41.3). Identification of an intracerebral hematoma on CT scan may be delayed for 8 hours, but in most patients, the hematoma can be identified within 2 days of admission.[36]

Frontal and temporal lobe hemorrhagic contusions should alert the physician to the potential for further deterioration from edema and brainstem compression (Figure 41.4).[75,101] Computed tomography scanning should also be repeated if the initial scan was performed within hours of the impact, or if the patient has documented coagulopathy. Less common localizations of intracranial hematomas are hemorrhages in the posterior

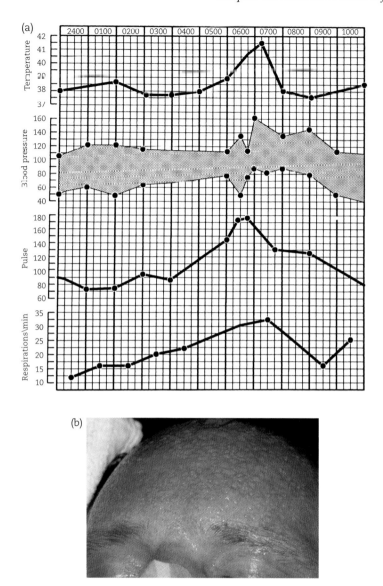

FIGURE 41.2. (a) Paroxysmal sympathetic hyperactivity. Alterations in core body temperature (in °C), blood pressure (in mm Hg), pulse (in beats per minute), and respiratory rate (in respirations per minute) during an episode. Note the increase in systolic pressure and decrease in diastolic pressure (with widening of pulse pressure) time-locked with the tachycardia. Hyperthermia occurred later and was not precisely time-locked with the hemodynamic changes. (b) Profuse pearls of sweat during this episode.

fossa, basal ganglia, or intraventricular compartment. However, in these patients, hemorrhagic contusions are found in other locations, all indicating a very significant traumatic impact.[5]

Many patients have small hemorrhages in both hemispheres, with only minimal shift of the midline structures. Tissue tear hemorrhages can also be seen in TBI, usually in the frontal cortex, white and gray matter interface, basal ganglia, thalamus, internal capsule,[124] and brainstem (Figure 41.5).

In 50% of these patients, additional traumatic subarachnoid or intraventricular blood occurs. When tissue tear hemorrhages are found in both the corpus callosum and the interpeduncular midbrain, the outcome is poor, but the predictive value of these shear lesions in other locations is much less clear.

It is important to look for the visibility of the basal cistern, an indicator of cerebral swelling, on CT scans. If a CT scan shows compressed or

TABLE 41.1. TYPES OF COMPUTED TOMOGRAPHY SCAN ABNORMALITIES IN TRAUMATIC BRAIN INJURY

Intraparenchymal
    Diffuse axonal injury
    Diffuse brain swelling
    Hemorrhagic contusion
    Tissue tear (shear) hemorrhage
    Brainstem hemorrhage
Extra-axial compartment
    Subarachnoid hemorrhage (sulci, vertex)
    Intraventricular
    Subdural hematoma
    Epidural hematoma
Secondary lesions
    Watershed, cortex, globi pallidi and thalami
        infarcts (anoxic–ischemic injury)
    Posterior cerebral artery territory infarct
        (brainstem displacement)
    Middle cerebral artery territory infarct (traumatic
        carotid dissection)

absent cisterns without a large intracranial mass lesion, or if the absence of cisterns is accompanied by marked midline shift, the outcome is poor. In the Traumatic Coma Data Bank study, however, these ominous CT scans were seen in only 32 of 746 (4%) patients.[62]

Computed tomography scans may show traumatic subarachnoid hemorrhage, usually located at the superficial cortical sulci. In patients with blood specifically localized in the sylvian fissure, trauma cannot be distinguished from aneurysmal rupture, and cerebral angiography is warranted.

Epidural hematomas appearing on CT scans are a neurosurgical emergency.[81,97] If the hematomas are small, they probably are associated with tear of a dural vessel rather than with rupture of a meningeal artery from a skull fracture (Figure 41.6). One study suggested that a radiolucent region (Figure 41.7) within a denser clot may be a sign of active bleeding and may prompt early evacuation.[49] Epidural hematomas in the posterior fossa are generally neurosurgical emergencies, and postponement of evacuation in clinically alert patients may be inappropriate (Figure 41.8)

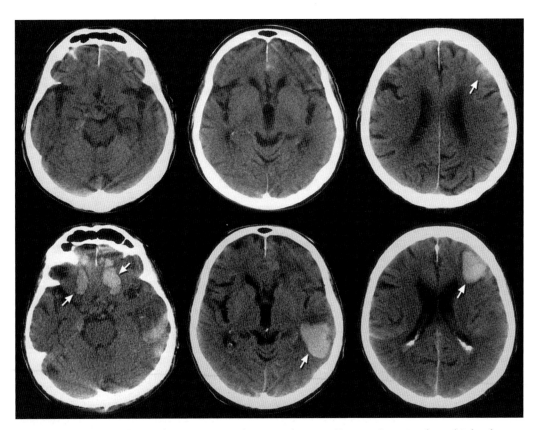

FIGURE 41.3: Delayed abnormalities on computed tomography scans. *Top row*: Contusion (*arrow*) is barely seen. *Bottom row*: Multiple lobar contusions (*arrows*) develop later.

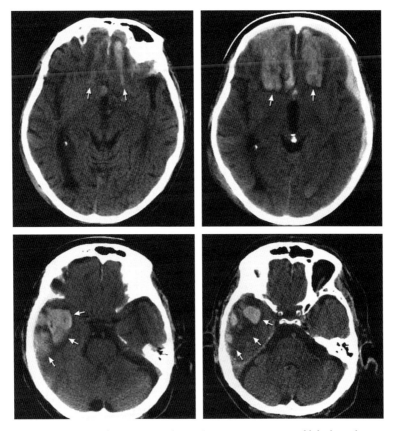

FIGURE 41.4. *Upper row*: Frontal lobe contusions (*arrows*). *Lower row*: Temporal lobe burst hematoma (*arrows*).

A subdural hematoma and its mass effect can usually be easily recognized on CT scans. However, when isodense and in patients with marked anemia, the size may be difficult to estimate (Figures 41.9 and 41.10). Bilateral subdural hematomas are common, but when they are isodense, the classic appearance of *hypernormal* CT scan may be apparent (Figure 41.11). (This descriptive term is derived from the fact that sulci are not visible and, together with the slit-like ventricular system, suggests a much younger patient.)

Any comatose patient with significant head trauma needs radiographs of the cervical spine.[41] Patients with cervical fractures may have double

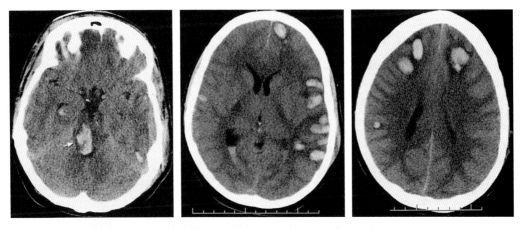

FIGURE 41.5: Multiple large contusional lesions with primary brainstem hemorrhage.

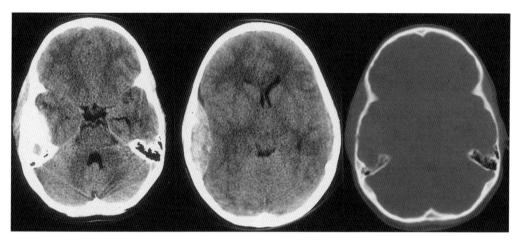

FIGURE 41.6: Epidural hematoma with associated skull fracture on bone window setting.

fractures in the cervical region or an additional lumbar body fracture; thus they require a full radiographic series of the spine. Cervical spine films should be carefully scrutinized for soft-tissue abnormalities, abnormalities in alignment, abnormalities in disk space and height, and fractures. Questionable plain film radiologic findings should prompt additional imaging with CT scan. However, important cervical spine fractures may be overlooked with 4- to 10-mm slices, because occasionally a segment is not displayed on CT scan. Discussion of cervical spine injuries are found in Chapter 36, and a more detailed overview with graphic display of the most common spine fractures is found in a companion monograph.[121]

Magnetic resonance imaging has a much higher sensitivity than conventional CT, but in the hectic ED setting should be deferred to a later stage. The clinical usefulness of MRI in acute brain injury remains unclear. Its contribution is mostly in the demonstration of diffuse injury and secondary abnormalities from anoxia or brain swelling.[32,100,122] The first prospective studies of MRI documented a higher frequency of abnormalities than that found on CT, and corpus callosum and brainstem lesions particularly seemed to predict poor outcome. Cognitive tasks were much worse in patients with MRI-documented lesions in the corpus callosum.[82] Magnetic resonance imaging could also be useful in confirming fat emboli to the brain. A case report suggested that a specific pattern of white spots on a dark background appears on diffusion-weighted imaging ("starfield" pattern).[80]

Laboratory tests in patients with severe head injury should include electrolytes, glucose, activated partial thromboplastin time, liver function tests, and urinalysis for hematuria. A blood sample must be sent to the blood bank for typing. An electrocardiogram should be obtained in all patients. In a young patient, it may detect additional cardiac contusion, although myocardial damage may be associated with increased circulating catecholamines. TBI progressing to brain death may be associated with cardiac stunning and significant wall motion abnormalities that can be diagnosed on echocardiograms; this condition currently precludes cardiac transplantation if the patient becomes an eligible donor (Chapter 65). Chest radiography should be repeated regularly for signs of possible aspiration or secondary bacterial infection after aspiration. There is a considerable risk of nosocomial pneumonia, usually within days of the impact, and for significant lung contusions, which may become more evident days after the impact.

FIRST STEPS IN MANAGEMENT

The management of TBI has been reviewed by the Brain Trauma Foundation. This review should be readily available in the NICU (see Part XIV, Guidelines).[12]

Many patients are stabilized in the ED, and often the decision is made there whether to transfer the patient to an NICU, a trauma unit, or an operating room. Transfer of a patient with severe head injury is fraught with potential danger. A study in the United Kingdom that audited transfer of conscious patients with head injury to a neurosurgical unit found that hypoxemia, hypotension, and failure to diagnose major extracranial injuries before transfer were prevalent.[31] In 25% of comatose patients, no endotracheal tube

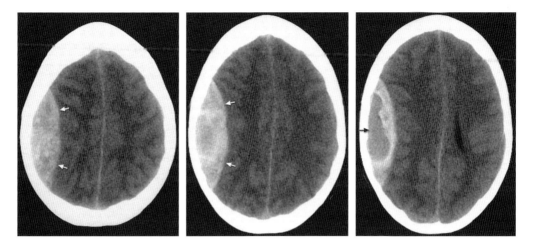

FIGURE 41.7: Epidural hematoma.

Typical convex configuration (*white arrows*) and hyperlucent area (*black arrow*).

was inserted, and many patients were transported supine. This landmark study in Glasgow pertained to patients admitted to the neurosurgical ICU from outside hospitals, but intrahospital transfer may pose the same threats.

The airway should be assessed immediately after the patient enters the NICU. The patient should be intubated if there is evidence of inadequate gas exchange on pulse oximetry or arterial blood gas determinations. Aspiration may already have occurred in patients with TBI, and acute respiratory distress syndrome (ARDS) may have developed. Neuromuscular blockade and sedation should be reserved only for this

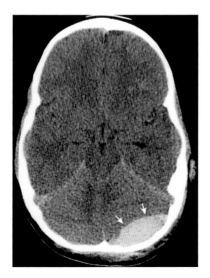

FIGURE 41.8: Epidural hematoma in the posterior fossa (*arrows*).

situation, because they make clinical monitoring impossible. Moreover, patients with TBI who are given neuromuscular blockade prophylactically have a higher incidence of pneumonia, more frequent sepsis, and longer intensive care stay. Neuromuscular blockade rarely has a place in the treatment of increased ICP and in general should be used sparingly. (It is a last resort in refractory increased ICP.) When neuromuscular blockade is used, ICP monitoring with an intraparenchymal fiberoptic device becomes essential to observe the patient's clinical status.

Securing adequate oxygenation throughout the clinical course is important. Episodes of hypoxemia, with PaO_2 less than 60 mm Hg, are frequently seen and must be immediately corrected. Mechanical ventilation in most patients is in the intermittent mandatory mode with pressure support. Breaths per minute vary from 8 to 10, and pressure support is usually set at 10 cm H_2O. Early tracheostomy (1–3 days) reduced length of stay in one study,[14] but many practices (excluding patients with marked facial fractures) would wait until 7–14 days. Moreover, the TracMan trial (not including many neurologic patients) found no benefit of "early" versus "late" tracheostomy.[130]

The ideal management of fluids in patients with severe TBI in the NICU is not exactly known. Currently, most investigators believe that adequate volume status with a maintenance dose of at least 3 L of isotonic saline a day is warranted.[67] There is no reason to believe that fluid restriction in TBI is beneficial. In addition, many patients receive mannitol for the control of ICP, and this, in combination with marginal fluid intake, may

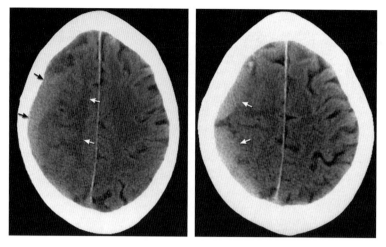

FIGURE 41.9: Acute subdural hematoma. No midline shift is seen, but there is compression of the white matter (*arrows*).

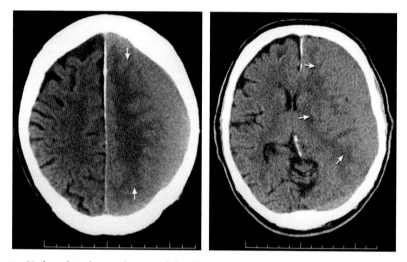

FIGURE 41.10: Unilateral isodense subacute subdural hematoma. Note compressed white matter (*arrows*). Note loss of sulcal definition and shift of septum pellucidum and pineal gland.

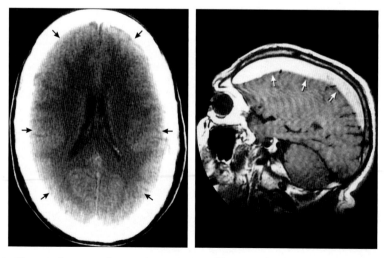

FIGURE 41.11: Computed tomography scan in an 85-year-old man with bilateral isodense subdural hematoma ("hypernormal") CT, better visualized by magnetic resonance imaging.

lead to rapid hypovolemia if urinary losses are not replaced by maintenance fluids.[28] Moreover, an analysis of fluid balance associated with poor outcome found a strong and independent correlation with a negative cumulative fluid balance of more than 500 mL over 4 days.[16]

Blood pressure should be titrated, if possible, to acceptable cerebral perfusion pressure (> 70 mm Hg) and ICP (< 20 mm Hg). Experimental data have also shown that the compensatory cardiovascular response to hypotension is, for some reason, significantly muted in patients with high ICP. Blood loss may more easily cause a shock syndrome in patients with increased ICP. The true mechanism is unclear.[48] A general guideline is avoidance of both hypotension, defined as systolic blood pressure of less than 100 mm Hg, and persistent hypertension, defined as mean arterial pressure greater than 130 mm Hg, particularly because the upper breakpoint of the autoregulation curve is situated at that level and brain edema may occur.[20] Persistent hypertension may be particularly deleterious in patients with diffuse brain swelling on CT scans. Most patients with TBI are young, and brief episodes of hypertension are well tolerated, but surges of hypertension may trigger plateau waves. However, treatment of hypertension may have the detrimental effect of decreasing cerebral perfusion pressure, particularly in areas with lost autoregulation. Blood pressure management should be titrated to a cerebral perfusion pressure of 70 mm Hg or higher. Patients with persistent hypertension are best treated with an intravenous bolus of labetalol because the duration of action is brief.

A randomized trial in 82 patients with a GCS score of 3–7 showed that initial 24-hour management with hypothermia (32°–33°C) and vecuronium and fentanyl to prevent shivering improved outcome.[60] The benefit could be demonstrated only in patients with coma scores of 5–7, with an approximately 50% reduction in death and poor outcome. Moreover, hypothermia reduced CSF glutamate, an effect suggesting an additional benefit through the reduction of central ischemia.[60] (Glutamate, an excitatory neurotransmitter released by ischemic neurons, results in calcium and sodium influx, leading to cell death.)

Another more defining trial found that hypothermia (cooling to a core temperature of 33°C within 8 hours after injury and for 2 days) did not result in improvement of outcome. However, active rewarming of moderately hypothermic

patients should be discouraged.[17,68] Hypothermia may remain an effective treatment for ICP management but a recent study found that cooling (32–35 degrees of Celcius) compared with conventional measures was equivalent in controlling intracranial pressure but cooling was associated with higher mortality and worse functional outcomes. Hypothermia resulted in a substantial decreased need for pentobarbital-induced coma.[1]

Insertion of an ICP monitor should be strongly considered.[19,69,72,78,103] Intracranial pressure monitoring has not been subjected to a prospective study to evaluate its effect on outcome but may help detect delayed hematomas,[96] limit the indiscriminate use of measures to lower ICP, and indicate lack of response and thus poor outcome. Studies with worse outcomes with monitoring represent a bias toward more severely affected patients.[96]

Use of the monitoring device may be limited to comatose patients after correction of confounding factors and in patients with a CT scan showing an intracranial hematoma[72] (especially in the temporal or frontal lobe) or brain edema. Patients in need of neuromuscular blockade for adequate ventilation (e.g., because of severe lung contusion or flail chest) almost certainly need ICP monitoring, because clinical neurologic signs, except for sudden pupillary changes, are lost.

The goals of management of increased ICP have not been well established, but 20 mm Hg should be considered the threshold above which treatment to lower ICP is initiated. Cerebral perfusion pressure should be maintained at more than 70 mm Hg.[88]

The ICP monitoring devices are discussed in Chapter 23. There is some debate about whether a ventricular catheter connected to an external strain gauge transducer is as accurate and reliable as a parenchymal fiberoptic transducer device.[93] The ventricular catheter has a comparatively low risk of infection, may not necessarily increase morbidity, and has the major advantage of withdrawal of CSF. The infection rate increases to 20% when these fluid-coupled ICP devices are irrigated, but bacterial colonization is low (5%).[64,99] The most compelling drawback of fluid-coupled ventricular catheters is malfunction from obstruction, particularly in patients with cerebral edema that compresses the lateral horns. Parenchymal fiberoptic probes are most often used, and clinical experience is very satisfactory.[93,126]

The treatment of increased ICP in the initial management of patients with severe head injury is guided toward changes in ICP and cerebral perfusion pressure.[34] The management of increased ICP includes control of hyperthermia, elevation of the head of the bed to 30 degrees in neutral position while avoiding obstruction of jugular venous outflow (generally, head elevation enhances jugular venous outflow and decreases ICP),[87] sedation in markedly combative patients, normal volume status, and adequate arterial oxygenation. Rigid collars may distort or compress neck veins and increase ICP.[43] Patients with increased ICP, a large mass, and no initial response to osmotic agents may need immediate neurosurgical evacuation of the contused brain.

Prophylactic hyperventilation should be avoided.[104] Titrating PCO_2 using end-tidal CO_2 may be useful, but hemodynamic instability and poor tissue perfusion may increase this value.[52] A prospective, randomized clinical study found that comatose patients who received prophylactic hyperventilation had significantly worse outcomes than patients with normocapnia.[66] Cerebral blood flow measurements in patients with severe TBI have shown that blood flow is decreased and may reach values consistent with ischemia.[6] Thus, the use of aggressive hyperventilation (defined as $PaCO_2$ < 30 mm Hg) may further reduce cerebral blood flow, and it is not certain whether this reduction is matched by increased cerebral oxygen extraction. In addition, the response to hyperventilation is muted in patients who have severe head injury, typically those with diffuse multiple hemorrhagic contusions and those with extra-axial hematomas.[90]

Although the use of hyperventilation as first-line treatment of increased ICP can be questioned, many patients have spontaneous hyperventilation, causing $PaCO_2$ to be in the lower 30s. Tachypnea in patients with a primary lung injury or aspiration often is simply a compensatory response to hypoxemia.

Patients with increased ICP probably should be treated first with osmotic agents. Administration of mannitol remains the preferred treatment.[115] How mannitol works remains a puzzle, and cerebral blood volume does change with mannitol doses.[23] Mannitol has an osmotic effect after 15–30 minutes of infusion. Mannitol should be administered in repeat boluses rather than by continuous infusion, because it may accumulate in the brain if infused for long periods. Serum osmolarity of 310–320 mOsm/L is considered the therapeutic goal. Reduction of ICP can be expected 20 minutes after a bolus, and the first-pass effect may last up to 6 hours.

Another method of osmotic diuresis is the use of hypertonic saline, probably equal to mannitol in effect.[24] Hypertonic saline of 23.4% has been used now in many practices.[35,51,73,111]

If patients with severe head injury cannot be managed with mannitol,[98] tromethamine,[128] hypertonic saline,[3,30,119,129] or propofol,[40] barbiturate treatment can be considered.[25,83,85,91,95,117] Barbiturate therapy lowers ICP and reduces mortality in patients with increased intracranial hypertension. However, the side effects are considerable, and include marked hypotension, hypocalcemia, hepatic and renal dysfunction, and sepsis.[91] Barbiturates may also depress lung mucociliary clearance, thereby accounting for an increased risk of pulmonary infections.[29] Corticosteroids are strongly discouraged,[7,92] except in patients with severe additional spinal cord injury seen within 8 hours (Chapter 36).[8]

The incidence of seizures after TBI can be significantly reduced in the first week by administration of phenytoin.[94,110] A 7-day course of antiepileptic agents is considered in patients with marked cerebral swelling on CT scan. Seizures may greatly increase ICP and trigger plateau waves. (Even in pharmacologically paralyzed patients, seizures may increase ICP.) Intravenous loading with fosphenytoin, 20 mg PE/kg, or levetiracetam (1 gram) are options.

Nimodipine may have a beneficial effect in patients with head injury, subarachnoid blood, and post-traumatic vasospasm.[74] A study of 130 patients with traumatic subarachnoid hemorrhage claimed to find delayed cerebral ischemia in 7%,[108] but the clinical relevance remains uncertain. Nimodipine 60 mg every 6 hours for 10 days[44] can be considered in patients with massive subarachnoid hemorrhage unless blood pressure is unstable (e.g., visceral trauma).

Early enteral nutrition is preferred but complicated.[71,79] The early use of parenteral nutrition in patients with marked catabolic response is controversial.[37] Glycemic control in traumatic head injury (Chapter 57) is advised but the ideal lowest tolerable serum glucose has not been defined, and aggressive control may cause cellular distress, as evidenced by changes in glutamate and lactate: pyruvate ratio on cerebral microdialysis studies.[113,114] The initial management of patients with severe TBI is summarized in Table 41.2.

The management of gunshot wounds (Capsule 41.1) is similar to that of any other type of nonpenetrating trauma. A large intracerebral hematoma with mass effect can be removed, but no further therapy can be offered to patients

TABLE 41.2. INITIAL MANAGEMENT OF TRAUMATIC BRAIN INJURY

Airway management	Intubation if patient has hypoxemia despite facemask with 10 L of 100% oxygen/minute, if abnormal respiratory drive or if abnormal protective reflexes (likely with motor response of withdrawal, or worse)
	Emergency tracheostomy in major facial injury
Mechanical ventilation	IMV/PS
	AC if pulmonary contusion or aspiration. Increasing PEEP if gas exchange is inadequate
	Chest tube in traumatic pneumothorax
Fluid management	0.9% NaCl, 3 L/day
Blood pressure management	Labetalol, 10–20 mg IV, for persistent hypertension (mean arterial pressure > 130 mm Hg); hydralazine 10–20 mg IV if bradycardia
Nutrition	Enteral nutrition with continuous infusion (on day 2)
	Blood glucose control (goal 140–180 mg/dL).
Prophylaxis	DVT prophylaxis with pneumatic compression devices and SC heparin 5,000 U t.i.d. Consider preventive IVC filter placement
	GI prophylaxis: pantoprazole 40 mg IV daily or lansoprazole 30 mg orally through nasogastric tube
ICP management	Placement of ICP monitoring device when comatose, ICH or brain swelling on CT or need for neuromuscular blockade.
	CPP > 70 mm Hg; ICP < 20 mm Hg
	Head elevation, 30°
	Mannitol, 0.25–1 g/kg, or hypertonic saline 23% 30 mL.
	Consider brief periods of hyperventilation
	Normothermia or induced hypothermia
Surgical management	Consider decompressive hemicraniectomy or bilateral frontal craniectomies with refractory ICP
	Consider evacuation of contusional mass
Additional measures	No corticosteroids (unless additional spinal cord lesion)
	Consider levetiracetam 1,000 mg IV over 15 minutes, 1,000 mg b.i.d. maintenance for 7 days
	Consider nimodipine, 60 mg q6h, for traumatic SAH
Access	Arterial catheter to monitor blood pressure (if IV antihypertensive drugs anticipated)
	Peripheral venous catheter or peripheral inserted central catheter

CPP, cerebral perfusion pressure; CT, computed tomography; DVT, deep vein thrombosis; GCS, Glasgow coma scale; GI, gastrointestinal; ICH, intracranial hemorrhage; ICP, intracranial pressure; IMV, intermittent mandatory ventilation; MAP, mean arterial pressure; NaCl, sodium chloride; PEEP, positive end-expiratory pressure; PS, pressure support; SAH, subarachnoid hemorrhage.

who, after initial resuscitation, remain comatose with absent upper brainstem reflexes, no motor responses to pain, and no major confounder such as drug ingestion. Reconstructive repair of the bone and dura should begin immediately. The wound is considered contaminated and broad-spectrum antibiotics (vancomycin with cefotaxime) should be administered early. When injury to the cerebral vasculature is anticipated, angiography can be performed, but therapeutic options other than endovascular or surgical occlusion are limited. A major problem is the early development of disseminated intravascular coagulation. Its occurrence is related to the amount of brain tissue damage; thus, it is frequent in gunshot wounds. Its appearance on laboratory tests (e.g., increased D-dimer or fibrinogen split products) denotes a poor outcome. If there is evidence of a full track throughout the brain, there appears to be very little benefit of aggressive ICP management. A bolus of mannitol, 1–2 g/kg, can be administered to determine whether improvement is possible; but if none is present, salvageability is unlikely.

DETERIORATION: CAUSES AND MANAGEMENT

The condition of patients with severe head injury may deteriorate from enlargement of

CAPSULE 41.1   GUNSHOTS TO THE HEAD

In the United States, gunshot wounds are a common cause of penetrating injury to the head. The impact to the brain when penetrated by a bullet is explosive and, due to its shock wave, enormously damaging. Not only do bullets penetrate the skull, brain, and vascular structures, but the great force and high pressure in the cavity of passage also damage the surrounding structures. The entrance wound often leaves unburned residues in the skin ("tattooing") and is typically smaller than the exit wound. The exit may be larger due to mushrooming of the bullet. Suicide wounds are often in the dominant temporal region or in the mouth. When multiple gunshot wounds are present, suicide is unlikely. The brainstem and deeper structures of the brain are frequent sites of hemorrhage, and ectopic bone fragments may be seen. Guns placed in the mouth may destroy the brainstem, or bullets may lodge under the skull base, damaging the carotid artery and cranial nerves. Gunshot wounds to the brain are complex injuries, with skull fracture, tracks of bone, and missile fragments (see accompanying illustration). Often, an associated intracerebral hematoma contributes to the initial clinical condition. Cerebral contusions may be seen at the entry and exit sites.

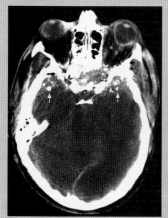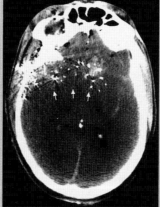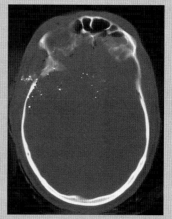

Computed tomography of gunshot wound. Gun was placed on temple and bullet cut through the brain horizontally, leaving a hemorrhage in its tracks (*arrows*).

hemorrhagic contusions, massive malignant cerebral edema, or further extension of an extra-axial hematoma.[26] Patients with traumatic subarachnoid hemorrhage alone are at risk of deterioration. The initial CT scan in patients susceptible to malignant diffuse brain swelling is more often abnormal, revealing diffuse shear injury and subarachnoid hemorrhage. In one study, approximately half the patients with severe head injury had an episode of hypoxemia and hypotension preceding diffuse cerebral edema; this finding emphasized the possible relationship between extracranial insults and the development of diffuse brain swelling. In another study, prominent leukocytosis that could not be explained by nosocomial infection was thought to be associated with a secondary increase in ICP from generalized brain swelling,[112] but the mechanism remains unexplained.

Malignant brain swelling often leads to brain death, and virtually no therapeutic option is available, other than aggressive ICP management with the previously mentioned pharmacologic agents.[50] Whether barbiturate treatment improves outcome in this situation is not known, and, as mentioned earlier, it is associated with complications of its own. Craniotomy with removal of frontoparietal bone flaps (often bilateral) and use of an expansile duraplasty is a last resort and has been successful in selected cases (Figure 41.12).[125]

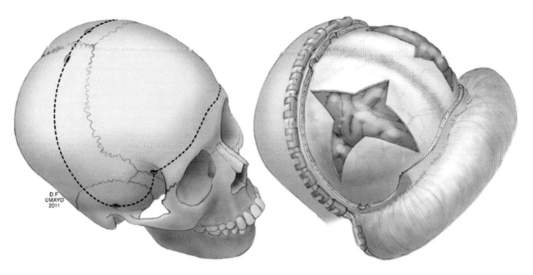

FIGURE 41.12: Bifrontal craniectomy for treatment of refractory increased intracranial pressure

Many patients have deterioration from enlargement of a hemorrhagic contusion. A bifrontal hematoma or temporal lobe hematoma increases the chance of marked deterioration. These patients, who typically "talk and deteriorate," need to be transported to the operating room at the first signs of deterioration.[86] If the temporal lobe is damaged, a lobectomy is done in the inferior segment of the damaged temporal lobe, and any other severely damaged brain tissue is resected.

Extra-axial hematomas can be watched closely, but the hematomas in most patients are evacuated before they are admitted to the NICU.[70] Initial management of acute subdural hematoma may remain conservative if the thickness of the hematoma is similar to the thickness of the skull bone and no midline shift is noted. However, if enlargement is associated with clinical deterioration, craniotomy must be timely for a potentially successful outcome. Delayed epidural hematoma has been noted in patients with hypotension whose condition deteriorated after correction of hypotension, which most likely increased cerebral perfusion pressure and thus caused recurrent bleeding.[9]

Patients with severe TBI may have clinical deterioration from a systemic complication. The risk of nosocomial pneumonia and ARDS is high. Rarely, disseminated coagulopathy or pulmonary embolus develops.

The treatment of paroxysmal sympathetic hyperactivity is needed to avoid cardiac arrhythmias, and several drugs can be tried. Propranolol has been used, but it may not be that successful.

Morphine (4 mg IV in multiple doses) may be more effective. Clonidine (0.1 mg up to 0.5 mg orally daily) or dexmedetomidine (0.2 mcg/kg/hr titrated up to 0.7 mcg/kg/hr) may be good options. In resistant cases, intrathecal baclofen may be needed, but there is some anecdotal evidence that high doses gabapentin (1,800–3,600 mg daily in 3 divided doses) may be helpful.

OUTCOME

Generally speaking, the most important factors with high predictive power are coma after adequate resuscitation, age of greater than 65 years, abnormal pupils (or abnormal pupils for at least one observation), shock on admission, persistently increased ICP, hypoxemia on admission, and CT scan abnormalities representing multiple contusions.[13,56,58,59,65,118,132]

Repeat CT or MRI imaging may show the ravages of secondary injury (Figure 41.13) and these findings can be taken into account with assessment of prognosis. There is, however, insufficient predictive value of routine MRI in TBI. A recent recommendation noted that MRI, more specifically the use of GRE and SWI sequences, was sensitive to microhemorrhages within the brain, but the number and volume of these microhemorrhages did not conclusively indicate injury severity or outcome.[127] In general, elderly patients do very poorly. In a series of patients older than 65 years, comatose patients had only a 10% chance of survival and a 4% chance of independent functional outcome.[61] Most likely, elderly patients more often have extradural hematomas, associated

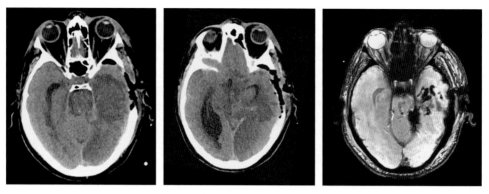

FIGURE 41.13: MRI showing secondary infarction in the PCA territory (thalamus and parietooccipital region) as a result of brain tissue shift (in this example, acute epidural hematoma).

vascular disease, or multitrauma that jeopardizes recovery.[84] Nonetheless, acute traumatic subdural hematoma alone remains associated with poor outcome in the elderly.[81,123] Two-thirds of comatose patients with an epidural hematoma are left disabled or die.[81] Outcome is excellent with posterior fossa epidural hematomas after immediate surgical evacuation.

The prediction of outcome in young patients without penetrating head injury is very difficult, with many examples of reasonable recovery when none of that appeared likely.

Permanent vegetative state is a much-feared outcome for family members confronted with a patient who is unresponsive after trauma. Patients can remain in a permanent vegetative state for 15–20 years, a situation that is extremely hard to bear for family members. However, in most patients, mortality for permanent vegetative state (defined as beginning 1 month after

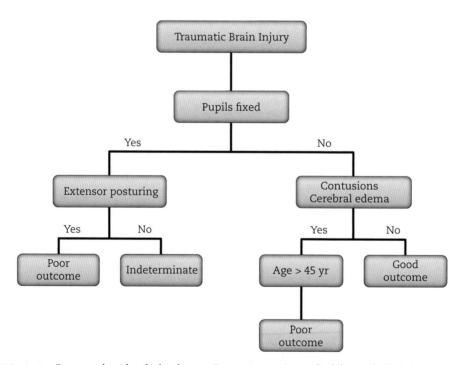

FIGURE 41.14: Outcome algorithm for head injury. Poor outcome: Severe disability or death. Indeterminate: Any statement would be a premature conclusion. Good outcome: No assistance needed, minor handicap may remain.

Data from Choi SC, Muizelaar JP, Barnes TY, et al. Prediction tree for severely head-injured patients. *J Neurosurg* 1991;75:251–255. With permission of the publisher.

trauma) is 82% at 3 years and 95% at 5 years. Mortality in permanent vegetative state is highly dependent on whether the family requests resuscitative efforts and antibiotic therapy for infections. Recovery from a vegetative state associated with TBI to a minimally conscious state or severely disabled state is common in the first year. Patients who become severely disabled after a severe head injury may be able to return to work in sheltered workplaces, usually with responsibilities far less challenging than those before injury. Only a minority are cared for in nursing homes. In many trauma data banks, prediction of good or poor outcome was more powerful than prediction of moderate disability (independent but with a significant handicap). Outcome in TBI [15] is shown in Figure 41.14, but data can be obtained using the IMPACT and CRASH studies, which have found several variables that consistently predict death or poor outcome. Calculators are found online. Both IMPACT and CRASH databanks have found strong predictors for outcome such as age, the motor response, pupil reactivity to light, and findings on an admission CT scan. Secondary insults that include hypotension and hypoxemia, and laboratory variables that include blood glucose and hemoglobin, have improved the model. One could argue against its use for prognostication, despite providing an excellent probabilistic estimate of outcome. Moreover, families may have difficulty interpreting percentages if they are close to 50/50 percentages. Details on prognostication can be found in other works.[57,120]

CONCLUSIONS

- Intracranial pressure monitoring is strongly indicated in comatose patients with TBI, who are usually patients with brain swelling or multiple contusions on CT scan, and in patients who need sedation or neuromuscular blockade to control mechanical ventilation.
- Mannitol or hypertonic saline are used to reduce ICP. Brief hyperventilation may be useful if ICP is not controlled. Alternatively, propofol, barbiturate treatment, or decompressive craniotomy are measures of last resort with unproven efficacy.
- Bilateral fixed, dilated pupils in patients with traumatic hematomas alone are a sign of poor prognosis, but 25% of patients may recover with independent function. Outcome is much worse in patients who additionally have bilateral extensor posturing.
- Poor outcome is expected in comatose elderly patients, and in those with abnormal pupils, hypoxemia or shock on admission, or multiple contusions on CT scans.
- Outcome is very difficult to predict accurately in young individuals.

REFERENCES

1. Andrews PJ, Sinclair HL, Rodriguez A, Harris BA, Battison CG, Rhodes JK, Murray GD. Eurotherm3235 Trial Collaborators Hypothermia for Intracranial Hypertension after Traumatic Brain Injury. *N Engl J Med* 2015;373:2403–2412.
2. Badjatia N, Carney N, Crocco TJ, et al. Guidelines for prehospital management of traumatic brain injury 2nd edition. *Prehosp Emerg Care* 2008;12 Suppl 1:S1–52.
3. Battison C, Andrews PJ, Graham C, Petty T. Randomized, controlled trial on the effect of a 20% mannitol solution and a 7.5% saline/6% dextran solution on increased intracranial pressure after brain injury. *Crit Care Med* 2005;33:196–202.
4. Boeve BF, Wijdicks EFM, Benarroch EE, Schmidt KD. Paroxysmal sympathetic storms ("diencephalic seizures") after severe diffuse axonal head injury. *Mayo Clinic Proc* 1998;73:148–152.
5. Boto GR, Lobato RD, Rivas JJ, et al. Basal ganglia hematomas in severely head injured patients: clinicoradiological analysis of 37 cases. *J Neurosurg* 2001;94:224–232.
6. Bouma GJ, Muizelaar JP. Cerebral blood flow, cerebral blood volume, and cerebrovascular reactivity after severe head injury. *J Neurotrauma* 1992;9 Suppl 1:S333–348.
7. Braakman R, Schouten HJ, Blaauw-van Dishoeck M, Minderhoud JM. Megadose steroids in severe head injury: results of a prospective double-blind clinical trial. *J Neurosurg* 1983;58:326–330.
8. Bracken MB, Shepard MJ, Collins WF, et al. A randomized, controlled trial of methylprednisolone or naloxone in the treatment of acute spinal-cord injury. Results of the Second National Acute Spinal Cord Injury Study. *N Engl J Med* 1990;322:1405–1411.
9. Bucci MN, Phillips TW, McGillicuddy JE. Delayed epidural hemorrhage in hypotensive multiple trauma patients. *Neurosurgery* 1986;19:65–68.
10. Bulger EM, Smith DG, Maier RV, Jurkovich GJ. Fat embolism syndrome: a 10-year review. *Arch Surg* 1997;132:435–439.
11. Bullard DE. Diencephalic seizures: responsiveness to bromocriptine and morphine. *Ann Neurol* 1987;21:609–611.

12. Bullock MR, Chesnut R, Ghajar J, et al. Guidelines for the surgical management of traumatic brain injury. *Neurosurgery* 2006;58 (Supplement):S1–S3.

13. Butcher I, McHugh GS, Lu J, et al. Prognostic value of cause of injury in traumatic brain injury: results from the IMPACT study. *J Neurotrauma* 2007;24:281–286.

14. Chesnut RM. What is wrong with the tenets underpinning current management of severe traumatic brain injury? *Ann N Y Acad Sci* 2014:1–9.

15. Choi SC, Muizelaar JP, Barnes TY, et al. Prediction tree for severely head-injured patients. *J Neurosurg* 1991;75:251–255.

16. Clifton GL, Miller ER, Choi SC, Levin HS. Fluid thresholds and outcome from severe brain injury. *Crit Care Med* 2002;30:739–745.

17. Clifton GL, Miller ER, Choi SC, et al. Lack of effect of induction of hypothermia after acute brain injury. *N Engl J Med* 2001;344:556–563.

18. Cooper DJ, Myles PS, McDermott FT, et al. Prehospital hypertonic saline resuscitation of patients with hypotension and severe traumatic brain injury: a randomized controlled trial. *JAMA* 2004;291:1350–1357.

19. Cremer OL, van Dijk GW, van Wensen E, et al. Effect of intracranial pressure monitoring and targeted intensive care on functional outcome after severe head injury. *Crit Care Med* 2005;33:2207–2213.

20. Czosnyka M, Smielewski P, Piechnik S, Steiner LA, Pickard JD. Cerebral autoregulation following head injury. *J Neurosurg* 2001;95:756–763.

21. Darrouzet V, Duclos JY, Liguoro D, et al. Management of facial paralysis resulting from temporal bone fractures: our experience in 115 cases. *Otolaryngol Head Neck Surg* 2001;125:77–84.

22. De Santis A, Cappricci E, Granata G. Early post traumatic seizures in adults: study of 84 cases. *J Neurosurg Sci* 1979;23:207–210.

23. Diringer MN, Scalfani MT, Zazulia AR, et al. Effect of mannitol on cerebral blood volume in patients with head injury. *Neurosurgery* 2012;70:1215–1218.

24. Doyle JA, Davis DP, Hoyt DB. The use of hypertonic saline in the treatment of traumatic brain injury. *J Trauma* 2001;50:367–383.

25. Eisenberg HM, Frankowski RF, Contant CF, Marshall LF, Walker MD. High-dose barbiturate control of elevated intracranial pressure in patients with severe head injury. *J Neurosurg* 1988;69:15–23.

26. Elsner H, Rigamonti D, Corradino G, Schlegel R, Jr., Joslyn J. Delayed traumatic intracerebral hematomas: "Spat-Apoplexie": report of two cases. *J Neurosurg* 1990;72:813–815.

27. Faul M, Xu L, Wald MM, Coronado VG. *Traumatic Brain Injury in the United States: Emergency Department Visits, Hospitalizations and Deaths 2002–2006*. Atlanta, GA: Centers for Disease Control and Prevention, National Center for Injury Prevention and Control;2010.

28. Feldman JA, Fish S. Resuscitation fluid for a patient with head injury and hypovolemic shock. *J Emerg Med* 1991;9:465–468.

29. Forbes AR, Gamsu G. Depression of lung mucociliary dlearance by thiopental and halothane. *Anesth Analg* 1979;58:387–389.

30. Freshman SP, Battistella FD, Matteucci M, Wisner DH. Hypertonic saline (7.5%) versus mannitol: a comparison for treatment of acute head injuries. *J Trauma* 1993;35:344–348.

31. Gentleman D, Jennett B. Audit of transfer of unconscious head-injured patients to a neurosurgical unit. *Lancet* 1990;335:330–334.

32. Gentry LR, Godersky JC, Thompson B. MR imaging of head trauma: review of the distribution and radiopathologic features of traumatic lesions. *AJR Am J Roentgenol* 1988;150:663–672.

33. Ghajar J. Traumatic brain injury. *Lancet* 2000;356:923–929.

34. Golding EM, Robertson CS, Bryan RM, Jr. The consequences of traumatic brain injury on cerebral blood flow and autoregulation: a review. *Clin Exp Hypertens* 1999;21:299–332.

35. Grande PO, Romner B. Osmotherapy in brain edema: a questionable therapy. *J Neurosurg Anesthesiol* 2012;24:407–412.

36. Gudeman SK, Kishore PR, Miller JD, et al. The genesis and significance of delayed traumatic intracerebral hematoma. *Neurosurgery* 1979;5:309–313.

37. Hadley MN, Grahm TW, Harrington T, et al. Nutritional support and neurotrauma: a critical review of early nutrition in forty-five acute head injury patients. *Neurosurgery* 1986;19:367–373.

38. Hartings JA, Vidgeon S, Strong AJ, et al. Surgical management of traumatic brain injury: a comparative-effectiveness study of 2 centers. *J Neurosurg* 2014;120:434–446.

39. Haug RH, Savage JD, Likavec MJ, Conforti PJ. A review of 100 closed head injuries associated with facial fractures. *J Oral Maxillofac Surg* 1992;50:218–222.

40. Herregods L, Verbeke J, Rolly G, Colardyn F. Effect of propofol on elevated intracranial pressure: preliminary results. *Anaesthesia* 1988;43 Suppl:107–109.

41. Holly LT, Kelly DF, Counelis GJ, et al. Cervical spine trauma associated with moderate and severe

head injury; incidence, risk factors, and injury characteristics. *J Neurosurg* 2002;96:285–291.

42. Holmes JM, Beck RW, Kip KE, Droste PJ, Leske DA. Predictors of nonrecovery in acute traumatic sixth nerve palsy and paresis. *Ophthalmology* 2001;108:1457–1460.

43. Hunt K, Hallworth S, Smith M. The effects of rigid collar placement on intracranial and cerebral perfusion pressures. *Anaesthesia* 2001;56:511–513.

44. Injury TESGoNiSH. A multicenter trial of the efficacy of nimodipine on outcome after severe head injury. *J Neurosurg* 1994;80:797–804.

45. Jalali R, Rezaei M. A comparison of the glasgow coma scale score with full outline of unresponsiveness scale to predict patients' traumatic brain injury outcomes in intensive care units. *Crit Care Res Pract* 2014;2014:289803.

46. Kern RC, Quinn B, Rosseau G, Farbman AI. Post-traumatic olfactory dysfunction. *Laryngoscope* 2000;110:2106–2109.

47. Kesinger MR, Nagy LR, Sequeira DJ, et al. A standardized trauma care protocol decreased in-hospital mortality of patients with severe traumatic brain injury at a teaching hospital in a middle-income country. *Injury* 2014;45:1350–1354.

48. Kirkeby OJ, Rise IR, Nordsletten L, Skjeldal S, Risoe C. Cardiovascular response to blood loss during high intracranial pressure. *J Neurosurg* 1995;83:1067–1071.

49. Knuckey NW, Gelbard S, Epstein MH. The management of "asymptomatic" epidural hematomas: a prospective study. *J Neurosurg* 1989;70:392–396.

50. Lang DA, Teasdale GM, Macpherson P, Lawrence A. Diffuse brain swelling after head injury: more often malignant in adults than children? *J Neurosurg* 1994;80:675–680.

51. Lazaridis C, Neyens R, Bodle J, DeSantis SM. High-osmolarity saline in neurocritical care: systematic review and meta-analysis. *Crit Care Med* 2013;41:1353–1360.

52. Lee SW, Hong YS, Han C, et al. Concordance of end-tidal carbon dioxide and arterial carbon dioxide in severe traumatic brain injury. *J Trauma* 2009;67:526–530.

53. Levi L, Guilburd JN, Lemberger A, Soustiel JF, Feinsod M. Diffuse axonal injury: analysis of 100 patients with radiological signs. *Neurosurgery* 1990;27:429–432.

54. Levy D. The fat embolism syndrome: a review. *Clin Orthop Relat Res* 1990:281–286.

55. Lobato RD, Sarabia R, Rivas JJ, et al. Normal computerized tomography scans in severe head injury: prognostic and clinical management implications. *J Neurosurg* 1986;65:784–789.

56. Maas AI, Hukkelhoven CW, Marshall LF, Steyerberg EW. Prediction of outcome in traumatic brain injury with computed tomographic characteristics: a comparison between the computed tomographic classification and combinations of computed tomographic predictors. *Neurosurgery* 2005;57:1173–1182.

57. Maas AI, Lingsma HF, Roozenbeek B. Predicting outcome after traumatic brain injury. *Handb Clin Neurol* 2015;128:455–474.

58. Maas AI, Marmarou A, Murray GD, Teasdale SG, Steyerberg EW. Prognosis and clinical trial design in traumatic brain injury: the IMPACT study. *J Neurotrauma* 2007;24:232–238.

59. Maas AI, Stocchetti N, Bullock R. Moderate and severe traumatic brain injury in adults. *Lancet Neurol* 2008;7:728–741.

60. Marion DW, Penrod LE, Kelsey SF, et al. Treatment of traumatic brain injury with moderate hypothermia. *N Engl J Med* 1997;336:540–546.

61. Marshall LF, Gautille T, Klauber MR, et al. The outcome of severe closed head injury. *J Neurosurg* 1991;75:S28–S36.

62. Marshall LF, Marshall SB, Klauber MR, et al. A new classification of head injury based on computerized tomography. *J Neurosurg* 1991;75: S14–S20.

63. Matsushita Y, Bramlett HM, Kuluz JW, Alonso O, Dietrich WD. Delayed hemorrhagic hypotension exacerbates the hemodynamic and histopathologic consequences of traumatic brain injury in rats. *J Cereb Blood Flow Metab* 2001;21: 847–856.

64. Mayhall CG, Archer NH, Lamb VA, et al. Ventriculostomy-related infections: a prospective epidemiologic study. *N Engl J Med* 1984;310:553–559.

65. McHugh GS, Engel DC, Butcher I, et al. Prognostic value of secondary insults in traumatic brain injury: results from the IMPACT study. *J Neurotrauma* 2007;24:287–293.

66. Muizelaar JP, Marmarou A, Ward JD, et al. Adverse effects of prolonged hyperventilation in patients with severe head injury: a randomized clinical trial. *J Neurosurg* 1991;75:731–739.

67. Myburgh J, Cooper DJ, Finfer S, et al. Saline or albumin for fluid resuscitation in patients with traumatic brain injury. *N Engl J Med* 2007;357:874–884.

68. Narayan RK. Hypothermia for traumatic brain injury: a good idea proved ineffective. *N Engl J Med* 2001;344:602–603.

69. Narayan RK, Kishore PR, Becker DP, et al. Intracranial pressure: to monitor or not to monitor? A review of our experience with severe head injury. *J Neurosurg* 1982;56:650–659.

70. Nelson AT, Kishore PR, Lee SH. Development of delayed epidural hematoma. *AJNR Am J Neuroradiol* 1982;3:583–585.

71. Norton JA, Ott LG, McClain C, et al. Intolerance to enteral feeding in the brain-injured patient. *J Neurosurg* 1988;68:62–66.

72. O'Sullivan MG, Statham PF, Jones PA, et al. Role of intracranial pressure monitoring in severely head-injured patients without signs of intracranial hypertension on initial computerized tomography. *J Neurosurg* 1994;80:46–50.

73. Oddo M, Levine JM, Frangos S, et al. Effect of mannitol and hypertonic saline on cerebral oxygenation in patients with severe traumatic brain injury and refractory intracranial hypertension. *J Neurol Neurosurg Psychiatry* 2009;80:916–920.

74. Oertel M, Boscardin WJ, Obrist WD, et al. Posttraumatic vasospasm: the epidemiology, severity, and time course of an underestimated phenomenon: a prospective study performed in 299 patients. *J Neurosurg* 2005;103:812–824.

75. Oertel M, Kelly DF, McArthur D, et al. Progressive hemorrhage after head trauma: predictors and consequences of the evolving injury. *J Neurosurg* 2002;96:109–116.

76. Okasha AS, Fayed AM, Saleh AS. The FOUR score predicts mortality, endotracheal intubation and ICU length of stay after traumatic brain injury. *Neurocrit Care* 2014;21:496–504.

77. Okie S. Traumatic brain injury in the war zone. *N Engl J Med* 2005;352:2043–2047.

78. Ostrup RC, Luerssen TG, Marshall LF, Zornow MH. Continuous monitoring of intracranial pressure with a miniaturized fiberoptic device. *J Neurosurg* 1987;67:206–209.

79. Ott L, Young B, Phillips R, et al. Altered gastric emptying in the head-injured patient: relationship to feeding intolerance. *J Neurosurg* 1991;74:738–742.

80. Parizel PM, Demey HE, Veeckmans G, et al. Early diagnosis of cerebral fat embolism syndrome by diffusion-weighted MRI (starfield pattern). *Stroke* 2001;32:2942–2944.

81. Phonprasert C, Suwanwela C, Hongsaprabhas C, Prichayudh P, O'Charoen S. Extradural hematoma: analysis of 138 cases. *J Trauma* 1980;20:679–683.

82. Pierallini A, Pantano P, Fantozzi LM, et al. Correlation between MRI findings and long-term outcome in patients with severe brain trauma. *Neuroradiology* 2000;42:860–867.

83. Rea GL, Rockswold GL. Barbiturate therapy in uncontrolled intracranial hypertension. *Neurosurgery* 1983;12:401–404.

84. Rivas JJ, Lobato RD, Sarabia R, et al. Extradural hematoma: analysis of factors influencing the courses of 161 patients. *Neurosurgery* 1988; 23:44–51.

85. Rockoff MA, Marshall LF, Shapiro HM. High-dose barbiturate therapy in humans: a clinical review of 60 patients. *Ann Neurol* 1979;6:194–199.

86. Rockswold GL, Leonard PR, Nagib MG. Analysis of management in thirty-three closed head injury patients who "talked and deteriorated." *Neurosurgery* 1987;21:51–55.

87. Ropper AH, O'Rourke D, Kennedy SK. Head position, intracranial pressure, and compliance. *Neurology* 1982;32:1288–1291.

88. Rosner MJ, Rosner SD, Johnson AH. Cerebral perfusion pressure: management protocol and clinical results. *J Neurosurg* 1995;83:949–962.

89. Sakas DE, Bullock MR, Teasdale GM. One-year outcome following craniotomy for traumatic hematoma in patients with fixed dilated pupils. *J Neurosurg* 1995;82:961–965.

90. Salvant JB, Jr., Muizelaar JP. Changes in cerebral blood flow and metabolism related to the presence of subdural hematoma. *Neurosurgery* 1993;33:387–393.

91. Sato M, Tanaka S, Suzuki K, Kohama A, Fujii C. Complications associated with barbiturate therapy. *Resuscitation* 1989;17:233–241.

92. Saul TG, Ducker TB, Salcman M, Carro E. Steroids in severe head injury: a prospective randomized clinical trial. *J Neurosurg* 1981;54:596–600.

93. Schickner DJ, Young RF. Intracranial pressure monitoring: fiberoptic monitor compared with the ventricular catheter. *Surg Neurol* 1992;37:251–254.

94. Schierhout G, Roberts I. Anti-epileptic drugs for preventing seizures following acute traumatic brain injury. *Cochrane Database Syst Rev* 2001:CD000173.

95. Schwartz ML, Tator CH, Rowed DW, et al. The University of Toronto head injury treatment study: a prospective, randomized comparison of pentobarbital and mannitol. *Can J Neurol Sci* 1984;11:434–440.

96. Shafi S, Diaz-Arrastia R, Madden C, Gentilello L. Intracranial pressure monitoring in brain-injured patients is associated with worsening of survival. *J Trauma* 2008;64:335–340.

97. Smith HK, Miller JD. The danger of an ultra-early computed tomographic scan in a patient with an evolving acute epidural hematoma. *Neurosurgery* 1991;29:258–260.

98. Smith HP, Kelly DL, Jr., McWhorter JM, et al. Comparison of mannitol regimens in patients with severe head injury undergoing intracranial monitoring. *J Neurosurg* 1986;65:820–824.

99. Smith RW, Alksne JF. Infections complicating the use of external ventriculostomy. *J Neurosurg* 1976;44:567–570.

100. Snow RB, Zimmerman RD, Gandy SE, Deck MD. Comparison of magnetic resonance imaging and computed tomography in the evaluation of head injury. *Neurosurgery* 1986,18:45–52.
101. Statham PF, Johnston RA, Macpherson P. Delayed deterioration in patients with traumatic frontal contusions. *J Neurol Neurosurg Psychiatry* 1989;52:351–354.
102. Stiell IG, Wells GA, Vandemheen K, et al. The Canadian CT Head Rule for patients with minor head injury. *Lancet* 2001;357:1391–1396.
103. Stocchetti N. Could intracranial pressure in traumatic brain injury be measured or predicted noninvasively? Almost. *Intensive Care Med* 2007;33:1682–1683.
104. Stocchetti N, Maas AI, Chieregato A, van der Plas AA. Hyperventilation in head injury: a review. *Chest* 2005;127:1812–1827.
105. Stocchetti N, Pagan F, Calappi E, et al. Inaccurate early assessment of neurological severity in head injury. *J Neurotrauma* 2004;21:1131–1140.
106. Sydenham E, Roberts I, Alderson P. Hypothermia for traumatic head injury. *Cochrane Database Syst Rev* 2009:CD001048.
107. Taber KH, Warden DL, Hurley RA. Blast-related traumatic brain injury: what is known? *J Neuropsychiatry Clin Neurosci* 2006;18:141–145.
108. Taneda M, Kataoka K, Akai F, Asai T, Sakata I. Traumatic subarachnoid hemorrhage as a predictable indicator of delayed ischemic symptoms. *J Neurosurg* 1996;84:762–768.
109. Teasdale GM, Murray G, Anderson E, et al. Risks of acute traumatic intracranial haematoma in children and adults: implications for managing head injuries. *BMJ* 1990;300:363–367.
110. Temkin NR, Dikmen SS, Wilensky AJ, et al. A randomized, double-blind study of phenytoin for the prevention of post-traumatic seizures. *N Engl J Med* 1990;323:497–502.
111. Torre-Healy A, Marko NF, Weil RJ. Hyperosmolar therapy for intracranial hypertension. *Neurocrit Care* 2012;17:117–130.
112. Unterberg A, Kiening K, Schmiedek P, Lanksch W. Long-term observations of intracranial pressure after severe head injury: the phenomenon of secondary rise of intracranial pressure. *Neurosurgery* 1993;32:17–23.
113. Vespa P, Boonyaputthikul R, McArthur DL, et al. Intensive insulin therapy reduces microdialysis glucose values without altering glucose utilization or improving the lactate/pyruvate ratio after traumatic brain injury. *Crit Care Med* 2006;34:850–856.
114. Vespa PM. Intensive glycemic control in traumatic brain injury: what is the ideal glucose range? *Crit Care* 2008;12:175.
115. Wakai A, Roberts I, Schierhout G. Mannitol for acute traumatic brain injury. *Cochrane Database Syst Rev* 2005:CD001049.
116. Wang BH, Robertson BC, Girotto JA, et al. Traumatic optic neuropathy: a review of 61 patients. *Plast Reconstr Surg* 2001;107:1655–1664.
117. Ward JD, Becker DP, Miller JD, et al. Failure of prophylactic barbiturate coma in the treatment of severe head injury. *J Neurosurg* 1985;62:383–388.
118. Wardlaw JM, Easton VJ, Statham P. Which CT features help predict outcome after head injury? *J Neurol Neurosurg Psychiatry* 2002;72:188–192.
119. Ware ML, Nemani VM, Meeker M, et al. Effects of 23.4% sodium chloride solution in reducing intracranial pressure in patients with traumatic brain injury: a preliminary study. *Neurosurgery* 2005;57:727–736.
120. Wijdicks EFM. *Communicating Prognosis.* New York: Oxford University Press; 2014.
121. Wijdicks EFM. *Neurologic Complications of Critical Illness.* 3rd ed. New York: Oxford University Press; 2009.
122. Wilberger JE, Jr., Deeb Z, Rothfus W. Magnetic resonance imaging in cases of severe head injury. *Neurosurgery* 1987;20:571–576.
123. Wilberger JE, Jr, Harris M, Diamond DL. Acute subdural hematoma: morbidity, mortality, and operative timing. *J Neurosurg* 1991;74:212–218.
124. Wilberger JE, Jr., Rothfus WE, Tabas J, Goldberg AL, Deeb ZL. Acute tissue tear hemorrhages of the brain: computed tomography and clinicopathological correlations. *Neurosurgery* 1990;27:208–213.
125. Williams RF, Magnotti LJ, Croce MA, et al. Impact of decompressive craniectomy on functional outcome after severe traumatic brain injury. *J Trauma* 2009;66:1570–1574.
126. Winfield JA, Rosenthal P, Kanter RK, Casella G. Duration of intracranial pressure monitoring does not predict daily risk of infectious complications. *Neurosurgery* 1993;33:424–430.
127. Wintermark M, Sanelli PC, Anzai Y, Tsiouris AJ, Whitlow CT. Imaging evidence and recommendations for traumatic brain injury: conventional neuroimaging techniques. *J Am Coll Radiol* 2015;12:e1–e14.
128. Wolf AL, Levi L, Marmarou A, et al. Effect of THAM upon outcome in severe head injury: a randomized prospective clinical trial. *J Neurosurg* 1993;78:54–59.
129. Worthley LI, Cooper DJ, Jones N. Treatment of resistant intracranial hypertension with hypertonic saline: report of two cases. *J Neurosurg* 1988;68:478–481.

130. Young D, Harrison DA, Cuthbertson BH, Rowan K. Effect of early vs late tracheostomy placement on survival in patients receiving mechanical ventilation: the TracMan randomized trial. *JAMA* 2013;309:2121–2129.

131. Yuan Q, Liu H, Wu X, Sun Y, Hu J. Comparative study of decompressive craniectomy in traumatic brain injury with or without mass lesion. *Br J Neurosurg* 2013;27:483–488.

132. Zink BJ. Traumatic brain injury outcome: concepts for emergency care. *Ann Emerg Med* 2001;37:318–332.

42

Guillain-Barré Syndrome

Guillain-Barré syndrome (GBS) is an acute, self-limiting, inflammatory, demyelinating polyneuropathy. The incidence has remained fairly constant at 1 per 100,000, but outbreaks, often of unknown cause, continue to occur.[6,74] Guillain-Barré syndrome is commonly precipitated by an infection, often a trivial viral respiratory infection. Certain pathogens predominate as triggers in GBS, mainly influenza virus, *Campylobacter jejuni*, cytomegalovirus, Epstein-Barr virus, and *Mycoplasma pneumoniae*.[42,57,102,115] Other, less robust, associations include vaccinations, surgery, and lymphoma.[89,122] An interesting finding is that no preceding illness can be identified in one-third of the patients.[97] Most recent outbreak is GBS associated with Zika virus.

The immunopathogenesis of GBS has remained elusive since its original description in 1916[40,48,49,127] (Figure 42.1). Some studies have suggested that complement activation triggers myelin destruction. Complement cascade activation is mediated by the binding of antibodies to the Schwann cells and results in vesicular myelin degeneration.[43] The axon may be a target as well, often after *Campylobacter jejuni* infection,[129] or may be involved in more severe manifestations of GBS ("the innocent bystander" theory). The proclivity of motor axonal involvement has led to the designation *acute motor axonal neuropathy* (AMAN). There might be a summer GBS (AMAN), but most GBS occurs in the winter.[119] Lack of demyelinization but the presence of macrophages within the periaxonal spaces of myelinated fibers in these patients is highly suggestive of direct macrophage invasion.[39] A competing explanation involves antibodies to ganglioside epitopes or myelin proteins.[49]

Campylobacter infection from undercooked poultry has been confirmed as a prominent trigger for severe forms of GBS, and the putative immunologic pathways have been characterized better than those of any other possible infection. The lipopolysaccharide of *Campylobacter* shows a homology with epitopes in gangliosides of the peripheral nerves, a suggestion of molecular mimicry. The risk of GBS developing after *Campylobacter* infection is very low, probably 1 in every 1,000 cases of *Campylobacter* infection.[71,72,80] The risk of GBS after influenza vaccination is low; in fact, the relative and attributable risks of Guillain-Barré syndrome after seasonal influenza vaccination are lower than the risks after a bout of influenza.[63]

First and foremost, patients with GBS can be managed on wards, but if their clinical condition is deteriorating, admission to the neurosciences intensive care unit (NICU) is justified. Generally, uncertainty about the progression of respiratory muscle weakness warrants brief admission to the neurologic unit for overnight monitoring of respiratory mechanics. This concern is particularly legitimate in a bed-bound patient with rapid onset of upper limb weakness, oropharyngeal involvement, bilateral facial palsy, and worsening pulmonary function.[65] Certain admission criteria are respiratory muscle failure, accumulating secretions from oropharyngeal weakness and poor coughing, and evolving aspiration pneumonia. Dysautonomia—usually onset of a cardiac arrhythmia or fluctuations in blood pressure—clearly should prompt admission to the NICU. Similarly, chest tightness or marked hypotension during the first course of plasma exchange necessitates transfer to the unit. Medical reasons for admission to a neurologic or medical ICU are sepsis syndrome, suspected pulmonary embolism, and gastrointestinal complications. In practice, most neurologists would prefer patients with evolving signs and symptoms of GBS to be in a safe, monitored environment and thus, quite rightly so, in any ICU.

CLINICAL RECOGNITION

To some extent, GBS is easy to diagnose.[31] The diagnosis becomes more difficult in circumstances in which the clinical presentation is more protean. Limb paresthesias, germane to typical GBS, are presenting signs. They often begin in the wrists and ankles and are experienced as a "tight band" or "nagging prickling sensation" but also as a "feeling

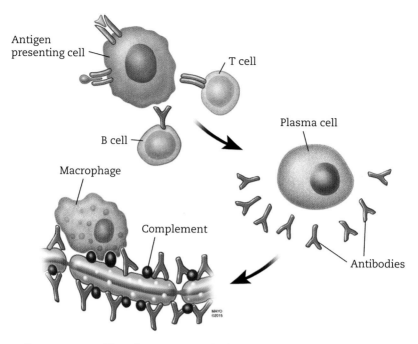

FIGURE 42.1: Current concept of demyelination as a result of macrophage and antibody attack.

of rocks in the shoes." The paresthesias gradually become scattered over the limbs and include the more proximal parts. Weakness is notable 1–2 days after the onset of paresthesias and begins in the more proximal muscles, causing difficulty with climbing stairs, getting out of a chair, and, if the disease progresses rapidly, lifting the arms. The tendon reflexes become absent or depressed in weak limbs, but may be initially spared in limbs that are not affected or are mildly weak and still can overcome the pull of gravity. Complete areflexia occurs in virtually all bed-bound patients. Thus, retained tendon reflexes in an otherwise seemingly clear-cut case of GBS may point to other causes, such as thallium or arsenic poisoning or to botulism.

Cramping, deep aching pain, and limb dysesthesias are accompanying symptoms in most patients, specifically in the proximal muscles, back, and buttocks (often referred to as "charley horse").[79,94] Shooting pain may occur when sudden movements are made and can be excruciating for several seconds.[79,94]

Facial weakness, very common in early GBS, does not necessarily imply further progression to bulbar involvement or ophthalmoplegia but is more commonly associated with respiratory failure and may precede it.[65] The emergence of ptosis, ophthalmoplegia, or oropharyngeal weakness during progression of limb weakness clearly suggests significant demyelination and a possibility of axonal damage with longer recuperation. Ptosis

may often be severe, up to a point that effort is needed to briefly open the eyelids.

Oropharyngeal weakness is manifested by difficulty in swallowing solid foods and clearing secretions, loss of vocal clarity, and some degree of dysarthria. Oropharyngeal weakness may occur in approximately one-third of hospitalized patients (Figure 42.2). Oropharyngeal weakness may coincide with neuromuscular respiratory weakness, but in some patients, clearing secretions is the only major concern next to muscle weakness. Intubation for airway protection alone is often imperative at this stage.

Respiratory failure occurs on average within 1 week after the onset of paresthesias. It is unusual for diaphragmatic failure to develop more than 2 weeks into the illness. The clinical signs and symptoms of neuromuscular failure have been detailed in Chapter 10. Again, respiratory failure in GBS is evident by interrupted speech; patients tend to speak with only a few syllables to each breath. In addition to increased respiratory rate and small tidal volumes, many patients have mild tachycardia and sweating on the forehead.[121] Rapid decline within the day of admission, including "crash intubation" (sudden respiratory distress), may occur quite unexpectedly. A pulmonary segmental collapse may also cause sudden worsening of respiration early in the course and bronchoscopy after intubation may detect a mucus plug. In our study, intubation between 6 P.M. and 8 A.M. was

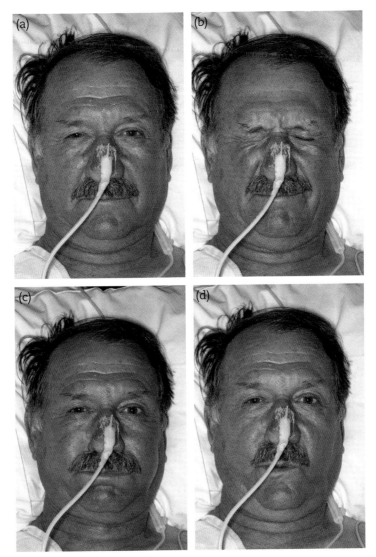

FIGURE 42.2: Guillain-Barré syndrome with marked oropharyngeal weakness. There is asymmetric ptosis and asymmetric facial palsy (a, b). Marked difficulties with blowing up cheeks and whistling (c, d).

common, a suggestion that the early signs of acute neuromuscular failure during the day were not recognized.[123] Nocturnal decompensation could also be due to impairment of central respiratory drive, along with poor pulmonary mechanics.[123] However, gradual decline (e.g., 30% reduction in vital capacity over more than 1 day) is much more common, and intubation can be planned.

Regional variants introduced by Ropper[92] include pharyngeal-cervical-brachial weakness, paraparetic weakness, bilateral facial weakness and paresthesias, sixth-nerve paresis with paresthesias, and lumbar plexopathy. Paraparetic weakness in GBS is uncommon, and patients have normal bladder function and no sensory level. The diagnosis

can only be made with a normal thoracolumbar MRI.[108,109,116] Other well-established, but no more frequent, clinical presentations are Fisher's variant, pure motor GBS without the classic presenting paresthesias, pure sensory GBS, and pure dysautonomia. The typical clinical findings in the Fisher's variant are characterized by various degrees of ophthalmoplegia, ptosis, gait ataxia, and areflexia and generally no limb, facial, or oropharyngeal weakness. Half the patients may have progression to a more generalized weakness, often within a week of presentation.[97] Whether any of these subtypes are defined by a certain infection trigger is not clear. Early data, however, suggest links between severe (axonal) GBS and *Campylobacter*

TABLE 42.1. CLINICAL FEATURES OF GBS, MFS AND THEIR SUBTYPES

Category	Clinical features		
	Pattern of weakness	Ataxia	Hypersomnolence
GBS			
Classic GBS	Four limbs	No or minimal	No
Pharyngeal–cervical–brachial weakness*	Bulbar, cervical and upper limbs	No	No
Acute pharyngeal weakness‡	Bulbar	No	No
Paraparetic GBS*	Lower limbs	No	No
Bifacial weakness with paraesthesias*	Facial	No	No
MFS			
Classic MFS	Ophthalmoplegia	Yes	No
Acute ophthalmoparesis§	Ophthalmoplegia	No	No
Acute ataxic neuropathy§	No weakness	Yes	No
Acute ptosis§	Ptosis	No	No
Acute mydriasis§	Paralytic mydriasis	No	No
BBE‖	Ophthalmoplegia	Yes	Yes
Acute ataxic hypersomnolence	No weakness	Yes	Yes

*Localized subtypes of GBS. ‡Incomplete form of pharyngeal–cervical–brachial weakness. §Incomplete forms of MFS. ‖CNS subtype of MFS. ¶Incomplete form of BBE. Abbreviations: BBE, Bickerstaff brainstem encephalitis; GBS, Guillain–Barré syndrome; MFS, Miller Fisher syndrome.
Adapted from Wakerly et al.[116,117]

and cytomegalovirus (CMV) with a fulminant form.[62,115] The variants and associated antibodies to gangliosides are shown in Tables 42.1 and 42.2.

Several, less frequent disorders may mimic Guillain-Barré syndrome. In patients with predominant ptosis, ophthalmoplegia, and oropharyngeal weakness at presentation, one should consider myasthenia gravis and other myasthenic syndromes, polymyositis, and botulism. Often the evaluation needs to be completed during their stay in the ICU. Careful clinical and electrodiagnostic examinations should suffice to differentiate the disorders. Although very uncommon in any patient with acute flaccid paralysis, the following can be considered: fulminant vasculitis, botulism, organophosphate poisoning, ingestion of the fruit of the buckthorn shrub, glue sniffing, and snake and spider bites. A remarkable presentation is tick paralysis, a disorder in children but also in young adults.[28,99,113] It is common in spring and summer and in the southeastern and northwestern parts of the United States. The ticks may settle in the scalp (young girls with long hair may be predisposed), axilla, or perineum. Within hours to days after neurotoxin from the female tick interferes with voltage-gated sodium channels of axons, ascending paralysis occurs. Recovery is spectacular within 24 hours after removal of the tick, baffling all description.[28,99,113]

Porphyria may be manifested by an acute flaccid paralysis and should certainly be suspected when barbiturates have recently been administered. In certain areas (e.g., Caribbean islands), ciguatera (eating reef fish) poisoning is endemic and a more common cause for paresthesias and rapid weakness than GBS. The most frequent diseases mimicking GBS and their distinguishing features are summarized in Table 42.3.[97,117]

TABLE 42.2. ANTIBODIES ASSOCIATED WITH CLINICAL VARIANTS OF GUILLAIN-BARRÉ SYNDROME

Clinical Manifestation	Ganglioside and Galactocerebroside Antibodies
Acute motor and axonal neuropathy (AMSAN)	GM, GM_{1b}, GD_{1a}
Acute motor axonal neuropathy (AMAN)	GM, GM_{1b}, GD_{1a}, Gal Nac-GD_{1a}
Acute sensory neuropathy	GD_{1b}
Ropper's regional variants	GT_{1a}
Fisher's variant	GD_{1b}, GT_{1a}

Adapted from Hughes RAC, Cornblath DR. Guillain-Barré syndrome. *Lancet* 2005; 366:1653–1666. With permission of publisher.

NEUROIMAGING AND LABORATORY TESTS

Exclusion of acute spinal cord disease or brainstem involvement may require neuroimaging studies, but they generally have a low priority in

TABLE 42.3. DISORDERS FREQUENTLY MIMICKING GUILLAIN-BARRÉ SYNDROME

Disease	Relevant Clinical Features	Helpful Laboratory Tests
Transverse myelitis	Sensory level Urinary incontinence No facial or bulbar involvement	MRI of spine with gadolinium CSF: pleocytosis (> 200 cells)
Myasthenia gravis	Marked fatiguing ptosis and ophthalmoplegia Intact tendon reflexes Masseter weakness No dysautonomia	EMG, NCV, repetitive stimulation Normal CSF Neostigmine test
Vasculitic neuropathy	History of PAN, SLE, WG, RA Pain without paresthesias Marked asymmetry of weakness	Chest and sinus radiographs or CT scan of thorax Nerve and muscle biopsies
Carcinomatous or lymphomatous meningitis	Cognitive changes or stupor Radicular pain Asymmetrical cranial nerve involvement	CSF cytology MRI with gadolinium MRI of spine or brain with gadolinium

CSF, cerebrospinal fluid; CT, computed tomography; EMG, electromyography; MRI, magnetic resonance imaging; NCV, nerve conduction velocity; PAN, polyarteritis nodosa; RA, rheumatoid arthritis; SLE, systemic lupus erythematosus; WG, Wegener's granulomatosis.

the evaluation of GBS. Magnetic resonance imaging of the spine is often performed in patients with atypical presentations, such as predominant paraparesis. Pronounced gadolinium enhancement (indicating breakdown of the blood–nerve barrier) of the anterior spinal nerve roots, conus medullaris, and cauda equina has been reported in GBS,[15,19,37,86] most often in the most severe cases.

Magnetic resonance imaging findings in the brain are normal, but cranial nerve enhancement has been noted.[33] In Fisher variant, a double dose of gadolinium enhanced the third, sixth, and seventh nerves.[35] Occasionally, a chronic inflammatory demyelinating polyneuropathy is manifested as acute GBS. Abnormal MRI findings of multifocal white matter lesions in periventricular and brainstem locations have been reported in patients with chronic inflammatory demyelinating polyneuropathy, but neither their diagnostic value nor their significance is known.[76]

Electrodiagnostic studies remain the most sensitive tests in the evaluation of GBS. The most common patterns are motor nerve conduction block (Figure 42.3), prolonged distal latency, temporal dispersion, slowing of nerve conduction, and increased F-wave latency.[7,41,96] Sural nerve conduction can be normal in combination with abnormal median sensory conduction.[7] Detection of these abnormalities is contingent on a competent and comprehensive electrophysiologic study. This could be arbitrarily defined as stimulation of at least two motor and sensory nerves

each in the arms or legs, assessment of conduction block, recording of F waves with attention to impersistence, determination of H reflex and blink reflexes, testing of the trigeminal and facial nerves, and needle examination in at least one distal and one proximal muscle, with confirmation in contralateral muscles when findings are abnormal. This protocol invariably produces abnormal

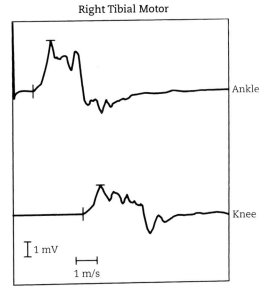

FIGURE 42.3: Conduction block (decline in compound motor action potential amplitude) in Guillain-Barré syndrome.

study results in patients with GBS who are several days into the illness. When study results appear normal, the electromyographer typically refocuses attention on early abnormalities, such as prolongation, dispersion, or absence of F waves.[96,120] The results of a comprehensive study in 113 consecutive patients at the Massachusetts General Hospital are summarized in Table 42.4.[96]

TABLE 42.4. ELECTRODIAGNOSTIC FINDINGS IN 113 CONSECUTIVE PATIENTS WITH GUILLAIN-BARRÉ SYNDROME*

Patient Findings	No.	%
PCB and DL	30	27
Isolated PCB	31	27
Generalized slowing	25	22
PCB and DCB	11	10
Isolated DL	6	5
PCB and ICB	4	4
Absent response	2	2
PCB, ICB, and DL	1	1
DL and ICB	1	1
Isolated ICB	1	1
Normal†	1	1
Total‡	113	

*The major motor nerve abnormalities were categorized as follows:
Distal lesion (DL): > 15% increase in duration of compound muscle action potential (CMAP) or increased distal motor latency on distal stimulation, with motor nerve conduction velocity > 80% of the lower limit of normal.
Distal conduction block (DCB): decreased CMAP amplitude (median or ulnar CMAP, < 4,000 mV; peroneal or tibial CMAP, < 2,000mV) in at least two nerves, with normal motor nerve conduction velocity, duration of CMAP, and distal motor latency.
Proximal conduction block (PCB): absent F waves or decreased F-wave persistence in the presence of motor nerve conduction velocity > 80% of the lower limit of normal, and no distal or intermediate block in the same nerve.
Intermediate conduction block (ICB): > 40% reduction between distal (D) and proximal (P) stimulation sites, specifically in the following ratio: [CMAP (D) − CMAP (P)]/[CMAP (D)] × 100, with < 10% difference in duration between sites without distal conduction block, increased duration, or distal motor latency in the same nerve.
Generalized slowing: maximum motor conduction velocity < 80% of the lower limit of normal in at least two of the median, ulnar, peroneal, or tibial nerves.
Absent response: no evoked motor response with distal stimulation sites in at least three nerves.
Multiple abnormalities: a combination of two or more of abnormalities 1 through 4, above.
Denervation: at least two muscles in the arms and two in the legs were examined for spontaneous activity in the form of fibrillation potentials or positive sharp deflections.
† Prolonged F-wave latencies were found on repeated testing 2 days later.
‡ Electromyography demonstrated extensive fibrillation in 10 patients.
Source: Ropper AH, Wijdicks EFM, Shahani BT. Electrodiagnostic abnormalities in 113 consecutive patients with Guillain-Barré syndrome. *Arch Neurol* 1990;47:881–887. With permission of the American Medical Association.

Prolonged phrenic nerve latency was common in one study (78%) but occurred in both ventilated and nonventilated patients with GBS. This study also emphasized that normal phrenic nerve conduction (the minority of the patients) was associated with normal respiratory mechanics.[133] Phrenic nerve conduction studies may help in establishing the diagnosis,[18] but whether a documented abnormality also predicts pending respiratory failure more reliably than abnormal clinical findings or respiratory function tests is uncertain.

Nerve biopsy in typical GBS is rarely performed and, as mentioned, the sural nerve may be spared in acute motor axonal variants.[70] Biopsy could be considered if the clinical suspicion of a rapidly progressive polyneuropathy from vasculitis is very strong, but usually other laboratory abnormalities point to the diagnosis.

Examination of the cerebrospinal fluid (CSF) typically shows normal cell counts and increased protein in the early days of the illness, but these abnormal findings level off after 1 month. When CSF of patients is examined in the first 3 days, protein is elevated in slightly more than 50% of cases.[97] It is very uncommon for typical GBS to be associated with increased cell counts of more than 10 cells, but marked pleocytosis (> 20 cells) may be a result of human immunodeficiency virus, infection, and Lyme disease, and if this abnormality is found, further serology and polymerase chain reaction testing should be done. Greatly increased protein values may be associated with papilledema. Papilledema is likely due to decreased CSF absorption from high protein concentration.[9] In patients with variants of GBS, CSF protein values tend to be normal, causing additional diagnostic confusion, but often electrophysiologic studies reveal the diagnosis.

Many other laboratory test results can be abnormal. These include liver function abnormalities that can be associated with coexisting hepatitis (A, B, or C), CMV, or Epstein-Barr virus. Liver function abnormalities are more often observed (up to several-fold more than the upper limits of normal) in patients treated with intravenous immunoglobulin (IVIG),[84] but may occur in 10%–20% of untreated patients.[84,97] Currently, pretreatment (including treatment with a solvent and detergent) of IVIG preparations to inactivate hepatitis C and other membrane-enveloped viruses excludes this possible explanation. The mechanism of liver function abnormalities in IVIG-treated GBS is unknown, but could be due to hepatic congestion associated with high protein load.

Patients with GBS may have a transient increase in sedimentation rate and increased white blood cell counts without concomitant infections. Because the creatine kinase level may become markedly elevated in patients with severe pain, some degree of muscle necrosis is suggested as a mechanism rather than a neurogenic cause for the increase.

Autoantibodies targeting gangliosides have been characterized and can be obtained by serologic tests. GM_1 is a major ganglioside that is diffusely located in either the myelin or the axon. Both clinically and in an animal model, antibody reactivity to GM_1 has been linked to a severe and pure motor variant of GBS. Anti-GM_{1b} antibodies were found more commonly in *Campylobacter*-associated GBS, and progression was more severe.[130,132] Antibodies to another ganglioside, GQ_{1b}, are highly specific for the Fisher variant and are found in high titers.[48,90,131] Measurement of these antibodies is not common practice but may have implications for prognosis and therapy. One unconfirmed study suggested that a subgroup with anti-GM_{1b}-positive antibodies had a better response with IVIG.[130]

Respiratory variables remain important, and serial measurements are very helpful in anticipating mechanical ventilation. Vital capacity of less than 20 mL/kg, maximum inspiratory pressure (PI_{max}) of less than 30 cm H_2O, and maximum expiratory pressure (PE_{max}) of less than 40 cm H_2O ("20–30–40 rule") or any reduction of more than 30% from baseline in any of these values highly predicts the need for endotracheal and mechanical ventilation.[65] A recent study[118] found rapid onset to quadriplegia and oropharyngeal weakness highly predictive of future intubation, but the study did not include any respiratory parameters.[118]

FIRST STEPS IN MANAGEMENT

The initial steps in the management of a patient with GBS depend on several clinical features. Pivotal factors at the bedside are severity of weakness or rapidity of progression, involvement of neuromuscular respiratory weakness, dysautonomia, an early systemic complication, and comorbid disease. Progression in symptoms usually is slow, reaching nadir in 75% of patients in the first 2 weeks. Extremely rapid progression (less than 48 hours from onset) has been recently reported in five patients, all with respiratory failure, but still with full functional recovery in three patients.[104]

The initial management in GBS is summarized in Table 42.5. Management in GBS, more than in any other neurologic critical illness, is guided by the physiologic changes during prolonged bed rest. These changes do not always pertain to dysautonomia. In any patient confined to bed, plasma volume tends to decrease by 10% in the first week and by 20% in the second week because of venous pooling in the lower extremities. Other cardiovascular alterations in bed rest are sinus tachycardia, an exaggerated increase in pulse rate, and decreased cardiac output with any type of exercise. The mechanism of orthostasis associated with bed rest may be related to decreased venous return and also to decreased baroreceptor responses.

Fluid intake in patients with GBS includes a 2 L infusion of isotonic saline, which should be adjusted when enteric feeding is started. Larger volumes are needed in patients receiving mechanical ventilation and in those with fever to compensate for imperceptible fluid loss. Hypotension commonly occurs in patients who are transferred to the NICU for mechanical ventilation. The sudden introduction of positive-pressure lung inflation diminishes venous return, and in patients who are relatively dehydrated, blood pressure may significantly decrease.

Bed rest alters gastrointestinal function, and the most salient changes are an almost two-thirds reduction in transit time through the stomach, reduced gastric bicarbonate secretion, and slowing of small bowel activity, rapidly leading to constipation. Enteral nutrition is started almost immediately after admission. In patients with diminished swallowing mechanics, a nasogastric tube is placed, and daily residuals (less than 50% of infused volume) are carefully monitored. At later stages, high-calorie feeding is contraindicated, because energy-rich formulas may seriously hamper weaning from the mechanical ventilator. Most patients need a stool softener such as docusate sodium 100 mg orally twice daily. Enteral feeding is contraindicated in patients with adynamic ileus. Selective decontamination has decreased time on the ventilator.[10]

The possible development of ileus must be monitored daily, but it occurs in only a minority of patients. Acute colonic pseudo-obstruction (Ogilvie syndrome) may occur early in the course of GBS[83] and during a bout of dysautonomia, but more commonly it occurs from secondary causes, including opiates given for pain.[14] One must be familiar with the early signs and symptoms of abdominal discomfort, thirst, and increase in pulse rate commensurate with the degree of distention.

TABLE 42.5. INITIAL MANAGEMENT OF GUILLAIN-BARRÉ SYNDROME

Airway management	Intubation with hypoxemia and rapid shallow breathing
	Intubation if vital capacity < 20 mL/kg and maximum inspiratory pressure ≤ −30 cm H_2O and maximum expiratory pressure < 40 cm H_2O
	Tracheostomy in most patients, but may defer if improvement is seen with PLEX or IVIG
Mechanical ventilation	IMV/PS or AC if severe atelectasis
Fluid management	2 L of 0.9% NaCl
Nutrition	Full strength enteral nutrition
	Early PEG in mechanically ventilated patients
	TPN with adynamic ileus
Sleep enhancement	Melatonin, zolpidem, doxylamine
Prophylaxis	DVT prophylaxis with pneumatic compression devices
	SC heparin 5,000 U t.i.d.
	GI prophylaxis: pantoprazole 40 mg daily IV or lansoprazole 30 mg orally through nasogastric tube
Specific management	IVIG, 0.4 g/kg/day for 5 days
	PLEX on 5 alternate days for a total of 250 mL/kg, if IVIG is not tolerated
Other measures	Oxycodone, fentanyl, or tramadol for pain
	Aggressive skin care
	Physical therapy and splinting to prevent contractures
Access	Arterial catheter to monitor blood pressures (if IV antihypertensive drugs anticipated)
	Peripheral venous catheter and place high flow catheter with PLEX

AC, assist control; DVT, deep vein thrombosis; GI, gastrointestinal; IMV, intermittent mandatory ventilation; IV, intravenously; IVIG, intravenous immunoglobulin; NaCl, sodium chloride; PLEX, plasma exchange; PS, pressure support; TPN, total parenteral nutrition; SC, subcutaneously.

Auscultation of the abdomen yields typical findings of silence interrupted by transmitted heart sounds. Ileus should be treated conservatively with continuous suctioning, liberal intravenous administration of fluids, and placement of a flatus tube. Neostigmine (2 mg IV), a parasympathomimetic agent that stimulates colonic contraction, has been considered in patients without response to conservative management.[87] Because of associated bradycardia, neostigmine is less attractive in GBS and in fact is contraindicated in patients with GBS and dysautonomia. Colonic perforation from acute colonic pseudo-obstruction is a potentially fatal complication but very uncommon. Decompressive colonoscopy can be performed in selected patients and may be more effective than promotility agents. Parenteral nutrition may be needed if the signs do not subside within days.

Bladder paralysis is not uncommon. Intermittent catheterization, although favored over an indwelling catheter, is impractical and time-consuming; careful attention to sterile handling of a closed system may be preferable. Voiding in patients with detrusor areflexia usually cannot be enhanced by pharmacologic agents.

The management of respiration is a major component of care in severe GBS. Any patient with GBS, and certainly one on the verge of diaphragmatic akinesis, is at considerable risk of atelectasis. The supine position relocates a large proportion of lung tissue into the most dependent third zone, resulting in a tendency toward the accumulation of interstitial fluid and closing of alveoli. Bed rest, therefore, produces a ventilation–perfusion mismatch, culminating in oxygen desaturation. It is prudent to monitor desaturation with a pulse oximeter in every patient with GBS.

Lung expansion techniques are important, and in patients with near-marginal tidal volume capacities, a rigorous protocol may prevent deterioration from progressive atelectasis, leading to intubation. Patients with GBS should be helped to perform incentive spirometry hourly. Aerosols are not very effective in nonintubated patients because most of the spray does not reach the most peripheral and lower parts of the respiratory tract. No benefit has been demonstrated with expectorants or aminophylline.

Noninvasive mechanical ventilation using bilevel positive-pressure airway pressure (BiPAP) has been considered in patients with marginal respiratory function who were not necessarily candidates for immediate intubation. Our attempt to use BiPAP in two consecutive patients was unsuccessful with emergency intubation. In both patients, marked clinical improvement was noted briefly and satisfactory tidal volumes were recorded, only to be interrupted by sudden cyanosis.[126] Noninvasive ventilation may produce thickened secretions due to loss of water vapor, but it is more likely that volume-triggered mechanical ventilation is needed in GBS with this severe degree of neuromuscular respiratory failure.[126]

The indications for endotracheal intubation and mechanical ventilation in patients with neuromuscular failure, including GBS, are summarized in Chapters 10 and 17. It is important to emphasize that the use of succinylcholine in paralyzed patients to facilitate endotracheal intubation is likely contraindicated. Massive potassium release may occur, leading to cardiac arrest. (However, the risk is most likely increased in patients with long-standing paralysis.)

Most patients are well served with an intermittent-mandatory ventilation mode and low settings of positive end-expiratory pressure (PEEP). Tracheostomy can be postponed for at least 3 weeks in many patients to await the effect of specific therapy,[67,68] as described in Chapter 17. Early tracheostomy can also be considered when a prolonged course seems inevitable, such as in severely affected patients. In these patients, quadriplegia has developed rapidly over several days, with electrodiagnostic findings of widespread fibrillations and low amplitudes or absent responses. In this circumstance, early tracheostomy allows significantly more comfort and much more effective respiratory care. Tracheostomy may also be considered for comfort in patients with marked bulbar weakness and pooling of secretions but normal respiratory function.[46] Percutaneous dilatory tracheostomy has clear advantages over traditional surgical tracheostomy. Cosmetic disfiguration, which can be substantial and may require later plastic surgery for correction,[124] is less profound in dilatory tracheostomy, which requires an incision of only 1–2 inches.

Skin, eye, and mouth care is crucial to the comfort of quadriplegic patients (Chapter 15). The skin must be kept dry, and after washing, lanolin cream should be applied. Special beds are required, but whether they prevent decubitus is not certain. Eyedrops are necessary in patients who cannot close their eyes completely. Patients with marked ptosis should be asked whether they want their eyes taped open for brief periods. Mouth care includes toothbrushing and careful inspection for oral candidiasis.

As discussed in Chapter 15, a semi-sitting (Fowler) position is preferred, and is alternated with a lateral recumbent position. The limbs should be maintained in a good anatomic position. Splints, foot boards, or sneakers are needed to prevent contractures. Patients with complete quadriplegia should be asked whether they are in a comfortable position, and a small change in alignment of the limbs and shoulders is often greatly appreciated.

Hot packs relieve pain in many patients, and they are certainly of use before the initiation of passive range of movements. Severe pain can be relieved by narcotics, nonsteroidal anti-inflammatory drugs (NSAIDs), and, in resistant cases, epidural morphine. In patients with excruciating pain and marginal diaphragmatic function, it is probably better to intubate and to treat pain aggressively. Brief, but significant, relief is possible by a single intramuscular injection of 60 mg of methylprednisolone sodium succinate. Burning pain (at the recovery stage) may be treated with amitriptyline or mexiletine (mexiletine is contraindicated in patients with dysautonomia). Carbamazepine, 100 mg three times a day, reduces the opiate requirement.[106] Pain control may also include increasing doses of gabapentin or pregabalin. There is a paucity of studies on pain control in GBS.[69]

Prophylaxis of deep vein thrombosis is important, although the true risk of deep vein thrombosis and pulmonary embolus is not exactly known.[55] It is not certain whether intermittent pneumatic compression devices on the calf are sufficient in bed-bound patients, and we have documented deep vein thrombosis within a week, despite intermittent pneumatic devices. In addition, many patients with GBS cannot tolerate these high-frequency devices. We continue to use heparin administered subcutaneously. However, in a recent series with heparin and warfarin prophylaxis in the majority of patients, 6% still developed deep vein thrombosis and 4% pulmonary emboli.[34]

Psychologic support must be provided. Some patients are calm and try to obtain adequate rest, but others are anxious, depressed, and dysphoric. High-strung persons may not accept complete immobility and complete dependence on others, and in the end they may put an almost unacceptable burden on family members. Discussions with the patient are necessary daily in the plateau phase, and patients with severe GBS should be told unequivocally that they have been hit hard but that improvement is expected. The future course should be projected as clearly as possible. Many patients need to master patience, and every time a gain in strength is made, even if subtle, some degree of enthusiasm is appreciated. Depression must be recognized, but the incidence is low in the earlier stages of GBS. Mirtazapine or Buspirone can be tried to relieve some anxiety. Sleep enhancement can be tried with melatonin or zolpidem.

IVIG or plasma exchange is the preferred treatment in typical GBS and in any other type of GBS that produces a bed-bound state or severe ataxia, such as Fisher's variant of GBS.[1,2,4,5,12,20,22,29,51,54,81,111,112] The mode of action of plasma exchange or IVIG has remained speculative. Plasma exchange may remove any of the mediators in the immune response, and IVIG could, by means of anti-idiotypic antibodies, block autoantibodies and neutralize their action on epitopes for nerve conduction.[13] IVIG typically costs less and is definitely much easier to use, but the therapy had been under serious scrutiny after several earlier reports of relapse and continued worsening after treatment. Corticosteroids alone in any dose are of no benefit,[3,50,53] but outcome is not negatively influenced when continued use is mandated (e.g., in asthma or immuno-suppressed patients).[50,53]

Evidence for a beneficial effect of plasma exchange is based on randomized studies, none of which compared plasma exchange with sham exchange.[2,4] North American and French studies, using independent raters, both showed an increase in the number of patients with significant functional improvement and a reduction in the number of days on the ventilator.[2,4] In the North American study, the median time to walking unassisted was reduced from 85 to 53 days, and in the French study, from 111 to 70 days, both statistically and clinically significant reductions in time to recovery. In approximately one-third to one-half of the patients on a mechanical ventilator who were treated by plasma exchange, effective weaning could be achieved within 2 weeks, obviating tracheostomy.

The benefits of plasma exchange are more pronounced in patients treated within 2 weeks of the onset of illness. The use of plasma exchange in patients who have not reached a bed-bound state has been investigated, because deferring plasma exchange in patients who have clear daily progression but who can still ambulate is too intimidating.

Two plasma exchanges significantly reduced clinical deterioration or placement on a mechanical ventilator.[1] Plasma exchange is recommended in any patient with a variant syndrome. In the Fisher variant of GBS, ataxia may resolve within weeks after a plasma exchange series (which makes the patient ambulant), but ophthalmoplegia may take considerably longer to abate.

Contraindications to plasma exchange are any ongoing major infection, recent myocardial infarction (6 months), marked dysautonomia, and active bleeding. Many surveys of large series of patients treated with plasma exchange have demonstrated that when plasma exchange is performed in hospitals with years of experience in exchange procedures, the incidence of serious complications is very low. The side effects are vasovagal reactions, hypovolemia, allergic reactions, hemolysis from kinking in the tubing, and, uncommonly, air embolization and large hematomas.[54] Adverse reaction to fresh frozen plasma accounts for a comparatively high incidence of anaphylactoid reactions, recognized by fever, rigors, urticaria, wheezing, and hypotension. Mostly, albumin 5% is used, with a much lower incidence of anaphylaxis. Generally, it is possible that differences in complication rates in the plasma exchange trials may be related to a higher proportion of small contributing centers with much less experience than the organizing major contributing center. Management strategies to avoid complications of plasma exchange[78] are summarized in Table 42.6.

Plasma exchange requires placement of a temporary high-flow catheter (Niagra™ or Mahurkar™). The actual amount of plasma removed varies from patient to patient but generally is 2 to 4 L, and the time ranges from 90 to 120 minutes. A total of five plasma exchanges on alternate days has remained standard.[2] Red blood cell loss must be minimized during one series of five total plasma exchanges. Again, the preferred replacement fluid is albumin 5% to provide the proper oncotic pressure.

Some positive effects of plasma exchange can be expected in the week after the series has been completed. Plasma exchange in patients with rapid quadriplegia with mechanical ventilation almost never leads to rapid clinically appreciable improvement. Progression to neuromuscular respiratory failure, resulting in the need for mechanical ventilation, has not been prevented with any of the currently available specific therapies.[65]

TABLE 42.6. COMPLICATIONS DURING AND AFTER PLASMA EXCHANGE

Complication	Potential Causes	Management
Hypocalcemia	Citrate	Prophylactic calcium administration ($CaCl_2$) 1 gram in 50 mL of normal saline, rate 30 minutes in central line
Hemorrhage	Depletion of coagulation factors by albumin	2 units of fresh frozen plasma (400–500 mL) at end of each exchange
Anaphylaxis or sensitivity	Anti-IgA antibodies Prekallikrein activator or bradykinin ACE-I*	Diagnostic evaluation after premedication with prednisone, 50 mg orally 13, 7, and 1 hour before treatment; diphenhydramine, 50 mg orally 1 hour before treatment; ephedrine, 25 mg orally 1 hour before treatment and before pheresis
Thrombocytopenia	Filter thrombosis Centrifugal methods	Plasma separation is substituted
Hypovolemia or hypotension	Inadequate or hypooncotic volume replacement Cardiac arrhythmia Dysautonomia	5% albumin, continuous flow separations with matched input and output
Hypothermia	Cold replacement fluids	Warming of fluids
Hypokalemia	Albumin devoid of potassium	Add 4 mEq of potassium to each liter of 5% albumin

IgA, immunoglobulin A.
* Angiotensin I—converting enzyme inhibitors (ACE-I) should be held 72 hours before plasma exchange

IVIG tested in two trials that compared plasma exchange with high doses of IVIG concluded that IVIG is as effective as plasma exchange[5,58,110] (Capsule 42.1). IVIG (0.4 g/kg/day for 5 days) should become the preferred treatment simply because of easy infusion through a peripheral catheter and lower costs.[22] Additionally, some hospitals cannot provide timely plasma exchange services. A small randomized trial of IVIG compared 3 days of therapy with 6 days.[88] A significantly shorter time to walking without assistance was found in mechanically ventilated patients in the 6-day group. However, the practical consequence of this study is not certain, and we continue to give IVIG for 5 days. An infusion guideline is shown in Table 42.7.

Possible disadvantages of IVIG have accumulated over the years. The adverse effects, all rare, are aseptic meningitis,[100,114] acute renal failure,[105] thromboembolic events (including ischemic stroke),[101] anaphylactic shock,[73] and pseudohyponatremia due to a laboratory artifact when an automated method does not correct for increased protein concentrations.[52,64] Anaphylaxis in patients with hereditary IgA deficiency is uncommon (1 in 1,000 individuals have the deficiency, but even then, only half have the antibodies implicated in the anaphylaxis). The measurement of serum IgA to detect a deficiency may considerably delay IVIG treatment and probably can be avoided in patients with no history of anaphylactic reactions to blood products and rapidly progressive weakness. Small anecdotal series have suggested a high relapse rate in patients receiving IVIG.[16,56] But a large comparative trial has not confirmed a higher relapse rate.[5,11]

The efficacy of IVIG is very comparable to that of plasma exchange, and results of a large British–North American trial suggest no difference in outcome at 48 weeks between IVIG and plasma exchange or between one alone and both together.[5] IVIG and plasma exchange can probably both be used in GBS, but not simultaneously; the choice is probably determined by availability (periodic

CAPSULE 42.1   IMMUNOGLOBULIN

Intravenous immunoglobulins (IVIGs) are highly purified products pooled from the serum of over 10,000 donors. Viral inactivation has been achieved with heat and pasteurization. The products differ in volume load, osmolarity, IgA content, and stabilizing agents (e.g., sucrose).[20,26,29,103] The costs of IVIGs are considerable, and there are periods with shortages. Sucrose content has been associated with renal failure and attributed to osmotic injury. Ischemic stroke has been predominantly in the elderly and tentatively has been linked to hyperviscosity, or formation of platelet-leukocyte aggregates.[20] IVIG contains pooled IgG and has multiple immune-modulating effects.[58] These effects can be categorized by segment of the IgG molecule. The F(ab')2 segment effects are neutralization of autoantibodies by anti-idiotypes, effects on cell adhesion and integrins, effects on cytokine levels, and antibodies to immunoregulatory molecules (TCR, CD4, CD5). The FC segment effects are inhibition of phagocytosis and blockade of access of immune complexes to FcR by IgG monomers and inhibition of antibody-dependent cellular cytotoxicity among other inhibitory effects. Intravenous immunoglobulin may also bind compliment components (C_1, C_3b, C_4), degrade C_3b, or bind to anaphylatoxins C_3a and C_5a.[58]

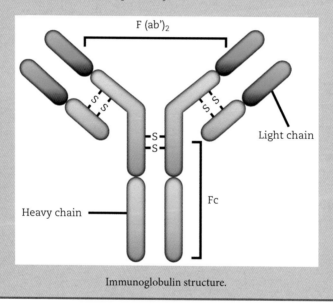

Immunoglobulin structure.

shortages are common in the United States) and provider costs (less for plasma exchange outside the United States).[26] A trial comparing IVIG with short-term use of methylprednisolone seemed to indicate better outcome with the combination, but the results require confirmation to become generally applicable.[51]

If one accepts the flaws of previous studies (none had placebo or sham exchange), the position that plasma exchange should be used first is untenable because of its obviously greater potential for serious complications. Patients very sensitive to IVIG should receive plasma exchange, but this is seldom seen.

A possible alternative to plasma exchange is CSF filtration. In some studies, up to six times, 30–50 mL of CSF was filtered and reinfused for several days. No difference in outcome was found compared with that of plasma exchange, but the study was underpowered, and the cost of this procedure has not been established.[128]

DETERIORATION: CAUSES AND MANAGEMENT

The typical course in GBS is progression to a maximal deficit within 3 weeks after onset of the first paresthesias, a plateau phase ranging from 1 day to 6 months (median, 2 weeks), and

TABLE 42.7. INFUSION GUIDELINE FOR INTRAVENOUS IMMUNOGLOBULIN (IVIG)*

Time (hour)	Rate of Infusion (mL/minute)	Total Dose (mL)
First 1/2	1	30
Second 1/2	3	90
Third 1/2	4	120
Fourth 1/2	5[†]	

* IVIG is contraindicated in patients with known anaphylaxis to blood products and in patients with immunoglobulin A deficiency. Usually, 10% IVIG is used; therefore, 0.4 g/kg becomes 4 mL/kg. For a 70-kg patient, the total volume infused would be 280 ml. The infusion dose is increased only if there is no persistent headache and no hypersensitivity reaction.
In case of anaphylaxis: (1) discontinue infusion; (2) epinephrine 1:1,000, 0.5 mL intramuscularly; (3) if no improvement, epinephrine 1:10,000, 3 mL intravenously; (4) if refractory bronchospasm, aminophylline, 0.5 mg/kg/hr-ideal body weight.
† Maximum rate (300 mL/hour) until infusion is completed.

gradual improvement in several months. Patients may have a halted progression, stuttering progression, virtually no identifiable plateau phase, recovery interrupted by a relapse that usually is less severe, or an intermittent course over weeks that suggests a chronic inflammatory demyelinating polyneuropathy. These clinical profiles were described before specific therapy, such as plasma exchange or IVIG, was introduced, but there is a possibility that plasma exchange or IVIG modifies the progression phase. Without a clear understanding of what plasma exchange and IVIG modify in the complex immunologic response, their effect on progression or relapse remains unknown.

Gradual progression may occur during plasma exchange or IVIG, suggesting treatment failure. This situation becomes especially urgent if deterioration continues and intubation and mechanical ventilation are imminent. Typically, symptoms progress rapidly, and there may be early electrophysiologic indicators of a severe form of GBS.

If motor function unexpectedly worsens after completion of a plasma exchange or IVIG that seemed to have halted progression, another 5-day series of plasma exchange or IVIG should be considered. Data are sparse, and it is not known whether IVIG should follow plasma exchange, or vice versa. The half-life of IVIG is 3–6 weeks, and there could be a concern that plasma exchange may wash out IVIG. Nonetheless, we have noted that worsening patients treated with IVIG improve days after plasma exchange (but not the reverse).

There is evidence that pharmacokinetics of IVIG are variable in GBS. The association between rapid clearance of IVIG and worse outcome implies that the current dose may be insufficient for some patients.[60] For the patient and family and treating physician, it may remain difficult to accept why improvement takes so long, and it is easy to order a second course of IVIG. Whether declining serial IgG levels should guide such a decision is unresolved. Additional treatment with another series of IVIG or plasma exchange may not change the course, but we have administered an additional second course of IVIG or plasma exchange in patients with prolonged plateau phase (more than a month). Corticosteroids may be considered (and also other immunosuppressive agents, such as cyclosporine[8] or mycophenolate mofetil[36]), but only when it becomes clear that chronic inflammatory demyelinating polyneuropathy (CIDP) is a more likely explanation than a single bout of GBS. Criteria for CIDP have been proposed.[98]

Another clinical course that should be clearly distinguished from the first one is relapse during improvement.[91] Relapse fortunately is limited, occurs in 5% of patients treated with plasma exchange, and very seldom is as severe as the previous state. A second series of plasma exchange or IVIG in these patients is successful, reversal is more rapid in onset, and the patient's condition returns to the baseline state. The cause of this relapse during improvement is not known. Intercurrent infections have been suggested.[91]

When GBS is worsening, specific expertise is required for management of dysautonomia. Dysautonomia most commonly occurs in patients with rapidly progressive GBS associated with ophthalmoplegia, but the autonomic nervous system may become involved in any degree of weakness. Dysautonomia is very uncommon in Fisher's syndrome and in CIDP beginning as GBS.

The most common manifestations are spontaneous blood pressure changes and cardiac arrhythmias. In our series of 114 patients with severe GBS admitted to the NICU, 15% had cardiac arrhythmias, 23% had marked blood pressure fluctuation, and 6% had hypotension, particularly during intubation.[44] Blood pressure changes may be caused by sepsis, pulmonary embolus, or severe electrolyte disturbances, but the appearance of wide fluctuations over minutes is characteristic for dysautonomia (Figure 42.4). These clinical manifestations are a result of impaired baroreceptor buffering.[95] (Baroreceptor function predominantly involves toning down acute changes in blood pressure. Baroreceptors in the carotid and aortic arch relay

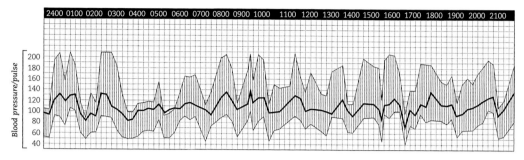

FIGURE 42.4: Labile blood pressures and pulse from dysautonomia.

to the nucleus solitarius, and vasoconstriction as well as increase in heart rate are seen after hypotensive episodes.) Spontaneous fluctuations in blood pressure are best ignored. Persistent hypotension may be treated by placement in the Trendelenburg position and administration of a bolus of albumin. The use of vasopressors is complicated because in some patients it may result in overcompensation to hypertension. Hypertension, which may lead to congestive heart failure in predisposed patients, can be treated with a morphine bolus of 10 mg, and preferably not with β-blockade (use of β-blockers has been linked to cardiac arrest). We and others have seen dysautonomia-associated posterior encephalopathy syndrome. A hypertensive surge was associated with generalized tonic-clonic seizures or even blindness and typical MRI imaging of T2 hyperintensity in bilateral occipital lobes.[17,32]

Another dysautonomic feature is cardiac arrhythmia. Arrhythmias are usually insignificant, consisting of sinus bradycardia and sinus tachycardia. More easily than usual, pressure on the eyeball may bring on bradycardia. The procedure is dangerous and we have seen bradycardia with many sinus pauses and believe that the test should be discouraged for diagnosis. In approximately 35% of severely affected patients, vagal spells are recognized. These episodes of sinus bradycardia, sinus arrest, and atrioventricular block are potentially life-threatening. Tracheal suctioning commonly provokes these arrhythmias. Complete heart block may occur, necessitating a temporary pacemaker.[24,25,38] It is prudent to have atropine readily available. In our experience, cardiac arrhythmias are not a common cause of sudden death or significant hypotension, and a pacemaker has not been placed recently in patients with severe GBS admitted to the Mayo Clinic. Other dysautonomic features are profuse sweating, increased bronchial secretion, and impaired salivation; none of these observed transient phenomena has been carefully studied.

Patients may not tolerate the ventilator initially, leading to fighting the ventilator. A combination of propofol (40–80 μg/kg/min) and fentanyl (50–75 μg/hr) may result in adequate sedation and pain control.

Long-term respiratory management in GBS is a complicated matter, and bronchopneumonia is a major cause of morbidity.[44] Most patients are well served with an intermittent-mandatory mode of ventilation and pressure support.[93] The intermittent-mandatory ventilation rate is determined by $PaCO_2$ and pH, and must secure normal alveolar ventilation. In many patients with GBS, 6–10 breaths per minute provide adequate support in conjunction with normal breathing at this stage of the disease. Only occasionally is a T-piece with pressure support alone sufficient; in many patients, switching to intermittent-mandatory ventilation is necessary, particularly at night.

Weaning from the ventilator in GBS can be expected within 20–30 days. The odds of prolonged ventilatory support are markedly increased if patients are not extubated 3 weeks after intubation. One recent study found vital capacity of greater than 20 mL/kg and a PI_{max} of –50 cm H_2O at extubation predictive of extubation success.[82] A change of ≥ 4 mL/kg of vital capacity measured after extubation and compared to intubation also indicated success (sensitivity 82%, positive predictive value of 90%).[82]

It is very important not to link diaphragmatic weakness with limb weakness. Patients with GBS who have prolonged mechanical ventilation generally first begin to have improvement in diaphragmatic function, often at a time when no signs of motor improvement in the limbs have been noticed for weeks.

Weaning should not be entertained when severe dysautonomia is still present, because the stress of weaning may trigger wide blood pressure fluctuations and cardiac arrhythmias.

Weaning trials in GBS have not been compared, but one approach is to reduce intermittent-mandatory ventilation and unload the ventilatory muscles with maximum pressure-support ventilation when vital capacity has reached 15 mL/kg and the patient can deliver tidal volumes of 10–12 mL/kg. Pressure support is gradually reduced to 5 cm H_2O, a necessary value for the decision to extubate (for laboratory weaning criteria, see Chapter 17).

OUTCOME

The recovery trajectory of severely affected patients is endlessly long. An example of one of our patients is shown in Table 42.8. It is often a reason to consider yet another course of IVIG, but there is no evidence of benefit. (I have occasionally used another 5-day course of IVIG in patients with a prolonged plateau [1–2 months] and have seen that this additional course started improvement.)

Guillain-Barré syndrome is a one-time event in the overwhelming majority of patients. Recurrence is very unusual, and patients should be unequivocally told that the risk of recurrence, even with a similar trigger (e.g., vaccination, documented infection), remains low. Because recurrences have been reported in patients receiving vaccinations, it is prudent to refrain from vaccinations, except when a premorbid condition (e.g., diabetes, emphysema) dictates vaccination or when the risk of infection is comparatively great (e.g., travel outside the United States). Avoidance of immunizations at least 1 year after the onset of GBS is good advice,[59] because most reported relapses have occurred within 1 year. Multiple influenza vaccinations have been tolerated in at least one patient after GBS.[122] When GBS has been associated with a specific vaccination, it is advised to avoid that type of vaccination.

Recurrence after a long asymptomatic interval (up to 36 years) has been reported, but again with full recovery.[61,125]

Poor outcome is related to previous serologic documentation of *Campylobacter jejuni* infection, older age, comorbidity (particularly underlying lung disease), and inexcitable motor potentials.[21] In ventilated patients with GBS, increasing age, upper limb paralysis, duration of ventilation (> 3 months), and delayed transfer to a tertiary institution were significantly more likely to result in poor functional outcome and even mortality.[30] Although repeated claims have been made in the literature, we did not find increased pulmonary morbidity in patients intubated emergently.[123] Mortality is more common in older patients and patients with underlying pulmonary disease, and may reach 20% in mechanically ventilated patients.[30,66,85] More recent cohorts have found nearly 3% mortality in first 6 months usually due to significant comorbidity, but circumstances remain unclear.[107] Chronic inflammatory demyelinating polyneuropathy may appear as GBS in fewer than 2% of patients, often with fluctuations, persistently elevated protein values, and, more important, very significant slowing of motor conduction velocity. The distinction between acute GBS and CIDP remains difficult, and even respiratory failure has been reported in exacerbations of chronic forms.[45] Most often, patients with GBS becoming CIDP have a relapse within 2 months of initial treatment.

Fatigue is a major component of disability, lasting for years.[23,77] Physical deconditioning and depression may have contributed, and these factors could be modified. Thyroid function and hemoglobin must be checked as well as cardiac function. Fatigue is more common in severely affected patients (axonal loss) but may persist despite significant improvement.

Patients with GBS recover completely, although examination will reveal that most have slight weakness and hyporeflexia that do not interfere with daily activities. In patients with persistent motor weakness (< 5% of the total population with GBS), improvement may continue up to 2 years after the initial symptoms.[30,97] Some patients who remain wheelchair-bound recover to walking with splints and braces, often, but not always, with full use of the arms. Factors that have been associated with an increased likelihood of permanent disabling weakness are mechanical ventilation for more than 4 months and quadriplegia within a week of onset.[97]

TABLE 42.8. TRAJECTORY OF RECOVERY IN A SEVERELY AFFECTED QUADRIPLEGIC MECHANICALLY VENTILATED PATIENT WITH GBS

---

1 week—quadriplegic, facial palsy
6 weeks—first upper limb movements
8 weeks—first speech Passy-Muir valve
9 weeks—off the ventilator and some movements
10 weeks—able to swallow food
12 weeks—able to transfer
13 weeks—tracheostomy removed
15 weeks—able to self-feed
21 weeks—able to stand
28 weeks—able to walk unassisted

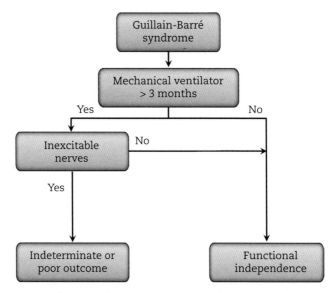

FIGURE 42.5: Outcome algorithm in Guillain-Barré syndrome. Indeterminate: Any statement would be a premature conclusion. Poor outcome: Severe disability and chance of fatal outcome from complications. Functional independence: No assistance needed, minor handicap may remain.

As noted earlier, a particularly severe course in GBS associated with rapid quadriplegia, cranial nerve involvement, dysautonomia, and anti-GM_1 antibodies has been linked to an axonal variant of GBS with very slow and often incomplete recovery.[27,39] Rapid disease progression to severe weakness (3 days after onset of tingling) predicts longer rehabilitation but also positive campylobacter jejuni and cytomegalovirus titers. About 75% of mechanically ventilated patients do regain the ability to walk independently, which is less common in those with severe quadriparesis.

The findings on electrodiagnostic examination have marginal long-term prognostic value, but a reduced mean compound muscle action potential amplitude of less than 20% of the lower limit of normal has been identified in a post hoc analysis as predictive of persistent weakness with a need for braces, splints, and wheelchair. Early randomly distributed fibrillations, multifocal conduction block, or inexcitable motor responses in a quadriplegic patient in need of mechanical ventilation suggests a protracted course. Another study found that the combination of early fibrillations with compound muscle action potential amplitude of 10% (or less) often predicts permanent disabling weakness.[75] Factors that do not necessarily indicate poor outcome are the total protein value in CSF, presence of pleocytosis in CSF, profound pain at onset, and time in plateau or critical illness.[47] The prediction of disability is summarized in Figure 42.5.

CONCLUSIONS

- Absolute indications for intensive care admission are recent 30% reduction in pulmonary function variables (vital capacity, PI_{max}, PE_{max}), oropharyngeal weakness, evidence of aspiration on chest radiographs, and dysautonomia.
- Intubation and mechanical ventilation are indicated in patients with vital capacity less than 20 mL, PI_{max} less than −30 cm H_2O, and PE_{max} less than 40 cm H_2O ("20–30–40 rule"); hypoxemia; and rapid shallow breathing.
- IVIG (0.4 g/kg/day for 5 days) or plasma exchange (albumin 5% as replacement fluid) of 250 mL/kg in five sessions on alternate days can be instituted, and they are equally effective.
- Tracheostomy may be delayed at least 2 weeks awaiting improvement from specific therapy. If there is evidence of the axonal form of GBS or significant bulbar weakness causing marked discomfort in handling secretions, tracheostomy can be placed earlier.
- Blood pressure changes could be a result of dysautonomia. Drugs used to treat blood pressure may cause exaggerated effects. Complete heart block is rare, and a temporary pacemaker may be necessary. Patients should be closely monitored for development of adynamic ileus.

REFERENCES

1. Appropriate number of plasma exchanges in Guillain-Barré syndrome. The French Cooperative Group on Plasma Exchange in Guillain-Barré Syndrome. *Ann Neurol* 1997;41:298–306.

2. Efficiency of plasma exchange in Guillain-Barré syndrome: role of replacement fluids. French Cooperative Group on Plasma Exchange in Guillain-Barré syndrome. *Ann Neurol* 1987;22:753–761.

3. Guillain-Barré Syndrome Steroid Trial Group. Double-blind trial of intravenous methylprednisolone in Guillain-Barré syndrome. *Lancet* 1993;341:586–590.

4. The Guillain-Barré syndrome Study Group. Plasmapheresis and acute Guillain-Barré syndrome. *Neurology* 1985;35:1096–1104.

5. Plasma Exchange/Sandoglobulin Guillain-Barré Syndrome Trial Group. Randomised trial of plasma exchange, intravenous immunoglobulin, and combined treatments in Guillain-Barré syndrome. *Lancet* 1997;349:225–230.

6. Alshekhlee A, Hussain Z, Sultan B, Katirji B. Guillain-Barré syndrome: incidence and mortality rates in US hospitals. *Neurology* 2008;70:1608–1613.

7. Bansal R, Kalita J, Misra UK. Pattern of sensory conduction in Guillain-Barré Syndrome. *Electromyogr Clin Neurophysiol* 2001;41:433–437.

8. Barnett MH, Pollard JD, Davies L, McLeod JG. Cyclosporin A in resistant chronic inflammatory demyelinating polyradiculoneuropathy. *Muscle Nerve* 1998;21:454–460.

9. Behan PO, Harrington H, Sekoni G. Papilloedema in the Landry-Guillain-Barré-Strohl syndrome. *Eur Neurol* 1981;20:62–63.

10. Bos Eyssen ME, van Doorn PA, Jacobs BC, et al. Selective digestive tract decontamination decreases time on ventilator in Guillain-Barré syndrome. *Neurocrit Care* 2011;15:128–133.

11. Bouget J, Chevret S, Chastang C, Raphael JC. Plasma exchange morbidity in Guillain-Barré syndrome: results from the French prospective, randomized, multicenter study. The French Cooperative Group. *Crit Care Med* 1993;21:651–658.

12. Bril V, Ilse WK, Pearce R, et al. Pilot trial of immunoglobulin versus plasma exchange in patients with Guillain-Barré syndrome. *Neurology* 1996;46:100–103.

13. Buchwald B, Ahangari R, Weishaupt A, Toyka KV. Intravenous immunoglobulins neutralize blocking antibodies in Guillain-Barré syndrome. *Ann Neurol* 2002;51:673–680.

14. Burns TM, Lawn ND, Low PA, Camilleri M, Wijdicks EFM. Adynamic ileus in severe Guillain-Barré syndrome. *Muscle Nerve* 2001;24:963–965.

15. Byun WM, Park WK, Park BH, et al. Guillain-Barré syndrome: MR imaging findings of the spine in eight patients. *Radiology* 1998;208:137–141.

16. Castro LH, Ropper AH. Human immune globulin infusion in Guillain-Barré syndrome: worsening during and after treatment. *Neurology* 1993;43:1034–1036.

17. Chen A, Kim J, Henderson G, Berkowitz A. Posterior reversible encephalopathy syndrome in Guillain-Barré syndrome. *J Clin Neurosci* 2015;22:914–916.

18. Chen R, Collins S, Remtulla H, Parkes A, Bolton CF. Phrenic nerve conduction study in normal subjects. *Muscle Nerve* 1995;18:330–335.

19. Crino PB, Zimmerman R, Laskowitz D, Raps EC, Rostami AM. Magnetic resonance imaging of the cauda equina in Guillain-Barré syndrome. *Neurology* 1994;44:1334–1336.

20. Dalakas MC. Intravenous immunoglobulin in autoimmune neuromuscular diseases. *JAMA* 2004;291:2367–2375.

21. Dhar R, Stitt L, Hahn AF. The morbidity and outcome of patients with Guillain-Barré syndrome admitted to the intensive care unit. *J Neurol Sci* 2008;264:121–128.

22. Donofrio PD, Berger A, Brannagan TH, 3rd, et al. Consensus statement: the use of intravenous immunoglobulin in the treatment of neuromuscular conditions report of the AANEM ad hoc committee. *Muscle Nerve* 2009;40:890–900.

23. Drenthen J, Jacobs BC, Maathuis EM, et al. Residual fatigue in Guillain-Barré syndrome is related to axonal loss. *Neurology* 2013;81:1827–1831.

24. Emmons PR, Blume WT, DuShane JW. Cardiac monitoring and demand pacemaker in Guillain-Barré syndrome. *Arch Neurol* 1975;32:59–61.

25. Favre H, Foex P, Guggisberg M. Use of demand pacemaker in a case of Guillain-Barré syndrome. *Lancet* 1970;1:1062–1063.

26. Feasby T, Banwell B, Benstead T, et al. Guidelines on the use of intravenous immune globulin for neurologic conditions. *Transfus Med Rev* 2007;21:S57–S107.

27. Feasby TE, Hahn AF, Brown WF, et al. Severe axonal degeneration in acute Guillain-Barré syndrome: evidence of two different mechanisms? *J Neurol Sci* 1993;116:185–192.

28. Felz MW, Smith CD, Swift TR. A six-year-old girl with tick paralysis. *N Engl J Med* 2000;342:90–94.

29. Fergusson D, Hutton B, Sharma M, et al. Use of intravenous immunoglobulin for treatment of neurologic conditions: a systematic review. *Transfusion* 2005;45:1640–1657.

30. Fletcher DD, Lawn ND, Wolter TD, Wijdicks EFM. Long-term outcome in patients with Guillain-Barré syndrome requiring mechanical ventilation. *Neurology* 2000;54:2311–2315.

31. Fokke C, van den Berg B, Drenthen J, et al. Diagnosis of Guillain-Barré syndrome and validation of Brighton criteria. *Brain* 2014;137:33–43.

32. Fugate JE, Wijdicks EFM, Kumar G, Rabinstein AA. One thing leads to another: GBS complicated by PRES and Takotsubo cardiomyopathy. *Neurocrit Care* 2009;11:395–397.

33. Fulbright RK, Erdum E, Sze G, Byrne T. Cranial nerve enhancement in the Guillain-Barré syndrome. *AJNR Am J Neuroradiol* 1995;16:923–925.

34. Gaber TA, Kirker SG, Jenner JR. Current practice of prophylactic anticoagulation in Guillain-Barré syndrome. *Clin Rehabil* 2002;16:190–193.

35. Garcia-Rivera CA, Rozen TD, Zhou D, et al. Miller Fisher syndrome: MRI findings. *Neurology* 2001;57:1755.

36. Garssen MP, van Koningsveld R, van Doorn PA, et al. Treatment of Guillain-Barré syndrome with mycophenolate mofetil: a pilot study. *J Neurol Neurosurg Psychiatry* 2007;78:1012–1013.

37. Gorson KC, Ropper AH, Muriello MA, Blair R. Prospective evaluation of MRI lumbosacral nerve root enhancement in acute Guillain-Barré syndrome. *Neurology* 1996;47:813–817.

38. Greenland P, Griggs RC. Arrhythmic complications in the Guillain-Barré syndrome. *Arch Intern Med* 1980;140:1053–1055.

39. Griffin JW, Li CY, Ho TW, et al. Pathology of the motor-sensory axonal Guillain-Barré syndrome. *Ann Neurol* 1996;39:17–28.

40. Guillain G, Barré J, Strohl A. Sur un syndrome de radiculo-neurite avec hyperalbuminose du liquide cephalo-rachidien sans reaction cellulaire: remarques sur les caracteres cliniques et graphiques des reflexes tendineux. *Rev Neurol* 1916;40:1462–1470.

41. Gupta D, Nair M, Baheti NN, Sarma PS, Kuruvilla A. Electrodiagnostic and clinical aspects of Guillain-Barré syndrome: an analysis of 142 cases. *J Clin Neuromuscul Dis* 2008;10:42–51.

42. Hadden RD, Karch H, Hartung HP, et al. Preceding infections, immune factors, and outcome in Guillain-Barré syndrome. *Neurology* 2001;56:758–765.

43. Hafer-Macko CE, Sheikh KA, Li CY, et al. Immune attack on the Schwann cell surface in acute inflammatory demyelinating polyneuropathy. *Ann Neurol* 1996;39:625–635.

44. Henderson RD, Lawn ND, Fletcher DD, McClelland RL, Wijdicks EFM. The morbidity of Guillain-Barré syndrome admitted to the intensive care unit. *Neurology* 2003;60:17–21.

45. Henderson RD, Sandroni P, Wijdicks EFM. Chronic inflammatory demyelinating polyneuropathy and respiratory failure. *J Neurol* 2005;252:1235–1237.

46. Herschman Z. Tracheostomy in Guillain-Barré syndrome. *Crit Care Med* 1991;19:743.

47. Ho D, Thakur K, Gorson KC, Ropper AH. Influence of critical illness on axonal loss in Guillain-Barré syndrome. *Muscle Nerve* 2009;39:10–15.

48. Hughes RA, Cornblath DR. Guillain-Barré syndrome. *Lancet* 2005;366:1653–1666.

49. Hughes RA, Hadden RD, Gregson NA, Smith KJ. Pathogenesis of Guillain-Barré syndrome. *J Neuroimmunol* 1999;100:74–97.

50. Hughes RA, Newsom-Davis JM, Perkin GD, Pierce JM. Controlled trial prednisolone in acute polyneuropathy. *Lancet* 1978;2:750–753.

51. Hughes RA, Swan AV, Raphael JC, et al. Immunotherapy for Guillain-Barré syndrome: a systematic review. *Brain* 2007;130:2245–2257.

52. Hughes RA, Swan AV, van Doorn PA. Intravenous immunoglobulin for Guillain-Barré syndrome. *Cochrane Database Syst Rev* 2014;9:CD002063.

53. Hughes RA, Swan AV, van Koningsveld R, van Doorn PA. Corticosteroids for Guillain-Barré syndrome. *Cochrane Database Syst Rev* 2006:CD001446.

54. Hughes RA, Wijdicks EFM, Barohn R, et al. Practice parameter: immunotherapy for Guillain-Barré syndrome: report of the Quality Standards Subcommittee of the American Academy of Neurology. *Neurology* 2003;61:736–740.

55. Hughes RA, Wijdicks EFM, Benson E, et al. Supportive care for patients with Guillain-Barré syndrome. *Arch Neurol* 2005;62:1194–1198.

56. Irani DN, Cornblath DR, Chaudhry V, Borel C, Hanley DF. Relapse in Guillain-Barré syndrome after treatment with human immune globulin. *Neurology* 1993;43:872–875.

57. Jacobs BC, Rothbarth PH, van der Meche FG, et al. The spectrum of antecedent infections in Guillain-Barré syndrome: a case-control study. *Neurology* 1998;51:1110–1115.

58. Jolles S, Sewell WA, Misbah SA. Clinical uses of intravenous immunoglobulin. *Clin Exp Immunol* 2005;142:1–11.

59. Juurlink DN, Stukel TA, Kwong J, et al. Guillain-Barré syndrome after influenza vaccination in adults: a population-based study. *Arch Intern Med* 2006;166:2217–2221.

60. Kuitwaard K, de Gelder J, Tio-Gillen AP, et al. Pharmacokinetics of intravenous immunoglobulin and outcome in Guillain-Barré syndrome. *Ann Neurol* 2009;66:597–603.

61. Kuitwaard K, van Koningsveld R, Ruts L, Jacobs BC, van Doorn PA. Recurrent Guillain-Barré

syndrome. *J Neurol Neurosurg Psychiatry* 2009;80:56–59.

62. Kuwabara S, Yuki N. Axonal Guillain-Barré syndrome: concepts and controversies. *Lancet Neurol* 2013;12:1180–1188.

63. Kwong JC, Vasa PP, Campitelli MA, et al. Risk of Guillain-Barré syndrome after seasonal influenza vaccination and influenza health-care encounters: a self-controlled study. *Lancet Infect Dis* 2013;13:769–776.

64. Lawn N, Wijdicks EFM, Burritt MF. Intravenous immune globulin and pseudohyponatremia. *N Engl J Med* 1998;339:632.

65. Lawn ND, Fletcher DD, Henderson RD, Wolter TD, Wijdicks EFM. Anticipating mechanical ventilation in Guillain-Barré syndrome. *Arch Neurol* 2001;58:893–898.

66. Lawn ND, Wijdicks EFM. Fatal Guillain-Barré syndrome. *Neurology* 1999;52:635–638.

67. Lawn ND, Wijdicks EFM. Post-intubation pulmonary function test in Guillain-Barré syndrome. *Muscle Nerve* 2000;23:613–616.

68. Lawn ND, Wijdicks EFM. Tracheostomy in Guillain-Barré syndrome. *Muscle Nerve* 1999;22:1058–1062.

69. Liu J, Wang LN, McNicol ED. Pharmacological treatment for pain in Guillain-Barré syndrome. *Cochrane Database Syst Rev* 2015;4:CD009950.

70. Lu JL, Sheikh KA, Wu HS, et al. Physiologic-pathologic correlation in Guillain-Barré syndrome in children. *Neurology* 2000;54:33–39.

71. McCarthy N, Andersson Y, Jormanainen V, Gustavsson O, Giesecke J. The risk of Guillain-Barré syndrome following infection with Campylobacter jejuni. *Epidemiol Infect* 1999;122:15–17.

72. McCarthy N, Giesecke J. Incidence of Guillain-Barré syndrome following infection with Campylobacter jejuni. *Am J Epidemiol* 2001;153:610–614.

73. McCluskey DR, Boyd NA. Anaphylaxis with intravenous gammaglobulin. *Lancet* 1990;336:874.

74. McGrogan A, Madle GC, Seaman HE, de Vries CS. The epidemiology of Guillain-Barré syndrome worldwide: a systematic literature review. *Neuroepidemiology* 2009;32:150–163.

75. McKhann GM, Griffin JW, Cornblath DR, et al. Plasmapheresis and Guillain-Barré syndrome: analysis of prognostic factors and the effect of plasmapheresis. *Ann Neurol* 1988;23:347–353.

76. Mendell JR, Kolkin S, Kissel JT, et al. Evidence for central nervous system demyelination in chronic inflammatory demyelinating polyradiculoneuropathy. *Neurology* 1987;37:1291–1294.

77. Merkies IS, Schmitz PI, Samijn JP, van der Meche FG, van Doorn PA. Fatigue in immune-mediated polyneuropathies. European Inflammatory Neuropathy Cause and Treatment (INCAT) Group. *Neurology* 1999;53:1648–1654.

78. Mokrzycki MH, Kaplan AA. Therapeutic plasma exchange: complications and management. *Am J Kidney Dis* 1994;23:817–827.

79. Moulin DE, Hagen N, Feasby TE, Amireh R, Hahn A. Pain in Guillain-Barré syndrome. *Neurology* 1997;48:328–331.

80. Nachamkin I, Allos BM, Ho T. Campylobacter species and Guillain-Barré syndrome. *Clin Microbiol Rev* 1998;11:555–567.

81. Netto AB, Kulkarni GB, Taly AB, et al. A comparison of immunomodulation therapies in mechanically ventilated patients with Guillain Barré syndrome. *J Clin Neurosci* 2012;19:1664–1667.

82. Nguyen TN, Badjatia N, Malhotra A, et al. Factors predicting extubation success in patients with Guillain-Barré syndrome. *Neurocrit Care* 2006;5:230–234.

83. Nowe T, Huttemann K, Engelhorn T, Schellinger PD, Kohrmann M. Paralytic ileus as a presenting symptom of Guillain-Barré syndrome. *J Neurol* 2008;255:756–757.

84. Oomes PG, van der Meche FG, Kleyweg RP. Liver function disturbances in Guillain-Barré syndrome: a prospective longitudinal study in 100 patients. Dutch Guillain-Barré Study Group. *Neurology* 1996;46:96–100.

85. Orlikowski D, Sharshar T, Porcher R, et al. Prognosis and risk factors of early onset pneumonia in ventilated patients with Guillain-Barré syndrome. *Intensive Care Med* 2006;32:1962–1969.

86. Perry JR, Fung A, Poon P, Bayer N. Magnetic resonance imaging of nerve root inflammation in the Guillain-Barré syndrome. *Neuroradiology* 1994;36:139–140.

87. Ponec RJ, Saunders MD, Kimmey MB. Neostigmine for the treatment of acute colonic pseudo-obstruction. *N Engl J Med* 1999;341:137–141.

88. Raphael JC, Chevret S, Harboun M, Jars-Guincestre MC. Intravenous immune globulins in patients with Guillain-Barré syndrome and contraindications to plasma exchange: 3 days versus 6 days. *J Neurol Neurosurg Psychiatry* 2001;71:235–238.

89. Re D, Schwenk A, Hegener P, et al. Guillain-Barré syndrome in a patient with non-Hodgkin's lymphoma. *Ann Oncol* 2000;11:217–220.

90. Rinaldi S, Brennan KM, Kalna G, et al. Antibodies to heteromeric glycolipid complexes in Guillain-Barré syndrome. *PLoS One* 2013;8:e82337.

91. Ropper AE, Albert JW, Addison R. Limited relapse in Guillain-Barré syndrome after plasma exchange. *Arch Neurol* 1988;45:314–315.

92. Ropper AH. Further regional variants of acute immune polyneuropathy. Bifacial weakness or sixth nerve paresis with paresthesias, lumbar polyradiculopathy, and ataxia with pharyngeal-cervical-brachial weakness. *Arch Neurol* 1994;51:671–675.

93. Ropper AH, Kehne SM. Guillain-Barré syndrome: management of respiratory failure. *Neurology* 1985;35:1662–1665.

94. Ropper AH, Shahani BT. Pain in Guillain-Barré syndrome. *Arch Neurol* 1984;41:511–514.

95. Ropper AH, Wijdicks EFM. Blood pressure fluctuations in the dysautonomia of Guillain-Barré syndrome. *Arch Neurol* 1990;47:706–708.

96. Ropper AH, Wijdicks EFM, Shahani BT. Electrodiagnostic abnormalities in 113 consecutive patients with Guillain-Barré syndrome. *Arch Neurol* 1990;47:881–887.

97. Ropper AH, Wijdicks EFM, Truax BT. *Guillain-Barré Syndrome*. Vol. 34. New York: Oxford University Press; 1991.

98. Saperstein DS, Katz JS, Amato AA, Barohn RJ. Clinical spectrum of chronic acquired demyelinating polyneuropathies. *Muscle Nerve* 2001;24:311–324.

99. Schaumburg HH, Herskovitz S. The weak child: a cautionary tale. *N Engl J Med* 2000;342:127–129.

100. Sekul EA, Cupler EJ, Dalakas MC. Aseptic meningitis associated with high-dose intravenous immunoglobulin therapy: frequency and risk factors. *Ann Intern Med* 1994;121:259–262.

101. Silbert PL, Knezevic WV, Bridge DT. Cerebral infarction complicating intravenous immunoglobulin therapy for polyneuritis cranialis. *Neurology* 1992;42:257–258.

102. Sivadon-Tardy V, Orlikowski D, Porcher R, et al. Guillain-Barré syndrome and influenza virus infection. *Clin Infect Dis* 2009;48:48–56.

103. Stangel M, Pul R. Basic principles of intravenous immunoglobulin (IVIg) treatment. *J Neurol* 2006;253 Suppl 5:V18–V24.

104. Steiner I, Wirguin I, Blumen SC, et al. 'Hyperacute' Guillain-Barré syndrome. *Eur Neurol* 2008;59:88–90.

105. Tan E, Hajinazarian M, Bay W, Neff J, Mendell JR. Acute renal failure resulting from intravenous immunoglobulin therapy. *Arch Neurol* 1993;50:137–139.

106. Tripathi M, Kaushik S. Carbamezapine for pain management in Guillain-Barré syndrome patients in the intensive care unit. *Crit Care Med* 2000;28:655–658.

107. van den Berg B, Bunschoten C, van Doorn PA, Jacobs BC. Mortality in Guillain-Barré syndrome. *Neurology* 2013;80:1650–1654.

108. van den Berg B, Fokke C, Drenthen J, van Doorn PA, Jacobs BC. Paraparetic Guillain-Barré syndrome. *Neurology* 2014;82:1984–1989.

109. van den Berg B, Walgaard C, Drenthen J, et al. Guillain-Barré syndrome: pathogenesis, diagnosis, treatment and prognosis. *Nat Rev Neurol* 2014;10:469–482.

110. van der Meche FG, Schmitz PI. A randomized trial comparing intravenous immune globulin and plasma exchange in Guillain-Barré syndrome. Dutch Guillain-Barré Study Group. *N Engl J Med* 1992;326:1123–1129.

111. van Der Meche FG, van Doorn PA. Guillain-Barré syndrome. *Curr Treat Options Neurol* 2000;2:507–516.

112. van Doorn PA, Ruts L, Jacobs BC. Clinical features, pathogenesis, and treatment of Guillain-Barré syndrome. *Lancet Neurol* 2008;7:939–950.

113. Vedanarayanan VV, Evans OB, Subramony SH. Tick paralysis in children: electrophysiology and possibility of misdiagnosis. *Neurology* 2002;59:1088–1090.

114. Vera-Ramirez M, Charlet M, Parry GJ. Recurrent aseptic meningitis complicating intravenous immunoglobulin therapy for chronic inflammatory demyelinating polyradiculoneuropathy. *Neurology* 1992;42:1636–1637.

115. Visser LH, van der Meche FG, Meulstee J, et al. Cytomegalovirus infection and Guillain-Barré syndrome: the clinical, electrophysiologic, and prognostic features. Dutch Guillain-Barré Study Group. *Neurology* 1996;47:668–673.

116. Wakerley BR, Uncini A, Yuki N. Guillain-Barré and Miller Fisher syndromes: new diagnostic classification. *Nat Rev Neurol* 2014;10:537–544.

117. Wakerley BR, Yuki N. Mimics and chameleons in Guillain-Barré and Miller Fisher syndromes. *Practi Neurol* 2015;15:90–99.

118. Walgaard C, Lingsma HF, Ruts L, et al. Prediction of respiratory insufficiency in Guillain-Barré syndrome. *Ann Neurol* 2010;67:781–787.

119. Webb AJ, Brain SA, Wood R, Rinaldi S, Turner MR. Seasonal variation in Guillain-Barré syndrome: a systematic review, meta-analysis and Oxfordshire cohort study. *J Neurol Neurosurg Psychiatry* 2015;86:1196–1201.

120. Weinberg DH. AAEM case report 4: Guillain-Barré syndrome. American Association of Electrodiagnostic Medicine. *Muscle Nerve* 1999;22:271–281.

121. Wijdicks EFM. Neurogenic paradoxical breathing. *J Neurol Neurosurg Psychiatry* 2013;84:1296.

122. Wijdicks EFM, Fletcher DD, Lawn ND. Influenza vaccine and the risk of relapse of Guillain-Barré syndrome. *Neurology* 2000;55:452–453.

123. Wijdicks EFM, Henderson RD, McClelland RL. Emergency intubation for respiratory failure in Guillain-Barré syndrome. *Arch Neurol* 2003;60:947–948.

124. Wijdicks EFM, Lawn ND, Fletcher DD. Tracheostomy scars in Guillain-Barré syndrome: a reason for concern? *J Neurol* 2001;248:527–528.

125. Wijdicks EFM, Ropper AH. Acute relapsing Guillain Barré syndrome after long asymptomatic intervals. *Arch Neurol* 1990;47:82–84.

126. Wijdicks EFM, Roy TK. BiPAP in early Guillain-Barré syndrome may fail. *Can J Neurol Sci* 2006;33:105–106.

127. Wijdicks EFM, Ropper AH. The Guillain-Barré syndrome. In: Koehler PJ, Bruyn GW, Pearce JMS, eds. *Neurological Eponyms*. Oxford: Oxford University Press; 2000:219–226.

128. Wollinsky KH, Hulser PJ, Brinkmeier H, et al. CSF filtration is an effective treatment of Guillain-Barré syndrome: a randomized clinical trial. *Neurology* 2001;57:774–780.

129. Yuki N. Campylobacter sialyltransferase gene polymorphism directs clinical features of Guillain-Barré syndrome. *J Neurochem* 2007;103 Suppl 1:150–158.

130. Yuki N, Ang CW, Koga M, et al. Clinical features and response to treatment in Guillain-Barré syndrome associated with antibodies to GM1b ganglioside. *Ann Neurol* 2000;47:314–321.

131. Yuki N, Hartung HP. Guillain-Barré syndrome *N Engl J Med* 2012;366:2294–2304.

132. Yuki N, Yamada M, Koga M, et al. Animal model of axonal Guillain-Barré syndrome induced by sensitization with GM1 ganglioside. *Ann Neurol* 2001;49:712–720.

133. Zifko U, Chen R, Remtulla H, et al. Respiratory electrophysiological studies in Guillain-Barré syndrome. *J Neurol Neurosurg Psychiatry* 1996;60:191–194.

43

Myasthenia Gravis

The neuromuscular junction is one of the targets for acute autoimmune neuromuscular disorders. Myasthenia gravis is such a disease, and the pathologic and biochemical processes have been well elucidated. Its pathogenesis can be briefly summarized as an antibody reaction at the antigen epitopes of the acetylcholine receptor (AChR), eventually leading to destruction and simplification of the junctional fold and widening of the synaptic cleft.[19,30,50,76] Defective neurotransmission leads to fatigable muscle weakness. Myasthenia gravis has an incidence of 0.5–5 per 100,000 population, occurs at all ages, and is more frequent in older men and younger women.[101,113] Many patients have lymphoid follicular hyperplasia or thymoma, cells of which, in culture, secrete immunoglobulins and AChR antibodies.[50]

Serious exacerbation of myasthenia gravis can be encountered in two clinical situations. First, a myasthenic crisis can cause imminent respiratory failure or impairment of swallowing. Important triggers for myasthenic crisis are a viral upper respiratory infection and, less common, recent use of medication that exacerbates the disease. In fact, the administration of certain pharmaceutical agents may be the first time that myasthenia gravis declares itself. Second, patients with myasthenia gravis have worsened while admitted to a surgical intensive care unit (ICU) after a surgical procedure, including thymectomy.

The most common reason for admission to the neurosciences intensive care unit (NICU) is a need to intervene for acute exacerbation, but often patients are admitted for overnight monitoring of respiratory function as a precautionary measure because their condition may unexpectedly worsen suddenly. The clinical diagnosis of myasthenia gravis is often well established before deterioration, and diagnostic evaluation for generalized muscle weakness is seldom a major focus of attention in the NICU. Myasthenia gravis leading to worsening with subsequent intubation may occur in one in three patients and then often within 2 years of diagnosis. Late onset (middle age) myasthenia is less severe but less likely to achieve full remission. Regrettably, many patients with myasthenia gravis in the NICU have had previous experience with deterioration during intercurrent respiratory infection.

CLINICAL RECOGNITION

Patients admitted to the NICU who are worsening from myasthenia gravis often have abnormal eye movements, oropharyngeal weakness, and proximal limb weakness. Progressive failure of neuromuscular transmission in the diaphragmatic muscle may occur in 30% of patients with myasthenia gravis at the time of diagnosis.

The archetypal clinical finding in myasthenia is fatigability of several muscles.[76,82,100] Documentation of the severity of weakness at admission is important, but when done, one must take into account and document the time of the last dose of pyridostigmine or neostigmine. The maximal effect can be expected up to 4 hours after administration of either drug, and weakness may not be noticed.

Cranial nerve examination should include assessment of the degree of ptosis and ophthalmoplegia.[112] Ptosis can be defined as a position of the eyelid just crossing the superior limbus. Ptosis is one of the clinical hallmarks in patients with myasthenia gravis, and several tests have been proposed to aggravate it.[112] Ptosis can be aggravated by upward gaze for 3 minutes (Figure 43.1) and can be relieved by cooling.[104] When an ice pack is placed over a closed eye for 2 minutes, ptosis can improve (Figure 43.2). The ice test is very specific and sensitive, with a positive result in 80% of patients with myasthenia gravis, and is not likely in patients without the disorder.[36,46] Resolution of ptosis can also be achieved with resting the eyelid from closure, also known as the "mini-sleep test,"[72] and patients themselves like to repeatedly close their eyes to open them better later. Interestingly, relief of ptosis on one side by elevation of the eyelid results in aggravation of ptosis on the contralateral side, explained by relaxation

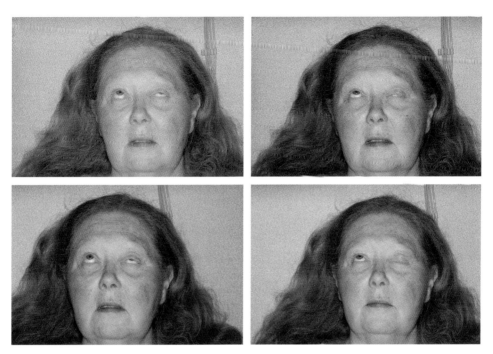

FIGURE 43.1: Worsening of ptosis ("curtain" phenomenon) with upgaze (left much more prominent).

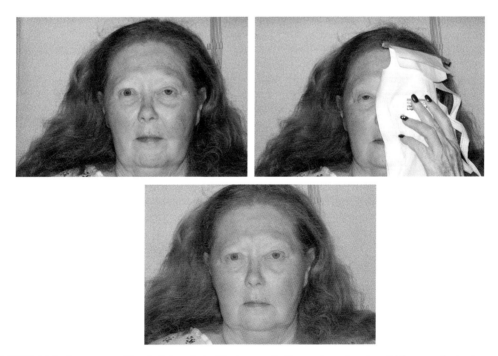

FIGURE 43.2: Improvement in ptosis is noted with placement of ice pack on closed eyelid for several minutes.

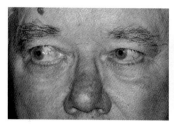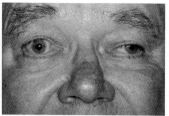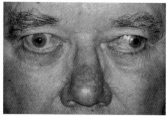

FIGURE 43.3: Myasthenia gravis with bilateral pseudo-internuclear ophthalmoplegia. There is bilateral failure of adduction. Asymmetric ptosis is also present.

of the contracted frontalis muscle. Chronic blinking mimicking blepharospasm, with a response to pyridostigmine, has been noted.[90] Orbicular oculi weakness may also be demonstrated. After gentle eyelid closure, the lid margins may rapidly separate, showing some sclera (the peek sign).[77]

Diplopia is difficult to assess. Fluctuating diplopia can be unmasked by sustained gaze to a fixed target, but at a considerable distance to eliminate convergence weakness. Pseudointernuclear ophthalmoplegia has been reported (Figure 43.3), but in most patients, ocular motility is limited in both vertical and horizontal directions, resulting in marked diplopia.

Bulbar function must be specifically assessed for fatigability and may determine the need for elective intubation. In patients with myasthenia gravis, muscle weakness occurs in the masseters, and jaw opening is typically stronger than jaw closure. The pterygoid muscles, which can be tested by resistance to lateral pressure against the jaw, can be normal. A few attempts at forceful biting on a tongue depressor eventually produces jaw weakness and the inability to bite, and the examiner can easily slide the blade out between the teeth. Nasopharyngeal weakness can be examined by carefully listening for slurring of speech and a nasal tone after the patient is asked to repeat brief sentences, or the dysarthria can be provoked by having the patient count to 100. After the patient is asked to puff out both cheeks and to attempt to resist pressure from the examiner's fingers, passage of air through the nose is typical. Bifacial weakness may be present, shown as a depressed grin or snarl. It is frequently associated with a frown as the patient attempts to alleviate ptosis by lifting the eyebrows. Whistling is impossible. These clinical tests are illustrated in Figure 43.4.

Dysphagia may be a presenting symptom and can be examined by having the patient take a few sips of water; nasal regurgitation or a flurry of weak and ineffective coughs may result. The gag reflex is often muted. However, careful history-taking may reveal a much longer period of choking on liquids or solid food.[52] When tested on videofluoroscopy, laryngeal elevation is incomplete, leading to aspiration.[44]

Isolated respiratory failure as the first manifestation of myasthenia gravis has been reported in a few patients, but unsurprisingly with bulbar or proximal muscle weakness found after a detailed examination.[28,68,70] As in acute neuromuscular respiratory failure of any other cause,

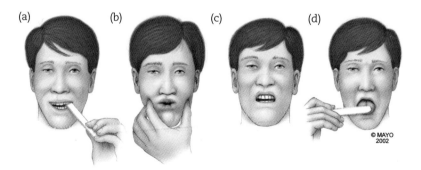

FIGURE 43.4: Clinical examination of pertinent features in myasthenia gravis. (a) Ptosis and typical snarl of bifacial weakness. (b) Puffing out cheeks and resisting pressure from examiner's fingers. (c) Biting on tongue depressor for masseter weakness. (d) Pushing away tongue depressor with tongue.

respiratory failure in the early stages of myasthenia gravis can be subtle. In most patients with generalized myasthenia gravis, spontaneous breathing is characterized by short inspiratory and expiratory times with a smaller tidal volume.[108] Reflex tachypnea may result in normal to low PCO_2. An additional primary pulmonary process may cause a mixed clinical picture, often with early hypoxemia.

Weakness in proximal muscle groups should be examined and documented because the findings are valuable clinical guidelines to assess the effects of specific treatment. A useful test is the "pump handle" test.[61] (The examiner repeatedly depresses the patient's abducted arm to the side while the patient strongly resists.) Other methods of testing muscle weakness include sitting up from the supine position without the use of the arms and rising from a sitting position. It is useful to grade proximal muscle strength in patients with myasthenia gravis. The Myasthenia Gravis Foundation of America published a grading scale of severity[47], based on the time in minutes a patient is able to hold the arms horizontally outstretched and to hold the legs above the plane of the bed while supine. The most useful components of this scale are summarized in Table 43.1.

Most patients are admitted to the NICU because of myasthenic crisis,[111] but attention should also be focused on cholinergic signs. A mixed clinical picture is certainly possible if patients have been overmedicated. Excessive salivation, thick bronchial secretions, and diarrhea are important clinical symptoms. Fasciculations may be the only symptom of cholinergic hyperactivity and not immediately evident.

TABLE 43.1. CLINICAL EXAMINATION OF MYASTHENIA GRAVIS

Examine for ptosis (60 sec)
Diplopia lateral gaze (60 sec)
Eyelid closure or total ptosis
Dysarthria counting 1–50
Biting on tongue depressor, pushing away with tongue
Swallowing ½ cup water
Arm outstretched at 90° supine (90 sec)
Head lift 45° supine (120 sec)
Legs outstretched at 45° supine (100 sec)
Counting one breath to 20
Accessory muscles used

* Partly based on quantitative myasthenia gravis score

NEUROIMAGING AND LABORATORY TESTS

The ocular or bulbar type of myasthenia gravis is usually confirmed by electrophysiologic studies.[8] However, it may be mimicked by many other rare progressive myopathies, brainstem compression from a vertebrobasilar aneurysm,[31] intracranial metastasis in the midbrain,[49] or a midbrain glioma.[11] In some of these curious cases, the results of edrophonium tests have also been claimed to be positive.[26] The diagnosis of myasthenia gravis should not pose insurmountable difficulties, but alternative diagnoses should be considered if any of these tests are nondiagnostic. Ocular myasthenia can be mimicked by mitochondrial cytopathy, oculopharyngeal muscular dystrophy, and thyroid ophthalmopathy. Generalized myasthenia can be mimicked by Lambert-Eaton myasthenic syndrome, botulism, venoms, and many other inflammatory myopathies or acquired neuromyotonia.[113] Magnetic resonance imaging (MRI) of the brain therefore seems warranted in patients with the bulbar or ocular type of myasthenia gravis if there is serious concern about the validity of the diagnosis.

Myasthenia gravis is a clinical diagnosis, but helpful tests with workable diagnostic accuracy include repetitive motor nerve stimulation testing; single-fiber electromyography (EMG); intravenous administration of a short-acting anticholinesterase drug, such as edrophonium chloride (Tensilon); and measurement of serum AChR antibody titers.[6,9,35]

The edrophonium test is simple to perform when objective markers are available, such as considerable limb weakness, diplopia, and ptosis. Intravenous injection of edrophonium should be contraindicated in patients with asthma or prior cardiac arrhythmias. The test is less useful in patients with only minor symptoms when improvement cannot be reliably judged. Limb weakness can be quantified by a dynamometer. Diplopia and its response are ideally documented by Lancaster green tests in the office,[116] but only virtually complete disappearance of diplopia has sufficient diagnostic value. Pulmonary function tests can also be performed before and after the edrophonium test.

The edrophonium test can be performed in a blind manner if the cause of deterioration is sufficiently uncertain.[21] Two syringes of 1 mL each are used, one filled with edrophonium, 10 mg/mL, and one with isotonic saline. The best technique is gradual injection of the contents of each syringe in five small increments and subsequent recording of improvement, which should continue for at least 5 minutes. Many patients have a response within minutes after 2 mg has been injected. Atropine should be administered in a dose of 0.5 mg in an intravenous bolus if abdominal cramps, bronchospasm, vomiting, or bradycardia occurs. If bradycardia remains and is associated with a reduction in blood pressure, an additional dose of 1 mg of atropine should be administered.[81]

Alternatively, neostigmine (1.5 mg IM), often in combination with atropine (0.4 mg SC), can be administered to test for myasthenia gravis. Its effect is present after 30 minutes and lasts for 1 hour, and although administration of neostigmine may allow more time for observation and additional testing, its delayed effect is not very useful for evaluation of a patient in a critical condition.

Electrodiagnostic studies are important for confirmation of the diagnosis, but the patient should ideally be without medication for 12 hours. Electrodiagnostic results are fairly reliable when testing is done on the day of plasma exchange (because significant improvement by plasmapheresis usually takes 2 or 3 days). The results are abnormal in all patients with severe generalized myasthenia gravis, but in only half of them if the disorder is limited to ocular signs.[73]

Surface electrodes are used for repetitive stimulation at a stimulation rate of 2–5 Hz before and after maximal voluntary contraction of the tested muscle.[30,93] Recording is from the abductor digiti minimi in a limb warmed to 37°C (low temperatures can mute the decremental response). An abnormal result is usually defined as a 10% or greater decrement of the compound muscle action potential amplitude between the first and the fourth responses with supramaximal stimulation (Figure 43.5). Response in testing of the proximal muscles is different, with better sensitivity in the deltoid than in the trapezius muscles.[99] Single-fiber EMG requires special expertise, and the recording surface of the fine concentric needle measures single-fiber action potentials. Single-fiber EMG has a sensitivity of 95% and typically demonstrates increased jitter and blocking.[35] Jitter, the variation in time intervals among the action potentials, increases with defective neuromuscular function; blocking occurs when nerve impulses fail to generate a muscle action

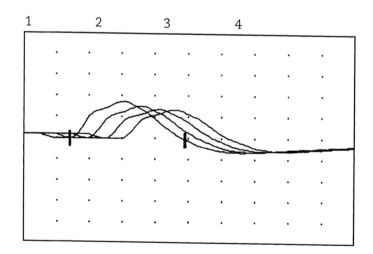

No.	Peak amp (mV)	Amp decr (%)	Area (mVms)	Area decr (%)	Stim level (mA)
1	1.75	0	7.01	0	73
2	1.54	12	6.11	13	73
3	1.40	20	5.50	22	73
4	1.37	22	5.39	23	73

Stimulus frequency 2 Hz, stimulus duration 0.1 ms

FIGURE 43.5: Repetitive stimulation of the ulnar nerve in a patient with myasthenia gravis and recording of decrement of the compound muscle action potential (CMAP).

potential.[93,96] Normal jitter in a weak muscle virtually excludes myasthenia gravis. A study suggested that the use of trans eyelid techniques to insert a needle in the superior rectus muscle has a high yield in the diagnosis of ocular myasthenia gravis.[88] Needle examination may demonstrate fibrillation, which may indicate functional denervation of the muscle fibers and is generally a marker for more severe disease.

Radioimmunoassay with purified human AChR antigen may demonstrate an AChR-binding antibody, which is positive in 86% of patients with generalized myasthenia.[9,94] In approximately 80% of patients with thymoma, striational antibodies against skeletal muscle proteins, such as titin, can be found. Titin antibodies have been associated with thymoma in patients younger than 60 years.[12] In patients with seronegative myasthenia gravis, antibodies against thyroid or gastric parietal cells may support the diagnosis. A recent study used a cell-based assay expressing AChRs on the surface of a human embryonic kidney (HEK) cell and clustering by co-expression with the intracellular anchoring protein rapsyn. This assay improves diagnostic sensitivity for myasthenia gravis, but also found that patients with these antibodies have a milder phenotype and a higher chance of later remission.[91]

Computed tomography scanning of the chest must be performed in every patient to screen for thymoma. Thymomas vary in their malignancy potential, and computed tomography (CT) scans may give a reasonable view of the invasive potential, a finding most often associated with well-differentiated thymic carcinoma. The essential laboratory tests in evaluation of myasthenia gravis are summarized in Table 43.2.

Autoantibodies to MuSK may be found in patients without antibodies to AChR, also known as "seronegative myasthenia gravis."[4,64,74] Focal weakness, in particular faciopharyngeal muscle weakness causing dysphagia, and developing tongue atrophy are clinical correlates of MuSK antibody myasthenia gravis. Treatment response to plasma exchange (PLEX) is more rapid than in other forms of myasthenia gravis.[97] The pathogenesis and involved proteins are discussed in Capsule 43.1.

Imminent respiratory failure is the most common reason for admission to the NICU, and the early clinical signs of diaphragmatic failure should be well known (Chapter 10). Measurement of vital capacity remains an important bedside test, although it may not accurately reflect

TABLE 43.2. DIAGNOSTIC TESTS IN MYASTHENIA GRAVIS

Electromyography, nerve conduction velocity, repetitive stimulation, single fiber study
Edrophonium or neostigmine test
Acetylcholine receptor blocking antibodies, titin antibodies, muscle antibodies
Thyroid, parietal cell antibodies
Thyroxine, triiodothyronine, thyrotropin
Computed tomography scan of the chest
Serial arterial blood gas determinations
Serial measurements of vital capacity and maximal inspiratory pressure
Preoperative pulmonary function test (with neostigmine provocation, optional)

diaphragmatic function. A useful additional maneuver is to measure vital capacity in the supine position. Typically, patients with diaphragmatic failure but no apparent clinical signs have a significant decrease (up to 60% from the baseline value in the erect position) in vital capacity when supine. In patients without neuromuscular failure, the decrease in vital capacity with position change is seldom more than 20% from baseline. The development of paradoxical breathing in a patient lying down is often a prelude to the need for endotracheal intubation and mechanical ventilation. A study performed in patients with myasthenia gravis found that these maximal static pressures were more sensitive in the early detection of neuromuscular failure and that pressures clearly improved after the administration of pyridostigmine.[67]

The frequency of measurements of vital capacity and inspiratory and expiratory pressures is often a matter of debate, but declining values must heighten the awareness of imminent respiratory failure. Risk factors for respiratory decline have not been studied prospectively, but it is prudent to measure vital capacity every 6 hours in a patient with myasthenic crisis. Unfortunately, the clinical course of myasthenia gravis is erratic, and repeated measurements of vital capacity with a documented decrease of 30% or more do not predict the need for intubation.[109]

However, patients with chest radiographic evidence of early atelectasis and right lower lobe infiltrates suggestive of aspiration are at considerable risk of worsening respiratory failure, as are patients with considerable bulbar dysfunction.

At the neuromuscular junction, myelinated axons divide to innervate muscle fibers and form unmyelinated boutons filled with multiple vesicles containing acetylcholine (see accompanying illustration). The synaptic cleft contains a regulating enzyme acetylcholine esterase that breaks down acetylcholine. The postsynaptic membrane has deep folds with acetylcholine receptor (AChR). When the nerve action potential reaches to the synaptic bouton, voltage-gated Ca^{2+} channels open on the presynaptic membrane and result in vesicle release. After binding to the receptor, this results in opening of the voltage-gated Na channels and muscle contraction. Several other proteins are in the muscle membrane (e.g., Rapsin, MuSk, Agrin, myotube-associated specificity component [MASC], rapsyn-associated transmembrane linker [RATL]). These proteins facilitate the clustering of AChRs. Muscle-specific tyrokinase is important for the assembly of the AChR.

Anti-acetyl receptor antibodies in myasthenia gravis lead to binding and activation of complement at the neuromuscular junction (membrane attack complex [MAC]), degradation of acetylcholine molecules, and functional AChR block. The deep folds disappear and a flat surface remains. The muscle-specific tyrokinase (MuSK) is an autoantigen in some patients (5%). Inhibition of MuSK synthesis leads to dispersion of the receptor and endplate disruption.

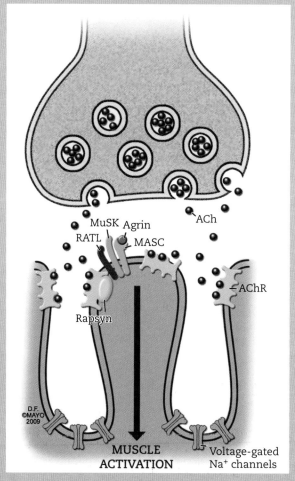

Structure of neuromuscular junction showing the axon synaptic cleft and muscle containing several proteins. Patients with myasthenia gravis may develop antibodies against MuSK or AChR.

Adapted from Conti-Fine BM, Milani M, Kaminski HJ. Myasthenia gravis: past, present, and future. *J Clin Invest* 2006;116:2843–2854. With permission of the publisher.

FIRST STEPS
IN MANAGEMENT

Patients with myasthenia gravis can become critically ill rapidly, and the severity of the exacerbation is commonly misjudged. The initial management is summarized in Table 43.3. Endotracheal intubation may be avoided with conservative measures, such as placing the patient in an erect position, using incentive spirometry and assisted coughing, and certainly can be avoided if PLEX is started promptly. However, conservative measures may fail, and one should probably electively intubate rather than procrastinate if the trend is a decline in respiratory function.

We have tried to avoid intubation in patients with myasthenic crises by using bilevel positive airway pressure ventilation (BiPAP) in our initial study. In 24 episodes, a BiPAP trial prevented intubation in 14 (58%), but not in patients with $PaCO_2$ values greater than 50 mm Hg. In these patients, hypercapnia reflected a more profound degree of respiratory failure that could not be assisted with positive pressure and thus needed a volume-and rate-controlled mode.[84] The mean duration of BiPAP was 4 days in a follow-up study.[102]

Elective intubation proceeds in an organized manner and is carefully explained to the patient. Patients should understand that mechanical ventilation is only a temporary supportive measure and that weaning is the rule. Neuromuscular blocking agents are discouraged during intubation, because patients with myasthenia gravis are very sensitive to these drugs. Several pharmaceutical agents have been reported to exacerbate myasthenia gravis (Table 43.4).[115]

Specific treatment in myasthenic crisis is PLEX or intravenous immunoglobulin (IVIG).[3,8,16,22,23,33,65] A trial in 87 patients with worsening myasthenia gravis showed similar benefits but a better safety profile for IVIG.[34] A randomized double-blind trial of IVIG found efficacy in myasthenia gravis with worsening symptoms. IVIG was not helpful in patients with mild weakness or only ocular symptoms, but the trial excluded patients admitted to NICU or with respiratory failure.[118] IVIG is reserved for patients with very difficult venous access, patients with possible sepsis as a trigger for myasthenic crisis, and, perhaps, children. Its effectiveness could be identical to that of PLEX. Similar outcome was demonstrated when PLEX were compared with IVIG, 0.4 g/kg/day for 3–5 days, but very few patients required mechanical ventilation during the crisis.[34] A retrospective

---

TABLE 43.3. INITIAL MANAGEMENT OF PATIENTS WITH MYASTHENIC CRISIS

Airway management	Endotracheal intubation in patients with impaired swallowing mechanism leading to inability to clear secretions, ineffective cough and nasal voice, signs of aspiration pneumonitis on chest radiograph, any patient with marginal Pao_2, widening A–a gradient, or any vital capacity near 15 mL/kg
	Tracheostomy deferred
Mechanical ventilation	BiPAP trial (if no hypercapnia)
	IMV/PS
Nutrition	Enteral nutrition with continuous infusion (day 2)
Prophylaxis	DVT prophylaxis with pneumatic compression devices
	SC heparin 5,000 U t.i.d.
	GI prophylaxis: Pantoprazole 40 mg IV daily or lansoprazole 30 mg orally through nasogastric tube
Specific management	Plasma exchange: 5 plasma exchanges or 5 days of IVIG, 0.4 g/kg/day; 2 consecutive days of plasma exchange are followed by three exchanges on alternate days
	Prednisone (60 mg/day) is given if no improvement after 5 days of plasma exchange
Other measures	Pyridostigmine is stopped during mechanical ventilation
	Pyridostigmine therapy is gradually reinstated intravenously or intramuscularly
Access	Peripheral venous catheter and place high-flow catheter with plasma exchange

A–a, alveolar–arterial; BiPAP, bilevel positive airway pressure ventilation; DVT, deep vein thrombosis; GI, gastrointestinal; IMV, intermittent mandatory ventilation; IV, intravenously; IVIG, intravenous immunoglobulin; PS, pressure support; SC, subcutaneously.

TABLE 43.4. PHARMACEUTICAL AGENTS WITH THE POTENTIAL TO AGGRAVATE MYASTHENIA GRAVIS

Antibiotics	*Cardiovascular agents*	*Miscellaneous*
Clindamycin	Quinidine	Penicillamine
Colistin	Propranolol	Chloroquine
Kanamycin	Procainamide	Succinylcholine
Neomycin	Practolol	Curare and other relaxants
Streptomycin	Lidocaine	Decamethonium
Tobramycin	Verapamil	Phenytoin
Tetracyclines	Nifedipine	Trimethadione
Gentamicin	Diltiazem	Carbamazepine
Polymyxin B	*Psychotropic agents*	
Bacitracin	Chlorpromazine	
Trimethoprim-sulfamethoxazole	Promazine	
Hormones	Phenelzine	
ACTH	Lithium	
Corticosteroids	Diazepam	
Thyroid hormone		
Oral contraceptives		

ACTH, adrenocorticotrophic hormone.

study, also limited by small patient numbers, suggested that intravenous IVIG was less effective in patients on a mechanical ventilator in a crisis episode.[83]

In our experience we have favored PLEX, and we could not liberate our patients from the mechanical ventilator with IVIG alone. We therefore start PLEX first in mechanically ventilated patients with myasthenic crises, and a high-flow temporary catheter is placed in the jugular vein (Niagra™ or Mahurkar™) (Figure 43.6). Administration of pyridostigmine (Mestinon) can be discontinued to facilitate mechanical ventilation and to improve bronchial suctioning.[8] Many patients have retained secretions from ineffective coughing, and have chest radiographic signs of early atelectasis.[110] Discontinuation of cholinesterase inhibitors leads to a considerable increase in muscle weakness, but some patients with severe myasthenic crisis, who are often exhausted, appreciate short-term mechanical ventilation and rest, and often accept the consequences of discontinuation of cholinesterase inhibitors. Moreover, when PLEX is started immediately, improvement is quickly notable after a series of exchanges. In some patients, PLEX is not fully effective, and only an increase in the intravenous dose of pyridostigmine with atropine or glycopyrrolate to counter hypersecretion results in weaning from the

ventilator. The risk of a cholinergic crisis from continuous infusion of pyridostigmine (initial infusion of 2 mg/hr, with a gradual titration in increments of 0.5–1 mg/hr to a maximum of 4 mg/hr) is considerable, but administration seems safe in patients with normal renal function.[10,92] In patients with considerable muscle weakness but no clinical or laboratory evidence of respiratory failure, it is reasonable to increase the dose of pyridostigmine in increments of 15–30 mg orally until a satisfactory response is apparent. In patients with difficulty swallowing, a syrup (60

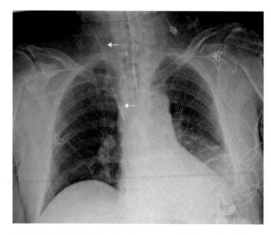

FIGURE 43.6: Mahurkar™ at cavoatrial junction (preferred position) to allow plasma exchange.

mg/5 mL) should be administered, or an intravenous dose can be tried[87] (dose equivalents are shown in Table 43.5). High doses of pyridostigmine (up to 50 mg IV in divided doses) may be required.

Patients recovering from a myasthenic crisis need pyridostigmine to improve, and a considerable dose in some instances. Neuromuscular respiratory failure is bellows failure, and pyridostigmine is essential to improve the mechanics. Underdosing leads to the pooling of secretions that may be misinterpreted as "hypersecretions" and mistakenly may lead to lowering the dose and a worsening of the clinical manifestations. We have seen patients transferred to us with failure to wean off the ventilator undergo rapid improvement with an increase in the dose of pyridostigmine.

Another complex management issue is preparation of the patient before thymectomy. The indications for thymectomy have been well outlined in several overviews.[41,54–56] A thymoma is an absolute indication for thoracotomy unless the tumor is malignant and significantly invades the mediastinum.[53,59,61] Thymoma, a slow-growing malignant lesion, has been staged by Masaoka[63] through modification of the Bergh[7] classification: stage I, tumor encapsulated, no invasion; stage II, macroscopic (IIa) or microscopic (IIb) invasion; stage III, invasion of the pericardium, great vessels, or lung; stage IV, pleural or pericardial dissemination (IVa) or metastasis (IVb).

Complete resection is associated with almost no recurrence, but cannot be achieved with stage III thymoma. Relapse has been reported in 20% of patients, with distant metastasis developing in 5%. Postoperative radiation and chemotherapy with a cisplatin regimen are needed in these cases.

TABLE 43.5. CHOLINESTERASE INHIBITOR DOSES IN MYASTHENIA GRAVIS

	Oral (mg)	Intravenous (mg)
Pyridostigmine bromide (Mestinon)	60	2.0
Neostigmine bromide (Prostigmin)	15	NA
Neostigmine methylsulfate (Prostigmin)	NA	0.5

NA, not available.

Absence of a thymoma on CT scan may guide the thoracic surgeon in deciding to proceed with transcervical thymectomy, which leaves a less deforming scar and reduces the risk of phrenic nerve damage. Many thoracic surgeons prefer the transsternal approach because this exposure almost certainly guarantees complete removal of the thymus. The thymus may have additional localizations within the mediastinum that are not in continuity with the bulk of its gland. A retrospective study of transcervical thymectomy in 53 patients with myasthenia gravis (but skewed toward milder disease) showed that 77% of the patients were in complete remission after 5 years of follow-up.[25] Only one patient had transsternal re-exploration for relapse; residual thymus tissue was found. It is not known whether less complete removal of thymus tissue, which is a possible consequence of limited surgical exposure, is as effective as complete removal. However, thymectomy has not been subjected to a rigorous controlled clinical trial. No randomized study comparing types of thymectomy or comparing thymectomy with the best medical treatment has been performed, and some remain doubtful about the benefit of the operation.[54,56] A recent systematic review using evidence-based criteria concluded that sufficient evidence of its benefit was lacking, and the need for thymectomy in myasthenia gravis was downgraded to "optional."[41,47] Others have argued persuasively that the course of myasthenia gravis is positively affected by surgery, and tentative evidence suggests that thymectomy improves the natural history in 50% of the patients, with the prospect of a complete remission. For now, thymectomy for myasthenia gravis without thymoma could be considered in patients with severe generalized myasthenia gravis, in younger patients, in patients who have a progressively decreasing response to medication, and in patients who have had several episodes of myasthenic crisis.[13,80] Patients selected for thymectomy should have a preoperative pulmonary function test evaluation with neostigmine provocation (2 mg IM). Patients with normal lung function can be expected to have an uncomplicated postoperative course and early extubation. In patients with marginal pulmonary function that cannot be further improved with neostigmine preoperatively, PLEX for 5 consecutive days before planned surgery should be scheduled. Preoperative PLEX to reduce the risk of prolonged postoperative ventilation probably is not needed in patients with normal lung function, but any deviation of pulmonary function test values from normal probably should prompt a complete course of PLEX. One unconfirmed study suggested the pre-operative administration of 60 mg of prednisone and found better postoperative respiration function after thymectomy.[48]

Cholinesterase inhibitors are discontinued the morning of surgery. Atropine is recommended to reduce secretions, and in patients with corticosteroid maintenance, preoperative protection from surgical stress response is very important (125 mg of hydrocortisone IV every 8 hours, beginning on the day before surgery and continuing for up to 3 days postoperatively).

DETERIORATION: CAUSES AND MANAGEMENT

Patients with myasthenia gravis are generally admitted because of a severe myasthenic crisis. A cholinergic crisis is rare in its pure form. The pertinent differences are shown in Table 43.6. The causes of myasthenic crisis are intercurrent infection, recent tapering or first administration of large doses of corticosteroids, and elective surgery. The condition of patients with myasthenic crisis may not improve or continues to deteriorate despite a series of plasma exchanges. It is reasonable practice to add prednisone (60 mg/day) if no hint of improvement appears after 5 days of plasma exchanges and an increase in the intravenous dose of pyridostigmine. The timing of the administration of corticosteroids remains arbitrary, and others may wait for at least 2 weeks after plasma exchange to start corticosteroid treatment. An additional 3-day plasma exchange series can be considered to cover the delay in the pharmaceutical effect of corticosteroids. The dose of corticosteroids is continued for 1 month, changed to alternate days, and then tapered to clinical response. At a later stage, azathioprine (50 mg/day orally, titrating to a goal of 2 mg/kg/day) can be added to reduce the side effects of corticosteroids[2] or to supplement prednisone if it is not adequately effective.[5] Some may even replace corticosteroids after several years of treatment.[79]

Some early experience suggests that high-dose intravenous methylprednisolone pulse therapy (1 g methylprednisolone administered in 250 mL of glucose, 50 mg/mL) for 2 consecutive days may reduce the long-term side effects of prednisone. Its effect was sustained for a mean of 2 months.[60] Before other immune-modulating therapies are considered, the effect of PLEX with corticosteroid supplementation must be observed for at least 2 weeks. Patients previously treated with IVIG who have deterioration should undergo a series of plasma exchanges, beginning with five exchanges. Alternative treatments have been studied in smaller populations, and their effects and side effects are less well known.

A recent experience in eight patients suggested refractory cases of MG could benefit from 6 cycles of 4 weekly IV cyclophosphamide infusion (0.75 g/m²), followed by oral maintenance. Six of eight patients showed marked clinical improvement, with four patients achieving remission later on maintenance therapy and three without need for corticosteroids.[15]

An alternative immunosuppressive therapy, administration of cyclosporine, has been evaluated in only two small controlled clinical trials.[37,111] Cyclosporine inhibits interleukin-2 production and helper T-cell release of cytokinesis but, most important, inhibits T-lymphocyte maturation. Its use (initially 5 mg/kg/day in two divided doses) is adjusted to maintain trough plasma levels of 100–150 ng/ml. In the initial trial, the administration of cyclosporine was discontinued in 25% of patients, mostly because of nephrotoxicity.

TABLE 43.6. DIFFERENTIATION OF CHOLINERGIC AND MYASTHENIC CRISES

	Cholinergic Crises	Myasthenic Crises
Frequency*	Rare	Common
Trigger	Overdose, drug therapy for MG	Infection, certain drugs, corticosteroids
Pupils	Miosis	Mydriasis
Respiration	Bronchus plugging and spasm, marked salivation	Diaphragm weakness
Fasciculations, cramps	Present	Absent
Diarrhea	Present	Absent

MG, myasthenia gravis.
* Combination of both crises is often clinically encountered.

In another retrospective analysis from Duke University Medical Center,[18] nephrotoxicity was also a limiting factor, and incidences of new-onset hypertension were similar, but control was good with antihypertensive agents. In an analysis of 57 patients treated with cyclosporine (mean use of 3.5 years), improvement began as early as 1 week but usually after 1 month and with maximal effect at approximately 6 months. Other side effects of cyclosporine were hirsutism, headache, tremor, gastrointestinal symptoms, and possibly increased risk of skin cancer. Pulsed intravenous cyclophosphamide (500 mg/m² body surface) has been considered in resistant cases.[24] Azathioprine (2.5 mg/kg) has often been combined with prednisone, allowing tapering of prednisone ("corticosteroid sparing effect"), but is now more often replaced by mycophenolate mofetil.

Another immunosuppressive agent, mycophenolate mofetil (CellCept), has been widely used in organ transplantation and has found its way to use in autoimmune disorders.[43] Mycophenolate mofetil has been tested in very few patients after a myasthenic crisis. The side effects may include hypertension and are similar to those of cyclosporine,[17,66,69] but the major advantage is that the incidence of side effects with this drug are low. Two trials of mycophenolate mofetil in combination with 20 mg/day prednisone did not improve outcome after 3 months, but its long-term effect remains unknown.[1,95,98] However, a recent prospective study in 11 patients used mycophenolate mofetil to replace azathioprine and found excellent results in most patients in up to 4 years' follow-up.[42] Rituximab (a monoclonal anti-CD20 B-cell antibody) has been successfully used in six patients with severe, treatment-refractory myasthenia gravis, but the drug needs further testing.[57] The pros and cons of these newer drugs compared with those of corticosteroids have been debated.[5,43,89] A major concern is high cost (300 times that of prednisone). A perioperative management protocol that includes careful evaluation of blood gas, breathing frequency reinstitution, or reintubation will reduce postoperative deterioration. Video-assisted thoracoscopic extended thymectomy has also minimized postoperative deterioration.[38] Therefore the most promising new approaches in immunotherapy are rituximab and, more recently, eculizumab.[45,106]

If available, a less often used option, immunoadsorption therapy, could be considered in patients with a particularly severe myasthenic crisis.[40,105] Immunoadsorption therapy uses a synthetic resin that adsorbs acetylcholine antibodies very effectively (e.g., tryptophan-linked polyvinyl alcohol gel). In a randomized study, this therapy had a striking effect on clinical response, and a 60% reduction in circulating acetylcholine antibodies was documented. Immunoadsorption therapy is accomplished with the exchange of one plasma volume during 5 consecutive days; the plasma separator consists of a cellulose diacetate membrane. Improvement can be expected in 48 hours, with a peak at 1–4 days after the last adsorption.[105]

One cause of in-hospital deterioration in myasthenia gravis is significant worsening within the first days of corticosteroid administration. Often, this clinical worsening is observed in patients exposed to corticosteroids for the first time, but it also can occur when the initial doses are high. We usually continue giving corticosteroids (in a lower starting dose) and treat the exacerbation with plasma exchange and increasing doses of pyridostigmine.

Another cause of deterioration in myasthenia gravis is a cholinergic crisis. Whether or not a cholinergic crisis causes weakness is unresolved, and its full-fledged manifestation is rarely observed. In clinical practice, both conditions are more commonly present at the same time. Typically, in patients with a continuing downhill clinical course, the dose of pyridostigmine has been incrementally increased, and although the clinically observed muscle weakness may be a manifestation of the myasthenic crisis itself, the other symptoms are related to gradual overdosing of the inhibiting cholinesterase drug. The common observation that generalized weakness becomes more severe after the discontinuation of drug therapy in patients with an alleged cholinergic crisis supports the contention that both conditions can exist at the same time.

The clinical signs of a cholinergic crisis are miosis (patients with a myasthenic crisis often tend to have some mydriasis); excessive, thick pulmonary secretions, rapidly leading to atelectasis, shunting, and hypoxemia; muscle fasciculations; abdominal cramping and diarrhea; sweating; and extreme tearing (Table 43.6). The cause of respiratory distress in a pure form of cholinergic crisis, therefore, may be bronchiolar spasm, aspiration, and difficulty clearing thick secretions, rather than diaphragmatic failure.

The treatment of patients with cholinergic crisis consists of respiratory care, most likely intubation, and mechanical ventilation, with discontinuation of medication until the symptoms have subsided. Bronchoscopy through the endotracheal tube to clear the major parts of the tracheobronchial tree may be needed regularly. Antibiotic coverage becomes important if fever and pulmonary infiltrates develop, and reinstitution of pyridostigmine therapy must be postponed to facilitate bronchial drainage. When the chest radiograph shows sufficient clearing, pyridostigmine is administered intravenously in half the initial total daily dose, and then the dose is gradually increased until the optimal clinical effect is obtained.

When laboratory weaning criteria are fulfilled, weaning can begin and can often be expedited. Extubation failure in our patients with myasthenia gravis was correlated to decreased vital capacity, but prediction in these patients remains very difficult.[103] Again, we found BiPAP helpful in some patients.[85]

After endotracheal extubation, swallowing must be assessed before soft food is allowed. Patients may still have considerable bulbar dysfunction despite recovery to fairly normal respiratory function, and premature feeding may lead to aspiration. When soft food is tolerated, the intravenous dose can be changed to an oral dose.

Postoperative deterioration following thymectomy in myasthenia gravis or failure to wean from the ventilator is less common with frequent use of preoperative plasma exchange[20,29] and meticulous preoperative pulmonary assessment. Several reports have highlighted risk factors for postoperative complications. Among these factors are duration of myasthenia gravis exceeding 6 years, preexisting respiratory illness, large doses of pyridostigmine before surgery, marginal pulmonary function measured by vital capacity, severity of bulbar dysfunction, and history of respiratory failure after any type of surgery with general anesthesia.[58,117]

Patients should not be extubated unless they can sustain a head lift for 5 seconds. Extension of the head in myasthenia is often much weaker than flexion and this discrepancy may confuse general internists if a patient still is unable to wean. Failure to wean from the ventilator may have several causes. The most significant complication is pneumothorax or hemothorax from transcervical thymectomy. With this operative approach, adherence of the thymus to the pleura and subsequent tearing after removal may cause right-sided pneumothorax. Immediate drainage is indicated.

In the transsternal approach, the phrenic nerve may become damaged, but this complication is rarely a reason for prolonged postoperative care. Seldom are parathyroid glands incidentally removed or the recurrent laryngeal nerve severed. Stridor after thymectomy may be an early lead, and difficulty breathing should not be immediately interpreted as worsening myasthenia.

Inadequate management of postsurgical pain may be one of the reasons for failure to wean early on. Pain management with epidural catheterization has significantly improved postoperative pulmonary care,[14] which often is hampered by disruption of the thoracic cage. None of the currently used narcotics is contraindicated in myasthenia gravis, and most patients benefit from fentanyl.

OUTCOME

In most patients, the symptoms of myasthenia gravis become most severe within approximately 3 years of onset.[62] Mortality in myasthenia crises was not caused by respiratory failure in one study from Norway.[78] Large surveys of the natural history of myasthenia gravis have also reported spontaneous, mostly short, remissions.[39,51,75] Extreme examples of remissions lasting more than a decade have been reported as well.[51,75] The remission of myasthenia gravis after standard transsternal thymectomy can be impressive, and complete, persistent remission can be achieved in 25%–40% of patients as early as 6 months.[32,71] In addition, studies of long-term outcome after thymectomy have shown continuing deterioration in only a very small proportion of patients.[27,71] The rate of remission may be lower with a transcervical approach.

Immunosuppressive therapy in patients who have not had a remission with thymectomy has improved life expectancy and remarkably improved quality of life.[27] Permanent tracheostomy and severe limb weakness, leading to a wheelchair-bound state, are currently unusual. However, associated neoplasms, mostly colorectal cancers, develop in approximately one-third of the patients.[114] Long-term use of immunosuppression leads to avascular hip necrosis and cataracts (corticosteroids) and hypertension (cyclosporin and corticosteroids).

One can expect that there is a median ICU stay of nearly 2 weeks (1–5 months of hospitalization in a recent UK experience). Mortality was low but related to sepsis.[107] In a Spanish experience the median time on the ventilator was 12 days.[86] In our experience prolonged ICU stay is often related to community-acquired pneumonia and difficulty weaning from the ventilator. An outcome algorithm is shown in Figure 43.7.

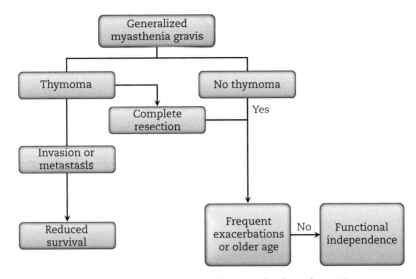

FIGURE 43.7: Outcome algorithm in myasthenia gravis. Functional independence: No assistance needed, minor handicap may remain.

CONCLUSIONS

- Myasthenic crisis is mostly triggered by intercurrent infection, tapering off or first-time initiation of corticosteroids, and elective surgery. Initial steps in the management of severe cases are endotracheal intubation, mechanical ventilation, discontinuation of pyridostigmine therapy, and plasma exchange. Bilevel positive airway pressure ventilation may prevent endotracheal intubation in some patients.

- Cholinergic symptoms are characterized by miosis, thick bronchial secretions, muscle fasciculations, abdominal cramping, diarrhea, and tearing. Bronchospasm, aspiration, or difficulty in clearing very thick secretions may cause respiratory failure.

- If a myasthenic crisis has not abated after 5 days of plasma exchange, prednisone (1 mg/kg/day) should be started or increased. Cyclosporine (5 mg/kg) or mycophenolate mofetil (1 gram bid) should be considered when treatment fails.

- Postoperative deterioration in myasthenia gravis can be largely eliminated by preoperative plasma exchange and postoperative pain control with fentanyl.

REFERENCES

1. Muscle Study Group. A trial of mycophenolate mofetil with prednisone as initial immunotherapy in myasthenia gravis. *Neurology* 2008;71:394–399.
2. Myasthenia Gravis Clinical Study Group. A randomised clinical trial comparing prednisone and azathioprine in myasthenia gravis: results of the second interim analysis. *J Neurol Neurosurg Psychiatry* 1993;56:1157–1163.
3. Arsura EL, Bick A, Brunner NG, Namba T, Grob D. High-dose intravenous immunoglobulin in the management of myasthenia gravis. *Arch Intern Med* 1986;146:1365–1368.
4. Bartoccioni E, Scuderi F, Minicuci GM, et al. Anti-MuSK antibodies: correlation with myasthenia gravis severity. *Neurology* 2006;67:505–507.
5. Bedlack RS, Sanders DB. Steroid treatment for myasthenia gravis: steroids have an important role. *Muscle Nerve* 2002;25:117–121.
6. Benatar M. A systematic review of diagnostic studies in myasthenia gravis. *Neuromuscul Disord* 2006;16:459–467.
7. Bergh NP, Gatzinsky P, Larsson S, Lundin P, Ridell B. Tumors of the thymus and thymic region. I: clinicopathological studies on thymomas. *Ann Thorac Surg* 1978;25:91–98.
8. Berrouschot J, Baumann I, Kalischewski P, Sterker M, Schneider D. Therapy of myasthenic crisis. *Crit Care Med* 1997;25:1228–1235.
9. Besinger UA, Toyka KV, Homberg M, et al. Myasthenia gravis: long-term correlation of binding and bungarotoxin blocking antibodies against acetylcholine receptors with changes in disease severity. *Neurology* 1983;33:1316–1321.
10. Borel CO. Management of myasthenic crisis: continuous anticholinesterase infusions. *Crit Care Med* 1993;21:821–822.

11. Brodsky MC, Boop FA. Lid nystagmus as a sign of intrinsic midbrain disease. *J Neuroophthalmol* 1995;15:236–240.

12. Buckley C, Newsom-Davis J, Willcox N, Vincent A. Do titin and cytokine antibodies in MG patients predict thymoma or thymoma recurrence? *Neurology* 2001;57:1579–1582.

13. Budde JM, Morris CD, Gal AA, Mansour KA, Miller JI, Jr. Predictors of outcome in thymectomy for myasthenia gravis. *Ann Thorac Surg* 2001;72:197–202.

14. Burgess FW, Wilcosky B, Jr. Thoracic epidural anesthesia for transsternal thymectomy in myasthenia gravis. *Anesth Analg* 1989;69:529–531.

15. Buzzard KA, Meyer NJ, Hardy TA, Riminton DS, Reddel SW. Induction IV cyclophosphamide followed by maintenance oral immunosuppression in refractory myasthenia gravis. *Muscle Nerve* 2015;52:204–210.

16. Chang I, Fink ME. Plasmapheresis in the treatment of myasthenic crisis. *Neurology* 1992;42 (Suppl 3):242.

17. Ciafaloni E, Massey JM, Tucker-Lipscomb B, Sanders DB. Mycophenolate mofetil for myasthenia gravis: an open-label pilot study. *Neurology* 2001;56:97–99.

18. Ciafaloni E, Nikhar NK, Massey JM, Sanders DB. Retrospective analysis of the use of cyclosporine in myasthenia gravis. *Neurology* 2000;55:448–450.

19. Conti-Fine BM, Milani M, Kaminski HJ. Myasthenia gravis: past, present, and future. *J Clin Invest* 2006;116:2843–2854.

20. d'Empaire G, Hoaglin DC, Perlo VP, Pontoppidan H. Effect of prethymectomy plasma exchange on postoperative respiratory function in myasthenia gravis. *J Thorac Cardiovasc Surg* 1985;89:592–596.

21. Daroff RB. The office Tensilon test for ocular myasthenia gravis. *Arch Neurol* 1986;43:843–844.

22. Dau PC. Plasmapheresis therapy in myasthenia gravis. *Muscle Nerve* 1980;3:468–482.

23. Dau PC, Lindstrom JM, Cassel CK, et al. Plasmapheresis and immunosuppressive drug therapy in myasthenia gravis. *N Engl J Med* 1977;297:1134–1140.

24. De Feo LG, Schottlender J, Martelli NA, Molfino NA. Use of intravenous pulsed cyclophosphamide in severe, generalized myasthenia gravis. *Muscle Nerve* 2002;26:31–36.

25. DeFilippi VJ, Richman DP, Ferguson MK. Transcervical thymectomy for myasthenia gravis. *Ann Thorac Surg* 1994;57:194–197.

26. Dirr LY, Donofrio PD, Patton JF, Troost BT. A false-positive edrophonium test in a patient with a brainstem glioma. *Neurology* 1989;39:865–867.

27. Durelli L, Maggi G, Casadio C, et al. Actuarial analysis of the occurrence of remissions following thymectomy for myasthenia gravis in 400 patients. *J Neurol Neurosurg Psychiatry* 1991;54:406–411.

28. Dushay KM, Zibrak JD, Jensen WA. Myasthenia gravis presenting as isolated respiratory failure. *Chest* 1990;97:232–234.

29. Eisenkraft JB, Papatestas AE, Kahn CH, et al. Predicting the need for postoperative mechanical ventilation in myasthenia gravis. *Anesthesiology* 1986;65:79–82.

30. Engel AG. Myasthenia gravis and myasthenic syndromes. *Ann Neurol* 1984;16:519–534.

31. Frisby J, Wills A, Jaspan T. Brain stem compression by a giant vertebrobasilar aneurysm mimicking seronegative myasthenia. *J Neurol Neurosurg Psychiatry* 2001;71:125–126.

32. Frist WH, Thirumalai S, Doehring CB, et al. Thymectomy for the myasthenia gravis patient: factors influencing outcome. *Ann Thorac Surg* 1994;57:334–338.

33. Gajdos P, Chevret S. Treatment of myasthenia gravis acute exacerbations with intravenous immunoglobulin. *Ann N Y Acad Sci* 2008;1132:271–275.

34. Gajdos P, Chevret S, Clair B, Tranchant C, Chastang C. Clinical trial of plasma exchange and high-dose intravenous immunoglobulin in myasthenia gravis. Myasthenia Gravis Clinical Study Group. *Ann Neurol* 1997;41:789–796.

35. Gilchrist JM, Massey JM, Sanders DB. Single fiber EMG and repetitive stimulation of the same muscle in myasthenia gravis. *Muscle Nerve* 1994;17:171–175.

36. Golnik KC, Pena R, Lee AG, Eggenberger ER. An ice test for the diagnosis of myasthenia gravis. *Ophthalmology* 1999;106:1282–1286.

37. Goulon M, Elkharrat D, Lokiec F, Gajdos P. Results of a one-year open trial of cyclosporine in ten patients with severe myasthenia gravis. *Transplant Proc* 1988;20:211–217.

38. Gritti P, Sgarzi M, Carrara B, et al. A standardized protocol for the perioperative management of myasthenia gravis patients: experience with 110 patients. *Acta Anaesthesiol Scand* 2012;56:66–75.

39. Grob D, Brunner NG, Namba T. The natural course of myasthenia gravis and effect of therapeutic measures. *Ann N Y Acad Sci* 1981;377:652–669.

40. Grob D, Simpson D, Mitsumoto H, et al. Treatment of myasthenia gravis by immunoadsorption of plasma. *Neurology* 1995;45:338–344.

41. Gronseth GS, Barohn RJ. Practice parameter: thymectomy for autoimmune myasthenia gravis (an evidence-based review): report of the Quality Standards Subcommittee of the American Academy of Neurology. *Neurology* 2000;55:7–15.

42. Hanisch F, Wendt M, Zierz S. Mycophenolate mofetil as second line immunosuppressant in Myasthenia gravis: a long-term prospective open-label study *Eur J Med Res* 2009;14:364–366.

43. Hart IK, Sharshar T, Sathasivam S. Immunosuppressant drugs for myasthenia gravis. *J Neurol Neurosurg Psychiatry* 2009;80:5–6.

44. Higo R, Nito T, Tayama N. Videofluoroscopic assessment of swallowing function in patients with myasthenia gravis. *J Neurol Sci* 2005;231:45–48.

45. Howard JF, Jr, Barohn RJ, Cutter GR, et al. A randomized, double-blind, placebo-controlled phase II study of eculizumab in patients with refractory generalized myasthenia gravis. *Muscle Nerve* 2013;48:76–84.

46. Jacobson DM. The "ice pack test" for diagnosing myasthenia gravis. *Ophthalmology* 2000;107:622–623.

47. Jaretzki A, 3rd, Barohn RJ, Ernstoff RM, et al. Myasthenia gravis: recommendations for clinical research standards. Task Force of the Medical Scientific Advisory Board of the Myasthenia Gravis Foundation of America. *Neurology* 2000;55:16–23.

48. Kaneda H, Saito Y, Saito T, et al. Preoperative steroid therapy stabilizes postoperative respiratory conditions in myasthenia gravis. *Gen Thorac Cardiovasc Surg* 2008;56:114–118.

49. Kao YF, Lan MY, Chou MS, Chen WH. Intracranial fatigable ptosis. *J Neuroophthalmol* 1999;19:257–259.

50. Katzberg HD, Aziz T, Oger J. In myasthenia gravis cells from atrophic thymus secrete acetylcholine receptor antibodies. *Neurology* 2001;56:572–573.

51. Kennedy FS, Moersch FP. Myasthenia gravis: a clinical review of eighty-seven cases observed between 1915 and the early part of 1932. *Can Med Assoc J* 1937;37:216–223.

52. Khan OA, Campbell WW. Myasthenia gravis presenting as dysphagia: clinical considerations. *Am J Gastroenterol* 1994;89:1083–1085.

53. Kim HK, Park MS, Choi YS, et al. Neurologic outcomes of thymectomy in myasthenia gravis: comparative analysis of the effect of thymoma. *J Thorac Cardiovasc Surg* 2007;134:601–607.

54. Kissel JT, Franklin GM. Treatment of myasthenia gravis: a call to arms. *Neurology* 2000;55:3–4.

55. Lacomis D. Myasthenic crisis. *Neurocrit Care* 2005;3:189–194.

56. Lanska DJ. Indications for thymectomy in myasthenia gravis. *Neurology* 1990;40:1828–1829.

57. Lebrun C, Bourg V, Tieulie N, Thomas P. Successful treatment of refractory generalized myasthenia gravis with rituximab. *Eur J Neurol* 2009;16:246–250.

58. Leventhal SR, Orkin FK, Hirsh RA. Prediction of the need for postoperative mechanical ventilation in myasthenia gravis. *Anesthesiology* 1980;53:26–30.

59. Lewis JE, Wick MR, Scheithauer BW, Bernatz PE, Taylor WF. Thymoma. A clinicopathologic review. *Cancer* 1987;60:2727–2743.

60. Lindberg C, Andersen O, Lefvert AK. Treatment of myasthenia gravis with methylprednisolone pulse: a double blind study. *Acta Neurol Scand* 1998;97:370–373.

61. Lisak RP, ed. *Handbook of Myasthenia Gravis and Myasthenic Syndromes*. New York: CRC Press; 1994. Neurological Disease and Therapy.

62. Mantegazza R, Beghi E, Pareyson D, et al. A multicentre follow-up study of 1152 patients with myasthenia gravis in Italy. *J Neurol* 1990;237:339–344.

63. Masaoka A, Monden Y, Nakahara K, Tanioka T. Follow-up study of thymomas with special reference to their clinical stages. *Cancer* 1981;48:2485–2492.

64. McConville J, Farrugia ME, Beeson D, et al. Detection and characterization of MuSK antibodies in seronegative myasthenia gravis. *Ann Neurol* 2004;55:580–584.

65. Meriggioli MN. IVIG in myasthenia gravis: getting enough "bang for the buck." *Neurology* 2007;68:803–804.

66. Meriggioli MN, Rowin J. Treatment of myasthenia gravis with mycophenolate mofetil: a case report. *Muscle Nerve* 2000;23:1287–1289.

67. Mier-Jedrzejowicz AK, Brophy C, Green M. Respiratory muscle function in myasthenia gravis. *Am Rev Respir Dis* 1988;138:867–873.

68. Mier A, Laroche C, Green M. Unsuspected myasthenia gravis presenting as respiratory failure. *Thorax* 1990;45:422–423.

69. Mowzoon N, Sussman A, Bradley WG. Mycophenolate (CellCept) treatment of myasthenia gravis, chronic inflammatory polyneuropathy and inclusion body myositis. *J Neurol Sci* 2001;185:119–122.

70. Nagappan R, Kletchko S. Myasthenia gravis presenting as respiratory failure. *N Z Med J* 1992;105:152.

71. Nieto IP, Robledo JP, Pajuelo MC, et al. Prognostic factors for myasthenia gravis treated by thymectomy: review of 61 cases. *Ann Thorac Surg* 1999;67:1568–1571.

72. Odel JG, Winterkorn JM, Behrens MM. The sleep test for myasthenia gravis: a safe alternative to Tensilon. *J Clin Neuroophthalmol* 1991;11:288–292.

73. Oh SJ, Kim DE, Kuruoglu R, Bradley RJ, Dwyer D. Diagnostic sensitivity of the laboratory tests in myasthenia gravis. *Muscle Nerve* 1992;15:720–724.

74. Ohta K, Shigemoto K, Kubo S, et al. MuSK antibodies in AChR Ab-seropositive MG vs AChR Ab-seronegative MG. *Neurology* 2004;62:2132–2133.

75. Oosterhuis HJ. Observations of the natural history of myasthenia gravis and the effect of thymectomy. *Ann N Y Acad Sci* 1981;377:678–690.

76. Oosterhuis HJGH. *Myasthenia Gravis.* Vol. 5. Edinburgh: Churchill Livingstone; 1984.

77. Osher RH, Griggs RC. Orbicularis fatigue: the 'peek' sign of myasthenia gravis. *Arch Ophthalmol* 1979;97:677–679.

78. Owe JF, Daltveit AK, Gilhus NE. Causes of death among patients with myasthenia gravis in Norway between 1951 and 2001. *J Neurol Neurosurg Psychiatry* 2006;77:203–207.

79. Palace J, Newsom-Davis J, Lecky B. A randomized double-blind trial of prednisolone alone or with azathioprine in myasthenia gravis. Myasthenia Gravis Study Group. *Neurology* 1998;50:1778–1783.

80. Papatestas AE, Genkins G, Kornfeld P, et al. Effects of thymectomy in myasthenia gravis. *Ann Surg* 1987;206:79–88.

81. Pascuzzi RM. The edrophonium test. *Semin Neurol* 2003;23:83–88.

82. Perlo VP, Poskanzer DC, Schwab RS, et al. Myasthenia gravis: evaluation of treatment in 1,355 patients. *Neurology* 1966;16:431–439.

83. Qureshi AI, Choudhry MA, Akbar MS, et al. Plasma exchange versus intravenous immunoglobulin treatment in myasthenic crisis. *Neurology* 1999;52:629–632.

84. Rabinstein A, Wijdicks EFM. BiPAP in acute respiratory failure due to myasthenic crisis may prevent intubation. *Neurology* 2002;59:1647–1649.

85. Rabinstein AA, Wijdicks EFM. Weaning from the ventilator using BiPAP in myasthenia gravis. *Muscle Nerve* 2003;27:252–253.

86. Ramos-Fransi A, Rojas-Garcia R, Segovia S, et al. Myasthenia gravis: descriptive analysis of life-threatening events in a recent nationwide registry. *Eur J Neurol* 2015;22:1056–1061.

87. Richman DP, Agius MA. Treatment of autoimmune myasthenia gravis. *Neurology* 2003;61:1652–1661.

88. Rivero A, Crovetto L, Lopez L, Maselli R, Nogues M. Single fiber electromyography of extraocular muscles: a sensitive method for the diagnosis of ocular myasthenia gravis. *Muscle Nerve* 1995;18:943–947.

89. Rivner MH. Steroid treatment for myasthenia gravis: steroids are overutilized. *Muscle Nerve* 2002;25:115–117.

90. Roberts ME, Steiger MJ, Hart IK. Presentation of myasthenia gravis mimicking blepharospasm. *Neurology* 2002;58:150–151.

91. Rodriguez Cruz PM, Al-Hajjar M, Huda S, et al. Clinical features and diagnostic usefulness of antibodies to clustered acetylcholine receptors in the diagnosis of seronegative myasthenia gravis. *JAMA Neurology* 2015;72:642–649.

92. Saltis LM, Martin BR, Traeger SM, Bonfiglio MF. Continuous infusion of pyridostigmine in the management of myasthenic crisis. *Crit Care Med* 1993;21:938–940.

93. Sanders DB. The electrodiagnosis of myasthenia gravis. *Ann N Y Acad Sci* 1987;505:539–556.

94. Sanders DB, Andrews I, Howard JF, Jr, Massey JM. Seronegative myasthenia gravis. *Neurology* 1997;48 (Suppl 5):S40–S45.

95. Sanders DB, Hart IK, Mantegazza R, et al. An international, phase III, randomized trial of mycophenolate mofetil in myasthenia gravis. *Neurology* 2008;71:400–406.

96. Sanders DB, Howard JF, Jr. AAEE minimonograph #25: single-fiber electromyography in myasthenia gravis. *Muscle Nerve* 1986;9:809–819.

97. Sanders DB, Juel VC. MuSK-antibody positive myasthenia gravis: questions from the clinic. *J Neuroimmunol* 2008;201–202:85–89.

98. Sanders DB, Siddiqi ZA. Lessons from two trials of mycophenolate mofetil in myasthenia gravis. *Ann N Y Acad Sci* 2008;1132:249–253.

99. Schady W, MacDermott N. On the choice of muscle in the electrophysiological assessment of myasthenia gravis. *Electromyogr Clin Neurophysiol* 1992;32:99–102.

100. Scherer K, Bedlack RS, Simel DL. Does this patient have myasthenia gravis? *JAMA* 2005;293:1906–1914.

101. Schon F, Drayson M, Thompson RA. Myasthenia gravis and elderly people. *Age Ageing* 1996;25:56–58.

102. Seneviratne J, Mandrekar J, Wijdicks EFM, Rabinstein AA. Noninvasive ventilation in myasthenic crisis. *Arch Neurol* 2008;65:54–58.

103. Seneviratne J, Mandrekar J, Wijdicks EFM, Rabinstein AA. Predictors of extubation failure in myasthenic crisis. *Arch Neurol* 2008;65:929–933.

104. Sethi KD, Rivner MH, Swift TR. Ice pack test for myasthenia gravis. *Neurology* 1987;37:1383–1385.

105. Shibuya N, Sato T, Osame M, et al. Immunoadsorption therapy for myasthenia gravis. *J Neurol Neurosurg Psychiatry* 1994;57:578–581.

106. Sieb JP. Myasthenia gravis: an update for the clinician. *Clin Exp Immunol* 2014;175:408–418.

107. Spillane J, Hirsch NP, Kullmann DM, Taylor C, Howard RS. Myasthenia gravis: treatment of acute severe exacerbations in the intensive care unit results in a favourable long-term prognosis. *Eur J Neurol* 2014;21:171–173.

108. Spinelli A, Marconi G, Gorini M, Pizzi A, Scano G. Control of breathing in patients with myasthenia gravis. *Am Rev Respir Dis* 1992;145:1359–1366.

109. Thieben MJ, Blacker DJ, Liu PY, Harper CM, Jr, Wijdicks EFM. Pulmonary function tests and blood gases in worsening myasthenia gravis. *Muscle Nerve* 2005;32:664–667.

110. Thomas CE, Mayer SA, Gungor Y, et al. Myasthenic crisis: clinical features, mortality, complications, and risk factors for prolonged intubation. *Neurology* 1997;48:1253–1260.

111. Tindall RS, Rollins JA, Phillips JT, et al. Preliminary results of a double-blind, randomized, placebo-controlled trial of cyclosporine in myasthenia gravis. *N Engl J Med* 1987;316:719–724.

112. Toyka KV. Ptosis in myasthenia gravis: extended fatigue and recovery bedside test. *Neurology* 2006;67:1524.

113. Vincent A, Drachman DB. Myasthenia gravis. *Adv Neurol* 2002;88:159–188

114. Wilkins KB, Sheikh E, Green R, et al. Clinical and pathologic predictors of survival in patients with thymoma. *Ann Surg* 1999;230:562–572.

115. Wittbrodt ET. Drugs and myasthenia gravis: an update. *Arch Intern Med* 1997;157:399–408.

116. Younge BR, Bartley GB. Lancaster test with Tensilon for myasthenia. *Arch Neurol* 1987;44:472–473.

117. Younger DS, Braun NM, Jaretzki A, 3rd, Penn AS, Lovelace RE. Myasthenia gravis: determinants for independent ventilation after transsternal thymectomy. *Neurology* 1984;34:336–340.

118. Zinman L, Ng E, Bril V. IV immunoglobulin in patients with myasthenia gravis: a randomized controlled trial. *Neurology* 2007;68:837–841.

PART VIII

Postoperative Neurosurgical
and Neurointerventional
Complications

44

Complications of Craniotomy and Biopsy

Practices vary, but both elective and emergency craniotomy are unchallenged indications for admission to a neurosciences intensive care unit (NICU). Tumor surgery is most often the indication for elective craniotomy; for many patients, a stay in the NICU is precautionary and brief.

Brain edema, seizures, and postoperative hemorrhage along the track of surgical excision constitute most of the complications. Other equally common complications, discussed in other chapters, include increased intracranial pressure (Chapter 22); status epilepticus, particularly focal status epilepticus (Chapter 40); and hyponatremia (Chapter 57). Neurosurgical problems in the perioperative period, such as wound infections, pseudomeningocele,[9,39,68,85] and cerebrospinal fluid (CSF) leaks are not discussed here. The organizing principle of this chapter is to provide a brief overview of some unusual complications. Most of these complications are handled by the neurosurgeon. However, neurointensivists may be consulted or may be asked to co-manage postoperative care.

GENERAL CARE AFTER CRANIOTOMY

Airway management remains an important priority after any type of craniotomy. Recovery of consciousness may be prolonged after extensive surgical procedures requiring brain retraction, and this may result in partial collapse of the airway. Reduced activation of the muscles of the upper airway may not keep the pharynx patent. Inability to maintain a normal airway then results in hypoxemia. Airway obstruction due to bilateral vocal cord paralysis after surgery in the posterior fossa that injures the vagal nerves (e.g., ependymoma, acoustic neuroma) may produce stridor. Temporary tracheostomy is needed if the cords remain fixed in position.

An abundance of seemingly mundane problems may occur after craniotomy. Refractory nausea and vomiting appear more commonly after removal of lesions in the posterior fossa.[17]

Effective therapeutic agents are ondansetron 1–4 mg intravenously and promethazine 12.5–25 mg intravenously. Unrest, anxiety, and discomfort are more common than profound agitation. Patients with these postoperative manifestations have a good response to infusion of dexmedetomidine (1 µg/kg IV over 10 minutes followed by 0.2–0.7 µg/kg/hr IV).[12–14] Because respiratory depression does not occur, the drug is ideal in patients who cannot tolerate the endotracheal tube (patients appear asleep but are quickly awakened). However, dexmedetomidine has a very narrow therapeutic range and hypotension, bradycardia, and nausea remain of concern as side effects (Chapter 16). Experience with dexmedetomidine is now substantial, and it has been approved for use on the first postoperative days.[12]

Postoperative hiccups can be difficult to manage. Placement of a nasogastric tube alone can be successful. Baclofen may be needed in resistant hiccups, and 10 mg three time a day may do wonders. In the postoperative period, success in European countries has also been claimed with the non-narcotic analgesic nefopam (10 mg slow intravenously).[5]

Craniotomy is a major surgical procedure and may be followed by significant facial swelling, unilateral soft tissue eyelid hematoma, and pain from transient removal of a bone flap. These discomforts subside gradually, but pain is traditionally handled with drugs such as codeine. A typical postcraniotomy order is shown in Table 44.1. Generally, drugs are avoided that potentially suppress megakaryopoiesis (for example, H_2 blockers and many antibiotics).

SPECIFIC COMPLICATIONS

Series involving craniotomy for glioma have reported mortality of 3% and morbidity approaching 10%.[10,18,66] Worsening brain tissue shift from postoperative edema is a substantial surgical risk, varying from 10% to 20% in most large series.[11,18,66] Specific complications may occur and

TABLE 44.1. EXAMPLE OF A STANDARD
POSTOPERATIVE CRANIOTOMY ORDER*

Codeine	30–60 mg IM, q4h p.r.n.
Cefazolin	1,000 mg IV, q8h
Dexamethasone	4 mg IV, q6h
Levetiracetam	1000 mg PO/IV, b.i.d.
Subcutaneous heparin	5,000 U, q8h

*Also includes swallowing precautions, incentive spirometry, crystalloid fluids, restriction of free water intake and continued treatment of increased intracranial pressure.

may include CSF leak, hemorrhage in the surgical bed, or vascular—arterial or venous—injury.[58,70]

Epilepsy surgery for intractable seizures has been established and proven.[77,80] The most frequent concerns are infectious complications, including wound infections that require bone flap removal.[4] Injury to the anterior choroidal artery in temporal lobectomy with radical medial resection may cause hemiplegia. Word-finding deficits can be present after left anterior temporal lobectomy.[4,42] An intracerebral hematoma with depth electrode implantation is uncommon, but the incidence may reach 3%.[56,74] In one experience with a total of 6,415 electrode implantations and 2,449 surgical procedures, major neurological morbidity was very low (0.5%) and mostly in multilobar resections. Complications included aseptic meningitis (mostly with temporal lobe resection) and intracranial hematomas (mostly in the extradural compartment).[73] Patients with early postoperative seizures have a slightly less favorable outcome, particularly if the seizures are similar in type to presurgical seizures. Isolated auras, however, do not predict a poor surgical result.[44]

Pituitary surgery may lead to neurologic, endocrine, and sinonasal complications.[26] Cerebrospinal fluid leaks, hemorrhage in the surgical site, diabetes insipidus, and panhypopituitarism are the best-known complications. Adrenal, thyroid, and gonadal deficiencies are often permanent.[26] Evaluation of postoperative endocrine status may show low thyroxine level and low free thyroxine index due to central hypothyroidism. Adrenal insufficiency may be difficult to detect clinically, but a random sample of cortisol less than 5 µg/dL is highly suggestive.

Diabetes insipidus is evident when polyuria occurs with increased serum tonicity, insufficient water intake, and hypotonic urine.

Transsphenoidal surgery for pituitary adenoma may cause hyponatremia (up to 2 weeks postoperatively),[37] and rapid correction in this situation has led, in a surprisingly high number of reported cases, to pontine or extrapontine myelinolysis.[7,27,64,76] The type of hyponatremia and hypernatremia associated with transsphenoidal surgery is further discussed in Chapter 57.

Remote Hemorrhages

Postoperative hemorrhages in the surgical bed are more common than hemorrhages at distant sites.[25,35,74] However, several cases have been described of intracranial hemorrhage occurring at a site remote from the craniotomy.[48,49,75,82] The hemorrhages may occur in the opposite hemisphere and in the cerebellum after surgery on, for example, one of the frontal lobes or after drainage of a subdural hematoma (Capsule 44.1).

Most remote hemorrhages become evident clinically and on computed tomography (CT) scan within the first 24 hours. A postoperative CT scan may document remote hemorrhages in a patient who does not awaken from general anesthesia. Postoperative headache may be a warning sign of a remote hemorrhage in the cerebellum. In several case reports in the literature, generalized tonic-clonic seizures signaled a hematoma involving a hemispheric location. Clinical features vary depending on the location. Hemorrhages in the cerebellar peduncles produce a tremor, and in the cerebellar hemisphere result in cerebellar ataxia and slurred speech. Nystagmus may change in direction with different positions of gaze (a typical feature of central nystagmus).

In cerebellar hematomas, the CT characteristics of the hemorrhage—much of the blood tracks through the folia—may suggest a venous hemorrhage from tearing of the superior vermian veins or any of their tributaries.[28,75,82]

Craniotomy for a traumatic intracranial lesion may be associated with a contralateral extradural hematoma. Failure to awaken after surgery is the most common presenting feature and is striking in some, with fixed, dilated pupils and bilateral extensor posturing.[83] However, remote hemorrhages after craniotomy for traumatic brain injury may be a result of the development of hemorrhagic contusions, rather than a consequence of the surgical procedure.[11]

Multiple intracerebral hemorrhages, a contralateral extradural hematoma,[48,49,83] and subarachnoid hemorrhages[41] have been described and may include supratentorial and intratentorial hemorrhages.[53,57] Examples of remote hemorrhages are shown in Figures 44.1–44.3.

With so few examples, the ideal management is not well established. When the hematoma

---

CAPSULE 44.1   PATHOPHYSIOLOGY OF REMOTE HEMORRHAGES AFTER CRANIOTOMY

The mechanism for these hemorrhages may be different in each location. Predisposing factors are coagulopathy; preoperative use of mannitol; prior alcohol abuse; use of valproic acid, which could interfere with anticoagulation;[75] and traumatic origin of the hematoma, but not postoperative hypertension.[8] These remote hemorrhages have been problematic, causing significant morbidity, but they can be small and may contribute little to the overall neurologic condition. The frequency is estimated to be 1 in 300 craniotomies.

Some data suggest that postoperative hemorrhage in the cerebellum is more likely with cerebrospinal fluid drainage during surgery, possibly a reflection of a mechanical shift of the cerebellum ("cerebellar sag").[21,31,82] These factors suggest that acute reduction in intracranial pressure from removal of a supratentorial mass can lead to a critical increase in transmural pressure in veins and venules, culminating in possible hemorrhage. Another hypothesis is that extension and rotation during positioning obstruct the veins of the cerebellum and result in a hemorrhagic infarct. Pterional craniotomy often involves various degrees of contralateral rotation and 20 degrees of extension of the neck that may predispose the patient to obstruction of the internal jugular vein. An examination of the biomechanics of this region confirmed that angulation and obstruction of the internal jugular vein at the transverse process of C1 on the same side as the craniotomy may be a contributing cause.[71]

---

involves the cerebellum and is causing mass effect, surgery is necessary to remove the mass effect, but this is very uncommon. Small hemorrhages in both hemispheres can probably be left alone. Most patients in cases reported in the literature have a predominantly poor outcome, often with serious

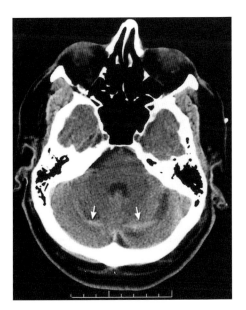

FIGURE 44.1: Remote cerebellar hematoma. Note tracking along folia (*arrows*) suggesting venous hemorrhage.

disability. Undoubtedly, outcome is determined by the time to recognition, and if a mass effect exists, surgical evacuation is necessary. Moreover, outcome may be determined by the initial lesion and not so much by this additional hemorrhage. Prevention of hemorrhage may be equally important. It is imperative to focus on type of drainage and perhaps to avoid intraoperative use of mannitol and valproic acid[28] (Figure 44.3).

Brain Biopsy or Ventriculostomy-Associated Hemorrhage

Biopsy-associated intracerebral hemorrhage (Figure 44.4) occurs in only a small percentage of patients.[1,19,34,40,67,79,86] (Table 44.2). A prospective study found neurologic deterioration in only a few patients (0.4%).[40] Silent hemorrhage was more common, occurring in more than half the studied cases. Multivariate analysis found an increased risk with a platelet count below 150×10^9/L or a lesion in the pineal gland due to the extreme vascularity of pinealomas and pinealoblastomas. There was also an increased risk with a higher number of biopsy specimens or postoperative hypertension.[19] One study of patients who had biopsy for presumed lymphoma after organ transplantation found an unexpectedly high incidence (four of six patients) of postbiopsy hemorrhage.[55]

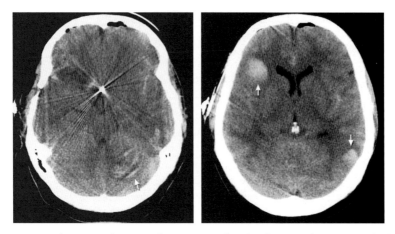

FIGURE 44.2: Computed tomography scan of supratentorial and infratentorial remote cerebral hemorrhages (*arrows*) after clipping of anterior communicating artery aneurysm.

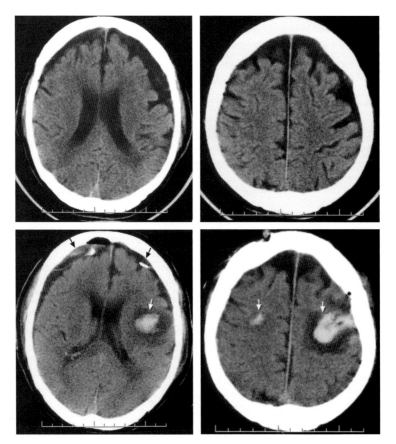

FIGURE 44.3: Bilateral frontal hematoma after drainage of subdural hygromas (*white arrows*) with burr holes and placement of a suction drains (*black arrows*).

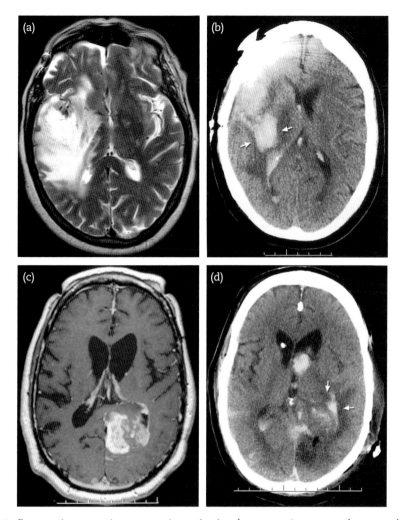

FIGURE 44.4: Preoperative magnetic resonance image (a, c) and postoperative computed tomography scan (b, d) in each of two patients with astrocytoma and postbiopsy intracerebral hematoma (*arrows*).

Evacuation of the hematoma is rarely needed and only if mass effect occurs (Figure 44.4). Intracerebral hematoma may also occur with ventriculostomy but is rarely observed or clinically of much relevance (Figure 44.5).[22,30,60,63,65]

Ventriculostomy is associated with higher in-hospital mortality, but this is a consequence of severity of illness.[62] Hemorrhagic complications with ventriculostomy placement varies from 0% to 32% (Table 44.3),[3] and may be dependent on many factors (coagulopathies and international normalized ratio before placement).[6]

Cerebral Infarction

Cerebral infarction is most commonly due to venous occlusion. This complication may occur after resection of a meningioma and is related to prior invasion of the dura and venous sinuses.

Convexity, parasagittal, and falcine meningiomas are close to the superior sagittal sinus, causing a particular risk of infarction.[36] In some instances, after resection the neurosurgeon has already attempted to reconstruct the cerebral venous sinus. Hemorrhagic infarction may incorporate the operative bed, but also may occur at a distance if the operation is to remove a tumor in the pineal region, or it may involve the deeper cerebral veins, causing bithalamic hemorrhagic infarcts.

A tentorial meningioma may require sacrifice of the transverse or sigmoid sinus, but if the torcula remains patent, venous cerebellar or supratentorial hemorrhage is less likely. Cerebellar infarction after the suboccipital approach has been used to remove an acoustic neuroma is a known complication to neurosurgeons. In some patients, cerebellar softening is already obvious before closure, and the

TABLE 44.2. LITERATURE REVIEW OF HEMORRHAGIC COMPLICATIONS AFTER STEREOTACTIC BRAIN BIOPSY

Authors (Year)	No. of Patients	Patients with Hemorrhage (%)
Voges et al., 1993[79]	338	2.4
Sawin et al., 1998[67]	225	3.6
Yu et al., 1998[86]	310	1.6
Field et al., 2001[19]	500	8.0

Modified from Field M, Witham TF, Flickinger JC, et al. Comprehensive assessment of hemorrhage risks and outcomes after stereotactic brain biopsy. *J Neurosurg* 2001;94:545–551. With permission of the American Association of Neurological Surgeons.

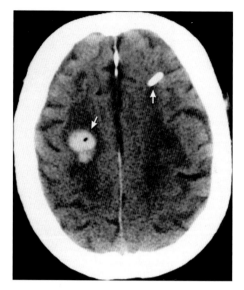

FIGURE 44.5: Ventriculostomy-associated intracerebral hematoma. Note air in hematoma. The ventriculostomy drain has been moved to the opposite side (*arrows*).

neurosurgeon resects the lateral part of the cerebellum. Postoperative CT scans may not be able initially to distinguish between edema and infarction, and magnetic resonance imaging (MRI) with magnetic resonance venography may be needed.

Arterial occlusion may occur because of the sacrifice of branches of the middle cerebral artery adherent to the sylvian fissure, for example, in patients who underwent surgery for a convexity meningioma. Cerebral infarction may be a consequence of the complicated repair of a cerebral aneurysm despite use of high-flow saphenous vein grafts. Resection of an arteriovenous malformation may cause retrograde thrombosis of the feeding arteries.[47]

Postoperative Cerebral Edema

Partial resection or stereotactic biopsy is more commonly associated with postoperative cerebral edema than gross total resection (Figure 44.6). Generally, prolonged retraction in the brain and an anesthetic regimen that increases cerebral blood volume may contribute. Opioids (leading to respiratory depression, high arterial carbon dioxide, and increased cerebral blood flow), isoflurane and nitrous oxide (vasodilators increasing cerebral blood volume), and enflurane and halothane (decreasing cerebral fluid resorption) can all increase intracranial pressure from edema.[78] Presurgical cerebral edema (e.g., in a large meningioma) may worsen with surgery

TABLE 44.3. VENTRICULOSTOMY ASSOCIATED HEMORRHAGES

Studies	Hemorrhages	Significant	EVDs
Guyot et al.[25]	9	2	274
Maniker et al.[45]	52	4	160
Paramore and Turner[54]	2	2	253
North and Reilly[52]	2	1	199
Rhodes et al.[59]	6	0	66
Wiesmann and Mayer[81]	6	0	92
Ehtisham et al.[15]	6	0	29
Khanna et al.[38]	0	0	106
Roitberg et al.[61]	1	0	103
Leung et al.[43]	1	0	133
Friedman et al.[21]	1	0	100
Narayan et al.[51]	4	1	207
Total	102 (5.7%)	11 (0.6%)	1,790

Modified from Binz DD, Toussaint G, Friedman JA. Hemorrhagic complications of ventriculostomy placement: a meta-analysis. *Neurocrit Care* 2009;10:253–256. With permission of Springer.

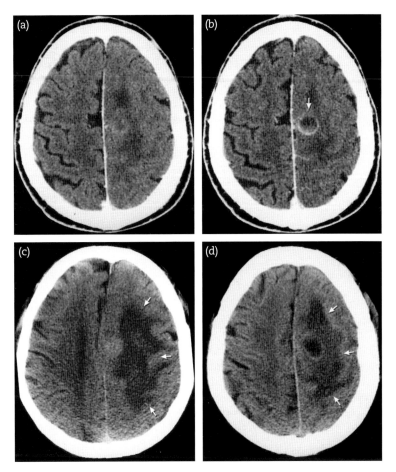

FIGURE 44.6. *Top row*: a, c Preoperative CT scan showing lesion before biopsy. *Bottom row*: b, d Postbiopsy CT scan with secondary brain edema (*arrows*). Cerebral edema presented with a new onset seizure.

and may considerably lengthen the stay in the NICU. Awakening may be protracted, and some patients need prolonged time on the ventilator and tracheostomy.

Dexamethasone (10–20 mg IV, followed by 4 mg every 6 hours in a 4-day taper) possibly reduces postoperative edema. Its use perioperatively in craniotomy is universally accepted, although not borne out by hard evidence.

Prevention (or treatment) of postoperative cerebral edema includes placement of the patient in a semirecumbent (30–40-degree) position to facilitate venous drainage, restriction of free water, and limitation of fluid intake to 2 L of isotonic saline. The role of blood pressure control is not known, and blood pressure goals in the perioperative period are not well established. Mannitol (1–2 g/kg bolus over 60 minutes) may be used temporarily, but most of the edema subsides spontaneously, and care is supportive only.

Syndrome of the Trephined

Unilateral or bilateral decompressive surgery may result in a late and rare complication known as syndrome of the trephined, or sinking scalp flap.[2,20,24,33,84] In a retrospective series of decompressive craniotomy, the incidence was 1% (2 patients in 164 craniotomies).[29] With intact skull, the ICP is negative in the upright position; but with a major deficit, ICP equalizes with atmospheric pressure. Clinical deterioration is not common but may result in marked decline in level of consciousness. Nursing in flat body position may improve clinical signs and improve CT scan findings. Cranioplasty is needed and will resolve the complication (Figure 44.7).

Seizures

Seizures may be due to a precipitous drop in antiepileptic drug level from failure to monitor levels in a patient with previous epilepsy or drug interactions. In other patients, high-risk situations,

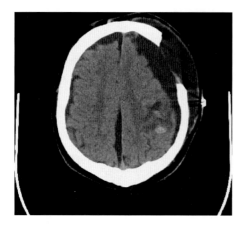

FIGURE 44.7: Marked brain sagging with bone defect.

TABLE 44.4. AIR EMBOLISM
AFTER NEUROSURGICAL PROCEDURES

Position	Incidence (%)
Sitting	25
Supine	15
Prone	10
Lateral	8

Modified from Albin MS, Carroll RG, Maroon JC. Clinical considerations concerning detection of venous air embolism. *Neurosurgery* 1978;3:380–384. With permission of the Congress of Neurological Surgeons.

such as the evacuation of subdural empyema and tumors abutting the primary motor cortex, may predispose to seizures. The prophylactic use of antiepileptic drugs (phenytoin or levetiracetam) in craniotomy is controversial because no effect on the prevalence of postoperative seizures has been demonstrated after surgery.[72] Focal seizures are most common and may be refractory to treatment. Electroencephalography should document epileptiform discharges. Aggressive management is needed, because some patients have prolonged hemiparesis, and partial status epilepticus lasting several days has been associated with permanent hemiparesis. Control may be achieved with the administration of phenobarbital 20 mg/kg (IV infusion rate at 25–50 mg/min). Intravenous administration of valproate, 15–30 mg/kg loading dose over 1 hour (max rate, 20 mg/min), may be successful. Management of focal status epilepticus has been further discussed in Chapter 11.

Air Embolus

The incidence of air embolization after posterior fossa surgery is difficult to estimate and depends on the detection methods. When Doppler ultrasonography is used for detection, air embolization is very common, particularly in a sitting position.[16] Table 44.4 shows that the incidences are variable and are related to neurosurgical positioning. However, a recent study found three cases in 187 patients in semi-sitting position monitored with perioperative transesophageal electrocardiogram (TEE).[32] Routine use of 10 cm of positive end-expiratory pressure (PEEP) during neurosurgery in the sitting position has no effect on the incidence of air embolization. One study documented significant adverse cardiovascular effects with the use of PEEP.[23] In most

patients, the symptoms are not clinically significant.[46,69] However, most dramatically, the clinical presentation of a paradoxical air embolus is a sudden decrease in arterial PO_2 or saturation (to low 50s), followed by a decrease in end-tidal PCO_2 (from 30s to single digits), almost immediately followed by hypotension and tachycardia. When air enters the coronary arteries, electrocardiographic changes, including widening of the QRS complex and ST-segment elevation or depression, can be seen, and cardiac arrest may occur. Air embolus entering the brain may cause a devastating injury. When anesthesiologists suspect air embolization, the surgeon should flood the wound with Ringer's solution and carefully inspect for open venous channels. The cut surfaces of the bone should be waxed and the open veins coagulated with bipolar forceps. In addition, the patient must be carefully moved to the right side to an upward position. Computed tomography scan in patients who have had air embolization may show black areas within the large arteries.

COMPLICATIONS OF CRANIOPLASTY

Cranioplasty often follows decompressive craniectomy, and this cosmetic repair increases patients' psychologic well-being and social contacts. A recent large series of 348 patients reported a very high and unusual complication rate of 31%,[87] which included postcranioplasty hydrocephalus reoperation for new hematomas and, most commonly, infections. Other "complications"—often not specifically mentioned—may include subgaleal fluid collection, bone resorption, and noninfectious wound dehiscence. Reoperation for hematoma evacuation significantly increased seizure risk, and these patients could benefit from preventive use of levetiracetam.

MEDICAL COMPLICATIONS

The available series on the medical complications of craniotomy have reported an incidence of 2%–8%. This approximation compares with an operative mortality of about 3%. As alluded to, most series involve patients who had craniotomy for brain tumors.[11,18,66] The complications after surgery, seldom specific, include deep vein thrombosis, pulmonary embolus, myocardial ischemia or cardiac arrhythmias, gastrointestinal bleeding, and pneumonia. (Each of these abnormalities is covered elsewhere in this book.) Several observations, however, are noteworthy. Medical complications were more likely to occur in patients who had two or more anatomic areas affected than in patients who had a lesion in only one area. Patients with a Karnofsky score of less than 80 had an increased risk of deep vein thrombosis or pulmonary embolus.[18] Gastrointestinal bleeding after craniotomy was observed in several studies, but the incidence appears to be comparatively low in comparison with incidences from other major surgical procedures. In one study of patients who underwent craniotomy, however, the incidence approached 10%.[50] There was no relationship to age, corticosteroid administration, or inconsistent use of prophylactic medication.

A prospective multicenter study of 2,944 patients found that 4% had infections at the surgical site, including wound infections, bone flap infections, osteitis, meningitis, and brain abscesses.[39] Risk factors identified were postoperative CSF leakage, recurrent surgery, emergency surgery, contaminated surgical fields, and operative time longer than 4 hours. Studies on the effect of antibiotics are conflicting. In one study, antibiotic prophylaxis decreased the risk of a postoperative wound infection.[39] Another randomized trial documented that postcraniotomy infections were virtually eliminated with prophylactic antibiotics.[56,85]

CONCLUSIONS

- A typical postcraniotomy order should include pain management with codeine, cefazolin, dexamethasone, phenytoin, and subcutaneous heparin; swallowing precautions; adequate fluids with crystalloids; and reduction of free water intake.
- Worsening after craniotomy may be due to hemorrhage in the surgical bed, remote hemorrhage, cerebral edema, or ischemic stroke from sacrifice of a large vein or artery.

- Careful evaluation of the endocrine axis (triiodothyronine, thyrotropin, cortisol, urine osmolarity) after pituitary surgery may detect panhypopituitarism.

REFERENCES

1. Air FI, Leach JL, Warnick RE, McPherson CM. Comparing the risks of frameless stereotactic biopsy in eloquent and noneloquent regions of the brain: a retrospective review of 284 cases. *J Neurosurg* 2009;111:820–824.
2. Annan M, De Toffol B, Hommet C, Mondon K. Sinking skin flap syndrome (or syndrome of the trephined): a review. *Br J Neurosurg* 2015;1–5.
3. Bauer DF, Razdan SN, Bartolucci AA, Markert JM. Meta-analysis of hemorrhagic complications from ventriculostomy placement by neurosurgeons. *Neurosurgery* 2011;69:255–260.
4. Behrens E, Schramm J, Zentner J, Konig R. Surgical and neurological complications in a series of 708 epilepsy surgery procedures. *Neurosurgery* 1997;41:1–9.
5. Bilotta F, Pietropaoli P, Rosa G. Nefopam for refractory postoperative hiccups. *Anesth Analg* 2001;93:1358–1360.
6. Binz DD, Toussaint LG, 3rd, Friedman JA. Hemorrhagic complications of ventriculostomy placement: a meta-analysis. *Neurocrit Care* 2009;10:253–256.
7. Boehnert M, Hensen J, Henig A, et al. Severe hyponatremia after transsphenoidal surgery for pituitary adenomas. *Kidney Int Suppl* 1998;64:S12–14.
8. Brisman MH, Bederson JB, Sen CN, et al. Intracerebral hemorrhage occurring remote from the craniotomy site. *Neurosurgery* 1996;39:1114–1121.
9. Brown LJ. Suprasellar tension pneumocyst after transsphenoidal surgery: case report. *J Neurosurg* 1998;89:146–148.
10. Bullock R, Hanemann CO, Murray L, Teasdale GM. Recurrent hematomas following craniotomy for traumatic intracranial mass. *J Neurosurg* 1990;72:9–14.
11. Cabantog AM, Bernstein M. Complications of first craniotomy for intra-axial brain tumour. *Can J Neurol Sci* 1994;21:213–218.
12. Coursin DB, Maccioli GA. Dexmedetomidine. *Curr Opin Crit Care* 2001;7:221–226.
13. De Wolf AM, Fragen RJ, Avram MJ, Fitzgerald PC, Rahimi-Danesh F. The pharmacokinetics of dexmedetomidine in volunteers with severe renal impairment. *Anesth Analg* 2001;93:1205–1209.
14. Ebert TJ, Hall JE, Barney JA, Uhrich TD, Colinco MD. The effects of increasing plasma

concentrations of dexmedetomidine in humans. *Anesthesiology* 2000;93:382–394.

15. Ehtisham A, Taylor S, Bayless L, Klein MW, Janzen JM. Placement of external ventricular drains and intracranial pressure monitors by neurointensivists. *Neurocrit Care* 2009;10:241–247.

16. Engelhardt M, Folkers W, Brenke C, et al. Neurosurgical operations with the patient in sitting position: analysis of risk factors using transcranial Doppler sonography. *Br J Anaesth* 2006;96:467–472.

17. Fabling JM, Gan TJ, Guy J, et al. Postoperative nausea and vomiting: a retrospective analysis in patients undergoing elective craniotomy. *J Neurosurg Anesthesiol* 1997;9:308–312.

18. Fadul C, Wood J, Thaler H, et al. Morbidity and mortality of craniotomy for excision of supratentorial gliomas. *Neurology* 1988;38:1374–1379.

19. Field M, Witham TF, Flickinger JC, Kondziolka D, Lunsford LD. Comprehensive assessment of hemorrhage risks and outcomes after stereotactic brain biopsy. *J Neurosurg* 2001;94:545–551.

20. Fodstad H, Love JA, Ekstedt J, Friden H, Liliequist B. Effect of cranioplasty on cerebrospinal fluid hydrodynamics in patients with the syndrome of the trephined. *Acta Neurochir* 1984;70:21–30.

21. Friedman JA, Piepgras DG, Duke DA, et al. Remote cerebellar hemorrhage after supratentorial surgery. *Neurosurgery* 2001;49:1327–1340.

22. Gardner PA, Engh J, Atteberry D, Moossy JJ. Hemorrhage rates after external ventricular drain placement. *J Neurosurg* 2009;110:1021–1025.

23. Giebler R, Kollenberg B, Pohlen G, Peters J. Effect of positive end-expiratory pressure on the incidence of venous air embolism and on the cardiovascular response to the sitting position during neurosurgery. *Br J Anaesth* 1998;80:30–35.

24. Grant FC, Norcross NC. Repair of cranial defects by cranioplasty. *Ann Surg* 1939;110:488–512.

25. Guyot LL, Dowling C, Diaz FG, Michael DB. Cerebral monitoring devices: analysis of complications. *Acta Neurochir Suppl* 1998;71:47–49.

26. Heilman CB, Shucart WA, Rebeiz EE, Gopal H. Endoscopic pituitary surgery. *Clin Neurosurg* 2000;46:507–514.

27. Hensen J, Henig A, Fahlbusch R, et al. Prevalence, predictors and patterns of postoperative polyuria and hyponatraemia in the immediate course after transsphenoidal surgery for pituitary adenomas. *Clin Endocrinol* 1999;50:431–439.

28. Honegger J, Zentner J, Spreer J, Carmona H, Schulze-Bonhage A. Cerebellar hemorrhage arising postoperatively as a complication of supratentorial surgery: a retrospective study. *J Neurosurg* 2002;96:248–254.

29. Honeybul S, Ho KM. Long-term complications of decompressive craniectomy for head injury. *J Neurotrauma* 2011;28:929–935.

30. Huyette DR, Turnbow BJ, Kaufman C, et al. Accuracy of the freehand pass technique for ventriculostomy catheter placement: retrospective assessment using computed tomography scans. *J Neurosurg* 2008;108:88–91.

31. Hyam JA, Turner J, Peterson D. Cerebellar haemorrhage after repeated burr hole evacuation for chronic subdural hematoma. *J Clin Neurosci* 2007;14:83–86.

32. Jadik S, Wissing H, Friedrich K, et al. A standardized protocol for the prevention of clinically relevant venous air embolism during neurosurgical interventions in the semisitting position. *Neurosurgery* 2009;64:533–538.

33. Janzen C, Kruger K, Honeybul S. Syndrome of the trephined following bifrontal decompressive craniectomy: implications for rehabilitation. *Brain Inj* 2012;26:101–105.

34. Josephson SA, Papanastassiou AM, Berger MS, et al. The diagnostic utility of brain biopsy procedures in patients with rapidly deteriorating neurological conditions or dementia. *J Neurosurg* 2007;106:72–75.

35. Kalfas IH, Little JR. Postoperative hemorrhage: a survey of 4992 intracranial procedures. *Neurosurgery* 1988;23:343–347.

36. Keiper GL, Jr., Sherman JD, Tomsick TA, Tew JM, Jr. Dural sinus thrombosis and pseudotumor cerebri: unexpected complications of suboccipital craniotomy and translabyrinthine craniectomy. *J Neurosurg* 1999;91:192–197.

37. Kelly DF, Laws ER, Jr., Fossett D. Delayed hyponatremia after transsphenoidal surgery for pituitary adenoma: report of nine cases. *J Neurosurg* 1995;83:363–367.

38. Khanna RK, Rosenblum ML, Rock JP, Malik GM. Prolonged external ventricular drainage with percutaneous long-tunnel ventriculostomies. *J Neurosurg* 1995;83:791–794.

39. Korinek AM, Golmard JL, Elcheick A, et al. Risk factors for neurosurgical site infections after craniotomy: a critical reappraisal of antibiotic prophylaxis on 4,578 patients. *Br J Neurosurg* 2005;19:155–162.

40. Kulkarni AV, Guha A, Lozano A, Bernstein M. Incidence of silent hemorrhage and delayed deterioration after stereotactic brain biopsy. *J Neurosurg* 1998;89:31–35.

41. Kuroda R, Nakatani J, Akai F, et al. Remote subarachnoid haemorrhage in the posterior fossa following supratentorial surgery: clinical observation of 6 cases. *Acta Neurochir* 1994;129:158–165.

42. Langfitt JT, Rausch R. Word-finding deficits persist after left anterotemporal lobectomy. *Arch Neurol* 1996;53.72 76.

43. Leung GK, Ng KB, Taw BB, Fan YW. Extended subcutaneous tunnelling technique for external ventricular drainage. *Br J Neurosurg* 2007;21:359–364.

44. Malla BR, O'Brien TJ, Cascino GD, et al. Acute postoperative seizures following anterior temporal lobectomy for intractable partial epilepsy. *J Neurosurg* 1998;89:177–182.

45. Maniker AH, Vaynman AY, Karimi RJ, Sabit AO, Holland B. Hemorrhagic complications of external ventricular drainage. *Neurosurgery* 2006;59:ONS419–424.

46. Matjasko J, Petrozza P, Cohen M, Steinberg P. Anesthesia and surgery in the seated position: analysis of 554 cases. *Neurosurgery* 1985;17:695–702.

47. Miyasaka Y, Yada K, Ohwada T, et al. Retrograde thrombosis of feeding arteries after removal of arteriovenous malformations. *J Neurosurg* 1990;72:540–545.

48. Mohindra S, Mukherjee KK, Gupta R, et al. Decompressive surgery for acute subdural hematoma leading to contralateral extradural haematoma: a report of two cases and review of literature. *Br J Neurosurg* 2005;19:490–494.

49. Moon KS, Lee JK, Kim TS, et al. Contralateral acute subdural hematoma occurring after removal of calcified chronic subdural hematoma. *J Clin Neurosci* 2007;14:283–286.

50. Muller P, Jirsch D, D'Sousa J, Kerr C, Knapp C. Gastrointestinal bleeding after craniotomy: a retrospective review of 518 patients. *Can J Neurol Sci* 1988;15:384–387.

51. Narayan RK, Kishore PR, Becker DP, et al. Intracranial pressure: to monitor or not to monitor? A review of our experience with severe head injury. *J Neurosurg* 1982;56:650–659.

52. North B, Reilly P. Comparison among three methods of intracranial pressure recording. *Neurosurgery* 1986;18:730–732.

53. Papanastassiou V, Kerr R, Adams C. Contralateral cerebellar hemorrhagic infarction after pterional craniotomy: report of five cases and review of the literature. *Neurosurgery* 1996;39:841–851.

54. Paramore CG, Turner DA. Relative risks of ventriculostomy infection and morbidity. *Acta Neurochir (Wien)* 1994;127:79–84.

55. Phan TG, O'Neill BP, Kurtin PJ. Posttransplant primary CNS lymphoma. *Neuro Oncol* 2000;2:229–238.

56. Pilcher WH, Roberts DW, Flanigin HF, et al. Complications of epilepsy surgery. In: Engel J, Jr, ed. *Surgical Treatment of the Epilepsies.* 2nd ed. New York: Raven Press; 1993:565–581.

57. Rapana A, Lamaida E, Pizza V. Multiple postoperative intracerebral hematomas remote from the site of craniotomy. *Br J Neurosurg* 1998;12:364–368.

58. Raymond J, Hardy J, Czepko R, Roy D. Arterial injuries in transsphenoidal surgery for pituitary adenoma; the role of angiography and endovascular treatment. *AJNR Am J Neuroradiol* 1997;18.655 665

59. Rhodes TT, Edwards WH, Saunders RL, et al. External ventricular drainage for initial treatment of neonatal posthemorrhagic hydrocephalus: surgical and neurodevelopmental outcome. *Pediatr Neurosci* 1987;13:255–262.

60. Roberts DW. Is good good enough? *Neurocrit Care* 2009;10:155–156.

61. Roitberg BZ, Khan N, Alp MS, et al. Bedside external ventricular drain placement for the treatment of acute hydrocephalus. *Br J Neurosurg* 2001;15:324–327.

62. Rosenbaum BP, Vadera S, Kelly ML, Kshettry VR, Weil RJ. Ventriculostomy: frequency, length of stay and in-hospital mortality in the United States of America, 1988–2010. *J Clin Neurosci* 2014;21:623–632.

63. Saladino A, White JB, Wijdicks EFM, Lanzino G. Malplacement of ventricular catheters by neurosurgeons: a single institution experience. *Neurocrit Care* 2009;10:248–252.

64. Salvesen R. Extrapontine myelinolysis after surgical removal of a pituitary tumour. *Acta Neurol Scand* 1998;98:213–215.

65. Savitz MH, Bobroff LM. Low incidence of delayed intracerebral hemorrhage secondary to ventriculoperitoneal shunt insertion. *J Neurosurg* 1999;91:32–34.

66. Sawaya R, Hammoud M, Schoppa D, et al. Neurosurgical outcomes in a modern series of 400 craniotomies for treatment of parenchymal tumors. *Neurosurgery* 1998;42:1044–1055.

67. Sawin PD, Hitchon PW, Follett KA, Torner JC. Computed imaging-assisted stereotactic brain biopsy: a risk analysis of 225 consecutive cases. *Surg Neurol* 1998;49:640–649.

68. Sawka AM, Aniszewski JP, Young WF, Jr., et al. Tension pneumocranium, a rare complication of transsphenoidal pituitary surgery: Mayo Clinic experience 1976–1998. *J Clin Endocrinol Metab* 1999;84:4731–4734.

69. Schaffranietz L, Gunther L. [The sitting position in neurosurgical operations. Results of a survey]. *Anaesthesist* 1997;46:91–95.

70. Semple PL, Laws ER, Jr. Complications in a contemporary series of patients who underwent transsphenoidal surgery for Cushing's disease. *J Neurosurg* 1999;91:175–179.

71. Seoane E, Rhoton AL, Jr. Compression of the internal jugular vein by the transverse process of the atlas as the cause of cerebellar hemorrhage after supratentorial craniotomy. *Surg Neurol* 1999;51:500–505.

72. Shaw MD, Foy PM. Epilepsy after craniotomy and the place of prophylactic anticonvulsant drugs: discussion paper. *J R Soc Med* 1991;84:221–223.

73. Tanriverdi T, Ajlan A, Poulin N, Olivier A. Morbidity in epilepsy surgery: an experience based on 2449 epilepsy surgery procedures from a single institution. *J Neurosurg* 2009;110:1111–1123.

74. Taylor WA, Thomas NW, Wellings JA, Bell BA. Timing of postoperative intracranial hematoma development and implications for the best use of neurosurgical intensive care. *J Neurosurg* 1995;82:48–50.

75. Toczek MT, Morrell MJ, Silverberg GA, Lowe GM. Cerebellar hemorrhage complicating temporal lobectomy: report of four cases. *J Neurosurg* 1996;85:718–722.

76. Tosaka M, Kohga H. Extrapontine myelinolysis and behavioral change after transsphenoidal pituitary surgery: case report. *Neurosurgery* 1998;43:933–936.

77. Van Buren JM. Complications of surgical procedures in the diagnosis and treatment of epilepsy. In: Engel J, Jr, ed. *Surgical Treatment of the Epilepsies*. New York: Raven Press; 1987:465–475.

78. Vender JR, Black P, Natter HM, Katsetos CD. Post-anesthesia uncal herniation secondary to a previously unsuspected temporal glioma. *J Forensic Sci* 1995;40:900–902.

79. Voges J, Schroder R, Treuer H, et al. CT-guided and computer assisted stereotactic biopsy: technique, results, indications. *Acta Neurochir* 1993;125:142–149.

80. Wiebe S, Blume WT, Girvin JP, Eliasziw M. A randomized, controlled trial of surgery for temporal-lobe epilepsy. *N Engl J Med* 2001;345:311–318.

81. Wiesmann M, Mayer TE. Intracranial bleeding rates associated with two methods of external ventricular drainage. *J Clin Neurosci* 2001;8:126–128.

82. Yacubian EM, de Andrade MM, Jorge CL, Valerio RM. Cerebellar hemorrhage after supratentorial surgery for treatment of epilepsy: report of three cases. *Neurosurgery* 1999;45:159–162.

83. Yague LG, Rodriguez-Sanchez J, Polaina M, et al. Contralateral extradural hematoma following craniotomy for traumatic intracranial lesion: case report. *J Neurosurg Sci* 1991;35:107–109.

84. Yamaura A, Makino H. Neurological deficits in the presence of the sinking skin flap following decompressive craniectomy. *Neurol Med Chir* 1977;17:43–53.

85. Young RF, Lawner PM. Perioperative antibiotic prophylaxis for prevention of postoperative neurosurgical infections: a randomized clinical trial. *J Neurosurg* 1987;66:701–705.

86. Yu X, Liu Z, Tian Z, et al. CT-guided stereotactic biopsy of deep brain lesions: report of 310 cases. *Chin Med J (Engl)* 1998;111:361–363.

87. Zanaty M, Chalouhi N, Starke RM, et al. Complications following cranioplasty: incidence and predictors in 348 cases. *J Neurosurg* 2015:1–7.

45

Complications of Carotid Endarterectomy and Stenting

Carotid endarterectomy is an established procedure in patients with symptomatic carotid artery stenosis of more than 70%, and surgical repair is considered in progressive asymptomatic stenosis of similar severity. The standard approach is carotid endarterectomy. Carotid stenting and angioplasty are another common type of intervention.[18,43,47] Stenting is currently limited to patients in whom carotid endarterectomy would be a "high-risk" procedure while under general anesthesia.[47] In keeping with many performance standards, patients who undergo carotid surgery for atherosclerotic carotid disease are briefly admitted to an intensive care unit (ICU). Depending on the surgeon, the patient is admitted to the neurosciences ICU (NICU) or a progressive care unit (PCU).

In-hospital mortality with carotid endarterectomy is 1% and may involve postoperative myocardial infarction.[51,57] Certain centers of expertise have reported very low frequency of complications (1.4% stroke and 0.2% mortality).[27] The medical complications of carotid endarterectomy are equally important, and respiratory compromise may occur, with a need for endotracheal reintubation. Whether these complications can be prevented or more effectively treated by having the patient in the NICU is uncertain. Moreover, the criteria for admission to the NICU have not been well defined, and some surgeons believe that routine admission leads to overutilization.[59] However, a survey of 91 carotid endarterectomies noted the use of intravenous vasoactive medication in more than two-thirds of the patients and three re-explorations, most occurring within 12 hours of the procedure.[75] Other surgeons believe that NICU admission should be restricted to patients who awaken with a stroke; who develop cardiac arrhythmias or early electrocardiographic changes; who have significant wound hemorrhage; who are reintubated in the recovery room; or, particularly, who require vasoactive medication more than 3 hours after surgery.[71] The implication is

that, for many other patients, the need for NICU admission is abrogated and an admission to a PCU may be appropriate.

Personal interaction with the neurointensivist to address complications amounts to a few cases a year. Nonetheless, because a sizable number of patients with carotid endarterectomy are admitted to the NICU, one must be familiar with the surgical procedure and its potential neurologic complications.

CAROTID ENDARTERECTOMY

Carotid endarterectomy (Capsule 45.1) is performed by vascular surgeons and neurosurgeons with additional expertise in vascular surgery.[10] Admission of these patients to our NICU is typically after surgery has been performed by neurosurgeons.

General anesthesia is commonly used for carotid endarterectomy. Regional (cervical block) anesthesia could become a feasible alternative, and preliminary studies have claimed reduced complications and hospital stay.[15] The recent GALA (General Anesthesia versus Local Anesthesia for Carotid Surgery) randomized controlled trial found no differences in outcome, although perioperative myocardial infarction was slightly higher in the local anesthesia group. In this study in the United Kingdom and Europe, 4.2% of patients with local anesthesia had complications that resulted in stroke from surgery, as opposed to 4.6% under general anesthesia.[53]

Standard variables recommended for monitoring by the American Society of Anesthesiologists are end-tidal carbon dioxide, oxygen saturation (pulse oximetry), electrocardiographic changes, temperature, and blood pressure. Many institutions apply full-channel electroencephalographic monitoring. Continuous transcranial Doppler monitoring may identify hyperperfusion states, microemboli, or an increase in middle cerebral

CAPSULE 45.1   CAROTID ENDARTERECTOMY

Carotid endarterectomy requires approximately 2–3 hours, with average cross-clamping time between 30–40 minutes. A sketch of the anatomy is shown in the accompanying illustration. The proximity of the cranial nerves predisposes them to injury during carotid exposure. Whether stretching from retraction or placement of the retractors can be implicated is uncertain. The common carotid artery is occluded with a vascular clamp, and smaller clamps or aneurysm clips are used to occlude the internal carotid artery and external carotid artery. The arteriotomy is made on the anterior surface of the internal carotid artery.

Intraoperative shunting is not a universal practice. Some practices have included placing a shunt in every patient and claim the benefits of improved cerebral protection.[84] Other surgeons, however, believe that shunting may increase stroke rate because of embolization from placement of the shunt or distal intimal damage, an injury that eventually may lead to embolization and carotid artery dissection. Others use the shunt only if electroencephalographic changes become apparent. In a few patients, shunt placement is technically not possible because of a high bifurcation, distal plaque, or diminutive internal carotid artery.

Another difference in technique is the use of vein patching, and typically, saphenous veins are used.[23] Some surgeons justify patching and claim reduced late restenosis in follow-up. Postoperative complications do not differ significantly between vein and polyethylene fiber (Dacron) patching.[39,77]

After removal of gross plaque, the artery is closed. A smooth arteriotomy bed is the best result, but may be difficult to attain in patients with stone-hard plaque. One of the most important parts of the surgical procedure is to reduce stray adventitial tacks or suture ends sewn into the lumen, because they may eventually produce thrombosis or dissection.

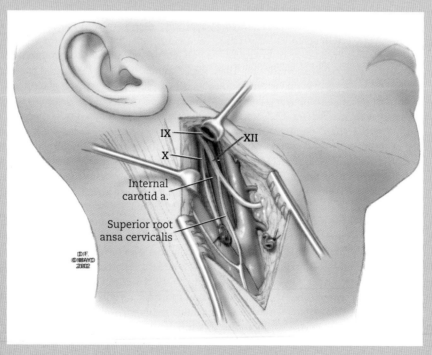

The proximity of cranial nerves to the carotid artery poses a risk of damage during carotid endarterectomy.

artery velocity during cross-clamping as signals of a developing postoperative stroke.[5,35] Somatosensory evoked potentials may show changes in scalp amplitudes with cross-clamping and could assist in determining the need for shunt insertion.[55] However, these tests may substantially increase the cost of the procedure and lack proof that complications are reduced.

CAROTID STENTING

There is a significant increase (and expertise) in carotid artery stenting.[66,89] Few patients come to the NICU and when they do mostly when the procedure was perceived complicated. Usually self-expanding stents with filter protection devices are used. Balloon dilatation is performed (Figure 45.1). Often intravenous atropine is administered before stenting to avoid bradycardia (or even asystole). Stent technology has evolved greatly, and many novel designs are available.[60] Both CREST and ICSS trials comparing the outcomes of carotid endarterectomy and carotid stenting have shown outcomes that are similar.[14,19]

NEUROLOGIC COMPLICATIONS

The American Heart Association guidelines imply that, to maintain accreditation, centers performing carotid endarterectomy must limit postoperative complications to a minimum of 3%.[62] Many of the major neurologic complications are immediately evident after surgery. Stroke is the most prevalent. In some patients, ischemic stroke becomes apparent in the recovery room. In others, a fatal intracranial hemorrhage occurs several days after surgery. Lesions of the cranial nerves are of considerable postoperative concern, and the difficulty with swallowing and coughing should be appreciated. Recommendations for management follow in separate sections.

Hyperperfusion Syndrome

Many patients have some increase in cerebral blood flow after a critically stenosed carotid artery

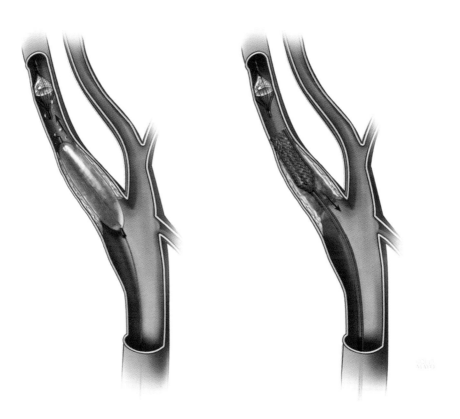

FIGURE 45.1: Stenting procedure with distal filter protection device, balloon dilatation followed by stent placement.

Adapted from Lanzino et al. Treatment of carotid artery stenosis: medical therapy, surgery, or stenting? *Mayo Clinic Proceedings* 2009;84:362–387.

is reopened,[85] but only a few symptoms occur. Hyperperfusion syndrome is very rare, estimated to occur in less than 0.5% of cases.[42,47,70,78,85] Risk factors include a large pressure gradient across the stenosis and contralateral carotid occlusion. Irritability, frontotemporal or, more characteristically, periorbital headache, acute confusional state, and seizures have been described, most occurring within hours but often at the end of the first postoperative week and even at 3 weeks. Intracerebral hematoma and ischemic stroke should be excluded. Neuroimaging modalities, such as transcranial Doppler ultrasonography and single-photon emission computed tomography, document major asymmetries in flow distribution.[25]

An interesting, but unconfirmed, study reported brain edema on computed tomography (CT) scans, with fatal outcome in one patient due to massive edema. Symptoms developed in each patient 5–8 days after carotid endarterectomy and, more worrisome, after an asymptomatic interval.[17] In another case example, the findings could represent edema associated with hemorrhagic infarction.[88] As expected in most cases of hyperperfusion, brain edema is not found on CT or magnetic resonance imaging (MRI).

The syndrome always is accompanied by greatly increased blood pressure (> 250 mm Hg systolic).[70,78] Treatment is judicious reduction of blood pressure with labetalol or nicardipine infusion.

Intracranial Hemorrhage

Intracranial hemorrhage following carotid endarterectomy is a very uncommon complication, and mortality and morbidity are high. It is estimated to occur in less than 1% of cases, and in the total of events after surgery, it may account for up to 25% of the complications. A recent study suggested the following predictive factors for intracerebral hemorrhage: young age, hypertension, and a high degree of ipsilateral and contralateral carotid stenosis or occlusion.[64] Mortality is very high, and many patients die within 72 hours of the hemorrhage.[21,37,40,46,64,67,68,81,82] More than one mechanism appears to contribute to the development of intracranial hemorrhage. We found that doubling of the cerebral blood flow at surgery significantly increased the chance of an intracerebral hematoma.[40] This finding argues that a hyperperfusion syndrome is present to a greater degree in patients with intracranial hematomas.

One of the mechanisms is that cerebral autoregulation is impaired in patients who have severe carotid artery stenosis. After endarterectomy, the increase in pressure in capillaries and vessels that are maximally dilated causes disruption of epithelial cells and breakdown of the blood–brain barrier. Loss of autoregulation reduces the necessary vasoconstriction that limits a downstream effect of increased blood flow. This event is most pronounced in the first week after carotid endarterectomy. Systemic hypertension by itself is not the only primary event leading to intracranial hemorrhage after carotid endarterectomy, because anticoagulation may also contribute.[30,40] In addition, an intracranial hematoma may extend within a cerebral infarct (Figure 45.2).

Massive hemorrhage commonly occurs with rapidly developing stupor or coma. Surgical evacuation of the hematoma thus can be seen as a salvaging procedure. Good recovery has been reported in patients in whom an intracerebral hematoma developed 7 weeks after the procedure and those in whom petechial hemorrhages were more common.[64]

Cranial Nerve Lesions

Cranial nerve lesions are uncommon, although frequency has varied significantly in prospective series.[1,2,6–9,11,16,26,32,33,41,56,76,93] The incidence of cranial or cervical nerve injuries is higher after repeat carotid endarterectomy. In one study, 21% of 89 consecutive patients who had repeat carotid endarterectomy had lesions of the hypoglossal nerve, vagal nerve, and laryngeal nerves, but most neurologic deficits were reversible.[1] Most frequently involved were the great auricular nerve, hypoglossal nerve (XII), mandibular branch of the facial nerve (VII), and vagus nerve (X). The recurrent laryngeal nerve was occasionally involved as well, but much less frequently than the superior glossopharyngeal nerve (IX) and accessory nerve (XI).[92] A review of the large European experience (European Carotid Surgery Trial [ECST]) showed 5.1% of 1,739 patients with cranial nerve deficits, but with 37% with residual deficits after 4 months (in this series, 27 patients had hypoglossal nerve, 17 had marginal mandibular nerve, 17 had recurrent laryngeal cranial nerve, one had accessory nerve, and three had Horner's syndrome).[24]

Clinical manifestations of each of these cranial nerve deficits are shown in Table 45.1. A major concern is a lesion of the recurrent laryngeal nerve with vocal cord paralysis. Hoarseness or dysphagia clearly improves within 6 months after carotid endarterectomy. In a few patients, the deficit is permanent.

Ischemic Stroke

The incidence of ischemic stroke after carotid endarterectomy has been estimated to be up to

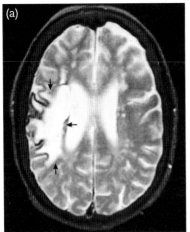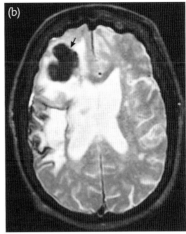

FIGURE 45.2: Magnetic resonance images of post–carotid endarterectomy cerebral hemorrhage (*arrows*). (a) Large right-sided middle cerebral artery infarct on pre-endarterectomy imaging. (b) An intracranial hematoma (*arrow*) developed into the area of infarction and surrounding brain tissue within 24 hours of right carotid endarterectomy (performed within 1 week of the infarction).

From Henderson RD, Phan TG, Piepgras DG, Wijdicks EFM. Mechanisms of intracerebral hemorrhage after carotid endarterectomy. *J Neurosurg* 2001;95:964–969. With permission of the American Association of Neurological Surgeons.

TABLE 45.1. CLINICAL FEATURES OF CRANIAL NERVE DEFICITS AFTER CAROTID ENDARTERECTOMY

Type	Symptoms	Mechanism	Permanent
Facial nerve (VII)	Mimics central VII Asymmetry of upper lip	Hyperextension Head rotation	Rare
Glossopharyngeal nerve (IX)	Dysphagia Nasal regurgitation Hemiparesis Reduced soft palate constriction Hypertension common (Hering nerve)	Shunt placement (more retraction) Subluxation of mandible	Up to 5%
Vagus nerve (X)	Hoarseness Reduced coughing Inability to produce high tones	Ligation or transection of superior thyroid artery	Infrequent after 3 months
Accessory nerve (XI)	Drooping shoulder Painful acromioclavicular joint	Retractor injury Electrical trauma	Unclear
Hypoglossal nerve (XII)	Deviation of tongue Dysarthria Chewing difficulties	Short neck after transection of digastric muscle	Infrequent after 6 months

5%.[28,29,38,45,48,50,58,73,86] A large study of 3,092 carotid endarterectomy patients in the New England area revealed a 30-day stroke or death rate of 1.8%.[36] Contralateral carotid artery occlusion and age over 70 years were important predictors of postoperative stroke.[36] Not all strokes are ipsilateral to carotid endarterectomy, and some even involve the posterior circulation.[3] Moreover, ischemic injury may remain silent.[13,34]

A recent study examining postoperative diffusion-weighted MRI found that carotid endarterectomy was associated with a significantly increased risk of small, scattered infarcts in the same territory.[61] The abnormalities were much more prevalent in patients who had carotid endarterectomy with shunting. However, one study of 1,001 carotid endarterectomies in which electroencephalography was used as a monitoring technique and selected shunting was done did not reveal an increased combined stroke and mortality rate (1%–3%).[38]

Ischemic stroke may be associated with acute occlusion of the carotid artery in the early postoperative period.[54,69,72] Occlusion can also occur during the surgical procedure, probably from embolization of atheromatous debris or thrombus. In other patients, however, an asymptomatic postoperative interval is followed by an acute severe neurologic deficit that involves hemiparesis of the face, arm, and leg, and gaze preference, all indicative of a stroke in a large arterial territory. Prompt surgical re-exploration has been done, but it is unclear whether thrombectomy or repair of the technical defect and patch angioplasty have had any effect on recovery of function.[4,69] Acute intraluminal thrombosis is shown in Figure 45.3. Immediate re-exploration was found to be successful in a study from the New York University Medical Center. This study found intraluminal thrombus in 15 of 18 re-explorations (83%), and it was possible to correct any technical defects. After 18 re-explorations in 12 patients, there was complete resolution or significant improvement in neurologic deficit.

Re-exploration may be tailored toward patients with a severe deficit.[31,74] Signs pertaining to large-territory stroke (gaze preference, hemianopia, and flaccid hemiplegia) warrant early exploration for occlusion of a major vessel. Isolated monoparesis can indicate a branch occlusion of the middle cerebral artery, which is treated by control of blood pressure surges or intravenous administration of dextran (20 mL bolus followed by infusion of dextran 40 at 20 mL/hr), but it may fall short, and many surgeons will still want to

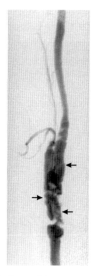

FIGURE 45.3: Patient with acute postoperative aphasia. Angiogram obtained after carotid endarterectomy showing typical rugged-shaped carotid artery but also contrast defects indicating thrombus (confirmed at re-exploration).

explore. Anecdotal reports of intraoperative infusion of thrombolytics have been published, but the risks of this intervention are unclear.[12,90]

Wall hematoma (carotid blowout) is rare but is often recognized by a rapidly growing neck mass. Extravasation leads to suffocation, and emergency intubation is needed, even if the neck mass is still small. It is a major error to obtain studies (CTA) before securing the airway (the trachea can become rapidly compressed).

Medical Complications

One of the reasons to monitor patients in an ICU setting is that considerable medical complications may occur after carotid endarterectomy.[65] A wound hematoma occurs from capillary oozing and, in approximately one-fourth of patients, arterial bleeding. Wound hematoma in the operated neck is uncommon, but the severity of airway compromise varies. Clinically obvious airway obstruction requiring reintubation is very uncommon, but obstruction may be more noticeable in patients studied by CT.[22] Major predictors of a wound hematoma are failure to reverse intravenous heparin, intraoperative hypotension (adequate hemostasis during hypotension may prove to be false after blood pressure is increased), and carotid shunt placement.[22] Postoperative coughing due to prior chronic obstructive pulmonary disease and brief hypertensive surges may contribute.[49,63] A large wound hematoma requires emergency evacuation, even at the bedside in some instances. Most of the time, compromise by the wound hematoma is transient and self-limiting. Corticosteroids, moist steam inhalers, and nursing care in a sitting position have been successful.[44] Dehiscence of the venous patch, caused by a tear in the middle of the vein graft, is obviously more serious.[79,80,94] Rupture may lead to hypoperfusion and massive cerebral infarction and also respiratory distress. A rupture with venous patching has been described, but the incidence of this serious complication is very low. At Mayo Clinic, five postoperative vein ruptures occurred after 2,888 carotid endarterectomies.[94] Reinforcing the vein patch with a synthetic mesh wrap may account for the infrequency of rupture.

Postoperative hypertension is a major concern and requires treatment with antihypertensive agents. Hypertension is a common manifestation of a lesion affecting the Hering nerve, a branch of the glossopharyngeal nerve.[91] Factors that increase the risk of postoperative hypertension are high-grade carotid stenosis, cardiac dysrhythmias, preoperative hypertension with a systolic blood pressure of more than 160 mm Hg, and evidence of renal failure. Postoperative hypertension can be expected in patients with preoperative hypertension, but in 20% of instances, the finding is new. Increased carotid baroreceptor sensitivity, in addition to true dysfunction after vagal nerve damage, is the proposed mechanism. The same mechanism accounts for bradycardia. Moreover, postoperative hypertension (systolic blood pressure of > 180 mm Hg, or 35 mm Hg from baseline) has been linked to cardiac complications, such as angina pectoris, congestive heart failure, myocardial infarction, and arrhythmias. Treatment of postoperative hypertension is mostly successful with labetalol 10–15 mg slowly, every 10 minutes, up to 100 mg (100 mg labetalol in 20 mL of normal saline). If the blood pressure stays high after 20 minutes and heart rate is less than 60/min, a switch to hydralazine 5 mg slowly, every 10 minutes, up to 10 mg is recommended (10 mg hydralazine in 10 mL of normal saline).[83]

Hemodynamic instability after carotid stenting is common. In a recent series, however, symptomatic hypotension was over 5%, and nearly 3% of patients developed symptomatic bradycardia.[89] However, overall perioperative hemodynamic instability (hypertension, hypotension, bradycardia) was found in 85% of 257 procedures.[87]

TABLE 45.2. TREATMENT FOR HYPOTENSION AND BRADYCARDIA AFTER CAROTID ARTERY STENTING

Atropine 0.5 mg with bradycardia

Fluid bolus 500 ml 0.9% NaCl

Phenylephrine bolus 200 mcg (repeat as needed or start 0.5 mcg/kg/minute infusion)

Keep MAP > 80 mm Hg

May start midodrine 10 mg t.i.d. before weaning phenylephrine

Adapted from Bujak et al. Dysautonomic responses during percutaneous carotid intervention: principles of physiology and management. *Catheter Cardiovasc Interv* 2015;85:282–291.

Baroreflex stretching during balloon angioplasty can be implicated. COPD, prior smoking, and diabetes seem to have a protective effect owing to preexisting baroreflex insensitivity. Increased risk has been found in patients with long lesions, ulcerated plaque, or calcifications. The effect may last for several hours to a day.[20] Treatment is summarized in Table 45.2.

CONCLUSION

- Adequate postoperative blood pressure control and discontinuation of anticoagulation may be justified in patients at high risk for intracerebral hematomas.
- Admission to the NICU is warranted to monitor for wound hematomas, hypertension, and cardiac stress.
- Re-exploration may be needed in stroke occurring after carotid endarterectomy.
- Carotid stenting may be briefly associated with symptomatic hypotension and bradycardia, and is treatable with vasopressors and atropine.

REFERENCES

1. AbuRahma AF, Choueiri MA. Cranial and cervical nerve injuries after repeat carotid endarterectomy. *J Vasc Surg* 2000;32:649–654.
2. AbuRahma AF, Lim RY. Management of vagus nerve injury afer carotid endarterectomy. *Surgery* 1996;119:245–247.
3. AbuRahma AF, Robinson P, Holt SM, Herzog TA, Mowery NT. Perioperative and late stroke rates of carotid endarterectomy contralateral to carotid artery occlusion: results from a randomized trial. *Stroke* 2000;31:1566–1571.
4. Aburahma AF, Robinson PA, Short YS. Management options for post carotid endarterectomy stroke. *J Cardiovasc Surg* 1996;37:331–336.

5. Ackerstaff RG, Moons KG, van de Vlasakker CJ, et al. Association of intraoperative transcranial doppler monitoring variables with stroke from carotid endarterectomy. *Stroke* 2000;31:1817–1823.

6. Aldoori MI, Baird RN. Local neurological complication during carotid endarterectomy. *J Cardiovasc Surg* 1988;29:432–436.

7. Assadian A, Senekowitsch C, Pfaffelmeyer N, et al. Incidence of cranial nerve injuries after carotid eversion endarterectomy with a transverse skin incision under regional anaesthesia. *Eur J Vasc Endovasc Surg* 2004;28:421–424.

8. Astor FC, Santilli P, Tucker HM. Incidence of cranial nerve dysfunction following carotid endarterectomy. *Head Neck Surg* 1983;6:660–663.

9. Ayari R, Ede B, Bartoli MI, Branchereau A. Neurologic complications of carotid surgery. In: Branchereau A, Jacobs M, eds. *Complications in Vascular and Endovascular Surgery: Part 1.* Armonk, NY: Futura Publishing; 2001:119–131.

10. Bailes JE. Carotid endarterectomy. *Neurosurgery* 2002;50:1290–1295.

11. Ballotta E, Da Giau G, Renon L, et al. Cranial and cervical nerve injuries after carotid endarterectomy: a prospective study. *Surgery* 1999;125:85–91.

12. Barr JD, Horowitz MB, Mathis JM, Sclabassi RJ, Yonas H. Intraoperative urokinase infusion for embolic stroke during carotid endarterectomy. *Neurosurgery* 1995;36:606–611.

13. Barth A, Remonda L, Lovblad KO, Schroth G, Seiler RW. Silent cerebral ischemia detected by diffusion-weighted MRI after carotid endarterectomy. *Stroke* 2000;31:1824–1828.

14. Bonati LH, Dobson J, Featherstone RL, et al. Long-term outcomes after stenting versus endarterectomy for treatment of symptomatic carotid stenosis: the International Carotid Stenting Study (ICSS) randomized trial. *Lancet* 2015;385:529–538.

15. Bowyer MW, Zierold D, Loftus JP, et al. Carotid endarterectomy: a comparison of regional versus general anesthesia in 500 operations. *Ann Vasc Surg* 2000;14:145–151.

16. Branchereau A, Ondo N'Dong F, Scotti L. Mécanismes des complications neurologiques postopératoires enhancement chirurgie carotidienne. In: Kieffer É, Natali J, eds. *Aspects Techniques de la Chirurgie Carotidienne* Paris: AERCV; 1987:317–331.

17. Breen JC, Caplan LR, DeWitt LD, et al. Brain edema after carotid surgery. *Neurology* 1996;46:175–181.

18. Brooks WH, McClure RR, Jones MR, Coleman TC, Breathitt L. Carotid angioplasty and stenting versus carotid endarterectomy: randomized trial in a community hospital. *J Am Coll Cardiol* 2001;38:1589–1595.

19. Brott TG, Hobson RW, 2nd, Howard G, et al. Stenting versus endarterectomy for treatment of carotid-artery stenosis. *N Engl J Med* 2010;363:11–23.

20. Bujak M, Stilp E, Meller SM, et al. Dysautonomic responses during percutaneous carotid intervention: principles of physiology and management. *Catheter Cardiovasc Interv* 2015;85:282–291.

21. Caplan LR, Skillman J, Ojemann R, Fields WS. Intracerebral hemorrhage following carotid endarterectomy: a hypertensive complication? *Stroke* 1978;9:457–460.

22. Carmichael FJ, McGuire GP, Wong DT, et al. Computed tomographic analysis of airway dimensions after carotid endarterectomy. *Anesth Analg* 1996;83:12–17.

23. Counsell CE, Salinas R, Naylor R, Warlow CP. A systematic review of the randomised trials of carotid patch angioplasty in carotid endarterectomy. *Eur J Vasc Endovasc Surg* 1997;13:345–354.

24. Cunningham EJ, Bond R, Mayberg MR, Warlow CP, Rothwell PM. Risk of persistent cranial nerve injury after carotid endarterectomy. *J Neurosurg* 2004;101:445–448.

25. Dalman JE, Beenakkers IC, Moll FL, Leusink JA, Ackerstaff RG. Transcranial Doppler monitoring during carotid endarterectomy helps to identify patients at risk of postoperative hyperperfusion. *Eur J Vasc Endovasc Surg* 1999;18:222–227.

26. Doig D, Turner EL, Dobson J, et al. Incidence, impact, and predictors of cranial nerve palsy and haematoma following carotid endarterectomy in the international carotid stenting study. *Eur J Vasc Endovasc Surg* 2014;48:498–504.

27. Duncan JM, Reul GJ, Ott DA, Kincade RC, Davis JW. Outcomes and risk factors in 1,609 carotid endarterectomies. *Tex Heart Inst J* 2008;35:104–110.

28. Enevoldsen EM, Torfing T, Kjeldsen MJ, Nepper-Rasmussen J. Cerebral infarct following carotid endarterectomy: frequency, clinical and hemodynamic significance evaluated by MRI and TCD. *Acta Neurol Scand* 1999;100:106–110.

29. Evans WE, Mendelowitz DS, Liapis C, Wolfe V, Florence CL. Motor speech deficit following carotid endarterectomy. *Ann Surg* 1982;196:461–464.

30. Fearn SJ, Parry AD, Picton AJ, Mortimer AJ, McCollum CN. Should heparin be reversed after carotid endarterectomy? A randomized prospective trial. *Eur J Vasc Endovasc Surg* 1997;13:394–397.

31. Findlay JM, Marchak BE. Reoperation for acute hemispheric stroke after carotid endarterectomy: is there any value? *Neurosurgery* 2002;50:486–492.

32. Forssell C, Kitzing P, Bergqvist D. Cranial nerve injuries after carotid artery surgery: a prospective study of 663 operations. *Eur J Vasc Endovasc Surg* 1995;10:445–449.

33. Forssell C, Takolander R, Bergqvist D, et al. Cranial nerve injuries associated with carotid endarterectomy: a prospective study. *Acta Chir Scand* 1985;151:595–598.

34. Gaunt M, Naylor AR, Lennard N, Smith JL, Bell PR. Transcranial Doppler detected cerebral microembolism following carotid endarterectomy. *Brain* 1998;121:389–390.

35. Ghali R, Palazzo EG, Rodriguez DI, et al. Transcranial Doppler intraoperative monitoring during carotid endarterectomy: experience with regional or general anesthesia, with and without shunting. *Ann Vasc Surg* 1997;11:9–13.

36. Goodney PP, Likosky DS, Cronenwett JL. Factors associated with stroke or death after carotid endarterectomy in Northern New England. *J Vasc Surg* 2008;48:1139–1145.

37. Hafner DH, Smith RB, 3rd, King OW, et al. Massive intracerebral hemorrhage following carotid endarterectomy. *Arch Surg* 1987;122:305–307.

38. Hamdan AD, Pomposelli FB, Jr., Gibbons GW, Campbell DR, LoGerfo FW. Perioperative strokes after 1001 consecutive carotid endarterectomy procedures without an electroencephalogram: incidence, mechanism, and recovery. *Arch Surg* 1999;134:412–415.

39. Hayes PD, Allroggen H, Steel S, et al. Randomized trial of vein versus Dacron patching during carotid endarterectomy: influence of patch type on postoperative embolization. *J Vasc Surg* 2001;33:994–1000.

40. Henderson RD, Phan TG, Piepgras DG, Wijdicks EFM. Mechanisms of intracerebral hemorrhage after carotid endarterectomy. *J Neurosurg* 2001;95:964–969.

41. Hertzer NR, Feldman BJ, Beven EG, Tucker HM. A prospective study of the incidence of injury to the cranial nerves during carotid endarterectomy. *Surg Gynecol Obstet* 1980;151:781–784.

42. Ho DS, Wang Y, Chui M, Ho SL, Cheung RT. Epileptic seizures attributed to cerebral hyperperfusion after percutaneous transluminal angioplasty and stenting of the internal carotid artery. *Cerebrovasc Dis* 2000;10:374–379.

43. Hobson RW, 2nd. Update on the Carotid Revascularization Endarterectomy versus Stent Trial (CREST) protocol. *J Am Coll Surg* 2002; 194:S9–14.

44. Hughes R, McGuire G, Montanera W, Wong D, Carmichael FJ. Upper airway edema after carotid endarterectomy: the effect of steroid administration. *Anesth Analg* 1997;84:475–478.

45. Jacobowitz GR, Rockman CB, Lamparello PJ, et al. Causes of perioperative stroke after carotid endarterectomy: special considerations in symptomatic patients. *Ann Vasc Surg* 2001;15:19–24.

46. Jansen C, Sprengers AM, Moll FL, et al. Prediction of intracerebral haemorrhage after carotid endarterectomy by clinical criteria and intraoperative transcranial Doppler monitoring. *Eur J Vasc Surg* 1994;8:303–308.

47. Jordan WD, Jr., Alcocer F, Wirthlin DJ, et al. High-risk carotid endarterectomy: challenges for carotid stent protocols. *J Vasc Surg* 2002;35:16–21.

48. Kieburtz K, Ricotta JJ, Moxley RT, 3rd. Seizures following carotid endarterectomy. *Arch Neurol* 1990;47:568–570.

49. Kunkel JM, Gomez ER, Spebar MJ, et al. Wound hematomas after carotid endarterectomy. *Am J Surg* 1984;148:844–847.

50. L'AURC, Becquemin JP, Souadka F. Risque opératoire actuel de la chirurgie carotidienne: expérience du groupe vasculaire de l'AURC. In: Kieffer É, Bousser MG, eds. *Indications et Résultats de la Chirurgie Carotidienne*. Paris: AERCV; 1988:41–50.

51. Lanska DJ, Kryscio RJ. In-hospital mortality following carotid endarterectomy. *Neurology* 1998;51:440–447.

52. Lanzino G, Rabinstein AA, Brown RD, Jr. Treatment of carotid artery stenosis: medical therapy, surgery, or stenting? *Mayo Clinic Proc* 2009;84:362–387.

53. Lewis SC, Warlow CP, Bodenham AR, et al. General anaesthesia versus local anaesthesia for carotid surgery (GALA): a multicentre, randomised controlled trial. *Lancet* 2008;372: 2132–2142.

54. Liapis CD, Satiani B, Florance CL, Evans WE. Motor speech malfunction following carotid endarterectomy. *Surgery* 1981;89:56–59.

55. Manninen PH, Tan TK, Sarjeant RM. Somatosensory evoked potential monitoring during carotid endarterectomy in patients with a stroke. *Anesth Analg* 2001;93:39–44.

56. Maroulis J, Karkanevatos A, Papakostas K, et al. Cranial nerve dysfunction following carotid endarterectomy. *Int Angiol* 2000;19:237–241.

57. McCrory DC, Goldstein LB, Samsa GP, et al. Predicting complications of carotid endarterectomy. *Stroke* 1993;24:1285–1291.

58. McKinsey JF, Desai TR, Bassiouny HS, et al. Mechanisms of neurologic deficits and

mortality with carotid endarterectomy. *Arch Surg* 1996;131:526–531.

59. Morasch MD, Hirko MK, Hirasa T, et al. Intensive care after carotid endarterectomy: a prospective evaluation. *J Am Coll Surg* 1996;183:387–392.

60. Morr S, Lin N, Siddiqui AH. Carotid artery stenting: current and emerging options. *Med Devices* 2014;7:343–355.

61. Muller M, Reiche W, Langenscheidt P, Hassfeld J, Hagen T. Ischemia after carotid endarterectomy: comparison between transcranial Doppler sonography and diffusion-weighted MR imaging. *AJNR Am J Neuroradiol* 2000;21:47–54.

62. O'Neill L, Lanska DJ, Hartz A. Surgeon characteristics associated with mortality and morbidity following carotid endarterectomy. *Neurology* 2000;55:773–781.

63. O'Sullivan JC, Wells DG, Wells GR. Difficult airway management with neck swelling after carotid endarterectomy. *Anaesth Intensive Care* 1986;14:460–464.

64. Ouriel K, Shortell CK, Illig KA, Greenberg RK, Green RM. Intracerebral hemorrhage after carotid endarterectomy: incidence, contribution to neurologic morbidity, and predictive factors. *J Vasc Surg* 1999;29:82–87.

65. Paciaroni M, Eliasziw M, Kappelle LJ, et al. Medical complications associated with carotid endarterectomy. North American Symptomatic Carotid Endarterectomy Trial (NASCET). *Stroke* 1999;30:1759–1763.

66. Perkins WJ, Lanzino G, Brott TG. Carotid stenting vs endarterectomy: new results in perspective. *Mayo Clinic Proc* 2010;85:1101–1108.

67. Piepgras DG, Morgan MK, Sundt TM, Jr., Yanagihara T, Mussman LM. Intracerebral hemorrhage after carotid endarterectomy. *J Neurosurg* 1988;68:532–536.

68. Pomposelli FB, Lamparello PJ, Riles TS, et al. Intracranial hemorrhage after carotid endarterectomy. *J Vasc Surg* 1988;7:248–255.

69. Radak D, Popovic AD, Radicevic S, Neskovic AN, Bojic M. Immediate reoperation for perioperative stroke after 2250 carotid endarterectomies: differences between intraoperative and early postoperative stroke. *J Vasc Surg* 1999;30:245–251.

70. Reigel MM, Hollier LH, Sundt TM, Jr., et al. Cerebral hyperperfusion syndrome: a cause of neurologic dysfunction after carotid endarterectomy. *J Vasc Surg* 1987;5:628–634.

71. Rigdon EE, Monajjem N, Rhodes RS. Criteria for selective utilization of the intensive care unit following carotid endarterectomy. *Ann Vasc Surg* 1997;11:20–27.

72. Riles TS, Imparato AM, Jacobowitz GR, et al. The cause of perioperative stroke after carotid endarterectomy. *J Vasc Surg* 1994;19:206–214.

73. Rockman CB, Cappadona C, Riles TS, et al. Causes of the increased stroke rate after carotid endarterectomy in patients with previous strokes. *Ann Vasc Surg* 1997;11:28–34.

74. Rockman CB, Jacobowitz GR, Lamparello PJ, et al. Immediate reexploration for the perioperative neurologic event after carotid endarterectomy: is it worthwhile? *J Vasc Surg* 2000;32:1062–1070.

75. Ross SD, Tribble CG, Parrino PE, et al. Intensive care is cost-effective in carotid endarterectomy. *Cardiovasc Surg* 2000;8:41–46.

76. Sajid MS, Vijaynagar B, Singh P, Hamilton G. Literature review of cranial nerve injuries during carotid endarterectomy. *Acta Chir Belg* 2007;107:25–28.

77. Scavee V, Viejo D, Buche M, et al. Six hundred consecutive carotid endarterectomies with temporary shunt and vein patch angioplasty: early and long-term results. *Cardiovasc Surg* 2001;9:463–468.

78. Schroeder T, Sillesen H, Sorensen O, Engell HC. Cerebral hyperperfusion following carotid endarterectomy. *J Neurosurg* 1987;66:824–829.

79. Scott EW, Dolson L, Day AL, Seeger JM. Carotid endarterectomy complicated by vein patch rupture. *Neurosurgery* 1992;31:373–376.

80. Self DD, Bryson GL, Sullivan PJ. Risk factors for post-carotid endarterectomy hematoma formation. *Can J Anaesth* 1999;46:635–640.

81. Shuaib A, Hunter KM, Anderson MA. Multiple intra-cranial hemorrhages after carotid endarterectomy. *Can J Neurol Sci* 1989;16:345–347.

82. Solomon RA, Loftus CM, Quest DO, Correll JW. Incidence and etiology of intracerebral hemorrhage following carotid endarterectomy. *J Neurosurg* 1986;64:29–34.

83. Stoneham MD, Thompson JP. Arterial pressure management and carotid endarterectomy. *Br J Anaesth* 2009;102:442–452.

84. Sundt TM, Jr., Ebersold MJ, Sharbrough FW, et al. The risk-benefit ratio of intraoperative shunting during carotid endarterectomy: relevancy to operative and postoperative results and complications. *Ann Surg* 1986;203:196–204.

85. Sundt TM, Jr., Sharbrough FW, Piepgras DG, et al. Correlation of cerebral blood flow and electroencephalographic changes during carotid endarterectomy: with results of surgery and hemodynamics of cerebral ischemia. *Mayo Clinic Proc* 1981;56:533–543.

86. Tretter MJ, Jr., Hertzer NR, Mascha EJ, et al. Perioperative risk and late outcome of non-elective carotid endarterectomy. *J Vasc Surg* 1999;30:618–631.

87. Ullery BW, Nathan DP, Shang EK, et al. Incidence, predictors, and outcomes of hemodynamic instability following carotid angioplasty and stenting. *J Vasc Surg* 2013;58:917–925.

88. van Harten B, van Gool WA, Bienfait HM, Stam J. Brain edema after carotid endarterectomy. *Neurology* 1997;48:544–545.

89. Wang J, Si Y, Li S, et al. Incidence and risk factors for medical complications and 30-day end points after carotid artery stenting. *Vasc Endovascular Surg* 2014;48:38–44.

90. Winkelaar GB, Salvian AJ, Fry PD, et al. Intraoperative intraarterial urokinase in early postoperative stroke following carotid endarterectomy: a useful adjunct. *Ann Vasc Surg* 1999;13: 566–570.

91. Wong JH, Findlay JM, Suarez-Almazor ME. Hemodynamic instability after carotid endarterectomy: risk factors and associations with operative complications. *Neurosurgery* 1997;41:35–41.

92. Woodward G, Venkatesh R. Spinal accessory neuropathy and internal jugular thrombosis after carotid endarterectomy. *J Neurol Neurosurg Psychiatry* 2000;68:111–112.

93. Yagnik PM, Chong PS. Spinal accessory nerve injury: a complication of carotid endarterectomy. *Muscle Nerve* 1996;19:907–909.

94. Yamamoto Y, Piepgras DG, Marsh WR, Meyer FB. Complications resulting from saphenous vein patch graft after carotid endarterectomy. *Neurosurgery* 1996;39:670–675.

46

Complications of Interventional Neuroradiology

The place of neuroendovascular procedures is clearly established. These procedures may have been performed for patients already admitted to the neurosciences intensive care unit (NICU), but procedural complications may have occurred that required close monitoring of patients who had elective neuroendovascular procedures. There are several other elective procedures (i.e., pipeline,[12] stenting) with the potential for complications in the management of acute stroke and aneurysmal subarachnoid hemorrhage.

These procedures are done by neuroradiologists, neurosurgeons, and neurologists and he often heard moniker is the *neurointerventionalist*. Depending on the complexity of the procedure and possibility of complications, patients may have to be admitted to the NICU under the care of a neurointensivist. Monitoring of patients after an elective endovascular procedure can be sufficient in an intermediate setting, but a large proportion of these complications occur during the period close to the time of the neuroendovascular procedure.[17] The decision to admit a patient to the NICU is usually at the behest of the neurointerventionalist.

Complications may be procedure-related and thus cause a neurologic deficit, or they may be from systemic complications or access site complications and thus cause changes in vital signs and laboratory values. These problems—fortunately incidental—are reviewed in this chapter.

ENDOVASCULAR TECHNIQUES

Neuroendovascular procedures most commonly involve coiling of a recently ruptured or incidentally discovered intracranial aneurysm, embolization of an arteriovenous malformation, balloon angioplasty for cerebral vasospasm, intra-arterial thrombolysis, and deployment of mechanical recanalization devices. These procedures are rapidly changing; moreover, a detailed review

is outside the scope of this book and, many will argue, outside the field of emergency and critical care neurology. A consensus statement from the Society for Neuroscience in Anesthesia and Critical Care has recently been published.[38]

Before any neurointerventional procedure, a brief perioperative evaluation is needed; however, this assessment can be curtailed in emergency situations (Table 46.1). Preparation is needed for patients with known contrast medium allergy and patients at risk for contrast nephropathy (those with an abnormal serum creatinine level of > 2 mg/dL, a glomerular filtration rate of ≤ 60 mL/min, and the presence of diabetes mellitus or multiple myeloma).

Many neurointerventionalists prefer that patients receive full anesthesia rather than conscious sedation during these procedures. General anesthesia provides much better airway protection in patients with a major neurologic deficit, and emergency intubation during the procedure may occur in 2%–3% of cases who elected not to proceed with general anesthesia. Some reports found worse outcome in patients converted to general anesthesia[1,3,16,26] and tentatively linked to pneumonitis with intubation or hypotension with anesthesia, but all were flawed by selection bias.[1,3,16,26] Most neurointerventionalists will proceed with intubation in agitated or uncooperative patients (e.g., aphasic), or patients with evolving brainstem stroke.

A common vascular access site is the right common femoral artery. The size of the introducer sheath varies and depends on the type of device used during the procedure (e.g., balloon-assisted coil embolization, mechanical embolectomy).

Neurointerventionalists introduce microcoils, balloons, stents, and mechanical embolectomy devices but also embolic material, such as *n*-butyl cyanoacrylate acid, Onyx liquid (Micro Therapeutics Inc., Irvine, CA), and polyvinyl alcohol particles. Any neurointerventional procedure

TABLE 46.1. PERINEUROINTERVENTIONAL MONITORING

Preinterventional evaluation

Concern for contrast medium allergy: methylprednisolone 80 mg IV or dexamethasone 16 mg IV 30 minutes before procedure, in combination with promethazine 12.5 mg IV (over 1 minute), ranitidine 100 mg IV, and montelukast sodium 10 mg PO

Concern for contrast-induced nephropathy: sodium bicarbonate 150 mEg/L IV solution at 3.5 ml/kg bolus over 1 hour, then 1.2 mL/kg/hr during procedure and for 6 hours after the procedure. N-acetylcysteine 600 mg orally at 24 hours and 12 hours before and after the procedure (total of 4 doses)

Platelet count, international normalized ratio

Consult anesthesia for monitored sedation or full anesthesia

Postinterventional monitoring

Completely immobilize the accessed leg for several hours

Maintain SAP at ≤ 140 mm Hg (24 hours)

Avoid use of heparin or LMWH

Perform a follow-up computed tomographic scan of the brain at 12 hours

IV, intravenous; LMWH, low-molecular-weight heparin; PO, by mouth; SAP, systolic arterial pressure

performed with full anesthesia requires later close monitoring in the NICU. Systolic blood pressure is carefully controlled during the first 24 hours postoperatively. The blood pressure targets are unknown, but systolic blood pressure is kept under 140 mm Hg; for patients at high risk for reperfusion injury (e.g., those with stenting for a near occluded carotid artery), it is kept at 120 mm Hg. Neurointerventionalists subsequently administer aspirin (325 mg) and load with clopidogrel (300 mg), followed by clopidogrel (75 mg), after stenting procedures and continue for 6 months.

PROCEDURAL COMPLICATIONS

Procedural complications can be divided into neurologic complications and access site complications. Local complications, although uncommon, may involve pseudoaneurysm, arteriovenous fistula, and extravasation around the sheath. Neurologic complications are caused by acute thrombus formation, acute flow limitation due to arterial dissection, and, most unfortunately, perforation of a cerebral artery.

The frequency of endovascular coiling of cerebral aneurysms has increased considerably, but the complication rate has been stable (Chapter 26). A meta-analysis of 1,248 ruptured cerebral aneurysms found that rupture during a procedure occurred in about 4% of the aneurysms; however, the mortality rate approached 2%, and death occurred in only 0.2% of cases.[8,18] Since this meta-analysis and a more recent analysis,[19] the incidence of procedure-associated rupture has further declined (Table 46.2).

Aneurysmal rupture during a coiling procedure may be due to a rebleed that occurs before the aneurysm is secured. This is simply because the risk of rebleeding is substantial in the hours after the initial rupture. Perforations of the aneurysm during coiling are not related to the timing of the coiling, the aneurysmal size, operator volume, or even years of operator experience.

TABLE 46.2. PROCEDURAL COMPLICATIONS AFTER CEREBRAL ANEURYSM COILING

Series, Year	No. of Patients	Rupture, %	Thromboembolism, %
Henkes et al., 2004[18]	1,034	5.0	4.7
Ross and Dhillon, 2005[32]	118	3.0	6.0
Van Rooij et al., 2006[41]	681	4.4	4.7
Elijovich et al., 2008[11]	299	5.0	
Yang et al., 2015[44]	243	1.6	2.3

Some studies have found that chronic obstructive pulmonary disease and African American and Asian descent increased the risk of rupture during endovascular procedures.[8,32,41] This tentative correlation has been explained by abnormalities of the arterial endothelium that could predispose patients to intraprocedural rupture, although prior smoking that resulted in chronic obstructive pulmonary disease could also be a variable. The use of adjunctive balloon remodeling has been considered a possible risk factor, but a search of the medical literature published between 1997 and 2006 found no evidence of an increased incidence of thromboembolic events or iatrogenic rupture.[34]

The management of a ruptured intracranial aneurysm during endovascular coil occlusion is uncertain. The neurointerventionalist notices a perforation because of the sudden appearance of contrast medium extravasation. In this problematic situation, the operator keeps the microcatheter in place, and when a balloon is in situ, it may be inflated to tamponade the bleeding. Some neurointerventionalists infuse n-butyl cyanoacrylate acid into the puncture site. When a large cerebral hematoma appears in an anesthetized patient, it may be clinically associated with sudden change in pupil size and acute hypertension. An emergent computed tomographic (CT) scan should be obtained, although the extent of the rupture might be difficult to distinguish from the amount of contrast medium administered during the procedure. A craniotomy to evacuate a new parenchymal hematoma may be needed. Rerupture may lead to an acute hydrocephalus that requires urgent ventriculostomy. Often, however, rupture occurs with placement of the last coil and, therefore, most of the aneurysm has been secured, requiring no further neurosurgical intervention. Later clipping of the aneurysm is rarely needed.

Thromboembolic complications may occur during the neuroendovascular procedure. These emboli may be from embolic (glue) material showering during the procedure or from catheter- or guidewire-induced arterial dissection. These complications are detected more often during imaging than from examination of the patient (most patients are briefly under full anesthesia).

Treatment of acute thromboembolic events during neuroendovascular procedures has changed with the use of abciximab (ReoPro®). An antigen-binding fragment of the monoclonal antibody directed against the glycoprotein IIb/IIIa receptor on the platelet surface, abciximab prevents platelet aggregation by blocking the binding of fibrinogen to receptors on platelets.[13,30]

Typically, abciximab is diluted in normal saline to 0.2 mg/mL and given as a bolus of 4–10 mg over 10–20 minutes.[36] It is usually administered intra-arterially through a microcatheter, with the catheter tip inserted in the thrombus. In some cases, the catheter tip is navigated distally to the thrombus. In a recent study of 31 patients, full thrombolysis of the new clot was achieved in 53% of the patients; 47% of the patients had partial thrombolysis. Improvement in neurologic deficit was significant for all patients.[28]

Severe thrombocytopenia is highly unusual during the use of abciximab. In 5% of the cases reviewed, abciximab-induced thrombocytopenia (platelet count, $< 100 \times 10^9/L$) was found.[20,42] Hemorrhagic complications, such as groin or pelvic hematomas or gastrointestinal bleeding, have not been observed but continue to be a considerable risk for patients treated with this drug. An unresolved issue is whether heparin should be reversed after the administration of abciximab.[14,27] Prior studies have not shown that this reversal reduced the rebleeding complication rate, and some investigators have found rebleeding despite reversal.[42] The half-life of abciximab is short—10 to 30 minutes—but platelet aggregation may take up to several days to normalize. Serial platelet counts are necessary, and platelet transfusion in patients with critical platelet counts ($< 50 \times 10^9/L$) may be needed in these very unusual situations.[20]

Recanalization can also be accomplished with intra-arterial thrombolysis, and one recently published study of six complications with neurovascular procedure found three of six middle cerebral arteries completely recanalized. In most patients, however, new cerebral infarcts were found on postprocedural neuroimaging.[2]

Another, often delayed, complication after coil occlusion of a cerebral aneurysm is the emergence of cerebral edema that surrounds the aneurysmal sac (Capsule 46.1). We recall a patient with an aneurysmal subarachnoid hemorrhage whose condition progressed rapidly into a minimally conscious state.[7] The patient was treated with intravenous corticosteroids, and improvement was gradual over several weeks. Return to alertness correlated closely with the progressive resolution of the cerebral edema, detected with magnetic resonance imaging (MRI) (Figure 46.1). This complication may also occur in smaller treated aneurysms and may be a cause of worsening.[9]

Flow diversion (pipeline) techniques are used for large, wide-necked, or fusiform aneurysms.[29] Blood flow is modified within the aneurysm in-flow zone.[12] Repair is expected after the

CAPSULE 46.1   PERICOIL EDEMA

Mild edema may form around a recently coil occluded aneurysm. In most cases, edema subsides and is clinically irrelevant.

The mechanism of pericoil edema is unexplained, but enlargement of the aneurysm with compaction of several coils is the principal cause. Thus, pericoil edema is mostly seen in patients with giant aneurysms who had a large number of coils placed. Explanations are venous congestion, inflammation due to the bioactive coil, and ischemia from compression of perianeurysmal vessels. Aneurysmal expansion is the most likely cause and may not be detected by visual inspection of the cerebral angiogram (Capsule Figure).

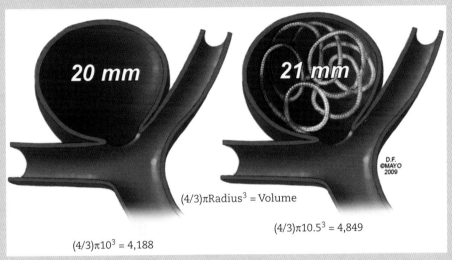

$$(4/3)\pi \text{Radius}^3 = \text{Volume}$$

$$(4/3)\pi 10.5^3 = 4,849$$

$$(4/3)\pi 10^3 = 4,188$$

The measurement of aneurysm size is deceptive, and a small change in diameter may translate into a much larger volume. In this example, 1 mm increase in diameter will translate to a 16% increase in volume.

appearance of neointimal endothelium. One systematic review found 3% postoperative subarachnoid hemorrhages and 3% perforator infarction rate. Ischemic stroke was 6% and higher with giant aneurysms.[5,10,43] Complete occlusion and a devastating stroke (despite prompt administration of abciximab and clopidrogel loading) may occur. A recent analysis of 279 cases in 2011–2013 found in-hospital mortality in 2 patients (0.7%), discharge to long-term care in 22 patients (7.9%), ischemic complications in 14 patients (5.0%), and hemorrhagic complications in 4 patients (1.4%).[25]

STENTING

Stents are used both to treat atherosclerotic high-grade stenosis in the extracranial and intracranial cerebral circulation and to assist with coil occlusion in complex aneurysms. The assumption is that the radial force of the stent struts facilitates the formation of new endothelium and thus causes a smooth lumen. Stent size differs depending on the site of deployment (smaller intracranially), and sirolimus-eluting stents have been introduced for vessels with a high risk of restenosis (e.g., vertebral artery). There is interest in using expandable stents for acute treatment of large vessel occlusion, but experience is insufficient to report complications (Chapter 27).

As alluded to in Chapter 45 carotid artery stenting after angioplasty has become an alternative to carotid endarterectomy.[15,23,40] The perioperative mortality rate is 1.2%; however, recent evidence suggests that the risk of periprocedural stroke is 40% higher than with carotid endarterectomy.[6] This risk is particularly high in patients older than 65 years.[31,37] Substantial complications with femoral catheterization have been reported in the Endarterectomy Versus Angioplasty in Patients with Symptomatic Severe Carotid Stenosis study from France. Femoral pseudo-aneurysm or

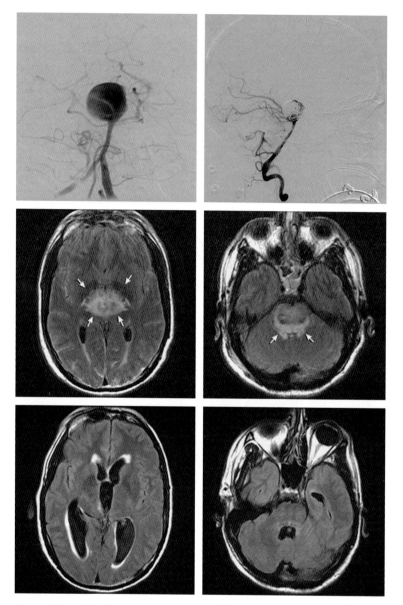

FIGURE 46.1: Ruptured giant basilar aneurysm and subsequent endovascular coil placement. The endovascular coiling involved 17 coils (*upper row*). The patient had thalamic edema, which caused stupor initially but worsened rapidly into a minimally conscious state (*middle row*). Gradual improvement was seen over 3 weeks, with full recovery in consciousness with commensurate improvement on magnetic resonance imaging (*lower row*).

From Burns J, Rabinstein AA, Cloft H, Lanzino G, Daniels DJ, Wijdicks EFM. Minimally conscious state after ruptured giant basilar aneurysm. *Arch Neurol* 2009;66:786–788. With permission of the publisher.

arteriovenous fistula occurred in 1.5% of patients. Cranial nerve injury (hypoglossal and recurrent laryngeal palsy) occurred with three of 261 stented arteries (1.1%).[24] The CAPTURE registry, with 3,500 patients, noted an overall stroke rate of 4.8%, with a rate of 2.9% for minor strokes.[13] Most strokes occurred after a stent was placed (< 24 hours from the procedure). Stroke may occur from emboli during stent deployment but also may be due to fractured plaque dislodged against side branches ("snowplow" effect).

Management of an ischemic complication is similar to that of any complication of a cerebral angiogram. Mechanical retrieval or intra-arterial thrombolysis can be considered if the identified clot is proximal and obstructing a large territory. Postcarotid stenting reperfusion hemorrhage (Figure 46.2) most likely occurs with an incidence similar to that in carotid endarterectomy (Chapter 45).

MECHANICAL CLOT RETRIEVAL

Procedural complications associated with mechanical retrieval devices[4,21,22,35] occurred in 5% of patients, with symptomatic hemorrhage in 9.8% of patients; the mortality rate was high at 34%.[36] Patients are usually treated within 8 hours of stroke onset. Current practices outside the ongoing trials are not known. Most neurointerventionalists attempt clot retrieval first, followed by intra-arterial administration of tissue plasminogen activator.[39] Use of both interventions makes it difficult to tease out the complications from the procedure versus those from thrombolysis.[33] Procedure-related complications were defined as death, a decline in the National Institutes of Health Stroke Scale, or groin complications requiring surgery or blood transfusion. Asymptomatic hemorrhages occurred in 30% of patients and in many instances (12 of 16 patients), the abnormality on CT scan showed hemorrhages with early swelling. Only one patient with vessel perforation was documented among 164 procedures.[36]

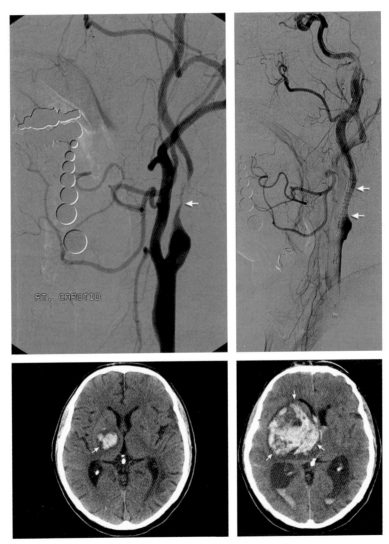

FIGURE 46.2: Reperfusion hemorrhage after carotid stenting. Patient had a rapid progression in volume and rapidly emerging coma (*arrows*).

CONCLUSIONS

- Most complications of interventional radiologic procedures are uncommon and usually are manageable.
- Abciximab, intra-arterial thrombolysis, or mechanical disruption are good options in acute procedure-related emboli.
- Pericoil edema in endovascular treated aneurysms may be a cause of neurologic deterioration.

REFERENCES

1. Abou-Chebl A, Lin R, Hussain MS, et al. Conscious sedation versus general anesthesia during endovascular therapy for acute anterior circulation stroke: preliminary results from a retrospective, multicenter study. *Stroke* 2010;41:1175–1179.
2. Arnold M, Fischer U, Schroth G, et al. Intra-arterial thrombolysis of acute iatrogenic intracranial arterial occlusion attributable to neuroendovascular procedures or coronary angiography. *Stroke* 2008;39:1491–1495.
3. Brekenfeld C, Mattle HP, Schroth G. General is better than local anesthesia during endovascular procedures. *Stroke* 2010;41:2716–2717.
4. Brekenfeld C, Schroth G, El-Koussy M, et al. Mechanical thromboembolectomy for acute ischemic stroke: comparison of the catch thrombectomy device and the Merci Retriever in vivo. *Stroke* 2008;39:1213–1219.
5. Brinjikji W, Murad MH, Lanzino G, Cloft HJ, Kallmes DF. Endovascular treatment of intracranial aneurysms with flow diverters: a meta-analysis. *Stroke* 2013;44:442–447.
6. Brott TG, Brown RD, Jr., Meyer FB, et al. Carotid revascularization for prevention of stroke: carotid endarterectomy and carotid artery stenting. *Mayo Clinic Proc* 2004;79:1197–1208.
7. Burns JD, Rabinstein AA, Cloft H, et al. Minimally conscious state after ruptured giant basilar aneurysm. *Arch Neurol* 2009;66:786–788.
8. Cloft HJ, Kallmes DF. Cerebral aneurysm perforations complicating therapy with Guglielmi detachable coils: a meta-analysis. *AJNR Am J Neuroradiol* 2002;23:1706–1709.
9. Craven I, Patel UJ, Gibson A, Coley SC. Symptomatic perianeurysmal edema following bare platinum embolization of a small unruptured cerebral aneurysm. *AJNR Am J Neuroradiol* 2009;30:1998–2000.
10. D'Urso PI, Lanzino G, Cloft HJ, Kallmes DF. Flow diversion for intracranial aneurysms: a review. *Stroke* 2011;42:2363–2368.
11. Elijovich L, Higashida RT, Lawton MT, et al. Predictors and outcomes of intraprocedural rupture in patients treated for ruptured intracranial aneurysms: the CARAT study. *Stroke* 2008;39:1501–1506.
12. Eller JL, Dumont TM, Sorkin GC, et al. The Pipeline embolization device for treatment of intracranial aneurysms. *Expert Rev Med Devices* 2014;11:137–150.
13. Gralla J, Rennie AT, Corkill RA, et al. Abciximab for thrombolysis during intracranial aneurysm coiling. *Neuroradiology* 2008;50:1041–1047.
14. Gupta V, Tanvir R, Garg A, Gaikwad SB, Mishra NK. Heparin-induced thrombocytopenia in a case of endovascular aneurysm coiling. *AJNR Am J Neuroradiol* 2007;28:155–158.
15. Hankey GJ. How I interpreted the randomised trials of carotid angioplasty/stenting versus endarterectomy. *Eur J Vasc Endovasc Surg* 2008;36:34–40.
16. Hassan AE, Chaudhry SA, Zacharatos H, et al. Increased rate of aspiration pneumonia and poor discharge outcome among acute ischemic stroke patients following intubation for endovascular treatment. *Neurocrit Care* 2012;16:246–250.
17. Heidenreich JO, Hartlieb S, Stendel R, et al. Bleeding complications after endovascular therapy of cerebral arteriovenous malformations. *AJNR Am J Neuroradiol* 2006;27:313–316.
18. Henkes H, Fischer S, Weber W, et al. Endovascular coil occlusion of 1811 intracranial aneurysms: early angiographic and clinical results. *Neurosurgery* 2004;54:268–280.
19. Hong Y, Wang YJ, Deng Z, Wu Q, Zhang JM. Stent-assisted coiling versus coiling in treatment of intracranial aneurysm: a systematic review and meta-analysis. *PLoS One* 2014;9:e82311.
20. Jones RG, Davagnanam I, Colley S, West RJ, Yates DA. Abciximab for treatment of thromboembolic complications during endovascular coiling of intracranial aneurysms. *AJNR Am J Neuroradiol* 2008;29:1925–1929.
21. Lutsep HL. Mechanical endovascular recanalization therapies. *Curr Opin Neurol* 2008;21:70–75.
22. Lutsep HL, Rymer MM, Nesbit GM. Vertebrobasilar revascularization rates and outcomes in the MERCI and multi-MERCI trials. *J Stroke Cerebrovasc Dis* 2008;17:55–57.
23. Mas JL, Chatellier G, Beyssen B, et al. Endarterectomy versus stenting in patients with symptomatic severe carotid stenosis. *N Engl J Med* 2006;355:1660–1671.
24. Mas JL, Trinquart L, Leys D, et al. Endarterectomy Versus Angioplasty in Patients with Symptomatic Severe Carotid Stenosis (EVA-3S) trial: results up to 4 years from a randomized, multicentre trial. *Lancet Neurol* 2008;7:885–892.

25. McDonald RJ, McDonald JS, Kallmes DF, Lanzino G, Cloft HJ. Periprocedural safety of Pipeline therapy for unruptured cerebral aneurysms: analysis of 279 patients in a multihospital database. *Interv Neuroradiol* 2015;21:6–10.

26. Nichols C, Carrozzella J, Yeatts S, et al. Is periprocedural sedation during acute stroke therapy associated with poorer functional outcomes? *J Neurointerv Surg* 2010;2:67–70.

27. Nogueira RG, Smith WS. Safety and efficacy of endovascular thrombectomy in patients with abnormal hemostasis: pooled analysis of the MERCI and multi MERCI trials. *Stroke* 2009;40:516–522.

28. Nonaka T, Oka S, Miyata K, et al. Prediction of prolonged postprocedural hypotension after carotid artery stenting. *Neurosurgery* 2005;57:472–477.

28. Nowakowski K, Rogers J, Nelson G, Gunalingam B. Abciximab-induced thrombocytopenia: management of bleeding in the setting of recent coronary stents. *J Interv Cardiol* 2008;21:100–105.

29. Papagiannaki C, Spelle L, Januel AC, et al. WEB intrasaccular flow disruptor-prospective, multicenter experience in 83 patients with 85 aneurysms. *AJNR Am J Neuroradiol* 2014;35:2106–2111.

30. Park JH, Kim JE, Sheen SH, et al. Intraarterial abciximab for treatment of thromboembolism during coil embolization of intracranial aneurysms: outcome and fatal hemorrhagic complications. *J Neurosurg* 2008;108:450–457.

31. Rhee-Moore SJ, DeRubertis BG, Lam RC, et al. Periprocedural complication rates are equivalent between symptomatic and asymptomatic patients undergoing carotid angioplasty and stenting. *Ann Vasc Surg* 2008;22:233–237.

32. Ross IB, Dhillon GS. Complications of endovascular treatment of cerebral aneurysms. *Surg Neurol* 2005;64:12–18.

33. Schulte-Altedorneburg G, Bruckmann H, Hamann GF, et al. Ischemic and hemorrhagic complications after intra-arterial fibrinolysis in vertebrobasilar occlusion. *AJNR Am J Neuroradiol* 2007;28:378–381.

34. Shapiro M, Babb J, Becske T, Nelson PK. Safety and efficacy of adjunctive balloon remodeling during endovascular treatment of intracranial aneurysms: a literature review. *AJNR Am J Neuroradiol* 2008;29:1777–1781.

35. Smith WS, Sung G, Saver J, et al. Mechanical thrombectomy for acute ischemic stroke: final results of the Multi MERCI trial. *Stroke* 2008;39:1205–1212.

36. Smith WS, Sung G, Starkman S, et al. Safety and efficacy of mechanical embolectomy in acute ischemic stroke: results of the MERCI trial. *Stroke* 2005;36:1432–1438.

37. Stingele R, Berger J, Alfke K, et al. Clinical and angiographic risk factors for stroke and death within 30 days after carotid endarterectomy and stent-protected angioplasty: a subanalysis of the SPACE study. *Lancet Neurol* 2008;7:216–222.

39. Taha MM, Toma N, Sakaida H, et al. Periprocedural hemodynamic instability with carotid angioplasty and stenting. *Surg Neurol* 2008;70:279–285.

38. Talke PO, Sharma D, Heyer EJ, et al. Society for Neuroscience in Anesthesiology and Critical Care Expert consensus statement: anesthetic management of endovascular treatment for acute ischemic stroke: endorsed by the Society of NeuroInterventional Surgery and the Neurocritical Care Society. *J Neurosurg Anesthesiol* 2014;26:95–108.

39. Tomsick TA. Mechanical embolus removal: a new day dawning. *Stroke* 2005;36:1439–1440.

42. Trocciola SM, Chaer RA, Lin SC, et al. Analysis of parameters associated with hypotension requiring vasopressor support after carotid angioplasty and stenting. *J Vasc Surg* 2006;43:714–720.

40. van der Vaart MG, Meerwaldt R, Reijnen MM, Tio RA, Zeebregts CJ. Endarterectomy or carotid artery stenting: the quest continues. *Am J Surg* 2008;195:259–269.

41. van Rooij WJ, Sluzewski M, Beute GN, Nijssen PC. Procedural complications of coiling of ruptured intracranial aneurysms: incidence and risk factors in a consecutive series of 681 patients. *AJNR Am J Neuroradiol* 2006;27:1498–1501.

42. Velat GJ, Burry MV, Eskioglu E, et al. The use of abciximab in the treatment of acute cerebral thromboembolic events during neuroendovascular procedures. *Surg Neurol* 2006;65:352–358.

43. Wong GK, Kwan MC, Ng RY, Yu SC, Poon WS. Flow diverters for treatment of intracranial aneurysms: current status and ongoing clinical trials. *J Clin Neurosci* 2011;18:737–740.

44. Yang H, Sun Y, Jiang Y, et al. Comparison of stent-assisted coiling vs coiling alone in 563 intracranial aneurysms: safety and efficacy at a high-volume center. *Neurosurgery* 2015;77:241–247.

PART IX

Emergency Consults in the General Intensive Care Unit

47

Neurology of Transplant Medicine

Ever since organ transplantation emerged as a viable surgical option for terminal disease, there has been a particular attention to a host of previously unknown neurologic complications. Organ transplantation has been associated with a distinct spectrum of neurologic complications. Complications can emerge during pretransplant preparation (e.g., hematopoietic stem cell transplantation and chemotherapy), perioperative support (e.g., cardiac transplantation with cardiopulmonary bypass), and postoperative management (e.g., newly introduced intravenous immunosuppression). Some neurologic complications, particularly peripheral nerve injury, are related to the surgical procedure and are less specific.

When large series are reported, neurologic complications from organ transplantation occur in approximately 5%–10% of patients, which is a rather substantial number.[1,13–15,19,20,27,38,44] Of course, the prevalence depends on the motivation of transplant teams to consult a neurologist and thus is a reflection of how relevant a neurologic complication is when seen in terms of the entire clinical picture—a situation over which consulting neurologists have no control. Prospective incidence studies never capture all the postoperative neurologic events and only if patients are carefully (and perhaps even serially) examined by neurologists. Nevertheless, it appears that over the years there has been a continuous and substantial decline in neurologic complications.[42] Neurologic complications are major when they involve recurrent seizures, postoperative failure to awaken, immunosuppression neurotoxicity, or acute disabling neuromuscular disease. Familiarity with the administration and dosing of the main intravenous immunosuppressive drugs has reduced the risk of major neurotoxicity—extreme manifestations with coma and seizures and neuroimaging showing diffuse white matter edema are now rarely seen.[26,41] In fact, neurologists may find it harder to convince the transplant teams that the MRI abnormalities justify a change in immunosuppressive drugs. Moreover, the nature of neurologic

complications may change with new treatment protocols and new drug approaches. Neurologic complications may result in an increased risk of early demise. Most instructively—when reviewed in more detail—the majority of patients with lung transplantation were found to have a neurologic manifestation or complication, with a third of these seriously affecting quality of life or resulting in a fatal outcome.[20] Thus the question remains of whether neurologic complications are sufficiently recognized and managed. There are also late neurologic complications after organ transplantation, and some are substantial, requiring ICU admission or even NICU admission (e.g., progressive multifocal leukoencephalopathy).

This field—neurology of organ transplantation—requires expertise and frequent reassessment of the spectrum of complications. Neurointensivists are in an ideal position to consult on these patients, and many intensivists have recognized their contribution in diagnosis and management. A considerable effort is still needed to manage some of these complications. This chapter concentrates on common and urgent consults in transplantation units.

GENERAL PRINCIPLES

There are some patterns. First, a patient with more elaborate surgery has a higher risk of an early neurologic complication. Much of it is ischemic or hemorrhagic stroke or drug neurotoxicity. Second, once the patient goes successfully through the first critical weeks, a later phase is entered, which includes a proclivity for CNS infections. Much later—although it may be only a few months—serious malignancies may appear.[29] Most dramatic is the appearance of post-transplant lymphoproliferative disease (PTLD), likely explained from introducing genetic material of an Epstein-Barr virus (EBV) seropositive donor into an EBV seronegative recipient. It may involve the central nervous system.[18]

There are several other considerations. Neurologic complications may be specific to the type of transplantation. Neurological complications associated with bone marrow transplantation are quite different from those in organ transplants, such as transplantation of a kidney or liver.[22] Severe sodium abnormalities and osmotic shifts can be seen after liver transplantation, causing demyelination in the pons and extrapontine locations.[8,35] Moreover, seizures are often drug related or, less commonly, due to a permanent structural lesion. It is a difficult task to implicate certain drugs, but some drugs lower the seizure threshold (calcineurin inhibitors, imipenem). Consulting neurologists should recognize that any structural lesion in the brain, whether it has the appearance of a cerebritis or is ring enhancing, is most often due to an infectious cause and requires immediate treatment.[23,36]

In actuality, there are some general issues that present themselves to the neurologist. The most commonly encountered reason for a consultation has to do with assessment of an "altered state of consciousness." The appearance of a new encephalopathy may be due to rejection causing dysfunction of the graft, or it may have other causes.

Acute confusional state remains difficult to define in transplant recipients and can be considered if it lasts more than 2–3 consecutive days.[44] Postoperative hyperactive delirium associated with hallucinations is common posttransplantation, and some circumstances should be recognized. If patients are seen in the immediate postoperative period, both hyperactive and hypoactive delirium after liver transplantation occurs in about a third of the patients.[6] This is more often in patients who had a pretransplant encephalopathy and is more often seen in alcoholic liver disease.

In evaluating patients with impaired consciousness, some guidance can be provided. All potential sedative drugs should be carefully scrutinized, and the time remaining to clearance should be calculated. Physicians should consider the administration of flumazenil or naloxone to eliminate the remaining effects. Neurotoxicity of immunosuppressive drugs is frequently implicated, and it continues to be a concern to be dealt with. None of these drugs causes structural disease, other than a leukoencephalopathy, which cannot be radiographically distinguished from posterior reversible encephalopathy syndrome (PRES). Clinically, there are often no other triggers than the immunosuppressant drugs; and there is evidence of high to very high drug levels. Whether MRI patterns have changed is not known, but white matter edema can be multifocal and widespread.

There are many causes that need to be considered in acute postoperative confusion, fogginess and stupor. These include the use of calcineurin inhibitors, opioid antagonists, beta-adrenergic blockers, and high-dose corticosteroids. All of these drugs can be implicated. Other commonly used drugs, such as midazolam and propofol, may impact level of consciousness, particularly because they have different pharmacokinetics in transplant patients. Midazolam, for example, although relatively short acting in comparison with other sedative agents, has a prolonged activity if the liver graft is not functioning fully. It is also highly protein bound, and preexisting low protein levels may increase its sedative effects. Clearance of propofol is dependent on hepatic blood flow and cardiac output; and if both are disturbed, awakening from propofol may be markedly delayed, and the patient may not characteristically awaken, as usually anticipated, 10–15 minutes after the discontinuation of infusion. Opioids may continue to linger after cardiac transplantation because typically very large doses are used during the procedure.

Neurotoxicity associated with cyclosporine or tacrolimus is often considered but now less often diagnosed. Breakdown of the blood–brain barrier is needed for cyclosporine to enter because no lipoprotein transport system exists. Cyclosporine is very lipophilic from aliphatic groups but will not cross the blood–brain barrier because of tight junctions. How crossing occurs remains unknown, and perhaps impairment of the blood–brain barrier is facilitated by surgery-associated ischemic insults due to inevitable brief periods of hypotension. The predilection of the posterior areas of the brain may also be related to a less-developed blood–brain barrier that quickly opens when challenged. Oligodendroglia is more susceptible than astrocytes. This characteristic fits nicely with the mostly white matter lesions on magnetic resonance imaging.

The pathway of neurotoxicity associated with cyclosporine or tacrolimus has not been resolved at a molecular level. Both immunosuppressive drugs bind to an immunophilin, a protein with an affinity for both drugs, and consequently trigger a cascade of actions that include blockade of calcineurin. Calcineurin is involved in cell signaling and maintenance of cytoskeletal protein function, particularly in oligodendrocytes. Inhibition of calcineurin activity, therefore, may lead to neuronal death or apoptosis. It remains very likely, however, that extremely high doses in the earlier days of transplantation, due to unfamiliarity with the drugs, has been the major driving factor. This possibility is also supported by the very low incidence of cyclosporine neurotoxicity using oral preparations, resulting in stable blood levels and avoidance of extreme blood levels during intravenous loading. The earliest abnormality seems to be neurotoxicity from fluid extravasation (vasogenic edema) and not cell destruction (cytotoxic edema). Very limited pathology studies are available, but some have found fields of demyelination.

One should obtain serum levels of cyclosporine or tacrolimus and trend the values. A marked increase in levels may indicate the development of neurotoxicity, but such an association is only plausible if it is seen outside the usual intravenous loading period that occurs within the first week of treatment. Many transplant teams titrate toward increasing plasma levels, and these levels should not be misinterpreted as indicative of neurotoxicity. Recent laboratory values should be obtained and should include electrolyte panel, liver and renal function tests, serum ammonia, arterial blood gas, and, where indicated, antiepileptic drug levels. A mistake is to label postoperative encephalopathy as multifactorial, which often does nothing to find the possible triggers. For example, a liver transplant recipient may have severe hyponatremia, rising creatinine and BUN, and may show signs of early rejection. Moreover, cefepime neurotoxicity may be the cause of decline in consciousness, with new myoclonus and improvement can be expected when the drug is discontinued.[12]

The threshold for cerebrospinal fluid examination should be low even if meningitis is not suspected. Because an infectious mass lesion may be present, a CT scan may need to be performed to exclude such a lesion. An acutely febrile patient with an abnormal level of consciousness should prompt an aggressive search for a central nervous system infection. Immunosuppressed transplant recipients have a proclivity for infections with *Listeria monocytogenes, Nocardia,* or *Aspergillus.*[36] Infections with *Cryptococcus neoformans* or *Toxoplasma gondii* are rarely seen within 6 months after transplantation. All of these infections present often with meningeal enhancement on a CT or MRI scan, solitary or multiple abscesses, or ring-lesions. None of them are specific and may need to be found by brain biopsy.[32,33]

ORGAN-SPECIFIC COMPLICATIONS

Lung transplant recipients, due to significant challenges in oxygenation, may have severe neurologic complications in about a third. Most severe complications are perioperative stroke, and when these neurologic complications occur there is a higher mortality. Acute hyperammonemia—an unexpected and not completely explained metabolic derangement in lung transplant recipients—has also been described, causing seizures and profound stupor.[16] Cyclosporin neurotoxicity is not a major cause of complications in lung transplant recipients.

Cardiac transplantations are obviously at risk of ischemic injury as a result of embolization from aortic atheroembolism, but they also are at risk of perioperative cardiogenic shock, requiring extreme measures such as intra-aortic balloon pump support or extracorporeal membrane oxygenation (ECMO). Intracerebral hemorrhage is rarely seen after cardiac transplantation, but prolonged extreme hypertension may cause a lobar or basal ganglia hemorrhage.

The most challenging category of patients is patients with fulminant hepatic failure. Magnetic resonance imaging (MRI) is helpful in assessing the severity of liver disease. In some patients with liver cirrhosis, increased symmetric T2 signal (FLAIR) abnormalities are seen along the corticospinal tracts, along with scattered white matter lesions, and these abnormalities disappear with improving liver function. More frequently—in approximately two-thirds of patients with advanced liver disease—hyper-intensity in the globus pallidus is found on T1-weighted images and disappears after liver transplantation. Hyperammonemia may cause diffuse restricted DWI in any patient with worsening liver disease. (Improvement of serum ammonia levels do show improvement of restricted diffusion; Figure 47.1.)

Fulminant hepatic failure can lead to rapid neurologic deterioration, attributed to brain edema. At some point during the course of time, a metabolic derangement (hepatic encephalopathy) progresses toward a structural lesion (cerebral edema) that causes permanent brainstem injury. Brain edema is more common in patients who have a short interval between the onset of jaundice and signs of encephalopathy, when there is an associated infection, need for vasopressors, or when there is associated renal failure. Increased arterial ammonia at presentation in fulminant hepatic failure is a strong predictor for more severe manifestations of cerebral edema.

The postoperative management of brain edema in patients who received a liver to replace an acutely necrotic liver is another major neurologic issue. Management starts in the

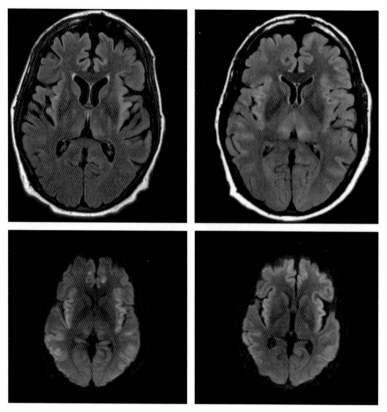

FIGURE 47.1: Serial MRI showing severe restricted diffusion in a patient with hyperammonemia and liver cirrhosis and varices hemorrhage. Improvement in DWI is associated with normalizing ammonia.

pretransplantation phase, but needs continuation in the days after transplantation.[2,9] Brain edema after fulminant hepatic failure is prominent in patients with stage III/IV hepatic encephalopathy;[11] in fact, those are usually the patients who are acutely listed for transplantation.[10,17]

Brain edema can be very rapid, causing a significant problem with management of increased intracranial pressure (ICP). Evaluation of a CT scan of the brain is very difficult, and ICP measurement does not always correlate with the degree of cerebral edema. Problems occur when brain edema is based on nonspecific signs such as smaller ventricles, poor gray white differentiation, and sulcal pattern. We have encountered patients with CT scans read as "brain edema" but with no evidence of MRI (Figure 47.2). Cerebral edema is best assessed when serial CT scans are available and we have used a score to systematically review these CT scans. The individual components are shown in Table 47.1. We found in some patients a major drop-off in score on CT scan with no parallel change yet in clinical examination, suggesting that ICP monitoring may be needed to pinpoint

this transition. The mechanism of brain edema in a fulminant hepatic failure is influenced by multiple factors (Capsule 47.1).

The management of fulminant hepatic failure and cerebral edema (Figure 47.3) has been summarized by some as quadruple H therapy. This includes hemodialysis (through MARS), hyperventilation, hypernatremia (from osmotic therapy), and hypothermia.[43] However, vasoconstriction induced by hypocapnia can decrease regional cerebral blood flow and inflict secondary ischemic brain injury. Not all patients are PCO_2 responders, and moreover the effect is short-lived. Using continuous infusion of hypertonic saline may create a new steady state, and additional osmotic gradients may be difficult to achieve with a bolus of hypertonic saline. Placement of an ICP monitoring device is necessary to control ICP during the perioperative phase. There is an understandable reluctance by neurosurgeons to place ICP monitors due to the associated coagulopathy with nearly absent liver function, but with the use of recombinant factor VIIa or prothrombin complex concentrate, coagulopathy can be controlled.[31] The risk of a clinically

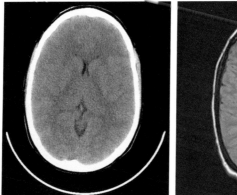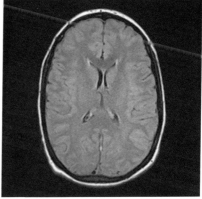

FIGURE 47.2: Serial CT scans in young patient with fulminant hepatic failure with suggestion of cerebral edema, but none on MRI.

relevant probe associated hemorrhage is approximately 10%–20%. On the other hand, losing a patient with rapid brain edema that could have been detected and controlled is equally problematic. Most experts in this field feel that ICP monitoring placement should be considered in a patient lapsing into stupor, necessitating intubation and mechanical ventilation. Monitoring ICP in fulminant hepatic failure may then remain essential to shepherd the patient through surgery.[5] A sudden increase in ICP has been noted during transplantation, and these surges of ICP do occur after reperfusion of the transplanted liver and may even extend through the first day after liver transplantation. Propofol may be useful and in small dosis has reduced intermittent increases in ICP. With a dosage of 1–3 mg/kg we were able to control ICP satisfactorily.[40]

Treatment of increased ICP is typically the use of osmotic drugs.[24,28] However, the use of mannitol may be initially problematic if the patient has developed a hepatorenal syndrome and hypertonic saline is a better option. There is a current interest in using hypothermia (33°–34°C) in combination with high-dose barbiturates.[34] Recent data found that using induced hypothermia in 97 patients did not improve overall and transplant-free survival when compared with historical controls, but there were no major side effects. Earlier concerns of inhibition of hepatic regeneration, increased infections, bleeding, or arrhythmias were not found.[17] What remains unclear is how many patients are able to be salvaged when frank edema and crowding of the basal cisterns appear on a repeat CT scan. In many of these patients, transplantation may come too late.

However, patients who have an ICP monitoring device placed and are treated aggressively do not have a better outcome or higher percentage of liver transplantation, and that could question the role of ICP-based management. Nonetheless, most centers place an intraparenchymal ICP. As mentioned earlier, preemptive administration of recombinant factor VIIa and use of prothrombin complex are important new developments in countering coagulopathy in fulminant hepatic

TABLE 47.1. CALCULATION OF BRAIN EDEMA SEVERITY SCORE (BESS), BASED ON COMPUTED TOMOGRAPHIC FINDINGS IN PATIENTS WITH FULMINANT HEPATIC FAILURE

Visibility of cortical sulci	
Visibility of cortical sulci	
3 CT scan slices of upper cerebral area (L/R)	6
Visibility of white matter	
Internal capsule (L/R)	2
Centrum semiovale (L/R)	2
Vertex (L/R)	2
Visibility of basal cisterns	
Sylvian fissure (horizontal-vertical, L/R)	4
Frontal interhemispheric fissure	1
Quadrigeminal cistern	1
Paired suprasellar cisterns (L/R)	2
Ambient cistern (L/R)	2
Maximal total BESS	22

CT, computed tomographic; L/R, left and right cerebral hemispheres.
From Wijdicks EFM, Plevak DJ, Rakela J, Wiesner RH. Clinical and radiologic features of cerebral edema in fulminant hepatic failure. *Mayo Clin Proc* 1995;70:119–124.

CAPSULE 47.1   MECHANISM OF BRAIN EDEMA IN FULMINANT HEPATIC FAILURE

Ammonia has been implicated in the pathogenesis of hepatic encephalopathy, perhaps through an imbalance between inhibitory and excitatory neurotransmitters. The GABA neurotransmitter system, an inhibitory system, possibly plays a prominent role. γ-aminobutyric acid (GABA) causes hyperpolarization of neuronal membrane through opening of chloride channel and influx of chloride inside the cells. It appears that the degree of hepatic encephalopathy is correlated with CSF levels of GABA. What is notably different is that acute liver failure is associated with the development of cerebral edema in the higher (III/IV) grades of encephalopathy. There are multiple pathophysiological mechanisms that play a role. One is a deficit in the ability of astrocytes to take up glutamate from the excess cellular space. That, in itself, leads to excitotoxicity of the neuronal glutamate receptors. Aquaporin-4, which is involved in brain water transport, may also play a role. In many situations, the abnormalities can be a result of alterations in cerebral hemodynamics, and this might be triggered by production of nitric oxide. Increase of nitric oxide and cerebral blood flow might be important in the development of cerebral edema and intracranial hypertension. Ammonia is detoxified by astrocytes through the synthesis of glutamine, and this may act as an osmolyte. Astrocyte swelling then leads to the formation of reactive oxygen and nitrogen oxygen species, and eventually to apoptosis. The current leading explanation is that there is an osmotic and oxidative stress neuronal damage. Glutamine has been the major responsible substance, and a significant increase of glutamine in the brain precedes increase in brain water in experimental models.

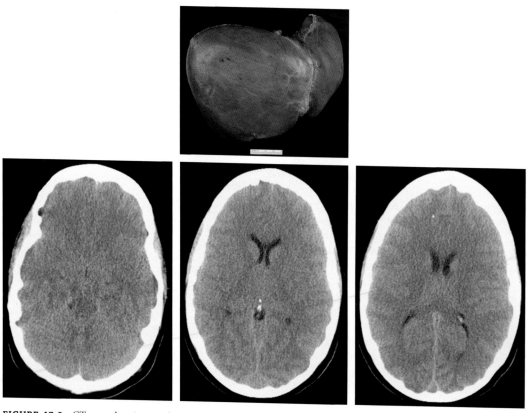

FIGURE 47.3: CT scan showing cerebral edema and massive liver swelling (note ICP monitor).

failure, and its use has significantly decreased the frequency of bleeding complications, of which most are catastrophic (Figure 47.4). A protocol for management of liver transplantation for fulminant hepatic failure is shown in Table 47.2.

Intestinal transplantation for a short bowel syndrome due to thrombosis, inflammatory bowel disease, or radiation enteritis has become another "organ" that can be transplanted, but experience is only in a few hundred patients. The initial experience is not sufficient to potentially identify specific complications, and most reported are in the known categories such as encephalopathy, CNS infection, seizures, stroke, and neuromuscular complications. Early assessment suggests that the rate of neurologic complications is much higher than that for solid organ transplants. One possible explanation is the higher immunosuppression as a result of relative lower resistance to rejection of the intestine.

Any transplant recipient is at risk of developing B-cell lymphomas or glioblastoma multiforme or progressive multifocal leukoencephalopathy (PML).[21,29] These disorders are extremely uncommon, but can present within months after transplantation. Most notorious is the occurrence of CNS lymphoma several weeks after transplantation (it may vary from a few weeks to more than 2 decades after transplantation). Most post-transplantation lymphomas are monoclonal B-cell lymphomas, but multiclonal B-cell lymphomas or T-cell lymphomas have been reported. Epstein-Barr virus infection has been linked to B-cell lymphoma. CNS lymphoma debuts with both brain and spinal cord involvement, but presentation is nonspecific, with new behavioral changes, visual hallucinations, or focal signs such as hemiparesis. In most patients a change in personality may be the only key sign. Meningeal involvement may produce headache. The diagnosis can only be considered if the CT scan shows a new mass lesion in the periventricular region and with proportionally large amount of perilesional edema. A biopsy might be necessary to make the diagnosis followed by aggressive treatment with radiation. Outcome, however, remains very poor, with ultimate demise in all patients.

Progressive multifocal leukoencephalopathy (PML) is caused by JC virus, and the disorder is usually relentless (Figure 47.5). Withdrawal of immunotherapy or highly active antiretroviral treatment is considered, with some good outcomes reported.[25,37] Behavioral change and dementia are common, due to demyelination of the frontal lobe. The MRI scan shows characteristic increased signal in the white matter, and brain

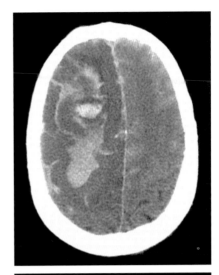

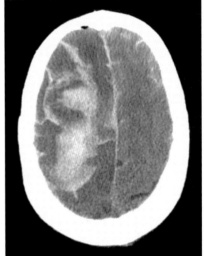

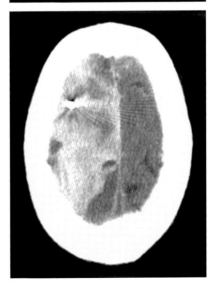

FIGURE 47.4: CT scan showing massive cerebral hematoma at ICP insertion site (INR at insertion was 1.2; at time of bleeding it was 4.5).

TABLE 47.2. TREATMENT OPTIONS
OF BRAIN EDEMA IN FULMINANT
HEPATIC FAILURE

Hemodiafiltration to reduce serum ammonia to less
than 60 micromol/L

Moderate hypothermia (33°–35°C) with cooling
device and control of shivering

Propofol infusion (start with 30 mcg/kg per minute
and may increase to 200 mcg/kg per minute for
brief periods of time)

Mannitol, 0.5–1 g/kg every 6 hr if plasma osmolality
is < 310 mOsm/L

Hypertonic saline bolus (10%–23%) to serum
sodium of 150–155 mmol/L

biopsy can demonstrate in situ hybridization for
JC virus. Cytarabine is used to temporize the
tumor growth, but with little success; and most
patients have not survived more than a year after
the diagnosis.

CNS INFECTIONS

CNS infections occur in patients with a complicated postoperative clinical course and already
long ICU stays. CNS infections present as a
meningoencephalitis with treatment refractory
headache, behavior changes, and, less commonly,
localizing signs such a hemiparesis. Intracerebral
hemorrhage may be associated with fungal infections. The most frequently encountered pathogen is *aspergillus fumigatus*, and it may be rapidly
invasive and fatal. The diagnosis is very difficult
to make intra vitam; more commonly, autopsy
will be able to show the widely disseminated
angioinvasive hyphae. Galactomannan is part of
the Aspergillus cell wall and a double sandwich
enzyme immunoassay detects the galactomannan antigen in serum when it is released. In our
experience, we have seen only sporadic cases in
liver transplant recipients, but when it occurred,
no patient survived the concomitant multiorgan
involvement. Systemic therapy for CNS aspergillosis is voriconazole 6 mg/kg intravenously every 12
hours initially and followed by 4 mg/kg IV every 12
hours. Other causes are *Cryptococcus neoformans*
and a variety of other fungal infections, but these
are mostly reported as anecdotes in the literature.
Treatment for cryptococcus meningitis is liposo-
mal amphotericin B (3–4 mg/kg per day IV) and
flucytosine (100 mg/kg per day in 4 divided doses)
for at least 2 weeks for the induction regimen.
Treatment of increased CSF pressure is key and
opening pressures during lumbar puncture may
be high without a clear hydrocephalus. A lumbar
drain is often needed (Part XIV, Guidelines).

MR imaging can be helpful in documenting
multiple small abscesses, but there are no distinguishing features. CSF will invariably show a
lymphocytic pleocytosis, and a biopsy or immu-
nodiffusion tests for the detection of antibodies.
CSF India Ink (with suspicion of *Cryptococcus
neoformans*) is frequently positive and is helpful
clinically.

Disseminated viral infections have also been
described with very high mortality rates, but
again, no systemic studies have been reported.
A viral encephalopathy that has emerged more
recently is a human herpes virus 6 (HHV6).[30] This
infection may be seen several weeks after transplantation and is not likely recognized or initially
is misdiagnosed as metabolic derangement or
neurotoxicity from immunosuppressive agents.
A confusional state with disorientation may be
the only clinical sign. Isolation by PCR is necessary, and expectedly no other tests, such as EEG

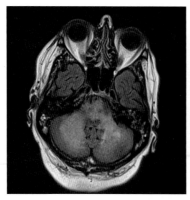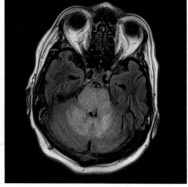

FIGURE 47.5: MRI in liver transplant patient with PML.

or MRI scan, have any key features. The mortality is high, with about 80% of the patients remaining comatose. Foscarnet has been tried in some cases, but there is yet little experience.

Another under-recognized infection is cytomegalovirus encephalopathy. Approximately 80% of liver recipients have reactivation of a latent CMV that may occur several weeks after transplantation. Again, the diagnosis of CMV encephalitis is notoriously difficult, with a presentation that is baffling to most clinicians. Some patients present with focal findings such as dysarthria, spasticity, rigidity, and tremor, and others develop fever and neck stiffness. CMV chorioretinitis may be demonstrated, but CMV encephalitis may occur without this manifestation. In all these opportunistic infections, the recent availability of PCR technology has increased recognition, but there is yet no evidence that early treatment improves outcome.

NEUROMUSCULAR COMPLICATIONS

Liver transplantation should spare muscle and nerve. However, neuropathies may occur due to cannulation, coagulation-induced compressive hematomas.[7,39] The relationship between immunosuppressive agents and development of a neuromuscular disorder has never been established and should be considered unlikely.

Most neuropathies are due to stretch with surgery or positioning and possibly are preventable. A brachial plexopathy can be due to a shoulder hyperabduction, but axillary vein cannulation is less commonly used in liver transplantation. Ulnar and radial neuropathies are uncommon after liver transplant surgery and are noticed by the patient usually as significant hand muscle weakness and more often painful tingling. Bilateral peroneal palsies are far more common after liver transplantation due to prolonged immobility during surgery in patients already predisposed as a result of marked weight loss. All these neuropathies have a good outcome over time. In our series, we found coagulopathy-associated psoas hematomas causing a femoral hematoma, but this may only be seen in the more severe cases with rejection after liver transplantation. Chronic inflammatory demyelinating polyneuropathy has been reported in patients after reduction of immunosuppressive drugs. The true incidence is not known, nor how an immunologic response to multiple nerves emerges.

Any patient that develops a postoperative sepsis is at risk of critical illness polyneuropathy. Patients are typically recognized by a severe quadriplegia with diffuse muscle wasting but no paresthesias or sensory loss. Rhabdomyolysis is also a presentation of severe sepsis but is less commonly seen after liver transplantation. In cases reported, certain drugs may have contributed (i.e., combination of statins and antibiotics). Patients may have considerable weakness and muscle pain. Muscles are tender to touch, but this may be an unreliable sign in a critically ill patient who just underwent a major transplantation procedure. Rhabdomyolysis cannot be clinically differentiated from critical illness myopathy that is more common in patients with sepsis, use of neuromuscular blockade and prolonged bed rest, and from corticosteroid-induced necrotic myopathy. In these cases, EMG will show a myopathic pattern (short-duration motor units and fibrillation potentials) and CPK values can be elevated. Outcome is favorable and rapid, and muscle biopsies are usually deferred. The outcome of patients with critical illness polyneuropathy after liver transplantation is not known, but likely not different from that of other clinical situations. There is generally little concern with neuromuscular disorders in liver transplant recipients, and they rarely impact mobility or function.

CONCLUSIONS

- CNS infections can be grouped in 6-month time periods, and each has specific risks for certain organisms.
- Comatose patients with fulminant hepatic failure need ICP control before, during, and after liver transplantation.
- Hematopoietic cell transplantation recipients have a high proclivity of drug neurotoxicity.
- Late neurologic complications may include CNS lymphoma or PML.

REFERENCES

1. Amodio P, Biancardi A, Montagnese S, et al. Neurological complications after orthotopic liver transplantation. *Dig Liver Dis* 2007;39:740–747.
2. Auzinger G, Wendon J. Intensive care management of acute liver failure. *Curr Opin Crit Care* 2008;14:179–188.
3. Blei AT. Brain edema in acute liver failure. *Crit Care Clin* 2008;24:99–114, ix.
4. Blei AT. Brain edema in acute liver failure: can it be prevented? Can it be treated? *J Hepatol* 2007;46:564–569.
5. Brandsaeter B, Hockerstedt K, Friman S, et al. Fulminant hepatic failure: outcome after listing for highly urgent liver transplantation: 12 years

experience in the nordic countries. *Liver Transpl* 2002;8:1055–1062.

6. Buis CI, Wiesner RH, Krom RA, Kremers WK, Wijdicks EFM. Acute confusional state following liver transplantation for alcoholic liver disease. *Neurology* 2002;59:601–605.

7. Campellone JV, Lacomis D, Giuliani MJ, Kramer DJ. Mononeuropathies associated with liver transplantation. *Muscle Nerve* 1998;21:896–901.

8. Cui R, Fayek S, Rand EB, et al. Central pontine myelinolysis: a case report and clinical-pathological review. *Pediatr Transplant* 2012;16:E251–E256.

9. Daas M, Plevak DJ, Wijdicks EFM, et al. Acute liver failure: results of a 5-year clinical protocol. *Liver Transpl Surg* 1995;1:210–219.

10. Emond JC, Aran PP, Whitington PF, Broelsch CE, Baker AL. Liver transplantation in the management of fulminant hepatic failure. *Gastroenterology* 1989;96:1583–1588.

11. Fraser CL, Arieff AI. Hepatic encephalopathy. *N Engl J Med* 1985;313:865–873.

12. Fugate JE, Kalimullah EA, Hocker SE, et al. Cefepime neurotoxicity in the intensive care unit: a cause of severe, underappreciated encephalopathy. *Crit Care* 2013;17:R264.

13. Ghaus N, Bohlega S, Rezeig M. Neurological complications in liver transplantation. *J Neurol* 2001;248:1042–1048.

14. Goldstein LS, Haug MT, 3rd, Perl J, 2nd, et al. Central nervous system complications after lung transplantation. *J Heart Lung Transplant* 1998;17:185–191.

15. Guarino M, Benito-Leon J, Decruyenaere J, et al. EFNS guidelines on management of neurological problems in liver transplantation. *Eur J Neurol* 2006;13:2–9.

16. Hocker S, Rabinstein AA, Wijdicks EFM. Pearls & Oysters: Status epilepticus from hyperammonemia after lung transplant. *Neurology* 2011;77:e54–e56.

17. Karvellas CJ,Stravitz RT, Battenhouse H, et al. Therapeutic hypothermia in acute liver failure: a multicenter retrospective cohort analysis. *Liver Transpl* 2015;21:4–12.

18. Knight JS, Tsodikov A, Cibrik DM, et al. Lymphoma after solid organ transplantation: risk, response to therapy, and survival at a transplantation center. *J Clin Oncol* 2009;27:3354–3362.

19. Lewis MB, Howdle PD. Neurologic complications of liver transplantation in adults. *Neurology* 2003;61:1174–1178.

20. Mateen FJ, Dierkhising RA, Rabinstein AA, van de Beek D, Wijdicks EFM. Neurological complications following adult lung transplantation. *Am J Transplant* 2010;10:908–914.

21. Mateen FJ, Muralidharan R, Carone M, et al. Progressive multifocal leukoencephalopathy in transplant recipients. *Ann Neurol* 2011;70:305–322.

22. Mour G, Wu C. Neurologic complications after kidney transplantation. *Semin Nephrol* 2015;35:323–334.

23. Munoz P, Valerio M, Palomo J, et al. Infectious and non-infectious neurologic complications in heart transplant recipients. *Medicine (Baltimore)* 2010;89:166–175.

24. O'Grady J. Modern management of acute liver failure. *Clin Liver Dis* 2007;11:291–303.

25. Ohara H, Kataoka H, Nakamichi K, Saijo M, Ueno S. Favorable outcome after withdrawal of immunosuppressant therapy in progressive multifocal leukoencephalopathy after renal transplantation: case report and literature review. *J Neurol Sci* 2014;341:144–146.

26. Pittock SJ, Rabinstein AA, Edwards BS, Wijdicks EFM. OKT3 neurotoxicity presenting as akinetic mutism. *Transplantation* 2003;75:1058–1060.

27. Pruitt AA, Graus F, Rosenfeld MR. Neurological complications of solid organ transplantation. *Neurohospitalist* 2013;3:152–166.

28. Raghavan M, Marik PE. Therapy of intracranial hypertension in patients with fulminant hepatic failure. *Neurocrit Care* 2006;4:179–189.

29. Schiff D, O'Neill B, Wijdicks EFM, Antin JH, Wen PY. Gliomas arising in organ transplant recipients: an unrecognized complication of transplantation? *Neurology* 2001;57:1486–1488.

30. Seeley WW, Marty FM, Holmes TM, et al. Post-transplant acute limbic encephalitis: clinical features and relationship to HHV6. *Neurology* 2007;69:156–165.

31. Shami VM, Caldwell SH, Hespenheide EE, et al. Recombinant activated factor VII for coagulopathy in fulminant hepatic failure compared with conventional therapy. *Liver Transpl* 2003;9:138–143.

32. Silveira FP, Husain S, Kwak EJ, et al. Cryptococcosis in liver and kidney transplant recipients receiving anti-thymocyte globulin or alemtuzumab. *Transpl Infect Dis* 2007;9:22–27.

33. Singh N. How I treat cryptococcosis in organ transplant recipients. *Transplantation* 2012;93:17–21.

34. Stravitz RT, Kramer AH, Davern T, et al. Intensive care of patients with acute liver failure: recommendations of the U.S. Acute Liver Failure Study Group. *Crit Care Med* 2007;35:2498–2508.

35. Uchida H, Sakamoto S, Sasaki K, et al. Central pontine myelinolysis following pediatric living donor liver transplantation: a case report and review of literature. *Pediatr Transplant* 2014;18:E120–E123.

36. van de Beek D, Patel R, Daly RC, McGregor CG, Wijdicks EFM. Central nervous system infections in heart transplant recipients. *Arch Neurol* 2007;64:1715–1720.

37. Weber SC, Uhlenberg B, Raile K, Querfeld U, Muller D. Polyoma virus-associated progressive multifocal leukoencephalopathy after renal transplantation: regression following withdrawal of mycophenolate mofetil. *Pediatr Transplant* 2011;15:E19–E24.

38. Wijdicks EFM, Hocker SE. Neurologic complications of liver transplantation. *Handb Clin Neurol* 2014;121:1257–1266.

39. Wijdicks EFM, Litchy WJ, Wiesner RH, Krom RA. Neuromuscular complications associated with liver transplantation. *Muscle Nerve* 1996;19:696–700.

40. Wijdicks EFM, Nyberg SL. Propofol to control intracranial pressure in fulminant hepatic failure. *Transplant Proc* 2002;34:1220–1222.

41. Wijdicks EFM, Wiesner RH, Krom RA. Neurotoxicity in liver transplant recipients with cyclosporine immunosuppression. *Neurology* 1995;45:1962–1964.

42. Wijdicks EFM. *Neurologic Complications in Organ Transplant Recipients.* Boston: Butterworth-Heinemann; 1999.

43. Warrillow SJ, Bellomo R. Preventing cerebral edema in acute liver disease: the case for quadruple-H therapy. *Anaesth Intensive Care* 2014;42:78–88.

44. Zhao CZ, Erickson J, Dalmau J. Clinical reasoning: agitation and psychosis in a patient after renal transplantation. *Neurology* 2012;79:e41–e44.

45. Zivkovic SA, Eidelman BH, Bond G, Costa G, Abu-Elmagd KM. The clinical spectrum of neurologic disorders after intestinal and multivisceral transplantation. *Clin Transplant* 2010;24:164–168.

48

Neurology of Cardiac and Aortic Surgery

Cardiac surgeries and major vascular repairs are performed in increasing numbers and largely due to improved anesthesia, technological innovations and advances in surgical skills. Undergoing cardiac surgery is with lower mortality when compared with previous decades. It is an undisputed fact that extensive repairs are commonly without major neurologic complications, or the neurologic presentation is fleeting and not concerning enough to the cardiac surgeon. Some of us may feel it is extraordinary that consults are not more often needed and perhaps cardiovascular surgeons know there is a problem and may not need a neurologist to be reminded of it. However, when new neurologic signs occur, they can be summarized as a consequence of invasive procedures (i.e., emboli associated with coronary angiogram or open heart surgery), repairs of aortic aneurysms (i.e., spinal cord injury), or complications due to prolonged general anesthesia (i.e., nerve injury). Vital signs may fairly quickly and substantially change during and after surgery, and this may include perioperative blood pressure fluctuations and cardiac arrhythmias. These changes are strangely enough rarely associated with major neurologic complications.

Some of the major complications after cardiac surgical procedures are discussed here, particularly those requiring urgent management. While neurologic complications of cardiac surgeries and procedures can occur in any age group, it has been proven that the higher risk group are older patients and those with significant comorbidities.[5,9,19,20,27,56,80,83] Some studies have identified specific risk factors for postoperative stroke[64] and postoperative cognitive impairment.[87]

Most of what we know is through reports of surgical series, built-up experiences, and systematically seeing these patients. The task for the consulting neurologist is to see if there is something to be gained by a specific intervention. Additionally, and to the satisfaction of the surgical team, a detailed communication with family members about expected recovery is often

initiated. Parenthetically, when there has been a major disabling complication, the neurologist may feel to nudge the cardiovascular team to stop escalating care. This chapter provides an overview and specifics where needed for best management. Consults in patients with vascular surgery involving the carotid artery are discussed in Chapter 45.

COMPLICATIONS WITH CARDIAC CATHETERIZATION

Cardiac catheterization-related strokes are expectedly embolic in origin.[58,99] Other mechanisms of cerebral infarction have included procedure-related acute arterial dissection and sudden hypotension, mostly as a result of myocardial failure.[20,65,101] A persistent occlusion in a large cerebral artery is unusual. Hemorrhagic stroke is also very uncommon.[20,58,75] Clinically apparent embolic strokes have been reported to occur during diagnostic cardiac catheterization procedures in 0.08%–0.4%.[13,25,30,46,61,83,86] With these extremely low numbers of procedure related strokes, cardiac catheterization is, however, not as innocuous as it may seem because asymptomatic cerebral infarction in patients undergoing diagnostic or interventional cardiac catheterization has been detected by diffusion-weighted (DWI) MRI in 15%–100% of patients.[14,37,59] There are conflicting data whether posterior circulation strokes are more common with the brachial artery approach and anterior circulation events are more common with the femoral artery approach.[13,19,55,86] There is no question that endovascular procedures such as stenting may cause miniscule emboli that are still large enough to be detected by DWI.

Risk factors predisposing to stroke with cardiac catheterization include patient characteristics such as age, and vascular comorbidities, but also procedure-related factors such as longer fluoroscopic time, use of large-caliber catheters, and introduction of emboli during catheter advancement.[5,20,55,83] Cerebral microemboli are predominantly detected during catheter advancement, catheter flushing, contrast injection, and ventriculography. There is also a significant correlation between the number of microemboli and the volume of contrast used.[59]

Transient cortical blindness after contrast media exposure is a well-described phenomenon during cardiac catheterization but is less common with non-ionic, low-osmolality radiocontrast agents. The mechanism is not fully clarified, but it has been thought to be due to a breakdown of the blood–brain barrier selective for the occipital cortex, with subsequent direct neurotoxicity of the contrast media.[77,93]

Another occasional complication is damage to peripheral nerves—plexus or single nerve. Peripheral nervous system complications have been divided into brachial plexopathy, median nerve injury, lumbosacral plexopathy, femoral nerve, or lateral femoral cutaneous nerve injury. Brachial plexopathy can occur due to prolonged fixed posture during the procedure. Median neuropathy is a rare complication of brachial artery catheterization and is thought to be due to direct injury in the antecubital region or hematoma formation. Brachial plexopathy has been described after axillary angiography and may be secondary to hematoma, pseudoaneurysm formation, or direct compression.[74]

The femoral nerve can be compressed by a hematoma at the groin puncture site or, rarely, by an arteriovenous fistula or pseudoaneurysm of the femoral profunda artery.[53] Groin, flank, or abdominal pain that radiates to the thigh, associated with numbness of the anterior thigh and medial calf, with a reduced or absent patellar reflex, should alert the clinician to discontinue any anticoagulation and investigate for retroperitoneal hematoma. The lateral femoral cutaneous nerve can be injured from tight compression bandages, resulting in meralgia paresthetica.[47]

COMPLICATIONS WITH CORONARY ARTERY BYPASS SURGERY

Clinically apparent strokes occur in approximately 0.8%–5% of patients undergoing coronary artery bypass grafting (CABG).[92] Using highly sensitive diffusion-weighted MRI increases the incidence of cerebral infarctions to 18%—again, about two-thirds of these infarcts are asymptomatic.[29] The occurrence of ischemic stroke is bimodal, and most strokes (61%) occur within the first 2 postoperative days, while the remainder occur in the second postoperative week (39%).[56] Embolic cerebral infarctions are the most common type of

stroke occurring in the perioperative period after CABG.[57,92] Cerebral infarctions involving watershed territories typically occur in the setting of prolonged hypotension, but they can also occur in patients without documented hemodynamic instability. The mechanism in these cases may be showers of microemboli that lodge in terminal branches, resulting in perfusion failure.[45] Clinical signs of lacunar infarction in this population is often mimicked by small emboli that occlude single perforating arteries.[56,57,60] "Late" ischemic strokes are more difficult to understand and are a surprising turn of events. An association with postoperative atrial fibrillation has been found, but in our experience an explanation is seldomly obvious. Aggressive control of atrial fibrillation with the use of ß-blockade, magnesium, amiodarone, statins, atrial pacing, or even posterior pericardiotomy has not convincingly reduced postoperative stroke rates, despite successful reduction of postoperative incidences of atrial fibrillation.[63]

Traditionally, atheromatous aorta and carotid artery disease are known predictors for stroke after CABG. Although pointed out as a major contender for postoperative stroke for many years, the role of high-grade asymptomatic carotid artery disease in postoperative stroke has not been substantiated, and there are very few cardiac surgeons who feel that preoperative treatment (carotid endarterectomy or stenting) is needed. The theory that has gained considerable traction is that, in some way or form, placement of catheters into a severe atheromatous arch (as part of cardiopulmonary bypass) plays a major role. Many leading cardiovascular surgeons would try to avoid such an injury ("no touch technique"). How this stroke could occur is shown in Figure 48.1.[31] Intraoperative use of epiaortic/transesophageal echocardiogram ultrasound to identify ascending and aortic atheromatous disease with appropriate surgical modifications, including, when possible, minimization of aortic manipulation and use of single aortic cross clamp for proximal grafts, no-touch aortic technique, and altered cannula placement, has been proposed. One study randomized patients to transcranial Doppler ultrasound of the middle cerebral arteries continuously before, during, and after aortic manipulation compared to control, and demonstrated that while epiaortic scanning did lead to modifications in intraoperative surgical management in 29% of patients, including adjustments of the cannulation site and avoidance of aortic cross-clamping, it did not lead to a reduced number of cerebral emboli.[24] Other explanations may

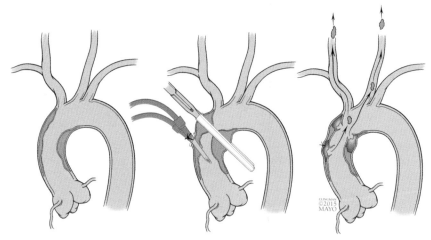

FIGURE 48.1: Ischemic stroke is likely caused by embolization out of damaged intravascular areas. Damage may be caused by clamping or catheter placement into severe atherosclerotic plaque.

relate to acid-base management of the cardiopulmonary bypass (Capsule 48.1).

Ischemic stroke after cardiac surgery usually presents with nursing staff noticing asymmetry of limb movement or if they are especially observant noting neglect (left side). Not uncommonly, aphasia is interpreted as "postoperative confusion," and this symptom also may—frustratingly for neurologists—delay detection. Patients with intraoperative strokes may be noted to have a failure to awaken from anesthesia and not as quickly as expected. Multiple ischemic strokes in both hemispheres may result in postoperative stupor, but only if extensive bihemispheric cortical areas are involved (Figure 48.2). A focal or generalized seizure may occur as a consequence of thromboembolic ischemic stroke, but it may also be caused by medication toxicity related to antibiotics or other perioperative drugs, such as high-dose tranexamic acid.[44]

The most worrisome complication, which is difficult to grapple with, is a postoperative

---

CAPSULE 48.1   CARDIOPULMONARY BYPASS AND CHANGES IN pH

There is a large body of literature on how the brain is damaged during cardiopulmonary bypass. The most important factor is embolic load, typically from microbubbles of air, the propagation of which may be influenced by changes in pH. Acid–base management during cardiopulmonary bypass can be accomplished with the pH-stat technique, which maintains a plasma pH of 7.4, regardless of temperature, by artificially increasing the carbon dioxide component of blood, resulting in hyperemia and possibly cerebral edema. With this technique, there is a mismatch in cerebral blood flow and metabolic rate; thus cerebral blood flow is pressure passive, and changes depending on cerebral perfusion pressure.

Alternatively, acid–base management can be accomplished with the "alpha-stat" technique, which permits relative alkalosis when the patient is cooled, preserving cerebral autoregulation, resulting in less cerebral blood flow, and probably decreased embolic load. In a randomized study of pH-stat versus alpha-stat management, cognitive dysfunction was significantly greater in the pH-stat group when bypass time was longer than 90 minutes.[100] A recent review addressing this question found that the best technique to follow in patients undergoing deep hypothermic circulatory arrest during cardiac surgery is dependent upon the age of the patient, with better results using pH-stat in the pediatric patient and alpha-stat in the adult patient.[2]

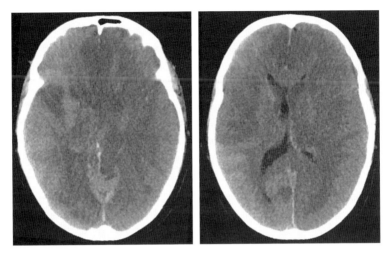

FIGURE 48.2: CT scan showing postcardiac surgery stroke.

encephalopathy defined as less attentiveness, poor memory retention, and disorientation in time and place. In most extreme circumstances, patients may not know they had surgery. Encephalopathy following CABG is typically clinically apparent following extubation and is frequently related to the effects of sedatives and analgesics administered during anesthesia or for comfort during mechanical ventilation or to metabolic disturbances. In patients without obvious drug-related or metabolic causes, there may be evidence of showers of microemboli. It seems reasonable to assume that stroke, coma, encephalopathy, and early and delayed cognitive impairment following CABG represent a continuum of conditions with the underlying mechanism of showers of embolic material (particulate matter, fat, thrombi, microbubbles) to the brain.[34,64,70] A longitudinal assessment of neurocognitive function after coronary artery bypass surgery by Newman et al. showed an incidence of neurocognitive decline of 53% at discharge, 36% at 6 weeks, 24% at 6 months, and 42% at 5 years.[70] Thus, there is evidence of cognitive decline after cardiac valve surgery in a substantial proportion of patients. Altered cognition was demonstrated by delayed P-300 auditory evoked responses at 7 days after valve replacement surgery.[108]

A devastating complication is acute postoperative blindness. Central retinal artery occlusion or branch retinal artery occlusion may occur with CABG. Patients are noted to have acute onset of complete visual loss in one eye (with central retinal artery occlusion) or acute onset of partial visual loss in one eye (with branch retinal artery occlusion).

Ischemic optic neuropathy is an extremely rare event after cardiac surgery, and the overall frequency is 0.06%.[72] Anterior ischemic optic neuropathy is characterized by sudden painless visual loss, involving mainly the lower part of the visual field in one eye, with optic disc swelling. Posterior ischemic optic neuropathy is characterized by unilateral or bilateral loss of visual acuity, visual fields, or blindness without disc swelling. Factors associated with visual loss after cardiopulmonary bypass are low hemoglobin concentration (< 8.5 g/dL), prior severe peripheral vascular disease, and—most revealingly—preoperative coronary angiogram within 48 hours of surgery.[72]

The most common nerves to be injured in cardiac surgery are the lower trunk of the brachial plexus. Patients with injured nerves have had longer operation times. Other nerves that may be damaged include the ulnar nerve, the recurrent laryngeal nerve, the saphenous nerve, the common peroneal nerve, and the cervical sympathetic chain. Brachial plexopathy may occur when the brachial plexus is stretched during a median sternotomy, when it is disrupted during surgery by the use of sternal retractors, or when there is direct trauma to the brachial plexus from pressure against the first rib.[16,89]

Phrenic nerve injury, resulting in unilateral or bilateral diaphragmatic paralysis, may result from direct manipulation of the nerve, but has become a rare complication.[23,48,89] Additionally, the left recurrent laryngeal nerve may have been injured in the past during internal mammary artery dissection and may be affected by ice water introduced to the pleural cavity,[89] but this complication is no longer commonly seen. Other mechanisms of damage may occur during endotracheal intubation, central venous catheter placement, or surgical dissection.[89]

The saphenous nerve may be injured during harvesting of the long saphenous vein, resulting in anesthesia, hyperesthesia, and pain in the distribution of the saphenous nerve. In about 0.19% of patients, the common peroneal nerve is affected during CABG, with damage to the nerve at the fibular head due to nerve ischemia from compression or stretching.[98] The cervical sympathetic chain, which lies medial to the inferior trunk of the brachial plexus, may be injured during sternal retraction with a posterior first rib fracture[89] and may present as Horner's syndrome.

COMPLICATIONS WITH VALVE SURGERY

The circumstances change when the heart is opened. Stroke is the most common neurologic complication of valvular heart surgeries. The incidence of postoperative stroke with these procedures has been estimated to be 1%–5%.[6,32,43,54,80] Combining vascular surgeries with cardiac surgery further increases the odds of a postoperative stroke, and it becomes impossible to point toward a single mechanism. If cardiac valve surgery is combined with CABG, repair of other cardiac abnormalities, or even carotid endarterectomy, the risk of stroke is higher.[28,95,104] Among all valve types stroke is more common with mitral valve surgeries, among all valve types. This has been attributed to an increased incidence of atrial fibrillation, left atrial enlargement, and possible endocardial damage from rheumatic disease of the mitral valve.[18] The incidence is considered to be equal between non-anticoagulated patients with bioprosthetic valves and anticoagulated patients with mechanical valves.[12,36]

Intraoperative strokes are commonly due to atherosclerotic emboli and hypoperfusion due to intraoperative hypotension or decreased cardiac output. Less common causes of intraoperative stroke include air embolism,[8] fat emboli,[3] and cardiopulmonary bypass or vessel clamping. In the postoperative period, valve thrombosis, left-atrial thrombi secondary to atrial fibrillation, and endocarditis are most common. Approximately 90% of patients with late-onset stroke had atrial fibrillation in one study. There was a significant difference in the stroke-free survival 15 years after valve surgery between those in normal sinus rhythm (90.7%) and those in chronic atrial fibrillation (73.8%).[9] One autopsy study of early death (between 1 and 60 days) found a 61% rate of left-atrial thrombus formation.[88] Since the ability of transesophageal echocardiography to detect atrial thrombi, and with the use of the Inoue technique,

which requires less left atrial manipulation, the incidence of systemic embolism has been lower with percutaneous mitral valvuloplasty.[35]

Methods for the prevention of neurologic complications before, during, and after the procedure have been proposed by McKhann and colleagues. The authors divide their proposed strategies into those used before, during, and after surgery. Protective methods to be used before surgery include identification of patients at high risk using established risk models and consideration of alternative surgical procedures (i.e., off-pump bypass), identification of symptomatic high grade carotid artery stenosis, and pharmacologic pretreatment of atrial fibrillation. Subsequent prospective work compared cognitive outcomes in patients with and without coronary artery disease after on-pump or off-pump bypass surgery and found that while patients with surgery had lower baseline cognitive performance and a greater degree of postoperative cognitive decline, this did not differ significantly whether they were in the on-pump or off-pump group.[87] Other intraoperative preventive strategies that may be appropriate in selected patients include the use of higher blood pressure during cardiopulmonary bypass, transfusion to keep the hematocrit greater than or equal to 30%, prevention of hyperglycemia, and use of arterial line filters. Two large studies evaluating the efficacy of thiopental loading for reducing the incidence of stroke and neuropsychologic deficits reached opposite conclusions, with Nussmeyer and colleagues reporting a decreased incidence of neurologic deficits and Zaidan and colleagues finding a higher incidence of neurologic complications in the thiopental-treated group.[71,106]

Following surgery, the clinician should prevent rewarming temperatures over 37°C, should monitor and intervene early for arrhythmias, and when stroke does occur, should implement early blood pressure intervention to minimize infarction size.[64] In patients with mechanical valves, occlusion of the left atrial appendage has been shown to be a potential alternative to warfarin in patients with atrial fibrillation who have contraindications to anticoagulation or who have had a hemorrhagic stroke.

Anticoagulation after valve surgery remains a dilemma. In general, patients with mechanical valves receive long-term anticoagulation, while patients with bioprosthetic valves receive a 3-month course of warfarin (target INR of 2.5), followed by antiplatelet therapy alone. The recommended INR value ranges for various cardiac valve replacements (i.e., bileaflet, aortic; tilting-disk, aortic; bileaflet, mitral; tilting-disk, mitral, caged-ball disk; etc.) are beyond the scope of this review. However, it is important to recognize that anticoagulation control has a dramatic and significant influence on survival after valve replacement surgery.[15]

Cerebral hematoma is rare and may be related to hematologic disturbances resulting from cardiopulmonary bypass. There may be consumption of platelets and coagulation factors, decreased platelet adhesiveness, and abnormal activation of the coagulation cascade.[4,50] Most instances of cerebral hematoma are in patients with valvular surgery after infective endocarditis. Anticoagulation-related hemorrhage is a risk with oral anticoagulant therapy in patients with valve replacements, but it is low (0.57 per 100 patient-years).[17] Spontaneous intracranial hemorrhages have been reported in patients without supra-therapeutic levels of anticoagulation following open heart surgery for valve replacement.[7,68,73]

COMPLICATIONS WITH CARDIAC SUPPORT DEVICES

The intra-aortic balloon pump (IABP) is a mechanical device that initially was used for perioperative cardiac failure; it is now also used for patients with pre-shock, severe congestive heart failure, and refractory angina. Patients who undergo insertion of intra-aortic balloon pumps can experience cerebrovascular events including ischemic stroke, transient ischemic attack (TIA), and intracranial hemorrhage, as well as peripheral nerve deficits.[38,40,42] The transthoracic route of IABP introduction may predispose to peripheral nerve deficits in the lower extremities, resulting from limb ischemia.[38] In one series of 39 patients with IABP, neurologic deficits ranged from a foot drop to almost total paralysis associated with the use of IABP. In these patients, IABP insertion was via the femoral artery; and the neurologic deficits have been hypothesized to occur secondary to obstruction to blood flow or thromboembolism in the femoral artery.[42]

Stroke has been reported to occur in 2.5% of patients with IABP.[38] Mechanisms associated with stroke in patients with IABP include thromboembolism associated with mobile atheroma in the thoracic aorta,[40] perioperatively and delayed spontaneous thromboembolism,[38] and cerebral air embolism.[22]

Ventricular assist devices are typically a bridging mechanism for patients with severe heart failure until heart transplantation; however, they can be used as permanent artificial hearts. Cerebral thromboembolism is the most common neurologic complication reported, the rate of which is varied, ranging from 3% to 47% in different series.[21,67,85,90,94] In another series of 23 patients with left ventricular assist devices (LVADs), the incidence of neurologic complications was 39%.[94] Acute intracranial hemorrhage is devastating, rapidly symptomatic, and has a high mortality in our experience (Figure 48.3).

Extracorporeal membrane oxygenation (ECMO) is an extracorporeal technique of providing both cardiac and respiratory support to patients whose heart and lungs are so severely diseased or damaged that they can no longer serve their function. CNS complications are the most serious and are primarily related to the degree of hypoxia and acidosis and to the use of anticoagulation. Neurologic complications have

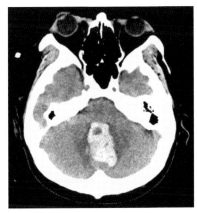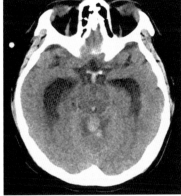

FIGURE 48.3: LVAD-associated hemorrhage in the vermis. Acute hydrocephalus with intraventricular hemorrhage after ventriculostomy was noted despite aggressive reversal of anticoagulation with platelets and PCC.

been reported to occur in up to 50% of patients undergoing treatment with ECMO, with a worse outcome observed in those having undergone cardiopulmonary resuscitation during their hospital course.[62,109] Once on ECMO, 59% died while on ECMO or within 7 days of discontinuation of ECMO.[62]

MANAGEMENT OF CARDIAC SURGERY COMPLICATIONS

Management of perioperative ischemic stroke in the setting of cardiac surgery is similar to that in other settings, except that use of intravenous rtPA is contraindicated in patients after cardiac surgery (Table 48.1).

At present, no standard treatment for ischemic stroke following cardiac catheterization exists; thus, there is variation in management strategies with intravenous or intra-arterial thrombolysis, as well as mechanical disruption interventions reported in the literature. Intra-arterial thrombolysis in pericoronary angiography has the advantage of direct visualization of the response to treatment and provides an opportunity for catheter-based mechanical clot disruption or clot retrieval. However, it has been associated with a higher rate of symptomatic intracerebral hemorrhage (14%) than that reported in clinical trials of intravenous thrombolysis (6%).[1,107]

In patients who have undergone open-heart surgery, systemic intravenous rtPA is contraindicated. While local intra-arterial thrombolysis has been used in selected patients in the postoperative period, prospective, randomized data regarding its use are limited.[66] Selected patients may undergo mechanical endovascular embolectomy using stent clot retrieval devices (Chapter 29).[91] If the etiology of cerebral infarction is presumed due to an massive air embolism, hyperbaric oxygen therapy should be administered early; the outcome may be excellent even with late treatments (5–7 total).[8]

A potential complication of cardiac surgery is postoperative bleeding, occurring up to 11% of the time. Recombinant factor VIIa (rFVIIa) has been increasingly used to control refractory hemorrhage in these cases. However, it may be associated with an increased risk of stroke in this setting. Pichon and colleagues reported a case of fatal bilateral thrombosis of the carotid arteries leading to brain death within 48 hours of administration of rFVIIa for refractory hemorrhagic shock after cardiothoracic surgery.[76]

Although the incidence of seizures remains low, clinicians should target their approach based on whether the seizures are focal or generalized, and based on a review of history and medications. Seizures can be managed acutely with benzodiazepines.

The management of cerebral hemorrhage in a patient with an LVAD is twofold. Small sulcal hemorrhages may be detected in patients with nonspecific symptoms such as presyncope or headaches[82] but rarely evolve into more robust hematomas. Also, some patients may have small layers of subdural hematomas of different age, and in both cases aggressive reversal of anticoagulation does not seem to be warranted.[102] In any other patient with an intracerebral hematoma, rapid administration of PCC (30 U/kg) and platelet infusion (2 units) may allow neurosurgical evacuation or ventriculostomy treatment. In a recent experience of 36 patients, intraparenchymal hemorrhage had the worst outcomes, with a mortality rate of 59% at one month.[103] Most of our patients with invariably large hematomas died despite aggressive management in some. Outcome may also be determined by family members deciding that this major complication should indicate finality of all aggressive care.

Conservative management remains the mainstay of therapy for peripheral nerve injury associated with cardiac procedures. Surgery is only recommended when there are coexisting complications (e.g., development of a large hematoma).

TABLE 48.1. MANAGEMENT OF POSTOPERATIVE STROKE FOLLOWING CARDIAC SURGERY

Ischemic	Obtain CTA/CTP
	Endovascular retrieval if MCA M1/M2 occlusion and large penumbra
	With large stroke avoid AC for 1–2 weeks
Hemorrhagic	Neurosurgical evacuation
	Correct INR with PCC
	Maintain INR < 1.3
	Platelet infusion if prior antiplatelet drugs
	Avoid antiplatelet agents
	Avoid AC for 1–2 weeks

CTA, computed tomography angiogram; CTP, computed tomography perfusion; M, middle cerebral artery; INR, international normalized ratio; AC, anticoagulation; PCC, prothrombin complex concentrate.

OUTCOME EXPECTATIONS

A retrospective review of 27 patients who suffered acute neurologic complications after cardiac catheterization or angioplasty found that 17 of 27 (63%) had complete resolution of neurologic deficits.[55] In a study of 23 patients with LVADs, ischemic strokes did not have a negative impact on outcome.[94] In patients who have undergone valve replacement surgery, the risk of stroke persists for the patient's lifetime. Approximately 20% of patients with heart valve prostheses have an embolic stroke within 15 years following surgery.[80] Intracranial and spinal bleeding have been reported to be 0.57 per 100 patient-years on oral anticoagulation among patients with mechanical heart valves.[17]

Seizures following cardiac surgery are typically self-limiting or easily controlled with benzodiazepines. Rarely, status epilepticus has been reported with associated findings of diffuse cerebral edema on neuroimaging.[84] Seizures are a poor prognostic indicator when they occur in patients with LVADs and are reportedly associated with 100% mortality.[94]

When visual loss occurs after cardiac surgery, the outcome is dependent on the mechanism. When the visual impairment is induced by contrast administration with normal-appearing optic nerves, the deficit is usually transient, with return of vision within 24–48 hours.[93] Visual loss due to anterior or posterior ischemic optic neuropathy following cardiac surgery is typically permanent.

Patients with delirium after cardiac surgery have a mixed outcome, which reflects the multifactorial nature of delirium. Neurocognitive decline is common after cardiac surgery, varying from 7% to 49% at 3 months and up to 33% after 1 year.[52,70,79,97] Patients with brachial or lumbosacral plexopathy following cardiac surgery can, in the majority of cases, expect full recovery with conservative management. While the severity of mononeuropathies following cardiac surgery can range from mild transient sensory neuropathy to disabling paralysis, symptoms almost always resolve completely.

COMPLICATIONS AFTER AORTIC SURGERY

Again, it remains surprising that with the major vascular repairs the incidence of paraplegia—at least in large experienced centers—is around 4%. It is the same reported incidence after carotid endarterectomy and stenting. There is some variability, with some centers reporting significantly higher numbers (10%–20%), but this can be explained by the heterogeneity of most reported surgical series.

Despite the low incidence, the handicap is devastating, and efforts should be in place to prevent ischemia of the spinal cord and brain.

There are emerging data on the best approach to prevent spinal cord injury after open or endovascular surgery.[41,81,96] Spinal cord injury may be present immediately or, more rarely, may emerge later.[69]

Spinal cord injury in aortic dissection is another precipitating vascular catastrophe, but whether or not paraplegia occurs is not related to the extent of intercostal artery involvement in the field of the dissection. A much more likely mechanism is hypoperfusion of the spinal cord associated with profound shock. Cardiogenic shock from aortic dissection is due to severe aortic regurgitation and cardiac tamponade with hemopericardium. Syncope is relatively common in aortic dissection and may be related to acute hypotension caused by cardiac tamponade or aortic rupture, cerebral vessel obstruction, or damage to the carotid baroreceptors. Outcome of paraplegia after dissection of the aorta is similarly poor. The reported incidences of spinal cord ischemia according to Crawford classification depends on surgical—open or endovascular—approach (Table 48.2).[26,81]

The vascularization of the spinal cord is described in Capsule 48.2. Initial assessment should involve determination of a complete spinal cord infarction, which involves the entire spinal cord. Involvement of the corticospinal, pyramidal, and spinothalamic tract and anterior horns results in flaccid paraplegia; and with absent pin prick, hot and cold sensation, but sparing of light touch and position sense, there is a reduced sensation to the level of the nipples at T4. There is a common loss of rectal sphincter tone. Paraplegia of the flaccid type may occur; but there may be paraplegia in extension of flexion, and this is often seen in partial lesions. When the spinal shock phase passes, the bladder is dysfunctional, and retention occurs, leading to renal failure with rising creatinine and prevented by immediate catheterization (more details are found in Chapter 9).

TABLE 48.2. INCIDENCE OF PARAPLEGIA

Crawford Classification	Incidence (Open Surgery)	Incidence (Endovascular)
I	7%	10%
II	24%	10%
III	22%	19%
IV	13%	5%
V	2%	3%

The blood supply to the spinal cord is provided by intercostal or lumbar arterial branches that give rise to anterior and posterior radicular arteries. These arteries branch to three longitudinal arterial trunks, the anterior spinal artery and both posterior spinal arteries, which regulate the blood supply to the entire spinal cord. The anterior spinal artery supplies approximately 75% of the blood to the cord. From this major contributing artery, sets of arteries pass through the central sulcus to the middle part of the cord. Each so-called sulcal artery supplies one side of the cord and provides flow to the gray matter, which harbors the cells of the origin of the ventral root fibers, preganglionic cells for the autonomic nervous system, and incoming posterior horn fibers.

In the longitudinal plane, a fairly consistent pattern of vascularization has been recognized. Three major segments of arterial organization of the spinal cord have been defined, but anatomical variations at various levels are the rule. The cervicothoracic territory includes the cervical cord and the first two or three thoracic segments. The anterior spinal artery and posterior spinal arteries are branches of the vertebral arteries and costocervical trunk. Below the T3 level, the intercostal arteries from the aorta supply the thoracic segments and are highly variable in number. The thoracolumbar territory derives its supply from the arteria radicularis magna or artery of Adamkiewicz, which typically originates between T5 and L2 but varies in its origin and in 75% of cases is identified between T9 and T12, in 15% between T5 and T8, and in 10% between L1 and L2. The terminal portions of the spinal cord and cauda equina depend on branches from the internal iliac or middle sacral artery (see accompanying figure).

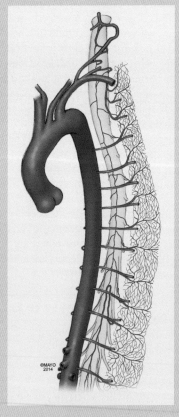

Vascular supply of the spinal cord.

TABLE 48.3. ACUTE SPINAL CORD ISCHEMIA

CSF diversion (lumbar drainage)

Aim at ICP 8–12 mm Hg

Increase MAP 10 mm Hg every 5 minutes until improvement of MAP of 130 mm Hg reached

MRI spine for epidural hematoma or assessment for ischemia

Maintain MAP for 2 days and wean and remove lumbar drain

See references 10 and 11.

MANAGEMENT OF COMPLICATIONS AFTER AORTIC SURGERY

Albeit with no proof of efficacy, many patients with a acute ischemic spinal cord injury will be treated with lumbar spinal drainage because it has a good physiologic underpinning.[10,39,49,51,105] A normal or limited infarction on MRI DWI of the spine may predict success of this intervention, and we have seen no change with multilevel spinal cord infarction. Lumbar drainage will reduce the intraspinal pressure and improve perfusion. Most of the time, the goal of CSF drainage is to maintain a spinal pressure of less than 10 mm Hg. Many institutions recommend a maximal drainage of 20 cc per hour. Drainage is continued for 24–48 hours, followed by clamping; and if the patient is asymptomatic or unchanged, the lumbar drain will be removed. Very few complications are seen with CSF drainage, but there have been incidental cases of subdural hematomas, meningitis, and spinal hematomas. Catheter-related morbidity is low—in the order of 4%. Delayed spinal cord injury is rare and more likely is delayed discovery. Nonetheless, convincing cases have been published; and systemic hypotension has frequently been implicated because some patients improve after improving blood pressure. Additional use of 1 gram of methylprednisolone has been recommended, but there are insufficient data to consider it standard of care.[11,33,78,109] Treatment is summarized in Table 48.3.

CONCLUSIONS

- Neurologic complications of cardiac and vascular surgery are not rare and remain an important cause of morbidity and mortality.
- Best evaluation of these complications requires a stat consult to the neurologist or neurosurgeon by the cardiac team.
- Spinal cord injury may be successfully treated with CSF diversion using a lumbar drain, but only if MRI of the entire spine is normal.

REFERENCES

1. Tissue plasminogen activator for acute ischemic stroke. The National Institute of Neurological Disorders and Stroke rt-PA Stroke Study Group. *N Engl J Med* 1995;333:1581–1587.
2. Abdul Aziz KA, Meduoye A. Is pH-stat or alpha-stat the best technique to follow in patients undergoing deep hypothermic circulatory arrest? *Interact Cardiovasc Thorac Surg* 2010;10:271–282.
3. Abend NS, Levine JM. Hypodense middle cerebral artery with fat embolus. *Neurocrit Care* 2007;6:147–148.
4. Addonizio VP, Jr., Smith JB, Strauss JF, 3rd, Colman RW, Edmunds LH, Jr. Thromboxane synthesis and platelet secretion during cardiopulmonary bypass with bubble oxygenator. *J Thorac Cardiovasc Surg* 1980;79:91–96.
5. Aggarwal A, Dai D, Rumsfeld JS, Klein LW, Roe MT. Incidence and predictors of stroke associated with percutaneous coronary intervention. *Am J Cardiol* 2009;104:349–353.
6. Akins CW. Results with mechanical cardiac valvular prostheses. *Ann Thorac Surg* 1995;60:1836–1844.
7. Aoyagi S, Kosuga T, Fukunaga S, Tayama E, Ueda T. Subdural hematoma after open-heart surgery. *J Heart Valve Dis* 2007;16:450–453.
8. Armon C, Deschamps C, Adkinson C, Fealey RD, Orszulak TA. Hyperbaric treatment of cerebral air embolism sustained during an open-heart surgical procedure. *Mayo Clinic Proc* 1991;66:565–571.
9. Bando K, Kobayashi J, Hirata M, et al. Early and late stroke after mitral valve replacement with a mechanical prosthesis: risk factor analysis of a 24-year experience. *J Thorac Cardiovasc Surg* 2003;126:358–364.
10. Bilal H, O'Neill B, Mahmood S, Waterworth P. Is cerebrospinal fluid drainage of benefit to neuroprotection in patients undergoing surgery on the descending thoracic aorta or thoracoabdominal aorta? *Interact Cardiovasc Thorac Surg* 2012;15:702–708.
11. Blacker DJ, Wijdicks EFM, Ramakrishna G. Resolution of severe paraplegia due to aortic dissection after CSF drainage. *Neurology* 2003;61:142–143.
12. Bloomfield P, Wheatley DJ, Prescott RJ, Miller HC. Twelve-year comparison of a Bjork-Shiley mechanical heart valve with porcine bioprostheses. *N Engl J Med* 1991;324:573–579.

13. Brown DL, Topol EJ. Stroke complicating percutaneous coronary revascularization. *Am J Cardiol* 1993;72:1207–1209.

14. Busing KA, Schulte-Sasse C, Fluchter S, et al. Cerebral infarction: incidence and risk factors after diagnostic and interventional cardiac catheterization—prospective evaluation at diffusion-weighted MR imaging. *Radiology* 2005;235:177–183.

15. Butchart EG, Payne N, Li HH, et al. Better anticoagulation control improves survival after valve replacement. *J Thorac Cardiovasc Surg* 2002;123:715–723.

16. Canbaz S, Turgut N, Halici U, et al. Brachial plexus injury during open heart surgery: controlled prospective study. *Thorac Cardiovasc Surg* 2005;53:295–299.

17. Cannegieter SC, Rosendaal FR, Wintzen AR, et al. Optimal oral anticoagulant therapy in patients with mechanical heart valves. *N Engl J Med* 1995;333:11–17.

18. Caswell J, O'Brien B, Schneck M. Risk of stroke following valve replacement surgery. *Seminars in Cerebrovascular Diseases and Stroke* 2003;3:214–218.

19. Cho L. Cerebrovascular complications in interventional cardiology. *Semin Cerebrovasc Dis Stroke* 2003;3:228–232.

20. Cline SL, Kalaria VG, Von Der Lohe E, Breall JA. Cerebrovascular complications of cardiac catheterization. *Semin Cerebrovasc Dis Stroke* 2003;3:194–199.

21. Copeland JG, Smith RG, Arabia FA, et al. Total artificial heart bridge to transplantation: a 9-year experience with 62 patients. *J Heart Lung Transplant* 2004;23:823–831.

22. Cruz-Flores S, Diamond AL, Leira EC. Cerebral air embolism secondary to intra-aortic balloon pump rupture. *Neurocrit Care* 2005;2:49–50.

23. Dimopoulou I, Daganou M, Dafni U, et al. Phrenic nerve dysfunction after cardiac operations: electrophysiologic evaluation of risk factors. *Chest* 1998;113:8–14.

24. Djaiani G, Ali M, Borger MA, et al. Epiaortic scanning modifies planned intraoperative surgical management but not cerebral embolic load during coronary artery bypass surgery. *Anesth Analg* 2008;106:1611–1618.

25. Dukkipati S, O'Neill WW, Harjai KJ, et al. Characteristics of cerebrovascular accidents after percutaneous coronary interventions. *J Am Coll Cardiol* 2004;43:1161–1167.

26. Etz DC, Luehr M, Aspern KV, et al. Spinal cord ischemia in open and endovascular thoracoabdominal aortic aneurysm repair: new concepts. *J Cardiovasc Surg (Torino)* 2014;55:159–168.

27. Fleck JD, Biller J. Cerebrovascular complications of cardiovascular interventions: coronary artery bypass graft procedures. *Semin Cerebrovasc Dis Stroke* 2003;3:207–213.

28. Fleck JD, O'Donnell JA, Biller J. Cardiac evaluation of patient with carotid artery stenosis and treatment strategies for coexisting disease. In: Loftus CM, Kresowik TF, eds. *Carotid Artery Surgery*. New York: Thieme Medical Publishers; 2000:121–129.

29. Floyd TF, Shah PN, Price CC, et al. Clinically silent cerebral ischemic events after cardiac surgery: their incidence, regional vascular occurrence, and procedural dependence. *Ann Thorac Surg* 2006;81:2160–2166.

30. Fuchs S, Stabile E, Kinnaird TD, et al. Stroke complicating percutaneous coronary interventions: incidence, predictors, and prognostic implications. *Circulation* 2002;106:86–91.

31. Gelman S. The pathophysiology of aortic cross-clamping and unclamping. *Anesthesiology* 1995;82:1026–1060.

32. Goldsmith I, Lip GY, Kaukuntla H, Patel RL. Hospital morbidity and mortality and changes in quality of life following mitral valve surgery in the elderly. *J Heart Valve Dis* 1999;8:702–707.

33. Goldstein LJ, Rezayat C, Shrikhande GV, Bush HL, Jr. Delayed permanent paraplegia after endovascular repair of abdominal aortic aneurysm. *J Vasc Surg* 2010;51:725–728.

34. Gootjes EC, Wijdicks EFM, McClelland RL. Postoperative stupor and coma. *Mayo Clinic Proc* 2005;80:350–354.

35. Guerios EE, Bueno R, Nercolini D, et al. Mitral stenosis and percutaneous mitral valvuloplasty (part 1). *J Invasive Cardiol* 2005;17:382–386.

36. Hammermeister KE, Sethi GK, Henderson WG, et al. A comparison of outcomes in men 11 years after heart-valve replacement with a mechanical valve or bioprosthesis. Veterans Affairs Cooperative Study on Valvular Heart Disease. *N Engl J Med* 1993;328:1289–1296.

37. Hamon M, Burzotta F, Oppenheim C, Morello R, Viader F. Silent cerebral infarct after cardiac catheterization as detected by diffusion weighted magnetic resonance imaging: a randomized comparison of radial and femoral arterial approaches. *Trials* 2007;8:15.

38. Hazelrigg SR, Auer JE, Seifert PE. Experience in 100 transthoracic balloon pumps. *Ann Thorac Surg* 1992;54:528–532.

39. Hnath JC, Mehta M, Taggert JB, et al. Strategies to improve spinal cord ischemia in endovascular thoracic aortic repair: outcomes of a prospective cerebrospinal fluid drainage protocol. *J Vasc Surg* 2008;48:836–840.

40. Ho AC, Hong CL, Yang MW, Lu PP, Lin PJ. Stroke after intraaortic balloon counterpulsation

associated with mobile atheroma in thoracic aorta diagnosed using transesophageal echocardiography. *Chang Gung Med J* 2002;25:612–616.

41. Hogendoorn W, Schlosser FJ, Muhs BE, Popescu WM. Surgical and anesthetic considerations for the endovascular treatment of ruptured descending thoracic aortic aneurysms. *Curr Opin Anaesthesiol* 2014;27:12–20.

42. Honet JC, Wajszczuk WJ, Rubenfire M, Kantrowitz A, Raikes JA. Neurological abnormalities in the leg(s) after use of intraaortic balloon pump: report of six cases. *Arch Phys Med Rehabil* 1975;56:346–352.

43. Horstkotte D, Schart RE, Schultheiss HP. Intracardiac thrombosis: patient-related and device-related factors. *J Heart Valve Dis* 1995;4:114–120.

44. Hunter GR, Young GB. Seizures after cardiac surgery. *J Cardiothorac Vasc Anesth* 2011;25:299–305.

45. Hupperts R, Wetzelaer W, Heuts-van Raak L, Lodder J. Is haemodynamical compromise a specific cause of border zone brain infarcts following cardiac surgery? *Eur Neurol* 1995;35:276–280.

46. Jackson JL, Meyer GS, Pettit T. Complications from cardiac catheterization: analysis of a military database. *Mil Med* 2000;165:298–301.

47. Karsli B, Cubukcu S. An unusual cause of meralgia paresthetica. *Pain Clinic* 2005;17:221–224.

48. Katz MG, Katz R, Schachner A, Cohen AJ. Phrenic nerve injury after coronary artery bypass grafting: will it go away? *Ann Thorac Surg* 1998;65:32–35.

49. Keith CJ, Jr, Passman MA, Carignan MJ, et al. Protocol implementation of selective postoperative lumbar spinal drainage after thoracic aortic endograft. *J Vasc Surg* 2012;55:1–8.

50. Kestin AS, Valeri CR, Khuri SF, et al. The platelet function defect of cardiopulmonary bypass. *Blood* 1993;82:107–117.

51. Khan SN, Stansby G. Cerebrospinal fluid drainage for thoracic and thoracoabdominal aortic aneurysm surgery. *Cochrane Database Syst Rev* 2012;10:CD003635.

52. Knipp SC, Matatko N, Schlamann M, et al. Small ischemic brain lesions after cardiac valve replacement detected by diffusion-weighted magnetic resonance imaging: relation to neurocognitive function. *Eur J Cardiothorac Surg* 2005;28:88–96.

53. Kuruvilla A, Kuruttukulam G, Francis B. Femoral neuropathy following cardiac catheterization for balloon mitral valvotomy. *Int J Cardiol* 1999;71:197–198.

54. Kvidal P, Bergstrom R, Malm T, Stahle E. Long-term follow-up of morbidity and mortality after aortic valve replacement with a mechanical valve prosthesis. *Eur Heart J* 2000;21:1099–1111.

55. Lazar JM, Uretsky BF, Denys BG, et al. Predisposing risk factors and natural history of acute neurologic complications of left-sided cardiac catheterization. *Am J Cardiol* 1995;75:1056–1060.

56. Libman RB, Wirkowski E, Neystat M, et al. Stroke associated with cardiac surgery: determinants, timing, and stroke subtypes. *Arch Neurol* 1997;54:83–87.

57. Likosky DS, Marrin CA, Caplan LR, et al. Determination of etiologic mechanisms of strokes secondary to coronary artery bypass graft surgery. *Stroke* 2003;34:2830–2834.

58. Liu XY, Wong V, Leung M. Neurologic complications due to catheterization. *Pediatr Neurol* 2001;24:270–275.

59. Lund C, Nes RB, Ugelstad TP, et al. Cerebral emboli during left heart catheterization may cause acute brain injury. *Eur Heart J* 2005;26:1269–1275.

60. Macdonald RL, Kowalczuk A, Johns L. Emboli enter penetrating arteries of monkey brain in relation to their size. *Stroke* 1995;26:1247–1250.

61. Mack MJ, Brown PP, Kugelmass AD, et al. Current status and outcomes of coronary revascularization 1999 to 2002: 148,396 surgical and percutaneous procedures. *Ann Thorac Surg* 2004;77:761–766.

62. Mateen FJ, Muralidharan R, Shinohara RT, et al. Neurological injury in adults treated with extracorporeal membrane oxygenation. *Arch Neurol* 2011;68:1543–1549.

63. McDonagh DL, Berger M, Mathew JP, et al. Neurological complications of cardiac surgery. *Lancet Neurol* 2014;13:490–502.

64. McKhann GM, Grega MA, Borowicz LM, Jr., Baumgartner WA, Selnes OA. Stroke and encephalopathy after cardiac surgery: an update. *Stroke* 2006;37:562–571.

65. Mehta R, Lee KJ, Chaturvedi R, Benson L. Complications of pediatric cardiac catheterization: a review in the current era. *Catheter Cardiovasc Interv* 2008;72:278–285.

66. Mullen MT, McGarvey ML, Kasner SE. Safety and efficacy of thrombolytic therapy in postoperative cerebral infarctions. *Neurol Clin* 2006;24:783–793.

67. Nabavi DG, Georgiadis D, Mumme T, et al. Clinical relevance of intracranial microembolic signals in patients with left ventricular assist devices: a prospective study. *Stroke* 1996;27:891–896.

68. Nakajima M, Tsuchiya K, Kanemaru K, et al. Subdural hemorrhagic injury after open heart surgery. *Ann Thorac Surg* 2003;76:614–615.

69. Nasr B, Schneider F, Marques da Fonseca P, Gouny P. Cholesterol crystal embolism and

delayed-onset paraplegia after thoracoabdominal aneurysm repair. *Ann Vasc Surg* 2014;28:1320 e1321–1323.

70. Newman MF, Kirchner JL, Phillips-Bute B, et al. Longitudinal assessment of neurocognitive function after coronary-artery bypass surgery. *N Engl J Med* 2001;344:395–402.

71. Nussmeier NA, Arlund C, Slogoff S. Neuropsychiatric complications after cardiopulmonary bypass: cerebral protection by a barbiturate. *Anesthesiology* 1986;64:165–170.

72. Nuttall GA, Garrity JA, Dearani JA, et al. Risk factors for ischemic optic neuropathy after cardiopulmonary bypass: a matched case/control study. *Anesth Analg* 2001;93:1410–1416, table of contents.

73. Oka K, Kamota T, Satou M, et al. [Subdural hematoma following cardiac surgery]. *Kyobu Geka* 2008;61:868–872.

74. Ozcakar L, Dincer F, Atalay A, et al. Compressive injury of the brachial plexus after axillary arteriography and its further consequences. *Joint Bone Spine* 2004;71:349–351.

75. Piatt JH, Jr. Massive intracerebral hemorrhage complicating cardiac catheterization with ergonovine administration. *Stroke* 1984;15:904–907.

76. Pichon N, Bellec F, Sekkal S, et al. Fatal thrombotic event after infusion of recombinant activated factor VII after cardiac surgery. *J Thorac Cardiovasc Surg* 2008;136:220–221.

77. Rama BN, Pagano TV, DelCore M, Knobel KR, Lee J. Cortical blindness after cardiac catheterization: effect of rechallenge with dye. *Cathet Cardiovasc Diagn* 1993;28:149–151.

78. Riess KP, Gundersen SB, 3rd, Ziegelbein KJ. Delayed neurologic deficit after infrarenal endovascular aortic aneurysm repair. *Am Surg* 2007;73:385–387.

79. Roach GW, Kanchuger M, Mangano CM, et al. Adverse cerebral outcomes after coronary bypass surgery. Multicenter Study of Perioperative Ischemia Research Group and the Ischemia Research and Education Foundation Investigators. *N Engl J Med* 1996;335:1857–1863.

80. Ruel M, Masters RG, Rubens FD, et al. Late incidence and determinants of stroke after aortic and mitral valve replacement. *Ann Thorac Surg* 2004;78:77–83.

81. Sadek M, Abjigitova D, Pellet Y, et al. Operative outcomes after open repair of descending thoracic aortic aneurysms in the era of endovascular surgery. *Ann Thorac Surg* 2014;97:1562–1567.

82. Sakaguchi M, Kitagawa K, Okazaki S, et al. Sulcus subarachnoid hemorrhage is a common stroke subtype in patients with implanted left ventricular assist devices. *Eur J Neurol* 2015; 22:1088–1093.

83. Sankaranarayanan R, Msairi A, Davis GK. Stroke complicating cardiac catheterization: a preventable and treatable complication. *J Invasive Cardiol* 2007;19:40–45.

84. Sansone V, Piazza L, Butera G, Meola G, Fontana A. Contrast-induced seizures after cardiac catheterization in a 6-year-old child. *Pediatr Neurol* 2007;36:268–270.

85. Schmid C, Weyand M, Nabavi DG, et al. Cerebral and systemic embolization during left ventricular support with the Novacor N100 device. *Ann Thorac Surg* 1998;65:1703–1710.

86. Segal AZ, Abernethy WB, Palacios IF, BeLue R, Rordorf G. Stroke as a complication of cardiac catheterization: risk factors and clinical features. *Neurology* 2001;56:975–977.

87. Selnes OA, Grega MA, Bailey MM, et al. Do management strategies for coronary artery disease influence 6-year cognitive outcomes? *Ann Thorac Surg* 2009;88:445–454.

88. Shachar GB, Vlodaver Z, Joyce LD, Edwards JE. Mural thrombosis of the left atrium following replacement of the mitral valve. *J Thorac Cardiovasc Surg* 1981;82:595–600.

89. Sharma AD, Parmley CL, Sreeram G, Grocott HP. Peripheral nerve injuries during cardiac surgery: risk factors, diagnosis, prognosis, and prevention. *Anesth Analg* 2000;91:1358–1369.

90. Slater JP, Rose EA, Levin HR, et al. Low thromboembolic risk without anticoagulation using advanced-design left ventricular assist devices. *Ann Thorac Surg* 1996;62:1321–1327.

91. Smith WS, Sung G, Starkman S, et al. Safety and efficacy of mechanical embolectomy in acute ischemic stroke: results of the MERCI trial. *Stroke* 2005;36:1432–1438.

92. Stamou SC. Stroke and encephalopathy after cardiac surgery: the search for the holy grail. *Stroke* 2006;37:284–285.

93. Sticherling C, Berkefeld J, Auch-Schwelk W, Lanfermann H. Transient bilateral cortical blindness after coronary angiography. *Lancet* 1998;351:570.

94. Thomas CE, Jichici D, Petrucci R, Urrutia VC, Schwartzman RJ. Neurologic complications of the Novacor left ventricular assist device. *Ann Thorac Surg* 2001;72:1311–1315.

95. Thourani VH, Weintraub WS, Guyton RA, et al. Outcomes and long-term survival for patients undergoing mitral valve repair versus replacement: effect of age and concomitant coronary artery bypass grafting. *Circulation* 2003;108:298–304.

96. Ullery BW, Cheung AT, Fairman RM, et al. Risk factors, outcomes, and clinical manifestations of spinal cord ischemia following thoracic endovascular aortic repair. *J Vasc Surg* 2011;54:677–684.

97. van Dijk D, Nierich AP, Jansen EW, et al. Early outcome after off-pump versus on-pump coronary bypass surgery: results from a randomized study. *Circulation* 2001;104:1761–1766.

98. Vazquez-Jimenez JF, Krebs G, Schiefer J, et al. Injury of the common peroneal nerve after cardiothoracic operations. *Ann Thorac Surg* 2002;73:119–122.

99. Weissman BM, Aram DM, Levinsohn MW, Ben-Shachar G. Neurologic sequelae of cardiac catheterization. *Cathet Cardiovasc Diagn* 1985;11:577–583.

100. Wijdicks EFM. Neurologic complications of cardiac surgery. In: *Neurologic Complications of Critical Illness*. 3rd ed. New York: Oxford University Press; 2009.

101. Wijman CA, Kase CS, Jacobs AK, Whitehead RE. Cerebral air embolism as a cause of stroke during cardiac catheterization. *Neurology* 1998;51:318–319.

102. Willey JZ, Demmer RT, Takayama H, Colombo PC, Lazar RM. Cerebrovascular disease in the era of left ventricular assist devices with continuous flow: risk factors, diagnosis, and treatment. *J Heart Lung Transplant* 2014;33:878–887.

103. Wilson TJ, Stetler WR, Jr., Al-Holou WN, Sullivan SE, Fletcher JJ. Management of intracranial hemorrhage in patients with left ventricular assist devices. *J Neurosurg* 2013;118:1063–1068.

104. Wolman RL, Nussmeier NA, Aggarwal A, et al. Cerebral injury after cardiac surgery: identification of a group at extraordinary risk. Multicenter Study of Perioperative Ischemia Research Group (McSPI) and the Ischemia Research Education Foundation (IREF) Investigators. *Stroke* 1999;30:514–522.

105. Wong CS, Healy D, Canning C, et al. A systematic review of spinal cord injury and cerebrospinal fluid drainage after thoracic aortic endografting. *J Vasc Surg* 2012;56:1438–1447.

106. Zaidan JR, Klochany A, Martin WM, et al. Effect of thiopental on neurologic outcome following coronary artery bypass grafting. *Anesthesiology* 1991;74:406–411.

107. Zaidat OO, Slivka AP, Mohammad Y, et al. Intra-arterial thrombolytic therapy in pericoronary angiography ischemic stroke. *Stroke* 2005;36:1089–1090.

108. Zimpfer D, Kilo J, Czerny M, et al. Neurocognitive deficit following aortic valve replacement with biological/mechanical prosthesis. *Eur J Cardiothorac Surg* 2003;23:544–551.

109. Zwischenberger JB, Nguyen TT, Upp JR, Jr, et al. Complications of neonatal extracorporeal membrane oxygenation. Collective experience from the Extracorporeal Life Support Organization. *J Thorac Cardiovasc Surg* 1994;107:838–848.

49

Neurology of Resuscitation Medicine

Well over 100,000 patients a year in the United States are admitted to intensive care units with anoxic–ischemic brain injury after cardiopulmonary resuscitation.[46] Although the pathophysiology of brain injury caused by cardiac arrest is reasonably well understood, less is known about effectively ameliorating the sometimes genuine onslaught of the anoxic–ischemic injury. For over a decade, there has been enthusiasm that modest induced hypothermia (33°–34°C) could not only improve survival rates but also improve neurological outcomes,[10] but this has recently been questioned.[41]

Neurologists (and particularly neurointensivists, as this book obviously argues) are in the best position to evaluate a comatose survivor after successful resuscitation for a cardiac or respiratory arrest. Early data on prognostication have been extracted from serial neurologic examinations by neurologists participating in and organizing prospective cohorts.[16,21–24,34,69,71] More recent data have been compiled from examinations done by general intensivists which could suggest a possible gap in accuracy.

The additional value of a neurointensivist is multifold: (1) comprehensive neurologic examination beyond the Glasgow Coma Score;[42,59] (2) assessment of seizures (or mimickers) and EEG patterns; (3) detailed reading of neuroimaging; (4) judging confounders on neurologic examination; and (5) discounting a prevailing notion that all prediction becomes self-fullfilling. Any global anoxic–ischemic injury to the brain is acutely profound, and more than 70% of patients die or remain comatose 24 hours after cardiopulmonary resuscitation (CPR);[49,76] but it is also important to avoid a misleading impression that recovery is not possible. Most patients are admitted after out-of-hospital cardiac arrest and, in many, documentation of rhythm disturbance is available. Other situations—not to be dismissed as insignificant—are cardiac or respiratory arrest associated with traumatic brain injury and poor grade subarachnoid hemorrhage. These dual injuries to the brain are more difficult to evaluate and may require magnetic resonance imaging (MRI).

This chapter critically evaluates the current knowledge of anoxic–ischemic brain injury after cardiopulmonary arrest. Studies have reported tools for predicting outcomes, and guidelines for the prediction of poor outcome have been developed by the American Academy of Neurology.[71] These predictors may have changed after the use of therapeutic hypothermia, and other predictors may have emerged. The topic of prognostication after targetted temperature management is a subject of ongoing investigations.

PATHOPHYSIOLOGICAL CONCEPTS

Anoxia describes the complete lack of oxygen delivery (e.g., during the cessation of blood flow due to cardiac arrest) while in contrast; hypoxia describes what may occur during times of decreased oxygen delivery but with some degree of continued flow. Hypoxic-ischemic brain injury—albeit less well defined and less clearly understood than anoxic–ischemic injury from cardiac arrest—can occur in patients with respiratory arrest or severe hypoxemia (e.g., asphyxia) and shock. Success of intervention in these conditions may be predicated on the early correction of hypoxemia and hypovolemia. The time interval until correction may be less important than the initial severity of the abnormality (Capsule 49.1).

One of the more vital questions for neuroscientists and clinicians is whether there is a specific period during which interventions can modify the degree of anoxic–ischemic brain injury and thus improve clinical outcomes. Is the damage to the brain permanent and present at ictus, or are there processes at work that could potentially be influenced and modulated? Several clinical facts are important. First, with cardiac arrest, whether due to asystole or ventricular fibrillation, there is no measurable flow to the brain. Moreover, even with standard CPR techniques, only one-third of the

---

CAPSULE 49.1   **NEURONAL DESTRUCTION FROM ANOXIC-ISCHEMIC INJURY**

After 2–4 minutes of anoxia, several biochemical mechanisms that result in irreversible neuronal damage become operative. Selective neuronal vulnerability to this type of injury involves areas in the hippocampus, the CA-1 sector, the thalami, the neocortex, and the cerebellar Purkinje cells. Necrosis of the cortex involves layers three, four, and five and is pathologically known as laminar necrosis. The vulnerability of these areas may be explained by the presence of receptors for excitatory neurotransmitters or the high metabolic demands of these neurons. The cell death cascade that involves several modulatory and degradation signals has been documented in global cerebral ischemia.[43] A caspase inhibitor did not affect neurological outcome after cardiopulmonary arrest in rats.[63]

Neuronal and glial damage may be due to excitatory brain injury. Glutamate efflux due to ischemic injury increases intracellular calcium concentration, and the excess release of calcium leads to the activation of catabolic enzymes and endonucleases. Glutamate excitotoxicity has remained the major hypothesis to explain the neuronal injury. Moreover, after resumption of circulation, there are major microcirculatory reperfusion deficits. Coagulation may occur within these reperfusion zones, with intravascular fibrin formation and microthrombosis; this concept is currently an incentive for experimental studies using recombinant tissue-type plasminogen activator (tPA).[17,26] Also, the use of hypertonic-hyperoncotic solutions improved these perfusion deficits.

---

pre-arrest cerebral blood flow can be attained.[37] In addition, the shockable rhythms (ventricular tachycardia and ventricular fibrillation) have a better outcome than "nonshockable" rhythms such as asystole, bradyarrhythmias or pulseless electrical activity (PEA). There might be a critical time period after which CPR may fail to restore neuronal function. This time interval is poorly defined; but we know that the neuronal oxygen stores are depleted within 20 seconds of cardiac arrest, and cerebral necrosis occurs as a result of ischemia. There is some uncertainty about whether hypoxemia alone could produce necrosis; although it certainly can cause damage (preferentially in the striatum), necrosis is rarely seen, even in patients with arterial PO_2 values less than 20 mm Hg.

CLINICAL EXAMINATION OF THE COMATOSE SURVIVOR

Early awakening after CPR, clinical signs that indicate localization of the pain stimuli, and following simple commands are indicators of a good outcome. However, the current clinical experience provides no criteria by which a good outcome can be reliably predicted. Most studies have specifically concentrated on identifying indicators of a poor outcome. An estimated 25% of patients remain comatose in the first 24 hours. In the pre-induced hypothermia era, the mortality rate in patients who have been resuscitated following cardiopulmonary arrest approaches 80%–90% when they have not awakened within the first 24 hours.[76]

Clinical neurological examination follows a standard procedure, with examination of the brainstem reflexes, motor response to pain, specific attention to myoclonus, and careful judgment of spontaneous or provoked eye movement abnormalities. Because the brainstem is far more resilient to anoxic–ischemic injury than the cortex, brainstem reflexes, including the pupillary reflex to light, are often normal. Absent pupil responses can be caused by a high dose of intravenous atropine used during resuscitation, although a pupil response can often still be found when examined under the magnifying glass. Fixed, dilated pupils presenting 6 hours after resuscitation are a sign of poor prognosis, but this is rarely present in isolation and is usually an indication that the brainstem has also been involved in the anoxic–ischemic injury. Corneal reflexes have been absent in about a third of patients, but they often reappear soon.

More important is the presence of eye movement abnormalities.[72] Sustained upward gaze is often indicative of a significant global bihemispheric injury which may include the thalamus. A proposed mechanism explaining this phenomenon is a complete disinhibition of the vestibulo-ocular reflexes from the ischemic cerebellar flocculus.[39] While forced upgaze is usually associated with poor outcomes, some found still compatible with survival in about 10% of cases.[18] In many patients, downward gaze can be elicited using rapid head shaking while attempting to elicit a vestibular ocular response.[29] Other eye abnormalities, including ping-pong gaze or periodic lateral gaze deviations, have not been specifically examined for their prognostic value[15] and probably are not very valuable as absolute prognosticators. Continuous blinking is often a common finding in comatose patients, although its anatomical substrate is unknown.

An important clinical sign is myoclonus status, defined as continuous and vigorous jerking movements involving facial muscles, limbs, and abdominal muscles.[65,75] These jerks can often be elicited or aggravated by touch or hand clap. Myoclonus may also involve the diaphragm, which complicates ventilation. Myoclonus status is a clinical sign which indicates a very poor prognosis. This sustained, diffuse, vigorous myoclonus should not be confused with occasional myoclonic jerks (which may not be predictive).[60] A high percentage of these patients have a burst suppression pattern on electroencephalogram (EEG) and computed tomography (CT), with early diffuse cerebral edema. Myoclonus status can be associated with frequent seizures on EEG and often on a suppressed background with no reactivity. This myoclonus status epilepticus is not neccessarily different in outcome from myoclonus status proper and there is no proof antiepileptic drugs would help the patient.

The motor response to pain should be classified and described as absent to pain, extensor response, pathological flexion response, withdrawal to pain, or localization. Lack of motor response to nail bed compression at the initial assessment does not necessarily predict poor outcome. It may represent the "man-in-the-barrel" syndrome that occurs after bilateral border-zone infarction in the anterior and middle cerebral watershed regions. Involvement in this territory will result in prolonged weakness of the arms with normal findings in the lower limbs. The outcome in these patients is often better than that for other patients with more global cortical ischemic–anoxic injury.

TABLE 49.1. CLINICAL SYNDROMES AFTER POSTANOXIC-ISCHEMIC ENCEPHALOPATHY

Clinical Syndrome	Mechanism	Outcome
"Man-in-the-barrel" syndrome	Bilateral watershed infarcts	Uncertain, may improve substantially
Parkinsonism	Infarcts in the striatum	Improvement possible
Action myoclonus	Cerebellar infarcts	In awake patients, could improve with medication

Awakening from coma can be protracted and prolonged, although the vast majority of patients awaken within the first 48 hours. In our series of patients, 94 of 101 patients with postanoxic-ischemic injury awoke within 3 days after cardiac arrest, and induced hypothermia did not seem to directly influence this.[19] However, awakening can occur even 3 months after onset, although rarely without a severe deficit such as an amnesic syndrome or other neurological findings (Table 49.1).

The neurological examination can be confounded by an additional systemic injury associated with CPR. Several patients may have an associated acute renal failure or liver injury. In addition, medications may have been administered to counter pain or to facilitate mechanical ventilation. Often patients have been treated with fentanyl and lorazepam, both of which have long elimination half-lives (Table 49.2). The use

TABLE 49.2. CONCERNS WHEN EVALUATING PATIENTS TREATED WITH HYPOTHERMIA

- Potentially confounded neurologic examination because hypothermia necessitates sedatives, neuromuscular blockers, and analgesics Motor response and corneal reflexes may not be reliable as early as day 3
- Decreased metabolism and clearance of sedative and analgesic medications related to hypothermia effects and kidney/liver injury
- Metabolic abnormalities and systemic shock
- Nonconvulsive seizures are possible during rewarming and require EEG for detection. Treatment is uncertain.

of therapeutic hypothermia may further prolong medication clearing in addition to abnormal hepatic metabolism and renal clearance.[47,57,58]

MANAGEMENT

The optimal management of anoxic–ischemic injury is unclear, and little guidance is available from clinical trials. Most of the initial treatment of patients with cardiac arrest is to stabilize blood pressure through fluid resuscitation. Protocols usually dictate the maintenance of normotension or the induction of hypertension with additional use of vasopressors. Prevention of hyperglycemia that may reduce regional cerebral blood flow is advised. This includes the avoidance of dextrose-containing solutions and initiation of an insulin drip to maintain a normoglycemic state. None of it is proven to change outcome of the comatose patient.

The practice of induced hypothermia—called *therapeutic hypothermia* (TH) and now *targeted temperature management*, in postcardiac arrest management has increased substantially over the previous 15 years, largely sparked by the publication of two influential trials in 2002.[1,7] Induced hypothermia targeting core temperature of 32°–34ºC has been recommended as standard therapy for patients with out-of-hospital cardiac arrests due to "shockable" rhythms in international guidelines. The early trials found improved survival, but details on the neurological condition of the patients were unclear because the neurological examinations reported in both trials were insufficient.[37] Several systematic reviews came to different conclusions regarding the effectiveness of TH.[20] The Cochrane systematic review and meta-analysis included 481 patients from four randomized controlled trials and indicated that induced hypothermia improves survival and neurological outcome after cardiac arrest.[5] However, a different systematic review and meta-analysis concluded that the quality of evidence was low and that the benefit from TH was inconclusive.[40] The beneficial effect of cooling has been challenged by two recent clinical trials. One showed that prehospital cooling did not improve outcomes, and the other found no benefit in targeting 33ºC compared to 36ºC.[31,41]

Cooling protocol is discussed in Chapter 21, but there are some important specific issues after CPR management. Cooling requires reduction in core temperature with ice packs, rapid infusion of cold intravenous fluids, and the use of external cooling devices or endovascular cooling systems.[27] Hypothermia is initiated within 2 to 3 hours to reduce core temperatures to 32°–34ºC and is maintained for 24 hours followed by gradual rewarming. Sedation and neuromuscular blockade are needed to control shivering. Major potential systemic complications include pneumonia, cardiac arrhythmias, pancreatitis, and hyperglycemia but are sometimes difficult to directly attribute to hypothermia, as these patients are systemically critically ill. The benefit of hypothermia has not been established in patients after in-hospital CPR or in those with initial cardiac rhythms other than ventricular fibrillation.

A more dubious situation is the comatose patient with post anoxic–ischemic brain edema. This may already occur within 24 hours after return of spontaneous circulation and may result in new neurologic findings, typically appearance of extensor posturing or loss of a motor response to stimuli or newly presenting loss of some brainstem reflexes such as new fixed and dilated pupils. There is no evidence that ICP monitoring or treatment of increased ICP (actually rarely high when monitored) improves outcome also because at this stage many patients may have lost brainstem reflexes or can be declared brain death. Global brain edema is just one extreme of anoxic–ischemic brain injury and not likely a treatable complication.

PREDICTION OF PROGNOSIS

In the pre-hypothermia era, the assessment of prognosis was summarized in a published algorithm in practice guidelines commissioned by the Quality Standard Subcommittee of the American Academy of Neurology.[71] This extensive literature review found that the circumstances surrounding CPR were not predictive of outcome. Several clinical features were highly predictive. The presence of myoclonus status within the first 24 hours in patients with circulatory arrest, absence of pupillary responses within day 1 to 3 after cardiopulmonary arrest, absence of corneal reflexes within day 1 to 3, and absent or extensor motor responses after day 3 were all associated with invariably poor neurological outcome. Eye movement abnormalities were insufficiently predictive, but clinical studies in these patients have not focused on the prediction of specific eye motor abnormalities. Each of these components is predictive, but decisions on outcome typically would call for a combination of sorts.

These guidelines were based on studies done prior to the routine use of induced hypothermia, and the reliability of predictors after cooling has been an area of great interest and investigation.

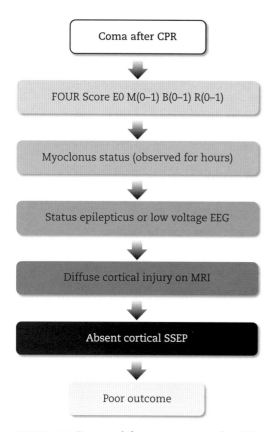

FIGURE 49.1: Framework for prognostication after CPR.

Neurologists need to consider key factors when prognosticating for patients treated with cooling protocols. Brainstem reflexes are crucial in the clinical evaluation of comatose patients after cardiac arrest. Because the brainstem is relatively resistant to anoxic–ischemic injury, the absence of pupil or corneal reflexes indicates a severe and often widespread injury that also involves much of the cortex. In a meta-analysis of 10 studies of prognostication after therapeutic hypothermia, the pupil response was tested in 566 patients at 72 hours. The absence of pupillary light reactivity remained a reliable predictor of poor outcome, with a false positive rate (FPR) of 0.004 (C.I. 0.001–0.03).[30] In contrast, after TH, the absence of corneal reflexes at 72 hours did not remain a reliable predictor of outcome with FPR of 0.02 (C.I. 0.002–0.13).

The reliability of the motor response at 72 hours after TH protocol also has been questioned.[3,51] Although it is still associated with outcome, an absent or extensor motor response at 72 hours after cardiac arrest after TH appears less reliable than in studies done in the pre-TH era.[51] In a meta-analysis, the motor response at 72 hours in 811 patients treated with TH had an unacceptably

high FPR of 0.21 (C.I. 0.08–0.43).[30] Again, patients treated with TH are more likely to receive sedation than those not treated with TH; and in studies with a "normothermia" comparison group, the motor response in patients sedated in that group also can be unreliable.[18,57,58] Thus it is crucial to ensure that there are no residual effects of sedative or analgesic medications used when assessing motor responses.

EEG has been used to provide some information on prognostication. So-called malignant EEG patterns include burst suppression, nonreactive alpha coma, and an isoelectric or markedly suppressed EEG. In a comprehensive review of pre-TH era literature, suppression or generalized epileptiform discharges predicted poor outcome; but the prognostic criteria were insufficiently accurate.[71] The presence of EEG background nonreactivity and discontinuity, however, may predict poor neurological outcomes,[52,64] even if it cannot be relied on fully in isolation. Some patients have periodic background patterns, such as generalized periodic epileptiform discharges (GPEDs) or bilateral periodic lateralized epileptiform discharges (BiPLEDs). These interictal patterns do not invariably indicate a poor outcome. Whether GPEDs can be considered seizures is controversial and some epileptologists define thresholds based on frequency (> 2–2.5 Hz) and evolution.

Continuous EEG monitoring during TH or rewarming has become more widely applied as it has become recognized that nonconvulsive seizures and nonconvulsive status epilepticus (NCSE) can occur.[2,33,55,64] Electrographic seizures have been found in 9%–33%[13,14,32,36,48,52,56] and NCSE in 2%–12%[14,33,48] of patients who are monitored during hypothermia protocols. While cEEG monitoring increases the detection of epileptiform activity, it has not been shown that earlier detection and treatment of seizures in this setting changes outcomes in this setting. The labor and resources needed for cEEG are substantial, and the added value and yield of cEEG compared to "spot" EEGs in this population is not clear.[4,14]

Of crucial importance are somatosensory evoked potentials (SSEP).[35] SSEPs are not influenced by drugs, temperature, or acute metabolic derangements and thus are a useful adjunct for prognostication.[11] SSEP requires stimulation of the median nerve that then results in a potential at the brachial plexus, cervical spinal cord, and finally bilateral cortex potentials (N20). For SSEP to be reliable, the cervical spine potential has to be recognized; and this could be of potential concern in patients with a severe anoxic–ischemic injury involving the cervical spinal cord. The bilateral absence of cortical potentials (N20 component) is nearly 100% specific in predicting unfavorable outcomes when performed between 1 and 3 days after cardiac arrest.[71] Evidence indicates that absent N20 responses during mild hypothermia after resuscitation maintains very acceptable accuracy in predicting a poor neurological outcome.[9,51] In a meta-analysis including 492 TH-treated post-arrest patients with bilaterally absent cortical responses on SSEP, the FPR was 0.007 (C.I. 0.001–0.047), which is comparable to that in patients not treated with TH.[30] In our practice, SSEP and clinical examination often provide enough information for prognostication.

Most studies of biomarkers in comatose survivors of cardiac arrest have examined serum neuron-specific enolase (NSE) and S100. NSE is a gamma isomer of enolase that is located in neurons, and S100[8,66,68] is a calcium-binding astroglial protein. In addition, earlier studies have looked at creatine kinase brain isoenzyme (CKBB). The usefulness of these biomarkers in prognostication may be more limited than the electrophysiological testing because none of these studies is automated, long laboratory turnaround times may be impractical, and standardization may not be optimal. In studies done prior to the routine use of hypothermia, CKBB and S100 were not reliable; and only NSE predicted outcome well, with a level > 33 μg/L at days 1–3 being associated with poor outcome. However, tempature modulation may have an effect on the metabolism and clearance of these biomarkers, clouding their prognostic value. Results of studies on the predictive value of NSE during or after hypothermia are conflicting, with some finding that NSE levels maintain prognostic accuracy,[44,53] while others find the prognostic value to be reduced.[18,62] With a cutoff value of 33 μg/L, FPRs have been reported as high as 22%–29% after TH protocols;[18,58] and one study found that an NSE level as high as 79 μg/L is needed to achieve a FPR of 0% for predicting unfavorable outcomes.[62] Differences in laboratory assays have made comparisons difficult, and at present there is not a strict threshold level of NSE that can be recommended for use in prognostication after cardiac arrest after hypothermia. Hemolysis of samples remains a problem in practice, as is quality control of commonly used assays. The most recent analysis of a large database found serial high NSE values predictive of outcome after out-of-hospital cardiac arrest. (Any increase between 24h and 48h samples was predictive, and any decrease of was predictive of good outcome.)[61]

The use of neuroimaging is growing as an adjunct to estimating neurological prognosis in comatose survivors of cardiac arrest, despite a lack of high-quality evidence (Figure 49.3).[25] Computed tomography (CT) imaging performed early is often normal and cannot determine the severity of anoxic–ischemic injury. After 1–3 days in more severe cases, global brain edema may be visualized. Several studies have found that the disappearance of the gray/white junction on non-contrast head CT has been associated with poor outcomes and failure to awaken.[28,67] Except for the obvious diffuse cerebral edema (Figure 49.2), findings should be interpreted cautiously because the literature regarding the use of CT imaging for prognosis is limited mostly to retrospective case series, and the timing of CT has ranged from minutes to nearly 3 weeks after the arrest.

Imaging with MRI holds promise as an adjunct to prognosis in comatose patients after cardiopulmonary arrest,[73] but there are still currently insufficient data to guide prognostication with MRI. Diffusion-weighted imaging (DWI) is particularly sensitive to ischemia, and ADC values can provide a quantitative measure of injury. Available literature is limited by heterogeneity of MRI timing and patient selection bias. MRI parameters associated with poor outcome include widespread and persistent cortical DWI abnormalities,[6,70] the combination of cortical and deep grey matter DWI/FLAIR abnormalities,[21,38] and severe global ADC reduction.[73,74] However, 20%–50% of patients with good outcomes have DWI abnormalities on MRI;[12,22,50] and some patients have poor outcomes despite a normal MRI (Figure 49.2). One study[45] was able to obtain MRI/DWI before initiation of therapeutic hypothermia and found good correlation of severe global DWI changes and poor outcome. The study importantly demonstrated that DWI may become more apparent on a second MRI scan. Another study found abnormal diffusion-weighted image findings had 93% sensitivity and 86% specificity for a poor neurologic outcome.[53] Thus, decisions on continuing medical care or withdrawal of life-sustaining treatments cannot be made on the basis of MRI findings alone.

There are several recent advisory statements and systematic reviews, but no new definitive prognosticators have been identified over last 2 decades.[23,59] The most recently published algorithm starts with evaluating patients with no motor response or extensor responses after excluding confounders. The use of a single value of NSE is discouraged. Multimodal prognosticating is advised.[59] This scientific statement attempted

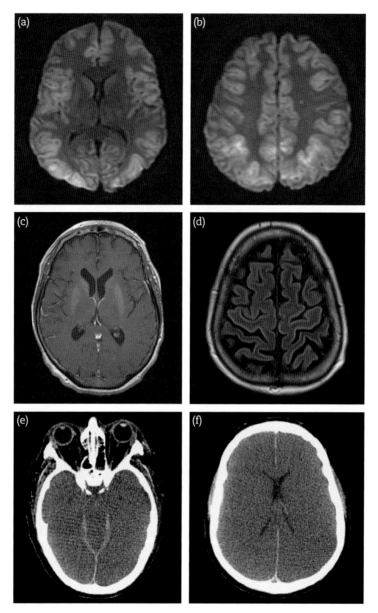

FIGURE 49.2: Spectrum of neuroimaging after CPR. Diffusion-weighted magnetic resonance images (MRI) in anoxic–ischemic injury show diffuse cortical hyperintensities indicative of likely laminar necrosis. (a, b) In a different patient, T1 post-gadolinium MRI shows contrast enhancement in the basal ganglia (c) and T2 hyperintensity involving the cortex (d), indicative of some anoxic injury despite clinical awakening. (e, f) shows effacement of the basal cisterns and a featureless CT (i.e. no gray-white matter differentiation and no sulci).

further precision by introducing "likely" or "very likely" poor outcome—determined by degree of false alarm or FPR—but key elements of prognostication have remained the same and neurologists recognize prediction in this condition is often imperfect. Many reviews fall short in advising neurologic expertise in prognostication and decision making.

CONCLUSION

- Repeat neurologic examination without confounders may identify poor outcome.
- MRI and SSEP are good (but not absolute) indicators of degree of acute brain injury.
- Therapeutic hypothermia is often associated with significant use of sedatives and analgesics, and clearance is poor.

- Absent brainstem reflexes (pupillary light and corneal reflex in particular) predicts poor outcome.
- Absent N20 peaks on SSEP predicts poor outcome.
- Serial NSE values may be valuable (poor outcome with increase, good outcome with decrease) but only when intergrated in a complete clinical assesment.

REFERENCES

1. Hypothermia after Cardiac Arrest Study Group. Mild therapeutic hypothermia to improve the neurologic outcome after cardiac arrest. *N Engl J Med* 2002;346:549–556.
2. Abend NS, Topjian A, Ichord R, et al. Electroencephalographic monitoring during hypothermia after pediatric cardiac arrest. *Neurology* 2009;72:1931–1940.
3. Al Thenayan E, Savard M, Sharpe M, Norton L, Young B. Predictors of poor neurologic outcome after induced mild hypothermia following cardiac arrest. *Neurology* 2008;71:1535–1537.
4. Alvarez V, Sierra-Marcos A, Oddo M, Rossetti AO. Yield of intermittent versus continuous EEG in comatose survivors of cardiac arrest treated with hypothermia. *Crit Care* 2013;17:R190.
5. Arrich J, Holzer M, Havel C, Mullner M, Herkner H. Hypothermia for neuroprotection in adults after cardiopulmonary resuscitation. *Cochrane Database Syst Rev* 2012;9:CD004128.
6. Barrett KM, Freeman WD, Weindling SM, et al. Brain injury after cardiopulmonary arrest and its assessment with diffusion-weighted magnetic resonance imaging. *Mayo Clinic Proc* 2007;82:828–835.
7. Bernard SA, Gray TW, Buist MD, et al. Treatment of comatose survivors of out-of-hospital cardiac arrest with induced hypothermia. *N Engl J Med* 2002;346:557–563.
8. Bottiger BW, Mobes S, Glatzer R, et al. Astroglial protein S-100 is an early and sensitive marker of hypoxic brain damage and outcome after cardiac arrest in humans. *Circulation* 2001;103:2694–2698.
9. Bouwes A, Binnekade JM, Zandstra DF, et al. Somatosensory evoked potentials during mild hypothermia after cardiopulmonary resuscitation. *Neurology* 2009;73:1457–1461.
10. Broccard A. Therapeutic hypothermia for anoxic brain injury following cardiac arrest: a "cool" transition toward cardiopulmonary cerebral resuscitation. *Crit Care Med* 2006;34:2008–2009.
11. Chen R, Bolton CF, Young B. Prediction of outcome in patients with anoxic coma: a clinical and electrophysiologic study. *Crit Care Med* 1996;24:672–678.
12. Choi SP, Park KN, Park HK, et al. Diffusion-weighted magnetic resonance imaging for predicting the clinical outcome of comatose survivors after cardiac arrest: a cohort study. *Crit Care* 2010;14:R17.
13. Cloostermans MC, van Meulen FB, Eertman CJ, Hom HW, van Putten MJ. Continuous electroencephalography monitoring for early prediction of neurological outcome in postanoxic patients after cardiac arrest: a prospective cohort study. *Crit Care Med* 2012;40:2867–2875.
14. Crepeau AZ, Rabinstein AA, Fugate JE, et al. Continuous EEG in therapeutic hypothermia after cardiac arrest: prognostic and clinical value. *Neurology* 2013;80:339–344.
15. Diesing TS, Wijdicks EFM. Ping-pong gaze in coma may not indicate persistent hemispheric damage. *Neurology* 2004;63:1537–1538.
16. Dragancea I, Horn J, Kuiper M, et al. Neurological prognostication after cardiac arrest and targeted temperature management 33 degrees C versus 36 degrees C: results from a randomised controlled clinical trial. *Resuscitation* 2015;93:164–170.
17. Echeverry R, Wu J, Haile WB, Guzman J, Yepes M. Tissue-type plasminogen activator is a neuroprotectant in the mouse hippocampus. *J Clin Invest* 2010;120:2194–2205.
18. Fugate JE, Wijdicks EFM, Mandrekar J, et al. Predictors of neurologic outcome in hypothermia after cardiac arrest. *Ann Neurol* 2010;68:907–914.
19. Fugate JE, Wijdicks EFM, White RD, Rabinstein AA. Does therapeutic hypothermia affect time to awakening in cardiac arrest survivors? *Neurology* 2011;77:1346–1350.
20. Geocadin RG, Wijdicks EFM, Armstrong MJ, et al. Evidence-based guideline summary: Reducing brain injury following cardiopulmonary resuscitation. *Neurology* 2016 in press.
21. Greer D, Scripko P, Bartscher J, et al. Serial MRI changes in comatose cardiac arrest patients. *Neurocrit Care* 2011;14:61–67.
22. Greer D, Scripko P, Bartscher J, et al. Clinical MRI interpretation for outcome prediction in cardiac arrest. *Neurocrit Care* 2012;17:240–244.
23. Greer DM, Rosenthal ES, Wu O. Neuroprognostication of hypoxic-ischaemic coma in the therapeutic hypothermia era. *Nat Rev Neurol* 2014;10:190–203.
24. Greer DM, Yang J, Scripko PD, et al. Clinical examination for outcome prediction in nontraumatic coma. *Crit Care Med* 2012;40:1150–1156.
25. Hahn DK, Geocadin RG, Greer DM. Quality of evidence in studies evaluating neuroimaging for neurologic prognostication in adult patients resuscitated from cardiac arrest. *Resuscitation* 2014;85:165–172.

26. Haile WB, Wu J, Echeverry R, et al. Tissue-type plasminogen activator has a neuroprotective effect in the ischemic brain mediated by neuronal TNF-alpha. *J Cereb Blood Flow Metab* 2012;32:57–69.

27. Holzer M, Mullner M, Sterz F, et al. Efficacy and safety of endovascular cooling after cardiac arrest: cohort study and Bayesian approach. *Stroke* 2006;37:1792–1797.

28. Inamasu J, Miyatake S, Suzuki M, et al. Early CT signs in out-of-hospital cardiac arrest survivors: temporal profile and prognostic significance. *Resuscitation* 2010;81:534–538.

29. Johkura K, Komiyama A, Kuroiwa Y. Vertical conjugate eye deviation in postresuscitation coma. *Ann Neurol* 2004;56:878–881.

30. Kamps MJ, Horn J, Oddo M, et al. Prognostication of neurologic outcome in cardiac arrest patients after mild therapeutic hypothermia: a meta-analysis of the current literature. *Intens Care Med* 2013;39:1671–1682.

31. Kim F, Nichol G, Maynard C, et al. Effect of prehospital induction of mild hypothermia on survival and neurological status among adults with cardiac arrest: a randomized clinical trial. *JAMA* 2014;311:45–52.

32. Knight WA, Hart KW, Adeoye OM, et al. The incidence of seizures in patients undergoing therapeutic hypothermia after resuscitation from cardiac arrest. *Epilepsy Res* 2013;106:396–402.

33. Legriel S, Bruneel F, Sediri H, et al. Early EEG monitoring for detecting postanoxic status epilepticus during therapeutic hypothermia: a pilot study. *Neurocrit Care* 2009;11:338–344.

34. Levy DE, Caronna JJ, Singer BH, et al. Predicting outcome from hypoxic-ischemic coma. *JAMA* 1985;253:1420–1426.

35. Madl C, Holzer M. Brain function after resuscitation from cardiac arrest. *Curr Opin Crit Care* 2004;10:213–217.

36. Mani R, Schmitt SE, Mazer M, Putt ME, Gaieski DF. The frequency and timing of epileptiform activity on continuous electroencephalogram in comatose post-cardiac arrest syndrome patients treated with therapeutic hypothermia. *Resuscitation* 2012;83:840–847.

37. Maramattom BV, Wijdicks EFM. Postresuscitation encephalopathy: current views, management, and prognostication. *Neurologist* 2005;11:234–243.

38. Mlynash M, Campbell DM, Leproust EM, et al. Temporal and spatial profile of brain diffusion-weighted MRI after cardiac arrest. *Stroke* 2010;41:1665–1672.

39. Nakada T, Kwee IL, Lee H. Sustained upgaze in coma. *J Clin Neuroophthalmol* 1984;4:35–37.

40. Nielsen N, Friberg H, Gluud C, Herlitz J, Wetterslev J. Hypothermia after cardiac arrest should be further evaluated: a systematic review of randomised trials with meta-analysis and trial sequential analysis. *Int J Cardiol* 2011;151:333–341.

41. Nielsen N, Wetterslev J, Cronberg T, et al. Targeted temperature management at 33 degrees C versus 36 degrees C after cardiac arrest. *N Engl J Med* 2013;369:2197–2206.

42. Oddo M, Rossetti AO. Early multimodal outcome prediction after cardiac arrest in patients treated with hypothermia. *Crit Care Med* 2014;42:1340–1347.

43. Ogawa S, Kitao Y, Hori O. Ischemia-induced neuronal cell death and stress response. *Antioxid Redox Signal* 2007;9:573–587.

44. Oksanen T, Tiainen M, Skrifvars MB, et al. Predictive power of serum NSE and OHCA score regarding 6-month neurologic outcome after out-of-hospital ventricular fibrillation and therapeutic hypothermia. *Resuscitation* 2009;80:165–170.

45. Park JS, Lee SW, Kim H, et al. Efficacy of diffusion-weighted magnetic resonance imaging performed before therapeutic hypothermia in predicting clinical outcome in comatose cardiopulmonary arrest survivors. *Resuscitation* 2015;88:132–137.

46. Peberdy MA, Kaye W, Ornato JP, et al. Cardiopulmonary resuscitation of adults in the hospital: a report of 14720 cardiac arrests from the National Registry of Cardiopulmonary Resuscitation. *Resuscitation* 2003;58:297–308.

47. Polderman KH. Mechanisms of action, physiological effects, and complications of hypothermia. *Crit Care Med* 2009;37:S186–202.

48. Rittenberger JC, Popescu A, Brenner RP, Guyette FX, Callaway CW. Frequency and timing of nonconvulsive status epilepticus in comatose postcardiac arrest subjects treated with hypothermia. *Neurocrit Care* 2012;16:114–122.

49. Rogove HJ, Safar P, Sutton-Tyrrell K, Abramson NS. Old age does not negate good cerebral outcome after cardiopulmonary resuscitation: analyses from the brain resuscitation clinical trials. The Brain Resuscitation Clinical Trial I and II Study Groups. *Crit Care Med* 1995;23:18–25.

50. Roine RO, Raininko R, Erkinjuntti T, Ylikoski A, Kaste M. Magnetic resonance imaging findings associated with cardiac arrest. *Stroke* 1993;24:1005–1014.

51. Rossetti AO, Oddo M, Logroscino G, Kaplan PW. Prognostication after cardiac arrest and hypothermia: a prospective study. *Ann Neurol* 2010;67:301–307.

52. Rossetti AO, Urbano LA, Delodder F, Kaplan PW, Oddo M. Prognostic value of continuous EEG monitoring during therapeutic hypothermia after cardiac arrest. *Crit Care* 2010;14:R173.

53. Ryoo SM, Jeon SB, Sohn CH, et al. Predicting outcome with diffusion-weighted imaging in cardiac arrest patients receiving hypothermia therapy: Multicenter retrospective cohort study. *Crit Care Med* 2015 Nov;43:2370–2377.

54. Rundgren M, Karlsson T, Nielsen N, et al. Neuron specific enolase and S-100B as predictors of outcome after cardiac arrest and induced hypothermia. *Resuscitation* 2009;80:784–789.

55. Rundgren M, Rosen I, Friberg H. Amplitude-integrated EEG (aEEG) predicts outcome after cardiac arrest and induced hypothermia. *Intens Care Med* 2006;32:836–842.

56. Sadaka F, Doerr D, Hindia J, Lee KP, Logan W. Continuous electroencephalogram in comatose postcardiac arrest syndrome patients treated with therapeutic hypothermia: outcome prediction study. *J Intensive Care Med* 2015;30:292–296.

57. Samaniego EA, Mlynash M, Caulfield AF, Eyngorn I, Wijman CA. Sedation confounds outcome prediction in cardiac arrest survivors treated with hypothermia. *Neurocrit Care* 2011;15:113–119.

58. Samaniego EA, Persoon S, Wijman CA. Prognosis after cardiac arrest and hypothermia: a new paradigm. *Curr Neurol Neurosci Rep* 2011;11:111–119.

59. Sandroni C, Cariou A, Cavallaro F, et al. Prognostication in comatose survivors of cardiac arrest: an advisory statement from the European Resuscitation Council and the European Society of Intensive Care Medicine. *Intens Care Med* 2014;40:1816–1831.

60. Seder DB, Sunde K, Rubertsson S, et al. Neurologic outcomes and postresuscitation care of patients with myoclonus following cardiac arrest. *Crit Care Med* 2015;43:965–972.

61. Stammet P, Collignon O, Hassager C, et al. Neuron-specific enolase as a predictor of death or poor neurological outcome after out-of-hospital cardiac arrest and targeted temperature management at 33 degrees C and 36 degrees C. *J Am Coll Cardiol* 2015;65:2104–2114.

62. Steffen IG, Hasper D, Ploner CJ, et al. Mild therapeutic hypothermia alters neuron specific enolase as an outcome predictor after resuscitation: 97 prospective hypothermia patients compared to 133 historical non-hypothermia patients. *Crit Care* 2010;14:R69.

63. Teschendorf P, Popp E, Motsh J. Effective inhibition of caspases on neuronal degeneration and outcome following global cerebral ischemia due to cardiocirculatory arrest in rats. *Anesthesiology* 2001;95:788 Abstract.

64. Thenayan EA, Savard M, Sharpe MD, Norton L, Young B. Electroencephalogram for prognosis after cardiac arrest. *J Crit Care* 2010;25:300–304.

65. Thomke F, Marx JJ, Sauer O, et al. Observations on comatose survivors of cardiopulmonary resuscitation with generalized myoclonus. *BMC Neurol* 2005;5:14.

66. Tiainen M, Roine RO, Pettila V, Takkunen O. Serum neuron-specific enolase and S-100B protein in cardiac arrest patients treated with hypothermia. *Stroke* 2003;34:2881–2886.

67. Torbey MT, Selim M, Knorr J, Bigelow C, Recht L. Quantitative analysis of the loss of distinction between gray and white matter in comatose patients after cardiac arrest. *Stroke* 2000;31:2163–2167.

68. Wang JT, Young GB, Connolly JF. Prognostic value of evoked responses and event-related brain potentials in coma. *Can J Neurol Sci* 2004;31:438–450.

69. Wijdicks EFM. From clinical judgment to odds: a history of prognostication in anoxic-ischemic coma. *Resuscitation* 2012;83:940–945.

70. Wijdicks EFM, Campeau NG, Miller GM. MR imaging in comatose survivors of cardiac resuscitation. *AJNR Am J Neuroradiol* 2001;22:1561–1565.

71. Wijdicks EFM, Hijdra A, Young GB, Bassetti CL, Wiebe S. Practice parameter: prediction of outcome in comatose survivors after cardiopulmonary resuscitation (an evidence-based review): report of the Quality Standards Subcommittee of the American Academy of Neurology. *Neurology* 2006;67:203–210.

72. Wijdicks EFM. *Neurologic Complications of Critical Illness*. 2nd ed. New York: Oxford University Press; 2002.

73. Wijman CA, Mlynash M, Caulfield AF, et al. Prognostic value of brain diffusion-weighted imaging after cardiac arrest. *Ann Neurol* 2009;65:394–402.

74. Wu O, Sorensen AG, Benner T, et al. Comatose patients with cardiac arrest: predicting clinical outcome with diffusion-weighted MR imaging. *Radiology* 2009;252:173–181.

75. Young GB, Doig G, Ragazzoni A. Anoxic-ischemic encephalopathy: clinical and electrophysiological associations with outcome. *Neurocrit Care* 2005;2:159–164.

76. Zandbergen EG, Hijdra A, Koelman JH, et al. Prediction of poor outcome within the first 3 days of postanoxic coma. *Neurology* 2006;66:62–68.

50

Neurology of Pregnancy

Pregnant and postpartum women may develop a critical illness with a neurologic complication or may develop a neurocritical illness while pregnant. NICU admissions as a result of pregnancy are uncommon, but so are medical or surgical ICU admissions. Pregnancy-specific disorders such as eclampsia, HELLP (hemolysis, elevated liver enzymes, and low platelet count) syndrome, and, very rarely, amniotic fluid embolism are some of the causes of admission to the ICU. Physicians then should immediately expect a very severe condition that requires critical intervention. Pregnancy-related ICU admissions remain uncommon and were estimated at 3.6/1,000 deliveries.[3] Pregnancy-specific causes such as choriocarcinoma, amniotic fluid embolization, or postpartum angiopathy are equally uncommon.[13] However, because pregnant patients occasionally present in the ICU, this chapter reviews the neurologic complications in the critically ill pregnant patient and options for managing a pregnant patient with a neurologic complication. It requires knowledge of specific treatment in the pregnant patient largely dependent on the trimester of pregnancy. Cerebral venous thrombosis—mostly postpartum—is discussed in Chapter 32 and reviewed elsewhere.[2]

GENERAL PRINCIPLES

Management or drug recommendations that could harm the fetus is a constant concern. In the United States and many other parts of the world, the general approach recommended by obstetricians is to give the health of the mother preference and to proceed with necessary and potentially lifesaving diagnostic procedures and interventions.

A first concern is to assess the effects of possible ionizing radiation on the fetus. Diagnostic imaging procedures expose the fetus to a level of radiation, but usually less than 0.05 Gy (5 rads). Radiation exposure over 0.05 Gy is associated with increased risk of congenital malformations, growth retardation, and intellectual disability. Thus, fetal radiation with exposure of a CT head is

minor (a single CT scan is less than 1 rad). Use of iodinated contrast should be completely avoided in pregnancy, and this also applies to gadolinium. (In the postpartum phase, miniscule amounts are excreted in breast milk.[5]) MRI scan and time-of-flight vascular images can be performed at any stage of pregnancy. The risk of cerebral angiogram can subject the fetus to radiation, but the procedure may be necessary to exclude or document an arteriovenous malformation in certain circumstances.

Several drugs and procedures may need to be carefully reconsidered in pregnancy. The FDA has issued pregnancy risk categories (Table 50.1) and has linked the categories to drugs. Certain drugs are potentially problematic in pregnancy, and this includes the use of mannitol as well as hypertonic saline because both can impact the osmotic status of the amniotic fluid. How to safely use these drugs is not conclusively known. Repeated use seems ill advised. Multiple epileptic agents have been identified that are problematic in pregnancy and can markedly increase the risk of fetal malformations. In general, valproic acid and phenobarbital have a high risk of major malformations. The types of fetal abnormalities are shown in Table 50.2.[16,19,27]

MAJOR CLINICAL SYNDROMES IN PREGNANCY

The neurointensivist—ideally—should be part of a multidisciplinary team caring for these patients. Some disorders are seen with some frequency (eclampsia); others are unique and new for most of us (postpartum angiopathy). Single-case experiences are very common in the field, thus limiting expertise. There likely is a spectrum of disorders with overlap in manifestations (Figure 50.1).

Eclampsia

Eclampsia is often seen in patients who are already predisposed with preexisting hypertension of renal disease. Preeclampsia is quite worrisome, with still a 10% maternal death frequency. Eclampsia

TABLE 50.1. FDA PREGNANCY RISK CATEGORIES

Category A	Controlled studies show no risk. Adequate, well-controlled studies in pregnant women have failed to demonstrate a risk to the fetus.
Category B	No evidence of risk in humans. Either animal study shows risk, but human findings do not, or if no adequate human studies have been done, animal findings are negative.
Category C	Risk cannot be ruled out. Human studies are lacking, and animal studies are either positive for fetal risk or lacking. However, potential benefits may justify potential risk.
Category D	Positive evidence of risk. Investigational or postmarketing data show risk to the fetus. Nevertheless, potential benefits may outweigh the potential risk.
Category X	Contraindicated in pregnancy. Studies in animals or humans or investigational or postmarketing reports have shown fetal risk, which clearly outweighs any possible benefit to the patient.
NA	FDA pregnancy category not available.

TABLE 50.2. ANTIEPILEPTIC DRUGS AND ASSOCIATED FETAL ANOMALIES

Antiepileptic Drugs	Fetal Anomalies
Carbamazepine	Neural tube defects, microcephaly, developmental delay, hypoplastic nails
Lamotrigine	Cleft lip, neural tube defects
Levetiracetam	Safety has not been established
Oxcarbazepine	Cleft lip, neural tube defects
Phenobarbital	Distal digital hypoplasia, low set ears, cleft lip, cleft palate, developmental delay, ptosis
Phenytoin	Cleft lip, cleft palate, heart malformations, and other minor birth defects (short fingers, widely spaced eyes)
Valproic acid	Neural tube defects, spina bifida, cleft lip, cleft palate, organ malformations, limb deficiencies, developmental delay

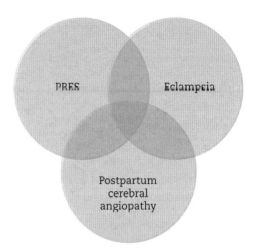

FIGURE 50.1: Overlap between posterior reversible encephalopathy syndrome (PRES), eclampsia, and angiopathy in pregnancy.

is usually defined as hypertension above 140/90 mm Hg on two occasions 4 hours apart.[9] The presence of proteinuria is defined as urinary secretion of protein exceeding 300 mg in 24 hours. Endothelial cell damage is considered the important component in the pathology of eclampsia (Capsule 50.1). The vascular injury results in the release of prostaglandins that increase thromboxane, causing vasoconstriction and clumping of platelets. Patients with eclampsia may present with generalized tonic-clonic seizures and, for that reason, may be admitted to the NICU. Mostly these patients may present virtually identical as posterior reversible encephalopathy syndrome (PRES), but usually with more extensive MRI scan abnormalities. MRI scan abnormalities may show multiple petechial hemorrhages in the white matter and significant white matter edema in predisposed areas such as the parietooccipital lobes, thalami, and cerebellar hemispheres.

The treatment is complex but should involve the immediate use of IV magnesium sulphate, which will improve outcome greatly.[7,18,23,24] Treating hypertension with a multiple dose of labetalol or hydralazine may not be sufficient, and a far more aggressive approach is needed. When patients are randomized using magnesium or diazepam, magnesium sulphate markedly reduced seizures up to 50% but only about a third of the patients with phenytoin. Usually magnesium sulphate is started with an IV load of 4–6 grams of magnesium sulphate (20 mL of a 20% solution), followed by an infusion of magnesium sulphate of 1–2 g/hour. The dose is determined by the number of seizures and must be increased with

---

CAPSULE 50.1   PUTATIVE MECHANISM OF ECLAMPSIA

The crucial component in the pathology of eclampsia is endothelial cell damage. In response to this vascular injury, a cascade of vasoconstriction and intravascular coagulation occurs involving renal, hepatic, and hematopoietic systems. The prostaglandins thromboxane (from trophoblastic tissue) and prostacyclin (from endothelial cells) work in opposite ways. Thromboxane causes vasoconstriction and clumping of platelets; prostacyclin causes vasodilation and inhibits platelet aggregation. A reversal of this normal balanced physiologic situation has been considered one of the possible mechanisms. Circulating human chorionic gonadotropin (hCG) and thrombomodulin may reflect the severity of endothelial injury. The changes in placental tissue are postulated to alter the syncytiotrophoblast and cytotrophoblast and thus alter hCG secretion. In addition, thrombomodulin, a soluble endothelial surface glycoprotein, is released after damage to the endothelium and is a cofactor for thrombin-catalyzed activation of protein. Magnesium antagonizes and suppresses seizures mediated by N-methyl-D-aspartate (NMDA). Neuronal burst firing and electroencephalographic spike generation are markedly suppressed. Magnesium sulfate also acts on the neuromuscular junction by decreasing the amount of acetylcholine liberated from the presynaptic junction, decreasing the sensitivity of the motor end plate to acetylcholine, and reducing the muscle membrane excitability. Magnesium sulfate dilates vessels, including the cerebral arteries. Magnesium sulfate opposes calcium-dependent arterial constriction and relieves vasospasm associated with this disorder. Other effects are increased production of the endothelial vasodilator prostacyclin and inhibition of platelet activation.

---

recurrence. The dose can be adjusted when the tendon reflexes disappear, and usually this clinical finding corresponds to a serum magnesium level of 8–12 mg/dL—one of the few instances a reflex hammer helps an obstetrician. Toxicity of magnesium sulphate is substantial and may lead to respiratory distress and need for intubation, but in most instances toxicity occurs if magnesium levels are allowed to go beyond 12 mg/dL. Mostly the administration of magnesium sulphate is continued for 24–48 hours and then gradually tapered. Very few other antihypertensives are effective or allowed. It is important to reemphasize that nitroprusside (Chapter 19) is a considerably concerning drug because it can lead to cyanide toxicity of the fetus, even if used for several hours. Angiotensin-converting enzyme inhibitors also are contraindicated.

The more severe manifestation of eclampsia is HELLP syndrome. The acronym "HELLP" (*h*emolysis, *e*levated *l*iver enzymes, and *l*ow *p*latelet count) was introduced to delineate a syndrome within the population of patients with eclampsia who in addition had hemolytic anemia, liver dysfunction, and thrombocytopenia. With an incidence of 3%–25%, the syndrome remains one of the most common causes of maternal mortality. The disorder may begin with nonspecific malaise, epigastric or right upper quadrant pain, and nausea and vomiting but without hypertension, which comes several days later. Early presentation with gum bleeding, gastrointestinal bleeding, hematuria, and jaundice may occur. The syndrome can be subclassified on the basis of platelet count, and studies have suggested that the actual platelet count may predict rapidity of recovery. The diagnosis is usually confirmed by thrombocytopenia (platelets less than $100/10^9$-L) and when there is an increased liver function tests and when there is hemolysis on blood smears. HELLP syndrome may be associated with subarachnoid hemorrhage and other coagulation-associated intracranial hemorrhages. There is little information available on the neurologic manifestations of HELLP syndrome. The best management for both conditions is, if possible, immediate delivery—most patients recover rapidly after that. Some patients may need a platelet transfusion if there is a significant decline of platelet counts. Infusion of platelet counts using 1–2 six-packs is needed if there is intracranial hemorrhage or if a neurosurgery evacuation is planned.

Neurologic manifestations are more profound and severe in HELLP syndrome. Seizures, cortical blindness, and reduced level of consciousness are the most common manifestations and reflect the PRES-like clinical picture. There is an increased risk for intracerebral hemorrhage due to severe hypertension and thrombocytopenia.

CT may show subarachnoid hemorrhage, but is located in sulci and rarely in the basal cisterns, a finding expected in a coagulation-associated subarachnoid hemorrhage and PRES-like radiologic picture. Serial CT scanning may show resolving features of white matter hypodensities and resorption of subarachnoid hemorrhage. If a subarachnoid hemorrhage is diagnosed by CT, it is not likely that aneurysmal rupture plays a role, and transfer for a cerebral angiogram may unnecessarily jeopardize patient safety and monitoring in the ICU.

Postpartum Angiopathy

This recently, better-defined entity may have an overlap with postpartum eclampsia (Figure 50.2).[12,13] In a series of 18 patients, important clinical descriptors were found. About half of the patients had proteinuria during pregnancy, two-thirds of the patients had at least one uneventful pregnancy, and one-third had a coagulopathy (e.g., protein S deficiency, antiphospholipid antibody syndrome). Pregnancy was complicated by preeclampsia or eclampsia in 39% of patients, and two patients were treated for HELLP. Severe headache (often thunderclap), focal neurologic deficit, and seizures were the most frequent presenting symptoms. CT scans showed intracranial hemorrhage[8,28] (cortical or subarachnoid) or parietooccipital hypodensities suggesting PRES. Diffuse cerebral edema was noted in one patient. Severe cerebral vasoconstriction was found about one week after onset (with normal initial cerebral angiogram in 5 patients).[12,13]

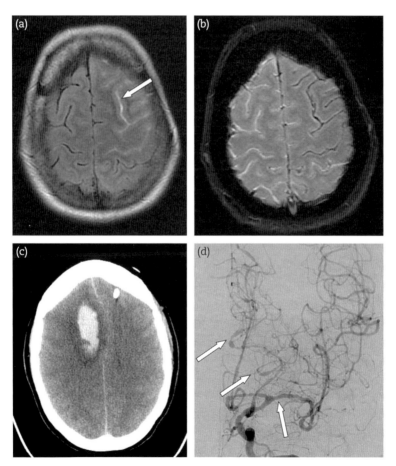

FIGURE 50.2: Axial Fluid-Attenuated Inversion Recovery (FLAIR) MRI 4 days after headache, seizures, and visual symptoms in a postpartum 32 year-old woman shows sulcal T2 hyperintensity over the left hemisphere consistent with sulcal subarachnoid hemorrhage (a, arrow), which subsequently involved both hemispheres (b). In another patient with fulminant course, noncontrast head CT shows right frontal intraparenchymal hemorrhage (c). Left carotid angiogram in this patient shows widespread vasculopathy (arrows, d). From reference 12.

Treatment remains poorly defined,[26,29] but patients have been treated with intra-arterial verapamil (with inconsistent improvement), balloon angioplasty, corticosteroids, and hemodynamic augmentation with vasopressors.[13] Intravenous magnesium has been considered a standard treatment, and doses are similar to those for eclampsia. Full recovery was only seen in half of the patients, and more relentless progression to catastrophic injury and brain death in 5 of 17 patients.[12]

Amniotic Fluid Embolism

One of the most catastrophic disorders of pregnancy (mortality approaches 80%) is amniotic fluid embolism, which may occur in 1 in 8,000 to 1 in 80,000 deliveries. The diagnosis is typically made at autopsy by demonstration of squamous cells or debris in the pulmonary artery vasculature.

At any time during pregnancy, amniotic fluid embolization may occur, varying from the first trimester to 48 hours postpartum. This critical condition immediately becomes apparent because of hypotension, depressed ventricular function, and profound hypoxemia. Hypoxemia is from initial pulmonary vasospasm and may result in death in 50% of the patients. If patients survive, a marked acute respiratory distress syndrome develops with major hemodynamic alterations. Disseminated intravascular coagulation often accompanies cardiorespiratory collapse. Approximately 50% of patients who survived may have suffered anoxic–ischemic brain injury. Coma after cardiopulmonary resuscitation due to amniotic fluid embolization has a very poor outcome despite urgent cesarean section. The fetus in all likelihood may have had an anoxic injury, too, and neonatal outcome is similarly poor. Resuscitation measures include mechanical ventilation, blood pressure support, and replacement of essential factors depleted by disseminated intravascular coagulation (use of cryoprecipitate or fresh frozen plasma).[14,20]

Anoxic–Ischemic Encephalopathy after Maternal Cardiac Arrest

Causes of maternal cardiac arrest are shown in Table 50.3. These are often very unfortunate situations and sad state of affairs. Anoxic–ischemic encephalopathy is a possible outcome in the patient who may carry a viable fetus. Patients may progress to brain death from cerebral swelling or may remain vegetative. If the fetus is 2 months preterm, prolonged care in patients in a vegetative state has been attempted with variable success. In

TABLE 50.3. MATERNAL CARDIAC ARREST (BEAU-CHOPS)

Bleeding/DIC
Embolism: coronary/pulmonary/amniotic fluid embolism
Anesthetic complications
Uterine atony
Cardiac disease (MI/ischemia/aortic dissection/cardiomyopathy)
Hypertension/preeclampsia/eclampsia
Other: differential diagnosis of standard ACLS guidelines
Placenta abruptio/previa
Sepsis

Adapted from reference 17.

a nonviable fetus, withdrawal of support is often requested by family members.[1]

Successful deliveries of newborns have been reported in mothers allegedly in a persistent vegetative state but experience is more often after traumatic brain injury and not obstetric emergencies).[4,25] The care of a brain-dead pregnant woman is more far complicated medically due to high probability of vasomotor loss, progressive hypotension, and cardiac arrest—an instability not seen in chronic disorders of unconsciousness. Since 1982, there have been over 25 successful reported deliveries with a mean gestational age at delivery of 29.5 weeks. No successful case associated with brain death has been reported in the United States in the last 20 years. Many of the reported "successful" cases failed to document all criteria for brain death, and some patients may not have progressed to brain death.[1,10] The conventional wisdom is that viability of the fetus is at a gestational age of 20–25 weeks, but neonates born after 20–21 weeks of pregnancy do not survive irrespective of resuscitative measures and it is also highly unlikely at 22–23 weeks.[22]

NEUROCRITICAL CARE IN A PREGNANT PATIENT

Disorders that should be considered in a pregnant patient with new neurologic findings are summarized in Table 50.4. Discussion of these disorders can be found in specific chapters in this book. In some instances, acute ischemic or hemorrhagic stroke may bring a pregnant patient to the intensive care unit. The management is not significantly different from any other patient, and again all attention is to the improvement of the mother. Hemorrhagic stroke may occur during

TABLE 50.4. MAJOR NEUROLOGIC
DISORDERS OF PREGNANCY
AND PUERPERUM

Eclampsia
Ischemic stroke
Lobar cerebral hematoma
Ruptured cerebral aneurysm or AVM
Postpartum angiopathy
Posterior reversible encephalopathy syndrome
Amniotic fluid embolism
Choriocarcinoma
Pituitary apoplexy
Thrombotic thrombocytopenic purpura
Glioma or other malignancy

pregnancy, and rupture of a cerebral aneurysm and arterial venous malformation have traditionally been found as the main causes. (In general, there is no increased risk of hemorrhage in patients with a cerebral AVM during pregnancy or in the puerperium.) Many cerebral hemorrhages—lobar or putaminal—in pregnancy are without a specific cause; but ruptured AVM, aneurysmal rupture, and hemorrhage into a choriocarcinoma should be considered, and MRI and MRA (time-of-flight sequence) are necessary tests. In principle, management should be similar as in nonpregnant patients, but neurosurgical procedures may be reconsidered or delayed due to the potential risk of general anesthesia. Treatment of cerebral hematoma is surgical removal when mass effect progresses. Lobar or putaminal hematoma with mass effect may be treated with repeated bolus of hypertonic saline accepting a certain risk to the fetus.

Pregnancy causes significant hemodynamic changes and includes increased intravascular volume, causing increased hemodynamic vascular stress. At the end of pregnancy, a hypercoagulable state occurs and extends into the puerperium. These changes may tip vulnerable patients out of balance. However, very few patients develop ischemic or hemorrhagic stroke. In one study (1996–2005) from Boston 17 ischemic strokes and 36 hemorrhagic strokes were seen in over 100,000 pregnancies.[11]

Thrombolysis with IV tPA has been successfully (tPA does not cross the placenta)[6,15,21] and with mostly uncomplicated fetal outcomes.[11] Endovascular retrieval is potentially associated with significant radiation exposure but there are no solid data on the consequences for the fetus.

Evaluation after treatment should focus on thrombophilia and paradoxical emboli. (Carotid or vertebral dissection is an uncommon cause of stroke in pregnancy and even after delivery).

CONCLUSIONS

- Endothelial dysfunction, hypersensitivity to angiotensin II resulting in acute hypertension, increased capillary permeability, and eventually brain edema are main components of eclampsia.
- Eclampsia does fall into the spectrum of posterior reversible encephalopathy syndrome, and MRI images can be identical.
- Postpartum angiopathy may be reversible or rapidly fatal.

REFERENCES

1. Burkle CM, Tessmer-Tuck J, Wijdicks EFM. Medical, legal, and ethical challenges associated with pregnancy and catastrophic brain injury. *Int J Gynaecol Obstet* 2015;129:276–280.
2. Cantu C, Barinagarrementeria F. Cerebral venous thrombosis associated with pregnancy and puerperium: review of 67 cases. *Stroke* 1993;24:1880–1884.
3. Chantry AA, Deneux-Tharaux C, Bonnet MP, Bouvier-Colle MH. Pregnancy-related ICU admissions in France: trends in rate and severity, 2006–2009. *Crit Care Med* 2015;43:78–86.
4. Chiossi G, Novic K, Celebrezze JU, Thomas RL. Successful neonatal outcome in 2 cases of maternal persistent vegetative state treated in a labor and delivery suite. *Am J Obstet Gynecol* 2006;195:316–322.
5. Cohan R. American College of Radiology Manual on Contrast Media. In: Medium ACoDaC, editor. *Sections on Pregnant and Breast-Feeding Women.* 7th ed. ACR; 2010:59–63.
6. Del Zotto E, Giossi A, Volonghi I, et al. Ischemic stroke during pregnancy and puerperium. *Stroke Res Treat* 2011;60678.
7. Duley L, Meher S, Abalos E. Management of pre-eclampsia. *BMJ* 2006;332:463–468.
8. Edlow BL, Kasner SE, Hurst RW, Weigele JB, Levine JM. Reversible cerebral vasoconstriction syndrome associated with subarachnoid hemorrhage. *Neurocrit Care* 2007;7:203–210.
9. Edlow JA, Caplan LR, O'Brien K, Tibbles CD. Diagnosis of acute neurological emergencies in pregnant and post-partum women. *Lancet Neurol* 2013;12:175–185.
10. Esmaeilzadeh M, Dictus C, Kayvanpour E, et al. One life ends, another begins: management of a

brain-dead pregnant mother: a systematic review. *BMC Med* 2010;8:74.

11. Feske SK, Singhal AB. Cerebrovascular disorders complicating pregnancy. *Continuum (Minneap Minn)* 2014;20:80–99.

12. Fugate JE, Ameriso SF, Ortiz G, Schottlaender LV, Wijdicks EFM, Flemming KD, Rabinstein AA. Variable presentations of postpartum angiopathy. *Stroke* 2012;43:670–676.

13. Fugate JE, Wijdicks EFM, Parisi JE, et al. Fulminant postpartum cerebral vasoconstriction syndrome. *Arch Neurol* 2012;69:111–117.

14. Gist RS, Stafford IP, Leibowitz AB, Beilin Y. Amniotic fluid embolism. *Anesth Analg* 2009;108:1599–1602.

15. Johnson DM, Kramer DC, Cohen E, et al. Thrombolytic therapy for acute stroke in late pregnancy with intra-arterial recombinant tissue plasminogen activator. *Stroke* 2005;36:e53–e55.

16. Kulaga S, Sheehy O, Zargarzadeh AH, Moussally K, Berard A. Antiepileptic drug use during pregnancy: perinatal outcomes. *Seizure* 2011;20:667–672.

17. Lipman S, Cohen S, Einav S, et al. The Society for Obstetric Anesthesia and Perinatology consensus statement on the management of cardiac arrest in pregnancy. *Anesth Analg* 2014;118:1003–1016.

18. Matthys LA, Coppage KH, Lambers DS, Barton JR, Sibai BM. Delayed postpartum preeclampsia: an experience of 151 cases. *Am J Obstet Gynecol* 2004;190:1464–1466.

19. Molgaard-Nielsen D, Hviid A. Newer-generation antiepileptic drugs and the risk of major birth defects. *JAMA* 2011;305:1996–2002.

20. Moore J, Baldisseri MR. Amniotic fluid embolism. *Crit Care Med* 2005;33:S279–S285.

21. Murugappan A, Coplin WM, Al-Sadat AN, et al. Thrombolytic therapy of acute ischemic stroke during pregnancy. *Neurology* 2006;66:768–770.

22. Raju TN, Mercer BM, Burchfield DJ, Joseph GF, Jr. Periviable birth: executive summary of a joint workshop by the Eunice Kennedy Shriver National Institute of Child Health and Human Development, Society for Maternal-Fetal Medicine, American Academy of Pediatrics, and American College of Obstetricians and Gynecologists. *Obstet Gynecol* 2014;123:1083–1096.

23. Shah AK, Rajamani K, Whitty JE. Eclampsia: a neurological perspective. *J Neurol Sci* 2008;271:158–167.

24. Sibai BM. Diagnosis, prevention, and management of eclampsia. *Obstet Gynecol* 2005;105:402–410.

25. Sim KB. Maternal persistent vegetative state with successful fetal outcome. *J Korean Med Sci* 2001;16:669–672.

26. Singhal AB, Hajj-Ali RA, Topcuoglu MA, et al. Reversible cerebral vasoconstriction syndromes: analysis of 139 cases. *Arch Neurol* 2011;68:1005–1012.

27. Tomson T, Battino D. Teratogenic effects of antiepileptic drugs. *Lancet Neurol* 2012;11:803–813.

28. Ursell MR, Marras CL, Farb R, et al. Recurrent intracranial hemorrhage due to postpartum cerebral angiopathy: implications for management. *Stroke* 1998;29:1995–1998.

29. Williams TL, Lukovits TG, Harris BT, Harker Rhodes C. A fatal case of postpartum cerebral angiopathy with literature review. *Arch Gynecol Obstet* 2007;275:67–77.

PART X

Critical Care Support

51

Shock

The term *shock* in a critically ill patient describes circulatory failure, poor oxygen delivery, and often unavoidably, organ failure. Hypotension and shock are two different entities, although both are intertwined. Most intensivists agree that shock is a combination of systemic arterial hypotension, often a systolic blood pressure ≤ 90 mm Hg or mean arterial pressure (MAP) ≤ 60 mm Hg, and clinical and laboratory signs of tissue hypoperfusion.[2,10,54] It becomes rapidly concerning with the development of severe vasoplegia, and the development of renal failure, defined as urinary output of < 0.5 mL/kg body weight/hour. Invariably, as a result of poor perfusion, serum lactate increases more than 4 mmol/L, and this value is an early laboratory predictor of poor outcome.[9]

As a major disease category, shock may be present in one of three patients in a general marquee ICU.[54] In the NICU, spiraling down hypotension and shock are less common, and causes are different. Nonetheless, most types of shock can be seen in critically ill neurologic patients. For example, we can expect vasodilatory shock in bacterial meningitis with septicemia, hypovolemic shock in patients with traumatic brain injury, and cardiogenic shock from severe neurogenic stress cardiomyopathy with status epilepticus or poor grade aneurysmal subarachnoid hemorrhage. Many neurointensivists know also very well that new hypotension in patients after catastrophic neurologic injury is often a defining sign of brain death.

As it is in many other intensive care units, the early recognition and treatment of shock determines outcome. Well thought-out treatment protocols are useful in prioritizing decisions, although they may not improve outcome in rapidly evolving complex conditions.[11,39] Moreover, traditional measurements such as serial lactate measurements, central venous oxygenation measurement, and activated protein C are all disputed indicators for success or failure.

Management of shock is a critical clinical problem, and this chapter briefly summarizes the evaluation and differential diagnosis of shock, mostly pertaining to patients with acute neurologic disorders, with best approaches modified to each pathophysiologic condition.

ASSESSMENT OF SHOCK STATES

Shock is a physiologic condition that leads to poor end-organ tissue perfusion. When tissues are hypoperfused, extremities become cool, skin bluish and mottled, and urine production stops or profoundly slows down.

Shock can be attributed to abnormal cardiac output, abnormal intravascular volume, and abnormal systemic vascular resistance.[55] With these anatomical components in mind, shock can be categorized in four types (Figure 51.1). Cardiogenic shock may be due to acute stress cardiomyopathy, acute myocardial infarction, or acute pulmonary (massive emboli) and, less commonly in the NICU, due to obstruction from pericardiac tamponade or acute valvular insufficiency. In cardiogenic shock, there is a cycle of injury because loss of cardiac stroke volume and cardiac output may reduce coronary perfusion and cause compensatory vasoconstriction, all leading to a downward spiral.[42] Moreover, the use of inotropes and vasopressors may increase myocardial oxygen demand. Decreased intravascular volume may occur with hemorrhage, hypovolemia, massive tension pneumothorax, or abdominal compartment syndrome. Decreased vascular resistance and vasodilation are characteristics of distributive shock and are mostly seen with sepsis or anaphylaxis. (The pathophysiology of septic shock is only partly understood, and current concepts are summarized in Capsule 51.1).

To get a general sense of what to expect in the general ICU, more than two-thirds of patients with shock are due to a vasodilatory, distributive septic shock; approximately one in five are due to hypovolemic shock and one in five due to cardiogenic shock.[54] Obstructive shock due to pericardial tamponade is an uncommon cause, in most series less

Introduction of bacteria into the bloodstream can cause an infinitude of signs and symptoms, eventually leading to multiorgan failure. Sepsis comes from the Greek word *sepo*, denoting decomposition. When bacteria enter the bloodstream, patients become sick, but even early use of antimicrobials cannot prevent a secondary, more severe onslaught in susceptible patients that is dominated by inflammatory mediators, cellular dysfunction, and tissue injury. There are multiple phases, with release of bacterial toxins that eventually lead to release of mediators. These toxins affect macrophage function and result in the reduction of mediators. The entire process involves Toll-like receptors.[37] Gram-negative bacteria require a lipopolysaccharide-binding protein before they are recognized by the microphage Toll receptor, and gram-positive bacteria require lipoteichoic asset for recognition. The next phase is that these proinflammatory mediators result in promoting endothelial cell leukocyte adhesion, the release of arachidonics and metabolites, and the activation of complements. Multi-proinflammatory mediators are involved that include tumor necrosis factor, interleukins, neutrophils, thromboxane, and vasoactive neuropeptides. A septic syndrome will eventually result from this excessive proinflammatory response and will lead to multiorgan failure (MOF).[12,15,30]

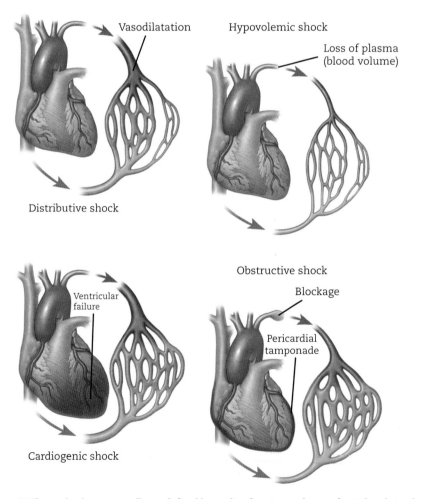

FIGURE 51.1: Different shock states usually are defined by cardiac function and state of peripheral circulation.

than 2%, and definitively uncommon in the NICU but slightly more common in trauma ICUs.

To the examiner, next to hypotension, patients in distributive shock show a hyperdynamic state, tachycardia, tachypnea, fever or hypothermia. Patient in hypovolemic or hemorrhagic shock show dry mucous membranes, poor skin turgor and decreased capillary refill or mottling. Patients in cardiogenic shock show acute respiratory failure, pulmonary edema and cardiac arrhythmias and elevated jugular venous pressure with cardiac tamponade.

Next to resuscitation, several important tests should be obtained, and these tests can assess the cause and severity of shock. Echocardiogram is a crucial test because the information may help in selecting therapy—IV fluids versus inotropes versus vasopressors. Echocardiogram measures left ventricular contractility and afterload, and cardiac output can be estimated by an echocardiogram. Normal cardiac chambers and preserved contractility are found in distributive shock and hypovolemic shock; however, increased ventricle size and poor contractility are seen in cardiogenic shock and obstructive shock. Sequential evaluation by echocardiogram shows the effects of treatment, but poor ejection fraction can be found in sepsis and cardiogenic shock, findings that may persist in an improving patient.

Lactate is elevated in shock (> 2 mmol/L) but in flux. Lactate measurement should be performed every 2 hours for a total of four. Some have argued that decreasing lactate by > 20% every 2 hours could guide management of fluid resuscitation ("lactate-based management").[25] Presence of a central venous catheter allows measurement of central venous oxygen saturation ($ScvO_2$), and outcome is better if oxygen transport is improved to values more than 70%. Moreover, the venoarterial carbon dioxide difference may be a marker of adequacy of resuscitation. (Values of the PCO_2 gap should be < 6 mm Hg.)[52] The mixed venous oxygen saturation (SVO_2) is decreased in patients in a low-flow state, but is normal or high in a distributive shock. Many resuscitation bundles do advise targeting at an SVO_2 of > 70% in the first hours of resuscitation.

MANAGEMENT OF SEPTIC SHOCK

Septic shock has been defined over the years, and some of the definitions that have been agreed upon are shown in Table 51.1.[17] A new 2016 consensus definition (part XIV Guidelines) identifies possible sepsis as hypotension requiring vasopressors with serum lactate of more than 2 mmol/L after adequate fluid resuscitation. As in many areas

TABLE 51.1. DEFINITIONS OF SYSTEMIC INFLAMMATORY RESPONSE SYNDROME (SIRS), SEPSIS, SEVERE SEPSIS, AND SEPTIC SHOCK

Term	Criteria
SIRS	Meets two of the following four:
	Temperature > 38°C or < 36°C
	Heart rate > 90 beats/min
	Respiratory rate > 30 breaths/min or arterial CO_2 < 32 mm Hg
	White blood cell count > 12,000 or < 4,000 cells/μL or >10% band forms
Sepsis	Documented or suspected infection plus systemic manifestations of infection (any of the SIRS criteria in addition other possible manifestations including elevations of procalcitonin, C-reactive protein, hyperglycemia in those without diabetes)
Severe sepsis	Sepsis plus evidence of organ dysfunction
	Arterial hypoxemia (PaO_2/FiO_2 < 300)
	Acute oliguria (urine output < 0.5 mL/kg per hour for at least 2 hours despite adequate fluid resuscitation)
	Increase in creatinine > 0.5 mg/dL
	Coagulation abnormalities (INR > 1.5, aPTT > 60 s, platelets < 100,000/μL)
	Hepatic dysfunction (elevated bilirubin)
	Paralytic ileus
	Decreased capillary refill or skin mottling
Septic shock	Sepsis with hypotension refractory to fluid resuscitation or hyperlactatemia
	Refractory hypotension persists despite resuscitation with bolus intravenous fluid of 30 mL/kg
	Hyperlactatemia > 2 mmol/L

aPTT, activated partial thromboplastin time; INR, international normalized ratio.

of critical care medicine, diagnosis is also based on an intervention, and most important is a fluid challenge.[46] Usually crystalloid solution is administered, infused rapidly, wide open with a pressure bag, and with 500 cc of fluids administered within 20 minutes. The major clinical clue of hypovolemia causing hypotension is a decrease in systemic arterial pressure with an increase in pulse rate, and these parameters will normalize after fluid resuscitation. Improving urinary output, however, may be delayed. Failure to correct hypotension with such a simple fluid challenge indicates a far more serious problem—and life-threatening shock—and vasopressor agents are now needed.

CAPSULE 51.2   FLUIDS AND SHOCK

If hypotension defines shock, fluid resuscitation is the first step in distributed and hypovolemic shock. Intensivists use 0.9% saline 90% of the time; others use albumin, knowing it stays longer in the intravascular volume. Unresolved issues are the type of fluid resuscitation, the amount of fluid resuscitation, and perhaps even the use of fluid resuscitation itself after a single fluid bolus. Saline causes—over time—metabolic acidosis and hypernatremia due to chlorine administration, and this effect might be harmful. Early fluid resuscitation, however, reduces tissue edema, likely through the prevention of reperfusion injury. Prolonged fluid resuscitation causes increased mortality, but the main variables are not known (the sickest refractory patients need more fluids). Most clinical trials have administered 2 liters in the first 6–8 hours.

Current discussion on early goal-directed therapy bundle and other measures of treatment with sepsis have found that bundle target resuscitation does not seem to improve outcome.[10,15–17,39] Such bundle therapy has included targets for central venous pressure (8–12 mmHg), mean arterial pressure (more than 65 mm Hg), urinary output (more than 0.5 ml/kg/hr), central venous oxygen saturation (more than 70%), arterial oxygen saturation (more than 93%), hematocrit (more than 30%), and, if available, cardiac index, and systemic oxygen consumption. The "standard care" has been defined as only using mean arterial blood pressure, central venous pressure, and urinary output, using a similar cutoff as in goal-directed care. None of these additional measures seems to have improved short- or long-term mortality in patients presenting with sepsis.[58]

Another concern is that septic shock often has a major hypovolemic component, and therefore large amounts of fluids may be necessary to adequately treat septic shock. Usually the response of central venous pressure to a fluid challenge given over 2 minutes may give an indication of a compliant venous system, and further fluid boluses may be necessary to increase the cardiac output. If there is a significant rise in pressure > 3 mm Hg, this would indicate that the right heart is noncompliant and that further fluids will overstress the right ventricle.[43]

The type of fluid resuscitation in septic shock is a matter of debate (Capsule 51.2). Generally, fluid resuscitation should not go beyond replacement of fluid lost, and serum sodium, osmolality and acid–base status should be considered when selecting a resuscitation fluid. Generally, oliguria is not a good marker of in adequate fluid resuscitation, particularly early in the postresuscitation.[43] Usually saline is preferred in patients with hypovolemia and alkalosis, and albumin can be considered during the early resuscitation of patients with

severe sepsis.[8] Albumin has been found to be problematic in patients with traumatic brain injury and may increase intracranial pressure.

Failure to respond to a change in blood pressure should prompt the initiation of vasopressor support (Table 51.2). Norepinephrine is the agent of choice in a patient with severe septic shock. This drug should be eventually be administered through a central venous line, but several doses can be administered through a peripheral catheter. If there is evidence of a severe cardiogenic shock with pulmonary edema, dobutamine is the agent of choice. A major concern with dobutamine is the increase in already existent tachycardia and arrhythmia and may worsen hypotension if there is inadequate preload.

To epitomize, it is reasonable to escalate care with three important steps; each are equally important.

First, fluid resuscitation remains important, but there is no benefit for colloids over crystalloids in the early resuscitation.[2,8] Some have used the definition of intravascular status using passive leg raise. With passive leg raise with legs raised to 45 degrees for several minutes, there is improved venous return, which could lead to improvement of blood pressure. Ultrasound has also been useful

TABLE 51.2. COMMON VASOACTIVE DRUGS IN SHOCK

Vasopressor	Dose	Effect
Epinephrine	0.07–1 mcg/kg/min	↑ SVR
Norepinephrine	0.04–1 mcg/kg/min	↑ SVR
Phenylephrine	0.5–5 mcg/kg/min	↑ SVR
Vasopressin	0.04 U/min	↑ SVR
Dopamine	5–20 mcg/kg/min	↑ SVR, ↑ CI
Milrinone	0.375–0.75 mcg/kg/min	↑ CI

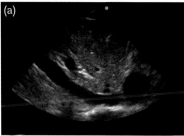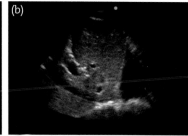

FIGURE 51.2: Ultrasound with subcostal view showing (a) normal IVC and (b) near 100% collapsibility.

in the evaluation of the inferior vena cava (IVC) and can examine for collapsibility. Minimally collapsed IVC is indicative of hypervolemia, and a highly collapsible IVC is associated with hypovolemia (Figure 51.2).

Second, and most essential, is an immediate administration of broad-spectrum antibiotic treatment and source control.[19,29] There is compelling evidence that delaying the administration of antibiotics—while actively resuscitating the patients—increases mortality and approximately 5% with each hour of delay in antibiotic administration. Antibiotic orders should come simultaneously with the order for fluid resuscitation, and blood cultures should come when other blood values are obtained. Care bundles may be very helpful in this respect. Two sets of cultures should be obtained immediately, and other source control should be immediately initiated with cultures from urine, tracheal secretions, and other body fluids.

There is no benefit of corticosteroids, nor is there any benefit of stimulation testing and initiating intravenous corticosteroids using hydrocortisone.[9] Similar recommendations are for bicarbonate therapy, which is not indicated in patients who have a pH of 7.15 or more. The emergence of multiorgan failure is problematic and may indicate higher mortality. This may include the development of acute respiratory distress syndrome or acute renal failure, often associated with acute kidney injury from hypotension.[26,30]

Third, norepinephrine is started earlier, and a second vasopressor is often needed to maintain a mean arterial blood pressure. The commonly used vasoactive drugs in shock are shown in Table 51.2. Norepinephrine has α-adrenergic action to increase vascular tone and β-adrenergic function to maintain cardiac output. A less optimal drug for sepsis is epinephrine, which only has α-adrenergic action and thus may decrease cardiac output and subsequently impair tissue blood flow. For the same reason, dopamine (mostly β-adrenergic) is

not ideal, and some studies found increased mortality in sepsis when dopamine was compared to norepinephrine.[13] The choice is often epinephrine or vasopressin; however, inotropic agents such as dobutamine may be used if there is evidence of myocardial dysfunction associated with sepsis.

MANAGEMENT OF ANAPHYLACTIC SHOCK

The response is a sudden systemic degranulation of mast cells or basophils.[7] Anaphylaxis is fortunately uncommon, but is acutely problematic because clinical presentation worsens quickly. Treatment requires a multisystem approach because respiratory and cardiovascular collapse can emerge within an hour. Immediate intervention is epinephrine 0.2–0.5 mg IM, possibly every 15 minutes, intubation, and immediate fluid replacement with 0.9% saline. Nebulized β2 agonist (albuterol) for bronchospasm and corticosteroids are needed. Treatment is summarized in Table 51.3.[1,4,32,38,49]

MANAGEMENT OF HEMORRHAGIC SHOCK

Bleeding will lead to a rapidly life-threatening condition as a result of hemodynamic instability and, finally, multisystem organ failure.[12,22] There have been many attempts to categorize the severity of hemorrhagic shock, and one is the shock index. A shock index of greater than 0.8 does indicate a compensated shock and may predict later hypotension, transfusion requirement, and cardiovascular collapse (Table 51.4). The shock index correlates the extent of hypovolemia with increased transfusion requirements; in more severely injured patients, an SI-based classification seems to discriminate the need for early blood product transfusion.[5,36,59] Isolated signs such as blood pressure or heart rate have very limited reliability in detecting hypovolemic shock. Therefore, the shock index is defined as

TABLE 51.3. THERAPEUTICS
FOR ANAPHYLAXIS
AFTER INTRAMUSCULAR EPINEPHRINE

Intervention	Dose and Route of Administration
Volume expansion	
0.9% saline	Adult: 1–2 L rapidly IV (5–10 ml/kg in first 5 min); child: 20 ml/kg in first hour
Epinephrine infusion	1 mg of 1:1,000 v/v (1 mg/ml) dilution added to 250 ml 5% dextrose in water (or NS) (i.e., 4 µg/ml concentration) infused at 1–4 µg/min (15–60 drops/min with microdrop), increasing to maximum 10 µg/min
Antihistamines	
Diphenhydramine	Adult: 25–50 mg IV; child: 1 mg/kg IV, up to 50 mg, infused over 10 min
Corticosteroids	
Methylprednisolone	1–2 mg/kg/day IV
Vasopressors	
Dopamine	400 mg in 500 ml 5% dextrose in water infused at 2–5 µg/kg/min
Glucagon	Initial dose, 1–5 mg slow IV, then 5–15 µg/min infusion
Methylene blue	Single-bolus 1.5–2 mg/kg in 100 ml 5% dextrose in water infused over 20 min has been used

Adapted from Kemp AM, Kemp SF. Pharmacotherapy in refractory anaphylaxis: when intramuscular epinephrine fails. *Curr Opin Allergy Clin Immunol* 2014;14:371–378.

TABLE 51.4. SHOCK INDEX

SHOCK INDEX (SI) = *HR/SBP*	
No shock	SI < 0.6
Mild shock	SI 0.6–0.9
Moderate shock	SI 1.0–1.3
Severe shock	SI ≥ 1.4

loss or more than 2 liters of blood volume loss, is associated with persistent hypotension and high mortality rate.

Key management is initial fluid resuscitation. A known concern with a significant fluid resuscitation is that it might be harmful in a patient who still needs control of a hemorrhage. Usually the common rule is to give enough fluid to maintain consciousness, but this might be difficult to assess if hemorrhagic shock is seen in a patient with multitrauma. Under no circumstances is hypotensive resuscitation recommended. A systolic blood pressure of at least 90 mm Hg must be maintained, likely higher. Rapid infusion can be secured with two large-bore (16-gauge or larger) peripheral intravenous catheters; and a pressure bag can be employed. Most patients also have developed marked hypothermia as the result of bleeding, and warm crystalloid solutions can be used as initial volume expanders. Initial management is a 1,000-cc bolus, repeated until the mean arterial blood pressure reaches 65 or shock index declines less than 0.8. The transient responders may have recurrent hypotension, and there are also nonrespondents who do not stabilize despite aggressive resuscitation efforts. An aggressive search for bleeding is initiated. This may include an abdominal angiogram. Control may only be achieved with a laparotomy, hepatic packing, and temporal abdominal closure with a vacuum pack. However, angiographic embolization has become more common, particularly in injury to the liver, spleen, pelvis, or chest. An important fact is that for each hour lost, mortality is increased by 47%, irrespective of the bleeding organ.[24] In more severe trauma, tranexamic acid 1 g IV until the bleeding stops can be considered.[44] Mostly crystalloids are administered, avoiding large amounts of colloids and generally less than 1,500 cc in the first 24 hours.[37] Resuscitation goals are shown in Table 51.5. Biochemical markers of hemorrhagic shock also include lactate and base deficit. Prothrombin time, international normalized ratio (INR), partial thromboplastic time, fibrinogen levels, and platelet counts are needed. Hemoglobin

the ratio of heart rate to systolic blood pressure. Other ways of classifying hemorrhagic shock is by blood loss percentage, but this classification has been criticized.[35] Class I shock is roughly 15% of blood loss, and there is a mild resting tachycardia. Class II shock is blood loss up to 30% and blood volume loss up to 1,500 cc, which leads to mild tachycardia, narrow pulse pressure, and delayed capillary refill. Class III shock is up to 40% blood loss and blood volume loss up to 2,000 cc resulting in hypotension and organ hypoperfusion, oliguria, and declining level of consciousness. Class IV shock, with more than 40% blood

TABLE 51.5. HEMORRHAGIC SHOCK

RESUSCITATION GOALS

SBP < 90 mm Hg

SPO2 > 96%

Hemoglobin 7–9 g/dL

Fibrinogen > 1.5g/L

INR ≤ 1.5

Platelets >50 g/L

From reference 12.

and hematocrit are poor indicators of early hemorrhage as a result of volume contraction.

Any coagulopathy should be treated with fresh frozen plasma, cryoprecipitate, or platelets, depending on drug used. Cryoprecipitate is used if fibrinogen levels are below 100 mg/dL and there is active bleeding.

MANAGEMENT OF CARDIOGENIC SHOCK

Usually a combination of inotropic or vasopressor agent is used, but the inotrope milrinone is a better alternative if inotropes or vasopressors cause arrhythmias.[33] Basic treatment remains using vasopressors (e.g., norepinephrine) and inotropes (e.g., dopamine) in combination.[47] Mechanical support is needed if inotropes and vasopressors have a limited effect and multiorgan failure emerges. Coronary revascularization may be needed, but this may not improve cardiac contractility quickly ("stunning"), and thus supportive devices may be needed. The mechanical devices are the intra-aortic balloon pump and extracorporal membrane oxygenation. The intra-aortic balloon pump is usually inserted during cardiac catheterization, and a balloon distal to the left subclaviar artery and proximal to the renal artery will inflate during diastole and actively deflate during systole.[28] The device is widely used, despite failure to improve 1-year mortality rates in large clinical trials[40] (IABP-shock II).[48] The intra-aortic balloon pump[56] improves coronary perfusion due to decrease in afterload with balloon deflation at the start of systole.

Extracorporeal membrane oxygenation (ECMO) may be considered in refractory cardiogenic shock (catheter in central vein draws blood, oxygenates it through an oxygenator, and returns it to arterial system).[20] This centrifugal pump may theoretically bridge a patient to a ventricular-assist device, but there is little experience with this scenario in critically ill neurologic patients.[45]

CONCLUSIONS

- The four major causes of shock are cardiac, vasodilatory, hypovolemic, and obstructive.
- The initial management is a fluid challenge with normal saline, but often vasopressor agents (norepinephrine) is norepinephrine is needed.
- Systolic blood pressure of at least 90 mm Hg must be maintained.
- Extracorporeal membrane oxygenation is needed in cardiogenic shock if inotropes and vasopressors have a limited effect and such aggressive management is warranted despite acute brain injury.

REFERENCES

1. Alrasbi M, Sheikh A. Comparison of international guidelines for the emergency medical management of anaphylaxis. *Allergy* 2007;62:838–841.
2. Angus DC, van der Poll T. Severe sepsis and septic shock. *N Engl J Med* 2013;369:840–851.
3. Bakker J, Perner A, Timsit JF. Evaluation of 7.5 years of Surviving Sepsis Campaign Guidelines. *Intensive Care Med* 2015;41:151–153.
4. Bauer CS, Vadas P, Kelly KJ. Methylene blue for the treatment of refractory anaphylaxis without hypotension. *Am J Emerg Med* 2013;31:264 e263–e265.
5. Birkhahn RH, Gaeta TJ, Terry D, Bove JJ, Tloczkowski J. Shock index in diagnosing early acute hypovolemia. *Am J Emerg Med* 2005;23:323–326.
6. Boyd JH, Forbes J, Nakada TA, Walley KR, Russell JA. Fluid resuscitation in septic shock: a positive fluid balance and elevated central venous pressure are associated with increased mortality. *Crit Care Med* 2011;39:259–265.
7. Brown SGA, Kemp SF, Lieberman PL. Anaphylaxis. In: Adkinson NF, Jr, Bochner BS, Burks W, et al., eds. *Middleton's Allergy: Principles and Practice.* Vol 1, 8th ed. Philadelphia: Elsevier Saunders; 2014.
8. Caironi P, Tognoni G, Masson S, et al. Albumin replacement in patients with severe sepsis or septic shock. *N Engl J Med* 2014;370:1412–1421.
9. Casserly B, Phillips GS,Schorr C et al. Lactate measurements in sepsis-induced tissue hypoperfusion: results from the surviving sepsis campaign database. *Crit Care Med* 2015; 43: 567–573.
10. Cawcutt KA, Peters SG. Severe sepsis and septic shock: clinical overview and update on management. *Mayo Clinic Proc* 2014;89:1572–1578.
11. Cecconi M, De Backer D, Antonelli M, et al. Consensus on circulatory shock and hemodynamic monitoring. Task force of the European

Society of Intensive Care Medicine. *Intens Care Med* 2014;40:1795–1815.

12. David JS, Spann C, Marcotte G, et al. Haemorrhagic shock, therapeutic management. *Ann Fr Anesth Reanim* 2013;32:497–503.

13. De Backer D, Aldecoa C, Njimi H, Vincent JL. Dopamine versus norepinephrine in the treatment of septic shock: a meta-analysis. *Crit Care Med* 2012;40:725–730.

14. De Backer D, Biston P, Devriendt J, et al. Comparison of dopamine and norepinephrine in the treatment of shock. *N Engl J Med* 2010;362:779–789.

15. Dellinger RP, Levy MM, Carlet JM, et al. Surviving Sepsis Campaign: international guidelines for management of severe sepsis and septic shock. *Intens Care Med* 2008;34:17–60.

16. Dellinger RP, Levy MM, Rhodes A, et al. Surviving Sepsis Campaign: international guidelines for management of severe sepsis and septic shock, 2012. *Intensive Care Med* 2013;39:165–228.

17. Dellinger RP, Levy MM, Rhodes A, et al. Surviving sepsis campaign: international guidelines for management of severe sepsis and septic shock: 2012. *Crit Care Med* 2013;41:580–637.

18. Deutschman CS, Tracey KJ. Sepsis: current dogma and new perspectives. *Immunity* 2014;40:463–475.

19. Ferrer R, Martin-Loeches I, Phillips G, et al. Empiric antibiotic treatment reduces mortality in severe sepsis and septic shock from the first hour: results from a guideline-based performance improvement program. *Crit Care Med* 2014;42:1749–1755.

20. Formica F, Avalli L, Redaelli G, Paolini G. Interhospital stabilization of adult patients with refractory cardiogenic shock by veno-arterial extracorporeal membrane oxygenation. *Int J Cardiol* 2011;147:164–165.

21. Glauser MP, Zanetti G, Baumgartner JD, Cohen J. Septic shock: pathogenesis. *Lancet* 1991;338:732–736.

22. Graham CA, Parke TR. Critical care in the emergency department: shock and circulatory support. *Emerg Med J* 2005;22:17–21.

23. Guly HR, Bouamra O, Little R, et al. Testing the validity of the ATLS classification of hypovolaemic shock. *Resuscitation* 2010;81:1142–1147.

24. Howell GM, Peitzman AB, Nirula R, et al. Delay to therapeutic interventional radiology postinjury: time is of the essence. *J Trauma* 2010;68:1296–1300.

25. Jones AE, Shapiro NI, Trzeciak S, et al. Lactate clearance vs central venous oxygen saturation as goals of early sepsis therapy: a randomized clinical trial. *JAMA* 2010;303:739–746.

26. Kellum JA, Bellomo R, Ronco C. The concept of acute kidney injury and the RIFLE criteria. *Contrib Nephrol* 2007;156:10–16.

27. Kemp AM, Kemp SF. Pharmacotherapy in refractory anaphylaxis: when intramuscular epinephrine fails. *Curr Opin Allergy Clin Immunol* 2014;14:371–378.

28. Krishna M, Zacharowski K. Principles of intra-aortic balloon pump counterpulsation. *Contin Educ Anaesth Crit Care Pain* 2009;9:24–28.

29. Kumar A, Roberts D, Wood KE, et al. Duration of hypotension before initiation of effective antimicrobial therapy is the critical determinant of survival in human septic shock. *Crit Care Med* 2006;34:1589–1596.

30. Legrand M, Dupuis C, Simon C, et al. Association between systemic hemodynamics and septic acute kidney injury in critically ill patients: a retrospective observational study. *Crit Care* 2013;17:R278.

31. Levy MM, Dellinger RP, Townsend SR, et al. The Surviving Sepsis Campaign: results of an international guideline-based performance improvement program targeting severe sepsis. *Intensive Care Med* 2010;36:222–231.

32. Lieberman P, Nicklas RA, Oppenheimer J, et al. The diagnosis and management of anaphylaxis practice parameter: 2010 update. *J Allergy Clin Immunol* 2010;126:477–480 e471–e442.

33. Lollgen H, Drexler H. Use of inotropes in the critical care setting. *Crit Care Med* 1990;18:S56–S60.

34. Monnet X, Rienzo M, Osman D, et al. Passive leg raising predicts fluid responsiveness in the critically ill. *Crit Care Med* 2006;34:1402–1407.

35. Mutschler M, Nienaber U, Brockamp T, et al. A critical reappraisal of the ATLS classification of hypovolaemic shock: does it really reflect clinical reality? *Resuscitation* 2013;84:309–313.

36. Mutschler M, Nienaber U, Munzberg M, et al. The Shock Index revisited: a fast guide to transfusion requirement? A retrospective analysis on 21,853 patients derived from the TraumaRegister DGU. *Crit Care* 2013;17:R172.

37. Nascimento B, Callum J, Rubenfeld G, et al. Clinical review: fresh frozen plasma in massive bleedings—more questions than answers. *Crit Care* 2010;14:202.

38. Nurmatov UB, Rhatigan E, Simons FE, Sheikh A. H2-antihistamines for the treatment of anaphylaxis with and without shock: a systematic review. *Ann Allergy Asthma Immunol* 2014;112:126–131.

39. Peake SL, Delaney A, Bailey M, et al. Goal-directed resuscitation for patients with early septic shock. *N Engl J Med* 2014;371:1496–1506.

40. Prondzinsky R, Lemm H, Swyter M, et al. Intra-aortic balloon counterpulsation in patients with acute myocardial infarction complicated by

cardiogenic shock: the prospective, randomized IABP SHOCK Trial for attenuation of multiorgan dysfunction syndrome. *Crit Care Med* 2010;38:152–160.

41. Remick DG. Pathophysiology of sepsis. *Am J Pathol* 2007;170:1435–1444.

42. Reynolds HR, Hochman JS. Cardiogenic shock: current concepts and improving outcomes. *Circulation* 2008;117:686–697.

43. Rochwerg B, Alhazzani W, Sindi A, et al. Fluid resuscitation in sepsis: a systematic review and network meta-analysis. *Ann Intern Med* 2014;161:347–355.

44. Shakur H, Roberts I, Bautista R, et al. Effects of tranexamic acid on death, vascular occlusive events, and blood transfusion in trauma patients with significant hemorrhage (CRASH-2): a randomized, placebo-controlled trial. *Lancet* 2010;376:23–32.

45. Sheu JJ, Tsai TH, Lee FY, et al. Early extracorporeal membrane oxygenator-assisted primary percutaneous coronary intervention improved 30-day clinical outcomes in patients with ST-segment elevation myocardial infarction complicated with profound cardiogenic shock. *Crit Care Med* 2010;38:1810–1817.

46. Seymour CW, Rosengart MR. Septic shock: Advances in diagnosis and treatment. *JAMA* 2015;314:708–717.

47. Thiele H, Ohman EM, Desch S, Eitel I, de Waha S. Management of cardiogenic shock. *Eur Heart J* 2015;3:1223–1230.

48. Thiele H, Zeymer U, Neumann FJ, et al. Intra-aortic balloon counterpulsation in acute myocardial infarction complicated by cardiogenic shock (IABP-SHOCK II): final 12 month

results of a randomized, open-label trial. *Lancet* 2013;382:1638–1645.

49. Thomas M, Crawford I. Best evidence topic report. Glucagon infusion in refractory anaphylactic shock in patients on beta-blockers. *Emerg Med J* 2005;22:272–273.

50. Trauma ACoSCo. *Advanced Trauma Life Support Program for Doctors*. 2004.

51. Unverzagt S, Machemer MT, Solms A, et al. Intra-aortic balloon pump counterpulsation (IABP) for myocardial infarction complicated by cardiogenic shock. *Cochrane Database Syst Rev* 2011:CD007398.

52. Vallet B, Pinsky MR, Cecconi M. Resuscitation of patients with septic shock: please "mind the gap"! *Intensive Care Med* 2013;39:1653–1655.

53. Vasselon T, Detmers PA. Toll receptors: a central element in innate immune responses. *Infect Immun* 2002;70:1033–1041.

54. Vincent JL, De Backer D. Circulatory shock. *N Engl J Med* 2013;369:1726–1734.

55. Wacker DA, Winters ME. Shock. *Emerg Med Clin North Am* 2014;32:747–758.

56. Webb CA, Weyker PD, Flynn BC. Management of intra-aortic balloon pumps. *Semin Cardiothorac Vasc Anesth* 2015;19:106–121.

57. Werdan K, Gielen S, Ebelt H, Hochman JS. Mechanical circulatory support in cardiogenic shock. *Eur Heart J* 2014;35:156–167.

58. Yealy DM, Kellum JA, Huang DT, et al. A randomized trial of protocol-based care for early septic shock. *N Engl J Med* 2014;370:1683–1693.

59. Zarzaur BL, Croce MA, Fischer PE, Magnotti LJ, Fabian TC. New vitals after injury: shock index for the young and age x shock index for the old. *J Surg Res* 2008;147:229–236.

52

Cardiopulmonary Arrest

In-hospital (and certainly ICU) cardiac arrest is very different from out-of-hospital arrest. It is more likely an indication of the severity of illness and reflecting a dying patient. In the hospital the potential responders are readily available, and immediate care after return of spontaneous circulation is more likely to be effective. Cardiopulmonary resuscitation (CPR) in the NICU is uncommon.[20] Cardiac arrest is very often a terminal event in unsurvivable brain injury, and patients are not resuscitated due to previously established do-not-resuscitate orders. This clinical setting is very different from CPR in general intensive care units, where often patients arrive in septic shock or with a pulmonary embolism that may lead to sudden cardiac arrest-condition where CPR could make a difference. Cardiac arrest in the setting of polytrauma dramatically increases mortality (50% within 24 hours) and certainly when associated with resuscitation from hemorrhagic shock. Some of these patients may rearrest soon after NICU admission. Similar scenarios may be seen in patients with poor-grade subarachnoid hemorrhage (SAH), and asystole (Chapter 56) increasing the probability of poor outcome, despite the fact that a considerable number of patients survive independently.[26]

Neurointensivists should also anticipate that occasionally patients may develop cardiac arrest as a result of pulmonary emboli,[15] or as a result of acute coronary syndrome associated with the sympathetic outburst of acute brain injury. Often the time for the evaluation of neurologic status is too short to assess the futility of cardiopulmonary resuscitation, and resuscitation may have started in patients developing terminal cardiac arrest when all brainstem reflexes are lost. Patients may remain comatose following cardiopulmonary resuscitation, but very little data on prognostication in this category are available.

CPR requires complex teamwork, leadership, and an obligation to generally adhere to American Heart Association algorithms (Figure 52.1), and this analytic approach remains successful in many instances.[8] The most recent guideline was published in 2015 (Part XIV, Guidelines). There have been several important initiatives to improve outcome after in-hospital arrest.[16]

The field of cardiopulmonary resuscitation is complex and vast, and this chapter can only provide a basic review of cardiopulmonary resuscitation. Unfortunately CPR in the NICU is rarely effective and this sums up the essence of the problem.

BASIC CARDIOPULMONARY RESUSCITATION

Cardiopulmonary resuscitation involves defibrillation and the administration of vasoactive drugs and it requires a team of responders who are well adjusted to each other. Many hospitals have simulation centers that provide this training. Immediate cardiopulmonary resuscitation is obviously essential because the likelihood of survival reduces quickly with delay. Technical skills and previous experience are necessary to provide an adequate resuscitation. Generally, family is present during cardiopulmonary resuscitation. A landmark study from France found that post-traumatic stress disorder following resuscitation was found to a lesser degree in family members if they were present during the efforts.[13,30]

The principles of management involve initial airway management, and ventilation is performed during CPR. GlideScope® video laryngoscope increases first-pass success rate significantly.[6] Bag-mask ventilation is performed while another team member provides chest compression. The 2010 resuscitation guideline from the American Heart Association provides an algorithm (Figure 52.1) that emphasizes accurately applied CPR (push hard/push fast), minimal interruptions, and taking no more than 10 seconds to check for a pulse. The key skill is to maintain a rate of 100 compressions per minute. The chest has to be compressed 5 cm (2 inches with each downward stroke), and the chest should recoil completely ("fast and hard").[24,27] In general, two ventilations after 30 compressions for the patient are provided, showing enough volume to see the chest rise.

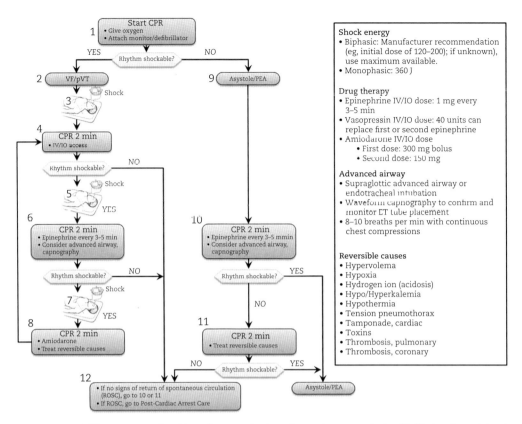

FIGURE 52.1: AHA consensus algorithms for resuscitation of asystole or ventricular fibrillation (copyright sign American Heart Association).

The next step is to assess cardiac rhythm (asystole or pulseless electrical activity) or a shockable rhythm (ventricle fibrillation, torsades de pointes, pulseless ventricular tachycardia). Asystole is the absence of electrical and mechanical cardiac activity. Pulseless electrical activity (PEA) is organized electrocardiographic rhythm without sufficient mechanical contraction of the heart in such a way that it does not produce a palpable pulse or noticeable and measureable blood pressure, and thus is a nonperfusing rhythm. Asystole and PEA are treated with vasopressors and start with administration of epinephrine 1 mg IV every 3–5 minutes. Vasopressin can be administered usually 40 units for the first 10 minutes after the first or second epinephrine dose.[25,28]

With ventricular fibrillation or pulseless fibrillation, at least one attempt at defibrillation is administered, but also epinephrine 1 mg IV is administered every 3–5 minutes. There is no evidence that three stacked shocks are better than one shock.[3] Antiarrhythmic drugs provide very little additional survival benefit, nor is the timing known. The second shock is administered after

five cycles of CPR (2 minutes). If a second defibrillation is unsuccessful, amiodarone 300 mg IV with a repeat dose of 150 mg IV is administered. Alternatively, lidocaine 1–1.5 mg/kg/IV, followed by 0.5–0.75 mg/kg every 5–10 minutes, can be used. In addition, magnesium sulfate 2g IV, followed by maintenance infusion, is necessary if the patient shows torsade de pointes.[11]

Additional cardiac arrhythmias are complex (Table 52.1) and treatment is discussed in Chapter 56. Generally, the pharmacological options for the complex post-arrest rhythms often include symptomatic bradycardia and ventricular tachycardia. Generally, bradycardia is treated with atropine 0.6 mg, repeated every 3–5 minutes. If atropine fails, dopamine and catecholamine with both α and β adrenergic action can be considered, and usually an infusion rate is started at 5 mcg/kg/min.

Patients with a narrow complex tachycardia, such as supraventricular tachycardia, can be terminated with a vagal maneuver or adenosine 6 mg IV push. When there is only short-lived conversion, amiodarone can be started and dosed at

TABLE 52.1. COMMON FIRST-DOCUMENTED RHYTHM IN ADULT CARDIAC ARREST*

Asystole	35%
PEA	32%
VF or pulseless VT	23%
VF	14%
Pulseless VT	9%

* In 10% there is no accurate documentation.
From Nadkarni et al. First documented rhythm and clinical outcome from in-hospital cardiac arrest among children and adults. *JAMA* 2006;295:50–57.
PEA, Pulseless electrical activity; VF, ventricular fibrillation; VT, ventricular tachycardia.

150 mg IV over 10 minutes, followed by 1 mg/min infusion over 6 hours.

In wide-complex tachycardia, defined as QRS more than 0.12 seconds, IV adenosine remains a safe drug for diagnosis and treatment. Alternative drugs for wide-complex tachycardia are procainamide and sotalol. Procainamide is dosed at 50 mg/min. Patients who displayed atrial fibrillation with rapid ventricular response can be treated with ß-blockade or calcium channel blockers and mostly diltiazem infusion.

The 2010 ACLS guidelines do mention termination of resuscitation efforts.[5,12,19] In general, the factor that influences this decision is the duration of resuscitation efforts of more than 30 minutes without a sustained perfusion rhythm; but in these circumstances, extracorporeal membrane oxygenation (ECMO) can be considered if the patient is eligible for such an intervention. The presence of an initial electrocardiographic reading of asystole is very problematic if this cannot be reversed. Patient age, severity of comorbid disease, and the presence of fixed pupils or absence of more brainstem reflexes, all in the setting of normothermia, can be acceptable endpoints of resuscitation. Worse outcomes are expected in resuscitated patients on chronic dialysis.[21] It has been shown that the best predictor of outcome is the end tidal CO_2 level following 20 minutes of resuscitation[2,10,14] (Capsule 52.1). A very low tidal CO_2 (< 10 mm Hg) following prolonged resuscitation of more than 20 minutes indicates absent circulation and is a high predictor of mortality. A

CAPSULE 52.1   FEEDBACK OF CPR WITH CAPNOGRAPHY

Success of CPR—particularly in a prolonged resuscitation attempt—can be measured by end-tidal carbon dioxide ($ETCO_2$). Capnography is also reflective of correct endotracheal tube placement. Failure to increase $ETCO_2$ during CPR may indicate suboptimal chest compression, cardiac tamponade, or pneumothorax. In one case, sustained CPR for 96 minutes with end tidal CO_2 values in the 28–36 mm Hg range and 12 shocks led to excellent outcome.[29] This value reflects cardiac output and less than 10 mm Hg seems a cut-off point. Abrupt increase in $ETCO_2$ may indicate return of spontaneous circulation. The device is placed between the endotracheal tube and the resuscitation bag.

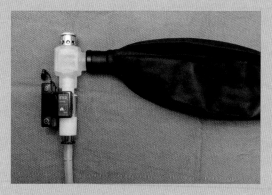

Capnograph placed between endotracheal tube and resuscitation bag.

greater end tidal CO_2 should encourage continuation of resuscitation. Echocardiography, if available, may be helpful.

POST–CARDIAC ARREST SYNDROME

After return of spontaneous circulation (ROSC), a complex pathophysiologic process is seen, which involves major organ systems.[7,15,18] Multisystem organ failure may be the cause of death and therefore its early recognition and care are important (Table 52.2). Early hemodynamic optimization is a major concern and involves fluid resuscitation (cardiac arrest with sepsis) and adequate oxygen delivery. Acute coronary syndromes may require emergent cardiac catheterization. Patients may need aortic balloon pump and multiple vasopressors and inotropes, may have additional liver injury, and may be anuric, requiring immediate dialysis.

This uncompromising complication, also called *post–cardiac arrest syndrome*, may occur in two-thirds of the patients resuscitated, and in essence is whole body ischemia followed by reperfusion. Timelines of different phases have been arbitrarily defined and it has been suggested that the interval of 20 minutes to 12 hours post-arrest may be the most likely period where interventions could work. The organs involved beside the brain are myocardium, kidney, liver, and adrenals. The

systemic ischemia-reperfusion response results in impaired vasoregulation, increased coagulation, adrenal suppression, and abnormal oxygen delivery. Patients are hemodynamically labile, but even patients with normal blood pressures have poor cardiac index. Hypotension despite use of multiple vasopressors and inotropes could exacerbate brain ischemia due to severely impaired cerebral autoregulation. How much of this relative hypotension can be tolerated is not known.

Renal replacement therapy and continuous dialysis for days or weeks may be needed. Most patients may have impaired liver function tests, and repeated studies will show a rise in the 1,000s. Oxygenation may be impaired from pulmonary edema (may be related to rib fractures and may be related to post-pneumothorax management). Hyperoxemia (prolonged oxygenation with 100% FIO_2) may increase hospital mortality post–cardiac arrest.

This rapidly unraveling syndrome may determine outcome and not so much brain injury. It is important to appreciate that there is such a post-resuscitation disease that involves cardiac stunning with hemodynamic instability and the need for either artificial support through a balloon pump or ECMO.[1,4,9,22] This intervention is needed because the stunning will lead to marked reduction in myocardial function and exacerbates the problem. In addition, these multiple periods of

TABLE 52.2. POST–CARDIAC ARREST SYNDROME: PATHOPHYSIOLOGY, CLINICAL MANIFESTATIONS, AND POTENTIAL TREATMENTS

Syndrome	Pathophysiology	Clinical Manifestation	Potential Treatments
Post–cardiac arrest myocardial dysfunction	Global hypokinesis (myocardial stunning) ACS	Reduced cardiac output Hypotension Dysrhythmias Cardiovascular collapse	Early revascularization of AMI Early hemodynamic optimization Intravenous fluid Inotropes IABP LVAD ECMO
Systemic ischemia/ reperfusion response	Systemic inflammatory response syndrome Impaired vasoregulation Increased coagulation Adrenal suppression Impaired tissue oxygen delivery and utilization Impaired resistance to infection	Ongoing tissue hypoxia/ ischemia Hypotension Cardiovascular collapse Pyrexia (fever) Hyperglycemia Multiorgan failure Infection	Early hemodynamic optimization IV fluid Vasopressors High-volume hemofiltration Temperature control Glucose control Antibiotics with documented infection

ACS indicates acute coronary syndrome; AMI, acute myocardial infarction; ECMO, extracorporeal membrane oxygenation; IABP, intra-aortic balloon pump; IV, intravenous; LVAD, left ventricular assist device.
Adapted from Neumar et al. Post-cardiac arrest syndrome: epidemiology, pathophysiology, treatment, and prognostication. *Circulation* 2008;118:2452–2483. Copyright ©2008, American Heart Association, Inc.

hemodynamic instability despite aggressive resuscitation can also lead to marked renal or acute hepatic failure. ECMO has significantly improved survival of cardiopulmonary resuscitation.[22,23]

CONCLUSIONS

- The important first decision is to start chest compression and ventilation (compression/ventilation 30:2 ratio).
- The important second decision is to determine rhythm and whether it is shockable.
- The important third decision is to treat remaining cardiac arrhythmia.
- Low end-tidal CO_2, prolonged effort in asystole, and absent brainstem reflexes in a normothermic patient may indicate failure of CPR.

REFERENCES

1. Abrams D, Combes A, Brodie D. Extracorporeal membrane oxygenation in cardiopulmonary disease in adults. *J Am Coll Cardiol* 2014;63: 2769–2778.
2. Ahrens T, Schallom L, Bettorf K, et al. End-tidal carbon dioxide measurements as a prognostic indicator of outcome in cardiac arrest. *Am J Crit Care* 2001;10:391–398.
3. Ali B, Zafari AM. Narrative review: cardiopulmonary resuscitation and emergency cardiovascular care: review of the current guidelines. *Ann Intern Med* 2007;147:171–179.
4. Avalli L, Maggioni E, Formica F, et al. Favourable survival of in-hospital compared to out-of-hospital refractory cardiac arrest patients treated with extracorporeal membrane oxygenation: an Italian tertiary care centre experience. *Resuscitation* 2012;83:579–583.
5. Berg RA, Hemphill R, Abella BS, et al. Part 5: adult basic life support: 2010 american heart association guidelines for cardiopulmonary resuscitation and emergency cardiovascular care. *Circulation* 2010;122:S685–705.
6. Bernhard M, Benger JR. Airway management during cardiopulmonary resuscitation. *Curr Opin Crit Care* 2015;21:183–187.
7. Binks A, Nolan JP. Post-cardiac arrest syndrome. *Minerva Anestesiol* 2010;76:362–368.
8. Bottiger BW. Cardiopulmonary resuscitation and postresuscitation care 2015: saving more than 200 000 additional lives per year worldwide. *Curr Opin Crit Care* 2015;21:179–182.
9. Chauhan S, Subin S. Extracorporeal membrane oxygenation, an anesthesiologist's perspective: physiology and principles. Part 1. *Ann Card Anaesth* 2011;14:218–229.
10. Grmec S, Klemen P. Does the end-tidal carbon dioxide (EtCO2) concentration have prognostic value during out-of-hospital cardiac arrest? *Eur J Emerg Med* 2001;8:263–269.
11. Hassan TB, Jagger C, Barnett DB. A randomised trial to investigate the efficacy of magnesium sulphate for refractory ventricular fibrillation. *Emerg Med J* 2002;19:57–62.
12. Hazinski MF, Nolan JP, Billi JE, et al. Part 1: Executive summary: 2010 international consensus on cardiopulmonary resuscitation and emergency cardiovascular care science with treatment recommendations. *Circulation* 2010;122:S250–275.
13. Jabre P, Belpomme V, Azoulay E, et al. Family presence during cardiopulmonary resuscitation. *N Engl J Med* 2013;368:1008–1018.
14. Kodali BS, Urman RD. Capnography during cardiopulmonary resuscitation: Current evidence and future directions. *J Emerg Trauma Shock* 2014;7:332–340.
15. Kurkciyan I, Meron G, Sterz F, et al. Pulmonary embolism as a cause of cardiac arrest: presentation and outcome. *Arch Intern Med* 2000;160:1529–1535.
16. Morrison LJ, Neumar RW, Zimmerman JL, et al. Strategies for improving survival after in-hospital cardiac arrest in the United States: 2013 consensus recommendations: a consensus statement from the American Heart Association. *Circulation* 2013;127:1538–1563.
17. Nadkarni VM, Larkin GL, Peberdy MA, et al. First documented rhythm and clinical outcome from in-hospital cardiac arrest among children and adults. *JAMA* 2006;295:50–57.
18. Neumar RW, Nolan JP, Adrie C, et al. Postcardiac arrest syndrome: epidemiology, pathophysiology, treatment, and prognostication. A consensus statement from the International Liaison Committee on Resuscitation (American Heart Association, Australian and New Zealand Council on Resuscitation, European Resuscitation Council, Heart and Stroke Foundation of Canada, InterAmerican Heart Foundation, Resuscitation Council of Asia, and the Resuscitation Council of Southern Africa); the American Heart Association Emergency Cardiovascular Care Committee; the Council on Cardiovascular Surgery and Anesthesia; the Council on Cardiopulmonary, Perioperative, and Critical Care; the Council on Clinical Cardiology; and the Stroke Council. *Circulation* 2008;118:2452–2483.
19. Neumar RW, Otto CW, Link MS, et al. Part 8: adult advanced cardiovascular life support: 2010 American Heart Association Guidelines for Cardiopulmonary Resuscitation and

Emergency Cardiovascular Care. *Circulation* 2010;122:S729–767.

20. Rabinstein AA, McClelland RL, Wijdicks EFM, Manno EM, Atkinson JL. Cardiopulmonary resuscitation in critically ill neurologic-neurosurgical patients. *Mayo Clinic Proc* 2004;79:1391–1395.

21. Saeed F, Adil MM, Malik AA, Schold JD, Holley JL. Outcomes of in-hospital cardiopulmonary resuscitation in maintenance dialysis patients. *J Am Soc Nephrol* 2015;26:3093–3101.

22. Shin TG, Choi JH, Jo IJ, et al. Extracorporeal cardiopulmonary resuscitation in patients with inhospital cardiac arrest: a comparison with conventional cardiopulmonary resuscitation. *Crit Care Med* 2011;39:1–7.

23. Shin TG, Jo IJ, Sim MS, et al. Two-year survival and neurological outcome of in-hospital cardiac arrest patients rescued by extracorporeal cardiopulmonary resuscitation. *Int J Cardiol* 2013;168:3424–3430.

24. Stiell IG, Brown SP, Christenson J, et al. What is the role of chest compression depth during out-of-hospital cardiac arrest resuscitation? *Crit Care Med* 2012;40:1192–1198.

25. Stiell IG, Hebert PC, Wells GA, et al. Vasopressin versus epinephrine for inhospital cardiac arrest: a randomized controlled trial. *Lancet* 2001;358:105–109.

26. Toussaint LG, 3rd, Friedman JA, Wijdicks EFM, et al. Survival of cardiac arrest after aneurysmal subarachnoid hemorrhage. *Neurosurgery* 2005;57:25–31.

27. Vadeboncoeur T, Stolz U, Panchal A, et al. Chest compression depth and survival in out-of-hospital cardiac arrest. *Resuscitation* 2014;85:182–188.

28. Warren SA, Huszti E, Bradley SM, et al. Adrenaline (epinephrine) dosing period and survival after in hospital cardiac arrest: a retrospective review of prospectively collected data. *Resuscitation* 2014;85:350–358.

29. White RD, Goodman BW, Svoboda MA. Neurologic recovery following prolonged out-of-hospital cardiac arrest with resuscitation guided by continuous capnography. *Mayo Clinic Proc* 2011;86:544–548.

30. Zavotsky KE, McCoy J, Bell G, et al. Resuscitation team perceptions of family presence during CPR. *Adv Emerg Nurs J* 2014;36:325–334.

53

Acute Kidney Injury

A problem to be dealt with from time to time is acute kidney injury (AKI), but patients with acute neurocritical illness and AKI are not quite like anyone else. Many patients have normal kidney function on admission to the NICU; a minority have chronic kidney disease, and even fewer have end-stage kidney disease—a conspicuous contrast with patients in general surgical and medical ICUs. When patients with critical neurologic illness develop kidney failure, noted by a sudden increase in serum creatine and fall in urine output, the commonly identified triggers are hypovolemia,[14] neuroimaging with contrast, and drug toxicity. In any patient with a nondominant hemispheric stroke and neglect, found down and unattended for some time, may have developed major muscle breakdown leading to rhabdomyolysis, which may seriously damage the kidney.[6]

However, patients admitted to the NICU are often elderly or may have preexisting kidney disease and thus may easily develop a secondary injury with temporary hypoperfusion. Later, as a result of prolonged bed rest, mechanical ventilation, and incremental polypharmacy, critically ill neurologic patients are also exposed to triggers for AKI that are common to the more general ICU population.

The prevalence of AKI in the NICU is not exactly known and is variable as a result of the patient mix, but one study suggested an unexpectedly high incidence of 9% in subarachnoid hemorrhage (SAH).[14] Although nephrologists are frequently consulted by intensivists, and major medical centers have ICU nephrology services, more than basic knowledge of a diagnostic approach to AKI is required. Particularly, physicians should be aware of drugs that may precipitate acute renal failure or that may worsen chronic renal failure. Most discouragingly, AKI may result in renal replacement therapy with increased risk of hospital mortality, and may increase risk for future development of chronic kidney disease, as improvement with dialysis is no guarantee. Close communication with the consulted nephrologist is needed to obtain insight into fluid removal and electrolyte replenishment. In the NICU, better management of osmotic fluid shifts with continuous renal replacement therapy has reduced incidences of surges in intracranial pressure, but it continues to be a concern. Prevention of AKI is key and requires the following: (1) identification of potential triggers; (2) avoidance of hypovolemia and nephrotoxic agents (e.g., angiotensin-converting enzyme inhibitors, NSAIDs); (3) prevention of contrast-induced nephropathy; and (4) drug monitoring and adjustment of dose as per estimated glomerular filtration rate. This chapter provides an approach specific to the NICU population.

DEFINITION OF ACUTE KIDNEY INJURY

Most intensivists define new acute kidney injury simply as a rise in creatinine and a decrease in urinary output. These two metrics are used in classification systems, and the commonly used RIFLE (Risk, Injury, Failure, Loss, and End-stage Kidney Disease) classification is shown in Table 53.1 The Acute Kidney Injury Network (AKIN) further fine-tuned the definition of risk as an abrupt reduction in kidney function with an absolute increase in serum creatinine of more or equal to 0.3 mg/dL, a 50% increase in serum creatinine or reduction in urinary output with oliguria, or less than 0.5 mL/kg/hr for more than 6 hours.[20] Most recently, KDIGO guidelines combined the parameters used in RIFLE and AKIN classification.[13] Once diagnosed, patients may progress further; and in general ICU populations (with a high prevalence of sepsis), about half of the patients progress to a far more serious injury or failure phase in the following days. Mortality is closely related to severity of kidney injury on the basis of RIFLE/AKIN classification. Barring any other approaches or modifications of the RIFLE classification, the recently proposed AKIN/KDIGO classification of acute kidney injury is currently the intensivist and nephrologist's framework and modus operandi.[18]

TABLE 53.1. RIFLE CRITERIA

	Creatinine	Urinary Output
Risk	Increase creatinine × 1.5 or acute rise ≥ 0.3 mg/dL	UO < 0.5 mL/kg/hr for 6 hours
Injury	Increased creatinine × 2	UO < 0.5 mL/kg/hr for 12 hours
Failure	Increased creatinine × 3 or creatinine > 4 mg/dL	UO < 0.3 mL/kg/hr for 24 hours or anuria for 12 hours
Loss		Complete loss of function > 4 weeks
ESRD	End-stage	Renal disease dialysis dependent

CAUSES OF ACUTE KIDNEY INJURY

The main causes of AKI are shown in Table 53.2 and mechanisms are found in Capsule 53.1. In a patient with established renal failure, it is important to differentiate between the acute and chronic nature of the kidney disease. History of underlying chronic hypertension, diabetes, kidney stone disease, with past history of renal dysfunction; evidence of chronic anemia and hyperphosphatemia; and small kidney sizes on imaging would suggest the chronic nature of kidney injury. For

TABLE 53.2. COMMON CAUSES OF ACUTE KIDNEY INJURY IN THE NICU

Acute blood loss in polytrauma
Drug induced hypotension
Hypovolemia
Vancomycin, acyclovir, NSAIDs
Rhabdomyolysis
Sepsis
Recent major surgery
Contrast dye

acute kidney injury, the most important thing to consider is looking for the reversible causes of renal dysfunction, such as hypovolemia and obstruction. One of the first concerns is to identify renal obstruction and exclude this possibility with a renal ultrasound. An obstructive urinary catheter with acute severe bladder retention may rapidly lead to significant increase in creatinine and is a commonly overlooked cause in acutely ill neurologic patients unable to signal a full bladder.

It is subsequently important to evaluate the intrinsic causes of the AKI. Urinary electrolytes (Na, K, urea, creatinine) and calculation of fractional excretion of sodium (FeNa) help to exclude prerenal azotemia from established renal injury with tubular damage. Urinalysis is needed to examine for hematuria,[25] proteinuria, and casts and then to differentiate between various causes of intrinsic renal failure. Granular, epithelial cell casts or free renal tubular epithelial cells are strongly suggestive of acute tubular necrosis which indicates some significant ischemic insult. Acute kidney injury may be due to new kidney infarction in a patient with multiple emboli including the brain. Increasing creatinine in a patient with a

---

CAPSULE 53.1   PATHOGENESIS OF ACUTE RENAL INJURY

When acute renal injury is caused by hypoperfusion, the main mechanism is hyperperfusion injury (Ischemia/reperfusion injury) resulting in tissue edema, decreased renal blood flow, tubular necrosis, tubular casting obstructing tubuli, and eventually loss of glomerular filtration. Fluids have got the attention. Excess fluids especially when given to patients who are not fluid deplete may result in renal interstitial edema, and thus worsening kidney failure. Furthermore, synthetic colloids are potentially nephrotoxic and chloride-rich solutions should be prescribed with caution. More paradoxically, in sepsis (approximately 50%–70% of cases, depending on ICU studied) the hyperdynamic state increases renal blood flow; but histology remains normal for a long time, despite marked pathophysiologic changes and increased creatinine.[4,10,15,16] Currently, biomarkers reflect severity of illness. Cystatin C relates to decreased glomerular filtration rate, and neutrophil gelatinase-associated lipocalin reflects tubular injury.[9]

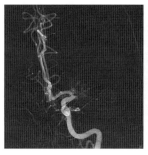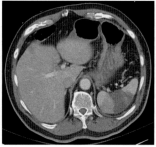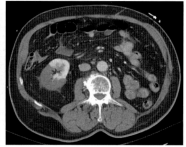

FIGURE 53.1: Acute embolus to the middle cerebral artery, spleen, and solitary kidney.

recent stroke may have its origin in ischemic kidney disease (Figure 53.1).

Glomerular or interstitial disease should be considered if there has not been a shock-induced trigger. The most commonly implicated drugs are antibiotics (nearly all), nonsteroidal anti-inflammatory drugs (NSAIDs), but also proton pump inhibitors have been implicated. The diagnosis is often tentative and a recent study has shown the poor correlation between urine eosinophils and eosinophilia and the presence of interstitial nephritis.[22]

Rhabdomyolysis may cause kidney injury, particularly if there are several aggravating factors—trauma plus seizures plus prior illicit drugs and alcohol. A large amount of muscle necrosis (CPKs in the 10,000 range) is needed for kidneys to become injured, and urine may become red-brown (myoglobin precipitates in renal tubules, obstructing and causing toxicity as a result of ferrous oxide). There is no absolute cutoff level of serum creatinine kinase above which the risk of acute kidney injury is markedly increased. The presence of low fractional excretion of sodium, reflecting tubular failure, is another characteristic.[6] Judging the severity of rhabdomyolysis-associated AKI requires serial serum creatine kinase levels and creatinine levels. While myoglobin is responsible for kidney injury in rhabdomyolysis, it has low sensitivity for the diagnosis because of rapid metabolism.[21] Monitoring consists of frequent checking of urinary output (> 200 ml per hour).

Toxicity needs to be considered next. Drugs that are notorious for acute kidney injury are amphotericin, aminoglycosides, angiotensin-converting enzyme inhibitors or angiotensin receptor blockers, β-lactam antibiotics, and vancomycin.

The most conspicuous cause for nephrotoxity in the NICU is intravenous contrast used in patients with multiple cerebral angiograms and contract CT scans. Nephrotoxicity is caused by iodinated contrast and theoretically is a preventable complication.[24] Known contrast allergy is pretreated with prednisone 50 mg orally in three doses, 12, 6, and 1 hour before administration, and combined with diphenhydramine 50 mg orally 1 hour before administration. It has been known for many years that hydration is critical for prevention of contrast-induced nephropathy, and when furosemide-based intervention is compared with saline hydration, there is a negative effect of the furosemide-based intervention.

Volume supplementation, therefore, is important and requires IV fluids for 12 hours pre-procedure and 12 hours post-procedure. Some protocols use 2 liters of normal saline within 12 hours before and after contrast media exposure. A protective effect of sodium bicarbonate has been demonstrated. One approach is to add 154 mEq/L of sodium bicarbonate in 5% dextrose and water, and to add 154 ml of 1,000 mEq/L sodium bicarbonate to 846 ml of 5% dextrose in H_2O, diluting the dextrose concentration to 4.23%. A recent meta-analysis of 20 randomized clinical trials found, however, sodium bicarbonate did not result in reduction of dialysis or mortality.[26]

Contrast osmolarity also may play a role, although the risk of developing acute renal failure is higher when patients receive an iso-osmolar, rather than a hypo-osmolar, agent. In general, high osmolar contrast and ionic contrast increase the risk of contrast medium–induced nephropathy. When cases are reviewed, there appear many other factors that can play an additional role, such as recent anemia and blood loss, the use of NSAIDs, intra-arterial balloon pump hypotension, and also reduced serum albumin, hypercholesterolemia, and hypercalcemia.

Gadolinium is a commonly used contrast medium to image the brain and its vessels, but it is excreted unchanged by the kidney. There are several hundred documented fatal cases of nephrogenic systemic fibrosis associated with gadolinium contrast use. The disorder appears as fibrotic nodules, gradually spread over extremities and trunk; but fibrosis also involves lungs, myocardium, pleura, and pericardium. Its particular concern is with patients with prior renal failure (even low-grade kidney disease) and has resulted in an FDA black box warning (the actual risk may be 5% in dialysis patients). Radiologists do not administer gadolinium in patients with a GFR < 30 ml/min per 1.73 m[2] or when on dialysis.[11,12]

The relationship between vancomycin and nephrotoxicity is well established and quite problematic due to the common use of vancomycin in hospitals.[7] Vancomycin use has increased due to an increase in methicillin-resistant *Staphylococcus aureus* (MRSA), and over time there may have been a rise in average vancomycin minimum inhibitory concentration. Vancomycin trough concentrations of more than 50 mcg/mL is a major risk factor for nephrotoxicity. When these concentrations are present, the risk is increased threefold.[23]

All β-lactam antibiotics can cause neurotoxicity. Cefepime may result in nephrotoxicity and neurotoxicity even after a renal-adjusted dosing. Routine assays for serum cefepime concentrations are not available; but cefepime levels can be considered increased in any patient who has a renal insufficiency.

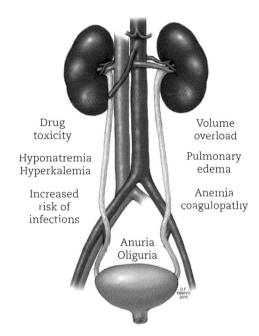

Drug toxicity
Hyponatremia
Hyperkalemia
Increased risk of infections
Anuria
Oliguria
Volume overload
Pulmonary edema
Anemia coagulopathy

FIGURE 53.2: Consequences of acute kidney injury in the NICU.

MANAGEMENT OF ACUTE RENAL FAILURE

The major systemic manifestations of AKI are shown in Figure 53.2 and Table 53.3. The most consequential are electrolyte shifts, causing escalating severe cardiac arrhythmias, and volume overload, causing pulmonary edema and acute respiratory distress syndrome. AKI causes acute lung injury due to increased pulmonary vascular permeability, leading to interstitial edema (with alveolar hemorrhages). Hypoxic-hypercarbic respiratory failure causes renal vasoconstriction; but once intubated, mechanical ventilation in some patients may also impact the kidney due to its positive pressure, reduced venous return, changes in cardiac preload and afterload—all factors that potentially further reduce renal blood flow.[24]

In the less severe cases, adequate hydration and preservation of diuresis are needed. Hydration to prevent kidney injury is the mainstay of therapy in rhabdomyolysis. There is no consensus for the composition of the replacement fluids, or use

of diuretics and mannitol in the management of acute kidney injury related to rhabdomyolysis. Alkalization with sodium bicarbonate when urine pH is < 6.5 is advised,[8] while also providing Lactated Ringer's or normal saline for hydration. Diuretics and mannitol should only be considered

TABLE 53.3. CLINICAL MANIFESTATIONS ASSOCIATED WITH ACUTE KIDNEY INJURY

Complication	Clinical Manifestation
Hyponatremia	Abnormal mentation and seizure
Hyperkalemia	Cardiac arrhythmias (including malignant types)
Volume overload	Pulmonary edema
	Pulmonary hemorrhage
	Acute hypertension
	Abdominal compartment syndrome
Anemia and thrombocythemia	Hemorrhage
Anion gap metabolic Acidosis	Cardiorespiratory abnormalities
Gut ischemia	Acute gastrointestinal hemorrhage
Uremia	Stupor, coma

in patients with adequate volume resuscitation. No randomized trial is available to support the use of mannitol, but expert opinion suggests the potential benefits due to osmotic diuretic effects. The major concern is the risk of osmotic nephrosis due to tubular damage and the vasoconstrictive effect of accumulated mannitol. Special attention should be given to electrolyte abnormalities (mostly hyperkalemia) during the management of rhabdomyolysis.[6]

In more severe cases of kidney failure, irrespective of the circumstances, patients become oliguric and develop abnormalities in serum electrolytes. Loop diuretics may be tried to obtain a diuretic response, but can be potentially harmful, not only causing blood volume in stability but also additional electrolyte depletion (hyponatremia, hypokalemia, hypomagnesemia), leading to potential cardiac dysrhythmias. A bolus of 80–140 mg of furosemide, followed by infusion of 1–5 mg/h, may be used. No response in a few hours is highly predictive of severe kidney injury and more furosemide is not beneficial. Failure to increase urinary output, worsening electrolytes, and fluid overload are the indications for renal replacement therapy. Hyperkalemia (more than 5.5 mmol/L) with or without elctrocardiographic (EKG) changes should be initially managed with calcium chloride (10 mL of 10% solution) or 10 units of insulin and 50 mL of D50 administered over 30 minutes, or high-dose nebulized albuterol (the effective dose of 10 mg is four times higher than that typically used for bronchodilation). The definitive therapy for hyperkalemia is removal of the body potassium, as opposed to shifting it to the cell, which can be achieved either by diuresis (in volume-depleted, non-oliguric patients by a single furosemide dose [40–80 mg]), by renal replacement therapy or by use of potassium-binding resins sodium polystyrene sulfonate (Kayexalate) enterally. Metabolic acidosis may require sodium bicarbonate supplementation if the pH is life-threating (pH < 7.1).

In patients with positive fluid balance and evidence of hypervolemia with respiratory decompensation, a high dose of IV furosemide (15–20 mg/h) may be needed to obtain a negative fluid balance. In some patients, pulmonary edema occurs, and transient ultrafiltration may be needed to remove excess fluids. However, in patients with refractory fluid overload and consequent cardiorespiratory failure, or hypercatabolic septic patients, considering renal replacement therapy, early is very essential.

TABLE 53.4. DRUGS THAT REQUIRE DECREASE OR AVOIDANCE IN ACUTE RENAL FAILURE

Drug	Adjustment with CLCR < 60 mL/min
Codeine	Up to 50%
Midazolam	Up to 50%
Acyclovir	Increase dosing interval or decrease 25%
Cephalosporins	Decrease
Vancomycin	Monitor serum level and adjust
Phenytoin	Monitor free drug level

An important next step is to "renally dose" all medications and drug adjustments are needed when creatinine clearance is less than 60 mL/min (Table 53.4). Adjustment may be extending the dose interval, which effectively reduces drug administration, or reducing the infusion rate. Loading doses of drugs generally does not affect concentration; however, due to its albumin binding, this does not apply to fosphenytoin. Close monitoring of free levels of fosphenytoin is needed.

Management of AKI in sepsis requires volume resuscitation or inotropic and vasopressor support. Mostly adequate fluid resuscitation to at least an MAP > 70 mm Hg may suffice (at least for the kidney), but vasopressors may be needed. There is likely complete loss of renal autoregulation, making renal perfusion passively dependent on blood pressure. There is a concern that low-dose dopamine worsens renal failure, and its use is not advised.[1,5,17] Use of diuretics is controversial and will not convert nonoliguric acute kidney failure, nor does it reduce the need for renal replacement therapy. Recently there has been ongoing debate over the ideal fluid for resuscitation for sepsis patients.[19] Concern has been raised about the potential of hyperchloremic metabolic acidosis with the use of 0.9% saline, and thus the use of a more balanced solution with low chloride content has been recommended. Despite the controversy, it is well accepted that patients with suspected sepsis should get early antimicrobials, vasopressor, and fluid resuscitation, but overhydration should be avoided.

Despite all these steps, renal replacement may be needed, and the indications of renal replacement are shown in Table 53.5. Different

TABLE 53.5. CRITERIA FOR THE
INITIATION OF RENAL REPLACEMENT
THERAPY (RRT) IN THE ICU

Anuria (no urine output for 6 hours)
Oliguria (urine output < 200 mL/12 hours)
BUN > 80 mg/dL or urea > 28 mmol/L
Creatinine > 3 mg/L or > 265 μmol/L
Serum potassium > 6.5 mmol/L or rapidly rising
Pulmonary edema unresponsive to diuretics
Uncompensated metabolic acidosis (pH < 7.1)
Uremic complications (encephalopathy/myopathy/
  neuropathy/pericarditis)

If one criterion is present, RRT should be considered. If two criteria
are simultaneously present, RRT is strongly recommended.

types are shown in Figure 53.3. Continuous renal replacement therapy (CRRT) is recommended in patients with hemodynamic instability and is now considered standard of care. CRRT maintains a constant intravascular volume due to slower fluid removal. Most studies in medical and general ICUs may not apply to the NICU population. But CRRT remains preferred in patients with a structural lesion accompanied by cerebral edema. CRRT allows a slower rate of urea and other uremic toxin clearance and thus reduces water shift. (Replacement fluid of isotonic saline is also preferred fluid management in critically ill neurologic patients.)

Renal replacement therapy may result in cerebral edema from osmotic changes, and several cases are on record (Capsule 53.2). Continuous renal replacement therapy is the best option in patients with cerebral edema because it has little impact on cerebral perfusion. Fluid overload should be avoided.

There are other concerns. Rapid correction of anion gap metabolic acidosis may increase CSF acidosis (the so-called paradoxical brain acidosis), and an osmotic gradient may be created.[2,3]

CONCLUSIONS

- Acute renal failure in the NICU is often related to hypotension, newly introduced antibiotics, and as a result of rhabdomyolysis.
- Contrast-induced nephropathy can be reduced with fluid therapy alone.
- Renal replacement therapy should be considered in patients with anuria, elevated potassium, and evidence of fluid overload.
- Renal replacement therapy (either intermittent or continuous) may lead to dialysis disequilibrium syndrome and consequently increase ICP, but less so with continuous mode.

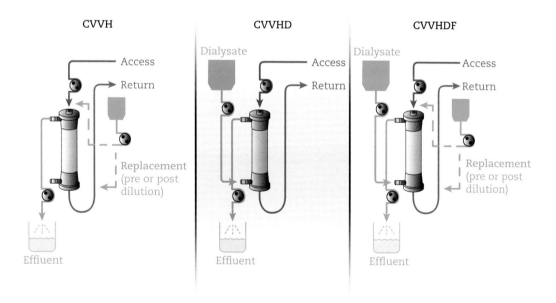

FIGURE 53.3: Types of renal replacement therapies: continuous veno-venous hemofiltration (CVVH), continuous veno-venous hemodialysis (CVVHD), and continuous venovenous hemodiafiltration (CVVHDF).

CAPSULE 53.2   OSMOTIC SHIFTS AND TREATMENT OF KIDNEY INJURY

Brain swelling may occur with dialysis, but the mechanism remains speculative. Earlier, the "reverse urea" hypothesis was introduced, suggesting that a significant urea gradient between blood and brain after dialysis results in water influx to the brain. In normal circumstances, urea diffuses more slowly than water across the blood–brain barrier; thus, when blood urea is rapidly increased, an osmotic difference is created, resulting in water extraction from the brain. Reversing this gradient with dialysis results in a higher brain-to-plasma urea concentration, and this phenomenon causes brain edema. It thus can be corrected by adding urea or mannitol or by increasing the sodium concentrate of the dialysate.

The "idiogenic osmole" hypothesis argues that brain swelling is promoted by the formation of idiogenic osmoles, possibly organic acids formed during rapid dialysis, leading to an increase in brain osmolality and water influx. Direct measurements of brain osmolality showed an increase in brain osmolality that cannot be explained by the sum of urea and electrolyte concentrations, suggesting a new formation of osmotically active particles (osmoles). Formation of organic osmoles in the brain during osmotic stress has been documented, but whether they formed after dialysis remains unknown.

REFERENCES

1. Argalious M, Motta P, Khandwala F, et al. "Renal dose" dopamine is associated with the risk of new-onset atrial fibrillation after cardiac surgery. *Crit Care Med* 2005;33:1327–1332.
2. Arieff AI, Guisado R, Massry SG, Lazarowitz VC. Central nervous system pH in uremia and the effects of hemodialysis. *J Clin Invest* 1976;58:306–311.
3. Arieff AI, Massry SG, Barrientos A, Kleeman CR. Brain water and electrolyte metabolism in uremia: effects of slow and rapid hemodialysis. *Kidney Int* 1973;4:177–187.
4. Bellomo R. Acute renal failure. *Semin Respir Crit Care Med* 2011;32:639–650.
5. Bellomo R, Chapman M, Finfer S, Hickling K, Myburgh J. Low-dose dopamine in patients with early renal dysfunction: a placebo-controlled randomized trial. Australian and New Zealand Intensive Care Society (ANZICS) Clinical Trials Group. *Lancet* 2000;356:2139–2143.
6. Bosch X, Poch E, Grau JM. Rhabdomyolysis and acute kidney injury. *N Engl J Med* 2009;361:62–72.
7. Bosso JA, Nappi J, Rudisill C, et al. Relationship between vancomycin trough concentrations and nephrotoxicity: a prospective multicenter trial. *Antimicrob Agents Chemother* 2011;55:5475–5479.
8. Cho YS, Lim H, Kim SH. Comparison of lactated Ringer's solution and 0.9% saline in the treatment of rhabdomyolysis induced by doxylamine intoxication. *Emerg Med J* 2007;24:276–280.
9. Devarajan P, Krawczeski CD, Nguyen MT, et al. Proteomic identification of early biomarkers of acute kidney injury after cardiac surgery in children. *Am J Kidney Dis* 2010;56:632–642.
10. Doi K, Leelahavanichkul A, Yuen PS, Star RA. Animal models of sepsis and sepsis-induced kidney injury. *J Clin Invest* 2009;119:2868–2878.
11. Evenepoel P, Zeegers M, Segaert S, et al. Nephrogenic fibrosing dermopathy: a novel, disabling disorder in patients with renal failure. *Nephrol Dial Transplant* 2004;19:469–473.
12. Gibson SE, Farver CF, Prayson RA. Multiorgan involvement in nephrogenic fibrosing dermopathy: an autopsy case and review of the literature. *Arch Pathol Lab Med* 2006;130:209–212.
13. KDIGO clinical practice guideline for acute kidney injury. *Kidney Int Suppl* 2012;2:1–138.
14. Kumar AB, Shi Y, Shotwell MS, Richards J, Ehrenfeld JM. Hypernatremia is a significant risk factor for acute kidney injury after subarachnoid hemorrhage: a retrospective analysis. *Neurocrit Care* 2015;22:184–191.
15. Langenberg C, Bellomo R, May CN, et al. Renal vascular resistance in sepsis. *Nephron Physiol* 2006;104:p1–p11.
16. Langenberg C, Wan L, Egi M, May CN, Bellomo R. Renal blood flow and function during recovery from experimental septic acute kidney injury. *Intensive Care Med* 2007;33:1614–1618.
17. Lauschke A, Teichgraber UK, Frei U, Eckardt KU. 'Low-dose' dopamine worsens renal perfusion

in patients with acute renal failure. *Kidney Int* 2006;69:1669–1674.

18. Li Z, Cai L, Liang X, et al. Identification and predicting short-term prognosis of early cardiorenal syndrome type 1: KDIGO is superior to RIFLE or AKIN. *PLoS One* 2014;9:e114369.

19. McDermid RC, Raghunathan K, Romanovsky A, Shaw AD, Bagshaw SM. Controversies in fluid therapy: type, dose and toxicity. *World J Crit Care Med* 2014;3:24–33.

20. Mehta RL, Kellum JA, Shah SV, et al. Acute Kidney Injury Network: report of an initiative to improve outcomes in acute kidney injury. *Crit Care* 2007;11:R31.

21. Mikkelsen TS, Toft P. Prognostic value, kinetics and effect of CVVHDF on serum of the myoglobin and creatine kinase in critically ill patients with rhabdomyolysis. *Acta Anaesthesiol Scand* 2005;49:859–864.

22. Muriithi AK, Nasr SH, Leung N. Utility of urine eosinophils in the diagnosis of acute interstitial nephritis. *Clin J Am Soc Nephrol* 2013;8:1857–1862.

23. Nolin TD, Himmelfarb J. Mechanisms of drug-induced nephrotoxicity. *Handb Exp Pharmacol* 2010:111–130.

24. Scheel PJ, Liu M, Rabb H. Uremic lung: new insights into a forgotten condition. *Kidney Int* 2008;74:849–851.

25. Waikar SS, Winkelmayer WC. Chronic or acute renal failure: long-term implications of severe acute kidney injury. *JAMA* 2009;302:1227–1229.

26. Zhang B, Liang L, Chen W, et al. The efficacy of sodium bicarbonate in preventing contrast-induced nephropathy in patients with pre-existing renal insufficiency: a meta-analysis. *BMJ Open*. 2015;5:e006989.

54

Endocrine Emergencies

By all accounts, the sudden appearance of these clinical states requires a multidisciplinary approach with endocrinologists and sometimes neurosurgeons. Apart from hyperglycemic crises, acute endocrinopathies are an uncommon cause of additional critical illness in the NICU. When they appear, they are the unexpected causes of coma, refractory seizures, and other neurologic manifestations mimicking an acute brain injury. The four most common endocrine disorders are diabetic ketoacidosis, hyperglycemic hyperosmolar coma, adrenal insufficiency, and thyroid storm.[17,18] Endocrinopathies may present a major—yet rewarding when recognized—challenge to the neurointensivist. The ultimate endocrine emergency is the presentation of pituitary apoplexy, which has a very specific management algorithm. Many endocrinopathies cause electrolyte abnormalities, and management is found in Chapter 57. Acute brain injury increases the susceptibility to marked hyperglycemia, but blood sugars are rarely above 200–300 mmol/L. General management of mild hyperglycemia as a result of neurocritical illness is also discussed in Chapter 57.[12,16,27] This chapter discusses noteworthy endocrine emergencies.

DIABETIC KETOACIDOSIS

Hyperglycemia becomes more concerning with higher values, particularly when acidosis appears. Acute brain injury can be an immediate trigger for a diabetic ketoacidosis, and both acute brain injury and derangement of a diabetic condition may coexist (Capsule 54.1). Classically, diabetic ketoacidosis presents with polyuria, polydipsia, weakness, and weight loss; but none of these symptoms is rapidly apparent. The hypovolemic state as a result of the osmotic effects of hyperglycemia will lead to clinical manifestations such as tachycardia, orthostatic hypotension, and marked decrease in level of consciousness. Hyperglycemia values are usually glucose levels that are between 500 and 1,000 mg/dL, and an anion gap metabolic acidosis is present. This metabolic acidosis is characteristic and diagnostic. A challenge is to differentiate between an undiagnosed hyperosmolar hypoglycemic state (HHS) or diabetic ketoacidosis (DKA) (Table 54.1). Differentiation is mostly in the level of serum glucose, which is much higher in HHS. Serum osmolality is markedly increased in HHS, and urinary ketones are absent.

The management is a series of important steps.[2,7,9,11,14] These are summarized and outlined in Figure 54.1. The first approach is to provide isotonic saline to improve intravascular status. This is immediately followed by correction of the potassium deficit, using 20–40 mEq of potassium.[24] Fluid replacement may be necessarily aggressive, defined as isotonic saline infused at 20 mL/kg, which may approach a liter per hour in most patients. The fluid replacement is then adjusted after serum electrolytes are known. The total amount of IV fluids are determined on the corrected sodium concentration. With corrected serum sodium concentrations less than 135 mmol/L, isotonic saline should be continued.

Other protocols exist and may include volume replacement with 2 liters of normal saline in the first 2 hours, followed by 2 liters of normal saline or 0.45% saline over the next 4 hours. This management is also accompanied by insulin therapy, typically starting at a continuous infusion of 0.1 units/k/hour. The best target is to have serum glucose levels fall by approximately 75 mg/dL/hour and to start 5% dextrose infusion once the levels are at 250–300 mg/dL. Only when the ketones are disappearing should subcutaneous insulin therapy be initiated. Several electrolytes will need to be replaced, such as potassium replacement, as mentioned earlier, which is simply a result of osmotic renal losses and shift of intracellular potassium to extracellular space. Oral replacement should continue even after DKA is corrected. Phosphate replacement is pertinent if serum phosphate is less than 1.5 mg/dL, and these patients will require 1,000 mg of phosphate over 12 hours. Bicarbonate replacement may not be necessary because acidosis will resolve with fluid replacement and insulin.

CAPSULE 54.1   GLUCOSE AND THE BRAIN

The brain needs glucose and lots of it. Glucose transporters—and not insulin—bring in about 80% of all available glucose. Acute brain injury results in a hypermetabolic state and causes hyperglycemia through the workings of the counter-regulatory catecholamines.[10] It results in insulin resistance and glucagon decrease. Hyperglycemia impairs endothelial function, causes mitochondrial injury, inhibits complement, but there are also indirect effects on the brain as a result of fluid depletion and hypoperfusion.[16] Hyperglycemia impairs astrocyte activity and causes neuronal stress. Another major injury (in stroke) comes from lactate acidosis, which impairs ion hemostasis. Lactate acidosis in the brain occurs as a result of anaerobically metabolized glucose.

Hypoglycemia, on the other hand, rarely damages the brain; and many diabetics can attest to good recovery. But most experienced neurologists have seen single cases of persistent vegetative state after a profound hypoglycemia. Hypoglycemia in an already damaged brain is also very consequential, with cellular distress and increased oxygen demand.[32,33]

Some have argued that bicarbonate replacement is needed with a pH less than 7.0, calculating a base deficit by the formula: bicarbonate (mmol) = base deficit × weight (kg) × 0.3.[29] In general, the use of 1,000 mEq of sodium bicarbonate and 400 mL of water with 20 mEq of potassium chloride is a safe way to correct a worsening and concerning acidosis (pH ≤ 7.0). Improving ketoacidosis is the best monitor of appropriate treatment with narrowing of the serum anion gap, which should be ≤ 12 mEq/L and a further decrease in plasma osmolality < 315 mOsmol/kg. Many patients will become far more alert, cooperative, and able to eat; and the patient would need multiple doses of subcutaneous insulin. This will require detailed recommendations by a consulting endocrinologist. Soon after DKA is under control, a search for a precipitating event is needed, which usually requires a thorough search for an infection. In the NICU, corticosteroids are a major contender. Neurointensivists will, on occasion, have to manage HHS and more rarely DKA; but both derangements may occur easily with the stressors of acute brain injury and ICU management.

HYPERGLYCEMIC HYPEROSMOLAR COMA

The classic features of HHC consist of progressive slipping into deep coma. Nonketotic hyperglycemic coma occurs with a sixfold to tenfold increase in serum glucose. Nonketotic hyperosmolar coma is associated with hypovolemia, which explains hyperglycemia (euvolemia would result in increased excretion of glucose and prevent high concentration in the blood). A crucial element in the treatment of HHC is rehydration with isotonic saline to establish refilling of the intravascular compartment. Insulin therapy can be withheld because of (unproven) concerns that the combination with rehydration will induce cerebral edema.

ACUTE HYPOTHYROIDISM

Myxedema is usually seen with severe hypothyroidism, and this is usually a long-standing issue in a patient with a known hypothyroidism where there has been an acute precipitant such as infection, cold exposure, or the administration of drugs, particularly opioids.[15,19,29] Patients with known hypothyroidism may worsen dramatically if opioids are used for pain medication, and potentially

---

TABLE 54.1. LABORATORY CRITERIA DIABETIC KETOACIDOSIS (DKA) AND HYPERGLYCEMIC HYPEROSMOLAR COMA (HHC)

Laboratory	DKA	HHC
Blood glucose	> 250 mg/dL	> 600 mg/dL
Arterial blood gas	pH < 7.3	pH > 7.3
	Bicarb < 18	Bicarb > 18
Anion gap	Increased	Mostly normal
Plasma osmolality	Normal to increased	Increased
Ketones in urine	++	±

Data from Keays R. Diabetic emergencies. In: Oh TE, Soni N, eds. *Oh's Intensive Care Manual*. 5th ed. Oxford: Butterworth-Heinemann, 2003; Kitabchi AE, Umpierrez GE, Murphy MB, et al. Hyperglycemic crises in patients with diabetes mellitus. *Diabetes Care* 2003;26 Suppl 1:S109–S117; Maletkovic J, Drexler A. Diabetic ketoacidosis and hyperglycemic hyperosmolar state. *Endocrinol Metab Clin N Am* 2013;42:677–695.

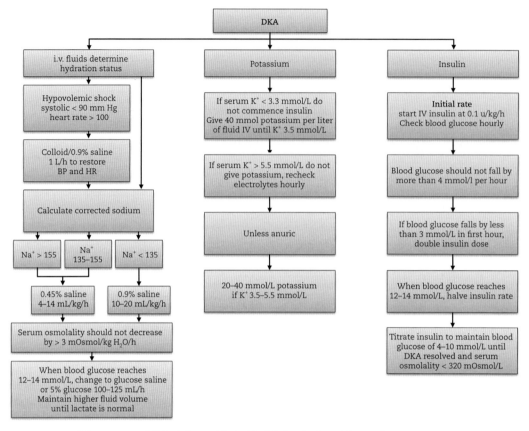

FIGURE 54.1: Management of diabetic ketoacidosis. Modified and adapted from references 14, 17, 18

could include patients who are admitted to the neurointensive care unit. Severe hypothyroidism has been associated with myxedematous coma and some patients may progress, but most will present with stupor alone. Myxedema coma is much more common in elderly females. Precipitating factors are shown in Table 54.2.

Hypothyroidism can be detected by subtle signs such as hypotension, bradycardia, hyponatremia, hypoglycemia, and hypoventilation. Most extremities are puffy, but there is puffiness of eyelids and significant hair loss in axillae and eyebrows. Severe hypothyroidism is often considered with unexplained hypothermia and constant need for warming blankets, hypoventilation, cardiovascular arrhythmias, and expectedly bradycardia as a result of decreased myocardial contractility. Seizures may occur and they can be focal, but mostly when there is severe hyponatremia or marked decline in sodium values. Nonconvulsive status epilepticus is a rare occurrence, and most EEGs in these patients will show diffuse slowing, triphasic waves, and no epileptiform discharges.

An immediate loading dose of levothyroxine (T4) is needed and includes 200–600 mcg T4 with a daily dose of 100 mg IV T4. It is not necessary to add T3 because this may cause an overshoot, leading to cardiac arrhythmias. The longer half-life of T4 (5–7 days) makes it the preferred approach. In many instances, a response in patients with myxedema can be additionally expected when methylprednisolone is used 500 mg/day for 5 days.

THYROID STORM

Hyperthyroidism is 10 times less common than hypothyroidism, and thyroid storm is even less

TABLE 54.2. PRECIPITATING FACTORS IN MYXEDEMATOUS COMA

General anesthesia

Narcotics

Sedatives

Amiodarone

Lithium carbonate

Infection

Hypothermia (incidental)

common than myxedema coma. Both conditions are rare because of better detection of thyroid disease. Acute hyperthyroidism is due to autoimmune Graves disease, where autoantibodies link to TSH receptors on the thyroid and cause toxic goiter. The clinical manifestation is not easy to distinguish from other common hyperthermia syndromes or even a psychotic break.[29,35,36] Patient is warm, febrile, sweaty, agitated and delirious, and tachycardic. We have only seen this clinical picture in a patient who had been administered ionized contrast, suddenly provoking a "storm" and prolonged flaccid quadriplegia.[8] Administration of propylthiouracil or methimazole, followed by potassium iodide solution sublingually, will inhibit synthesis and release of thyroid hormones T4 and T3. Tachycardia must be immediately treated with intravenous labetalol (bolus or infusion). Many endocrinologists add a short course of corticosteroids.[1]

ADRENAL INSUFFICIENCY

Recognition of renal insufficiency in a patient with acute brain injury is usually considered in patients who have been on corticosteroids and usually at a high dose.[5,13,22,26,30,37] Sudden discontinuation of a high dose of dexamethasone may be a trigger, and patients may become hypotensive. Some patients may evolve into a significant hypotensive shock and may become comatose. Typical electrolyte abnormalities are hyponatremia combined with hyperkalemia. Acute adrenal insufficiency can also be seen in any infection or in a patient who has been treated with thrombolytics or anticoagulants. The treatment is immediate administration of hydrocortisone 75–100 mg every 6–8 hours and dexamethasone 3–4 mg every 6–8 hours. Significant fluid and electrolyte replacement is necessary to maintain adequate vascular volume.

PITUITARY APOPLEXY

This condition is usually apparent in a patient with a known pituitary adenoma. Usually vascular stasis and clotting ischemia may cause necrosis and hemorrhagic infarction. These patients may present with a thunderclap headache, usually retro-orbital, that is persistently excruciating and needs to be recognized. These symptoms are followed with some delay with visual field defects and oculomotor abnormalities.[3,5,6,23,25,31] Patients may become rapidly drowsy and comatose if this is unrecognized (Table 54.3). In addition patients may develop hypotension and hyponatremia from glucocorticoid deficiency. Therefore corticosteroids need to be immediately administered if there is a high suspicion. A diagnosis made on CT scan

TABLE 54.3. PRESENTING SIGNS OF PITUITARY APOPLEXY (IN ORDER OF FREQUENCY)

Thunderclap (or acute) headache
Nausea and vomiting
Visual field defect
Third-nerve palsy
Sixth-nerve palsy
Multiple cranial nerve palsies
Facial pain

showing a tumor with a hyperintensity in the center is often confirmed on MRI scan. The MRI scan is important to show the compression of diencephalon and optic chiasm (Figures 54.2 and 54.3). Endocrinology consult is necessary to further treat long-standing pituitary hormone replacement. This would require glucocorticoid (hydrocortisone 50 mg twice daily), thyroid hormone (L-thyroxine 100–125 mcg daily), sex hormones (cyclic estrogens or testosterone), growth hormone (usually by daily subcutaneous injection), and vasopressin using DDAVP nasal spray if diabetes insipidus occurs. Not infrequently, the sudden enlargement of the pituitary tumor will jeopardize vision, and the appearance of visual fields defect or visual loss is an immediate indication for decompressive surgery. This is usually a combined surgical procedure with otorhinolaryngology and neurosurgery.

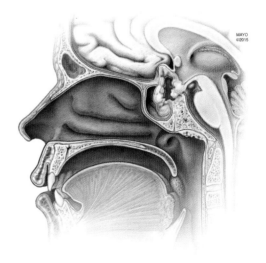

FIGURE 54.2: Pressure effects of pituitary apoplexy on the optic chiasm.

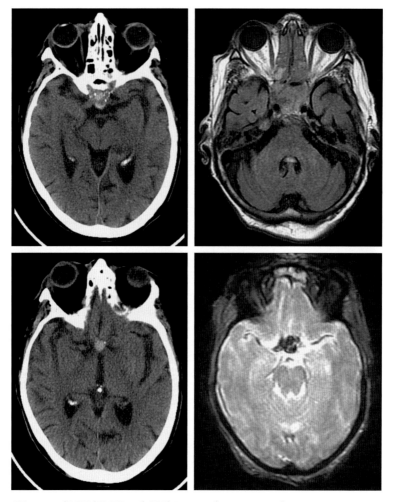

FIGURE 54.3. CT scan and MRI (FLAIR and GRE) images of pituitary apoplexy.

A recent large series of 55 patients[4] from the United Kingdom accentuated that surgery is indicated with progressive decline in visual acuity and visual field and decline in responsiveness, but the clinical course may be very unpredictable. Isolated ophthalmoplegia is not an absolute indication for surgery because conservative management has shown spontaneous resolution.[4] The MRI findings (Figure 54.3) may sway surgeons to surgery, particularly if there is significant compression and lifting of the optic chiasm. Some patients (10%) may undergo delayed elective surgery with good outcomes, also arguing for an initially conservative approach. The degree of hypopituitarism is up to 80% in operated cases, with hypogonadism in 50%, hypothyroidism in 60%, and ACTH deficiency in 80%. In a series from Mayo Clinic, 70% of 87 patients had surgery within 10 days (as early

as 3 days) and a minority had delayed (2 months and beyond) surgery. Intensive care admission was needed in 40% of patients.[34]

CONCLUSIONS

- Treatment of both DKA and HHS is adequate fluid administration with isotonic saline and correction of potassium deficit.
- Major thyroid abnormalities may lead to impaired consciousness with good response to replacement of T3 or blocking with propylthiouracil.
- Unexpected hypothermia and bradycardia may indicate severe hypothyroidism.
- Initially, most patients with pituitary apoplexy are not urgent surgical candidates and not endocrine crises but may worsen quickly.

REFERENCES

1. Angell TE, Lechner MG, Nguyen CT, et al. Clinical features and hospital outcomes in thyroid storm: a retrospective cohort study. *J Clin Endocrinol Metab* 2014:jc20142850.

2. Brenner ZR. Management of hyperglycemic emergencies. *AACN Clin Issues* 2006;17:56–65; quiz 91–53.

3. Briet C, Salenave S, Bonneville JF, et al. Pituitary apoplexy. *Endocr Rev* 2015;36:622–645.

4. Bujawansa S, Thondam SK, Steele C, et al. Presentation, management and outcomes in acute pituitary apoplexy: a large single-centre experience from the United Kingdom. *Clin Endocrinol (Oxf)* 2014;80:419–424.

5. Capatina C, Inder WJ, Karavitaki N, Wass JA. Management of endocrine disease: pituitary tumour apoplexy. *Eur J Endocrinol* 2015;172:R179–R190.

6. Cardoso ER, Peterson EW. Pituitary apoplexy: a review. *Neurosurgery* 1984;14:363–373.

7. Chiasson JL, Aris-Jilwan N, Belanger R, et al. Diagnosis and treatment of diabetic ketoacidosis and the hyperglycemic hyperosmolar state. *CMAJ* 2003;168:859–866.

8. Couillard P, Wijdicks EFM. Flaccid quadriplegia due to thyrotoxic myopathy. *Neurocrit Care* 2014;20:296–297.

9. De Beer K, Michael S, Thacker M, et al. Diabetic ketoacidosis and hyperglycaemic hyperosmolar syndrome: clinical guidelines. *Nurs Crit Care* 2008;13:5–11.

10. Egi M, Finfer S, Bellomo R. Glycemic control in the ICU. *Chest* 2011;140:212–220.

11. Fulop M, Tannenbaum H, Dreyer N. Ketotic hyperosmolar coma. *Lancet* 1973;2:635–639.

12. Godoy DA, Di Napoli M, Rabinstein AA. Treating hyperglycemia in neurocritical patients: benefits and perils. *Neurocrit Care* 2010;13:425–438.

13. Gonzalez H, Nardi O, Annane D. Relative adrenal failure in the ICU: an identifiable problem requiring treatment. *Crit Care Clin* 2006;22:105–118, vii.

14. Gosmanov AR, Gosmanova EO, Dillard-Cannon E. Management of adult diabetic ketoacidosis. *Diabetes Metab Syndr Obes* 2014;7:255–264.

15. Hampton J. Thyroid gland disorder emergencies: thyroid storm and myxedema coma. *AACN Adv Crit Care* 2013;24:325–332.

16. Jeremitsky E, Omert LA, Dunham CM, Wilberger J, Rodriguez A. The impact of hyperglycemia on patients with severe brain injury. *J Trauma* 2005;58:47–50.

17. Keays R. Diabetic emergencies. In: Oh TE, Soni N, eds. *Oh's Intensive Care Manual.* 5th ed. Oxford: Butterworth-Heinemann; 2003.

18. Kitabchi AE, Umpierrez GE, Murphy MB, et al. Hyperglycemic crises in patients with diabetes mellitus. *Diabetes Care* 2003;26 Suppl 1:S109–S117.

19. Klubo-Gwiezdzinska J, Wartofsky L. Thyroid emergencies. *Med Clin N Am* 2012;96:385–403.

20. Latif KA, Freire AX, Kitabchi AE, Umpierrez GE, Qureshi N. The use of alkali therapy in severe diabetic ketoacidosis. *Diabetes Care* 2002;25:2113–2114.

21. Maletkovic J, Drexler A. Diabetic ketoacidosis and hyperglycemic hyperosmolar state. *Endocrinol Metab Clin N Am* 2013;42:677–695.

22. Marik PE, Pastores SM, Annane D, et al. Recommendations for the diagnosis and management of corticosteroid insufficiency in critically ill adult patients: consensus statements from an international task force by the American College of Critical Care Medicine. *Crit Care Med* 2008;36:1937–1949.

23. Murad-Kejbou S, Eggenberger E. Pituitary apoplexy: evaluation, management, and prognosis. *Curr Opin Ophthalmol* 2009;20:456–461.

24. Murthy K, Harrington JT, Siegel RD. Profound hypokalemia in diabetic ketoacidosis: a therapeutic challenge. *Endocr Pract* 2005;11:331–334.

25. Nawar RN, AbdelMannan D, Selman WR, Arafah BM. Pituitary tumor apoplexy: a review. *J Intens Care Med* 2008;23:75–90.

26. Nerup J. Addison's disease: clinical studies: a report of 108 cases. *Acta Endocrinol* 1974;76:127–141.

27. Oddo M, Schmidt JM, Mayer SA, Chiolero RL. Glucose control after severe brain injury. *Curr Opin Clin Nutr Metab Care* 2008;11:134–139.

28. Papi G, Corsello SM, Pontecorvi A. Clinical concepts on thyroid emergencies. *Front Endocrinol* 2014;5:102.

29. Popoveniuc G, Chandra T, Sud A, et al. A diagnostic scoring system for myxedema coma. *Endocr Pract* 2014;20:808–817.

30. Rao RH, Vagnucci AH, Amico JA. Bilateral massive adrenal hemorrhage: early recognition and treatment. *Ann Intern Med* 1989;110:227–235.

31. Sibal L, Ball SG, Connolly V, et al. Pituitary apoplexy: a review of clinical presentation, management and outcome in 45 cases. *Pituitary* 2004;7:157–163.

32. Sieber FE, Koehler RC, Derrer SA, Saudek CD, Traystman RJ. Hypoglycemia and cerebral autoregulation in anesthetized dogs. *Am J Physiol* 1990;258:H1714–1721.

33. Simpson IA, Carruthers A, Vannucci SJ. Supply and demand in cerebral energy metabolism: the role of nutrient transporters. *J Cereb Blood Flow Metab* 2007;27:1766–1791.

34. Singh TD, Valizadeh N, Meyer FB, et al. Management and outcomes of pituitary apoplexy. *J Neurosurg* 2015:1–8.

35. Swee DS, Chng CL, Lim A. Clinical characteristics and outcome of thyroid storm: a case series and review of neuropsychiatric derangements in thyrotoxicosis. *Endocr Pract* 2014:1–21.

36. Tenner AG, Halvorson KM. Endocrine causes of dangerous fever. *Emerg Med Clin N Am* 2013;31:969–986.

37. Xarli VP, Steele AA, Davis PJ, et al. Adrenal hemorrhage in the adult. *Medicine* 1978;57: 211–221.

PART XI

Management of Systemic Complications

55

Management of Pulmonary Complications

Acute pulmonary disease is a complicating factor in acutely ill neurologic patients, whereas in other medical intensive care units (ICUs), exacerbation of long-standing pulmonary disease is often the primary reason for admission.[8,66] Acute respiratory distress from pulmonary disease in the neurosciences intensive care unit (NICU) can be due to aspiration pneumonia, pulmonary emboli, and nosocomial pneumonia. Polytrauma rarely spares the lung, resulting in rapidly blossoming contusions, and some patients require immediate chest tube placement for traumatic pneumothorax.

Outcome from critical neurologic illness may be determined in many patients by whether or not major pulmonary complications arise. More worrisome is that certain modes of mechanical ventilation in traumatic brain injury have been implicated, with high tidal volumes as a main culprit.[43] Better outcomes can be expected with closer attention to the prevention, recognition, and management of potentially fatal pulmonary complications. Impaired arousal or defective swallowing mechanism most likely is an important factor in the development of aspiration pneumonia. Pulmonary embolism from immobilization, particularly in patients not protected by subcutaneous heparin, can surprisingly emerge as early as several days after admission.[69]

This chapter describes two important issues: the general pathophysiologic principles of acute respiratory failure, and the most significant respiratory complications in patients with acute neurologic catastrophes. The goal in any of these patients is to improve oxygenation or hypercapnia, or both. Mechanical ventilation is often required (Chapter 17).

PATHOPHYSIOLOGY OF ACUTE RESPIRATORY FAILURE

Respiration is often understood in terms of ventilation–perfusion match. The parts of the lung that do not participate in respiration are known as the *physiologic dead space*, the sum of *anatomical dead space* (the part of the airway system not connected with the alveoli, possibly including the tubing between the Y connector and the patient, the pharynx, and the major conduction airways) and *alveolar dead space* (the part of the airway system that does not permit gas exchange, in which inspired gas is similar to exhaled gas). This component of the respiratory system is 20%–30% of total ventilation.

Several formulas are helpful at the bedside. (Calculators are available at www.medcalc.com.) The first measure is dead space assessment. The ratio of dead-space gas volume to tidal gas volume (V_D/V_T) can be measured in two ways. The respiratory therapist may collect expired gas from several tidal volumes exhaled over 5 minutes into a collection bag, and this sample is analyzed together with an arterial sample. Currently, most often an infrared light device can measure mixed expired PCO_2 ($PECO_2$). This simple device is connected to the exhalation hose, and end-tidal carbon dioxide is measured just before the arterial blood gas is obtained. The dead space (normal range, 0.2 to 0.3) can then be measured from the following formula:

$$V_D/V_T = \frac{PaCO_2 - PECO_2}{PaCO_2}$$

Increasing dead space over time is an indicator of worsening pulmonary function and mortality (highest when > 0.57).[46]

The second measure of bedside assessment of gas exchange is the alveolar–arterial oxygen difference (A–a gradient). The alveolar PO_2 (PAO_2) is calculated from the following formula:

$$PAO_2 = \frac{FIO_2 \times 713 - PaCO_2}{0.8}$$

The difference between PAO_2 and PaO_2 is 10–20 mm Hg. An A–a gradient greater than 20 mm

Hg indicates abnormal diffusion or a ventilation perfusion defect.

A third measure is the oxygenation index (OI), with high values (> 20) indicating poor oxygenation. The OI is calculated using mean airway pressure (MAP), inspired oxygen fraction (FIO_2), and PAO_2 as follows,

$$OI = \frac{MAP \times (FIO_2 \times 100)}{PaO_2}$$

The OI might be the best surrogate for the presence of an intrapulmonary shunt.

The fourth measure is PaO_2/FIO_2. Patients with severe acute respiratory distress syndrome have a ratio of < 300.

The fifth important measure is maximum inspiratory pressure (PI_{max}). Maximum inspiratory pressure can be used (together with vital capacity) and maximum expiratory pressure to differentiate a neuromuscular cause from other causes of respiratory failure.

Measurement of one set of arterial blood gases determines the seriousness of respiratory impairment. It is convenient to divide acute respiratory failure into acute hypoxemia (PaO_2 < 50 mm Hg) and acute hypercapnia ($PaCO_2$ > 50 mm Hg). Hypoxemia occurs in conditions causing alveolar hypoventilation or in instances of perfusion directed toward lung areas in which the ratio of alveolar ventilation ($\dot{V}A$) to perfusion ($\dot{Q}$) is less than 1.0. The hallmarks of bedside evaluation of acute hypoxemic respiratory failure are determination of the A–a gradient, whether hypoxemia is corrected by 100% oxygen, and if the PI_{max} has changed from the norm.

The most common clinical disorders in the NICU associated with acute hypoxemic respiratory failure and ventilation–perfusion mismatch are atelectasis, aspiration pneumonitis, pulmonary embolism, and pulmonary edema (cardiac or neurogenic). The clinical features of acute hypoxemia are fairly consistent and include impaired arousal, restlessness, tachypnea, tachycardia, and, sometimes, hypertension and peripheral vasoconstriction.

Similarly, acute hypercapnic respiratory failure is delineated by both the A–a gradient and PI_{max}. Decreased PI_{max} identifies many of the neuromuscular disorders, including those of motor neurons (e.g., amyotrophic lateral sclerosis), neuromuscular junction (e.g., myasthenia gravis, Lambert-Eaton syndrome, botulism, neuromuscular junction blockade by specific paralytic agents), peripheral nerve (e.g., Guillain-Barré

TABLE 55.1. INITIAL BEDSIDE APPROACH TO ACUTE HYPOXEMIC RESPIRATORY FAILURE

A–a Gradient	Other Variable	Disorder
Normal	PI_{max} decreased	Neuromuscular cause of hypoventilation
	PI_{max} normal	Central cause of hypoventilation
Increased	Correction with 100% O_2	Ventilation–perfusion mismatch
	No correction with 100% O_2	Right-to-left shunt, intraparenchymal or intracardiac

A–a, alveolar-arterial; PI_{max}, maximum inspiratory pressure.

syndrome, critical illness polyneuropathy), and muscle (e.g., polymyositis, acid maltase deficiency). When the respiratory muscles fail, alveolar ventilation is insufficient to eliminate carbon dioxide, and the result is increased tidal volume or respiratory rate.[70] A normal PI_{max} often indicates central hypoventilation (e.g., primary brainstem lesion) or increased carbon dioxide production by sepsis or from a flurry of generalized tonic-clonic seizures. A bedside approach to hypoxemia and hypercapnia is shown in Tables 55.1 and 55.2.

ACUTE RESPIRATORY DISTRESS IN MECHANICALLY VENTILATED PATIENTS

As discussed in Chapter 10, acute respiratory distress—at its simplest—denotes concerns with an open airway, adequacy of oxygenation, or air movement. Agitated patients with an acute

TABLE 55.2. INITIAL BEDSIDE APPROACH TO ACUTE HYPERCAPNIC RESPIRATORY FAILURE

A–a Gradient	Other Variable	Disorder
Normal	PI_{max} decreased PI_{max} normal	Neuromuscular
	Increased CO_2 production	Sepsis, seizures
	Normal CO_2 production	Central hypoventilation
Increased		Cardiopulmonary

A–a, alveolar-arterial; PI_{max}, maximum inspiratory pressure.

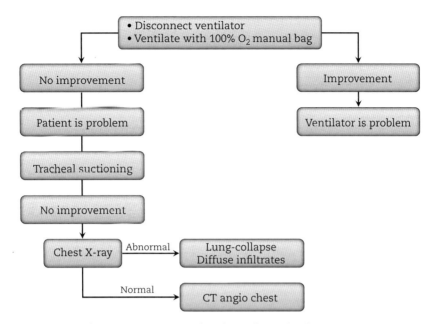

FIGURE 55.1: Algorithm for initial management of mechanically ventilated patients in acute respiratory distress.

central nervous system catastrophe may have an increased respiratory drive, culminating in large minute volumes asynchronous with the mechanical ventilator. In other mechanically ventilated patients, a quasi-stable situation is abruptly disturbed by tachypnea, or complete arrhythmic breathing, often with use of the accessory respiratory muscles.

Important initial clinical signs to look for in a mechanically ventilated patient with acute respiratory distress and a sudden increase in respiratory rate are hypotension, hypoxemia, and cardiac arrhythmias, all possibly connected with one another. An analytic approach is imperative to resolve the causes of acute critical respiratory distress in mechanically ventilated patients (Figure 55.1). The patient is disconnected from the ventilator and connected to a manual bag with 100% oxygen. This bypasses any problem in the machine, and immediate clinical improvement with 100% oxygen unmasks a ventilator-related cause (e.g., leak in the system connections). If the pulse oximeter does not indicate immediate improvement in oxygenation, the next step is to check the patency of the airway. If secretions are heard, tracheal suctioning must be performed immediately. In addition, if asymmetrical breath sounds are heard on auscultation of the lungs, main stem intubation or obstruction may be present. One should acknowledge, however, that asymmetrical breath sounds are not specific, and many conditions can produce these findings,

including acute pneumothorax, pleural effusions, and atelectasis of large segments.

Failure to resolve respiratory distress after an attempt at tracheobronchial suctioning is followed by emergency chest radiography to determine the position of the tube and the existence of a primary pulmonary problem (pneumothorax, pulmonary infiltrates) or abdominal distention (gastric distention, bowel perforation), which is suggested by diaphragmatic elevation. Fiberoptic bronchoscopy may follow in patients with diminished breath sounds to clear excess secretions or remove a foreign body[68] (Capsule 55.1).

Acute pneumothorax is probable in patients who have unilateral absence of breath sounds and certainly when there is additional sudden hypotension (Figure 55.2).[14] Pneumothorax in a mechanically ventilated patient, fortunately rare (5%), most likely is caused by large tidal volumes (> 12 mL/kg) and high positive end-expiratory pressure (PEEP) values (> 15 cm H_2O) in patients with known obstructive lung disease. It is also— and perhaps more commonly—a complication of placement of a subclavian venous catheter. Tension pneumothorax may develop quickly and a tube thoracostomy is placed immediately.

However, patients with persistent hypoxemia and normal findings on initial chest radiography pose a diagnostic challenge. The differential diagnosis includes pulmonary embolism, acute bronchospasm, and microatelectasis. It is important to consider pulmonary emboli and, when

CAPSULE 55.1   BRONCHOSCOPY IN THE NICU

Diagnostic bronchoscopy is usually performed with a flexible endoscope through the endotracheal tube (see accompanying illustration). The procedure has an established role in the ICU to evaluate lung infiltrates, particularly in immunocompromised patients. The procedure often includes transbronchial biopsies[67] and bronchoalveolar lavage. Mucus obstruction due to mechanical ventilation is an overriding reason to proceed with bronchoscopy. Mucous plugs may cause atelectasis, and distal bronchial lavages and aspirations may improve atelectasis more rapidly than physiotherapy or nebulizers.[41] Insufflation has been used in addition to lavage, using different methods including oxygen gas at 40 cm H_2O pressures to accomplish lung re-expansion. Aggressive chest physiotherapy and multiple inflations with a 1–2 L anesthesia bag may be equally effective in atelectasis resolution.

A major concern is the observation that bronchoscopy may increase intracranial pressure, and at least one study found increases to 38 mm Hg and, more worrisome, these sudden increases occurred also in sedated patients.[36] Other complications have included cardiac arrhythmias, marked hypoxemia (> 50% decline) with protracted return to baseline, and these are potential additional injurious factors to the brain.

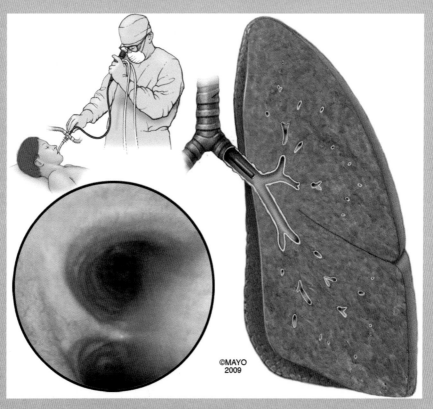

©MAYO
2009

Technique of bronchoscopy.

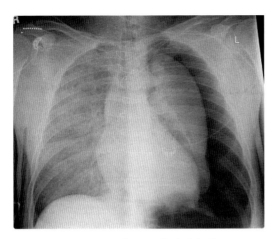

FIGURE 55.2: Pneumothorax only the left after attempt at subclavian catheter placement.

clinical suspicion is high, to obtain a helical computed tomography (CT) scan of the chest, duplex ultrasound examination of the legs, and D-dimer assay.

If the laboratory findings are normal and no other cause is evident, the ventilator settings should be adjusted. Inappropriate ventilator settings may underlie a maladaptation of the patient-to-ventilator timing (patient–ventilator asynchrony).[56] Patients with reduced respiratory drive may insufficiently trigger the ventilator if the trigger threshold is insensitive. Flow triggering could be different from pressure triggering, and adjustments may have to be made. A high proportion of mandatory breaths with synchronous intermittent-mandatory ventilation or a high-pressure support level may cause problems.

Auto-PEEP (a condition of air trapping), a very important phenomenon, must be considered. Auto-PEEP occurs in patients with obstructed airways, often in those with underlying bronchospastic disease. Auto-PEEP is the difference between the alveolar pressure and the pressure at the airway opening at end-expiration. Exhalation is incomplete in patients with airway obstruction from whatever cause, and the alveolar pressure remains positive at end-expiration. Auto-PEEP increases mean intrapleural pressure and decreases venous return, and the result may be hypotension. In addition, auto-PEEP increases the threshold at which the ventilator is triggered, and this diminished sensitivity may become particularly distressing for acutely ill neurologic patients with decreased levels of consciousness. In this clinical situation, the typical sequence of events is inability to trigger the

ventilator, a controlled breath completely asynchronous with the patient's respiratory pattern, increase in the work of breathing, discomfort, and agitation. When suspicion of auto-PEEP is high—because of otherwise unexplained sudden hypotension and increased work of breathing auto-PEEP can be resolved by increasing the respiratory flow rate to increase the expiratory time, by decreasing the respiratory rate in patients with spontaneous efforts, and by decreasing the tidal volume in assist-control ventilation.[65]

Agitation with markedly increased respiratory drive also must be considered and is best treated with sedation (Chapter 16). It may be difficult to separate pain from agitation, and opioids may be needed in addition. Remifentanil hydrochloride can be considered because of its short half-life and brevity of action[55] (initial dose, 0.5–1 µg/kg/min IV; maintenance, 0.05–2 µg/kg/min IV), but dexmedetomidine can be used in doses of 0.2–0.4 µg/kg/hr.

In the NICU, acute aspiration pneumonitis, bronchus obstruction, and pulmonary embolus are most common. A more extensive list of causes of acute respiratory distress in mechanically ventilated patients is provided in Table 55.3.

PLEURAL EFFUSIONS

Pleural effusions develop frequently in patients admitted to the NICU. Mostly they become apparent on a chest X-ray, which will show blunting or disappearance of a costophrenic angle—it can occur with as little as 100 mL of fluid, and sometimes it appears as if the diaphragm is elevated (the so-called veiling effect). CT of the chest is often more diagnostic (Figure 55.3) The pleural effusion

TABLE 55.3. DIFFERENTIAL DIAGNOSIS OF ACUTE RESPIRATORY DISTRESS IN MECHANICALLY VENTILATED PATIENTS

Acute main bronchus obstruction
Pneumothorax
Atelectasis
Pulmonary embolus
Pulmonary edema
Dislodgment of tracheostomy
Endotracheal malposition
Inappropriate ventilator setting
Ventilator dysfunction
Abdominal distention

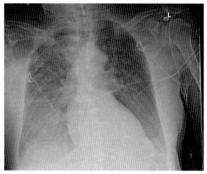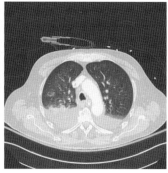

FIGURE 55.3: Pleural effusions confirmed on CT scan of the chest.

does cause atelectasis and eventually poor alveolar transport, shunting, and hypoxemia.

However, it may go both ways. Atelectasis causes a decrease in pleural pressure and allows transudate into the pleural space. Larger pleural effusions then cause atelectasis from pressure. Pleural effusions are commonly a result of prolonged hospitalization and are found in patients with anasarca (marked hypoalbuminemia), in patients with pneumonia progressing into an empyema, and in patients with chronic renal failure. Pleural effusions are mostly transudate and may improve with improvement of atelectasis and thus PEEP—transiently increasing to 15 cm water. If this is not helpful and oxygen supplementation remains high (FiO$_2$ more than 0.7), a thoracocentesis is considered and sometimes leaving a pigtail catheter behind to allow drainage.

ASPIRATION PNEUMONIA

Altered level of consciousness alone is a major risk factor for aspiration, but many other factors coincide (Chapter 59). The gastric reservoir, presence of gastroesophageal reflux (common in mechanically ventilated patients), and position of the patient may contribute.[52] In a randomized trial, when patients were placed in a semirecumbent position (45°), a 75% reduction in the rate of nosocomial pneumonia and a fourfold reduction in the rate per 1,000 ventilator days were found.[18]

Clinical Features and Management

Aspiration is often subclinical, and very rarely a fulminant aspiration syndrome is observed. Overspill of large amounts of gastric acid into the airways may cause acute hypoxemia, wheezing, cyanosis, and shock.[9] Many patients have no clinical symptoms or transient hypoxemia before a chest radiograph uncovers infiltrates. In others, hypoxemia can be profound, with PaO$_2$ values in the 40 mm Hg range. Hypoxemia associated with aspiration is explained by a large intrapulmonary shunt, and pulmonary artery pressures may increase because of hypoxemic vasoconstriction. Pulmonary edema from acid-induced damage to capillaries eventually may lead to a more concerning clinical course.

The radiologic features are pivotal in the evaluation because the clinical symptoms can be attenuated. The most consistent findings in adults are right lower lobe infiltrates (the left main stem bronchus has a more angular course) (Figure 55.4), atelectasis, and air bronchogram in

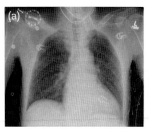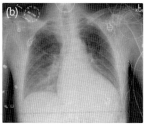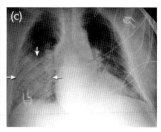

FIGURE 55.4: Aspiration pneumonia. (a, b) Evolving aspiration pneumonia. (c) Matured aspiration pneumonitis in right lower lobe (*arrows*).

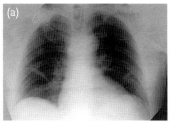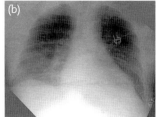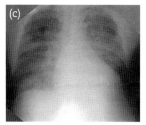

FIGURE 55.5: Serial chest radiographs of developing diffuse aspiration pneumonitis. (a) Plate-like atelectasis. (b, c) Gradual appearance of whiteout-like infiltrates.

large-segment aspiration. Infiltrates can be bilateral and more diffuse when restricted to the lower lobes, and usually repeat chest radiography demonstrates these abnormalities (Figure 55.5).

Conservative treatment is indicated in many patients, and the radiographic abnormalities usually subside rapidly. Corticosteroids are of no benefit and are potentially harmful. The emergence of fever may signal aspiration pneumonitis, but antibiotic coverage must not await the demonstration of a likely pathogen.[57] Cultures containing anaerobes such as *Bacteroides melaninogenicus, Fusobacterium nucleatum, Peptostreptococcus, Bacteroides fragilis,* and *Streptococcus* species suggest active infection from aspiration.[41] (A more comprehensive discussion of antibiotic management is found in the subsection on nosocomial pneumonia in Chapter 49.) Mechanical ventilation may be indicated if progressive infiltrative abnormalities are demonstrated. Standard modes of mechanical ventilation may not provide adequate ventilatory support, and occasionally the mode of mechanical ventilation must be switched to a more aggressive mode of pressure-support ventilation with, at times, inverse ratio in patients with fulminant aspiration pneumonitis or acute respiratory distress syndrome (ARDS). As a last resort, a prone (face down) position can be tried.[21] In earlier studies it has been shown to improve oxygenation, regional changes in ventilation, and ventilation-perfusion match.[21] Change in pulmonary mechanics in this position may also account for improvement in oxygenation. Disappointingly, a recent randomized controlled clinical trial found that prone positioning in ARDS, despite improving oxygenation, did not change high mortality rates (around 50%–60%).[63]

NEUROGENIC PULMONARY EDEMA

Acute injury to the brain or brainstem may cause diffuse pulmonary edema, but the true frequency seems very low.[6,9,15,19] Conditions that have been associated with neurogenic pulmonary edema are ganglionic hemorrhage,[10] subarachnoid hemorrhage (SAH),[1,45,72] medulla oblongata hemorrhage,[33,44] seizures and status epilepticus,[20] traumatic brain injury,[13] and cerebellar hematoma.[73]

In its full presentation, the clinical picture is very specific, almost always appearing soon after the initial brain injury. The clinical entity may be mistaken for other pulmonary conditions, such as massive aspiration pneumonia or pulmonary contusion.

Recent observations in SAH[62] and traumatic brain injury[4] have raised provocative questions about the underlying mechanism and have challenged the classic explanation that pulmonary edema is of neurogenic origin. Traditionally, neurogenic pulmonary edema is attributed to a massive sympathetic discharge, probably mediated by the anterior hypothalamus and triggered by an initial increase in intracranial pressure during the aneurysmal rupture. The increased sympathetic activity leads to generalized vasoconstriction, hypertension, and direct damage to endothelial cells, which may result in increased permeability (capillary leak) and subsequent airspace flooding, commonly known as "blast injury."

However, there is increasing evidence that pulmonary edema in SAH may have a cardiogenic origin.[4] Structural damage to the myocardium has been amply documented, and contraction bands and focal and subendocardial myocardial injury are characteristic histologic features. There is sufficient clinical evidence that myocardial dysfunction is common in poor-grade SAH. Hemodynamic measurements demonstrated significant reduction in ventricular performance as measured by left ventricular stroke index, cardiac index, and echocardiogram in patients with SAH, and often abnormal serum markers are found (Chapter 56). The true incidence of cardiogenic diffuse pulmonary edema in SAH is not known, and we have observed dramatic pulmonary edema without any echocardiographic evidence of ventricular dysfunction. In one study that obtained pleural fluid and compared pulmonary edema fluid with plasma protein, hydrostatic edema was found in more than half the patients.[62] This result suggested either myocardial dysfunction with increase in left cardiovascular pressures or, alternatively, profound venoconstriction. Pulmonary venoconstriction may force fluid into the lungs.

Clinical Features and Management

The clinical picture is striking. Excessive sweating, hypertension, tachypnea, and production of frothy sputum are typical. The diagnosis of neurogenic pulmonary edema is supported by the combination of marked hypoxemic respiratory failure (hypoxemia, greatly increased A–a gradient). Chest radiography demonstrates diffuse pulmonary infiltrates (Figure 55.6).

Management of neurogenic pulmonary edema is focused on the recruitment of collapsed alveoli with PEEP to correct the marked ventilation–perfusion mismatch. Mechanical ventilation with PEEP nearly always reverses the condition, and definite radiographic improvement is evident after several hours. Ventilation in a prone position was successful in one case.[42] In most severe cases, extracorporeal membrane oxygenation (ECMO) has been advocated with variable success in the more severe, refractory cases.[7]

Positive end-expiratory pressure is titrated by maximizing oxygen delivery at the lowest FIO_2 settings, usually possible at a level of 10–15 cm H_2O. Positive end-expiratory pressure ventilation alone should be sufficient to resolve neurogenic pulmonary edema, and weaning can be achieved fairly rapidly in many patients when the effect of the acute impact has subsided. If the origin of pulmonary edema is not clear or is possibly confounded by cardiac injury and dysfunction, inotropes to improve ventricular forward flow could be considered.

CHEST TRAUMA

Thoracic injuries may be observed in a significant number of trauma patients admitted to the NICU. Chest wall injuries vary from a single rib fracture without significant impairment to major pulmonary contusion. Fracture of a first rib, however, is indicative of major trauma[54] and may involve vascular structures. Most instances of chest trauma can be managed nonsurgically. Emergency thoracotomy is indicated for cardiac tamponade, control of air embolization, and shock not responding to aggressive resuscitation.[34,35] This section does not further consider mediastinal trauma or great-vessel injury, but focuses on pulmonary lesions.

Pulmonary trauma can be life-threatening if it produces such conditions as pneumothorax, flail chest, and tracheobronchial injury.

Clinical Features and Management

Usually, a consecutive series of ribs is fractured, and in patients with marked flail chest, paradoxical motion of the chest wall occurs with spontaneous breathing (Figure 55.7) and gas exchange rapidly becomes compromised.[5]

Pulmonary contusion from blunt trauma may not be immediately noticeable, but in most patients becomes apparent within hours. Serial chest radiographs or CT scans already often taken on the same day show evolution of patchy, often ill-defined parenchymal densities that do not coincide with the anatomical division of the lung.[53,60] Post-traumatic pneumatoceles (thin-walled air sacs) develop hours to days later. The differentiation from aspiration pneumonia is that the density

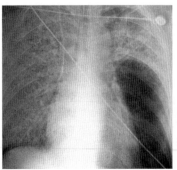
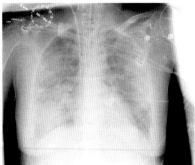

FIGURE 55.6: Two patients with neurogenic pulmonary edema on chest X-ray.

(a)

(b)

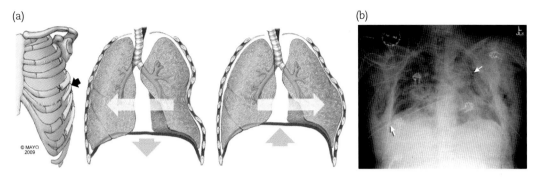

FIGURE 55.7. (a) Paradoxical movement with flail chest. Note rib fracture (*left*), inspiration (*middle*), and expiration (right). (b) Chest tube placement (*arrows*).

is more centrally located in aspiration pneumonia and limited to a bronchial distribution.

Treatment of a pulmonary contusion is conservative. Flail chest does not necessarily warrant intubation or mechanical ventilation if gas exchange is within normal limits, and relief of pain suffices.[53,60]

Traumatic pneumothorax should be treated with thoracotomy tube drainage,[11] and in patients with progressive deterioration from tension pneumothorax, drainage is preceded by needle decompression. Many patients with tension pneumothorax have hyperresonance, hypotension, distended neck veins, and tracheal deviation on examination.

PULMONARY EMBOLISM

Patients with acute neurologic diseases are susceptible to deep vein thrombosis.[16,17] In a craniotomy series, venous thromboembolism was 3.5% and pulmonary emboli 1.4%.[37] Asymptomatic deep vein thrombosis may be quite common (24% in a recent series of patients following subarachnoid hemorrhage).[51] Pulmonary emboli may occur in the first week after initial presentation of any acute stroke and are not necessarily the consequence of prolonged immobilization.[61,69] Deep vein thrombosis is significantly more common in a paralyzed leg.[69] Large proximal veins in the thigh may clot, and the risk of pulmonary embolization is considerably higher than in patients with calf vein thrombosis alone (40% vs. 15%).[36] In addition, one should appreciate that postoperative neurosurgical patients have an incidence of pulmonary embolism similar to that with hip and knee surgery (1%–3% fatal pulmonary embolism).[26,31] High-risk patients are those who undergo craniotomy for glioma[2] (cumulative risk of 23% at 1-year follow-up). A discussion on deep vein thrombosis prophylaxis appears in Chapter 15.

Clinical Features and Management

The clinical presentation of pulmonary embolism is never straightforward, and data from the classic Prospective Investigation of Pulmonary Embolism Diagnosis (PIOPED) study have confirmed the widely held conception that pulmonary embolism is often silent and not easy to diagnose on clinical grounds alone.[3]

Pulmonary embolism is likely if patients have two or three typical manifestations: low-grade fever, sudden tachypnea (respiratory rate of ≥ 20), and pleuritic pain together with hypocapnia from hyperventilation and marginal PO_2 (which may be only positional).[27] However, the clinical examination may not be helpful; rales, wheezing, and signs of pleural effusion are absent in many patients. Massive pulmonary embolism is often dramatic and may cause sudden death. When this occurs, pulmonary embolism may superficially resemble rebleeding in SAH. (However, in our patients with SAH, pulmonary emboli occurred mostly after surgical clipping of the aneurysm.)

The most startling presentation of pulmonary embolus is right ventricular failure, usually developing only if more than two-thirds of the pulmonary circulation is obstructed. Acute dilatation of the right ventricle causes increased ventricular pressure that is transmitted to the right atrium and is clinically detected by pronounced neck veins, right-sided S_3 gallop, and, rarely, parasternal lift.[25,29]

The clinical features of pulmonary embolism have a moderate specificity. In one study, the highest specificities were in tachypnea (0.80), hemoptysis (0.76), and pleuritic chest pain (0.64). Laboratory support for the diagnosis of pulmonary embolism is summarized in Table 55.4. Electrocardiographic abnormalities may have some value. The most frequently seen abnormalities are T-wave inversions

TABLE 55.4. LABORATORY TEST
RESULTS SUPPORTIVE OF PULMONARY
EMBOLISM AND INCREASING
THE PROBABILITY OF A DIAGNOSTIC
HELICAL CT OF THE CHEST

Hypocapnia and hypoxemia
Electrocardiographic abnormalities
T-wave inversion in the right precordial leads, III,
    and aVF
ST depression (nonreciprocal)
T-wave inversion (patients with history of
    cardiopulmonary disease)
Sudden atrial fibrillation
P pulmonale
Right bundle-branch block
D-dimer increase (> 500 μg/L)
Increased right ventricular dimension or dilated
    right pulmonary artery on echocardiography

and a nonreciprocal ST depression. A sudden new onset of any type of cardiac arrhythmia should in any immobilized patient raise the suspicion of a pulmonary embolus.

The use of serum D-dimer values has generated considerable interest.[38,39] D-dimers are fibrin breakdown products that become measurable when the fibrin matrix of fresh emboli fragments. D-dimer assay of whole blood agglutination has a reported sensitivity of 96% but a very low specificity of 48%. The negative predictive value of serum D-dimer (values < 500 μg/L) was 100% in a recent study from Duke University Medical Center and thus is a useful additional test to rule out segmental or massive pulmonary embolism.[24]

A combination of a normal serum D-dimer and normal alveolar dead-space fraction was associated with a probability of less than 1% in a multicenter study.[38] However, the threshold of obtaining a helical CT of the chest in the NICU remains low and is performed with any trace of suspicion.

Bedside echocardiography could be useful in a few instances. The indirect demonstration of increased right ventricular dimension, a dilated right pulmonary artery, and flattening of the intraventricular septum may be more supportive of pulmonary emboli.

Helical CT scans miss subsegmental emboli with standard 3-mm sections, but detection increases 40% with 1-mm scans. These small peripheral emboli most likely are also clinically relevant, as they may cause pulmonary hypertension.[49,50,58]

Helical CT scans have a false-negative rate of 5% in patients with clinically suspected pulmonary embolus, increased D-dimer (> 500 μg/L), and normal leg ultrasound findings.[49] Pulmonary angiogram is rarely, if ever, performed nowadays.[64] A prior Canadian cost–benefit analysis suggested that helical CT can replace pulmonary angiography when ventilation–perfusion scans and leg ultrasound findings are negative.[48] There have been multiple attempts to scale back diagnostic tests to arrive at a diagnosis, and currently D-dimer assay, helical multislice CT, and leg ultrasonography should provide sufficient information.

Treatment of pulmonary embolism depends on the size of the embolus. Patients with massive pulmonary embolus most often are in shock from acute cor pulmonale, which justifies aggressive treatment with thrombolytic agents.

Studies with thrombolytic agents have indeed shown improvement in hemodynamic variables.[23] Tissue plasminogen activator, 0.6 mg/kg (maximum dose of 50 mg) over 15 minutes, can be administered.[71] A retrospective study in France of patients treated with thrombolysis for massive pulmonary emboli and associated right ventricular dilatation found three patients with intracranial hemorrhage but no benefit over heparin.[25] Another trial found no fatal hemorrhages but benefit from alteplase.[40] There is no published experience in patients with an acute ischemic or hemorrhagic stroke and recent pulmonary emboli, and undoubtedly the administration of thrombolytics may substantially increase the probability of hemorrhage in a recent hemispheric infarct. As a last resort, emergency embolectomy or ECMO may be indicated in patients when there is no improvement in hemodynamic measurements.[7] A recent metaanalysis showed lower rates of mortality but also increased risk of major bleeding and cerebral hemorrhage.[12]

Supportive treatment therefore remains the mainstay of management in patients with pulmonary emboli. Correcting hypoxemia with FIO_2 of 0.6–1.0 is effective. Patients with low cardiac output are best served by norepinephrine in a continuous infusion of 0.1 μg/kg/min in an attempt to improve right ventricular performance. Volume expansion in patients in shock from massive pulmonary embolization is indicated only for those who need additional volume to counter the effects of positive-pressure ventilation; in many other patients, fluid loading may cause further right ventricular distention and more ventricular strain.

Heparin treatment is initiated immediately. A weight-based nomogram with partial thromboplastin time at two times the normal value is used[30]

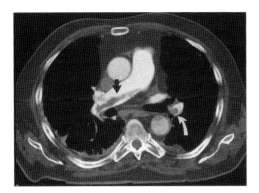

FIGURE 55.8: Helical computed tomography scan demonstrates thrombus within the right pulmonary artery (*black arrow*) and within the left descending trunk (*white arrow*).

(Chapter 20). Heparin treatment should not be adjusted to a lower level for fear of hemorrhagic conversion of ischemic stroke—albeit real— because failure to give a bolus or, worse, failure to provide adequate anticoagulation—particularly in patients with massive consumption of heparin associated with widespread embolization—may increase mortality from pulmonary embolism. Administration of warfarin can begin 48 hours after the start of heparinization. Patients are not mobilized until warfarin is therapeutic, and administration is continued for 6 months.[59]

Filter devices (e.g., Greenfield) should be placed in patients with an absolute contraindication to anticoagulation and in patients with recurrent episodes despite adequate anticoagulation[32,47] (Figure 55.8). Absolute contraindications

are patients with a recent cerebral hematoma or substantial hemorrhagic conversion of a cerebral infarct. Retrievable inferior vena cava filters (Günther-Tulip filter) are commonly used. Long-term anticoagulation is warranted in patients with a considerable pulmonary clot burden, and anticoagulation probably can be started 2 weeks ("low and slow" warfarin) after the ictus (Figure 55.9).[22,28]

CONCLUSIONS

- The most common cause of acute hypoxemic respiratory failure in the NICU is ventilation–perfusion mismatch from atelectasis, aspiration, pulmonary edema, or pulmonary embolism.
- Sudden respiratory distress in a mechanically ventilated patient should prompt disconnection (to demonstrate machine failure), tracheal suctioning or bronchoscopy (to demonstrate bronchial obstruction), chest radiography (to demonstrate pulmonary infiltrates or pneumothorax), and helical CT scan (to demonstrate pulmonary emboli). Inappropriate ventilator settings may cause patient–ventilator asynchrony.

REFERENCES

1. Ahrens J, Capelle HH, Przemeck M. Neurogenic pulmonary edema in a fatal case of subarachnoid hemorrhage. *J Clin Anesth* 2008;20:129–132.
2. Anderson F, Huang W, Sullivan C, al. e. The continuing risk of venous thromboembolism following operation for glioma: findings from the Glioma Outcomes Project. *Thromb Haemost* 2001;86 (Suppl):OC902.
3. Anderson GB. Noninvasive testing in the diagnosis of pulmonary embolism. PIOPED revisited. *Chest* 1996;109:5–6.
4. Bahloul M, Chaari AN, Kallel H, et al. Neurogenic pulmonary edema due to traumatic brain injury: evidence of cardiac dysfunction. *Am J Crit Care* 2006;15:462–470.
5. Bastos R, Calhoon JH, Baisden CE. Flail chest and pulmonary contusion. *Semin Thorac Cardiovasc Surg* 2008;20:39–45.
6. Baumann A, Audibert G, McDonnell J, Mertes PM. Neurogenic pulmonary edema. *Acta Anaesthesiol Scand* 2007;51:447–455.
7. Beiderlinden M, Eikermann M, Boes T, Breitfeld C, Peters J. Treatment of severe acute respiratory distress syndrome: role of extracorporeal gas exchange. *Intens Care Med* 2006;32:1627–1631.

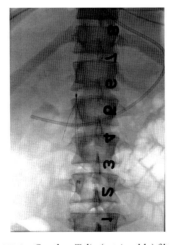

FIGURE 55.9: Gunther-Tulip (retrievable) filter in inferior vena cava.

8. Brun-Buisson C, Minelli C, Bertolini G, et al. Epidemiology and outcome of acute lung injury in European intensive care units: results from the ALIVE study. *Intens Care Med* 2004;30:51–61.

9. Busl KM, Bleck TP. Neurogenic pulmonary edema. *Crit Care Med* 2015;43:1710–1705.

10. Carlson RW, Schaeffer RC, Jr., Michaels SG, Weil MH. Pulmonary edema following intracranial hemorrhage. *Chest* 1979;75:731–734.

11. Casos SR, Richardson JD. Role of thoracoscopy in acute management of chest injury. *Curr Opin Crit Care* 2006;12:584–589.

12. Chatterjee S, Chakraborty A, Weinberg I, et al. Thrombolysis for pulmonary embolism and risk of all-cause mortality, major bleeding, and intracranial hemorrhage: a meta-analysis. *JAMA* 2014;311:2414–2421.

13. Chen HI, Sun SC, Chai CY. Pulmonary edema and hemorrhage resulting from cerebral compression. *Am J Physiol* 1973;224:223–229.

14. Chiles C, Ravin CE. Radiographic recognition of pneumothorax in the intensive care unit. *Crit Care Med* 1986;14:677–680.

15. Colice GL. Neurogenic pulmonary edema. *Clin Chest Med* 1985;6:473–489.

16. Cook D, Meade M, Guyatt G, et al. Clinically important deep vein thrombosis in the intensive care unit: a survey of intensivists. *Crit Care* 2004;8:R145–152.

17. Crowther MA, Cook DJ, Griffith LE, et al. Deep venous thrombosis: clinically silent in the intensive care unit. *J Crit Care* 2005;20:334–340.

18. Drakulovic MB, Torres A, Bauer TT, et al. Supine body position as a risk factor for nosocomial pneumonia in mechanically ventilated patients: a randomised trial. *Lancet* 1999;354:1851–1858.

19. Fein IA, Rackow EC. Neurogenic pulmonary edema. *Chest* 1982;81:318–320.

20. Fredberg U, Botker HE, Romer FK. Acute neurogenic pulmonary oedema following generalized tonic clonic seizure: a case report and a review of the literature. *Eur Heart J* 1988;9:933–936.

21. Gattinoni L, Tognoni G, Pesenti A, et al. Effect of prone positioning on the survival of patients with acute respiratory failure. *N Engl J Med* 2001;345:568–573.

22. Given MF, McDonald BC, Brookfield P, et al. Retrievable Gunther Tulip inferior vena cava filter: experience in 317 patients. *J Med Imaging Radiat Oncol* 2008;52:452–457.

23. Goldhaber SZ. Thrombolysis in pulmonary embolism: a large-scale clinical trial is overdue. *Circulation* 2001;104:2876–2878.

24. Gupta RT, Kakarla RK, Kirshenbaum KJ, Tapson VF. D-dimers and efficacy of clinical risk estimation algorithms: sensitivity in evaluation of acute pulmonary embolism. *AJR Am J Roentgenol* 2009;193:425–430.

25. Hamel E, Pacouret G, Vincentelli D, et al. Thrombolysis or heparin therapy in massive pulmonary embolism with right ventricular dilation: results from a 128-patient monocenter registry. *Chest* 2001;120:120–125.

26. Hamilton MG, Hull RD, Pineo GF. Venous thromboembolism in neurosurgery and neurology patients: a review. *Neurosurgery* 1994;34:280–296.

27. Hoellerich VL, Wigton RS. Diagnosing pulmonary embolism using clinical findings. *Arch Intern Med* 1986;146:1699–1704.

28. Hoff WS, Hoey BA, Wainwright GA, et al. Early experience with retrievable inferior vena cava filters in high-risk trauma patients. *J Am Coll Surg* 2004;199:869–874.

29. Huet Y, Lemaire F, Brun-Buisson C, et al. Hypoxemia in acute pulmonary embolism. *Chest* 1985;88:829–836.

30. Hull RD, Raskob GE, Rosenbloom D, et al. Optimal therapeutic level of heparin therapy in patients with venous thrombosis. *Arch Intern Med* 1992;152:1589–1595.

31. Inci S, Erbengi A, Berker M. Pulmonary embolism in neurosurgical patients. *Surg Neurol* 1995;43:123–128.

32. Ingber S, Geerts WH. Vena caval filters: current knowledge, uncertainties and practical approaches. *Curr Opin Hematol* 2009;16:402–406.

33. Inobe JJ, Mori T, Ueyama H, Kumamoto T, Tsuda T. Neurogenic pulmonary edema induced by primary medullary hemorrhage: a case report. *J Neurol Sci* 2000;172:73–76.

34. Jones NS. An audit of the management of 250 patients with chest trauma in a regional thoracic surgical centre. *Arch Emerg Med* 1989;6:97–106.

35. Keel M, Meier C. Chest injuries: what is new? *Curr Opin Crit Care* 2007;13:674–679.

36. Kerwin AJ, Croce MA, Timmons SD, et al. Effects of fiberoptic bronchoscopy on intracranial pressure in patients with brain injury: a prospective clinical study. *J Trauma* 2000;48:878–882.

37. Kimmell KT, Jahromi BS. Clinical factors associated with venous thromboembolism risk in patients undergoing craniotomy. *J Neurosurg* 2014:1–8.

38. Kline JA, Israel EG, Michelson EA, et al. Diagnostic accuracy of a bedside D-dimer assay and alveolar dead-space measurement for rapid exclusion of pulmonary embolism: a multicenter study. *JAMA* 2001;285:761–768.

39. Kline JA, Nelson RD, Jackson RE, Courtney DM. Criteria for the safe use of D-dimer testing in emergency department patients with suspected

pulmonary embolism: a multicenter US study. *Ann Emerg Med* 2002;39:144–152.

40. Konstantinides S, Geibel A, Heusel G, Heinrich F, Kasper W. Heparin plus alteplase compared with heparin alone in patients with submassive pulmonary embolism. *N Engl J Med* 2002;347:1143–1150.

41. Kreider ME, Lipson DA. Bronchoscopy for atelectasis in the ICU: a case report and review of the literature. *Chest* 2003;124:344–350.

42. Marshall SA, Nyquist P. A change of position for neurogenic pulmonary edema. *Neurocrit Care* 2009;10:213–217.

43. Mascia L, Zavala E, Bosma K, et al. High tidal volume is associated with the development of acute lung injury after severe brain injury: an international observational study. *Crit Care Med* 2007;35:1815–1820.

44. Matsuyama T, Okuchi K, Nishiguchi T, Seki T, Murao Y. Neurogenic pulmonary edema caused by a medulla oblongata lesion after head trauma. *J Trauma* 2007;63:700–702.

45. Muroi C, Keller E. Treatment regimen in patients with neurogenic pulmonary edema after subarachnoid hemorrhage. *J Neurosurg Anesthesiol* 2009;21:68.

46. Nuckton TJ, Alonso JA, Kallet RH, et al. Pulmonary dead-space fraction as a risk factor for death in the acute respiratory distress syndrome. *N Engl J Med* 2002;346:1281–1286.

47. Palareti G. How I treat isolated distal deep vein thrombosis (IDDVT). *Blood* 2014;123:1802–1809.

48. Paterson DI, Schwartzman K. Strategies incorporating spiral CT for the diagnosis of acute pulmonary embolism: a cost-effectiveness analysis. *Chest* 2001;119:1791–1800.

49. Perrier A, Howarth N, Didier D, et al. Performance of helical computed tomography in unselected outpatients with suspected pulmonary embolism. *Ann Intern Med* 2001;135:88–97.

50. Rathbun SW, Raskob GE, Whitsett TL. Sensitivity and specificity of helical computed tomography in the diagnosis of pulmonary embolism: a systematic review. *Ann Intern Med* 2000;132:227–232.

51. Ray WZ, Strom RG, Blackburn SL, et al. Incidence of deep venous thrombosis after subarachnoid hemorrhage. *J Neurosurg* 2009;110:1010–1014.

52. Rebuck JA, Rasmussen JR, Olsen KM. Clinical aspiration-related practice patterns in the intensive care unit: a physician survey. *Crit Care Med* 2001;29:2239–2244.

53. Richardson JD, Adams L, Flint LM. Selective management of flail chest and pulmonary contusion. *Ann Surg* 1982;196:481–487.

54. Richardson JD, McElvein RB, Trinkle JK. First rib fracture: a hallmark of severe trauma. *Ann Surg* 1975;181:251–254.

55. Rosow CE. An overview of remifentanil. *Anesth Analg* 1999;89:S1–3.

56. Sassoon CS, Foster GT. Patient-ventilator asynchrony. *Curr Opin Crit Care* 2001;7:28–33.

57. Scheld WM, Mandell GL. Nosocomial pneumonia: pathogenesis and recent advances in diagnosis and therapy. *Rev Infect Dis* 1991;13 Suppl 9:S743–751.

58. Schoepf UJ, Holzknecht N, Helmberger TK, et al. Subsegmental pulmonary emboli: improved detection with thin-collimation multi-detector row spiral CT. *Radiology* 2002;222:483–490.

59. Schulman S, Rhedin AS, Lindmarker P, et al. A comparison of six weeks with six months of oral anticoagulant therapy after a first episode of venous thromboembolism: duration of Anticoagulation Trial Study Group. *N Engl J Med* 1995;332:1661–1665.

60. Shorr RM, Crittenden M, Indeck M, Hartunian SL, Rodriguez A. Blunt thoracic trauma: analysis of 515 patients. *Ann Surg* 1987;206:200–205.

61. Silver FL, Norris JW, Lewis AJ, Hachinski VC. Early mortality following stroke: a prospective review. *Stroke* 1984;15:492–496.

62. Smith WS, Matthay MA. Evidence for a hydrostatic mechanism in human neurogenic pulmonary edema. *Chest* 1997;111:1326–1333.

63. Taccone P, Pesenti A, Latini R, et al. Prone positioning in patients with moderate and severe acute respiratory distress syndrome: a randomized controlled trial. *JAMA* 2009;302:1977–1984.

64. Teigen CL, Maus TP, Sheedy PF, 2nd, et al. Pulmonary embolism: diagnosis with contrast-enhanced electron-beam CT and comparison with pulmonary angiography. *Radiology* 1995;194:313–319.

65. Tobin MJ. Respiratory monitoring in the intensive care unit. *Am Rev Respir Dis* 1988;138:1625–1642.

66. Treggiari MM, Martin DP, Yanez ND, et al. Effect of intensive care unit organizational model and structure on outcomes in patients with acute lung injury. *Am J Respir Crit Care Med* 2007;176:685–690.

67. Turner JS, Willcox PA, Hayhurst MD, Potgieter PD. Fiberoptic bronchoscopy in the intensive care unit: a prospective study of 147 procedures in 107 patients. *Crit Care Med* 1994;22:259–264.

68. Weiss YG, Deutschman CS. The role of fiberoptic bronchoscopy in airway management of the critically ill patient. *Crit Care Clin* 2000;16:445–451, vi.

69. Wijdicks EFM, Scott JP. Pulmonary embolism associated with acute stroke. *Mayo Clinic Proc* 1997;72:297–300.
70. Wijdicks EFM. Short of breath, short of air, short of mechanics. *Practical Neurology* 2002;2:208–213.
71. Wood KE. Major pulmonary embolism: review of a pathophysiologic approach to the golden hour of hemodynamically significant pulmonary embolism. *Chest* 2002;121:877–905.
72. Yabumoto M, Kuriyama T, Iwamoto M, Kinoshita T. Neurogenic pulmonary edema associated with ruptured intracranial aneurysm: case report. *Neurosurgery* 1986;19:300–304.
73. Young YR, Lee CC, Sheu BF, Chang SS. Neurogenic cardiopulmonary complications associated with spontaneous cerebellar hemorrhage. *Neurocrit Care* 2007;7:238–240.

56
Management of Cardiac Complications

Myocardial injury may be attributable to acute brain injury and can result in cardiac arrhythmias and cardiac failure. When seen in the neurosciences intensive care unit (NICU), cardiac abnormalities can be grouped into three categories. First, left ventricular dysfunction occurs in some patients with acute central nervous system (CNS) catastrophes, and this phenomenon is known as *stress cardiomyopathy*.[49] Second, cardiac arrhythmias are prevalent. The most common causes are underlying structural heart disease, associated drug therapy, left ventricular strain, pulmonary embolism, fever, and anemia. Third, although traumatic injury to the heart is uncommon, possible considerations in patients with polytrauma include traumatic aortic dissection; damage to the right ventricle, septum, and tricuspid valve (susceptible because of proximity to the sternum); and pericardial effusion. Laceration of the left anterior descending coronary artery and right ventricular wall contusion have been diagnosed in isolated cases.[68]

The presence of acute myocardial ischemia has important repercussions if patients need neurosurgical intervention. In some patients, evolving cardiac failure may result in pulmonary edema that compromises gas exchange. In other critical neurologic illnesses, cardiac arrhythmias are life-threatening, and a temporary pacemaker may be indicated. This chapter considers frequently observed cardiac abnormalities and provides practical basic knowledge.

PATHOPHYSIOLOGIC MECHANISMS OF CARDIAC ABNORMALITIES

Cardiac injury and arrhythmias have been linked to transient sympathetic hyperactivity, which may result in objective myocardial damage, mostly in the form of dispersed areas of hemorrhages and myocytolysis, myofibrillar degeneration, myocyte eosinophilia, and contraction bands, but not necrosis[23,31,39] (Capsule 56.1).

In acute lesions of the CNS, sympathetic preponderance is clinically noted as sustained hypertension, dilatation of pupils, fever, profuse sweating, and, at times, peripheral cutaneous vasoconstriction, resulting in characteristically cold fingers and toes. The alleged anatomical site associated with sympathetic stimulation is the anterior hypothalamus.[5,39] Other structures besides the diencephalon possibly involved in sympathetic response are neurons in the ventrolateral medulla oblongata and right-sided insular cortex.[38,52,66] The role of the right insula in sudden death due to tachyarrhythmias has been suggested in clinical studies.[16] Pressure, stretch, or hypoxemia may trigger depolarization of these sensitive neurons, leading to a persistent sympathetic tone.

In acute lesions of the peripheral nervous system, cardiac arrhythmias may also occur, particularly Guillain-Barré syndrome (GBS). Life-threatening cardiac arrhythmias in GBS are very uncommon, and the pathologic substrate of cardiac arrhythmias in GBS has not been elucidated. Clinicopathologic studies, however, have demonstrated scattered lymphocytic infiltrates in ganglia and in parasympathetic and sympathetic branches. In GBS, sinus tachycardia is the most common cardiac arrhythmia and may be related to lesions of the afferent baroreceptors.[74]

In general, the cardiac manifestations can be considered to result from triggers of the central or peripheral nervous system, but in some conditions, the pathophysiologic state truly originates from the heart in an NICU population with a high proclivity for coronary artery disease. Examples of primary cardiac causes are acute myocardial infarction complicated by embolic ischemic stroke, and the occasional situation in which endocarditis is associated with intracranial hematoma from a ruptured infectious aneurysm. Electrolyte disorders or drug toxicity can be implicated in some patients with cardiac arrhythmias. A correlation between prolonged PR interval and hypomagnesemia has been found in aneurysmal subarachnoid hemorrhage (SAH).[79] In addition,

CAPSULE 56.1   AUTONOMIC NERVOUS SYSTEM AND THE HEART

The presynaptic cell bodies of the autonomic nervous system originate in the gray matter of the spinal column. The sympathetic part is located between T1 and L2 and L3. The parasympathetic parts originate from the medulla oblongata and sacral portion (S2–S4) of spinal cord. The sympathetic segments project to the cardiac plexus (see accompanying illustration). The right sympathetic branch targets the sinoatrial node; the left sympathetic tract targets the atrioventricular node and ventricles. The parasympathetic portion starts in the nucleus ambiguus and descends via the superior and inferior cervical and thoracic rami, and ends in the cardiac plexus.[43] The normal resting portion produces a tonic level of vagal activity (sleep, rest). Many nerves follow the pathways of coronary arteries and may end up in epicardial regions, mostly in ventricles. However, in ventricles, the distribution is more concentrated at the base than apex. Parasympathetic representation in ventricles is much less than sympathetic innervation.

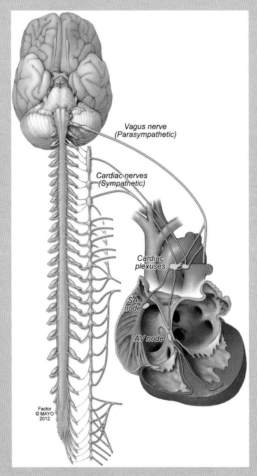

Autonomic innervation of the heart.

multifocal atrial tachycardia (often mistaken for atrial fibrillation) may occur in response to a brief hypoxemic event, particularly in patients with pulmonary disease.

CARDIAC MANIFESTATIONS IN SPECIFIC NEUROLOGIC CIRCUMSTANCES

The fascinating link between acute lesions to the brain and the heart has been investigated clinically for many years by both cardiologists and neurologists.[42]

This section reviews cardiac arrhythmias and the most pertinent electrocardiogram (EKG) abnormalities in acute neurologic disorders.

Aneurysmal Subarachnoid Hemorrhage

The incidence of cardiac arrhythmias in aneurysmal SAH is difficult to estimate. Most likely, differences in the recording of abnormalities result in varying incidences of EKG abnormalities and arrhythmias. The incidence of cardiac arrhythmias may also be inaccurate because sudden death in SAH (approximately 10% of all patients) is possibly associated with asystole of Pulseless electrical activity (PEA) arrest (Capsule 56.2).

The most common cardiac rhythm disturbances in SAH are sinus bradycardia and sinus tachycardia, but both are nonspecific and can be associated with multiple causes. Possible causes for sinus bradycardia are administration of opioids, increased vagal tone from vomiting, and use of β-blockers. Potential causes of sinus tachycardia are fever, the combination of hypovolemia with anemia (a frequently overlooked cause of tachycardia), and sympathomimetic drugs such as dopamine (or other inotropes).

The incidence of life-threatening tachyarrhythmias varies considerably in studies.[2,65] Tachyarrhythmias are observed significantly more often in patients with SAH and massive intraventricular hemorrhage. When Holter monitoring was used within 48 hours of admission in patients with SAH, 41% of the patients had transient life-threatening arrhythmias, such as torsades de pointes, ventricular flutter, and ventricular fibrillation.[22] This high incidence of potentially life-threatening arrhythmias is unusual and was not found in another series of patients with serial EKG recordings and daily bedside monitoring.[12] Other SAH-associated cardiac arrhythmias are runs of ventricular premature complexes, sustained ventricular tachycardia, and bradyarrhythmias,

mostly transient idioventricular rhythm and atrioventricular block.[2,19,22,28]

Morphologic EKG changes are common in SAH.[12] One study suggested that frequencies of EKG abnormalities were higher in patients with blood in the right sylvian fissure and quadrigeminal cistern, a finding that may argue for irritation of the insular cortex.[38] The significance of EKG changes remains unclear; they do not affect overall outcome, and studies have not been able to separate out patients with higher risks of cardiac death.[89]

The most common EKG changes are shown in Table 56.1. Most frequently, the morphologic abnormalities are related to changes in the QRS complex. Very often, ST-segment sagging appears (leads I, aVL); T waves are deeply inverted, and the QT interval is prolonged (Figure 56.1). (The QT interval varies with the heart rate, and a corrected QT [QT_c] is calculated by dividing the QT interval by the square root of the interval between two R waves; normal is 0.41 second in women and 0.39 second in men.)

One retrospective study found ST- and T-wave abnormalities, most commonly T-wave inversions and ST elevations, in 27% of patients with EKG readings. None of these abnormalities predicted fatal arrhythmias.[89] Echocardiographic studies have repeatedly shown ventricular dysfunction in these patients. Corresponding regional wall motion abnormalities have been found in patients with transient ST segment elevation.[70] Another study found that inverted T waves and QT-segment prolongation were significantly correlated with left ventricular function.[56]

Tako-tsubo cardiomyopathy (apical ballooning) has been reported in aneurysmal SAH, but can occur after any major acute overwhelming stressful event ("broken heart syndrome").[87] Subarachnoid hemorrhage and stress cardiomyopathy both occur often in middle-aged women, linking the two together simply by age and overwhelming ictus. The diagnosis of Tako-tsubo cardiomyopathy is based on several criteria: (1) a major acute unexpected stressful event or acute brain injury; (2) transient left ventricular wall motion abnormalities involving the apical or mid-ventricular myocardial segments but with wall motion abnormalities extending beyond the single epicardial coronary distribution; (3) absence of obstructive coronary artery disease or angiographic evidence of acute plaque rupture that could be responsible for the observable wall motion abnormality; and (4) new EKG

CAPSULE 56.2 ASYSTOLE AND ANEURYSMAL RUPTURE

The leading theories behind the mechanism for cardiac arrest include (1) massive catecholamine release and sympathetic surge leading to cardiac stunning, or (2) sudden massive ICP increase leading to brainstem dysfunction with respiratory arrest and hypoxia. Moreover, the hypercapnic, hypoxic respiratory acidosis that follows respiratory arrest results in release of endogenous adenosine and nitric oxide, both of which cause bradycardia. The acidosis acts on central and peripheral chemoreceptors to result in profound bradycardia and subsequent asystole. Hypoxia has also been shown to decrease calcium release from cardiac myocytes resulting in a loss of cardiac contractile force. This in turn results in ventricular motion with a lack of palpable pulse, known as Pulseless electrical activity (PEA). In contrast, focal ischemia causes regional electrophysiological abnormalities and disorganized reentry, resulting in ventricular fibrillation. The prognosis of these patients is very poor, with mortality rates as high as 96–100% and many patients are braindeath after they have been resuscitated.[4,59,88]

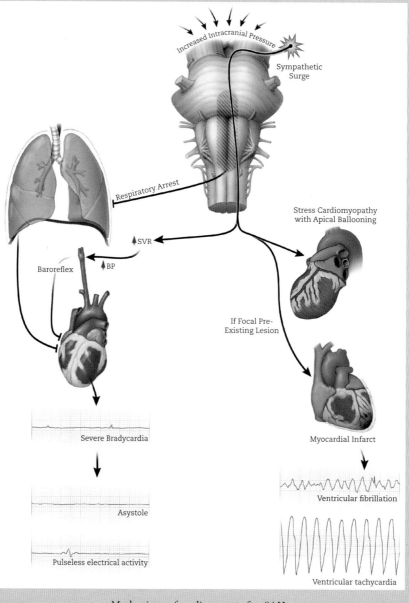

Mechanisms of cardiac arrest after SAH.

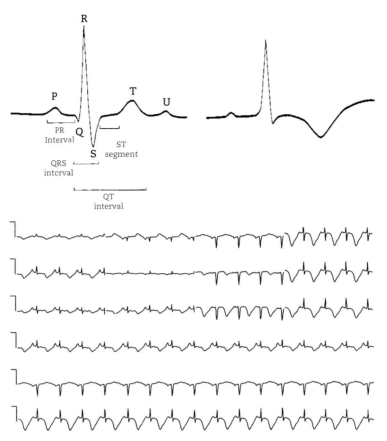

FIGURE 56.1: Typical morphologic changes in electrocardiographic tracing associated with acute severe brain injury. Note these changes in EKG. *Left*: Normal tracing. *Right*: Abnormal tracing with ST-segment depression, marked T-wave inversion, and QT interval prolongation.

TABLE 56.1. ELECTROCARDIOGRAPHIC CHANGES IN SUBARACHNOID HEMORRHAGE*

	No. of Patients
Ischemic ST segment	44
Ischemic T wave	41
Prominent U wave	39
QT$_c$ interval prolongation	34
Flat or isoelectric T wave	24
Short PR interval	14
Long PR interval	13
Transient pathologic Q wave	11
Peaked P wave	10
Tall T wave	10
Broad P wave	4

*Based on findings in 61 patients with serial electrocardiograms. Modified from Brouwers PJ, Wijdicks EFM, Hasan D, et al. Serial electrocardiographic recording in aneurysmal subarachnoid hemorrhage. *Stroke* 1989;20:1162–1167. With permission of the American Heart Association.

abnormalities such as transient ST-elevation or diffuse T-wave inversion or troponin elevations. Marked apical akinesia can be found on echocardiography but is reversible[21,47,48] (Figure 56.2).

Cardiac involvement is mostly expected in more severe manifestations of SAH.[32,57,58] Pathologically, myocardial damage in SAH is sub-endocardial in the form of small, scattered hemorrhages. In an important study of 72 patients with aneurysmal SAH without prior cardiac disease, abnormal left ventricular wall motion was found in only 9 (13%) and was directly linked to high creatine kinase MB levels and troponin levels.[30,56,67]

Echocardiographic abnormalities could persist for weeks, although spontaneous reversibility has been described.[83,90] An echo-cardiogram may demonstrate significant regional wall motion abnormalities that, unlike acute myocardial infarction, may be reversible as early as 4 days later.[34] Serial EKGs and echocardiography are important because "acute myocardial infarction

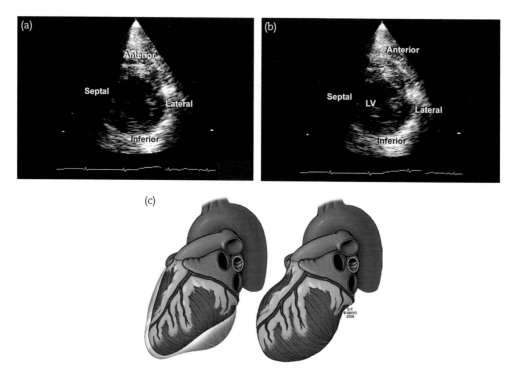

FIGURE 56.2: Transthoracic echocardiograms in a patient with aneurysmal subarachnoid hemorrhage. End-diastolic (a) and end-systolic (b) phases are shown in short-axis views. Note electrocardiographic tracing below, showing the view in relation to the cardiac cycle. Global severe hypokinesis is shown as virtually no change in left chamber size from end-diastole to end-systole. (c) Graphic representation of normal contraction (*left*) and tako-tsubo cardiomyopathy (*right*) (named after octopus fishing pot due to its resemblance).

LV, left ventricle.

patterns" may dramatically change, even within 1 day.[12,55] A recent meta-analysis concluded that cardiac abnormalities in SAH (EKG changes, echocardiographic abnormalities, and markers for myocardial injury) are related to poor outcome and delayed cerebral ischemia.[80] However, the nature of this relationship remains unexplained.

Real-time myocardial perfusion contrast echocardiography (RTP-CE) is a new technique that allows for simultaneous assessment of wall motion and perfusion (Figure 56.3). It uses microbubbles behaving similarly to red blood cells, which work as tracers for blood flow.[47] The assessment of gradual refill of microbubbles into the myocardial microcirculation is key for the evaluation of perfusion using RTP-CE. In our clinical study, we documented normal myocardial perfusion despite regional wall motion abnormalities.[1] With quantitative RTP-CE, we showed higher myocardial blood flow velocity and myocardial blood flow in patients with regional wall motion abnormalities versus those with normal wall motion, suggesting reperfusion after initial hypoperfusion.[1]

Clinical management of tako-tsubo cardiomyopathy is close observation and if cardiogenic shock is part of the presentation (about 10–15%) dopamine is administered at a dose of 5–20 mcg/kg/min.[77] Dopamine increases contractility and heart rate through activation of the β-adrenergic receptors but also results in vasoconstriction through the activation of α-receptors in the periphery. Alternatively Milrinone (a phosphodiesterase inhibitor) can significantly increase cardiac output through peripheral vasodilatation and reduction in cardiac afterload.

Head Injury
Cardiac arrhythmias have been studied less frequently in head injury.[40] Cardiac arrhythmias have been reported in patients with acute subdural hematoma. In a study of 100 patients, 41% had new rhythm disturbances, half with ventricular arrhythmias.[81] Confounding factors could exist, particularly in patients with multitrauma who may have direct cardiac trauma.[33] Electrocardiographic abnormalities in closed head injury may indicate pericardial effusion,

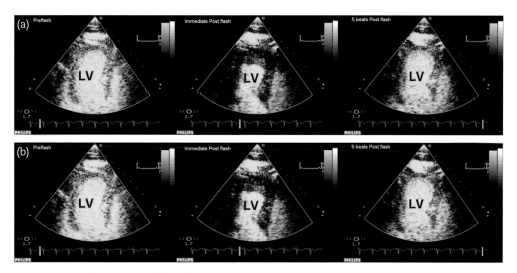

FIGURE 56.3: Real-time myocardial perfusion contrast echocardiography.

(a) A 73-year-old woman with subarachnoid hemorrhage and ST-T wave abnormalities on electrocardiogram and elevated cardiac enzymes. Resting RTP-CE in apical four-chamber view showing homogenous myocardial contrast enhancement at five beats after microbubble destruction (flash). (b) For comparison, a case of ST-segment elevation myocardial infarction (STEMI) showing resting real-time myocardial perfusion contrast echocardiography (RTP-CE) in the apical long axis view of the left ventricle. Regional wall motion abnormality in the apical segments with transmural myocardial perfusion defect (*arrows*).

From Abdelmoneim SS, Wijdicks EFM, Lee VH, et al. Real time myocardial perfusion contrast echocardiography in regional wall motion abnormalities after aneurysmal subarachnoid hemorrhage. *J Neurosurg* 2009;111:1023–1028. Used with permission from the *Journal of Neurosurgery.*

myocardial infarction from laceration of coronary arteries, or ventricular wall motion abnormalities from stress cardiomyopathy. If the EKG findings are normal 3 hours after trauma, the chance of later complications is greatly reduced. The diagnosis of myocardial contusion is facilitated by echocardiographic findings of regional wall motion abnormalities and, most important, pericardial effusion. Cardiogenic shock is uncommon, and left ventricular ejection fraction usually is not reduced, because the right ventricle is preferentially involved in blunt trauma.[68] Cardiac tamponade is most impressive in its presentation, with hypotension, cyanosis of the upper chest and face, and distended neck veins.

Acute Ischemic or Hemorrhagic Stroke

Patients with a major stroke in arterial territory often have previous evidence of underlying heart disease. Therefore, in this clinical category, cardiac arrhythmias may be a cause rather than a result of stroke.[44] In one prospective study, asymptomatic coronary artery disease was found in approximately one-third of the patients with stroke.[73] We reported on a patient with a pristine coronary angiogram, new regional wall motion abnormalities on echocardiography, and transient EKG abnormalities after a hemorrhage damaging the rostral ventrolateral medulla oblongata.[72]

The prevailing rhythm abnormality in acute ischemic stroke is atrial fibrillation, but sinus tachycardia, premature ventricular complexes, and premature atrial complexes are almost as frequent.[11,20] In a retrospective study, only patients with right-sided hemispheric stroke had supraventricular tachycardia, whereas patients with left-sided hemispheric stroke more often had multiform premature ventricular complexes, couplets, and ventricular tachycardia—findings that suggested differences in influence of the hemispheres.[46] Whether aggressive monitoring is indicated in patients with left hemispheric strokes, whose cardiac arrhythmias seem more life-threatening, remains unresolved and doubtful.

Life-threatening arrhythmias in acute stroke are very unusual and should point to other causes, particularly acute myocardial infarction. Most often patients need management of atrial fibrillation with a transient rapid ventricular response.

Status Epilepticus

Cardiac arrhythmias are possibly more often present in status epilepticus than truly recognized. In our review of patients admitted to the emergency department with status epilepticus, cardiac arrhythmias occurred in 15 of 38 (39%). Sinus tachycardia was found in the vast majority, but two patients had ventricular tachycardia and a brief asystole after sudden bradycardia. No relationship was found with respiratory or metabolic (lactic) acidosis, a common occurrence in this condition.[84] Another study found bradycardia during seizures but only in the context of associated brief apnea.[62] In a pathology study from the Mayo Clinic, a high percentage (72%) of patients with fatal status epilepticus had pathologic evidence of contraction band necrosis,[53] and that finding could point toward increased sympathetic activity. These contraction bands are a reflection of a hypercontracted state causing myocytolysis, followed by a mononuclear infiltrate and calcification ("stone heart"). A more recent study found over 50% stress cardiomyopathy after status epilepticus but with rapid recovery.[9] An interesting question is whether patients with status epilepticus and cardiac arrhythmias need β-blockers for myocardial protection and we have been paying close attention to it and treat when needed.

Guillain-Barré Syndrome

The entire gamut of cardiac arrhythmias can be seen in Guillain-Barré syndrome (GBS), including complete heart block. In the large plasma exchange trials conducted by the GBS study group and the French Cooperative Group, fatal cardiac arrest occurred in three of the combined total of 445 patients. Fortunately, pacemaker intervention is very rarely necessary in GBS.[74]

Sinus tachycardia and so-called vagal bradycardia spells are most frequent in patients with GBS. Persistent sinus tachycardia invariably occurs in patients with complete quadriplegia and mechanical ventilation; it may appear at any time during the illness and generally is not associated with hypotension or angina pectoris. Slowing of rate is indicated with signs of myocardial ischemia on EKG.

Vagal spells are brief salvos of bradycardia or sinus arrest, and tracheal suctioning is a common trigger. Vagal spells are usually a feature seen in the plateau phase but may extend into the recovery phase. When these episodes occur, EKG monitoring should continue until the patient becomes ambulant.

Bradycardia has been associated with reversible stress cardiomyopathy in a young woman with GBS.[8] The mechanism of stress cardiomyopathy in GBS may be more complicated. A sympathetic overdrive in GBS may result in marked reduction in ejection fraction from sudden ventricular strain with hypertension. In one of our patients, stress cardiomyopathy and posterior reversible encephalopathy syndrome (PRES) did occur simultaneously and resolved spontaneously.[29]

Morphologic EKG abnormalities are uncommon and nonspecific in GBS, but when they are present, ST-segment abnormalities are frequent.[74] It is uncertain whether they represent myocardial damage.

Brain Death

Cardiac arrhythmias may occur in patients who fulfill the criteria for brain death. Sinus tachycardia is frequent and possibly a combination of vasopressors and hypovolemia.

During apnea testing, cardiac arrhythmia may occur with severe acidosis (pH < 7.0), and it is commonly ventricular tachyarrhythmia. This arrhythmia may be associated with hypotension, which has the potential to jeopardize organ recovery if it is not rapidly corrected. Only when acidosis becomes severe and PCO_2 approaches 90 mm Hg can cardiac arrhythmias be expected despite adequate preoxygenation. In general, connection to the ventilator corrects the arrhythmia.

Myocardial dysfunction after catastrophic brain injury leading to brain death is common and often is associated with ventricular arrhythmias. Myocardial dysfunction is more severe in patients with traumatic head injury than in those with SAH or intraparenchymal hemorrhage. In our study of 66 patients, myocardial dysfunction in brain death from SAH was more regional, and ejection fraction more marginally abnormal and was not accompanied by histologic changes in the ventricular myocardium. However, a very significant reduction in ejection fraction and global hypokinesis interspersed with large akinetic segments was found in patients with head trauma who had progression to brain death. Ventricular arrhythmias occurred in 30% of brain dead patients with severe echocardiographic abnormalities and in none with normal echocardiographic findings.[25,60]

Echocardiography is routinely used to screen brain-dead donors. Patients who fulfill the clinical criteria of brain death have an invariant heart rate due to autonomic uncoupling. Cardiac arrest is an inevitable consequence of brain death. Lack of autonomic nervous system input results in a decrease in contractility and coronary perfusion and in terminal cardiac rhythms, such as sinus bradycardia, or isolated atrial activity.[36,37,50]

CARDIAC ARRHYTHMIAS

The most commonly observed cardiac arrhythmias in CNS catastrophes and their management options are systematically described in this section for easy reference. In the acute phase of cardiac arrhythmias, pharmacologic management is often not indicated in patients with acute neurologic illness because many of the manifestations are very brief and the agents may reduce blood pressure to unwanted levels. Not infrequently, cardiac arrhythmias may occur in patients on rate control drugs that have been discontinued temporarily to maintain acceptable blood pressures (e.g., β-blockade in patients with prior atrial fibrillation). Nonetheless, some cardiac arrhythmias are immediately life-threatening or are warning signals of malignant arrhythmia to come. Arrhythmias may arise from certain regions in the brain, including the insular cortex, cingulate cortex, and the amygdala; but this link is not so clear in clinical practice, where there is often more widespread or multifocal hemispheric involvement (Figure 56.4). The initial strategy is described; further management and evaluation of triggers other than those from the CNS should be left to the judgment of the consulting cardiologist.[13,87] The most commonly used antiarrhythmic agents and their potential side effects are listed in Table 56.2.

Sinus Tachycardia

Sinus tachycardia remains the most common rhythm disturbance in acutely ill neurologic patients. The EKG abnormalities are not very difficult to detect. P waves are uniform, PR intervals are fixed, and the rate is regular, with an increase only above 100–150 beats/minute.

Sinus tachycardia should not be considered a mundane rhythm disturbance. Sustained sinus tachycardia may cause a significant decrease in cardiac output, but often only if ventricular rates reach more than 200 beats/minute. Causes of sudden onset of sinus tachycardia are fever, hypovolemia, anxiety, pain, pulmonary embolism, and

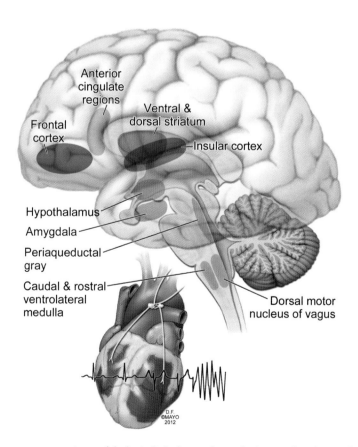

FIGURE 56.4: Areas of the brain linked to cardiac arrhythmias when damaged.

TABLE 56.2. INTRAVENOUS ANTIARRHYTHMIC DRUGS

Drug	Dose	Side Effects
Atropine	0.5–1.0 mg as a rapid bolus, max 3 mg	Sinus tachycardia
Adenosine	6 mg in 2 minutes; if no effect, 12 mg	Profound hypotension, facial flushing, bradycardia
Diltiazem	0.25 mg/kg (actual body weight) bolus over 2 minutes; maintenance 5–15 mg per hour	Hypotension, heart block, headache
Verapamil	5–10 mg bolus over 3 minutes; repeated if necessary may be followed by continuous infusion of 0.005 mg/kg per minute	Headache, nausea, constipation, hypotension, heart block
Lidocaine	0.7–1.4 mg/kg bolus over 3 minutes followed by 1–4 mg/minute constant infusion	Seizures, respiratory arrest, dizziness, heart block (usually associated with preexisting abnormal His-Purkinje conduction), sinoatrial arrest
Procainamide	100 mg IV slowly (25 mg/minute) to maximum 1,000 mg	Hypotension, prolonged AV and His-Purkinje conduction
Metoprolol	5 mg every 5 minutes up to 15 mg	Hypotension, bradycardia, prolonged AV conduction and heart block, myocardial depression
Propranolol	1 mg/minute every 5 minutes up to 10 mg	Hypotension, bradycardia, prolonged AV conduction and heart block, myocardial depression, bronchospasm
Esmolol	0.5 mg/kg bolus, 0.05–0.2 mg/kg per minute infusion	Hypotension, bradycardia, bronchoconstriction
Magnesium sulfate	1 g in 10 mL of normal saline over 20 minutes or 1–4 g/hour infusion	Diarrhea, flushing

AV, atrioventricular; IV, intravenously.

any type of infection. The rate should be slowed, because myocardial oxygen consumption is directly related to rate, and myocardial ischemia may develop under these conditions (especially if there is underlying coronary disease). In addition, persistent sinus tachycardia may produce congestive heart failure.

In most patients, catecholamine excess is the main culprit, so that β-blockade seems the most appropriate treatment. (A study of severe head injury indeed showed a reduction in cardiac necrosis after prophylactic β-blockade.)[17] Esmolol 0.5 mg/kg given in 1 minute, followed by 0.05–0.2 mg/kg/min as a maintenance dose, or metoprolol 5–10 mg intravenously may control this rhythm.

Sinus Bradycardia

Sinus bradycardia arrhythmia often develops in patients with acute lesions in the posterior fossa and in patients with brainstem displacement from supratentorial masses. Both conditions result in brainstem shift or compression, and bradycardia therefore may be part of the Cushing response.[18]

Bradycardia is also seen in the NICU after the use of morphine for pain control, after profuse vomiting in patients due to increased vagal tone, and in patients with β-blockade. Bradycardia in massive hemispheric strokes may be prominent in the first days but usually normalizes spontaneously. Therefore, treatment of sinus bradycardia is usually postponed, but in patients with sustained bradycardia and a decrease in blood pressure, atropine in a 0.5 mg bolus, or isoproterenol, 1 mg in 250 mL normal saline, at a rate of 2–10 μg per minute (the solution contains 4 μg/mL), is administered.

Atrial Fibrillation

Acute atrial fibrillation can be observed in acute brain injury, but it often portends underlying heart disease. Potential causes of atrial fibrillation in the NICU are acute myocardial infarction, alcohol withdrawal, pulmonary embolus, and any other acute pulmonary disease. Thyrotoxicosis may underlie atrial fibrillation, especially in elderly patients. The physical examination in patients with atrial fibrillation is notable for a completely irregular pulse and a pulse deficit (more beats heard at the heart than felt at the radial pulse).

Atrial fibrillation is relatively easily recognized on EKG, except when it is associated with a rapid ventricular response. The characteristic findings on EKG examination are the absence of P waves between the T waves and the QRS complexes (Figure 56.5a). Typically, F waves are clearly visible in the precordial leads. F waves are continuous undulating lines, may vary in amplitude during respiration, and may depend on left atrial pressure. In patients with a rapid response, carotid massage may stimulate the vagal input to the atrioventricular node and uncover the F waves. The QRS complexes are irregular but have a normal configuration.

Treatment of atrial fibrillation, as in many of the supraventricular arrhythmias, is dictated by a tendency toward hypotension and by the early development of pulmonary edema, clinical situations that are often associated with a rapid ventricular rate. Carotid sinus pressure, a common procedure, slows the ventricular rate and often

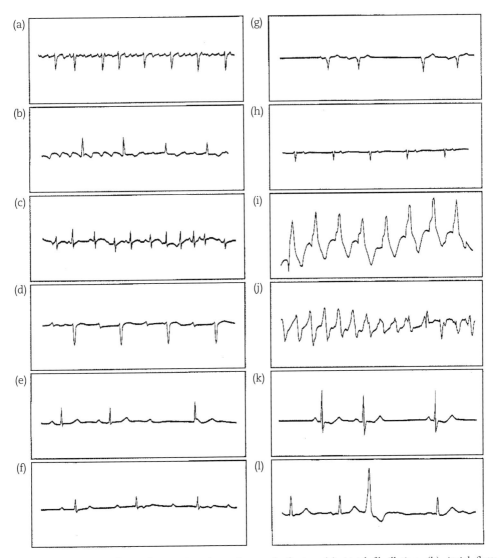

FIGURE 56.5: Electrocardiographic tracings in various arrhythmias. (a) Atrial fibrillation. (b) Atrial flutter. (c) Multifocal atrial tachycardia. (d) Junctional rhythm. (e) First-degree atrioventricular block. (f) Second-degree atrioventricular block (Mobitz type I). (g) Second-degree atrioventricular block (Mobitz type II). (h) Third-degree atrioventricular block. (i) Ventricular tachycardia. (j) Torsades de pointes. (k) Premature atrial complex. (l) Premature ventricular complex.

makes atrial fibrillation easier to recognize but virtually never converts atrial fibrillation into sinus rhythm.

Calcium channel blockers and β-blockers are the drugs of choice to reduce the ventricular rate.[26] Verapamil intravenously in a bolus of 5–10 mg over 2 minutes, followed by an additional dose of 5 mg after 15 minutes, converts atrial fibrillation in many patients. If this attempt at conversion fails, one can resort to a low dose of diltiazem (10 mg bolus or infusion of 5 mg/hr), procainamide (100 mg IV every 5 minutes to a maximum of 1 g), or esmolol (0.5 mg/kg IV gradually over several minutes). Digitalis is reserved for patients with atrial fibrillation and normal ventricular response or underlying left ventricular dysfunction (1.0–1.5 mg IV in 3 divided doses over 24 hours).[26]

Another option for converting atrial fibrillation, especially in the hemodynamically unstable patient, is electrical cardioversion, which is effective in more than 50% of patients. Positive predictive factors for successful cardioversion are recent onset of atrial fibrillation, coarse or large F waves on the EKG, and, possibly, normal-sized left atrium on echocardiography or routine chest radiography. Cardioversion is performed with 50–100 J after sedation with propofol or midazolam. A higher power (200 J) can be used if the first shock is not effective or if atrial fibrillation recurs. Typically, anticoagulation is required for 3–4 weeks after cardioversion, but this may not be possible in some patients. In these patients, a combination of aspirin and clopidogrel could be considered.

Disopyramide, amiodarone, quinidine, or sotalol can be used to maintain sinus rhythm.[63] Ablation of the atrioventricular node and pacemaker implantation are a last resort.[86]

Atrial Flutter

Atrial flutter often occurs in combination with atrial fibrillation. The characteristics on EKGs are P waves resembling a picket fence or sawteeth. They are best seen in inferior leads II, III, and aVF (Figure 56.5b). The rhythm is regular or irregular, depending on whether the degree of atrioventricular block varies. Atrial flutter is very often rapid, with ventricular responses up to 300 beats/min, and the risk of pulmonary edema, hypotension, and myocardial ischemia is very significant. More often, however, flutter is associated with 2:1 block and much lower ventricular rates (150 beats/min). The characteristic sawtooth features may be unrecognized in tachyarrhythmias, and a Valsalva maneuver, carotid massage, or gradual

administration of a single dose of verapamil (5 mg) may sufficiently slow the rhythm. Electrical cardioversion remains the preferred management strategy. Long-term administration of antiarrhythmic drugs is needed to reduce the risk of recurrence. Currently, flecainide and propafenone are widely used but perhaps should be reserved for patients with normal underlying left ventricular function.

Multifocal Atrial Tachycardia

This tachyarrhythmia is frequent in acutely ill patients but remains comparatively rare in hospital populations. As noted previously, the clinical findings of an irregular rapid rhythm may initially suggest atrial fibrillation. Patients with acute pulmonary disease are particularly at risk when treated with high doses of isoproterenol or aminophylline. Multifocal atrial tachycardia also recurs more frequently in susceptible patients after a major procedure (e.g., neurosurgical evacuation of an intracranial hematoma, neuroradiologic intervention) and in patients with sepsis, diabetes mellitus, or magnesium deficiency.

The EKG criteria are tachycardia; multiform (three or more) P waves indicating ectopic foci (upright, inverted, biphasic, and peaked), most evident in leads II, III, and V_1; and irregular PP, PR, and RR intervals (Figure 56.5c). Occasionally, a P wave is blocked when it coincides with the refractory period of the previous beat.

The treatment of multifocal atrial tachycardia is very complex and may not be effective without special attention to potential triggers. Cardioversion is seldom successful. The drug of choice is verapamil. Metoprolol in a dose of 5 mg IV every 5 minutes may be successful, but its use is limited if multifocal atrial tachycardia occurs in bronchospastic disease. Low doses of esmolol may be successful. Intravenous administration of magnesium in patients with normal magnesium levels may be tried as well (1 g of magnesium sulfate in 10 mL of normal saline over 20 minutes) because it suppresses ectopic activity. This cardiac arrhythmia should be considered one of the malignant arrhythmias.

Junctional Rhythm

In the NICU, junctional rhythm can occur after pronounced hypoxic episodes, digitalis intoxication, and the relatively unusual situation of acute myocardial infarction (Figure 56.5d). Junctional rhythm originates in the bundle of His, and the rhythm may vary. The characteristic feature of this often transient rhythm is the absence of P waves, or the presence of continuously changing PR intervals with relatively narrow QRS complexes. The P waves may be captured in the QRS complex or appear just before or after the QRS complex (as shown in Figure 56.5d). The difference from atrioventricular dissociation is that the atria and ventricles beat independently with a slow ventricular rate.

Specific treatment is not indicated in many patients, but in accelerated junctional rhythm, atropine (1 mg bolus IV) can restore sinus rhythm. Cardioversion is not successful.

Atrioventricular Block

This rhythm disturbance, uncommon in the NICU, is most often seen in GBS. First-degree atrioventricular block is characterized by a prolonged PR interval above the normal limit of 0.2 second. The interval may become more significantly prolonged with bradycardia, but the rhythm remains regular (Figure 56.5e).

Mobitz type I second-degree atrioventricular block, or Wenckebach type of block, is typically recognized by a progressively longer PR interval until the ventricular response drops, a pause ensues, and the cycle resumes (Figure 56.5f). In Mobitz type II second-degree atrioventricular block, a more serious abnormality, the ventricle suddenly fails to respond to atrial stimulation (Figure 56.5g). It occurs in anterior wall infarction. In third-degree atrioventricular block (complete block), rhythm is regular but usually slow (20–60 beats/min), and atrial and ventricular beats are independent (Figure 56.5h). Cardiac pacing is the ultimate treatment in patients with rapid progression of atrioventricular block and episodes of cardiac arrest.

Ventricular Tachycardia

Ventricular tachycardia is one of the most frequently observed tachycardias in acute CNS injury. Many patients have nonsustained tachycardia.

The diagnostic hallmark of ventricular tachycardia is a wide QRS complex of 140 msec or more. The P waves are mostly obscured within the ST segment and are difficult to detect at high rates[15,76] (Figure 56.5i). This type of tachycardia can be mistaken for supra-ventricular tachycardia, but intravenous administration of adenosine, which converts reentry supraventricular tachycardia (rarely seen in NICUs), can be used for differentiation. In fact, adenosine gives information similar to that of the vagal maneuver by blocking atrioventricular nodal conduction.

Treatment depends on the level of blood pressure. Cardioversion is indicated in patients with a significant reduction in blood pressure. Lidocaine is indicated in patients with normal blood pressure.

Miscellaneous Cardioarrhythmias

Occasionally, torsades de pointes arrhythmias appear in patients with poor-grade aneurysmal SAH, typically in association with bradyarrhythmia and prolonged QT interval. The wide QRS complexes twist around the baseline, continuously change in shape, are extremely rapid, with rates around 300 beats/min, and are brief[7] (Figure 56.5j). Hypokalemia and hypomagnesemia are risk factors, as are many drugs (antipsychotic and antidepressant agents, antibiotics, and many cardiovascular drugs).

Cardiac arrhythmias of no consequence are single premature atrial complex (Figure 56.5k) and premature ventricular complex (Figure 56.5l). The management of cardiac arrhythmias is summarized in Table 56.3.

MANAGEMENT OF CARDIAC ABNORMALITIES

Cardiac abnormalities of any sort may signal myocardial injury or dysfunction. Cardiac wall motion abnormalities are frequently found but generally do not pose a particular management problem. Their potential to be present in poor-grade SAH and traumatic brain injury should be recognized, but significant hemodynamic instability is uncommon. Dobutamine (5 μg/kg/min

TABLE 56.3. GUIDELINES FOR THE INITIAL MANAGEMENT OF COMMON CARDIAC ARRHYTHMIAS

Arrhythmia	Therapy
Sinus tachycardia	Esmolol
Sinus bradycardia	Atropine, cardiac pacing
Atrial fibrillation (RVR)	Diltiazem, verapamil
Atrial flutter (RVR)	Diltiazem, verapamil
Multifocal atrial tachycardia	Verapamil or metoprolol
Junctional rhythm	Atropine
Atrioventricular block	Cardiac pacing
Ventricular tachycardia	Cardioversion
Torsades de pointes	Magnesium sulfate

RVR, rapid ventricular response.

starting dose) can be helpful if blood pressure decreases and pulmonary edema occurs.[41]

In every patient with cardiac arrhythmia and an EKG abnormality, a full 12-lead EKG and echocardiography are warranted. Management becomes highly complex in patients with new EKG abnormalities suggesting myocardial infarction. In particular, the decision to evaluate these patients with EKG abnormalities for possible coronary artery disease is difficult, as alluded to earlier. Any pattern of myocardial infarction can be observed, but when infarction is truly present, a subendocardial pattern is most common, with large T waves and a major ST segment decrease, often exceeding 2 or 3 mm. ST elevation in the precordial leads (predominantly V_4 through V_6) has been associated with acute brain injury (particularly SAH) without angiographic evidence of coronary artery disease.[45] In addition, acute myocardial infarction causes a major increase in creatine kinase, in contrast to the minor increases from cerebral creatine kinase. Creatine kinase MB samples obtained every 8–12 hours for at least 24–48 hours should generate reliable information. The ratio of myocardial isoenzyme (creatine kinase MB fraction) to total creatine kinase, however, is only marginally increased in patients with nonsignificant EKG abnormalities associated with acute CNS disease.

Troponin (T or I) is not detectable in healthy persons and is a better marker for cardiac injury because isoforms expressed in skeletal muscle are not detected by current assays. The sensitivity and specificity of cardiac troponin I for myocardial dysfunction, at least in aneurysmal SAH, is much higher than those of creatine kinase MB.[69] The cTnT assay is very sensitive, and only mild increases can be detected after cardioversion[10] or in mimicking disorders such as pulmonary embolism due to acute right ventricular strain, dilation, and injury.[24]

Troponin elevations vary in degree, but one large study found that admission cardiac troponin T (cTnT) more than 0.01 µg/L already predicted mortality in critically ill patients and appeared as an independent variable.[6] The usefulness of this sensitive cardiac assay in acute brain injury warrants more study. Increased troponin I correlates with EKG abnormalities, gallop rhythm, and pulmonary edema—relationships not found with increased MB fraction of creatine kinase. Cardiac troponin has been studied in aneurysmal SAH and was related to cardiopulmonary complications and predicted poor outcome.[61] Whether troponin increases predict outcome in cerebral

hemorrhage is unclear, and there are conflicting results.[34,54]

Factors that should influence the decision to further investigate significant coronary artery disease are history of myocardial infarction, angina pectoris, and older age. Emergency cardiology consultation is imperative, certainly when EKGs suggest critical proximal left anterior descending coronary stenosis (ST segment elevation in precordial leads and progressive symmetrical T-wave inversion without pathologic precordial Q waves). In addition, bundle branch block or hemiblock in association with acute myocardial infarction increases the risk of early death. However, despite these discriminating signs, coronary angiography and possibly angioplasty should be considered in patients with a high likelihood of acute myocardial infarction.

A detailed review of the perioperative cardiac risks and guidelines have been published by the American College of Cardiology and American Heart Association (ACC/AHA) task force on practice guidelines.[27,51] Craniotomy should be considered an intermediate surgical risk, with a reported cardiac death and nonfatal myocardial infarction rate of less than 5%.[27] Generally, the risk of perioperative myocardial infarction in patients with no coronary disease (by EKG, history of angina, or coronary angiogram) is low. However, cardiac complications are up to five times more common in emergency procedures, such as evacuation of a traumatic intracerebral hematoma. This increase most likely reflects the inclusion of patients with significant coronary disease who were not evaluated because of the brief time between ictus and surgery.

The risk increases significantly in patients with unstable coronary syndromes, decompensated congestive heart failure, arrhythmias, and severe valvular disease. A full cardiologic evaluation, if time allows, is needed, often with noninvasive testing. New wall motion abnormalities within one or two coronary vessel territories on echocardiography or abnormal findings on dobutamine stress echocardiography justify coronary angiography or aggressive medical management. No data on whether preoperative percutaneous transluminal coronary angioplasty or bypass grafting in the event of coronary artery disease reduces the perioperative risk are available in patients with acute neurologic illness, although this benefit seems likely.

Perioperative management in patients with suspected myocardial ischemia probably should include more aggressive monitoring during anesthesia (12-lead EKG) and intravenous administration of nitroglycerin intraoperatively, or intraoperative administration of diltiazem, or oral administration of metoprolol. Clonidine may have potential and seems beneficial, but further evaluation in a prospective trial is needed.[64] The management of ST-elevation myocardial infarction or other coronary syndromes is outside the scope of this book, but guidelines have been published by ACC/AHA (see Part XIV, Guidelines).

Postoperative EKG studies are needed on the first and second days, and cardiac enzymes are studied only in patients with demonstrated EKG abnormalities.[27]

The approach to stress cardiomyopathy is complex. The diagnosis of stress cardiomyopathy is based on several criteria: (1) a major acute unexpected stressful event or acute brain injury; (2) transient left ventricular wall motion abnormalities involving the apical or mid-ventricular myocardial segments but with wall motion abnormalities extending beyond the single epicardial coronary distribution; (3) absence of obstructive coronary artery disease or angiographic evidence of acute plaque rupture that could be responsible for the observable wall motion abnormality; and (4) new EKG abnormalities such as transient ST-elevation or diffuse T-wave inversion or troponin elevations.[14] Clinical management is the consideration of early treatment with β-blockade, but also inotropes. The treatment of stress cardiomyopathy is largely determined by its presentation. Mostly, patients have a decreased ventricular function but are not in shock. In these patients, close observation and avoidance of fluid overload and cardiac rhythm control, if needed, are sufficient, and the abnormalities will reverse.

If shock occurs, patients would need to be treated immediately and aggressively. If the patient has developed acute heart failure with congestion, intravenous vasodilators are used with diuretics. Vasodilators, however, cannot be used if there is symptomatic hypotension. In patients with cardiogenic shock, defined as significant hypotension of systolic blood pressure < 90 mm Hg due to impaired contractility, high intracardiac filling pressures, and marked tissue hyperperfusion, intravenous inotropes should be administered acutely. Mostly dopamine is administered at a dose of 5–20 mcg/kg/min. Dopamine increases contractility and heart rate through activation of the β-adrenergic receptors and also mediates vasoconstriction through the activation of α-receptors in the periphery. In stress cardiomyopathy it is important to look for left ventricular outflow obstruction (LOTV), and inotropes actually can worsen shock (this is described in about

1 in 10 patients). Generally, a much less attractive option is IV norepinephrine due to increasing afterload without significantly increasing cardiac output, but in this situation with LVOT, low-dose norepinephrine may be used.

In certain circumstances, dopamine and milrinone (a phosphodiesterase inhibitor) can significantly increase cardiac output through peripheral vasodilatation and reduction in cardiac afterload. Milrinone reduces right and left ventricular filling pressures but also mean arterial pressure. Therefore, there is a risk of hypotension with milrinone; moreover, the drug also has a long half-life, making it a somewhat complicated drug in this setting. In extreme instances, a severe stress cardiomyopathy with hypotension has been treated with intra-aortic balloon counterpulsation pumps (IABP).

Approach to an acute coronary syndrome is even more complex in patients with acute brain injury. STEMI (ST-segment elevation myocardial infarction) is a life-threatening clinical syndrome that—in neurologic patients—may not be associated with chest pain or pressure but may manifest itself with shortness of breath, nausea, and vomiting in comatose patients with acute brain injury. Many EKG changes falsely suggest STEMI and turn out to be transient repolarization disturbances not related to myocardial injury. Patients with coronary artery disease who develop an acute brain injury, however, may have an acute or partial occlusion of the coronary artery as a result of activation of the sympathetic nervous system, resulting in catecholamine circulation.

STEMI criteria are well defined by the American College of Cardiology and the American Heart Association (ACC/AHA).[3] After the diagnosis is established by EKG, troponin, echocardiography, or coronary angiogram, the therapy of acute coronary syndromes is reasonably well established; and all patients should immediately receive 325 mg of chewable aspirin. Aspirin reduces mortality by 25% and blocks β-activation by limiting thromboxane production via the cyclooxygenase pathway. Current guidelines recommend against the routine use of β-blockers for acute STEMI. The administration of β-blockers to patients with acute coronary syndromes may lead to increased incidence of cardiogenic shock and may nullify the reduction of recurrent ischemia and reinfarction following reperfusion therapy. It is important to rapidly establish if the patient is a candidate for revascularization, either through administration of fibrinolytic therapy or primary percutaneous coronary intervention. In patients with acute neurologic disease, fibrinolytic therapy is often contraindicated because of the presence of an intracranial hemorrhage, recent ischemic stroke, recent traumatic head injury, or even the presence of a brain tumor. The common presence of hypertension, with a diastolic blood pressure > 100 mm Hg in patients with acute brain injury, also is a relative contraindication. Therefore, it is imperative in these patients to provide immediate reperfusion therapy and percutaneous coronary intervention (PCI) in a cardiac catheterization laboratory.[71,78,85] A major problem is that the PCI may be contraindicated in acute brain injury (recent cerebral hemorrhage, large territorial cerebral infarction, hemorrhagic contusions, ventriculostomy in situ, and so forth), given the need for high-dose anticoagulation to maintain stent patency.

CONCLUSIONS

- Most cardiac arrhythmias in acute CNS disorders are transient and do not require therapeutic intervention.
- Atrial fibrillation with rapid ventricular rate is common in patients admitted to the NICU and responds well to diltiazem infusion.
- The most common morphologic EKG changes in acute CNS catastrophes are prolonged QT interval, ST-segment sagging, and deeply inverted T waves. They may be difficult to distinguish from patterns seen in acute myocardial infarction.
- Echocardiography may be a useful noninvasive tool for the early diagnosis of cardiac anatomical or functional abnormalities that may underlie the arrhythmias.
- The risk of cardiac mortality and nonfatal myocardial infarction with craniotomy is less than 5% but increases in patients with unstable angina, congestive heart failure, cardiac arrhythmias, or valvular disease.

REFERENCES

1. Abdelmoneim SS, Wijdicks EFM, Lee VH, et al. Real-time myocardial perfusion contrast echocardiography and regional wall motion abnormalities after aneurysmal subarachnoid hemorrhage: clinical article. *J Neurosurg* 2009;111:1023–1028.
2. Andreoli A, di Pasquale G, Pinelli G, et al. Subarachnoid hemorrhage: frequency and severity of cardiac arrhythmias: a survey of 70 cases studied in the acute phase. *Stroke* 1987;18:558–564.
3. Antman EM, Hand M, Armstrong PW, et al. 2007 focused update of the ACC/AHA 2004 guidelines for the management of patients with ST-elevation myocardial infarction: a report of the American College of Cardiology/American Heart Association Task Force on Practice Guidelines. *J Am Coll Cardiol* 2008;51:210–247.
4. Arnaout M, Mongardon N, Deye N, et al. Out-of-hospital cardiac arrest from brain cause: epidemiology, clinical features, and outcome in a multicenter cohort. *Crit Care Med* 2015;43:453–460.
5. Attar HJ, Gutierrez MT, Bellet S, Ravens JR. Effect of stimulation of hypothalamus and reticular activating system on production of cardiac arrhythmia. *Circ Res* 1963;12:14–21.
6. Babuin L, Vasile VC, Rio Perez JA, et al. Elevated cardiac troponin is an independent risk factor for short- and long-term mortality in medical intensive care unit patients. *Crit Care Med* 2008;36:759–765.
7. Ben-David J, Zipes DP. Torsades de pointes and proarrhythmia. *Lancet* 1993;341:1578–1582.
8. Bernstein R, Mayer SA, Magnano A. Neurogenic stunned myocardium in Guillain-Barre syndrome. *Neurology* 2000;54:759–762.
9. Belcour D, Jabot J, Grard B, et al. Prevalence and Risk Factors of Stress Cardiomyopathy After Convulsive Status Epilepticus in ICU Patients. *Crit Care Med* 2015;43:2164–2170.
10. Boriani G, Biffi M, Cervi V, et al. Evaluation of myocardial injury following repeated internal atrial shocks by monitoring serum cardiac troponin I levels. *Chest* 2000;118:342–347.
11. Britton M, de Faire U, Helmers C, et al. Arrhythmias in patients with acute cerebrovascular disease. *Acta Med Scand* 1979;205:425–428.
12. Brouwers PJ, Wijdicks EFM, Hasan D, et al. Serial electrocardiographic recording in aneurysmal subarachnoid hemorrhage. *Stroke* 1989;20:1162–1167.
13. Brugada P, Gursoy S, Brugada J, Andries E. Investigation of palpitations. *Lancet* 1993;341:1254–1258.
14. Bybee KA, Prasad A. Stress-related cardiomyopathy syndromes. *Circulation* 2008;118:397–409.
15. Campbell RW. Ventricular ectopic beats and non-sustained ventricular tachycardia. *Lancet* 1993;341:1454–1458.
16. Cheung RT, Hachinski V. The insula and cerebrogenic sudden death. *Arch Neurol* 2000;57:1685–1688.
17. Cruickshank JM, Neil-Dwyer G, Degaute JP, et al. Reduction of stress/catecholamine-induced

cardiac necrosis by beta 1-selective blockade. *Lancet* 1987;2:585–589.

18. Cushing H. The blood-pressure reaction of acute cerebral compression, illustrated by cases of intracranial hemorrhage: a sequel to the Mütter Lecture for 1901. *Am J Med Sci* 1903;125:1017–1043.

19. Davies KR, Gelb AW, Manninen PH, Boughner DR, Bisnaire D. Cardiac function in aneurysmal subarachnoid hemorrhage: a study of electrocardiographic and echocardiographic abnormalities. *Br J Anaesth* 1991;67:58-63.

20. Davis TP, Alexander J, Lesch M. Electrocardiographic changes associated with acute cerebrovascular disease: a clinical review. *Prog Cardiovasc Dis* 1993;36:245–260.

21. Deininger MH, Radicke D, Buttler J, et al. Takotsubo cardiomyopathy: reversible heart failure with favorable outcome in patients with intracerebral hemorrhage: case report. *J Neurosurg* 2006;105:465–467.

22. Di Pasquale G, Pinelli G, Andreoli A, et al. Holter detection of cardiac arrhythmias in intracranial subarachnoid hemorrhage. *Am J Cardiol* 1987;59:596–600.

23. Doshi R, Neil-Dwyer G. Hypothalamic and myocardial lesions after subarachnoid hemorrhage. *J Neurol Neurosurg Psychiatry* 1977;40:821–826.

24. Douketis JD, Crowther MA, Stanton EB, Ginsberg JS. Elevated cardiac troponin levels in patients with submassive pulmonary embolism. *Arch Intern Med* 2002;162:79–81.

25. Dujardin KS, McCully RB, Wijdicks EFM, et al. Myocardial dysfunction associated with brain death: clinical, echocardiographic, and pathologic features. *J Heart Lung Transplant* 2001;20:350–357.

26. Falk RH. Atrial fibrillation. *N Engl J Med* 2001;344:1067–1078.

27. Fleisher LA, Beckman JA, Brown KA, et al. ACC/AHA 2007 guidelines on perioperative cardiovascular evaluation and care for noncardiac surgery: a report of the American College of Cardiology/American Heart Association Task Force on Practice Guidelines (Writing Committee to Revise the 2002 Guidelines on Perioperative Cardiovascular Evaluation for Noncardiac Surgery): developed in collaboration with the American Society of Echocardiography, American Society of Nuclear Cardiology, Heart Rhythm Society, Society of Cardiovascular Anesthesiologists, Society for Cardiovascular Angiography and Interventions, Society for Vascular Medicine and Biology, and Society for Vascular Surgery. *Circulation* 2007;116:e418–499.

28. Frangiskakis JM, Hravnak M, Crago EA, et al. Ventricular arrhythmia risk after subarachnoid hemorrhage. *Neurocrit Care* 2009;10:287–294.

29. Fugate JE, Wijdicks EFM, Kumar G, Rabinstein AA. One thing leads to another: GBS complicated by PRES and Takotsubo cardiomyopathy. *Neurocrit Care* 2009;11:395–397.

30. Garrett MC, Komotar RJ, Starke RM, et al. Elevated troponin levels are predictive of mortality in surgical intracerebral hemorrhage patients. *Neurocrit Care* 2010;12:199–203.

31. Goldstein B, Toweill D, Lai S, Sonnenthal K, Kimberly B. Uncoupling of the autonomic and cardiovascular systems in acute brain injury. *Am J Physiol* 1998;275:R1287–1292.

32. Greenhoot JH, Reichenbach DD. Cardiac injury and subarachnoid hemorrhage: a clinical, pathological, and physiological correlation. *J Neurosurg* 1969;30:521–531.

33. Hackenberry LE, Miner ME, Rea GL, Woo J, Graham SH. Biochemical evidence of myocardial injury after severe head trauma. *Crit Care Med* 1982;10:641–644.

34. Handlin LR, Kindred LH, Beauchamp GD, Vacek JL, Rowe SK. Reversible left ventricular dysfunction after subarachnoid hemorrhage. *Am Heart J* 1993;126:235–240.

35. Hays A, Diringer MN. Elevated troponin levels are associated with higher mortality following intracerebral hemorrhage. *Neurology* 2006;66:1330–1334.

36. Herijgers P, Borgers M, Flameng W. The effect of brain death on cardiovascular function in rats. Part I: is the heart damaged? *Cardiovasc Res* 1998;38:98–106.

37. Herijgers P, Flameng W. The effect of brain death on cardiovascular function in rats. Part II: the cause of the in vivo haemodynamic changes. *Cardiovasc Res* 1998;38:107–115.

38. Hirashima Y, Takashima S, Matsumura N, et al. Right sylvian fissure subarachnoid hemorrhage has electrocardiographic consequences. *Stroke* 2001;32:2278–2281.

39. Hockman CH, Mauck HP, Jr., Hoff EC. ECG changes resulting from cerebral stimulation. II: a spectrum of ventricular arrhythmias of sympathetic origin. *Am Heart J* 1966;71:695–700.

40. Jacobson SA, Danufsky P. Marked electrocardiographic changes produced by experimental head trauma. *J Neuropathol Exp Neurol* 1954;13:462–466.

41. Jain R, Deveikis J, Thompson BG. Management of patients with stunned myocardium associated with subarachnoid hemorrhage. *AJNR Am J Neuroradiol* 2004;25:126–129.

42. Katsanos AH, Korantzopoulos P, Tsivgoulis G, et al. Electrocardiographic abnormalities and cardiac arrhythmias in structural brain lesions. *Int J Cardiol* 2013;167:328–334.

43. Kawano H, Okada R, Yano K. Histological study on the distribution of autonomic nerves in the human heart. *Heart Vessels* 2003;18:32–39.

44. Kishore A, Vail A, Majid A, et al. Detection of atrial fibrillation after ischemic stroke or transient ischemic attack: a systematic review and meta-analysis. *Stroke* 2014;45:520–526.

45. Kono T, Morita H, Kuroiwa T, et al. Left ventricular wall motion abnormalities in patients with subarachnoid hemorrhage: neurogenic stunned myocardium. *J Am Coll Cardiol* 1994;24:636–640.

46. Lane RD, Wallace JD, Petrosky PP, Schwartz GE, Gradman AH. Supraventricular tachycardia in patients with right hemisphere strokes. *Stroke* 1992;23:362–366.

47. Lee VH, Abdelmoneim SS, Daugherty WP, et al. Myocardial contrast echocardiography in subarachnoid hemorrhage-induced cardiac dysfunction: case report. *Neurosurgery* 2008;62:E261–262.

48. Lee VH, Connolly HM, Fulgham JR, et al. Tako-tsubo cardiomyopathy in aneurysmal subarachnoid hemorrhage: an underappreciated ventricular dysfunction. *J Neurosurg* 2006;105:264–270.

49. Lee VH, Oh JK, Mulvagh SL, Wijdicks EFM. Mechanisms in neurogenic stress cardiomyopathy after aneurysmal subarachnoid hemorrhage. *Neurocrit Care* 2006;5:243–249.

50. Logigian EL, Ropper AH. Terminal electrocardiographic changes in brain-dead patients. *Neurology* 1985;35:915–918.

51. Mangano DT, Goldman L. Preoperative assessment of patients with known or suspected coronary disease. *N Engl J Med* 1995;333:1750–1756.

52. Manning JW, deV. Cotton M. Mechanism of cardiac arrhythmias induced by diencephalic stimulation. *Am J Physiol* 1962;203:1120–1124.

53. Manno EM, Pfeifer EA, Cascino GD, Noe KH, Wijdicks EFM. Cardiac pathology in status epilepticus. *Ann Neurol* 2005;58:954–957.

54. Maramattom BV, Manno EM, Fulgham JR, Jaffe AS, Wijdicks EFM. Clinical importance of cardiac troponin release and cardiac abnormalities in patients with supratentorial cerebral hemorrhages. *Mayo Clinic Proc* 2006;81:192–196.

55. Marion DW, Segal R, Thompson ME. Subarachnoid hemorrhage and the heart. *Neurosurgery* 1986;18:101–106.

56. Mayer SA, LiMandri G, Sherman D, et al. Electrocardiographic markers of abnormal left ventricular wall motion in acute subarachnoid hemorrhage. *J Neurosurg* 1995;83:889–896.

57. Mayer SA, Lin J, Homma S, et al. Myocardial injury and left ventricular performance after subarachnoid hemorrhage. *Stroke* 1999;30:780–786.

58. Miss JC, Kopelnik A, Fisher LA, et al. Cardiac injury after subarachnoid hemorrhage is independent of the type of aneurysm therapy. *Neurosurgery* 2004;55:1244–1250.

59. Mitsuma W, Ito M, Kodama M, et al. Clinical and cardiac features of patients with subarachnoid haemorrhage presenting with out-of-hospital cardiac arrest. *Resuscitation* 2011;82:1294–1297.

60. Mohamedali B, Bhat G, Tatooles A, Zelinger A. Neurogenic stress cardiomyopathy in heart donors. *J Card Fail* 2014;20:207–211.

61. Naidech AM, Kreiter KT, Janjua N, et al. Cardiac troponin elevation, cardiovascular morbidity, and outcome after subarachnoid hemorrhage. *Circulation* 2005;112:2851–2856.

62. Nashef L, Walker F, Allen P, et al. Apnoea and bradycardia during epileptic seizures: relation to sudden death in epilepsy. *J Neurol Neurosurg Psychiatry* 1996;60:297–300.

63. Nichol G, McAlister F, Pham B, et al. Meta-analysis of randomised controlled trials of the effectiveness of antiarrhythmic agents at promoting sinus rhythm in patients with atrial fibrillation. *Heart* 2002;87:535–543.

64. Nishina K, Mikawa K, Uesugi T, et al. Efficacy of clonidine for prevention of perioperative myocardial ischemia: a critical appraisal and meta-analysis of the literature. *Anesthesiology* 2002;96:323–329.

65. Oppenheimer SM, Cechetto DF, Hachinski VC. Cerebrogenic cardiac arrhythmias: cerebral electrocardiographic influences and their role in sudden death. *Arch Neurol* 1990;47:513–519.

66. Oppenheimer SM, Gelb A, Girvin JP, Hachinski VC. Cardiovascular effects of human insular cortex stimulation. *Neurology* 1992;42:1727–1732.

67. Oras J, Grivans C, Dalla K, et al. High-sensitive troponin T and N-terminal pro B-type natriuretic peptide for early detection of stress-induced cardiomyopathy in patients with subarachnoid hemorrhage. *Neurocrit Care* 2015;23:233–242.

68. Orliaguet G, Ferjani M, Riou B. The heart in blunt trauma. *Anesthesiology* 2001;95:544–548.

69. Parekh N, Venkatesh B, Cross D, et al. Cardiac troponin I predicts myocardial dysfunction in aneurysmal subarachnoid hemorrhage. *J Am Coll Cardiol* 2000;36:1328–1335.

70. Pollick C, Cujec B, Parker S, Tator C. Left ventricular wall motion abnormalities in subarachnoid hemorrhage: an echocardiographic study. *J Am Coll Cardiol* 1988;12:600–605.

71. Riczebos RK, Tijssen JG, Verheugt FW, Laarman GJ. Percutaneous coronary intervention for non ST-elevation acute coronary syndromes: which, when and how? *Am J Cardiol* 2011;107:509–515.

72. Rogers ER, Phan TG, Wijdicks EFM. Myocardial injury after hemorrhage into the lateral medulla oblongata. *Neurology* 2001;56:567–568.

73. Rokey R, Rolak LA, Harati Y, Kutka N, Verani MS. Coronary artery disease in patients with cerebrovascular disease: a prospective study. *Ann Neurol* 1984;16:50–53.

74. Ropper AH, Wijdicks EFM, Truax BT. *Guillain-Barré Syndrome.* Vol. 34. Oxford: Oxford University Press; 1991.

75. Samuels MA. The brain-heart connection. *Circulation* 2007;116:77–84.

76. Shenasa M, Borggrefe M, Haverkamp W, Hindricks G, Breithardt G. Ventricular tachycardia. *Lancet* 1993;341:1512–1519.

77. Templin C, Ghadri JR, Diekmann LC, et al. Clinical features and outcomes of takotsubo (stress). cardiomyopathy *N Engl J Med* 2015;373:929–938.

78. Trost JC, Lange RA. Treatment of acute coronary syndrome. Part 1: non-ST-segment acute coronary syndrome. *Crit Care Med* 2011;39:2346–2353.

79. van den Bergh WM, Algra A, Rinkel GJ. Electrocardiographic abnormalities and serum magnesium in patients with subarachnoid hemorrhage. *Stroke* 2004;35:644–648.

80. van der Bilt IA, Hasan D, Vandertop WP, et al. Impact of cardiac complications on outcome after aneurysmal subarachnoid hemorrhage: a meta-analysis. *Neurology* 2009;72:635–642.

81. VanderArk GD. Cardiovascular changes with acute subdural hematoma. *Surg Neurol* 1975;3:305–308.

82. Waldo AL, Wit AL. Mechanisms of cardiac arrhythmias. *Lancet* 1993;341:1189–1193.

83. Wells C, Cujec B, Johnson D, Goplen G. Reversibility of severe left ventricular dysfunction in patients with subarachnoid hemorrhage. *Am Heart J* 1995;129:409–412.

84. Wijdicks EFM, Hubmayr RD. Acute acid-base disorders associated with status epilepticus. *Mayo Clinic Proc* 1994;69:1044–1046.

85. Wong CK, White HD. Medical treatment for acute coronary syndromes. *Curr Opin Cardiol* 2000;15:441–462.

86. Wood MA, Brown-Mahoney C, Kay GN, Ellenbogen KA. Clinical outcomes after ablation and pacing therapy for atrial fibrillation: a meta-analysis. *Circulation* 2000;101:1138–1144.

87. Yoshikawa T. Takotsubo cardiomyopathy, a new concept of cardiomyopathy: clinical features and pathophysiology. *Int J Cardiol* 2015;182:297–303.

88. Yamashina Y, Yagi T, Ishida A, et al. Differentiating between comatose patients resuscitated from acute coronary syndrome-associated and subarachnoid hemorrhage-associated out-of-hospital cardiac arrest. *J Cardiol* Jun 2015;65:508–513.

89. Zaroff JG, Rordorf GA, Newell JB, Ogilvy CS, Levinson JR. Cardiac outcome in patients with subarachnoid hemorrhage and electrocardiographic abnormalities. *Neurosurgery* 1999;44:34–39.

90. Zaroff JG, Rordorf GA, Ogilvy CS, Picard MH. Regional patterns of left ventricular systolic dysfunction after subarachnoid hemorrhage: evidence for neurally mediated cardiac injury. *J Am Soc Echocardiogr* 2000;13:774–779.

57

Management of Acid–Base Disorders, Sodium and Glucose Handling

Most of the laboratory derangements that neurointensivists are concerned with are acid–base disorders, electrolyte abnormalities, and hyperglycemia. Although frequent in medical and surgical intensive care units (ICUs), life-threatening acid–base disorders are uncommon in patients with acute neurologic disorders. When they occur, they are often transient (e.g., metabolic acidosis in status epilepticus), or even purposely induced (respiratory alkalosis to treat increased intracranial pressure). But in any other instances a persistent acid–base disorder more often indicates a complicating major medical problem.

The most commonly encountered electrolyte abnormalities in the neurosciences intensive care unit (NICU) are hyponatremia and hypernatremia.[1,2] These derangements in sodium and water balance are very common in the NICU and are, if not managed promptly, consequential.

Additionally, aggressive glucose control has become standard in many ICUs around the world, but this practice has now been challenged by the results of a large clinical trial.[24,27,28,40]

This chapter presents a foundation of the basic principles and interpretation of these three categories of derangements. Insights into the pathophysiology and practical advice for management are provided here.

GENERAL CONSIDERATIONS

Critically ill patients develop electrolyte imbalances, and in some measure, these aberrations occur in patients with acute neurologic illnesses. Replacement orders are daily practice, but severe electrolyte abnormalities are unusual. The most commonly encountered abnormalities, next to abnormalities in serum sodium values, are hypokalemia, hypomagnesemia, and hypophosphatemia.

Potassium depletion has many causes, and often patients have more than one. It is associated with diuretic agents, vomiting, and diarrhea related to gastrointestinal feeding. Hypokalemia may be a result of profound sweating, and skin losses may be substantial in patients with paroxysmal sympathetic hyperactivity (e.g., traumatic brain injury). Severe hypokalemia not only produces electrocardiographic abnormalities (prominent U waves, ST segment changes), but also atrial and ventricular arrhythmias. Muscle weakness is seldom seen in patients admitted to the NICU, and can only be expected when serum potassium is less than 2 mEq/L.

Hypomagnesemia is also fairly common in the NICU, albeit rarely severe enough to become symptomatic (myoclonus, postural tremor, and seizures). A deficit is commonly seen in patients with chronic alcohol abuse, but it also may be caused by the use of antibiotics, parenteral nutrition, and acute renal disorders.[71]

Phosphate metabolism is disturbed in patients with profound vomiting and sepsis, and with the use of some of the antiepileptic drugs, but any critical illness may deplete phosphate and calcium stores. Renal loss due to frequent use of mannitol can be implicated in some patients with hypophosphatemia.

The electrolyte abnormalities far more common in medical or surgical ICUs are described in more detail in a companion monograph on neurologic complications of critical illness.[112] Table 57.1 provides a guide for replacement therapy.

ACID–BASE ABNORMALITIES

This section explores the mechanisms underlying acidosis and alkalosis. Clinically, these derangements—when deviation from the normal range is severe—are important because the level of consciousness may decrease and cardiac arrhythmias can result. A useful acid–base nomogram is shown in Figure 57.1.

TABLE 57.1. REPLACEMENT THERAPY IN ELECTROLYTE ABNORMALITIES OTHER THAN SODIUM DISORDER

Electrolyte Abnormality	Cause	Consequences	Treatment*
Hypomagnesemia	Gastrointestinal and renal loss, drug interaction	Cardiac arrhythmias, muscle weakness	1–2 g of magnesium sulfate in 20 mL of normal saline over 5–20 minutes
Hypermagnesemia	Renal failure, antacids, enemas	Muscle weakness, hypotension, asystole	1–2 grams of calcium gluconate IV over 15 minutes
Hypercalcemia	Diabetes insipidus, malignancy, hyper parathyroidism	Seizures, coma, cardiac arrhythmias	Hydration, 0.9% NaCl, 500 mL/hour
Hypocalcemia	Critical illness, hypoparathyroidism, fat-deficient diet	Cardiac arrhythmias, tetanus, seizures, laryngospasm	1–2 g of calcium gluconate IV over 15 minutes; then 6 g of calcium gluconate in 500 mL normal saline with infusion for 4–6 hours
Hypophosphatemia	Parenteral nutrition, preexisting alcoholism, renal failure	Congestive cardiomyopathy, respiratory failure, rhabdomyolysis	Potassium phosphate, 0.08 mmol/kg IV in 500 mL of 0.45% saline over 6 hours
Hyperphosphatemia	Rare	Similar to those with hypocalcemia	Phosphate binders, 1 g of calcium PO t.i.d.
Hypokalemia	Vomiting, prolonged starvation, gastrointestinal loss	Ventricular fibrillation, quadriplegia	KCL 10 mEq/hour IV infusion
Hyperkalemia	Crush injury, hemolysis, renal failure	Cardiac arrest	1 gram of calcium gluconate IV over 5 minutes

IV, intravenously.
*When markedly abnormal.
Data from Singer GG. Fluid and electrolyte management. In Ahya SN, Flood K, Paranjothi S, eds. *Washington Manual of Medical Therapeutics*. 30th ed. Philadelphia: Lippincott Williams & Wilkins; 2001: 43–75. With permission of the publisher.

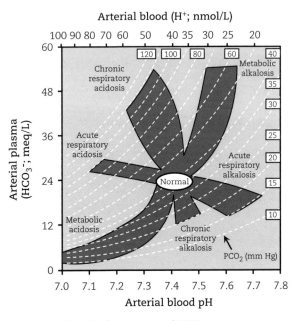

FIGURE 57.1: Acid–base nomogram. Boxed values are arterial PCO_2.

Modified from DuBose TD Jr. Acid-base disorders. In Brenner BM, ed., *Brenner & Rector's The Kidney,* 6th ed. Vol. 1. Philadelphia: W. B. Saunders, 2000: 925–997. With permission of the publisher.

Principles of Acid–Base Physiology and Interpretation

The H^+ concentration in body fluids is held constant by buffers. Changes in H^+ concentration and reciprocal pH concentration are important, because vital cellular enzyme systems depend on a constant milieu for functioning. The most important buffer in the extracellular fluid is the HCO_3^-/CO_2 system, although other buffers (H_2PO_4, NH_3) are recruited to maintain the balance.

Changes in the acid–base balance are reflected by changes in arterial PCO_2 (respiratory acidosis with an increase in PCO_2, respiratory alkalosis with a decrease in PCO_2) or changes in arterial HCO_3^- concentration (metabolic acidosis with a decrease in HCO_3^- metabolic alkalosis with an increase in HCO_3^-). Changes of this nature result in an appropriate compensatory response. To maintain a constant ratio of arterial PCO_2 to arterial, HCO_3^- a change must be in the same direction: an increase in arterial PCO_2, an increase in arterial HCO_3, and, vice versa—a decrease in arterial PCO_2 and a decrease in arterial HCO_3^-. Blood gas interpretation remains complex, even for experienced clinicians in critical care. Before an attempt is made to interpret a blood gas, an erroneous result should be excluded. A well-known cause for acidosis is related to heparin used to anticoagulate the sample before transport to the laboratory. This is often recognized by extreme reductions in values, approaching a pH of 6.5, not fitting with the clinical manifestations. Venous blood sampling may occur and actually is rather common, and it has resulted in inappropriate admission to the NICU of patients with suspected acute neuromuscular failure. Usually, oxygen saturation is in the 70s, and a marked discrepancy with pulse oximetric values is noted. Another helpful method is to compare oxygen content with that of hemoglobin (the oxygen content of arterial blood is greater than that of hemoglobin). Obtaining blood gases from an arterial catheter eliminates this error.

Blood gas interpretation is usually guided by changes in arterial pH and arterial PCO_2. A change in pH defines acidosis or alkalosis. Given a decrease in arterial pH, metabolic acidosis is present when the arterial PCO_2 is normal or decreased. Metabolic acidosis is then differentiated into metabolic acidosis with a normal or high anion gap HCO_3^- (anion gap = $Na^+ - [Cl^- +]$ = 10 to 12 mEq/L). An increased anion gap occurs in lactic acidosis (e.g., status epilepticus), uremic acidosis, diabetic or alcoholic ketoacidosis, and intoxication (ethylene glycol, methanol, and salicylate), situations that are uncommon in critically ill neurologic patients but are occasionally causes for coma of unexplained origin or contribute to impaired arousal. A normal anion gap identifies loss of alkali from the gastrointestinal tract (e.g., diarrhea), which also results in compensatory reciprocal change in chloride and bicarbonate or renal acidosis. Given a decrease in arterial pH, respiratory acidosis is present when arterial PCO_2 is increased. Conversely, given an increase in arterial pH, metabolic alkalosis is present when arterial PCO_2 is normal or increased. Respiratory alkalosis is present when arterial PCO_2 is decreased (Figure 57.1).

Treatment of acid–base disorders requires correction of the trigger and, less often, additional active intervention.[7,86] Metabolic or respiratory acidosis is mostly asymptomatic until the pH reaches 7.2. The systemic effects of metabolic acidosis usually warrant correction. These systemic effects begin with tachycardia, which is replaced by bradycardia when the blood pH approaches 7.1. Ventricular contractility is markedly reduced with these degrees of acidosis. The risk of acute ventricular fibrillation increases significantly at these levels. Patients with previous cardiac disease may be predisposed.

Metabolic Acidosis

The most probable conditions that produce metabolic acidosis in patients with central or peripheral nervous system disorders are shown in Table 57.2. Metabolic acidosis is not frequently observed in acutely ill neurologic patients and must alert neurologists to other, unrelated, conditions. The most common conditions that must be excluded are diabetic ketoacidosis, renal failure, and cardiogenic or hypervolemic shock (Chapter 51).[47] Lactic acidosis from a series of tonic-clonic seizures or status epilepticus, however, is comparatively more common. Ethylene glycol intoxication should be considered in patients with an increased anion gap. These patients may present

---

TABLE 57.2. COMMON CAUSES OF METABOLIC ACIDOSIS IN THE NICU

Lactic acidosis (status epilepticus)
Ketoacidosis (diabetes, alcoholism, malnourishment)
Septic shock
Rhabdomyolysis
Diarrhea
Hyperalimentation

---

with status epilepticus and increased anion gap that initially are falsely attributed to lactic acidosis from seizures. However, an osmolar gap should increase the clinical suspicion.

Rhabdomyolysis should be considered in patients with greatly increased creatine kinase values. Although the condition is uncommon, it may be observed after status epilepticus and in patients with a major stroke, in whom it is discovered after days of muscular ischemia from prolonged compression of a hemiplegic limb. No treatment of the metabolic acidosis is indicated, because spontaneous correction can be expected after rehydration. Bicarbonate infusion in status epilepticus (up to 90 mEq initially) may be considered when the pH is lower than 7.0. However, when cardiac arrhythmias are absent, bicarbonate supplementation can be postponed. Replenishment may lead to marked metabolic alkalosis, which lowers the seizure threshold. Large fluid volumes are necessary in diabetic ketoacidosis, and bicarbonate is administered cautiously if severe hyperkalemia is present. Hemodialysis is virtually always indicated in patients with methanol or ethylene glycol intoxication.

Metabolic Alkalosis

The causes of metabolic alkalosis are listed in Table 57.3. Most patients with metabolic alkalosis have lost sodium and water from excessive use of diuretic agents (contraction alkalosis), excessive vomiting, or, particularly, nasogastric suctioning. Typically, urinary chloride concentration is less than 15 mEq/L. Metabolic alkalosis with increased urinary loss of chloride (and potassium) often identifies hyperaldosteronism, which may be causing hypertension. Metabolic alkalosis can cause a significant decrease in level of consciousness and can be a possible reason for clinical deterioration in any patient with an acute brain injury. Management is directed toward judicious repletion of the volume deficit.

Respiratory Acidosis

Respiratory acidosis remains the most frequent acid–base disorder in patients requiring mechanical ventilation. In patients with acute respiratory acidosis, additional laboratory evidence of hypercapnia and decreased pH is present, often with associated hypoxemia. The most likely causes of respiratory acidosis in critically ill neurologic patients are summarized in Table 57.4. The obvious first considerations are aspiration and acute pulmonary edema. Particularly in patients with underlying pulmonary disease, a single bout of aspiration or aspiration pneumonitis compromises their condition. Acute pulmonary edema triggered by acute brain injury alone (neurogenic pulmonary edema) is uncommon. It most commonly occurs in patients with poor-grade subarachnoid hemorrhage (SAH), particularly a ruptured basilar artery aneurysm, and in patients who meet the clinical criteria for brain death within hours after the insult.

Patients with an acute neuromuscular disorder may have rapid progression to acute hypercapnia if the initial clinical signs of air hunger, tachycardia, brow sweating, and use of accessory muscles (sternocleidomastoid) are not appreciated as signals of imminent danger. These patients often are markedly hypoxemic; in some patients, more often those with long-standing neuromuscular disease, correction with only 1–2 L of oxygen may substantially increase PCO_2 (and reduce alertness) without measures to increase alveolar ventilation. In addition, in patients with long-standing carbon dioxide retention and hypoxemia drive, removal of the stimulus with oxygen therapy eliminates the drive, reduces ventilation, and intensifies hypercapnia.

In general, the treatment of respiratory acidosis consists of mechanical ventilation and correction of the more relevant life-threatening hypoxemia.

TABLE 57.3. COMMON CAUSES OF METABOLIC ALKALOSIS IN THE NICU

Excessive vomiting
Gastrointestinal losses
Diuretics (loop or thiazide)
Massive blood transfusion in multitrauma
Severe hypokalemia
Sodium bicarbonate infusion

TABLE 57.4. COMMON CAUSES OF RESPIRATORY ACIDOSIS IN THE NICU

Aspiration pneumonitis
Adult respiratory distress syndrome
Acute pulmonary edema
Pneumothorax
Neuromuscular respiratory failure (end stage)

Respiratory Alkalosis

Induced hyperventilation is the most common reason for respiratory alkalosis, but patients may have an increased ventilatory drive after a major acute brain injury. The causes are found in Table 57.5. In newly admitted patients with unexplained coma, aspirin poisoning, amphetamines, and cocaine should be considered when appropriate. Hyperventilation in an attempt to overcome hypoxemia must be excluded. Respiratory alkalosis is common in patients with mechanical ventilation because of large tidal volumes, and can easily be corrected if necessary. Treatment is directed to the cause and may vary from mild sedation to correction of hypoxemia and its underlying cause.

DISORDERS OF SODIUM AND WATER HOMEOSTASIS

Critically ill neurologic patients are exposed to multiple factors that can perturb sodium and volume homeostasis. Many factors stimulate secretion of the antidiuretic hormone. Mechanical ventilation with positive end-expiratory pressure, overwhelming pain and stress, and medications may all result in abnormal water retention and dilutional hyponatremia. At the other extreme, hypernatremia is less frequent, but most commonly is due to diabetes insipidus and osmotic diuretics.

Possible routes for additional fluid and electrolyte losses are the skin in patients with high fever and profuse diaphoresis, the lung in patients with induced hyperventilation, and the stomach from gastric suctioning.

Some unifying principles must be understood. The absolute value of the electrolyte abnormality is less important than the rate of change. Furthermore, the accompanying change

---

TABLE 57.5. COMMON CAUSES OF RESPIRATORY ALKALOSIS IN THE NICU

Induced hyperventilation
Mechanical ventilation
Intracranial pressure management
Compensatory response to hypoxemia
Adult respiratory distress syndrome
Pulmonary embolism
Central neurogenic hyperventilation
Early sepsis
Postoperative pain and anxiety

---

in intravascular status is more relevant than the absolute serum sodium level.

Hypotonic and Hypertonic States

The most common disorders of tonicity or effective osmolality are hyponatremia and hypernatremia. Plasma sodium values should be monitored daily, sometimes hourly. Management, particularly of hyponatremia, is often difficult, and rapid correction of the abnormalities could prove disastrous.

Evaluation of Hyponatremia

Hyponatremia (serum sodium ≤ 134 mmol/L) is classified on the basis of serum osmolality. Hyponatremia may be associated with normal or increased osmolality when additional solutes are present, such as in hyperglycemia or with recent administration of a hypertonic solution such as mannitol. Hyperglycemia reduces plasma sodium because an extracellular shift of water driven by glucose cannot emanate from the extracellular space. A correction factor of a decrease of 2.4 mEq/L in sodium concentration per 100 mg/dL increase in glucose concentration has been recommended.[38] With recent administration of mannitol, calculation of serum osmolality demonstrates lower serum osmolality. (Blood urea nitrogen [BUN] and glucose values are expressed as milligrams per deciliter. The calculated value should be at least 10 mOsm/kg lower than the measured value.)

Normal serum osmolality with hyponatremia (pseudohyponatremia) may indicate severe hyperlipemia (e.g., in patients with known brittle diabetes admitted with acute stroke), severe hyperproteinemia (e.g., in patients with multiple myeloma admitted with CNS infection), or the use of intravenous immunoglobulin.[51] Intravenous administration of immunoglobulin increases the protein-containing nonaqueous phase of plasma. The ion-selective electrodes measure sodium concentration per liter of serum but do not correct for increased protein or lipid concentration. Sodium is present only in the aqueous phase; each unit volume of plasma measured has less sodium-containing water. When measured after infusion of intravenous immunoglobulin, serum protein concentration is increased. However, most hospital laboratories have measures in place to adjust for this abnormality.

The three major categories of hyponatremia can be distinguished on clinical grounds and are associated with volume depletion (relative tachycardia, orthostasis, marginal skin turgor), volume expansion (edema, weight gain), or normal volume (lack of edema, normal blood pressure and pulse).[88–90]

Hypovolemic hyponatremia may result from extrarenal spills (vomiting, diarrhea, and third-space fluid losses in trauma) or from nephrotic syndrome, cirrhosis, or cardiac failure. A random urine specimen with a urine sodium concentration below 20 mEq/L is useful because it indicates hypovolemia.

Hyponatremia can be generated when water is excessive in relation to sodium. This physiologic state of hypo-osmolality prompts an appropriate response of reduced antidiuretic hormone (ADH) secretion, which results in excess excretion of water, dilution of urine, and decrease in urine osmolality. Conversely, in patients with hypovolemia and hyponatremia, the volume-sensitive carotid sinus baroreceptors stimulate the paraventricular neurons to secrete ADH and cause water to be retained in an attempt to restore the depleted volume (a marked ADH response is seen after blood volume depletion of more than 20%).

Many other nonosmotic stimuli of ADH have been identified. Pain, nausea, and drugs such as morphine and carbamazepine[49] may profoundly stimulate ADH secretion. However, when carefully studied, oxcarbazepine (an analogue of carbamazepine) was not associated with increased ADH, but hyponatremia occurred with failure to excrete a water load, suggesting an effect on collecting tubules by the drug itself.[79]

Traditionally, the syndrome of inappropriate antidiuretic hormone (SIADH) has been a major cause of hyponatremia in patients with acute brain injury. The diagnostic criteria for SIADH include hyponatremia with hypo-osmolar serum, inappropriately concentrated urine, continued sodium excretion (urinary sodium of > 25 mEq/L), and exclusion of renal or endocrine disease (hypothyroidism or hypoadrenalism). There must also be no stimuli that could produce a non-osmotic release of ADH, such as hypovolemia, hypotension, pain, stress, or nausea, a precondition that is difficult to exclude in any critically ill patient.[84] It should also be noted that increased urine sodium concentration is difficult to interpret. Unfortunately, it is commonly explained as indicative of SIADH, particularly when found in combination with increased urine osmolality. However, increased urinary sodium concentration may also have its origin in cerebral salt wasting or large sodium intake. Increased concentration may also occur in dehydrated patients with metabolic

TABLE 57.6. POTENTIAL CAUSES OF HYPO-OSMOLAR HYPONATREMIA IN THE NICU

Hypovolemia	Normovolemia or Hypervolemia
Diuretics (thiazide, loop)	SIADH
Addison's disease (acute corticosteroid withdrawal)	Acute renal failure Congestive heart failure
Gastrointestinal and skin losses	
Dietary sodium restriction (with excess hypotonic fluid intake)	Hepatic failure
Cerebral salt wasting	

SIADH, syndrome of inappropriate antidiuretic hormone.

alkalosis from profuse vomiting. (The increased load on the renal tubules from sodium bicarbonate produced by the stomach results in increased excretion of sodium to neutralize the load.)

Other laboratory tests that may be helpful in further determination of hyponatremia are serum uric acid concentration (increased in volume depletion, decreased in volume expansion and euvolemia) and blood urea nitrogen (increased in volume depletion, normal in volume expansion). It now appears that cerebral salt wasting syndrome is more likely in many CNS disorders,[4,16,35,56,70,99] although some disagree with this concept.[65] The possible causes of hyponatremia in neurologic disease are listed in Table 57.6. The following sections discuss hyponatremia associated with specific clinical neurologic disorders. A recent guideline has been developed (Part XIV, Guidelines).[74]

Hyponatremia in Aneurysmal Subarachnoid Hemorrhage

Hyponatremia is the most common electrolyte disturbance after aneurysmal SAH. The precise physiologic changes in hyponatremia associated with SAH have yet to be elucidated. Early studies noted that only 10% of patients with SAH had hyponatremia, but later studies showed sodium values below 134 mmol/L in 34% of patients with SAH.[108] Severe hyponatremia (serum sodium level < 120 mmol/L) is not frequently seen in SAH; as a consequence, neurologic deterioration can seldom be attributed to hyponatremia alone. Hyponatremia can usually be expected within the first week after the initial hemorrhage and closely parallels the period of cerebral vasospasm.[108]

For many years, neurosurgeons viewed the development of hyponatremia as a marker for impending cerebral ischemia in SAH, but the relationship had never been systematically studied. In a post hoc analysis of a prospectively acquired series of patients with SAH, cerebral infarction occurred significantly more often in patients with hyponatremia (61%) than in patients with normal serum sodium values (21%).[108]

Initially, hyponatremia in patients with SAH was attributed to SIADH, and it was believed that excessive water retention led to dilutional hyponatremia.[22] Nelson and colleagues should be credited for initially challenging the concept of SIADH in intracranial disease.[63] Both human and animal studies suggested that hypovolemic hyponatremia was caused by excessive natriuresis and diuresis, rather than hypervolemic or euvolemic hyponatremia from water retention. These studies first suggested that cerebral salt wasting more accurately explained hyponatremia after SAH than SIADH. Later, a prospective study of 21 patients with aneurysmal SAH demonstrated that plasma volume was decreased in most patients with hyponatremia. Hyponatremia was preceded by a negative sodium balance in all instances. Blood ADH levels were increased or normal on admission, but had decreased by the time hyponatremia occurred. The ADH levels remained slightly higher than those in controls, but this increase could have been a response to hypovolemia.[109]

Later data in patients with SAH, however, suggested that ADH remains increased despite the prevention of volume contraction.[21,34] In a prospective study of 19 patients who received hypervolemic therapy, volume contraction was prevented, but ADH levels were detectable during a hypo-osmolar state. Whether critically ill patients with recent aneurysmal rupture have an additional disturbance in vasopressin regulation remains to be defined. As alluded to earlier, non-osmolar stimuli to ADH may cause an increase in ADH and may be difficult to ferret out in clinical studies.

Certain computed tomography (CT) scan characteristics may predict the development of hyponatremia. The risk of hyponatremia developing after aneurysmal rupture is significantly increased in patients with enlargement of the third ventricle, with or without dilatation of the lateral ventricles, on initial CT scanning.[107] The relationship between enlargement of the third ventricle and hyponatremia tentatively suggests that pressure on the hypothalamus produces

hyponatremia by the release of natriuretic peptide stimulating factors located in the anteroventral region of the third ventricle.

Much of the recent research has concentrated on the role of natriuretic factors. These are digoxin-like immunoreactive substance (endogenous ouabain), natriuretic peptides, and adrenomedullin. In a preliminary study of a digoxin-like substance, enlargement of the third ventricle and the lateral ventricles and, particularly, location of the center of the hemorrhage in the frontal interhemispheric fissure in association with rupture of the anterior communicating artery increased the detection of this natriuretic substance, but no clear relationship to hyponatremia was detected.[110] Although the source and nature of digitalis-like circulating factors (endogenous ouabain) are largely unknown, these substances inhibit Na^+, K^+ –ATPase and cause natriuresis. These factors are very limited in effect, but they may also have a role in maintaining increased blood pressure.[33] Their role in SAH remains unclear, and interest has waned.[35,116]

The putative role of another, better characterized natriuretic substance, atrial natriuretic peptide (ANP), in clinical deterioration after SAH, has been extensively studied.[20,23,42,102,104] Several studies, using single daily measurements of ANP, found marked elevation of serum ANP levels but no association with the development of hyponatremia or the net sodium balance. A study with diurnal measurements of ANP and ADH found a second surge of ANP followed by natriuresis and net sodium loss. In addition, ANP peaks were accompanied by a reciprocal decrease in ADH levels, allowing diuresis. All patients with cerebral infarction after SAH had a brief natriuresis associated with an ANP peak in the previous day.[104]

The possible role of other members of the natriuretic peptide family was recently studied in SAH.[42,44,95,106] The natriuretic peptide family now consists of ANP, brain natriuretic peptide (BNP), C-type natriuretic peptide (CNP), and dendroaspis natriuretic peptide (DNP). BNP is also markedly increased in SAH, but both BNP and ANP increase after SAH and seem to be regulated differently.[94,95,102,106] The natriuretic properties of CNP are few, if any, and it may be more involved with vasodilatation. It usually is released by endothelial cells. In a preliminary study, a possible vasoregulatory role for CNP was suggested because it was more often increased in patients in whom cerebral vasospasm developed.[103] DNP (discovered in the venom of the green mamba snake)[85] is increased in the serum of patients with congestive heart failure and found in human atrial myocardium. Injected into rat ventricles, it increased renal water excretion.[52] It has not yet been fully characterized to prove its genuine endogenous origin,[54,55,85] nor has it been systematically studied in aneurysmal SAH, but in our pilot study, we found a relative increase, particularly in patients with hyponatremia.[46] A loop similar to that of a comparable amino acid sequence is shared (Figure 57.2). C-type natriuretic peptide has very little natriuretic activity, and DNP is markedly diuretic; thus, the major differences appear in the tail. The relationship of the natriuretic peptide system with renin angiotensin and ADH has been carefully delineated. ANP not only causes natriuresis but also reduces ADH and inhibits renin aldosterone release.[44,114] How these natriuretic factors—particularly ANP and BNP, secreted respectively from atrium and ventricle—increase is not known. The time course of these changes in SAH is depicted in Figure 57.3.

Recently, adrenomedullin, an endogenous peptide with both vasodilatory and natriuretic properties, was discovered.[60,103] Adrenomedullin is structurally related to calcitonin, and thus its main biologic action is vasodilatation. When administered, it decreases peripheral vascular resistance, reduces blood pressure, and vasodilates cerebral arteries. Its effects seem uncoupled from

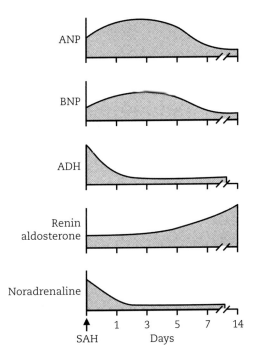

FIGURE 57.3: Time course of plasma levels of natriuretic peptides, antidiuretic hormone (ADH), and renin-aldosterone after subarachnoid hemorrhage (SAH).

ANP, atrial natriuretic peptide; BNP, brain natriuretic peptide.

the natriuretic system effects but significantly correlated with vasospasm, so that it may play a role in countering vasoconstriction and inhibiting vasoconstrictor hormone production.

The relevance of these studies to the pathophysiology of cerebral vasospasm remains to be determined. One possible explanation for development into symptomatic vasospasm could be the additional reduction of cerebral perfusion from a simultaneous hypovolemic state due to natriuresis. Current management reflects that concept.

Hyponatremia in Head Injury

Severe traumatic brain injury has also been linked to SIADH, but both its prevalence and its mechanism have been poorly studied. The preliminary impression is that, as in SAH, blood volume is decreased with appropriately increased ADH levels. Reports of patients with hyponatremia and natriuresis resistant to fluid restriction have appeared. Hyponatremia could only be corrected after expansion with hypertonic saline or an increase in the daily sodium load.[69,72,99] These patients may also be susceptible to cerebral vasospasm, which may be more common in those with traumatic subarachnoid bleeding. Hyperosmolarity and possible hypernatremia

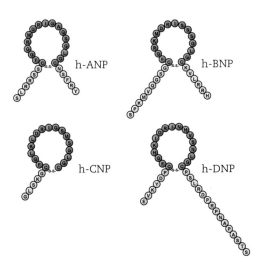

FIGURE 57.2: Natriuretic peptide system amino acid sequences of human atrial natriuretic peptide (h-ANP), human brain natriuretic peptide (h-BNP), human C-type natriuretic peptide (h-CNP), and human dendroaspis natriuretic peptide (h-DNP). One-letter amino acid code. Note 17-amino acid disulfide ring structure in all types. DNP has the longest C-terminus amino acid "tail."

after severe head injury, however, are far more common in clinical practice. In fact, most physicians deliberately induce a hyperosmolar state by administering mannitol to treat increased intracranial pressure.

Hyponatremia in Meningitis

Studies, mainly in children, have found that SIADH is present in bacterial, tuberculous, and aseptic meningitis.[17,26,58] In one large study, 32% of 300 pediatric patients with bacterial meningitis had serum sodium values between 122 and 133 mmol/L.[101] Another study[26] found that 88% of 50 children with *Haemophilus influenzae* meningitis had evidence of increased secretion of ADH. Although some reports in children suggest a role for initial water restriction after meningitis, experience in adults is very limited.

One study suggested a possible role for ANP,[62] challenging the concept of SIADH. Plasma levels of ADH have been increased, most likely appropriately so because of dehydration and hypovolemia. Prophylactic fluid restriction in patients with developing cerebral edema remains controversial, is possibly detrimental, and should be avoided.[58]

Hyponatremia in Guillain-Barré Syndrome

Hyponatremia occurs in up to 30% of patients with GBS, but severe, symptomatic hyponatremia is rare.[76] The risk of hyponatremia developing is much greater in mechanically ventilated patients.

In a prospective series, symptomatic mild hyponatremia appeared at an average of 10 days after intubation (range, 1–23 days).[76] Hyponatremia occurred in 42% of ventilated patients and in 19% of nonventilated patients with GBS and responded well to fluid restriction. Hyponatremia in mechanically ventilated patients with GBS probably results from SIADH. In a study of 12 consecutive patients with GBS, plasma ADH levels were higher than in nonventilated patients and controls. In ventilated patients, secretion of ADH is stimulated by impaired venous return, particularly when positive end-expiratory pressure is applied. Atrial natriuretic peptide levels were increased only in patients with extreme blood pressure changes from dysautonomia, possibly simply as a reflection of atrial stretch from increased blood volume.[105]

Syndrome of inappropriate antidiuretic hormone may also result from abnormalities in afferent nerves of volume receptors. Osmotic resetting due to afferent defect has been suggested, but this mechanism has not been carefully studied.[68]

Hyponatremia after Pituitary Surgery

After transsphenoidal surgery, almost 50% of patients have a disorder of water homeostasis within the first 2 postoperative weeks. Several patterns may occur (Figure 57.4), but early postoperative polyuria is most common. This phenomenon can be attributed to the unloading of large amounts of perioperative fluid, or to the depletion of ADH induced by surgical trauma. More interesting are the biphasic or triphasic patterns of polyuria and hyponatremia.[37,66] Hyponatremia can be severe, with values less than 125 mmol/L. A higher risk of hyponatremia seems more likely in patients operated on for microadenomas. The tentative explanation is possible involvement of the stalk or upward displacement of the posterior lobe outside the surgical field. Hyponatremia can possibly be linked to cortisol deficiency, a stimulus from one of the natriuretic peptides, unregulated vasopressin secretion from the damaged posterior pituitary body, or prolonged treatment with desmopressin (delayed hyponatremia). Continuous monitoring of plasma sodium is imperative, together with reduction of free water intake.

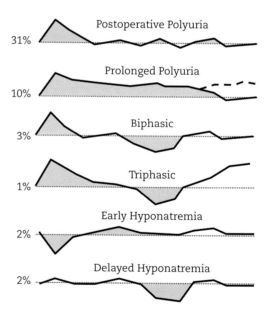

FIGURE 57.4: Patterns and frequency of postoperative polyuria (> 2,500 mL). Hypernatremia, upward movement, and hyponatremia, downward movement, after transsphenoidal surgery in 1,571 patients.

From Hensen J, Henig A, Fahlbusch R, et al. Prevalence, predictors and patterns of postoperative polyuria and hyponatremia in the immediate course after transsphenoidal surgery for pituitary adenomas. *Clin Endocrinol (Oxf)* 1999;50:431–439. With permission of Blackwell Science.

Miscellaneous Neurologic Disorders Associated with Hyponatremia

Syndrome of inappropriate antidiuretic hormone or any other cause of hyponatremia has been reported after chronic subdural hematoma, stroke, carotid endarterectomy,[57] obstructive hydrocephalus, and fulminant multiple sclerosis.[41] In patients infected with human immunodeficiency virus who have recent cytomegalovirus (CMV) encephalitis, hyponatremia could point to CMV-induced adrenalitis (Chapter 33).

Treatment of Hyponatremia

The treatment of asymptomatic hyponatremia is focused on correction of the volume derangement alone; the absolute serum sodium value has much less clinical relevance.[2] The management of asymptomatic hyponatremia, irrespective of severity, should be conservative. If hyponatremia is associated with the contraction of intravascular volume (and secondary release of ADH), treatment should consist of volume replacement with isotonic saline. Once the intravascular volume is normalized, the stimulus to ADH release is eliminated and the patient excretes excess water to correct hyponatremia. If the cause is SIADH, the restriction of free water alone slowly corrects hyponatremia. Syndrome of inappropriate antidiuretic hormone is self-limited in neurologic patients; therefore, a brief period of free water restriction may be definitive therapy. Traditionally, in resistant cases, lithium carbonate has been used because it inhibits the renal response to ADH. (The recommended initial dose is 900–1,200 mg/day.) Demeclocycline hydrochloride also inhibits the renal response to ADH.[29] (The recommended initial dose is 1,200 mg/day, in two divided doses, which should be reduced to the lowest effective dose.) Both agents are very rarely used in neurologic patients with acute hyponatremia and are more often administered in patients with long-standing hyponatremia.[87–89,98]

The management of symptomatic hyponatremia is more controversial, and an osmotic demyelination syndrome or central pontine myelinolysis demyelination[14,91,92,96] can occur if hyponatremia is corrected by more than 12–24 mmol/L in 24 hours or to values greater than the upper limit of normal.[11,61,92] Most cases of acute severe symptomatic hyponatremia that require correction result from excessive water; therefore, facilitating the excretion of water is the appropriate therapy. This is best achieved with furosemide-induced diuresis (20 mg) and a hypertonic saline solution

(3%) or a vasopressin antagonist conivaptan[8,19] (Capsule 57.1). The diuretic produces renal loss of free water (hypotonic diuresis), and the excreted sodium is returned in a smaller volume with a hypertonic solution.

Conventional formulas calculate the sodium requirement by multiplying total body water by the difference between the desired serum sodium concentration and the current sodium concentration. An elegant approach introduced by Adrogué and Madias[2] uses a formula that projects the change in serum sodium after infusion and retention of 1 L of a previously chosen infusate, mostly 3% sodium chloride (Table 57.7).

In SAH, volume status is more important than hyponatremia per se. Volume resuscitation is achieved with normal saline or 5% albumin alone. Oral administration of salt, tomato juice, or vegetable juice (V8) may further increase sodium intake to balance natriuresis. If the fluid balance remains negative, fludrocortisone (0.2 mg orally b.i.d.) is effective[36,59,111,115] (Capsule 57.2). The effect of fludrocortisone is apparent within hours and may last for days. Often, administration for more than 5 days may have little merit because of a "mineralocorticoid escape" phenomenon. (Sodium retention is overcome by renal mechanisms, including an increase in plasma ANP and a decrease in renin and sympathetic nerve activity, and no further positive sodium balance is observed.) Fludrocortisone remains a useful adjunct in the management of resistant hyponatremia and negative fluid balance.[117] Recommendations are given in Table 57.7.

Hypernatremia

Hypernatremia is defined as sodium values exceeding 145 mEq/L. The conditions associated with increased serum sodium concentration are listed in Table 57.8.

Hypernatremia is commonly associated with acute neurologic events, often from dehydration in patients unable to obtain water. It may occur in patients with persistent vomiting, causing hypotonic fluid loss. The clinical manifestations of acute hypernatremia appear only when serum osmolalities approach 400 mOsm/kg of water and may lead to a decrease in level of consciousness and generalized tonic-clonic seizures. Hypernatremia in the NICU is due commonly to diabetes insipidus,[10] pure water loss, and, less commonly, to an artificially administered large dose of sodium (e.g., hypertonic saline enemas or feeding preparations), causing a gain in hypertonic sodium.[1]

CAPSULE 57.1   THE VAPTANS

The secretion of antidiuretic hormone reduces free-water excretion, and mostly interacts with V_2 receptors in the renal collecting tube.[18] Antagonists at the V_2 receptor site have been developed, and these create water diuresis, or aquaresis. Aquaresis is a highly hypotonic diuresis without electrolyte loss that occurs with the use of diuretics. Conivaptan is an orally active derivative of vasopressin (see accompanying illustration) and approved by the US Food and Drug Administration.[19] The drug is administered in a 20 mg IV bolus over 30 minutes followed by a continuous infusion of 20 mg over 24 hours for a few days (insufficiently treated hyponatremia has been noted with a single dose). Usually 1.5% saline infusion is maintained as fluid intake. Conivaptan is mostly used in difficult to manage euvolemic or hypervolemic hyponatremia when serum sodium levels are 125 mmol/L or less (e.g., in patients with advanced cardiac failure). Mild cases of phlebitis and hypotension have been reported, and thirst may occur. Serum sodium usually does rise outside the 24 mmol/L/day limit, and osmotic demyelination syndromes have not been documented.

Conivaptan (YM-087)

The chemical structure of conivaptan.

TABLE 57.7. TREATMENT OF SYMPTOMATIC HYPONATREMIA

Volume Contraction	Volume Dilution
0.9% NaCl (or 1.5%)	Calculate need to normalize serum sodium by using
3% NaCl*	3% NaCl (513 mmol/L) in the formula
Fludrocortisone acetate, 0.4 mg/day	$\dfrac{513 - \text{current serum Na}}{0.5 \times \text{body weight (kg)} + 1}$
	to provide total millimoles per liter
	Rate: raise serum sodium 1 mmol/L/hr

*Patient needs a central venous catheter placed.
A calculator is available on www.medcalc.com.
Data from Adrogué HJ, Madias NE. Hyponatremia. *N Engl J Med* 2000;342:1581-1589. With permission of the Massachusetts Medical Society.

Evaluation of Hypernatremia

Hypernatremia is similarly categorized by the volume of extracellular fluid. Loss of proportionally more water than salt causes hypernatremia in most patients if water is not replenished. Examples of acute severe hypernatremia are correction of lactic acidosis by intravenously administered sodium bicarbonate and excessive doses of hypertonic saline to achieve hypervolemic therapy. The combination of hypernatremia, hypovolemia, and hypotonic urine indicates that the patient is not conserving water. In the NICU, the cause of hypernatremia is often defective central release of ADH (diabetes insipidus) or induced osmotic diuresis.

Nephrogenic diabetes insipidus is very uncommon but can be acquired through drug toxicity (e.g., amphotericin B). It can be differentiated from neurogenic diabetes insipidus by lack of response to the administration of ADH.[1,10]

CAPSULE 57.2   CEREBRAL SALT WASTING SYNDROME AND FLUDROCORTISONE

Treatment of cerebral salt wasting syndrome (CSW) is replacement of water and salt loss. However more fluid intake will lead to more water and salt loss—the hole in the bucket phenomenon—and only fixing the holes with fludrocortisone, so to speak, will result in more effective treatment (see accompanied figure). Fludrocortisone acetate is a synthetic glucocorticoid with potent mineralocorticoid activity and moderate glucocorticoid activity. It stimulates Na-K-ATPase activity and increases the potassium secretion from the gastrointestinal tract. When used in the dose range of 0.2–0.4 mg/day, it reduces serum potassium but rarely causes profound hypokalemia. In large doses, it inhibits endogenous adrenal cortical secretion, thymic activity, and pituitary corticotropin excretion. Fludrocortisone produces an increase in extracellular and plasma fluid volume and may sensitize adrenergic receptors to circulating catecholamines.

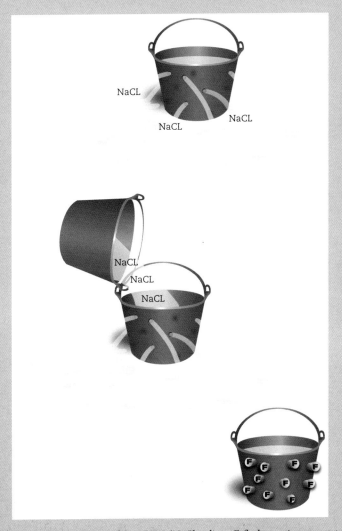

The way fludrocortisone works in CSW. (NaCl, saline; F, fludrocortisone acetate).

TABLE 57.8. CAUSES
OF HYPERNATREMIA IN THE NICU

Hypovolemia	Normovolemia or Hypervolemia
Gastrointestinal loss	Hypertonic sodium solutions
Diuretics (e.g., mannitol) Diabetes insipidus Increased insensible fluid loss	Corticosteroid excess

Patients with traumatic brain injury, massive cerebral edema, or rapid central brainstem displacement injuring the stalk, and certainly patients with the clinical criteria for brain death[81] are prone to develop diabetes insipidus. Therefore, fluid balance, urine specific gravity, and serum sodium concentration must be carefully monitored. Obviously, increased urine output has multiple potential causes. In traumatic brain injury, for example, diuresis may be an appropriate response to fluid administered during resuscitation from trauma, or the output may be a result of osmotic diuresis from the administration of mannitol.

TABLE 57.9. TREATMENT
OF SYMPTOMATIC HYPERNATREMIA

Pure Water Loss or Hypotonic Hypernatremic	Hypertonic Hypernatremia
Calculate need to normalize serum sodium by using 5% dextrose in the formula:	Furosemide, 40–80 mg IV; switch to electrolyte-free water infusion (5% dextrose)

$$\frac{0 - current\ plasma\ Na}{0.5 \times body\ weight + 1}$$

Or

0.45% NaCl in the formula:

$$\frac{77 - current\ plasma\ Na}{0.5 \times body\ weight + 1}$$

to provide total millimoles per liter

Rate: reduce serum sodium 10 mmol/L in 24 hours

Desmopressin, 2–4 mcg IV in 2 divided doses

A calculator is available on www.medcalc.com
Data from Adrogué HJ, Madias NE. Hypernatremia. N Engl J Med 2000;342:1493–1499. With permission of the Massachusetts Medical Society.

Diabetes insipidus is characterized by hypotonic urine (osmolality < 300 mOsm/kg or specific gravity < 1,010) and polyuria (> 30 mL/kg per day).[10,75] Clinically significant polyuria does not develop until approximately 75% of the ADH-secreting neurons are destroyed; in most patients, therefore, the impairment of ADH release is incomplete. The disruption of ADH secretion is transient in 50%–60% of patients with traumatic brain injury. Normal osmoregulation returns in 3 to 5 days.

Treatment of Hypernatremia

Hypernatremic dehydration is best corrected by the judicious use of intravenous fluids. In very rare clinical situations of overt shock, colloids are administered.

The water deficit can be calculated (Part XIII Formulas and Scales). The rate of correction is not exactly known, but water deficits are best corrected within 48 hours. If the clinical situation allows, half the water deficit is restored within 24 hours and the rest over 48 hours. Preferably a formula similar to that in hyponatremia can be used, typically using hypotonic fluids.[1] Recommendations are given in Table 57.9.

In general, patients unable to sense thirst require careful monitoring of fluid balance, urine specific gravity, body weight, and serum sodium concentration. If urine volume is not excessive, replacement of urine output and insensible losses with intravenous fluids may be sufficient. Treatment of acute diabetes insipidus requires meticulous management. Intravenous fluids or aqueous vasopressin may be used if the polyuria and polydipsia are difficult to manage. Hormonal replacement with vasopressin in acute diabetes insipidus should be considered if urine output is more than 300 mL/hr for 2 consecutive hours. Therapy should begin with desmopressin, 2–4 mcg intravenously in two divided doses.

GLUCOSE HANDLING

A major acute brain injury of any sort may result in rapid increase of serum glucose. Uptake of glucose by neurons is a direct reflection of the glucose availability and is not regulated by insulin. Normoglycemia, hyperglycemia, or hypoglycemia may each further injure the injured brain.[6,25,43,78,118] Increased glucose utilization and increase in glucose transport are common in diffuse brain injury.[45] Associations of hyperglycemia with other medical and surgical conditions have been established as a marker of poor outcome.[39]

Serum glucose is an indicator of potential supply, but the ideal value is not known. Normoglycemia may be an insufficient supply and may reduce cerebral tissue glucose, followed by peri-ischemic cortical depolarization. Hypoglycemia has been known to cause rapid and permanent injury in diencephalic and cortical structures. Decreased serum glucose increases glutamate concentration in the brain and also elevates the lactate pyruvate ratio as measured by cerebral microdialysis.[100] These signs of "metabolic distress" have been seen in aggressive glycemic control with insulin. Hyperglycemia may increase oxidative stress and subsequently increases toxic derivatives, including reactive oxygen species and inflammatory cytokines.[73]

The mere presence of hyperglycemia in the early clinical course of acute stroke, traumatic head injury, or acute encephalitis increases the chance of a poor outcome.[5] For example, hyperglycemia may worsen the ischemia-induced anaerobic glycolysis, resulting in even more tissue acidosis. Magnetic resonance spectroscopy (MRS) studies have confirmed transition of ischemic penumbra to infarction when hyperglycemia is present. Acute lactate production on MRS is correlated with worsening infarction in patients with hyperglycemia.[67] In addition, persistent hyperglycemia may increase the risk of hospital acquired pneumonia.

Hyperglycemia is usually defined as more than 140 mg/dL and severe hyperglycemia—mostly hyperosmolar and nonketotic—as more than 800 mg/dL. Early "mild" hyperglycemia does not produce additional clinical signs. Hyperosmolar hyperglycemia may result in seizures and in coma.

Whether aggressive blood glucose control is necessary in critically ill neurologic patients remains unresolved. Tight glucose control (defined as normoglycemia of 80–110 mg/dL) has become a mainstay of management since prospective clinical trials (the Leuven Trials) have shown improved outcome or reduced length of ICU stay.[97] The results of the Normoglycemia in Intensive Care Evaluation–Survival Glucose Algorithm Regulation (NICE–SUGAR) trial surprisingly showed a much different result and higher mortality and severe hypoglycemia (≤ 40 mg/dL) in the tightly controlled patient group (80–110 mg/dL).[27]

The unblinded clinical trials in Leuven also documented a high mortality in the control group with most patients treated with parenteral nutrition. It has been alleged that parenteral nutrition may have increased glucose load (2–3 L of 10% glucose daily) and harm to the control patient, with less harm to the insulin-managed patient, thereby explaining the results of the Leuven trials.

Most ICUs throughout the United States and elsewhere have computerized treatment algorithms.[13] The impact of these disappointing findings cannot be evaluated at this point, but they may lead to less strict control, and perhaps less attentive practices. A recent study found, even more surprisingly, that after rapid adoption of strict glucose control there was little to no de adoption following the NICE–SUGAR trial that demonstrated harm.[64] In medically and surgically critically ill patients, conventional glucose control (140–180 mg/dL) may be appropriate and will avoid unnecessary hypoglycemic episodes. The benefit of strict control in acute neurologic conditions remains unclear. Most studies in the NICU are retrospective, and in studies with alleged benefit of glucose control, the care of the control group (including withdrawal of care) may be substantially different.[3] The current evidence, or lack thereof,[118] in each of these conditions is reviewed here.

Acute Stroke

Hyperglycemia is present early after the onset of stroke.[15,53,93,113] Several feasibility studies of intense glucose control have been reported in acute ischemic and hemorrhagic stroke. A recent prospective study from Spain (glycemia in acute stroke [GLIAS]) identified a serum glucose level of 155 mg/dL as a cutoff level for poor outcome, independently of the presence of preexisting diabetes.[30]

The recent Treatment of Hyperglycemia in Ischemic Stroke (THIS) trial found very satisfactory control with an intravenous insulin.[12] One randomized trial—albeit underpowered, with 899 patients—the UK Glucose Insulin Stroke Trial (GIST–UK) was prematurely stopped due to poor enrollment but found no improvement in outcome in ischemic and hemorrhage stroke.[31,32] Currently, there is no evidence that aggressive glucose control improves outcome in stroke, and hypoglycemia in these studies remains prevalent (15%–35%).[31,32] A recent randomized study in acute stroke found that intensive insulin therapy in the first 24 hours was associated with growth of infarct size.[77]

Current recommendation of blood glucose control varies among organizations. The European Stroke Initiative Guidelines recommends insulin treatment with glucose of 180 mg/dL or higher; the Stroke Council of the American Stroke Association recommends a target of 140 to 185 mg/dL (Part XIV Guidelines).

Aneurysmal Subarachnoid Hemorrhage

A recent meta-analysis of studies reporting admission glucose levels in aneurysmal SAH found a correlation of poor outcome with hyperglycemia.[48]

A large retrospective study from Massachusetts General Hospital found no difference between patients treated with insulin infusion protocols or insulin sliding scales but only improved outcome in the subset of patients with good glucose control. Hypoglycemia was noted in 13% of the aggressively treated patients.[50] Microdialysis studies in aneurysmal SAH have found a decrease in cerebral glucose, but without consistent evidence of metabolic distress.[45,48,82,83]

Traumatic Brain Injury

Outcome is worse in patients with hyperglycemia and traumatic head injury.[80] One randomized clinical trial in severe traumatic head injury found no difference in outcome with insulin treatment. The study also noted that all patients in the intensive insulin therapy group developed at least two hypoglycemia episodes. The mean glucose in the intensive insulin group was 92 mg/dL.[9] These observations are concerning, and the long-lasting effect of hypoglycemia may remain difficult to demonstrate in comatose patients after traumatic brain injury.

CONCLUSIONS

- Most patients with metabolic acidosis in the NICU have transient lactic acidosis after seizures. A major systemic illness should be considered in other circumstances.
- Hyponatremia must be viewed against volume status. Cerebral salt wasting (hypovolemic hyponatremia) is more common in certain CNS disorders than SIADH (normovolemic hyponatremia). The laboratory criteria are virtually identical. Differentiation from SIADH is possible with serial body weight (decrease), fluid balance (negative), and with clinical signs of early dehydration, relative tachycardia, orthostasis, and marginal skin turgor.
- Hypernatremia from dehydration is most common with diabetes insipidus from traumatic brain injury, at the time of diagnosis of brain death, or with the use of osmotic diuretic agents.
- Hyperglycemia is a stress response after any major acute neurologic illness. Treatment of severe hyperglycemia is warranted, aiming at glucose values between 140 and 180 mg/dL.

REFERENCES

1. Adrogue HJ, Madias NE. Hypernatremia. *N Engl J Med* 2000;342:1493–1499.
2. Adrogue HJ, Madias NE. Hyponatremia. *N Engl J Med* 2000;342:1581–1589.
3. Anger KE, Szumita PM. Barriers to glucose control in the intensive care unit. *Pharmacotherapy* 2006;26:214–228.
4. Audibert G, Steinmann G, de Talance N, et al. Endocrine response after severe subarachnoid hemorrhage related to sodium and blood volume regulation. *Anesth Analg* 2009;108:1922–1928.
5. Bagshaw SM, Egi M, George C, Bellomo R. Early blood glucose control and mortality in critically ill patients in Australia. *Crit Care Med* 2009;37:463–470.
6. Baird TA, Parsons MW, Phan T, et al. Persistent poststroke hyperglycemia is independently associated with infarct expansion and worse clinical outcome. *Stroke* 2003;34:2208–2214.
7. Berend K, de Vries AP, Gans RO. Physiological approach to assessment of acid-base disturbances. *N Engl J Med* 2014;371:1434–1445.
8. Bhardwaj A. Neurological impact of vasopressin dysregulation and hyponatremia. *Ann Neurol* 2006;59:229–236.
9. Bilotta F, Caramia R, Cernak I, et al. Intensive insulin therapy after severe traumatic brain injury: a randomized clinical trial. *Neurocrit Care* 2008;9:159–166.
10. Blevins LS, Jr., Wand GS. Diabetes insipidus. *Crit Care Med* 1992;20:69–79.
11. Brunner JE, Redmond JM, Haggar AM, Kruger DF, Elias SB. Central pontine myelinolysis and pontine lesions after rapid correction of hyponatremia: a prospective magnetic resonance imaging study. *Ann Neurol* 1990;27:61–66.
12. Bruno A, Kent TA, Coull BM, et al. Treatment of hyperglycemia in ischemic stroke (THIS): a randomized pilot trial. *Stroke* 2008;39:384–389.
13. Butcavage K. Glycemic control and intensive insulin protocols for neurologically injured patients. *J Neurosci Nurs* 2012;44:E1–E9.
14. Calakos N, Fischbein N, Baringer JR, Jay C. Cortical MRI findings associated with rapid correction of hyponatremia. *Neurology* 2000;55:1048–1051.
15. Christensen H, Boysen G. Blood glucose increases early after stroke onset: a study on serial measurements of blood glucose in acute stroke. *Eur J Neurol* 2002;9:297–301.
16. Cort JH. Cerebral salt wasting. *Lancet* 1954;266:752–754.
17. Cotton MF, Donald PR, Schoeman JF, et al. Plasma arginine vasopressin and the syndrome of inappropriate antidiuretic hormone secretion in tuberculous meningitis. *Pediatr Infect Dis J* 1991;10:837–842.
18. Day RE, Kitchen P, Owen DS, et al. Human aquaporins: regulators of transcellular water flow. *Biochim Biophys Acta* 2014;1840:1492–1506.

19. Decaux G, Soupart A, Vassart G. Non-peptide arginine-vasopressin antagonists: the vaptans. *Lancet* 2008;371:1624–1632.

20. Diringer M, Ladenson PW, Stern BJ, Schleimer J, Hanley DF. Plasma atrial natriuretic factor and subarachnoid hemorrhage. *Stroke* 1988;19:1119–1124.

21. Diringer MN, Wu KC, Verbalis JG, Hanley DF. Hypervolemic therapy prevents volume contraction but not hyponatremia following subarachnoid hemorrhage. *Ann Neurol* 1992;31:543–550.

22. Doczi T, Bende J, Huszka E, Kiss J. Syndrome of inappropriate secretion of antidiuretic hormone after subarachnoid hemorrhage. *Neurosurgery* 1981;9:394–397.

23. Dorhout Mees SM, Hoff RG, Rinkel GJ, Algra A, van den Bergh WM. Brain natriuretic peptide concentrations after aneurysmal subarachnoid hemorrhage: relationship with hypovolemia and hyponatremia. *Neurocrit Care* 2011;14: 176–181.

24. Fahy BG, Sheehy AM, Coursin DB. Glucose control in the intensive care unit. *Crit Care Med* 2009;37:1769–1776.

25. Farrokhnia N, Bjork E, Lindback J, Terent A. Blood glucose in acute stroke, different therapeutic targets for diabetic and non-diabetic patients? *Acta Neurol Scand* 2005;112:81–87.

26. Feigin RD, Stechenberg BW, Chang MJ, et al. Prospective evaluation of treatment of Hemophilus influenzae meningitis. *J Pediatr* 1976;88:542–548.

27. Finfer S, Chittock DR, Su SY, et al. Intensive versus conventional glucose control in critically ill patients. *N Engl J Med* 2009;360:1283–1297.

28. Finfer S, Delaney A. Tight glycemic control in critically ill adults. *JAMA* 2008;300:963–965.

29. Forrest JN, Jr., Cox M, Hong C, et al. Superiority of demeclocycline over lithium in the treatment of chronic syndrome of inappropriate secretion of antidiuretic hormone. *N Engl J Med* 1978;298:173–177.

30. Fuentes B, Castillo J, San Jose B, et al. The prognostic value of capillary glucose levels in acute stroke: the GLycemia in Acute Stroke (GLIAS) study. *Stroke* 2009;40:562–568.

31. Gray CS, Hildreth AJ, Alberti GK, O'Connell JE. Poststroke hyperglycemia: natural history and immediate management. *Stroke* 2004;35:122–126.

32. Gray CS, Hildreth AJ, Sandercock PA, et al. Glucose-potassium-insulin infusions in the management of post-stroke hyperglycaemia: the UK Glucose Insulin in Stroke Trial (GIST-UK). *Lancet Neurol* 2007;6:397–406.

33. Hamlyn JM, Hamilton BP, Manunta P. Endogenous ouabain, sodium balance and blood pressure: a review and a hypothesis. *J Hypertens* 1996;14:151–167.

34. Hannon MJ, Behan LA, O'Brien MM, et al. Hyponatremia following mild/moderate subarachnoid hemorrhage is due to SIAD and glucocorticoid deficiency and not cerebral salt wasting. *J Clin Endocrinol Metab* 2014;99:291–298.

35. Harrigan MR. Cerebral salt wasting syndrome: a review. *Neurosurgery* 1996;38:152–160.

36. Hasan D, Lindsay KW, Wijdicks EFM, et al. Effect of fludrocortisone acetate in patients with subarachnoid hemorrhage. *Stroke* 1989;20:1156–1161.

37. Hensen J, Henig A, Fahlbusch R, et al. Prevalence, predictors and patterns of postoperative polyuria and hyponatraemia in the immediate course after transsphenoidal surgery for pituitary adenomas. *Clin Endocrinol (Oxf)* 1999;50:431–439.

38. Hillier TA, Abbott RD, Barrett EJ. Hyponatremia: evaluating the correction factor for hyperglycemia. *Am J Med* 1999;106:399–403.

39. Hirshberg E, Lacroix J, Sward K, Willson D, Morris AH. Blood glucose control in critically ill adults and children: a survey on stated practice. *Chest* 2008;133:1328–1335.

40. Inzucchi SE, Siegel MD. Glucose control in the ICU: how tight is too tight? *N Engl J Med* 2009;360:1346–1349.

41. Ishikawa E, Ohgo S, Nakatsuru K, et al. Syndrome of inappropriate secretion of antidiuretic hormone (SIADH) in a patient with multiple sclerosis. *Jpn J Med* 1989;28:75–79.

42. Isotani E, Suzuki R, Tomita K, et al. Alterations in plasma concentrations of natriuretic peptides and antidiuretic hormone after subarachnoid hemorrhage. *Stroke* 1994;25:2198–2203.

43. Jauch-Chara K, Oltmanns KM. Glycemic control after brain injury: boon and bane for the brain. *Neuroscience* 2014;283:202–209.

44. Johnston CI, Phillips PA, Arnolda L, Mooser V. Modulation of the renin-angiotensin system by atrial natriuretic peptide. *J Cardiovasc Pharmacol* 1990;16 Suppl 7:S43–46.

45. Kerner A, Schlenk F, Sakowitz O, Haux D, Sarrafzadeh A. Impact of hyperglycemia on neurological deficits and extracellular glucose levels in aneurysmal subarachnoid hemorrhage patients. *Neurol Res* 2007;29:647–653.

46. Khurana VG, Wijdicks EFM, Heublein DM, et al. A pilot study of dendroaspis natriuretic peptide in aneurysmal subarachnoid hemorrhage. *Neurosurgery* 2004;55:69–75.

47. Kraut JA, Madias NE. Lactic acidosis. *N Engl J Med* 2014;371:2309–2319.

48. Kruyt ND, Biessels GJ, de Haan RJ, et al. Hyperglycemia and clinical outcome in

aneurysmal subarachnoid hemorrhage: a meta-analysis. *Stroke* 2009;40:e424–430.

49. Lahr MB. Hyponatremia during carbamazepine therapy. *Clin Pharmacol Ther* 1985;37:693–696.

50. Latorre JG, Chou SH, Nogueira RG, et al. Effective glycemic control with aggressive hyperglycemia management is associated with improved outcome in aneurysmal subarachnoid hemorrhage. *Stroke* 2009;40:1644–1652.

51. Lawn N, Wijdicks EFM, Burritt MF. Intravenous immune globulin and pseudohyponatremia. *N Engl J Med* 1998;339:632.

52. Lee J, Kim SW. Dendroaspis natriuretic peptide administered intracerebroventricularly increases renal water excretion. *Clin Exp Pharmacol Physiol* 2002;29:195–197.

53. Lindsberg PJ, Roine RO. Hyperglycemia in acute stroke. *Stroke* 2004;35:363–364.

54. Lisy O, Jougasaki M, Heublein DM, et al. Renal actions of synthetic dendroaspis natriuretic peptide. *Kidney Int* 1999;56:502–508.

55. Lisy O, Lainchbury JG, Leskinen H, Burnett JC, Jr. Therapeutic actions of a new synthetic vasoactive and natriuretic peptide, dendroaspis natriuretic peptide, in experimental severe congestive heart failure. *Hypertension* 2001;37:1089–1094.

56. Maesaka JK, Gupta S, Fishbane S. Cerebral salt-wasting syndrome: does it exist? *Nephron* 1999;82:100–109.

57. Magovern JA, Sieber PR, Thiele BL. The syndrome of inappropriate secretion of antidiuretic hormone following carotid endarterectomy: a case report and review of the literature. *J Cardiovasc Surg (Torino)* 1989;30:544–546.

58. Moller K, Larsen FS, Bie P, Skinhoj P. The syndrome of inappropriate secretion of antidiuretic hormone and fluid restriction in meningitis: how strong is the evidence? *Scand J Infect Dis* 2001;33:13–26.

59. Mori T, Katayama Y, Kawamata T, Hirayama T. Improved efficiency of hypervolemic therapy with inhibition of natriuresis by fludrocortisone in patients with aneurysmal subarachnoid hemorrhage. *J Neurosurg* 1999;91:947–952.

60. Nagaya N, Nishikimi T, Horio T, et al. Cardiovascular and renal effects of adrenomedullin in rats with heart failure. *Am J Physiol* 1999;276:R213–R218.

61. Narins RG. Therapy of hyponatremia: does haste make waste? *N Engl J Med* 1986;314:1573–1575.

62. Narotam PK, Kemp M, Buck R, et al. Hyponatremic natriuretic syndrome in tuberculous meningitis: the probable role of atrial natriuretic peptide. *Neurosurgery* 1994;34:982–988.

63. Nelson PB, Seif SM, Maroon JC, Robinson AG. Hyponatremia in intracranial disease: perhaps not the syndrome of inappropriate secretion of antidiuretic hormone (SIADH). *J Neurosurg* 1981;55:938–941.

64. Niven DJ, Rubenfeld GD, Kramer AA, Stelfox HT. Effect of published scientific evidence on glycemic control in adult intensive care units. *JAMA Intern Med* 2015;175:801–809.

65. Oh MS, Carroll HJ. Cerebral salt-wasting syndrome: we need better proof of its existence. *Nephron* 1999;82:110–114.

66. Olson BR, Gumowski J, Rubino D, Oldfield EH. Pathophysiology of hyponatremia after transsphenoidal pituitary surgery. *J Neurosurg* 1997;87:499–507.

67. Parsons MW, Barber PA, Desmond PM, et al. Acute hyperglycemia adversely affects stroke outcome: a magnetic resonance imaging and spectroscopy study. *Ann Neurol* 2002;52:20–28.

68. Penney MD, Murphy D, Walters G. Resetting of osmoreceptor response as cause of hyponatremia in acute idiopathic polyneuritis. *Br Med J (Clin Res Ed)* 1979;2:1474–1476.

69. Penney MD, Walters G, Wilkins DG. Hyponatremia in patients with head injury. *Intensive Care Med* 1979;5:23–26.

70. Peters JP, Welt LG, Sims EA, Orloff J, Needham J. A salt-wasting syndrome associated with cerebral disease. *Trans Assoc Am Physicians* 1950;63:57–64.

71. Polderman KH, Bloemers FW, Peerdeman SM, Girbes AR. Hypomagnesemia and hypophosphatemia at admission in patients with severe head injury. *Crit Care Med* 2000;28:2022–2025.

72. Poon WS, Mendelow AD, Davies DL, et al. Secretion of antidiuretic hormone in neurosurgical patients: appropriate or inappropriate? *Aust N Z J Surg* 1989;59:173–180.

73. Prakash A, Matta BF. Hyperglycaemia and neurological injury. *Curr Opin Anaesthesiol* 2008;21:565–569.

74. Rahman M, Friedman WA. Hyponatremia in neurosurgical patients: clinical guidelines development. *Neurosurgery* 2009;65:925–935.

75. Robertson GL. Differential diagnosis of polyuria. *Annu Rev Med* 1988;39:425–442.

76. Ropper AH, Wijdicks EFM, Truax BT. *Guillain-Barré Syndrome*. Vol. 34. Oxford: Oxford University Press; 1991.

77. Rosso C, Corvol JC, Pires C, et al. Intensive versus subcutaneous insulin in patients with hyperacute stroke: results from the randomized INSULINFARCT trial. *Stroke* 2012;43:2343–2349.

78. Rostami E. Glucose and the injured brain-monitored in the neurointensive care unit. *Front Neurol* 2014;5:91.

79. Sachdeo RC, Wasserstein A, Mesenbrink PJ, D'Souza J. Effects of oxcarbazepine on sodium

concentration and water handling. *Ann Neurol* 2002;51:613–620.

80. Salim A, Hadjizacharia P, Dubose J, et al. Persistent hyperglycemia in severe traumatic brain injury: an independent predictor of outcome. *Am Surg* 2009;75:25–29.

81. Sazontseva IE, Kozlov IA, Moisuc YG, et al. Hormonal response to brain death. *Transplant Proc* 1991;23:2467.

82. Schlenk F, Graetz D, Nagel A, Schmidt M, Sarrafzadeh AS. Insulin-related decrease in cerebral glucose despite normoglycemia in aneurysmal subarachnoid hemorrhage. *Crit Care* 2008;12:R9.

83. Schlenk F, Nagel A, Graetz D, Sarrafzadeh AS. Hyperglycemia and cerebral glucose in aneurysmal subarachnoid hemorrhage. *Intensive Care Med* 2008;34:1200–1207.

84. Schwartz WB, Bennett W, Curelop S, Bartter FC. A syndrome of renal sodium loss and hyponatremia probably resulting from inappropriate secretion of antidiuretic hormone. *Am J Med* 1957;23:529–542.

85. Schweitz H, Vigne P, Moinier D, Frelin C, Lazdunski M. A new member of the natriuretic peptide family is present in the venom of the green mamba (Dendroaspis angusticeps). *J Biol Chem* 1992;267:13928–13932.

86. Seifter JL. Integration of acid-base and electrolyte disorders. *N Engl J Med* 2014;371:1821–1831.

87. Sood L, Sterns RH, Hix JK, Silver SM, Chen L. Hypertonic saline and desmopressin: a simple strategy for safe correction of severe hyponatremia. *Am J Kidney Dis* 2013;61:571–578.

88. Spasovski G, Vanholder R, Allolio B, et al. Clinical practice guideline on diagnosis and treatment of hyponatraemia. *Nephrol Dial Transplant* 2014;29 Suppl 2:i1–i39.

89. Spasovski G, Vanholder R, Allolio B, et al. Clinical practice guideline on diagnosis and treatment of hyponatraemia. *Eur J Endocrinol* 2014;170:G1–47.

90. Sterns RH. Disorders of plasma sodium: causes, consequences, and correction. *N Engl J Med* 2015;372:55–65.

91. Sterns RH. The management of hyponatremic emergencies. *Crit Care Clin* 1991;7:127–142.

92. Sterns RH, Riggs JE, Schochet SS, Jr. Osmotic demyelination syndrome following correction of hyponatremia. *N Engl J Med* 1986;314:1535–1542.

93. Stollberger C, Exner I, Finsterer J, Slany J, Steger C. Stroke in diabetic and non-diabetic patients: course and prognostic value of admission serum glucose. *Ann Med* 2005;37:357–364.

94. Sviri GE, Feinsod M, Soustiel JF. Brain natriuretic peptide and cerebral vasospasm in subarachnoid hemorrhage: clinical and TCD correlations. *Stroke* 2000;31:118–122.

95. Tomida M, Muraki M, Uemura K, Yamasaki K. Plasma concentrations of brain natriuretic peptide in patients with subarachnoid hemorrhage. *Stroke* 1998;29:1584–1587.

96. Tormey WP. Central pontine myelinolysis and changes in serum sodium. *Lancet* 1990;335:1169.

97. Vanhorebeek I, Langouche L, Van den Berghe G. Tight blood glucose control with insulin in the ICU: facts and controversies. *Chest* 2007;132:268–278.

98. Verbalis JG, Goldsmith SR, Greenberg A, et al. Diagnosis, evaluation, and treatment of hyponatremia: expert panel recommendations. *Am J Med* 2013;126:S1–42.

99. Vespa P. Cerebral salt wasting after traumatic brain injury: an important critical care treatment issue. *Surg Neurol* 2008;69:230–232.

100. Vespa P, Boonyaputthikul R, McArthur DL, et al. Intensive insulin therapy reduces microdialysis glucose values without altering glucose utilization or improving the lactate/pyruvate ratio after traumatic brain injury. *Crit Care Med* 2006;34:850–856.

101. von Vigier RO, Colombo SM, Stoffel PB, et al. Circulating sodium in acute meningitis. *Am J Nephrol* 2001;21:87–90.

102. Weinand ME, O'Boynick PL, Goetz KL. A study of serum antidiuretic hormone and atrial natriuretic peptide levels in a series of patients with intracranial disease and hyponatremia. *Neurosurgery* 1989;25:781–785.

103. Wijdicks EFM, Heublein DM, Burnett JC, Jr. Increase and uncoupling of adrenomedullin from the natriuretic peptide system in aneurysmal subarachnoid hemorrhage. *J Neurosurg* 2001;94:252–256.

104. Wijdicks EFM, Ropper AH, Hunnicutt EJ, Richardson GS, Nathanson JA. Atrial natriuretic factor and salt wasting after aneurysmal subarachnoid hemorrhage. *Stroke* 1991;22:1519–1524.

105. Wijdicks EFM, Ropper AH, Nathanson JA. Atrial natriuretic factor and blood pressure fluctuations in Guillain-Barre syndrome. *Ann Neurol* 1990;27:337–338.

106. Wijdicks EFM, Schievink WI, Burnett JC, Jr. Natriuretic peptide system and endothelin in aneurysmal subarachnoid hemorrhage. *J Neurosurg* 1997;87:275–280.

107. Wijdicks EFM, Van Dongen KJ, Van Gijn J, Hijdra A, Vermeulen M. Enlargement of the

third ventricle and hyponatraemia in aneurysmal subarachnoid haemorrhage. *J Neurol Neurosurg Psychiatry* 1988;51:516–520.

108. Wijdicks EFM, Vermeulen M, Hijdra A, van Gijn J. Hyponatremia and cerebral infarction in patients with ruptured intracranial aneurysms: is fluid restriction harmful? *Ann Neurol* 1985;17:137–140.

109. Wijdicks EFM, Vermeulen M, ten Haaf JA, et al. Volume depletion and natriuresis in patients with a ruptured intracranial aneurysm. *Ann Neurol* 1985;18:211–216.

110. Wijdicks EFM, Vermeulen M, van Brummelen P, den Boer NC, van Gijn J. Digoxin-like immunoreactive substance in patients with aneurysmal subarachnoid hemorrhage. *Br Med J (Clin Res Ed)* 1987;294:729–732.

111. Wijdicks EFM, Vermeulen M, van Brummelen P, van Gijn J. The effect of fludrocortisone acetate on plasma volume and natriuresis in patients with aneurysmal subarachnoid hemorrhage. *Clin Neurol Neurosurg* 1988;90:209–214.

112. Wijdicks EFM. *Neurologic Complications of Critical Illness*. 3rd ed. New York: Oxford University Press; 2009.

113. Williams LS, Rotich J, Qi R, et al. Effects of admission hyperglycemia on mortality and costs in acute ischemic stroke. *Neurology* 2002;59:67–71.

114. Williams TD, Walsh KP, Lightman SL, Sutton R. Atrial natriuretic peptide inhibits postural release of renin and vasopressin in humans. *Am J Physiol* 1988;255:R368–R372.

115. Woo MH, Kale-Pradhan PB. Fludrocortisone in the treatment of subarachnoid hemorrhage-induced hyponatremia. *Ann Pharmacother* 1997;31:637–639.

116. Yamada K, Goto A, Nagoshi H, Hui C, Omata M. Role of brain ouabainlike compound in central nervous system-mediated natriuresis in rats. *Hypertension* 1994;23:1027–1031.

117. Yee AH, Burns JD, Wijdicks EFM. Cerebral salt wasting: pathophysiology, diagnosis, and treatment. *Neurosurg Clin N Am* 2010;21: 339–352.

118. Yoder J. Con: tight glucose control after brain injury is unproven and unsafe. *J Neurosurg Anesthesiol* 2009;21:55–57.

58

Management of Gastrointestinal Complications

Gastrointestinal disorders seen in the neurosciences intensive care unit (NICU) are not unique, but they may be of a different nature from those seen in medical or surgical ICUs. For example, the gastrointestinal complications associated with sepsis (acute pancreatitis, acalculous cholecystitis), often observed in medical or surgical ICUs, are less prevalent in the NICU. The single most important gastrointestinal complication in the NICU is bleeding and adynamic ileus.

Gastrointestinal discomfort is rarely voiced by patients with acute brain injury and consequently these disorders may easily go unnoticed. Impaired level of consciousness often precludes an adequate history of abdominal pain, and, in trauma, there may be distracting painful injuries.[28] Generally, the risk of gastrointestinal bleeding is increased in comatose patients, and in those with mechanical ventilation, coagulopathy, or sepsis.[2,14,18,66] Often, significant laboratory changes, such as a decrease in hematocrit, point to a gastrointestinal complication. In addition, disorders of bowel motility may occur; of these, diarrhea associated with enteral nutrition is common in hospitalized patients.[33]

This chapter summarizes the important principles in the recognition and management of acute conditions in the gastrointestinal tract, complicating acute neurologic illness. Bowel care in spinal cord injury, which is complicated because of neurogenic bowel disorder, receives attention here. Although there may be a tendency to underreport gastrointestinal complications, the true incidence after any acute neurologic illness is, in reality, low.

GASTROINTESTINAL BLEEDING

Acute central nervous system disorders may induce lesions in the lining of the gastrointestinal tract, which generally appear at multiple sites (Capsule 58.1). They may be confined to the mucosa (erosions) or extend into the submucosa or beyond (ulcers).[7,21,40,51]

Gastrointestinal hemorrhages from stress-associated erosions are minor and seldom lead to massive, life-threatening situations or require frequent blood transfusions.[48,51,56,60,75] Nonetheless, a measurable risk remains in patients in the NICU, and this risk is greater in anticoagulated patients, patients with previous use of nonsteroidal anti-inflammatory drugs (NSAIDs),[87] and patients with underlying coagulopathies.[13] For patients with red blood in gastric aspirate or red blood from the rectum, mortality may be as high as 30%.[4,49]

Clinical Features and Evaluation

Mucosal lesions in patients with a catastrophic central nervous system event have become more evident since the introduction of endoscopy.[29,30,47] Appreciable bleeding, however, occurs in less than 5% of the patients and reaches the clinical stage of shock in a much smaller percentage.[44]

The clinical signs of gastrointestinal bleeding can be dangerously subtle. Feelings of oppression, nausea associated with excessive sweating, relative tachycardia, and pale facial features may soon be followed by oozing of blood or, at times, massive production of blood. Gastrointestinal bleeding can first be signaled by a coffee-ground color in aspirate.

The clinical presenting signs that should be recognized as possible indicators of severe hemorrhage are orthostatic hypotension and, eventually, decrease in hemoglobin and hematocrit concentrations. Clinically, orthostatic hypotension is the most reliable forerunner of hypovolemic shock. After the head of the bed is changed to at least 60 degrees, with the patient's legs in a dependent position, sequential measurement of systolic blood pressure and pulse provides a reasonable estimate of the volume of blood loss.

CAPSULE 58.1   STRESS-RELATED MUCOSAL DISEASE

The gastric mucosa has an intrinsic defense mechanism that prevents ulceration and bleeding. Acute brain lesions, especially those associated with increased intracranial pressure, have been reported to produce ulcers, but any stress may challenge these defense mechanisms. An ulcer caused by acute brain injury or after craniotomy (particularly posterior fossa surgery) is known as *Cushing's ulcer.*[21]

Most of the injury can be explained by a combination of local ischemia and acid (see accompanying illustration).[36] Blood flow may be compromised by marked episodes of hypotension, but mechanical ventilation may already have caused reduced splanchnic hypoperfusion. Increased parasympathetic nervous system activation (vagal nerve) may play a crucial role, but also the sympathoadrenal response with angiotensin constricting the gastric vasculature. The end effect of hypoperfusion is diminished mucus production and compromise of the mucus barrier, exposing the epithelial layer to acidic material.[51]

Stress-related ulcers are thus expectedly in the acid-producing areas such as the fundus and upper body. The vulnerability of the mucosa may also be increased by substances such as acetylcholine, histamine, and endogenous thyrotropin-releasing hormone. Disruption of the mucus gel overlying the gastric epithelium may also be a consequence of previous bile reflux, uremia, alcohol, aspirin, and nonsteroidal anti-inflammatory drugs (NSAIDs).

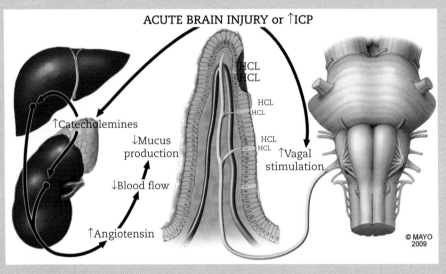

The brain–stomach connection.

New-onset tachycardia without change in systolic blood pressure indicates a fractional loss of blood volume of 15% or less. Tachycardia with a change in systolic blood pressure of 10 mm Hg when position is changed indicates a blood volume depletion of at least 20%, and a spontaneous change in blood pressure to systolic levels below 100 mm Hg indicates a loss of 25% or more.[4,67] At this juncture, oliguria (urine volume, < 15 mL/hr) is invariably present. With loss of whole blood, the hematocrit does not change immediately because the percentage of erythrocyte mass to total blood mass remains similar. Decrease in hematocrit lags behind and appears after redistribution of plasma to the intravascular space. Replacement of fluid with saline or volume expanders decreases the hematocrit further, and the decrease should not be misinterpreted as an indicator of continuing gastrointestinal bleeding. In this circumstance, active gastrointestinal bleeding is suggested only when hypotension persists and the hematocrit does not increase after infusion of whole blood or packed cells. Hematemesis or sudden appearance of large fresh clots per rectum is also a sign of active bleeding in the gastrointestinal tract, but does not indicate whether the site is in the upper or the lower part of the tract.

Gastrointestinal bleeding after acute stroke could present with hematemesis or melena and occasionally with a sudden decrease in hemoglobin value. However, in our study, orthostatic hypotension and massive hematemesis developed in a minority of patients.[87] Others found more severe gastrointestinal hemorrhages after acute stroke and hypotension, or a decrease in hemoglobin in 50% of the patients.[22] In a recent large study of the registry of the Canadian Stroke Network, 1.5% of patients had gastrointestinal hemorrhage after stroke, but a third had blood transfusions. This study could not report on the use of prophylactic therapy with H_2 antagonists or proton-pump inhibitors, which could explain such a low prevalence.[69] Minor (and probably less clinically significant) gastrointestinal hemorrhages may not be noticed, and some patients may have only a transient tinge of blood with nasogastric return, possibly related to mucosal damage from the nasogastric tube alone.

The source of gastrointestinal bleeding should be actively sought. Intuitively, stress ulcers are implicated as a cause of gastrointestinal bleeding, but many other causes should be pursued. Hemorrhage from the nasopharynx should be investigated in any patient with prolonged intubation or tracheostomy. Proper inspection of the mouth may sporadically identify damage to the mucosa of the oral pharynx incurred during placement of the endotracheal tube. Bleeding is common in nasally intubated patients (even occasionally excessive), and may lead to accumulation in the dependent portions of the stomach. Bleeding from a tracheostomy can appear minimal because the blood is swallowed. Massive bleeding at the tracheostomy site from erosion of the brachiocephalic artery is fortunately rare (< 1%) but often is fatal, appearing much more commonly with hemoptysis.

Mallory-Weiss tears should be considered in patients with profound vomiting. Associated conditions with profound vomiting are acute cerebellar stroke and aneurysmal subarachnoid hemorrhage (SAH). Repeated retching and vomiting may cause a circumferential mucosal laceration in the cardia portion of the stomach, or longitudinally in the proximal esophagus[35]

(Figure 58.1). However, it can occur in any situation that increases abdominal pressure, such as repeated bucking and coughing with tracheostomy in situ. An important predisposing factor for Mallory-Weiss tears is a history of alcohol or aspirin abuse. Hemorrhage from Mallory-Weiss tears ceases spontaneously, and half the patients do not require blood transfusion. An underlying profound gastritis is often confirmed by endoscopy. Definitive treatment with multipolar electrocoagulation is needed in only a few patients with these complications.

Some form of esophagitis occurs in 50% of patients receiving mechanical ventilation. The cause is mechanical irritation from nasogastric tubes or induction of gastroenteric reflux from interference with sphincter function.[35]

An autopsy study of gastrointestinal bleeding in intracranial disease found significant occurrences of gastric petechiae (50%) and gastric or duodenal ulcers (30%), but some of these lesions may have represented agonal changes.[42] A retrospective review in neurosurgical patients found that 7% of 526 had gastrointestinal bleeding, mostly from superficial mucosal erosions (Figure 58.2).[13] Comatose patients with acute ulcers were at significantly higher risk for life-threatening complications. Lower gastrointestinal bleeding is much less common in acutely ill neurologic patients, and in many is related to local mucosal trauma. However, in one study of 14 patients who had gastrointestinal hemorrhage in acute stroke, the most common associated possible causes were long-term use of aspirin, other NSAIDs, and anticoagulation.[87] These alternative explanations for

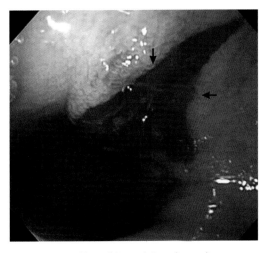

FIGURE 58.1: Typical linear injury (*arrows*) at gastroesophageal junction (Mallory-Weiss).

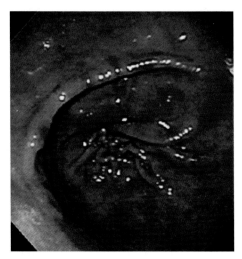

FIGURE 58.2: Typical endoscopic view of superficial erosion and ulcerations in acute brain injury.

gastrointestinal bleeding suggest that medication-induced gastrointestinal bleeding, at least in acute stroke, may be underappreciated.

Enteral nutrition is insufficient as a measure to prevent stress ulcers.[59,71] The use of prophylactic medication (antacids or H_2-blockers) for gastrointestinal bleeding in traumatic brain injury has been addressed in prospective studies. Cimetidine prophylaxis was effective in a single controlled trial.[37] The use of the more expensive drug ranitidine in "high-risk" neurosurgical patients significantly reduced gastrointestinal bleeding.[12] However, alkalization of gastric contents may result in colonization with gram-negative organisms.

Proton-pump inhibitors act by selectively inhibiting H^+/K^+ adenosine triphosphatase in the stimulated parietal cells of the stomach, thus decreasing acid secretion.[20,76,88,89] This new class of drugs is considered equally efficacious and less expensive. However, proton-pump inhibitors have not been compared with histamine receptor antagonists.[38,43] Lansoprazole is better and easier to use than ranitidine and is administered through the nasogastric tube.[55] Lansoprazole is dissolved in 10 mL of water and administered in the morning.[45,52,53] Omeprazole should not be administered via nasogastric tube because it may clog the tube. Pantoprazole has become available in an intravenous formulation, and costs are comparable to, if not less than, those of alternatives. Generally, our practice is to use Pantoprazole 40 mg intravenously once a day, or lansoprazole (crushed and dissolved) 30 mg orally per nasogastric tube.

The policy of prophylaxis in acutely ill neurologic patients remains to be determined. One should appreciate the significant hospital expenses of stress ulcer prophylaxis. Practice guidelines can reduce the inappropriate use of costly drugs but have not been developed for NICU patients.[58,64] If one extrapolates the results of studies in other intensive care units to NICUs, the administration of proton-pump inhibitors is reasonable in patients who have used aspirin or other NSAIDs, are taking anticoagulants, have a history of peptic ulcer, or are receiving mechanical ventilation. Specific neurologic conditions associated with a comparatively high risk of gastrointestinal bleeding and for which prophylaxis is indicated are pontine hemorrhage, traumatic head injury, poor-grade subarachnoid hemorrhage, and acute spinal cord injury.[44,65,78,81,86]

Management of Gastrointestinal Bleeding

The order of priority and the problems in the management of patients with an underlying neurologic disorder and acute gastrointestinal bleeding are not much different from those in other intensive care populations. However, there is a need for more stringent control of blood pressure. Immediate stabilization of blood pressure is important in any patient, but more so in a patient with an acute brain injury. Blood pressure–dependent areas in the acutely injured brain and a shift in cerebral autoregulation in patients with chronic hypertension imply that hypotension may not be well tolerated. In patients with large vessel occlusions, a precipitous decrease in blood pressure may extend (or at least threaten) the ischemic area to surrounding tissue. Fortunately, most gastrointestinal bleeding in critically ill neurologic patients is minor and stops even before endoscopy is performed.

Volume replacement is the first line of treatment, and pharmacologic support with vasopressors is usually not indicated.[5,67] At least two short peripheral venous catheters should be inserted. If the primary goal is to improve infusion rate, cannulation of central veins is not recommended and may complicate matters further from its high incidence of iatrogenic complications in an emergency situation.

Replacement fluid usually consists of isotonic saline. Massive gastrointestinal hemorrhages should be treated with whole blood alone to replace loss of both components of blood volume (Chapter 51 for hemorrhagic shock). When to begin infusion of whole blood or red blood cells depends on the ability of the patient to tolerate acute anemia but should be ordered with hemoglobin < 9 g/dL. Patients with signs of imminent cardiac failure or transient electrocardiographic changes should have blood transfusion immediately. Transfusion guidelines are discussed in Chapter 60. One unit of fresh frozen plasma after 4 units of packed erythrocytes replaces lost coagulation factors.[85] When gastrointestinal bleeding is associated with a coagulopathy, fresh frozen plasma (2–4 units) or platelet infusion (platelet count < 50 × 10⁹/L) is needed for correction.

Empirical treatment with a continuous intravenous infusion of histamine₂-receptor antagonists or proton-pump blockers is advised because of tenable evidence of a reduced incidence of recurrent bleeding and, more important, of reduced mortality in randomized trials.[53] Despite its costs, ranitidine infusion at 0.30 mg/kg/hr can be used in gastrointestinal bleeding after a loading dose of 0.5 mg/kg, but proton-pump inhibitors are preferred.[11] Pantoprazole 80 mg IV loading dose followed by 8 mg/hr for 3 days and 40 mg orally b.i.d. later is the most appropriate approach.

After initial resuscitation, fiberoptic endoscopy should be considered to localize the bleeding site.[6,19,24,32,54] Emergency endoscopy localizes the source of bleeding in 95% of patients and, more relevant, determines the activity of the bleeding.[17] Localization of a bleeding ulcer with a visible vessel (estimated prevalence, 25%) and localization of an ulcer with an adherent clot (estimated prevalence, 10%) have risks of rebleeding of, respectively, 50% and 20%.[25,80] At least half the patients with active bleeding, including oozing and spurting, observed during the procedure have rebleeding. A low risk (< 5%) of rebleeding can be expected when a clean base is found containing only old blood or pigments that can be washed away without effort.[25]

Several direct therapeutic approaches can be tried at the time of endoscopy. Multipolar electrocoagulation and heater probes are the most common and have reduced the need for early surgery.[50]

After hemodynamic stabilization and identification of the most likely source, specific treatment in most neurologically ill patients is medical. Suggested management tailored to the cause of gastrointestinal hemorrhage is summarized in Table 58.1. Continued bleeding without an identified source after several endoscopic attempts should prompt angiography or colonoscopy.

The decision to surgically intervene in bleeding stress ulcers is not difficult in extreme circumstances, such as failure to control active bleeding endoscopically, shock associated with an endoscopically visible artery, and increasing transfusion needs. Recommendations for surgical management in other clinical situations are more complicated and usually are guided by the age of the patient and the existence of comorbid disease.

TABLE 58.1. MANAGEMENT OF ACUTE UPPER GASTROINTESTINAL BLEEDING

Mallory-Weiss syndrome	Volume resuscitation
	Endoscopic confirmation
	Observation or electrocoagulation
Peptic ulcer, erosions	Volume resuscitation
	Endoscopic confirmation
	Proton-pump inhibitors
	Surgery if at increased risk for rebleeding

Before surgery is planned, arteriography for localization, possibly followed by arterial embolization or vasopressin infusion, is often considered.

Lower gastrointestinal tract bleeding is usually associated with angiodysplasia and diverticulitis, which are very unusual causes of bleeding in the NICU.[46] Localization can be difficult, and radionuclide scanning with technetium-labeled red blood cells may provide information (sensitivity of 91% and specificity of 100%) before angiography is performed.[8]

Disordered Intestinal Motility
Bed rest, medication, and enteral alimentation change bowel movement. Constipation may develop in patients confined to bed, but in many others, diarrhea or frequent loose stools complicate the acute neurologic illness.

Diarrhea
Hospital diarrhea is a serious problem in acutely ill neurologic patients. It is often self-limiting and is related to fecal impaction, which in turn is associated with narcotic analgesics, reduced oral intake, and mild dehydration. In patients with Guillain-Barré syndrome (GBS), early onset of diarrhea may indicate that *Campylobacter jejuni* infection has triggered GBS (certainly if the diarrhea is associated with mucus or blood). It is important to consider bacterial enteritis from *C. difficile*, but in most instances the causes are more mundane, and a change in gut flora alone may cause diarrhea.

Most often, clindamycin, penicillins, and cephalosporins are implicated in diarrhea. Theophylline in toxic doses, digoxin, and most central-acting antihypertensive agents can produce diarrhea.

Initiation of enteral nutrition alone probably is the most common reason for diarrhea in the NICU (Table 58.2). Most often, sudden exposure

TABLE 58.2. CAUSES OF DIARRHEA
IN NICU

Hyperosmolar enteral nutrition

Enteral feeding at high infusion rates

Antacids, clindamycin, cephalosporins, histamine$_2$-receptor antagonists, angiotensin-converting enzyme inhibitors, theophylline

Hypoalbuminemia

Clostridium difficile infection

TABLE 58.3. POSSIBLE CAUSES
OF PARALYTIC ILEUS AND OGILVIE
SYNDROME

Neurologic disorders

Guillain-Barré syndrome

Meningitis

Spinal cord injury

Surgical procedures

Abdominal exploration for blunt trauma and shock

Drugs

Opioids

Tricyclic antidepressants

Phenothiazines

See also Vanek VW, Al-Salti M. Acute pseudo-obstruction of the colon (Ogilvie's syndrome): an analysis of 400 cases. *Dis Colon Rectum* 1986;29:203–210.

of the gut to undiluted enteral formula results in frequent loose stools or diarrhea. High infusion rate (> 50 mL per hour), certainly when hyperosmolar enteral formulas are used, is a possible factor. Another possible cause is lactose intolerance. Better adaptation can be achieved by a very gradual increase in the amount and by substitution of lactose-free formulas. Dilution of hyperosmolar solutions reduces diarrhea, but dilution of iso-osmolar solutions does not.

In any event, analysis of the stool is warranted, and the examination should include determination of pH, leukocytes, muscle fibers, fat, pathogenic bacteria, osmolality, occult blood, and 24-hour volume. Specific attention is needed to identify a possible *C. difficile* infection.

Adynamic Ileus

Adynamic ileus may be mild or commonly may progress to significant cecal distention. It occurs invariably in GBS, after exploratory abdominal surgery in patients with multi-trauma, and as a side effect of medication (opioids).[10]

The typical presentation is great discomfort but little pain from distention. Vomiting may occur. No visible peristalsis and absolute silence on auscultation are characteristic. In a few patients, the disorder progresses to life-threatening acute colonic pseudo-obstruction (Ogilvie syndrome).[23,67,73,74,84] Pain, distention, and tympany are more likely to be evident on physical examination. Perforation may occur, but in most patients recovery is possible without surgical intervention.

The possible causes of adynamic ileus are summarized in Table 58.3, and potential triggers should be eliminated. (For a complete overview of causes, see an analysis of 400 cases.[83])

The pathophysiologic explanation remains unclear. In GBS, as well as in other etiologic disorders, sympathetic overdrive may be operative as a form of dysautonomia. The incidence in GBS is low (2%–5%), and cecal perforation is rare,

although it was documented in the Massachusetts General Hospital series.[72] In our series of patients with severe GBS, adynamic ileus developed in 15%, but only a few instances seemed correlated with dysautonomia (Figure 58.3). Preexisting conditions, such as abdominal surgery, and incremental doses of opioids for pain management, were dominant causes.[9]

Abdominal films-plain or CT confirm the diagnosis (Figure 58.4), usually showing involvement of the cecum and ascending or transverse colon. Air–fluid levels are present. Management consists of discontinuing the administration of opioids[31] or any anticholinergic agents, placement of oral and rectal tubes, adequate hydration, no oral intake, and correction of electrolyte abnormalities if they arise.[27] Total parental nutrition may be needed for several days (Chapter 18).

The recent discovery of the remarkable effect of neostigmine may result in its acceptance as a first-line agent, particularly since a colonic decompression tube is technically difficult to use.[26] Because neostigmine may slow conduction of the atrioventricular node, it is contraindicated in patients with bradycardia, hypotension, recent myocardial infarction, previous β-blocker therapy, bronchospasm, or renal failure. Neostigmine increases parasympathetic stimulation, which enhances colonic activity through binding to the motilin receptor. A single intravenous dose of 2 mg of neostigmine may restore colonic function. The dose is repeated, or a scheduled dose is needed. It is prudent to have 1 mg of atropine available should bradycardia occur.[1,63,70,82]

If symptoms persist for more than 2–3 days, decompressive colonoscopy may be indicated.

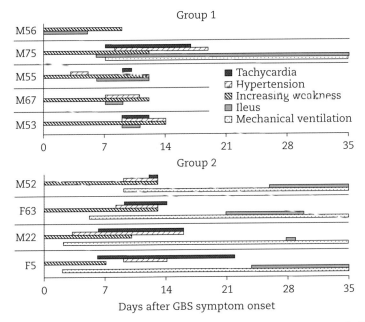

FIGURE 58.3: Adynamic ileus in Guillain-Barré syndrome (GBS). Group 1, patients with GBS and worsening strength. Note the relation of ileus onset to dysautonomic features; group 2, patients with GBS in the phase of improving strength.

F, female; M, male; age in years.

From Burns TM, Lawn ND, Low PA, et al. Adynamic ileus in severe Guillain-Barré syndrome. *Muscle Nerve* 2001; 24:963–965. With permission of John Wiley & Sons.

Tube cecostomy (Figure 58.4c) is considered if cecal distention persists.[15] Perforation is imminent when cecal dilatation reaches 10 cm on plain abdominal films.

Neurogenic Bowel in Spinal Cord Injury

Neurogenic bowel disorder in acute spinal cord injury results in reduced reflex-mediated defecation. The gastrocolic reflex (feeding triggering intestinal peristalsis) may be muted, colon transit time is slowed, and anorectal dyssynergia (anal sphincter contraction with rectal contraction) may occur.[34,79]

Bowel dysfunction may have different patterns related to the level of spinal injury. Injury above the sacral segments of the spinal cord results in reflexic (upper motor neuron) bowel, and defecation cannot be initiated by voluntary relaxation of the external anal sphincter. Injury at the sacral segments or cauda equina results in areflexic (lower motor neuron) bowel, causing fecal incontinence and hypotonic sphincter. Bowel care is different in each of these types.

Bowel management for reflexic bowel includes insertion of a glycol-based suppository or a small volume of bisacodyl in a saline enema,[40] followed by digital stimulation with gentle rolling of a finger while the patient is upright or lying on one side. In contrast, the routine for areflexic bowel is a Valsalva maneuver and manual evacuation of the entire rectum. This technique is preferred for patients in the spinal shock phase.

Major parts of bowel care also include a diet of at least 15 g of fiber daily and an additional 500 mL of fluid to improve stool consistency. Prokinetic agents may cause serious side effects and are generally not effective.

Abdominal Trauma

Patients with closed head injury may have obvious or occult chest, urogenital, or abdominal trauma.[5] A detailed discussion is beyond the scope of this book and outside the purview of the neurointensivist. The issues are highly complex, and trauma may involve many intra-abdominal structures. It is mentioned here only to alert attending neurologists to the possibility of its existence.

It is important to consider abdominal trauma in traumatic brain injury. Abdominal findings on examination could be minimal in patients with profound lesions, such as small bowel perforation, hepatic lacerations, pancreatic transection,

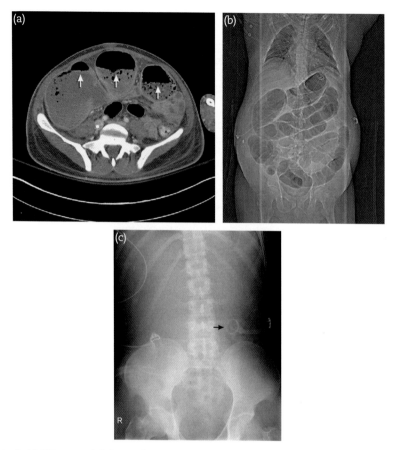

FIGURE 58.4. (a, b) CT scan and abdominal X-ray in a patient with Guillain-Barré syndrome with adynamic ileus. (c) Tube cecostomy.

and gallbladder injuries.[3,16,39,41,77] Abdominal trauma causing extreme changes in blood pressure and a decrease in hematocrit is most often identified in the emergency department, and patients are transferred to an operating room for surgical exploration. It has been emphasized that signs of blood loss and hollow viscus injury may be subtle, and a normal ultrasound scan does not exclude injury.[41]

Without question, frequent clinical assessment of the abdomen in a recently admitted patient with traumatic brain injury is essential. Baseline liver function tests and serum amylase levels could be helpful. In many patients with a history of possible intra-abdominal injury, ultrasonography or abdominal computed tomography (CT) scanning is needed. Hemodynamically unstable patients require diagnostic peritoneal lavage or laparotomy. In general, increasing abdominal tenderness and a marked decrease in hematocrit without an obvious source of bleeding should prompt CT scanning. Computed tomography is valuable for detecting free intraperitoneal blood and completely images

of the intra-abdominal solid organs. Considerable amounts of free fluid, but absent solid organ injury on CT, increase the probability of finding organ injury, and exploratory laparotomy is needed.[61,68] Contrast medium may be administered, but its additional diagnostic value is uncertain. Administration of a contrast agent may complicate the interpretation of CT scans of the brain, because traumatic subarachnoid blood, if present, may not be differentiated from hyperdense contrast material. Ultrasound evaluation is also useful and cost-effective, but the identification of parenchymal injury is more difficult. With multiple views, sensitivity may reach 90% and specificity 98%.[62] Some of the detected findings, such as small hematomas in the liver, may be clinically irrelevant. One study suggested that repeat abdominal examination and normal abdominal CT findings beyond the first day sufficiently exclude major injury.[57] An algorithm is shown in Figure 58.5.[3]

Trauma surgeons should be consulted if there is any doubt about whether abdominal injury is present.

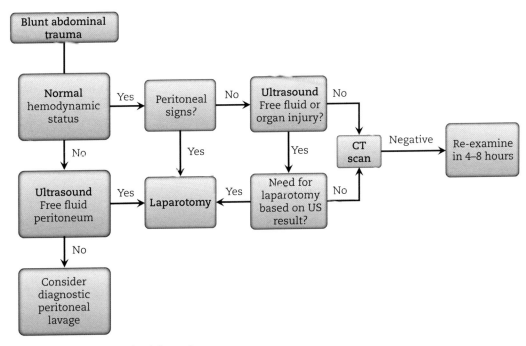

FIGURE 58.5: Algorithm for abdominal trauma.

CT, computed tomography; US, ultrasound.

Modified from Amoroso TA. Evaluation of the patient with blunt abdominal trauma: an evidence based approach. *Emerg Med Clin N Am* 1999;17:63–75. With permission of W. B. Saunders Company.

CONCLUSIONS

- The severity of gastrointestinal hemorrhage should be assessed immediately. Potentially ominous clinical signs are orthostatic hypotension and tachycardia with change in position. Tachycardia with position change but without change in blood pressure indicates a 15% loss of volume, and decrease in blood pressure to 100 mm Hg with position change indicates a 25% or greater volume loss.
- Endoscopy is indicated in patients with gastrointestinal bleeding and need for transfusion.
- Management in gastrointestinal hemorrhage is focused on volume resuscitation and preservation of adequate blood pressure. Proton-pump inhibitors should be administered early.
- Diarrhea is most commonly associated with enteral nutrition and release of fecal impaction related to narcotic analgesics or dehydration.
- Adynamic ileus is usually treated with oral and rectal tubes, no oral intake, and intravenous neostigmine.

- Traumatic abdominal injury may be subtle, and CT scanning and repeat examination for abdominal tenderness are needed within the first day of admission. Laparotomy is required in hemodynamically unstable patients.

REFERENCES

1. Abeyta BJ, Albrecht RM, Schermer CR. Retrospective study of neostigmine for the treatment of acute colonic pseudo-obstruction. *Am Surg* 2001;67:265–268.
2. Ali T, Harty RF. Stress-induced ulcer bleeding in critically ill patients. *Gastroenterol Clin N Am* 2009;38:245–265.
3. Amoroso TA. Evaluation of the patient with blunt abdominal trauma: an evidence based approach. *Emerg Med Clin N Am* 1999;17:63–75.
4. Bardou M, Quenot JP, Barkun A. Stress-related mucosal disease in the critically ill patient. *Nat Rev Gastroenterol Hepatol* 2015;12:98–107.
5. Bent C, Iyngkaran T, Power N, et al. Urological injuries following trauma. *Clin Radiol* 2008;63:1361–1371.
6. Birkett DH. Gastrointestinal tract bleeding: common dilemmas in management. *Surg Clin N Am* 1991;71:1259–1269.

7. Bresalier RS. The clinical significance and patho-physiology of stress-related gastric mucosal hemorrhage. *J Clin Gastroenterol* 1991;13 Suppl 2:S35–S43.

8. Browder W, Cerise EJ, Litwin MS. Impact of emergency angiography in massive lower gastro-intestinal bleeding. *Ann Surg* 1986;204:530–536.

9. Burns TM, Lawn ND, Low PA, Camilleri M, Wijdicks EFM. Adynamic ileus in severe Guillain-Barre syndrome. *Muscle Nerve* 2001;24:963–965.

10. Carlson GL, Dark P. Acute intestinal failure. *Curr Opin Crit Care* 2010;16:347–352.

11. Cash BD. Evidence-based medicine as it applies to acid suppression in the hospitalized patient. *Crit Care Med* 2002;30:S373–S378.

12. Chan KH, Lai EC, Tuen H, et al. Prospective double-blind placebo-controlled randomized trial on the use of ranitidine in preventing postoperative gastroduodenal complications in high-risk neuro-surgical patients. *J Neurosurg* 1995;82:413–417.

13. Chan KH, Mann KS, Lai EC, et al. Factors influ-encing the development of gastrointestinal complications after neurosurgery: results of mul-tivariate analysis. *Neurosurgery* 1989;25:378–382.

14. Cheon JH, Kim JS, Ko SJ, et al. Risk fac-tors for upper gastrointestinal rebleeding in critically ill patients. *Hepatogastroenterology* 2007;54:766–769.

15. Chevallier P, Marcy PY, Francois E, et al. Controlled transperitoneal percutaneous cecos-tomy as a therapeutic alternative to the endo-scopic decompression for Ogilvie's syndrome. *Am J Gastroenterol* 2002;97:471–474.

16. Chiang WK. Isolated jejunal perforation from nonpenetrating abdominal trauma. *Am J Emerg Med* 1993;11:473–475.

17. Clason AE, Macleod DA, Elton RA. Clinical fac-tors in the prediction of further haemorrhage or mortality in acute upper gastrointestinal haemor-rhage. *Br J Surg* 1986;73:985–987.

18. Cook DJ, Fuller HD, Guyatt GH, et al. Risk fac-tors for gastrointestinal bleeding in critically ill patients. Canadian Critical Care Trials Group. *N Engl J Med* 1994;330:377–381.

19. Cook DJ, Guyatt GH, Salena BJ, Laine LA. Endoscopic therapy for acute nonvariceal upper gastrointestinal hemorrhage: a meta-analysis. *Gastroenterology* 1992;102:139–148.

20. Cote GA, Howden CW. Potential adverse effects of proton pump inhibitors. *Curr Gastroenterol Rep* 2008;10:208–214.

21. Cushing H. Peptic ulcer and the interbrain. *Surg Obst* 1932;55:1–34.

22. Davenport RJ, Dennis MS, Warlow CP. Gastrointestinal hemorrhage after acute stroke. *Stroke* 1996;27:421–424.

23. De Giorgio R, Knowles CH. Acute colonic pseudo-obstruction. *Br J Surg* 2009;96:229–239.

24. Eastwood GL. Endoscopy in gastrointestinal bleeding: are we beginning to realize the dream? *J Clin Gastroenterol* 1992;14:187–191.

25. Elmunzer BJ, Young SD, Inadomi JM, Schoenfeld P, Laine L. Systematic review of the predictors of recurrent hemorrhage after endoscopic hemo-static therapy for bleeding peptic ulcers. *Am J Gastroenterol* 2008;103:2625–2632.

26. Elsner JL, Smith JM, Ensor CR. Intravenous neostigmine for postoperative acute colonic pseudo-obstruction. *Ann Pharmacother* 2012;46:430–435.

27. Fazel A, Verne GN. New solutions to an old prob-lem: acute colonic pseudo-obstruction. *J Clin Gastroenterol* 2005;39:17–20.

28. Ferrera PC, Verdile VP, Bartfield JM, Snyder HS, Salluzzo RF. Injuries distracting from intraab-dominal injuries after blunt trauma. *Am J Emerg Med* 1998;16:145–149.

29. Fleischer D. Endoscopic therapy of upper gastro-intestinal bleeding in humans. *Gastroenterology* 1986;90:217–234.

30. Fleischer DE. Endoscopic control of upper gastrointestinal bleeding. *J Clin Gastroenterol* 1990;12 Suppl 2:S41–S47.

31. Frantzides CT, Cowles V, Salaymeh B, Tekin E, Condon RE. Morphine effects on human colonic myoelectric activity in the postoperative period. *Am J Surg* 1992;163:144–148.

32. Fromm D. Endoscopic coagulation for gastroint-estinal bleeding. *N Engl J Med* 1987;316:1652–1654.

33. Fruhwald S, Holzer P, Metzler H. Intestinal motil-ity disturbances in intensive care patients patho-genesis and clinical impact. *Intens Care Med* 2007;33:36–44.

34. Gore RM, Mintzer RA, Calenoff L. Gastrointestinal complications of spinal cord injury. *Spine (Phila Pa 1976)* 1981;6:538–544.

35. Graham DY, Schwartz JT. The spectrum of the Mallory-Weiss tear. *Medicine (Baltimore)* 1978;57:307–318.

36. Gudeman SK, Wheeler CB, Miller JD, Halloran LG, Becker DP. Gastric secretory and muco-sal injury response to severe head trauma. *Neurosurgery* 1983;12:175–179.

37. Halloran LG, Zfass AM, Gayle WE, Wheeler CB, Miller JD. Prevention of acute gastrointestinal complications after severe head injury: a con-trolled trial of cimetidine prophylaxis. *Am J Surg* 1980;139:44–48.

38. Heidelbaugh JJ, Goldberg KL, Inadomi JM. Overutilization of proton pump inhibitors: a review of cost-effectiveness and risk. *Am J Gastroenterol* 2009;104 Suppl 2:S27–S32.

39. Horst HM, Bivins BA. Pancreatic transection: a concept of evolving injury. *Arch Surg* 1989;124:1093–1095.
40. House JG, Stiens SA. Pharmacologically initiated defecation for persons with spinal cord injury: effectiveness of three agents. *Arch Phys Med Rehabil* 1997;78:1062–1065.
41. Jansen JO, Yule SR, Loudon MA. Investigation of blunt abdominal trauma. *BMJ* 2008;336:938–942.
42. Kamada T, Fusamoto H, Kawano S, Noguchi M, Hiramatsu K. Gastrointestinal bleeding following head injury: a clinical study of 433 cases. *J Trauma* 1977;17:44–47.
43. Kantorova I, Svoboda P, Scheer P, et al. Stress ulcer prophylaxis in critically ill patients: a randomized controlled trial. *Hepatogastroenterology* 2004;51:757–761.
44. Karch SB. Upper gastrointestinal bleeding as a complication of intracranial disease. *J Neurosurg* 1972;37:27–29.
45. Khuroo MS, Yattoo GN, Javid G, et al. A comparison of omeprazole and placebo for bleeding peptic ulcer. *N Engl J Med* 1997;336:1054–1058.
46. Kim BC, Cheon JH, Kim TI, Kim WH. Risk factors and the role of bedside colonoscopy for lower gastrointestinal hemorrhage in critically ill patients. *Hepatogastroenterology* 2008;55:2108–2111.
47. Kohler B, Riemann JF. Upper GI-bleeding: value and consequences of emergency endoscopy and endoscopic treatment. *Hepatogastroenterology* 1991;38:198–200.
48. Krag M, Perner A, Wetterslev J, Wise MP, Hylander Moller M. Stress ulcer prophylaxis versus placebo or no prophylaxis in critically ill patients: a systematic review of randomized clinical trials with meta-analysis and trial sequential analysis. *Intens Care Med* 2014;40:11–22.
49. Kupfer Y, Cappell MS, Tessler S. Acute gastrointestinal bleeding in the intensive care unit: the intensivist's perspective. *Gastroenterol Clin N Am* 2000;29:275–307.
50. Laine L. Multipolar electrocoagulation in the treatment of active upper gastrointestinal tract hemorrhage: a prospective controlled trial. *N Engl J Med* 1987;316:1613–1617.
51. Laine L, Takeuchi K, Tarnawski A. Gastric mucosal defense and cytoprotection: bench to bedside. *Gastroenterology* 2008;135:41–60.
52. Lasky MR, Metzler MH, Phillips JO. A prospective study of omeprazole suspension to prevent clinically significant gastrointestinal bleeding from stress ulcers in mechanically ventilated trauma patients. *J Trauma* 1998;44:527–533.
53. Laterre PF, Horsmans Y. Intravenous omeprazole in critically ill patients: a randomized, crossover study comparing 40 with 80 mg plus 8 mg/hour on intragastric pH. *Crit Care Med* 2001;29:1931–1935.
54. Lau JY, Barkun A, Fan DM, et al. Challenges in the management of acute peptic ulcer bleeding. *Lancet* 2013;381:2033–2043.
55. Levy MJ, Seelig CB, Robinson NJ, Ranney JE. Comparison of omeprazole and ranitidine for stress ulcer prophylaxis. *Dig Dis Sci* 1997;42:1255–1259.
56. Liolios A, Oropello JM, Benjamin E. Gastrointestinal complications in the intensive care unit. *Clin Chest Med* 1999;20:329–345.
57. Livingston DH, Lavery RF, Passannante MR, et al. Admission or observation is not necessary after a negative abdominal computed tomographic scan in patients with suspected blunt abdominal trauma: results of a prospective, multi-institutional trial. *J Trauma* 1998;44:273–280.
58. Lu WY, Rhoney DH, Boling WB, Johnson JD, Smith TC. A review of stress ulcer prophylaxis in the neurosurgical intensive care unit. *Neurosurgery* 1997;41:416–425.
59. MacLaren R, Jarvis CL, Fish DN. Use of enteral nutrition for stress ulcer prophylaxis. *Ann Pharmacother* 2001;35:1614–1623.
60. Marik PE, Vasu T, Hirani A, Pachinburavan M. Stress ulcer prophylaxis in the new millennium: a systematic review and meta-analysis. *Crit Care Med* 2010;38:2222–2228.
61. McAnena OJ, Moore EE, Marx JA. Initial evaluation of the patient with blunt abdominal trauma. *Surg Clin N Am* 1990;70:495–515.
62. McKenney MG, McKenney KL, Hong JJ, et al. Evaluating blunt abdominal trauma with sonography: a cost analysis. *Am Surg* 2001;67:930–934.
63. McNamara R, Mihalakis MJ. Acute colonic pseudo-obstruction: rapid correction with neostigmine in the emergency department. *J Emerg Med* 2008;35:167–170.
64. Mostafa G, Sing RF, Matthews BD, et al. The economic benefit of practice guidelines for stress ulcer prophylaxis. *Am Surg* 2002;68:146–150.
65. Muller T, Barkun AN, Martel M. Non-variceal upper GI bleeding in patients already hospitalized for another condition. *Am J Gastroenterol* 2009;104:330–339.
66. Mutlu GM, Mutlu EA, Factor P. GI complications in patients receiving mechanical ventilation. *Chest* 2001;119:1222–1241.
67. Nanni G, Garbini A, Luchetti P, Ronconi P, Castagneto M. Ogilvie's syndrome (acute colonic pseudo-obstruction): review of the literature (October 1948 to March 1980) and report of four additional cases. *Dis Colon Rectum* 1982;25:157–166.

68. Ng AK, Simons RK, Torreggiani WC, et al. Intra-abdominal free fluid without solid organ injury in blunt abdominal trauma: an indication for laparotomy. *J Trauma* 2002;52:1134–1140.

69. O'Donnell MJ, Kapral MK, Fang J, et al. Gastrointestinal bleeding after acute ischemic stroke. *Neurology* 2008;71:650–655.

70. Ponec RJ, Saunders MD, Kimmey MB. Neostigmine for the treatment of acute colonic pseudo-obstruction. *N Engl J Med* 1999;341:137–141.

71. Quenot JP, Thiery N, Barbar S. When should stress ulcer prophylaxis be used in the ICU? *Curr Opin Crit Care* 2009;15:139–143.

72. Ropper AH, Wijdicks EFM, Truax BT. *Guillain-Barré Syndrome*. Vol. 34. Oxford: Oxford University Press; 1991.

73. Saunders MD, Kimmey MB. Colonic pseudo-obstruction: the dilated colon in the ICU. *Semin Gastrointest Dis* 2003;14:20–27.

74. Saunders MD, Kimmey MB. Systematic review: acute colonic pseudo-obstruction. *Aliment Pharmacol Ther* 2005;22:917–925.

75. Schirmer CM, Kornbluth J, Heilman CB, Bhardwaj A. Gastrointestinal prophylaxis in neurocritical care. *Neurocrit Care* 2012;16:184–193.

76. Sesler JM. Stress-related mucosal disease in the intensive care unit: an update on prophylaxis. *AACN Adv Crit Care* 2007;18:119–126.

77. Sharma O. Blunt gallbladder injuries: presentation of twenty-two cases with review of the literature. *J Trauma* 1995;39:576–580.

78. Spirt MJ, Stanley S. Update on stress ulcer prophylaxis in critically ill patients. *Crit Care Nurse* 2006;26:18–20, 22–18.

79. Stiens SA, Bergman SB, Goetz LL. Neurogenic bowel dysfunction after spinal cord injury: clinical evaluation and rehabilitative management. *Arch Phys Med Rehabil* 1997;78:S86–S102.

80. Swain CP, Storey DW, Bown SG, et al. Nature of the bleeding vessel in recurrently bleeding gastric ulcers. *Gastroenterology* 1986;90:595–608.

81. Tanaka S, Mori T, Ohara H, Takaku A, Suzuki J. Gastrointestinal bleeding in cases of ruptured cerebral aneurysms. *Acta Neurochir (Wien)* 1979;48:223–230.

82. Turegano-Fuentes F, Munoz-Jimenez F, Del Valle-Hernandez E, et al. Early resolution of Ogilvie's syndrome with intravenous neostigmine: a simple, effective treatment. *Dis Colon Rectum* 1997;40:1353–1357.

83. Vanek VW, Al-Salti M. Acute pseudo-obstruction of the colon (Ogilvie's syndrome): an analysis of 400 cases. *Dis Colon Rectum* 1986;29:203–210.

84. Vantrappen G. Acute colonic pseudo-obstruction. *Lancet* 1993;341:152–153.

85. Villanueva C, Colomo A, Bosch A, et al. Transfusion strategies for acute upper gastrointestinal bleeding. *N Engl J Med* 2013;368:11–21.

86. Watts CC, Clark K. Gastric acidity in the comatose patient. *J Neurosurg* 1969;30:107–109.

87. Wijdicks EFM, Fulgham JR, Batts KP. Gastrointestinal bleeding in stroke. *Stroke* 1994;25:2146–2148.

88. Yang YX, Lewis JD. Prevention and treatment of stress ulcers in critically ill patients. *Semin Gastrointest Dis* 2003;14:11–19.

89. Zed PJ, Loewen PS, Slavik RS, Marra CA. Meta-analysis of proton pump inhibitors in treatment of bleeding peptic ulcers. *Ann Pharmacother* 2001;35:1528–1534.

59

Management of Nosocomial Infections

A nosocomial infection is arbitrarily defined as any infection developing 48 hours after admission. This definition implies that there is no clinical or laboratory evidence of infection in the first 2 days and no infection incubating on admission. An infection manifested earlier is considered community-acquired.[47] Nosocomial infections are much more likely in intensive care units (ICUs) because of the severity of the underlying illness, and the multiplicity of devices and instruments. Published epidemiologic surveys have unequivocally shown that healthcare-associated infection contributes greatly to morbidity, mortality, and, often, length of stay in the ICU, with attendant extravagant costs.[12] Cross-contamination from patient to patient by the hands of medical staff ultimately remains a common and possibly most preventable cause. Adherence to the use of masks, gowns, and gloves remains suboptimal.[19]

Prevalence studies of nosocomial infections in the neurosciences intensive care unit (NICU) are few, and it is clear that the results of available prevalence studies in other medical ICUs cannot be extrapolated to acutely ill neurologic patients.[74] For example, a prospective study in 208 critically ill patients admitted to a medical–surgical ICU in Spain reported a 25% rate of nosocomial pneumonia, mostly from *Staphylococcus aureus*. In contrast, a survey in a neurosurgery department that included intensive care beds reported much lower incidences (approximately 10%), but a five-fold increase in nosocomial pneumonia in comatose patients.[63]

The Centers for Disease Control National Healthcare Safety Network (NHSN) publishes a semiannual report (www.cdc.gov) that includes healthcare-associated infections reported voluntarily by NHSN facilities. Increased use of electronic medical records may improve surveillance.[79]

This chapter discusses the prophylaxis, recognition, and treatment of nosocomial infections in patients with an acute neurologic disorder.

NOSOCOMIAL PNEUMONIA

In immunocompetent patients, nosocomial pneumonias are most often caused by bacterial pathogens. In the NICU, bacterial pneumonias are typically caused by gastric and oropharyngeal colonization with aerobic bacteria and repeated small-volume aspiration during sleep, certainly in patients with impaired gag reflexes.[70] The pharynx can be colonized by gram-negative bacilli (*Escherichia coli, Klebsiella, Enterobacter, Proteus, Pseudomonas aeruginosa, Serratia, Acinetobacter, Legionella pneumophila*), gram-positive cocci (*Staphylococcus aureus, Streptococcus pneumoniae*), and, less often, gram-negative cocci (*Haemophilus influenzae, Branhamella catarrhalis*).[15,16,65,66] Although anaerobic bacteria are frequently isolated in cultures, in critically ill neurologic patients the anaerobic presence in the oropharynx often changes into a predominance of gram-negative rods. *Legionella pneumophila* typically strikes in epidemics and particularly in surgical patients. This very virulent pathogen may hide in humidifiers, nebulizers, ventilation bags, tracheostomy tubes, and tap water.[68]

In neurologic patients, the cause of nosocomial pneumonia is often aspiration associated with impaired swallowing mechanism. The distinction between aspiration pneumonia and nosocomial pneumonia, therefore, often is academic. Other risk factors for nosocomial pneumonia are age over 70 years, mechanical ventilation, colonization of the oropharynx, use of H_2-blockers with or without antacids,[70] daily change of ventilator circuits, underlying chronic lung disease, and reintubation.[69] Infections are predictors of poor outcome in acute stroke. Clinical trials to investigate the effect of prophylactic antibiotics (particularly ceftriaxone with potential additional neuroprotective effects) were considered.[73] But two recent clinical trials found antibiotics neither reduced the frequency of pneumonia nor improved outcome after stroke when administered preemptively.[38,75]

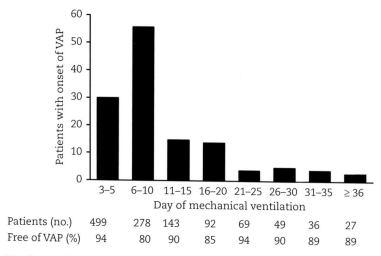

	3–5	6–10	11–15	16–20	21–25	26–30	31–35	≥ 36
Patients (no.)	499	278	143	92	69	49	36	27
Free of VAP (%)	94	80	90	85	94	90	89	89

FIGURE 59.1: Distribution of onset of ventilator-associated pneumonia (VAP).

From Ibrahim EH, Tracy L, Hill C, et al. The occurrence of ventilator-associated pneumonia in a community hospital: risk factors and clinical outcomes. *Chest* 2001;120:555–561. With permission of the American College of Chest Physicians.

A major cause of morbidity in ventilated patients is the development of ventilator-associated pneumonia, which is related to ventilator days[31,37] (Figure 59.1). A prospective study of 132 patients with ventilator-associated pneumonia found that tracheostomy, multiple central venous catheter insertions, reintubation, and the use of antacids were associated factors. *P. aeruginosa* and *S. aureus* were common pathogens. Ventilator-associated pneumonia was frequent within 2 weeks of intubation.[37] Increased mortality has been linked to *P. aeruginosa*, inappropriate antibiotic therapy, and age, but data are derived from medical intensive care units.

The prevention of nosocomial pneumonia in mechanically ventilated patients is very important.[28,34,38] Guidelines for the prevention of nosocomial pneumonia have been published and are regularly updated (see Part XIV, Guidelines).[56] Selective digestive decontamination has been suggested,[14,44] and indeed gram-negative colonization decreased with a suspension of polymyxin 100 mg, tobramycin 80 mg, and amphotericin 500 mg in 10 mL delivered by nasogastric tube and cefotaxime 4–6 grams/day in 4 divided doses for 4 days given intravenously.[20] No difference in the incidence of nosocomial pneumonia or mortality was found in one study.[26] Topical antimicrobial prophylaxis with gentamicin-colistin vancomycin 2% in Orabase every 6 hours significantly reduced oropharyngeal colonization and reduced ventilator-associated pneumonia in a prospective, randomized study.[4] A promising and simple method is continuous aspiration of subglottic secretions, which theoretically may decrease the volume of colonized secretions aspirated into the bronchial tree. A randomized trial in 76 mechanically ventilated patients found a significant reduction in pneumonia and reduction in attributable mortality.[72] A major recent trial in 13 intensive care units (5,939 patients) found either selective digestive decontamination (4 days of cefotaxime, topical tobramycin, colistin, and amphotericin B in the oropharynx and stomach) or selective oropharyngeal decontamination (application of these antibiotics in the oropharynx) reduced mortality, albeit by only 3 percentage points.[20]

Nebulized antibiotics to treat ventilator-associated pneumonia is an attractive new concept (e.g., nebulized colistin) but there is insufficient data to support its use in practice.[82]

CLINICAL FEATURES AND EVALUATION

The clinical diagnosis of nosocomial bronchopneumonia is undisputedly difficult. Fever is a key sign, but the most salient findings remain increased sputum production with a change in its quality to thick, purulent mucus.[10,53] The chest film may be supportive if peripheral infiltrates are demonstrated (Figure 59.2), but the sensitivity and specificity of radiographic abnormalities are low. *P. aeruginosa* is responsible for many of the ventilator-associated pneumonias, with substantial morbidity from acute respiratory distress syndrome (ARDS). The radiographic findings are

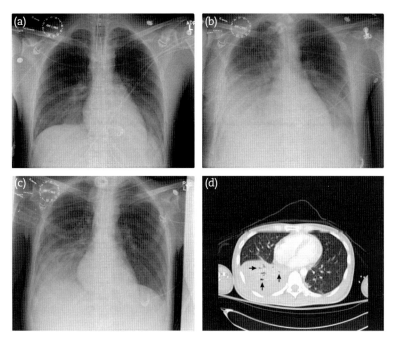

FIGURE 59.2: Development of pulmonary abscess in a patient in prolonged coma.

(a) Bilateral infiltrates. (b) Consolidation of infiltrates. (c) Developing pleural effusion. (d) Pulmonary abscess and air (*arrows*).

nonspecific, typically consisting of bilateral multifocal and diffuse opacities with occasional air-space disease cavities, indicating microabscesses. However, although typical for *P. aeruginosa*, microabscesses were found in only five of 56 studied patients with ventilator-associated pneumonia.[76] The diagnosis in clinical practice is based on the microbiologic diagnosis of a sample obtained by intratracheal suctioning, but the results are often inaccurate. Surveillance definitions for ventilator-associated pneumonia have been published[41] (Table 59.1). Because cultures have an overpowering number of gram-negative bacteria, Gram's stain becomes important. Even if large numbers of single or multiple morphologic types are seen on the sputum Gram stain, only more than 25 polymorphonuclear leukocytes and fewer than 10 contaminating epithelial cells (indicative of the oral cavity rather than the airways) per lower power field suggest nosocomial pneumonia.[49] Alveolar macrophages and elastic fibers suggest that the specimen was obtained from a lung undergoing necrosis. Bronchoalveolar lavage during bronchoscopy in patients on mechanical ventilators may increase detection if the clinical diagnosis is uncertain.[11] The yield of blood cultures in nosocomial pneumonias is only 5%. Open lung biopsy or transthoracic needle aspiration is a measure of last resort. Routine microbiologic cultures of aspirates before the onset of ventilator pneumonia may identify microorganisms that mostly are not involved with later pneumonia and cannot be used to guide antimicrobial agents.[2,35]

Treatment

The decision to treat pulmonary infiltrates is problematic. The empirical use of antibiotics to avoid missing an infection has unfortunately almost become a "traditional approach." A useful scoring system (the clinical pulmonary infection score) has been proposed by Pugin and colleagues[58]

TABLE 59.1. COMMONLY FOUND ORGANISMS IN ASPIRATION PNEUMONIA

Community Acquired	Healthcare Acquired
Haemophilus influenzae	Anaerobes *Streptococcus*
Streptococcus pneumonia	Other otopharyngeal
Anaerobes	*Streptococcus aureus*
Other otopharyngeal	*Enterobacteriaceae*
Streptococcus	*Pseudomonas aeruginosa*

TABLE 59.2. THE MODIFIED PULMONARY INFECTION SCORE

CPIS Points	0	1	2
Tracheal secretions	Rare	Abundant	Abundant + purulent
Chest X-ray infiltrates	No infiltrate	Diffuse	Localized
Temperature, °C	≥ 36.5 and ≤ 38.4	≥ 38.5 and ≤ 38.9	≥ 39 or ≤ 36
Leukocytes count, per mm^3	$\geq 4,000$ and $\leq 11,000$	$< 4,000$ or $> 11,000$	$< 4,000$ or $>11,000$ + band forms $\geq 50\%$
PaO$_2$/FIO$_2$ mm Hg	> 240 or ARDS		≤ 240 and no evidence of ARDS
Microbiology	Negative		Positive

Definitions of abbreviations: ARDS, acute respiratory distress syndrome; CPIS, clinical pulmonary infection score.
The modified CPIS at baseline was calculated from the first five variables. The CPIS Gram and CPIS culture were calculated from the CPIS baseline score by adding two more points when Gram stains or culture were positive. A score of more than 6 at baseline or after incorporating the Gram stains (CPIS gram) or culture (CPIS culture) results was considered suggestive of pneumonia.
Fartoukh M, Maître B, Honoré S, et al. Diagnosing pneumonia during mechanical ventilation: the Clinical Pulmonary Infection Score revisited. *Am J Respir Crit Care Med* 2003;168:173–179.

(Table 59.2). This scoring system (requiring microbiology data) found originally a sensitivity of 93% and specificity of 100%, but not in subsequent studies. A revision of the clinical pulmonary infection score is shown in Table 59.2. Other scoring systems are currently being developed.[81]

In most patients, a broad spectrum of empirical treatment is initiated.[1] Some recommended empirical treatment regimens start with a third-generation cephalosporin with an aminoglycoside, but a third- or fourth-generation cephalosporin alone is sufficient, avoiding the toxicity of many of the amino-glycosides.[63,67] Cefepime may be preferred in *P. aeruginosa*. The broad-spectrum quinolones can be very useful, largely because they penetrate well into secretions and to double cover resistant pseudomonas. The suggested treatment is summarized in Table 59.3.[47] Vancomycin is the preferred drug if *S. aureus* pneumonia is suspected. (Dosing of vancomycin should be

carefully monitored. Vancomycin dose of more than 4 grams a day increases nephrotoxicity and need for dialysis.[46]) The treatment of anaerobic pneumonias is best initiated with the use of ertapenem. Poor outcome after hospital-acquired pneumonia can be predicted using certain clinical factors.[24]

INFECTIONS RELATED TO INTRAVENOUS CATHETERS

Transient bacteremias are often related to placement of catheters in ICUs, including NICUs. Mortality attributed to nosocomial bloodstream infections is high, and a study also found that time in the ICU was significantly prolonged in survivors.[54,55,80] The risk of catheter infection seems greater in internal jugular catheters than in subclavian catheters. In addition, an analysis of the potential risk factors in catheter-related infections emphasized that transparent dressings were associated with a significantly higher risk than gauze dressings,[51,59,60] but the link remains inconclusive. Central venous catheter infections may be prevented if catheter insertion is done with maximal aseptic techniques, topical mupirocin,[36] antibiotic-coated catheters,[39] and obsessional use of cutaneous antiseptics. Recent prospective trials suggested that impregnating catheters with minocycline and rifampin significantly prevents colonization and catheter-related bacteremia,[17,61] with a low likelihood of antibiotic resistance.

Frequent manipulations increase the incidence of catheter-related infections to approximately 10%. Prevention guidelines have diverged on whether to replace the catheter with a new puncture or to change the guidewire. Proponents of guidewire change argue that a new puncture only introduces new unnecessary risks of

TABLE 59.3. INITIAL ANTIMICROBIAL TREATMENT FOR HOSPITAL-ACQUIRED OR VENTILATOR-ASSOCIATED PNEUMONIA

Antipseudomonal cephalosporin

Cefepime	1–2 gram every 8–12 hours
Ceftazidime	2 gram every 8 hours

or

β-lactam/β-lactamase inhibitor

Piperacillin/tazobactam plus	4.5 gram every 6 hours

Antipseudomonal fluoroquinolone

Ciprofloxacin	400 mg every 8 hours
Levofloxacin	750 mg every day

complications and that infection rates between guidewire exchange and new puncture are similar in prospective studies. Indeed, a controlled clinical study found that replacement of central venous catheters every 3 days did not prevent infection but rather, as expected, increased medical complications.[13] Catheter-related sepsis is more common in patients with triple-lumen catheters, which are usually considered when multiple sites for venous access are required. Typically, these catheters are needed in patients with frequent administration of electrolytes, blood products, and parenteral alimentation. The risk of catheter-related infections increases threefold when these types of catheters are used.[64]

Coagulase-negative staphylococci (*Staphylococcus epidermidis* accounts for more than 70%) are most frequently isolated from cultures, followed by *S. aureus, Enterococcus* species, *P. aeruginosa, Candida* species, *Enterobacter* species, *Acinetobacter* species, and *Serratia* species. *S. aureus* infection is extremely dangerous and can appear fulminantly, with bacteremia terminating in endocarditis and osteomyelitis.

The clinical diagnosis of infection from intravascular catheters usually is based on new-onset fever and colonization of more than 15 colony-forming units in cultures of the catheter tip. Local inflammation may be diagnostic, but only in peripheral catheters.

The diagnosis of catheter-related sepsis is based on two positive blood cultures and is confirmed by semiquantitative catheter cultures obtained by rolling the catheter tip back and forth across the agar plate. Additional blood cultures (two samples not drawn through the catheter) may be helpful.[9] Treatment is guided by the results of the cultures. For empirical treatment of suspected intravenous catheter sepsis, vancomycin and a third-generation cephalosporin are advisable (Table 59.4). Amphotericin or fluconazole may be needed if blood cultures are positive for *Candida* infection.

Phlebitis, one of the most common nosocomial infections, has the potential to become serious. Well-recognized causes of phlebitis are antibiotic infusions (e.g., vancomycin) and placement of a peripheral line into the antecubital vein. The risk is also increased when peripheral catheters are inserted in an emergency, because antisepsis could be less guarded. Early phlebitis is suggested by pain, tenderness, erythema, and swelling; later stages by purulence and a palpable cord. Changing the catheter to another site and treating the phlebitis with wet, cold compresses usually are sufficient. Suppurative peripheral phlebitis, fortunately rare, is a medical emergency, and surgical intervention to remove the infected vein is needed.

NOSOCOMIAL URINARY TRACT INFECTIONS

Of all ICU populations, acutely ill neurologic and neurosurgical patients are at the highest risk for urinary tract infections (Table 59.5). Nosocomial urinary tract infection sharply increases in comatose patients with in-dwelling catheters. Urinary tract infections may potentially cause sepsis syndrome, but bacteremia is often asymptomatic. However, urinary catheterization should keep the urine sterile in most patients. Bacteriuria takes place when catheters have been inserted for weeks. Urinary catheters impregnated with minocycline and rifampin reduce gram-positive infections but not gram-negative bacteria. Routine use is also discouraged because of cost.[17,18] More likely, nosocomial urinary tract infections can be reduced if the prolonged use of catheters can be avoided, which is achievable only by constant questioning of the need for catheterization and consideration of alternative methods, such as condom drainage.

Proper separation of infection from colonization is difficult. Suprapubic or flank pain or

TABLE 59.4. ANTIMICROBIAL TREATMENT OF CATHETER-RELATED BACTEREMIA OR SEPSIS

Vancomycin	15–20 mg/kg IV 12 h
with cefotaxime	1–2 g q6h IV
or	
Vancomycin	2 g q12h IV
with gentamicin	1.5–1.7 mg/kg q8h IV

TABLE 59.5. ANTIMICROBIAL TREATMENT OF NOSOCOMIAL URINARY TRACT INFECTION

Gentamicin	1–1.3 mg/kg q8h IV
or	
Ceftriaxone	1–2 g q24h IV
or	
Ciprofloxacin	0.2–0.4 g q12h IV
or	
Ampicillin	0.5 g q6h IV
with gentamicin	1 mg/kg q8h IV

dysuria has additional diagnostic value but is uncommon in this patient population. The laboratory criteria for urinary tract infection are unclear. Cultures alone may not determine whether significant bacteriuria is present, although 100,000 colony-forming units are at least indicative. New-onset fever and a leukocyte count exceeding 10 cells/mm^3 are highly suggestive of urinary tract infection, and white blood cell casts more strongly indicate involvement of the upper urinary tract.

Urine culture should be repeated if no response is seen in 2 days. Nosocomial urinary tract infections are often caused entirely by *E. coli* and *Proteus mirabilis*, but in patients who earlier received a course of antibiotics, *P. aeruginosa*, *Serratia marcescens*, and *Enterobacter* species are important contenders, with an occasional, far more complicated, emergence of antibiotic-resistant organisms.

Treatment is guided by sensitivity tests or, if the results are not yet available, by the outcome of Gram's stain. Uncomplicated urinary tract infection can be treated with trimethoprim 100 mg orally twice a day for 7 days, or with oral fluoroquinolones. In uncomplicated catheter-associated sepsis, antibiotics are usually administered for 10 days. In most patients, aminoglycosides are effective (Table 59.5), but in patients with gram-positive cocci, vancomycin is the preferred choice. In immunocompromised patients with neutropenia, an aminoglycoside with ceftazidime or cefepime is recommended.

An unusual occurrence in immunocompromised patients with in-dwelling catheters is the emergence of candiduria. Topical irrigation of the bladder with infusions of amphotericin B (50 mg/L of sterile distilled water) or miconazole (50 mg/L) at a rate of 40 mL/hr for 5 days should eradicate candidal cystitis.

NOSOCOMIAL GASTROINTESTINAL INFECTIONS

Nosocomial gastroenteritis is manifested by diarrhea, but the appearance of diarrhea does not imply an infectious cause.

Clostridium difficile has been most often implicated. The presenting features of antibiotic-associated colitis can be subtle, with only a minor increase in the number, weight, and liquid content of stools and in fever, but occurrence is also frequently suggested by leukocytosis, severe abdominal cramping, and abdominal tenderness.[32] Watery diarrhea is much more common

TABLE 59.6. ANTIMICROBIAL TREATMENT OF NOSOCOMIAL GASTROINTESTINAL INFECTIONS*

Discontinuation of antibiotics	
and	
Metronidazole[†]	500 mg q8h PO
or	
Vancomycin	125–250 mg q6h PO

* Virtually always caused by *Clostridium difficile*.
† Drug of choice.

than bloody diarrhea. *Clostridium difficile* can be diagnosed from the stool by an assay for its cytotoxin and may be recovered from the stool in 30%–60% of cultures. Endoscopic confirmation of inflammatory colitis is more specific. However, the prototypical pseudomembranous lesions scattered throughout the bowel mucosa are infrequent, and mild inflammatory changes are more often expected in antibiotic-related diarrhea.

An important risk factor for nosocomial diarrhea is combination antimicrobial therapy.[6,48] In a survey, exposure to second- and third-generation cephalosporins emerged as the major risk factor for nosocomial diarrhea, more frequent than exposure to clindamycin.[48]

Treatment of nosocomial diarrhea associated with *C. difficile* includes the discontinuation of antibiotic therapy, unless it is critical to the patient's survival. The preferred approach is to begin treatment orally with metronidazole; oral vancomycin is reserved for unresponsive infections (Table 59.6). In very mild but persistent cases, cholestyramine (4 g three times a day) is a reasonable approach.

NOSOCOMIAL INFECTIONS IN IMPLANTABLE CENTRAL NERVOUS SYSTEM DEVICES

Patients with a ventriculostomy are at risk for ventriculitis, which has potentially serious consequences. The incidence of ventriculitis in the NICU has decreased, most likely because of the increased use of fiberoptic parenchymal intracranial pressure monitors,[77] and remains very low. Risk factors for ventriculostomy-associated infections are ventricular catheterization lasting more than 5 days, intracerebral hemorrhage with intraventricular extension, and irrigation of the device.[62] The most frequently isolated bacterial agents in ventriculitis are *S. epidermidis* and *aureus*.

TABLE 59.7. COMBINATIONS
OF ANTIMICROBIAL AGENTS
FOR TREATMENT OF NOSOCOMIAL
INFECTIONS ASSOCIATED
WITH IMPLANTABLE CENTRAL
NERVOUS SYSTEM DEVICES

Vancomycin	15–20 mg/kg IV q12h IV
with cefotaxime	2 g q4–6h IV
or	
Vancomycin	2 g q12h IV
with gentamicin	2 mg/kg q8h*

*May result in low cerebrospinal fluid levels.

Ventriculitis is typically asymptomatic early in the course and may become evident only with clinical signs of meningeal irritation and fever. Cultures of the CSF confirm infection, and blood cultures often become positive. Definition of ventriculitis is not entirely clear. Some have suggested any positive CSF culture with fever and reduced glucose.[33] Ventriculostomies may easily cause increased WBC, and some have suggested using CSF lactate level. Once infected, vancomycin with cefotaxime is preferred (Table 59.7).

Impregnating the ventricular catheter with rifampin and clindamycin has been suggested to prevent infection. Early studies suggest benefit.[33,50,78] Most neurosurgeons agree that subcutaneous tunneling and prophylactic administration of antibiotics with IV cefazolin 2g every 8 hours may prevent infections, but firm data are not known. Removal of the catheter after 5 days and meticulous aseptic techniques are probably equally effective.

CHOOSING ANTIBIOTICS

There are some general guidelines that can be used in determining the appropriate antibiotic (Capsule 59.1 and Table 59.8). Penicillins act against gram-positive and gram-negative bacilli. The gram-positive bacilli are *Bacillus anthracis, Clostridium perfringens,* or *Clostridium tetani.* There are many penicillinase-resistant penicillins, and these agents are oxacillin, nafcillin, and dicloxacillin. Its spectrum of activity is for methicillin-sensitive *Staphylococcus aureus* (MSSA). It is active against most streptococci but has no gram-negative or anaerobic activity. The β-lactam and β-lactamase inhibitor combinations are commonly used. They have a good anaerobic activity and increased activity against β-lactamase-producing organisms such as MSSA.

It is not active against methicillin-resistant *Staphylococcus aureus* (MRSA) or penicillin-resistant *Streptococcus pneumoniae.*

First-generation cephalosporins are mostly used. Cefepime is very active against *Pseudomonas aeruginosa,* has an improved gram-positive activity toward *Staphylococcus aureus* and pneumococci, is less likely to induce β-lactamase of *Enterobacter* species, and has very good CNS penetration.

The fluoroquinolones include ciprofloxacin and levofloxacin. These drugs have an excellent tissue penetration with high enteric absorption. It is most active against aerobic gram negative bacteria including the Enterobacteriaceae and active against *Pseudomonas aeruginosa.* It is not reliable against streptococci such as *Streptococcus pneumoniae.*

Vancomycin is the drug of choice for multiple-resistant gram-positive organisms. Vancomycin has significant toxicity that includes infusion-related pruritus and erythematous rash involving face, neck, and upper body, producing a "red man" syndrome.

Linezolid has excellent tissue-distribution but has significant adverse effects that include thrombocytopenia, anemia, and long-term peripheral. It is primarily used to treat MRSA and VRE. Tigecycline is a new agent derived from minocycline and is active against many gram-positive, gram-negative, aerobic, and atypical species. It is very important to note that it is inactive against *Pseudomonas aeruginosa.*

ANTIBIOTIC-RESISTANCE PROBLEM

Experts in infectious disease have recognized the six so-called ESKAPE pathogens. These are *Enterococcus faecium, Staphylococcus aureus, Klebsiella pneumoniae, Acinetobacter baumannii, Pseudomonas aeruginosa,* and *Enterobacter* species. Of all these organisms, gram-negative bacilli (*Klebsiella pneumoniae, Acinetobacter baumannii, Pseudomonas aeruginosa,* and *Enterobacter* species) remain the most challenging microbials to keep in check or even eradicate.

Strains resistant to antibiotics have become more prevalent in recent years.[23,25,29,30,43,45,52] Examples are gram-negative bacilli resistant to third-generation cephalosporins or aminoglycosides, pneumococci resistant to penicillins, and, more significant, enterococci resistant to multiple antibiotics.[7] Important factors are horizontal spread in hospitals, excessive use of antibiotics in intensive care units, and world travel.

CAPSULE 59.1   ANTIBIOTIC TEMPLATE

Despite the culture of over-prescribing, there has been a concern about delay in initiating antibiotic treatment. Tests of antibiotic susceptibility usually report minimum inhibitory concentration semiquantitatively as sensitive, intermediate, or resistant. The carbapenems (imipenem and meropenem) have the broadest antibacterial activity of any antibiotic class and have excellent activity against MSSA, streptococcus, and enterococcus species. The carbapenems are very effective but not preferred, and possibly are contraindicated in patients with acute brain injury at risk of seizures. These antibiotics lower the seizure threshold. The imipenem seizure rates are much higher (3%–33%) than meropenem rates, which are less than 1%, and even the newer carbapenems such as ertapenem may have low risk of seizures. The most common pathogens are shown for easy reference.[27,40,57] The general susceptibility of bacteria to commonly prescribed antibiotics is known and is summarized in the accompanying illustration.

Antibiotic	Staph. Aureus (penicillin-resistant)	Staph. Aureus (methicillin-resistant)	Strep. pneumoniae	Strep. pyogenes	Ent. Faecalis	N. meningitidis	H. influenzae	Escherichia coli	Klebsiella spp.	Proteus mirabilis	Serratia spp.	Pseudomonas aeruginosa	Bacteroides fragilis
Penicillin	●	●	○	◐	○	◐	○	●	●	●	●	●	●
Ampicillin/amoxicillin	●	●	○	◐	○	◐	○	○	●	◐	●	●	●
Amoxicillin/clavulanate	○	●	○	◐	○	●	○	◐	○	◐	○	●	◐
Flucloxacillin	○	●	○	◐	●	●	●	●	●	●	●	●	●
Cefuroxime	◐	●	○	◐	●	●	○	○	○	○	●	●	●
Cefotaxime	◐	●	○	◐	●	◐	◐	○	○	○	●	●	●
Ceftazidime	●	●	○	◐	●	◐	◐	○	○	○	○	◐	●
Erythromycin	○	○	○	○	●	●	●	●	●	●	●	●	◐
Clindamycin	◐	○	○	○	●	●	●	●	●	●	●	●	○
Tetracyclines	○	●	○	◐	●	●	○	○	◐	●	○	●	○
Vancomycin/telcoplanin	○	◐	○	◐	◐	●	●	●	●	●	●	●	●
Linezolid	●	◐	○	◐	○	●	●	●	●	●	●	●	●
Gentamicin/tobramycin/ netilmicin/amikacin	●	○	●	◐	◐	●	●	●	○	○	○	○	●
Co-trimoxazole	●	○	◐	○	◐	●	○	○	◐	○	○	●	◐
Trimethoprim	●	○	○	○	◐	◐	○	○	◐	○	○	●	●
Ciprofloxacin	○	○	○	●	●	●	◐	○	○	◐	○	○	●

◐ Sensitive
● Resistant
● Sensitive but not appropriate therapy
○ Some strains resistant

Template for antibiotics in the NICU.

Gram-negative bacilli are becoming resistant not only to aminoglycosides but also to third-generation cephalosporins and aztreonam. Treatment with imipenem or ciprofloxacin may be effective. *P. aeruginosa* may therefore be treated with these agents, but tobramycin has been successful as well.

Penicillin-resistant pneumococci, consisting of up to 15% of US strains, may be a major problem in the NICU in patients with pneumonia and meningitis. More comprehensive susceptibility testing is needed. Often, pneumococcal strains have a minimal inhibitory concentration of greater than 2 μg/mL and are resistant

Organism	Antimicrobial Agent of Choice	Alternative Agents
Gram-positive cocci (aerobic)		
Staphylococcus aureus		
Non-penicillinase-producing	Penicillin	Vancomycin, cephalosporin
Penicillinase-producing	Nafcillin, oxacillin	Vancomycin, cephalosporin
α-Streptococci (*S. viridans*)	Penicillin	Erythromycin, clindamycin, cephalosporin
β-Streptococci (A, B, C, G)	Penicillin	Cephalosporin, erythromycin
Streptococcus faecalis		
Serious infection	Penicillin or ampicillin and aminoglycoside	Vancomycin and aminoglycoside
Uncomplicated urinary tract infection	Ampicillin	Vancomycin
Streptococcus bovis	Penicillin	Cephalosporin, vancomycin
Streptococcus pneumoniae	Penicillin	Erythromycin, vancomycin, cephalosporin
Gram-positive bacilli (aerobic)		
Corynebacterium, group JK	Vancomycin	
Gram-negative bacilli (aerobic)		
Acinetobacter sp.	Imipenem	Penicillin and gentamicin, aminoglycoside, ceftazidime, trimethoprim-sulfamethoxazole
Campylobacter sp.	Erythromycin or quinolone	Tetracycline, gentamicin
Enterobacter sp.	Imipenem	Cefotaxime, ceftriaxone, ceftazidime, aminoglycoside
Haemophilus influenzae	Third- or fourth-generation cephalosporin	Aminoglycoside, extended-spectrum penicillin
Escherichia coli	Third- or fourth-generation cephalosporin	Trimethoprim-sulfamethoxazole
Klebsiella pneumoniae	Third- or fourth-generation cephalosporin	Aminoglycoside, aztreonam, extended-spectrum penicillin
Legionella sp.	Erythromycin and rifampin	Ciprofloxacin
Proteus mirabilis	Ampicillin	Aminoglycoside, cephalosporin
Other *Proteus* sp.	Cefotaxime, ceftriaxone, ceftazidime	Aminoglycoside, aztreonam, imipenem
Providencia sp.	Cefotaxime, ceftriaxone, ceftazidime	Aminoglycoside, imipenem, extended-spectrum penicillin
Pseudomonas aeruginosa	Aminoglycoside and extended-spectrum penicillin	Ceftazidime, aztreonam, imipenem, cefepime
Salmonella sp.	Cefotaxime, ceftriaxone, quinolone	Ampicillin, trimethoprim-sulfamethoxazole
Serratia marcescens	Cefotaxime, ceftriaxone, ceftazidime	Aminoglycoside, imipenem, aztreonam
Shigella sp.	Quinolone	Cefotaxime, ceftriaxone, ceftazidime
Anaerobes		
Anaerobic streptococci	Penicillin	Clindamycin
Bacteroides sp.		
Oropharyngeal strains	Penicillin or clindamycin	Metronidazole

(*continued*)

TABLE 59.8. CONTINUED

Organism	Antimicrobial Agent of Choice	Alternative Agents
Gastrointestinal strains	Metronidazole	Cefoxitin, clindamycin, imipenem, ticarcillin-clavulanic acid, piperacillin-tazobactam
Clostridium sp. (except *C. difficile*)	Penicillin	Clindamycin, metronidazole, imipenem
Clostridium difficile	Metronidazole	Vancomycin
Other bacteria		
Actinomyces and *Arachnia*	Penicillin G	Tetracycline, clindamycin
Nocardia sp.	Trimethoprim-sulfamethoxazole	Tetracycline, imipenem
Mycobacterium tuberculosis	Isoniazid and rifampin and pyrazinamide and ethambutol	Streptomycin, ciprofloxacin, cycloserine, capreomycin, ethionamide

Modified from Abramowicz M, ed. The choice of antibacterial drugs. *Med Lett Drugs Ther* 1996;38:25–34. With permission of *The Medical Letter*.

to third- and fourth-generation cephalosporins. Management may begin with cefotaxime if the minimal inhibitory concentration is less than 0.25 µg/mL, but in most cases, vancomycin with rifampin, imipenem, or chloramphenicol is required.

Multiple antibiotic-resistant enterococci are less common in NICUs because wound and intra-abdominal infections are less prevalent. MRSA reported to the US Centers for Disease Control (CDC) has shown to be increased in bloodstream infections associated with central venous catheters. Swabs from axillae, nose, and perineum detected 60% of MRSA in a critically ill population, but throat and rectal swabs have a higher sensitivity (76%).[3,7] Vancomycin is the first-line therapy for MRSA (15–20 mg/kg dose IV every 12 hours). Vancomycin trough levels need to be monitored, aiming at concentrations between 15 and 20 mcg/mL. Management remains highly complex because many strains are resistant to penicillin, ampicillin, aminoglycosides, and vancomycin. The newer antibiotics linezolid and quinupristin-dalfopristin have both been approved for MRSA and vancomycin-resistant enterococci. Linezolid (Zyvox) is administered intravenously (600 mg every 12 hours for up to 4 weeks).[22] Headache remains a side effect in one of 10 patients and is more common than diarrhea and nausea. The dalfopristin-quinupristin combination (Synercid) is also used for treatment of vancomycin-resistant enterococcus infections (7.5 mg/kg/dose infused IV over 1 hour every 8–12 hours). Other, yet unproven, strategies are antibiotic cycling (withdrawal for a defined period and reintroduction later); hospital formulary restrictions; and use of narrow-spectrum, and older, more established antibiotics. The involvement of infectious disease specialists is needed in many instances and improves choice and dosage of antibiotics.[8] Several reviews with more detailed discussions are available.[5,8,21,39,42,44,66]

CONCLUSIONS
- New-onset fever often indicates infection but may be caused by resorption of blood (relative bradycardia), thromboembolism (persistent tachycardia, painful calves), or drugs (incremental increase in temperature within several days).
- Nosocomial pneumonia is typically recognized by fever, peripheral infiltrates on chest radiographs, change in sputum quality to purulent mucus, and ≥ 25 polymorphonuclear leukocytes on Gram's stain.
- Phlebitis remains the most common catheter-related infection. Changing the catheter site and applying cold, wet compresses are often sufficient. Catheter-associated bacteremia is an emergency that should be treated by intravenous administration of vancomycin and a cephalosporin.
- Nosocomial urinary tract infections in catheterized patients are diagnosed by increased leukocyte counts (> 10 cells/mm^3) and cultures. When gram-positive cocci are suspected, vancomycin is preferred.

- Nosocomial gastrointestinal infections are invariably caused by *C. difficile*. Metronidazole is given orally.
- Ventriculitis can be effectively treated with vancomycin and cefotaxime intravenously, assuming that *S. epidermidis* and *aureus* are the causative agents.

REFERENCES

1. Aoun M, Klastersky J. Drug treatment of pneumonia in the hospital: what are the choices? *Drugs* 1991;42;962–973.
2. Bassi GL, Ferrer M, Marti JD, Comaru T, Torres A. Ventilator-associated pneumonia. *Semin Respir Crit Care Med* 2014;35:469–481.
3. Batra R, Eziefula AC, Wyncoll D, Edgeworth J. Throat and rectal swabs may have an important role in MRSA screening of critically ill patients. *Intensive Care Med* 2008;34:1703–1706.
4. Bergmans DC, Bonten MJ, Gaillard CA, et al. Prevention of ventilator-associated pneumonia by oral decontamination: a prospective, randomized, double-blind, placebo-controlled study. *Am J Respir Crit Care Med* 2001;164:382–388.
5. Bergogne-Berezin E. Current guidelines for the treatment and prevention of nosocomial infections. *Drugs* 1999;58:51–67.
6. Brown E, Talbot GH, Axelrod P, Provencher M, Hoegg C. Risk factors for Clostridium difficile toxin-associated diarrhea. *Infect Cont Hosp Epidem* 1990;11:283–290.
7. Burton DC, Edwards JR, Horan TC, Jernigan JA, Fridkin SK. Methicillin-resistant Staphylococcus aureus central line-associated bloodstream infections in US intensive care units, 1997–2007. *JAMA* 2009;301:727–736.
8. Byl B, Clevenbergh P, Jacobs F, et al. Impact of infectious diseases specialists and microbiological data on the appropriateness of antimicrobial therapy for bacteremia. *Clin Infect Dis* 1999;29:60–66.
9. Cercenado E, Ena J, Rodriguez-Creixems M, Romero I, Bouza E. A conservative procedure for the diagnosis of catheter-related infections. *Arch Intern Med* 1990;150:1417–1420.
10. Chastre J, Fagon JY. Invasive diagnostic testing should be routinely used to manage ventilated patients with suspected pneumonia. *Am J Respir Crit Care Med* 1994;150:570–574.
11. Chastre J, Fagon JY, Domart Y, Gibert C. Diagnosis of nosocomial pneumonia in intensive care unit patients. *Eur J Clin Microbiol Infect Dis* 1989;8:35–39.
12. Chen YY, Wang FD, Liu CY, Chou P. Incidence rate and variable cost of nosocomial infections in different types of intensive care units. *Infect Cont Hosp Epidem* 2009;30:39–46.
13. Cobb DK, High KP, Sawyer RG, et al. A controlled trial of scheduled replacement of central venous and pulmonary-artery catheters. *N Engl J Med* 1992;327:1062–1068.
14. Cockerill FR, 3rd, Muller SR, Anhalt JP, et al. Prevention of infection in critically ill patients by selective decontamination of the digestive tract. *Ann Intern Med* 1992;117:545–553.
15. Craven DE, Barber TW, Steger KA, Montecalvo MA. Nosocomial pneumonia in the 1990s: update of epidemiology and risk factors. *Semin Respir Infect* 1990;5;157–172.
16. Craven DE, Steger KA. Nosocomial pneumonia in the intubated patient: new concepts on pathogenesis and prevention. *Infect Dis Clin N Am* 1989;3:843–866.
17. Darouiche RO, Raad, II, Heard SO, et al. A comparison of two antimicrobial-impregnated central venous catheters. Catheter Study Group. *N Engl J Med* 1999;340:1–8.
18. Darouiche RO, Smith JA, Jr., Hanna H, et al. Efficacy of antimicrobial-impregnated bladder catheters in reducing catheter-associated bacteriuria: a prospective, randomized, multicenter clinical trial. *Urology* 1999;54:976–981.
19. Daugherty EL, Perl TM, Needham DM, et al. The use of personal protective equipment for control of influenza among critical care clinicians: a survey study. *Crit Care Med* 2009;37: 1210–1216.
20. de Smet AM, Kluytmans JA, Cooper BS, et al. Decontamination of the digestive tract and oropharynx in ICU patients. *N Engl J Med* 2009;360:20–31.
21. den Hertog HM, van der Worp HB, van Gemert HM, et al. The Paracetamol (Acetaminophen) In Stroke (PAIS) trial: a multicentre, randomised, placebo-controlled, phase III trial. *Lancet Neurol* 2009;8:434–440.
22. Diekema DJ, Jones RN. Oxazolidinone antibiotics. *Lancet* 2001;358:1975–1982.
23. Doron S, Davidson LE. Antimicrobial stewardship. *Mayo Clin Proc* 2011;86:1113–1123.
24. Esperatti M, Ferrer M, Giunta V, et al. Validation of predictors of adverse outcomes in hospital-acquired pneumonia in the ICU. *Crit Care Med* 2013;41:2151–2161.
25. Felmingham D. Antibiotic resistance: do we need new therapeutic approaches? *Chest* 1995;108:70S-78S.
26. Ferrer M, Torres A, Gonzalez J, et al. Utility of selective digestive decontamination in mechanically ventilated patients. *Ann Intern Med* 1994;120:389–395.

27. File TM, Jr., Solomkin JS, Cosgrove SE. Strategies for improving antimicrobial use and the role of antimicrobial stewardship programs. *Clin Infect Dis* 2011;53 Suppl 1:S15–22.

28. Flaherty JP, Weinstein RA. Infection control and pneumonia prophylaxis strategies in the intensive care unit. *Semin Respir Infect* 1990;5:191–203.

29. Flaherty JP, Weinstein RA. Nosocomial infection caused by antibiotic-resistant organisms in the intensive-care unit. *Infect Control Hosp Epidemiol* 1996 ;17:236–48.

30. Friedland IR, McCracken GH, Jr. Management of infections caused by antibiotic-resistant Streptococcus pneumoniae. *N Engl J Med* 1994;331:377–382.

31. George DL. Epidemiology of nosocomial ventilator-associated pneumonia. *Infect Cont Hosp Epidem* 1993;14:163–169.

32. Gerding DN, Olson MM, Peterson LR, et al. Clostridium difficile-associated diarrhea and colitis in adults: a prospective case-controlled epidemiologic study. *Arch Intern Med* 1986;146:95–100.

33. Gozal YM, Farley CW, Hanseman DJ, et al. Ventriculostomy-associated infection: a new, standardized reporting definition and institutional experience. *Neurocrit Care* 2014;21:147–151.

34. Hamer DH, Barza M. Prevention of hospital-acquired pneumonia in critically ill patients. *Antimicrob Agents Chemother* 1993;37:931–938.

35. Hayon J, Figliolini C, Combes A, et al. Role of serial routine microbiologic culture results in the initial management of ventilator-associated pneumonia. *Am J Respir Crit Care Med* 2002;165:41–46.

36. Hill RL, Fisher AP, Ware RJ, Wilson S, Casewell MW. Mupirocin for the reduction of colonization of internal jugular cannulae: a randomized controlled trial. *J Hosp Infect* 1990;15:311–321.

37. Ibrahim EH, Tracy L, Hill C, Fraser VJ, Kollef MH. The occurrence of ventilator-associated pneumonia in a community hospital: risk factors and clinical outcomes. *Chest* 2001;120:555–561.

38. Kalra l, Irshad S, Hodsoll J, et al. Prophylactic antibiotics after acute stroke for reducing pneumonia in patients with dysphagia (STROKE-INF): a prospective, cluster-randomized, open-label, masked endpoint, controlled clinical trial. *Lancet* 2015;386:1835–1844.

39. Kamal GD, Pfaller MA, Rempe LE, Jebson PJ. Reduced intravascular catheter infection by antibiotic bonding: a prospective, randomized, controlled trial. *JAMA* 1991;265:2364–2368.

40. Kanj SS, Kanafani ZA. Current concepts in antimicrobial therapy against resistant gram-negative organisms: extended-spectrum beta-lactamase-producing Enterobacteriaceae, carbapenem-resistant Enterobacteriaceae, and multidrug-resistant Pseudomonas aeruginosa. *Mayo Clinic Proc* 2011;86:250–259.

41. Klompas M, Magill S, Robicsek A, et al. Objective surveillance definitions for ventilator-associated pneumonia. *Crit Care Med* 2012;40:3154–3161.

42. Kollef MH. Optimizing antibiotic therapy in the intensive care unit setting. *Crit Care* 2001;5:189–195.

43. Kollef MH, Fraser VJ. Antibiotic resistance in the intensive care unit. *Ann Intern Med* 2001;134:298–314.

44. Korinek AM, Laisne MJ, Nicolas MH, et al. Selective decontamination of the digestive tract in neurosurgical intensive care unit patients: a double-blind, randomized, placebo-controlled study. *Crit Care Med* 1993;21:1466–1473.

45. Kunin CM. Resistance to antimicrobial drugs: a worldwide calamity. *Ann Intern Med* 1993;118:557–561.

46. Lodise TP, Lomaestro B, Graves J, Drusano GL. Larger vancomycin doses (at least four grams per day) are associated with an increased incidence of nephrotoxicity. *Antimicrob Agents Chemother* 2008;52:1330–1336.

47. Mandell LA, Wunderink RG, Anzueto A, et al. Infectious Diseases Society of America/American Thoracic Society consensus guidelines on the management of community-acquired pneumonia in adults. *Clin Infect Dis* 2007;44 Suppl 2:S27–S72.

48. McFarland LV, Mulligan ME, Kwok RY, Stamm WE. Nosocomial acquisition of Clostridium difficile infection. *N Engl J Med* 1989;320:204–210.

49. Meduri GU. Ventilator-associated pneumonia in patients with respiratory failure: a diagnostic approach. *Chest* 1990;97:1208–1219.

50. Mikhaylov Y, Wilson TJ, Rajajee V, et al. Efficacy of antibiotic-impregnated external ventricular drains in reducing ventriculostomy-associated infections. *J Clin Neurosci* 2014;21:765–768.

51. Moro ML, Vigano EF, Cozzi Lepri A. Risk factors for central venous catheter-related infections in surgical and intensive care units. The Central Venous Catheter-Related Infections Study Group. *Infect Cont Hosp Epidem* 1994;15:253–264.

52. Murray BE. New aspects of antimicrobial resistance and the resulting therapeutic dilemmas. *J Infect Dis* 1991;163:1184–1194.

53. Nathens AB, Chu PT, Marshall JC. Nosocomial infection in the surgical intensive care unit. *Infect Dis Clin N Am* 1992;6:657–675.

54. O'Grady NP, Alexander M, Dellinger EP, et al. Guidelines for the prevention of intravascular

catheter-related infections. *Infect Cont Hosp Epidem* 2002;23:759–769.

55. Pittet D, Tarara D, Wenzel RP. Nosocomial bloodstream infection in critically ill patients. Excess length of stay, extra costs, and attributable mortality. *JAMA* 1994;271:1598–1601.

56. Prevention CfDCa. Guidelines for prevention of nosocomial pneumonia. *MMWR Recomm Rep* 1997;46:1–79.

57. Prowle JR, Heenen S, Singer M. Infection in the critically ill: questions we should be asking. *J Antimicrob Chemother* 2011;66 Suppl 2:ii3–10.

58. Pugin J, Auckenthaler R, Mili N, et al. Diagnosis of ventilator-associated pneumonia by bacteriologic analysis of bronchoscopic and nonbronchoscopic "blind" bronchoalveolar lavage fluid. *Am Rev Respir Dis* 1991;143:1121–1129.

59. Putterman C. Central venous catheter related sepsis: a clinical review. *Resuscitation* 1990;20:1–16.

60. Raad, II, Bodey GP. Infectious complications of indwelling vascular catheters. *Clin Infect Dis* 1992;15:197–208.

61. Raad II, Darouiche R, Hachem R, Mansouri M, Bodey GP. The broad-spectrum activity and efficacy of catheters coated with minocycline and rifampin. *J Infect Dis* 1996;173:418–424.

62. Rebuck JA, Murry KR, Rhoney DH, Michael DB, Coplin WM. Infection related to intracranial pressure monitors in adults: analysis of risk factors and antibiotic prophylaxis. *J Neurol Neurosurg Psychiatry* 2000;69:381–384.

63. Rello J, Ausina V, Ricart M, et al. Nosocomial pneumonia in critically ill comatose patients: need for a differential therapeutic approach. *Eur Respir J* 1992;5:1249–1253.

64. Richet H, Hubert B, Nitemberg G, et al. Prospective multicenter study of vascular-catheter-related complications and risk factors for positive central-catheter cultures in intensive care unit patients. *J Clin Microbiol* 1990;28:2520–2525.

65. Rodriguez JL. Hospital-acquired gram-negative pneumonia in critically ill, injured patients. *Am J Surg* 1993;165:34S–42S.

66. Scheld WM, Mandell GL. Nosocomial pneumonia: pathogenesis and recent advances in diagnosis and therapy. *Rev Infect Dis* 1991;13 Suppl 9:S743–S751.

67. Schentag JJ. Antimicrobial management strategies for Gram-positive bacterial resistance in the intensive care unit. *Crit Care Med* 2001;29:N100–N107.

68. Septimus EJ. Nosocomial bacterial pneumonias. *Semin Respir Infect* 1989;4:245–252.

69. Torres A, Gatell JM, Aznar E, et al. Re-intubation increases the risk of nosocomial pneumonia in patients needing mechanical ventilation. *Am J Respir Crit Care Med* 1995;152:137–141.

70. Tryba M. The gastropulmonary route of infection: fact or fiction? *Am J Med* 1991;91:135S–146S.

71. Trzeciak S, Dellinger RP, Abate NL, et al. Translating research to clinical practice: a 1-year experience with implementing early goal directed therapy for septic shock in the emergency department. *Chest* 2006;129:225–232.

72. Valles J, Artigas A, Rello J, et al. Continuous aspiration of subglottic secretions in preventing ventilator-associated pneumonia. *Ann Intern Med* 1995;122:179–186.

73. van de Beek D, Wijdicks EFM, Vermeij FH, et al. Preventive antibiotics for infections in acute stroke: a systematic review and meta-analysis. *Arch Neurol* 2009;66:1076–1081.

74. Weinstein RA. Epidemiology and control of nosocomial infections in adult intensive care units. *Am J Med* 1991;91:179S–184S.

75. Westendorp WF, Vermeij JD, Zock E, et al. The Preventive Antibiotics in Stroke Study (PASS): a pragmatic randomized open-label masked endpoint clinical trial. *Lancet* 2015;385, 1519–1526.

76. Winer-Muram HT, Jennings SG, Wunderink RG, Jones CB, Leeper KV, Jr. Ventilator-associated Pseudomonas aeruginosa pneumonia: radiographic findings. *Radiology* 1995;195:247–252.

77. Winfield JA, Rosenthal P, Kanter RK, Casella G. Duration of intracranial pressure monitoring does not predict daily risk of infectious complications. *Neurosurgery* 1993;33:424–430.

78. Wright K, Young P, Brickman C, et al. Rates and determinants of ventriculostomy-related infections during a hospital transition to use of antibiotic-coated external ventricular drains. *Neurosurg Focus* 2013;34:E12.

79. Wright MO, Fisher A, John M, et al. The electronic medical record as a tool for infection surveillance: successful automation of device-days. *Am J Infect Control* 2009;37:364–370.

80. Yoshida J, Ishimaru T, Fujimoto M, et al. Risk factors for central venous catheter-related bloodstream infection: a 1073-patient study. *J Infect Chemother* 2008;14:399–403.

81. Zahar JR, Nguile-Makao M, Francais A, et al. Predicting the risk of documented ventilator-associated pneumonia for benchmarking: construction and validation of a score. *Crit Care Med* 2009;37:2545–2551.

82. Zampieri FG, Nassar AP Jr, Gusmao-Flores D, et al. Nebulized antibiotics for ventilator-associated pneumonia: A systematic review and meta-analysis. *Crit Care* 2015;19:150.

60

Management of Hematologic Complications and Transfusion

Predictably, hematologic complications are not commonly a manifestation in patients with an acute neurologic illness. Most changes in hematologic laboratory values are key indicators of a new systemic illness, a response to fluid management, or a side effect of a newly introduced medication, rather than a consequence of neurologic injury. In some presenting patients, however, acute neurologic manifestations are a continuation of an oncologic emergency with abnormal hemostasis. Another notable exception is a patient with traumatic brain injury, particularly one with lesions from projectiles or gunshot wounds, because severe neuronal injury causes the release of a thromboplastin, triggering the development of disseminated intravascular coagulation.[55]

This chapter discusses the most important hematologic complications in patients with a prolonged stay in the neurosciences intensive care unit (NICU) and concentrates on the management of anemia and thrombocytopenia. Acute or rapidly emerging anemia may require blood transfusion, but the threshold for blood transfusion has not been clearly defined in patients with critical neurologic illness. Guidelines for red blood cell transfusions in critically ill patients have been recently published[37] (Part XIV, Guidelines).

ANEMIA

A hematocrit level of 30%–40% (normal 46% in males, 38% in females) or a hemoglobin value less than 10 g/dL is common in any critically ill patient.[14] The decrease in hematocrit level is related to age, severity of injury, and the presence of acute renal failure or multiorgan failure, or of an evolving infection, such as pneumonia and sepsis.[46] The mechanism in sepsis may be related to blunting of the erythropoietin response. Some studies have suggested that critically ill patients have decreased levels of both serum iron and total iron-binding capacity and an elevated serum ferritin level, next to a reduced erythropoietin response.[31] These parameters might result from multiorgan failure.

Any severe anemia should prompt aggressive investigation into blood loss. Laboratory tests that are needed include mean cell volume (MCV), smear, and serum iron and ferritin concentrations. Traditionally, anemia in critical illness can be divided into anemia from marrow underproduction (normocytic anemia due to renal disease, endocrine crisis, undernutrition, iron deficiency), maturation deficiency (microcytic or macrocytic anemia due to drug toxicity, folate and vitamin B_{12} deficiency), hemolysis, or blood loss.

In the NICU, exploration into the most common causes of anemia is tailored toward acutely ill patients with neurologic disease (Table 60.1). Anemia is common because frequent phlebotomy and blood sampling may remove, on average, more than 40 mL per day. During neurosurgical procedures, patients may have intraoperative blood loss, which is certainly more prevalent in patients with multitrauma, penetrating scalp injuries, and acute thoracic spine stabilization. Albeit rare, side effects of certain drugs may be related to myelosuppression. Retroperitoneal hematoma is a known complication of cerebral angiography. It may be signaled as abdominal pain or tenderness, and increased girth may be detected.

Generally, the development of anemia is potentially problematic for the simple reason that the body's oxygen-carrying capacity is decreased.[53] The relationship between the hematocrit level, cerebral oxygen delivery, and cerebral perfusion pressure is based on the Hagen-Poiseuille equation:

$$\Delta V = \pi/8 \cdot 1/L \cdot 1/\eta \cdot \Delta P \cdot r4$$

in which P is the pressure gradient; r, the radius of the vessel; L, the length of the vessel; η, the blood viscosity, and V, the blood flow. Therefore, a high hematocrit level may decrease cerebral blood flow and increase the risk of ischemia (Capsule 60.1).

Blood transfusion maintains optimal tissue oxygenation, but possibly also causes congestive heart failure and pulmonary edema, resulting in

TABLE 60.1. CAUSES OF ANEMIA IN THE NICU	
Blood loss	Frequent sampling
	Multitrauma
	Neurosurgical intervention
	Retroperitoneal hematoma
Reduced red blood cell production	Drug-induced sepsis or multiorgan failure
	Adverse drug reaction
	Myelosuppression
	Carbamazepine
	Furosemide
	Indomethacin
	Phenobarbital
	Phenothiazine
	Phenytoin
Hemolysis	Phenobarbital
	Phenytoin
	Cephalosporins
	Erythromycin
	NSAIDs
	Omeprazole
	Ketoconazole

NSAIDs, nonsteroidal anti-inflammatory drugs.

poor oxygenation.[16,32,62,73] Blood transfusion is considered in patients with falling hemoglobin levels, but the benefit of blood transfusion in acute neurologic illness is an area of uncertainty.[11,15]

Data from patients with aneurysmal subarachnoid hemorrhage have been conflicting, with one group's data suggesting that postoperative blood transfusion increases the risk of cerebral vasospasm.[52] Other investigators have found that a higher hemoglobin level was related to better outcome, with red blood cell transfusion increasing cerebral oxygenation.[36] One preliminary study in 20 comatose patients with poor-grade subarachnoid hemorrhage, monitored with brain tissue oxygen monitoring and microdialysis, found evidence of metabolic distress (reduced brain tissue oxygen and increased extracellular lactate/pyruvate ratio) with hemoglobin levels of less than 9 g/dL.[38] Little is known on whether blood transfusion improves these early parameters of secondary injury, or if this applies only to more severely affected patients.

Most neurosurgeons have voiced reserve about the use of frequent blood transfusions in traumatic brain injury.[45] Anemia with traumatic brain injury is a major predictor of morbidity and death, and blood transfusion was found to be an important factor in these outcomes. However, aggressive blood transfusions have not resulted in a measurable improvement of outcome in head injury.[20] Other studies have found that patients with traumatic brain injury are able to tolerate a considerable degree of anemia (hematocrit level, < 30%).[45] This evidence has led to a more conservative transfusion practice and to the acceptance of low hemoglobin values. One systematic review found one in three patients with traumatic brain injury had red blood cell transfusions but found no significant association between transfusion and in-hospital mortality. Increased risk of unfavorable outcome after transfusion was observed in patients with higher hemoglobin values. Pretransfusion hemoglobin level was observed as a potentially important predictor of clinical outcomes including mortality and neurologic outcome.[9]

Anemia has been correlated to poor outcome in many critically ill patients with neurologic disease, but anemia could also be a confounding variable and the result of multiple fluid boluses to augment intravascular volume in patients with unstable blood pressures, or a result of frequent laboratory measurements in a very sick patient.[10]

These circumstances may make daily practice decisions difficult.[40] Blood transfusion should be ordered in any patient with substantial blood loss. Other guidelines are best applied to those who do not have active bleeding.[1,13,26,37] A restrictive strategy of red blood cell transfusion (transfuse when Hb < 7 g/dL) is currently recommended in most critically ill patients. In the NICU patients, a more liberal transfusion policy may apply, with consideration of transfusion with Hb < 9 g/dL. Transfusion for patients with hemoglobin levels of less than 10 g/dL are considered only for patients with acute coronary syndromes and early sepsis.[42,63,64,66] A recent study of (recombinant human erythropoietin) epoetin alpha[12] in the ICU did not reduce transfusion requirements, but there were more often clinically relevant thrombotic vascular events (pulmonary emboli, deep vein thrombosis, and myocardial infarction).

THROMBOCYTOPENIA

In medical ICUs, thrombocytopenia is common and may reach 50% when defined as a platelet count of less than 100,000 per cubic millimeter.[2,6,17,19] Contributing factors are uremia or medications used in the NICU. Thrombocytopenia is a concerning complication in critically ill patients with neurologic disease, but in many cases its cause is indeterminate.[35,49,54,56,61] Thrombocytopenia usually is associated with critical illness or is drug induced and results in a slow decline. The likelihood of drug-induced thrombocytopenia is increased when platelet counts drop precipitously

CAPSULE 60.1   ANEMIA AND BRAIN PHYSIOLOGY

The hemodynamic adaptation to acute anemia (or an abrupt decrease in hematocrit level) is largely related to compensatory changes in cerebral blood flow (CBF). The accompanying figure illustrates the body's capacity to compensate for a change in blood viscosity and a decrease in hematocrit level. The regulatory system is exhausted when the hematocrit level is less than 15%, at which point oxygen consumption becomes entirely dependent on arterial oxygen content, and cerebral tissue hypoxemia and lactic acidosis result.[25,43,44] Therefore, extreme hemodilution (hematocrit, < 10%) cannot be overcome with an increase in either CBF or cerebral oxygen extraction. Reduced blood viscosity and reduced arterial oxygen content equally increase CBF, but vasodilation seems to be the overriding mechanism of compensation.[57,58] Data show that nitric oxide mediates CBF regulation. Neuronal nitric oxide synthetase expression, but not endothelial nitric oxidase expression, increases during anemia, suggesting that it may be the main stimulant during these changed conditions.

These regulatory mechanisms may not be as operational in an injured brain, and experimental studies have shown that hemoglobin levels of less than 9 g/dL may cause cerebral hypoxemia.[25]

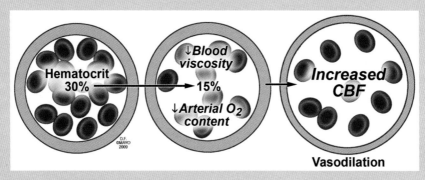

Changes in cerebral blood flow associated with reduced hematocrit.

and to values less than 50,000 per cubic millimeter.[5] The most common causes of thrombocytopenia in the NICU are shown in Table 60.2.

A major concern is rapid-onset thrombocytopenia associated with heparin use, also known as heparin-induced thrombocytopenia (HIT).[21,27,28,67–69,71] Heparin-induced thrombocytopenia is a serious disorder that may occur with use of any type of heparin, unfractionated heparin, and low-molecular-weight heparin.[3] It may also be associated with frequent heparin flushes and is not necessarily associated with prolonged heparin administration. Patients with thrombocytopenia may have evidence of new thrombosis, skin necrosis, or thrombosis in the arterial or venous system.

The laboratory diagnosis of HIT is based on criteria that include a platelet count decrease of more than 50–75%, often with onset at 5–10 days after IV administration of heparin. The diagnosis of HIT is unlikely if heparin was administered more than 30 days since the onset of thrombocytopenia.

Laboratory assays for HIT antibodies are currently available, and platelet factor 4-dependent enzyme-linked immunosorbent assays can detect all antibody classes (i.e., IgA, IgG, and IgM to the platelet factor 4-heparin complexes).

TABLE 60.2. CAUSES OF NEW-ONSET THROMBOCYTOPENIA

Sepsis
Diffuse intravascular coagulation
Massive transfusions (> 50% of blood volume)
Heparin use (unfractionated, low-molecular weight heparin)
Drug use (e.g., rifampin, sulfonamides, vancomycin, carbamazepine, phenytoin, valproic acid, cimetidine, famotidine, acetaminophen, chlorothiazide)

The diagnosis can be confirmed with anti-PF4/heparin EIA-IgG or platelet serotonin-release essay (Chapter 20). Enzyme-linked immunosorbent assay has a high sensitivity and continues to be an important test in the diagnosis of this disorder.[48,70,74] Therefore, when thrombocytopenia is associated with heparin use, heparin administration should be immediately discontinued, including heparin used for flushing intravascular catheters. Platelet transfusions are problematic, particularly because the transfused platelets will be destroyed by the HIT antibodies.

Heparin-induced thrombocytopenia can be treated with danaparoid sodium, 750 units subcutaneously q12h. For patients with severe renal impairment, the dose should be reduced by 30%. An alternative thrombin inhibitor is lepirudin.[23,24] For this recombinant bivalent thrombin inhibitor, the initial dose of 0.4 mg/kg is followed by a continuous infusion of 0.15 mg/kg/hr.[34] We prefer Argatroban, 25 mcg/kg/min IV infusion to a maximum dose of 40 mcg/kg/min.

Platelet transfusions are considered for any other patients with marked thrombocytopenia.[4,7,47] Published guidelines have suggested that platelet transfusion is necessary when platelet counts are less than 50×10^9/L, particularly when invasive procedures are anticipated.[4,7]

RISKS ASSOCIATED WITH TRANSFUSION

One of the greatest risks of transfusion-transmitted disease is bacterial and viral contamination of platelets, which is more common in platelet transfusions than in red blood cell transfusions[33,39,72] (Table 60.3). Studies have found that bacterial contamination of platelet concentrates occurs in concentrations of approximately 1:1,000 to 1:2,000 units.[8] Other concerns are transfusion-related acute lung injury (TRALI),[18,22,29,30,50,51] which is likely when acute hypoxemia and acute

TABLE 60.3. ESTIMATED BLOOD TRANSFUSION RISKS

Transfusion associated related lung injury (1 in 5,000)
Bacterial contamination (1 in 15,000)
Hepatitis B (1 in 130,000)
Severe hemolytic reaction (1 in 600,000)
Hepatitis C (1 in 1,000,000)
Human immunodeficiency virus (1 in 1,200,000)
West Nile virus (minimal)

lung injury occur in proximity to a blood transfusion with no evidence of circulatory overload. Signs emerging within 6 hours of transfusion are a commonly used parameter.[60] Although this disorder has been estimated to occur in 1 in 5,000 transfusions, it may be a cause of the rapid onset of hypoxemia associated with marked pulmonary edema (Figure 60.1).[41]

In most instances, plasma alone causes TRALI, and it appears that reactive lipid products from donor blood cell membranes may be the main mechanism of this disorder.[59,60] These substances may result in damage to the pulmonary capillary endothelium and in an acute respiratory distress syndrome (ARDS). Many patients need mechanical ventilation for several days, and death has been described in 50% of cases.[65] Most concerning is that fresh frozen plasma may damage the heart and lungs.

There is a risk of transfusion-associated cardiac overload syndrome (TACO), and it usually is a consequence of rate of infusion and the total volume of blood product that has been transfused. Typically patients develop dyspnea, hypertension, and tachypnea and, on auscultation, have significant crackles and rales. A chest X-ray often shows development of pulmonary edema and also other features of congestive heart

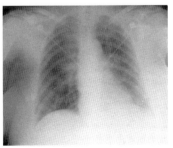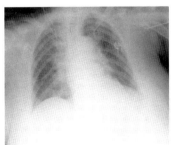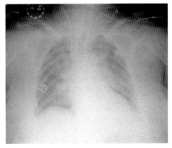

FIGURE 60.1: Series of chest radiographs showing development of pulmonary edema within hours after plasma infusion. (Each radiograph was taken 4 hours apart).

failure. TACO occurs on average in patients who have received 4 or more units of fresh frozen plasma and when the average rate was approximately 600 ml/hour. There is a quick response to aggressive diuresis that may require short-term furosemide infusion.

CONCLUSIONS

- Anemia may be an indicator of critical illness alone, and blood transfusion is advised when the hemoglobin level is 7–9 g/dL. Transfusion strategy in the NICU is not well defined.
- Thrombocytopenia may be related to heparin use, including IV heparin flushes, or to subcutaneously administered heparin. HIT antibodies can be easily detected by enzyme-linked immunosorbent assay.
- Blood product use is associated with risks varying from minor febrile reaction to fatal lung injury.

REFERENCES

1. Guidelines for the use of platelet transfusions. *Br J Hematol* 2003;122:10–23.
2. Akca S, Haji-Michael P, de Mendonca A, et al. Time course of platelet counts in critically ill patients. *Crit Care Med* 2002;30:753–756.
3. Arepally GM, Ortel TL. Clinical practice: heparin-induced thrombocytopenia. *N Engl J Med* 2006;355:809–817.
4. Arnold DM, Crowther MA, Cook RJ, et al. Utilization of platelet transfusions in the intensive care unit: indications, transfusion triggers, and platelet count responses. *Transfusion* 2006;46:1286–1291.
5. Aster RH, Bougie DW. Drug-induced immune thrombocytopenia. *N Engl J Med* 2007;357:580–587.
6. Baughman RP, Lower EE, Flessa HC, Tollerud DJ. Thrombocytopenia in the intensive care unit. *Chest* 1993;104:1243–1247.
7. Beale E, Zhu J, Chan L, et al. Blood transfusion in critically injured patients: a prospective study. *Injury* 2006;37:455–465.
8. Brecher ME, Holland PV, Pineda AA, Tegtmeier GE, Yomtovian R. Growth of bacteria in inoculated platelets: implications for bacteria detection and the extension of platelet storage. *Transfusion* 2000;40:1308–1312.
9. Boutin A, Chassé M, Shemilt M, et al. Red blood cell transfusion in patients with traumatic brain injury: A systematic review and meta-analysis. *Transfus Med Rev* 2016;30:15–24.
10. Carson JL, Noveck H, Berlin JA, Gould SA. Mortality and morbidity in patients with very low postoperative Hb levels who decline blood transfusion. *Transfusion* 2002;42:812–818.
11. Chandrasekhar J, Dara SI, Bahurlingam S, et al. RBC Transfusion threshold and outcomes in the medical intensive care unit. *Chest* 2003;124:125S-b-126S.
12. Corwin HL, Gettinger A, Fabian TC, et al. Efficacy and safety of epoetin alfa in critically ill patients. *N Engl J Med* 2007;357:965–976.
13. Corwin HL, Gettinger A, Pearl RG, et al. The CRIT Study: anemia and blood transfusion in the critically ill—current clinical practice in the United States. *Crit Care Med* 2004;32:39–52.
14. Corwin HL, Krantz SB. Anemia of the critically ill: "acute" anemia of chronic disease. *Crit Care Med* 2000;28:3098–3099.
15. Corwin HL, Surgenor SD, Gettinger A. Transfusion practice in the critically ill. *Crit Care Med* 2003;31:S668–S671.
16. Corwin HL, Napolitano LM. Anemia in the critically ill: do we need to live with it? *Crit Care Med* 2014;42:2140–2141.
17. Crowther MA, Cook DJ, Meade MO, et al. Thrombocytopenia in medical-surgical critically ill patients: prevalence, incidence, and risk factors. *J Crit Care* 2005;20:348–353.
18. Dellinger EP, Anaya DA. Infectious and immunologic consequences of blood transfusion. *Crit Care* 2004;8 Suppl 2:S18–S23.
19. Drews RE, Weinberger SE. Thrombocytopenic disorders in critically ill patients. *Am J Respir Crit Care Med* 2000;162:347–351.
20. George ME, Skarda DE, Watts CR, Pham HD, Beilman GJ. Aggressive red blood cell transfusion: no association with improved outcomes for victims of isolated traumatic brain injury. *Neurocrit Care* 2008;8:337–343.
21. Gettings EM, Brush KA, Van Cott EM, Hurford WE. Outcome of postoperative critically ill patients with heparin-induced thrombocytopenia: an observational retrospective case-control study. *Crit Care* 2006;10:R161.
22. Goodnough LT. Risks of blood transfusion. *Crit Care Med* 2003;31:S678–S686.
23. Greinacher A. Lepirudin: a bivalent direct thrombin inhibitor for anticoagulation therapy. *Expert Rev Cardiovasc Ther* 2004;2:339–357.
24. Greinacher A, Eichler P, Lubenow N, Kwasny H, Luz M. Heparin-induced thrombocytopenia with thromboembolic complications: meta-analysis of 2 prospective trials to assess the value of parenteral treatment with lepirudin and its therapeutic aPTT range. *Blood* 2000;96:846–851.
25. Hare GM. Anaemia and the brain. *Curr Opin Anaesthesiol* 2004;17:363 369.
26. Hill SR, Carless PA, Henry DA, et al. Transfusion thresholds and other strategies for guiding

allogeneic red blood cell transfusion. *Cochrane Database Syst Rev* 2002:CD002042.

27. Hrushesky WJ. Subcutaneous heparin-induced thrombocytopenia. *Arch Intern Med* 1978;138:1489–1491.

28. Kim GH, Hahn DK, Kellner CP, et al. The incidence of heparin-induced thrombocytopenia Type II in patients with subarachnoid hemorrhage treated with heparin versus enoxaparin. *J Neurosurg* 2009;110:50–57.

29. Kleinman S, Caulfield T, Chan P, et al. Toward an understanding of transfusion-related acute lung injury: statement of a consensus panel. *Transfusion* 2004;44:1774–1789.

30. Kopko PM, Marshall CS, MacKenzie MR, Holland PV, Popovsky MA. Transfusion-related acute lung injury: report of a clinical look-back investigation. *JAMA* 2002;287:1968–1971.

31. Krafte-Jacobs B, Levetown ML, Bray GL, Ruttimann UE, Pollack MM. Erythropoietin response to critical illness. *Crit Care Med* 1994;22:821–826.

32. Leal-Noval SR, Rincon-Ferrari MD, Marin-Niebla A, et al. Transfusion of erythrocyte concentrates produces a variable increment on cerebral oxygenation in patients with severe traumatic brain injury: a preliminary study. *Intensive Care Med* 2006;32:1733–1740.

33. Leiby DA, Kerr KL, Campos JM, Dodd RY. A retrospective analysis of microbial contaminants in outdated random-donor platelets from multiple sites. *Transfusion* 1997;37:259–263.

34. Levine RL, Hursting MJ, McCollum D. Argatroban therapy in heparin-induced thrombocytopenia with hepatic dysfunction. *Chest* 2006;129:1167–1175.

35. Moreau D, Timsit JF, Vesin A, et al. Platelet count decline: an early prognostic marker in critically ill patients with prolonged ICU stays. *Chest* 2007;131:1735–1741.

36. Naidech AM, Drescher J, Ault ML, et al. Higher hemoglobin is associated with less cerebral infarction, poor outcome, and death after subarachnoid hemorrhage. *Neurosurgery* 2006;59:775–779.

37. Napolitano LM, Kurek S, Luchette FA, et al. Clinical practice guideline: red blood cell transfusion in adult trauma and critical care. *Crit Care Med* 2009;37:3124–3157.

38. Oddo M, Milby A, Chen I, et al. Hemoglobin concentration and cerebral metabolism in patients with aneurysmal subarachnoid hemorrhage. *Stroke* 2009;40:1275–1281.

39. Pealer LN, Marfin AA, Petersen LR, et al. Transmission of West Nile virus through blood transfusion in the United States in 2002. *N Engl J Med* 2003;349:1236–1245.

40. Pendem S, Rana S, Manno EM, Gajic O. A review of red cell transfusion in the neurological intensive care unit. *Neurocrit Care* 2006;4:63–67.

41. Perrotta PL, Snyder EL. Non-infectious complications of transfusion therapy. *Blood Rev* 2001;15:69–83.

42. Rana R, Afessa B, Keegan MT, et al. Evidence-based red cell transfusion in the critically ill: quality improvement using computerized physician order entry. *Crit Care Med* 2006;34:1892–1897.

43. Rebel A, Lenz C, Krieter H, et al. Oxygen delivery at high blood viscosity and decreased arterial oxygen content to brains of conscious rats. *Am J Physiol Heart Circ Physiol* 2001;280:H2591–H2597.

44. Rebel A, Ulatowski JA, Kwansa H, Bucci E, Koehler RC. Cerebrovascular response to decreased hematocrit: effect of cell-free hemoglobin, plasma viscosity, and CO2. *Am J Physiol Heart Circ Physiol* 2003;285:H1600–1608.

45. Salim A, Hadjizacharia P, DuBose J, et al. Role of anemia in traumatic brain injury. *J Am Coll Surg* 2008;207:398–406.

46. Scharte M, Fink MP. Red blood cell physiology in critical illness. *Crit Care Med* 2003;31:S651–657.

47. Schiffer CA, Anderson KC, Bennett CL, et al. Platelet transfusion for patients with cancer: clinical practice guidelines of the American Society of Clinical Oncology. *J Clin Oncol* 2001;19:1519–1538.

48. Selleng K, Warkentin TE, Greinacher A. Heparin-induced thrombocytopenia in intensive care patients. *Crit Care Med* 2007;35:1165–1176.

49. Shalansky SJ, Verma AK, Levine M, Spinelli JJ, Dodek PM. Risk markers for thrombocytopenia in critically ill patients: a prospective analysis. *Pharmacotherapy* 2002;22:803–813.

50. Shander A. Emerging risks and outcomes of blood transfusion in surgery. *Semin Hematol* 2004;41:117–124.

51. Smith KM, Jeske CS, Young B, Hatton J. Prevalence and characteristics of adverse drug reactions in neurosurgical intensive care patients. *Neurosurgery* 2006;58:426–433.

52. Smith MJ, Le Roux PD, Elliott JP, Winn HR. Blood transfusion and increased risk for vasospasm and poor outcome after subarachnoid hemorrhage. *J Neurosurg* 2004;101:1–7.

53. Smith MJ, Stiefel MF, Magge S, et al. Packed red blood cell transfusion increases local cerebral oxygenation. *Crit Care Med* 2005;33:1104–1108.

54. Strauss R, Wehler M, Mehler K, et al. Thrombocytopenia in patients in the medical intensive care unit: bleeding prevalence, transfusion requirements, and outcome. *Crit Care Med* 2002;30:1765–1771.

55. Talving P, Benfield R, Hadjizacharia P, et al. Coagulopathy in severe traumatic brain injury: a prospective study. *J Trauma* 2009;66:55–61.

56. Taylor RW, Manganaro L, O'Brien J, et al. Impact of allogenic packed red blood cell transfusion on nosocomial infection rates in the critically ill patient. *Crit Care Med* 2002;30:2249–2254.

57. Tomiyama Y, Brian JE, Jr., Todd MM. Plasma viscosity and cerebral blood flow. *Am J Physiol Heart Circ Physiol* 2000;279:H1949-H1954.

58. Tomiyama Y, Jansen K, Brian JE, Jr., Todd MM. Hemodilution, cerebral O2 delivery, and cerebral blood flow: a study using hyperbaric oxygenation. *Am J Physiol* 1999;276:H1190–H1196.

59. Toy P, Popovsky MA, Abraham E, et al. Transfusion-related acute lung injury: definition and review. *Crit Care Med* 2005;33:721–726.

60. Triulzi DJ. Transfusion-related acute lung injury: current concepts for the clinician. *Anesth Analg* 2009;108:770–776.

61. Vanderschueren S, De Weerdt A, Malbrain M, et al. Thrombocytopenia and prognosis in intensive care. *Crit Care Med* 2000;28:1871–1876.

62. Vincent JL, Baron JF, Reinhart K, et al. Anemia and blood transfusion in critically ill patients. *JAMA* 2002;288:1499–1507.

63. Vincent JL, Sakr Y, Sprung C, Harboe S, Damas P. Are blood transfusions associated with greater mortality rates? Results of the Sepsis Occurrence in Acutely Ill Patients study. *Anesthesiology* 2008;108:31–39.

64. Wahl WL, Hemmila MR, Maggio PM, Arbabi S. Restrictive red blood cell transfusion: not just for the stable intensive care unit patient. *Am J Surg* 2008;195:803–806.

65. Wallis JP, Lubenko A, Wells AW, Chapman CE. Single hospital experience of TRALI. *Transfusion* 2003;43:1053–1059.

66. Walsh TS, Garrioch M, Maciver C, et al. Red cell requirements for intensive care units adhering to evidence-based transfusion guidelines. *Transfusion* 2004;44:1405–1411.

67. Warkentin TE. Heparin-induced thrombocytopenia in critically ill patients. *Semin Thromb Hemost* 2015;41:49–60.

68. Warkentin TE. Heparin-induced thrombocytopenia: pathogenesis and management. *Br J Hematol* 2003;121:535–555.

69. Warkentin TE, Greinacher A, Koster A, et al. The treatment and prevention of heparin-induced thrombocytopenia: the 8th ACCP Conference on Antithrombotic and Thrombolytic Therapy. *Chest* 2008;133:340S–380S.

70. Warkentin TE, Heddle NM. Laboratory diagnosis of immune heparin-induced thrombocytopenia. *Curr Hematol Rep* 2003;2:148–157.

71. Warkentin TE, Levine MN, Hirsh J, et al. Heparin-induced thrombocytopenia in patients treated with low-molecular-weight heparin or unfractionated heparin. *N Engl J Med* 1995;332:1330–1335.

72. Yomtovian R, Lazarus HM, Goodnough LT, et al. A prospective microbiologic surveillance program to detect and prevent the transfusion of bacterially contaminated platelets. *Transfusion* 1993;33:902–909.

73. Zilberberg MD, Stern LS, Wiederkehr DP, Doyle JJ, Shorr AF. Anemia, transfusions and hospital outcomes among critically ill patients on prolonged acute mechanical ventilation: a retrospective cohort study. *Crit Care* 2008;12:R60.

74. Zwicker JI, Uhl L, Huang WY, Shaz BH, Bauer KA. Thrombosis and ELISA optical density values in hospitalized patients with heparin-induced thrombocytopenia. *J Thromb Haemost* 2004;2:2133–2137.

61

Management of Complications Associated with Vascular Access

Venous access through vascular cannulation is ubiquitous in any population of critically ill patients. Differences in utilization of catheters between specialized intensive care units are expected, and these mostly pertain to the indication for access and indirectly reflect the degree of hemodynamic instability. Similarly, critically ill neurologic patients, and certainly those with prolonged stay in the neurosciences intensive care unit (NICU), will have a central venous access catheter placed at some point. Central venous access is also necessary for certain infusates such as osmotic diuretics (e.g., hypertonic saline), vasopressors (e.g., norepinephrine), and many antimicrobials (e.g., vancomycin).

Any in-dwelling lines predisposes for adverse events.[12,41] The complications with central venous catheter placement are not always unavoidable, but common wisdom dictates that these complications are less common with supervision during placement, and in general, with clinician experience.[37] A recent large study of 1,794 catheterizations in critically ill patients found mechanical complications in 7% and arterial puncture in 3%, including four arterial cannulations and pneumothorax (0.6%).[35] This study found that the occurrence of complications was not reduced with clinician experience, and the complications were more common after two failed cannulation attempts. Most studies have documented that risk of complications increased sixfold after three failed attempts.[21]

This chapter deals mainly with common complications of catheter placement. Techniques of placement of commonly used access catheters are outside the scope of this chapter, and teaching videos have been published.[5,15]

VASCULAR CANNULATION AND PROCEDURE COMPLICATIONS

Central venous access can be obtained through a peripherally inserted central venous catheter (PICC), a subclavian catheter, or an internal jugular catheter[3,4] (Figure 61.1). Placement for each of these catheters requires a certain level of competency, and simulation programs may be helpful in teaching (Capsule 61.1). A preferred catheterization location continues to be the subclavian vein because it retains its diameter in hypotension due to its attachment to surrounding tissue, and head movements in restless patients do not jeopardize its placement. Subclavian catheter placement requires knowledge of variations of anatomy and structures that may be damaged during insertion.[3] Complications related to the placement procedure include puncture of the subclavian artery and, more seriously, of the ascending aorta, which causes a hemopericardium. Any punctured artery may cause a hemothorax that in extreme circumstances requires urgent thoracostomy. Even with appropriate precautions, a venous air embolus (for insertion sites vertically higher than the heart) may occur, causing sudden desaturation and hypotension when air lodges in the pulmonary artery. Also, brachial plexus and phrenic nerve injury may cause long-standing motor and sensory deficits and, often, persistent paralysis of one side of the diaphragm. Dysrhythmias and pneumothorax are the most common complications; chylothorax (injury to the lymphatic duct) and hydrothorax (intravenous leakage into the pleural space) are unusual complications.[3,4]

Insertion of the catheter into the right internal jugular vein is usually without difficulty. Placement is typically 2 cm above the clavicle, but higher puncture sites can be equally safe.[29] Complications similar to those in subclavian catheter placement are expected with insertion of an internal jugular catheter, but other more specific complications exist. Horner's syndrome is an unusual but well-known complication associated with damage of the sympathetic chain.[40] Injury to the vagus nerve may occur during placement, resulting in hoarseness because the recurrent

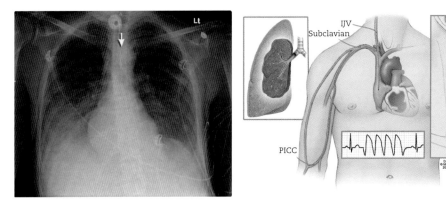

FIGURE 61.1. *Left*: Proper placement of a peripherally inserted central catheter (*arrow*). *Right*: Central vein catheterization and internal jugular vein catheter with potential complications (inserts show cardiac arrhythmias, pneumothorax, damage to sympathetic nerve causing Horner's syndrome).

IJV, internal jugular vein.

laryngeal branch is located directly posterior to the internal jugular vein. A recent systematic review of patients who received internal jugular versus subclavian catheter insertions found more arterial punctures with internal jugular placement than with subclavian access, but no difference in the occurrence of pneumothorax between the two approaches.[9]

Thromboembolic events have been reported in endovascular catheter, particularly when anticoagulation was not possible or not administered. Catheter-related thrombosis was found in 15% in recent series.[22,25,32] Peripherally inserted central venous catheters (PICC) could potentially provide adequate venous access for many patients and allow extended intravenous therapy. The PICC lines are inserted through a peripheral vein and advanced to float freely at the distal third of the superior vena cava or close to the superior vena cava junction with the right atrium.[36] One prospective trial found that among the PICCs audited, 7% were in distal position (i.e., in the right atrium and farther downstream).[36] Radiographic catheter position verification continues to be essential before the infusion is started and, in particular, when aspiration of venous blood is doubtful.[30]

Malpositioning is common with central venous catheters, but depends on the type of catheter. Recently, a Swedish study of central venous catheters found catheter-tip malposition in 3% of catheters, as documented in radiologic studies.[30] Malposition in catheterizations of the right subclavian vein occurred in 9% of catheterizations, compared with 1% of catheterizations of the right

---

CAPSULE 61.1   TEACHING PROCEDURES

Bedside teaching has been a traditional way of teaching central line placement, and it has remained the only way to reliably teach the technique. Many placements are needed to attain an acceptable level of proficiency. The slogan "see one, do one, teach one" never had merit and, if applied, may result in high complication rates. Skills have been taught using manikins (e.g., CentralLineman), and this process has led to an increased comfort level in performing these procedures. Performance measures can be defined and graded on each step in the procedure, including preparation (draping, Trendelenburg position), identification of landmarks, the correct angle of approach, number of attempts and technique of passing line over the wire, ultrasound demonstration of puncture of internal jugular vein, and transducing pressure to confirm adequate catheter position. Complications can also be simulated. Proficiency standards have been developed.[2,18,42] How these simulated skills translate to practice (safety and quality) is not yet known. Increased supervision may already lead to improved safety of placement.[33]

internal jugular vein. Ultrasound imaging of catheter placement is often used at the bedside, and a randomized controlled trial of neck ultrasonography after PICC line insertion identified catheter malpositioning in virtually all instances.[36] The presence of a saline push leading to a swirl in the right atrium on bedside echocardiography may also confirm correct placement.[39] Malpositioning still can occur when catheterization is performed by experienced clinicians, with a reported 14% occurrence rate in one study[14] and only 3% in another.[11]

Complications of central venous catheter placement are also more significant in patients who have thrombocytopenia. However, a recent study found that these complications can be minimized with platelet transfusions.[1] The investigators found that in cases of severe thrombocytopenia, minor complications occurred in 50% of the internal jugular catheter group, as opposed to 6% of the subclavian catheter group. In such patients, a single catheterization attempt is warranted, because complications markedly increase with additional attempts.[1] Risk of hemothorax in subclavian catheterization is low, and subcutaneous hematoma associated with numerous punctures is more common in patients with an international normalized ratio between 2 and 3.[10]

In summary, the optimal site for catheter insertion varies. The subclavian approach may not be available in certain cases, and a jugular site is recommended for patients with a high body mass index. Contraindications for the placement of central lines are skin lesions (due to infection or burn), rib fracture (especially of the clavicle), and severe coagulopathy.[1] Iatrogenic complications are more often seen in the sickest patients and require more frequent catheter placement and replacement. In one large prospective study in France of 360 iatrogenic complications in the ICU, human errors were found in two-thirds of the complications. Patients with multiorgan failure were at increased risk of iatrogenic complication.[13]

Finally, femoral artery puncture as a result of cerebral angiogram may lead to pseudo aneurysm, and they are usually detected 48 hours after removal of the sheath (Figure 61.2). Obesity, large sheath size, poor postprocedural compression, and peripheral arterial disease are some of the risk factors. Most small size (less than 2 cm) aneurysms resolve spontaneously. The risk of rupture increases when greater than 3 cm. Thrombin injection can be injected under ultrasound guidance and is highly effective. When recurrence occurs, surgical repair is needed.

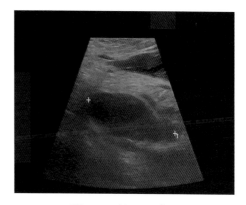

FIGURE 61.2: Ultrasound image of a pseudoaneurysm associated with a cerebral angiogram.

CENTRAL VENOUS CATHETER-RELATED THROMBOSIS

Venous thrombosis and its more dangerous complication, pulmonary embolus, are rare and are estimated to occur in approximately 0.1% of all catheter placements.[17,23,31] Nonetheless, catheter placement continues to be an important risk factor for symptomatic venous occlusive disease.[26,31] Patients with underlying malignancy may be at increased risk of thrombosis when an in-dwelling central venous catheter is placed. Venous thrombosis has been documented in up to 20% of patients who have a chemotherapy-associated catheter placement. Several studies have shown an increased incidence of central vein catheter–related thrombosis among patients in general ICUs, estimated to be as high as 4%. This incidence is likely underestimated because most patients continue to be asymptomatic, and ultrasonography in these studies was predicated on recently documented pulmonary embolus.[7,20] Central vein thrombosis is less frequently observed in patients who have received anticoagulation therapy, but only when the therapy is associated with a prolonged prothrombin time or activated partial thromboplastin time. The risk of thrombosis might also be decreased for patients who receive heparin flushes in addition to intravenous fluids. Theoretically limited use of subcutaneous heparin in patients with a recent neurosurgical procedure may place these patients at a comparatively high risk of thrombosis.

A recent randomized controlled trial on complications of femoral and subclavian venous catheterization found that femoral venous catheterization was associated with higher risk of thromboembolic complications. In this prospective study, thrombosis rate was approximately 2% at the subclavian site and 21% at the femoral catheter site.[23] Risk of pulmonary emboli associated with upper-limb venous thrombosis has been estimated at between 9% and 36%, and at a lower level than the estimated 50% risk of proximal lower-limb venous thrombosis.[24] A recent study of critically ill neurologic patients and PICC placement have a higher risk of symptomatic catheter-related deep vein thrombosis compared to jugular or subclavian catheters, but pulmomary emboli are very infrequent. The best treatment for PICC related thrombus is removal of the catheter and follow up ultrasound to monitor propagation of clot.[11]

Complications associated with PICC lines have been insufficiently studied, but the clinical impression is that they are uncommon. Increased occurrence of complications was found in patients who had PICC placement for chemotherapy, and this finding undoubtedly relates to the underlying coagulopathy. Using prophylactic anticoagulation with low-dose (4 mg) warfarin could decrease the prevalence of deep vein thrombosis, but using low-dose (1 mg) unmonitored warfarin therapy does not decrease the risk of thrombosis in patients with malignancy and central venous catheters.[16,27] The clinical manifestations of upper-extremity deep vein thrombosis are typically pain, swelling, and skin changes.[38] However, deep vein thrombosis is mostly detected incidentally.

CENTRAL VENOUS CATHETER INFECTION

Any intravascular catheter increases the risk of infection, and maintenance and replacement are discussed in Chapter 59. This remains a major area for quality control studies and safety programs that have proven to be effective.[19] In one study of patients receiving intensive care, the risk of catheter infection in colonization was low, at approximately 3%.[9] Strict sterile technique may have decreased the occurrence of bloodstream infection from central venous catheters, and another study suggested a 66% decrease with such technique and improved operator training.[8]

One study suggested that jugular venous catheterization access did not increase bacterial colonization compared with femoral catheterization.[34] In a randomized trial of 750 patients, the incidence of catheter colonization remained high among catheters inserted for 5 days or less. Gram-negative bacteria and fungi were predominant in

cultures from femoral catheters in this study.[28] Studies in other populations could be extrapolated to the NICU population, but in other ICUs most of these patients are in poorer health and often have multiorgan failure. There is interest in developing catheter devices with antimicrobial caps that would reduce contamination.[6]

CONCLUSIONS

- Most complications of venous access catheters include extravasation, thrombus formation, and infection. Many of the complications are infrequent, but they are often unavoidable.
- Ultrasound detection of catheter insertions has become an important additional tool.
- Training programs (simulation centers) using catheter insertions may improve skills and reduce real-life complications.

REFERENCES

1. Barrera R, Mina B, Huang Y, Groeger JS. Acute complications of central line placement in profoundly thrombocytopenic cancer patients. *Cancer* 1996;78:2025–2030.
2. Barsuk JH, McGaghie WC, Cohen ER, O'Leary KJ, Wayne DB. Simulation-based mastery learning reduces complications during central venous catheter insertion in a medical intensive care unit. *Crit Care Med* 2009;37:2697–2701.
3. Boon JM, van Schoor AN, Abrahams PH, Meiring JH, Welch T. Central venous catheterization: an anatomical review of a clinical skill. Part 2: internal jugular vein via the supraclavicular approach. *Clin Anat* 2008;21:15–22.
4. Boon JM, van Schoor AN, Abrahams PH, et al. Central venous catheterization: an anatomical review of a clinical skill. Part 1: subclavian vein via the infraclavicular approach. *Clin Anat* 2007;20:602–611.
5. Braner DA, Lai S, Eman S, Tegtmeyer K. Videos in clinical medicine. Central venous catheterization—subclavian vein. *N Engl J Med* 2007;357:e26.
6. Buchman AL, Spapperi J, Leopold P. A new central venous catheter cap: decreased microbial growth and risk for catheter-related bloodstream infection. *J Vasc Access* 2009;10:11–21.
7. Chin EE, Zimmerman PT, Grant EG. Sonographic evaluation of upper extremity deep venous thrombosis. *J Ultrasound Med* 2005;24:829–838; quiz 839–840.
8. Coopersmith CM, Rebmann TL, Zack JE, et al. Effect of an education program on decreasing catheter-related bloodstream infections in

the surgical intensive care unit. *Crit Care Med* 2002;30:59–64.

9. Deshpande KS, Hatem C, Ulrich HL, et al. The incidence of infectious complications of central venous catheters at the subclavian, internal jugular, and femoral sites in an intensive care unit population. *Crit Care Med* 2005;33:13–20.

10. Fisher NC, Mutimer DJ. Central venous cannulation in patients with liver disease and coagulopathy: a prospective audit. *Intens Care Med* 1999;25:481–485.

11. Jeffrey J, Fletcher JJ, Wilson TJ, Rajajee V, et al. A randomized trial of central venous catheter type and thrombosis in critically ill neurologic patients. *Neurocrit Care* 2016, in press.

12. Garrouste Orgeas M, Timsit JF, Soufir L, et al. Impact of adverse events on outcomes in intensive care unit patients. *Crit Care Med* 2008;36:2041–2047.

13. Giraud T, Dhainaut JF, Vaxelaire JF, et al. Iatrogenic complications in adult intensive care units: a prospective two-center study. *Crit Care Med* 1993;21:40–51.

14. Gladwin MT, Slonim A, Landucci DL, Gutierrez DC, Cunnion RE. Cannulation of the internal jugular vein: is postprocedural chest radiography always necessary? *Crit Care Med* 1999;27:1819–1823.

15. Graham AS, Ozment C, Tegtmeyer K, Lai S, Braner DA. Videos in clinical medicine: central venous catheterization. *N Engl J Med* 2007;356:e21.

16. Heaton DC, Han DY, Inder A. Minidose (1 mg) warfarin as prophylaxis for central vein catheter thrombosis. *Intern Med J* 2002;32:84–88.

17. Horattas MC, Wright DJ, Fenton AH, et al. Changing concepts of deep venous thrombosis of the upper extremity: report of a series and review of the literature. *Surgery* 1988;104:561–567.

18. Hoskote SS, Khouli H, Lanoix R, et al. Simulation-based training for emergency medicine residents in sterile technique during central venous catheterization: impact on performance, policy, and outcomes. *Acad Emerg Med* 2015;22:81–87.

19. Hsu YJ, Marsteller JA. Influence of the comprehensive unit-based safety program in ICUs: evidence from the Keystone ICU Project. *Am J Med Qual* 2015.

20. Huisman MV, Buller HR, ten Cate JW, et al. Unexpected high prevalence of silent pulmonary embolism in patients with deep venous thrombosis. *Chest* 1989;95:498–502.

21. Mansfield PF, Hohn DC, Fornage BD, Gregurich MA, Ota DM. Complications and failures of subclavian-vein catheterization. *N Engl J Med* 1994;331:1735–1738.

22. Maze R, Le May MR, Froeschl M, et al. Endovascular cooling catheter related thrombosis in patients undergoing therapeutic hypothermia for out of hospital cardiac arrest. *Resuscitation* 2014;85:1354–1358.

23. Merrer J, De Jonghe B, Golliot F, et al. Complications of femoral and subclavian venous catheterization in critically ill patients: a randomized controlled trial. *JAMA* 2001;286: 700–707.

24. Monreal M, Lafoz E, Ruiz J, Valls R, Alastrue A. Upper-extremity deep venous thrombosis and pulmonary embolism: a prospective study. *Chest* 1991;99:280–283.

25. Muller A, Lorenz A, Seifert B, Keller E. Risk of thromboembolic events with endovascular cooling catheters in patients with subarachnoid hemorrhage. *Neurocrit Care* 2014;21:207–210.

26. Ong B, Gibbs H, Catchpole I, Hetherington R, Harper J. Peripherally inserted central catheters and upper extremity deep vein thrombosis. *Australas Radiol* 2006;50:451–454.

27. Paauw JD, Borders H, Ingalls N, et al. The incidence of PICC line-associated thrombosis with and without the use of prophylactic anticoagulants. *JPEN J Parenter Enteral Nutr* 2008;32:443–447.

28. Parienti JJ, Thirion M, Megarbane B, et al. Femoral vs jugular venous catheterization and risk of nosocomial events in adults requiring acute renal replacement therapy: a randomized controlled trial. *JAMA* 2008;299:2413–2422.

29. Park HS, Kim YI, Lee SH, et al. Central venous infusion port inserted via high versus low jugular venous approaches: retrospective comparison of outcome and complications. *Eur J Radiol* 2009;72:494–498.

30. Pikwer A, Baath L, Davidson B, Perstoft I, Akeson J. The incidence and risk of central venous catheter malpositioning: a prospective cohort study in 1619 patients. *Anaesth Intensive Care* 2008;36:30–37.

31. Prandoni P, Polistena P, Bernardi E, et al. Upper-extremity deep vein thrombosis: risk factors, diagnosis, and complications. *Arch Intern Med* 1997;157:57–62.

32. Reccius A, Mercado P, Vargas P, Canals C, Montes J. Inferior vena cava thrombosis related to hypothermia catheter: report of 20 consecutive cases. *Neurocrit Care* 2015;23:72–77.

33. Roux D, Reignier J, Thiery G, et al. Acquiring procedural skills in ICUs: a prospective multicenter study. *Crit Care Med* 2014;42:886–895.

34. Ruesch S, Walder B, Tramer MR. Complications of central venous catheters: internal jugular

versus subclavian access: a systematic review. *Crit Care Med* 2002;30:454–460.

35. Schummer W, Schummer C, Rose N, Niesen WD, Sakka SG. Mechanical complications and malpositions of central venous cannulations by experienced operators: a prospective study of 1794 catheterizations in critically ill patients. *Intens Care Med* 2007;33:1055–1059.

36. Schweickert WD, Herlitz J, Pohlman AS, et al. A randomized, controlled trial evaluating postinsertion neck ultrasound in peripherally inserted central catheter procedures. *Crit Care Med* 2009;37:1217–1221.

37. Sznajder JI, Zveibil FR, Bitterman H, Weiner P, Bursztein S. Central vein catheterization: failure and complication rates by three percutaneous approaches. *Arch Intern Med* 1986;146: 259–261.

38. Timsit JF, Farkas JC, Boyer JM, et al. Central vein catheter-related thrombosis in intensive care patients: incidence, risks factors, and relationship with catheter-related sepsis. *Chest* 1998;114:207–213.

39. Weekes AJ, Johnson DA, Keller SM, et al. Central vascular catheter placement evaluation using saline flush and bedside echocardiography. *Acad Emerg Med* 2014;21:65–72.

40. Weinstein M. Severe soft-tissue injury following intravenous infusion of phenytoin. *Arch Intern Med* 1989;149:1905.

41. Wijdicks EFM. *Neurologic Complications of Critical Illness*. 3rd ed. Oxford: Oxford University Press; 2009.

42. Ziv A, Rubin O, Sidi A, Berkenstadt H. Credentialing and certifying with simulation. *Anesthesiol Clin* 2007;25:261–269.

62

Management of Drug Reactions

Drug administration in critically ill neurologic patients is generally different from patients on the ward and also different from patients in general medical and surgical ICUs. First, IV administration of medication is preferred to circumvent absorption problems in acute brain injury. Second, acute hepatic and renal failure is less common in the NICU, and adjustment in dosing is less frequently needed. Third, therapeutic drug monitoring for commonly used antiepileptic drugs that have a narrow therapeutic range is often needed, and these drugs may blend over into toxicity. Fourth, the safety profile of any drug is different in the elderly and the actively cooled patient; both are relatively more commonly seen in the NICU.

Drug-related events in the NICU are likely common, but they are rarely accurately tabulated. Skin rash remains most common; but even if drug reactions are suspected, it may not be clear that a certain drug can be attributable or if the dermatological reaction can be sufficiently characterized.

Any NICU will see adverse drug reactions, some of which are minimal and easily spotted, such as increase in liver function tests after recent introduction of a new agent. There are major adverse effects with a potential dramatic course that requires immediate action besides discontinuation of the drug. Recognition that a certain drug causes a certain clinical syndrome remains for some reason difficult, and many physicians need to be reminded of it by pharmacists. This is understandable because ICU physicians cannot have extensive knowledge of drug side effects or even complex pharmacodynamics or kinetics.

The most concerning adverse drug reaction is DRESS (drug reaction with eosinophilia and systemic symptoms) syndrome. For the neurointensivist, it is pertinent to know that antiepileptic drugs are a recognized cause of DRESS.[6] There are several other drugs in the NICU that can cause undesirable side effects. This chapter will discuss and show the most pertinent drug reactions, but excludes drug administration errors or major toxicity and recognizes the myriad drug side effects can be found in on-line drug databases.

PRINCIPLES OF PHARMACODYNAMICS AND PHARMACOKINETICS

The application of pharmacodynamic principles is relevant in the NICU. With any drug, distribution is most important and dependent on absorption (potentially disturbed by gastrointestinal motility disturbances), distribution (potentially affected by obesity or lean body mass), metabolism (potentially delayed by liver failure), and elimination (potentially impaired by renal failure). Pharmacodynamics studies the relationship between the drug concentration and its efficacy. The study of pharmacodynamics has qualitative aspects (e.g., specific chemical receptors, active sites of enzymes, and selective target tissue sites) and quantitative aspects (e.g., dose responsiveness, potency, therapeutic efficacy, and tolerance).

The qualitative component of pharmacodynamics mostly pertains to drug attachment to receptors (e.g., generally used anesthetic agents act unselectively or by binding to receptors). Important receptors in the pharmacodynamics of anesthetic drugs are γ-aminobutyric acid (GABA), N-methyl-D-aspartate (NMDA), and opioids (μ, δ, and κ). Barbiturates, benzodiazepines, and propofol bind to the GABA receptors and activate them because they resemble the natural transmitter. The number of receptors changes from exposure and may decrease with continuous exposure (down-regulation), resulting in a loss of efficacy (tachyphylaxis). This so-called acquired tolerance is especially known with opioids at their receptor sites. They may also have an increased effect from prolonged contact with antagonists (up-regulation). For example, when a benzodiazepine is administered, tolerance may occur with excessive doses and extended duration. Most typically, patients who are tolerant of the effects of alcohol have a similar physiologic response to benzodiazepines and barbiturates so that a higher dose is required to achieve sedation.

The quantitative aspects of pharmacodynamics include potency and efficacy. Potency is the amount of drug in relation to its effect, and therapeutic efficacy is the capacity of a drug to produce an often maximum effect. An important concept is the therapeutic index, which, simplified, is the maximum tolerated dose divided by the minimum desired therapeutic effect. Drugs with a small therapeutic window cause adverse effects well below the amount that produces the maximum effect and often have a minimal difference between toxic and therapeutic doses.

Pharmacokinetics studies the relationships of dose administration, concentration of the drug over time, and rate at which the drug enters, diffuses within, and leaves the body. Most drugs are subject to first-order processes of absorption, distribution within the central compartment (predominantly the blood volume and any highly vascularized organ), metabolism, and excretion. The rate at which these occur is directly proportional to the concentration of the drug. In first-order (exponential) processes, it can be predicted that, for example, a 50% increase in dose will lead to an increase in steady-state plasma concentration by the same percentage.

Zero-order processes (saturation) are much slower than first-order processes, and elimination occurs independent of concentration. This process requires enzymatic elimination and thus is limited in speed. Many drugs exhibit saturation, or zero-order, kinetics when a high enough dose is administered, and this effect explains delay in recovery from drug overdose. Phenytoin is a typical example. At low doses, elimination can match an increase in dose; but gradually with higher doses, the enzymatic process reaches saturation and the plasma concentration rises disproportionately into toxic territory.

Many drugs are administered intravenously. In about five times the half-life, the mean plasma concentration is constant and at a plateau; the plasma concentration decreases to zero in five times the half-life when infusion is stopped.

Altered protein binding remains a crucial component in hepatic drug metabolism associated with critical illness and may last up to 4 weeks after the critical illness has been controlled. With hypoalbuminemia, a greater proportion of benzodiazepines is unbound and thus active. Finally, after liver transplantation, liver function (monitored by bile output and liver function tests) can

be marginal; and accumulation of benzodiazepines can be very rapid. Thus, hepatic dysfunction in critically ill patients is a major contributor to prolonged sedation and may be underappreciated.

Renal failure predominantly affects the clearance of morphine and midazolam metabolites. Commonly, the proposed mechanism is reduced perfusion of the kidney; but metabolic acidosis and respiratory alkalosis in this condition may also change the pH difference between tissue and plasma compartments, leading to a change in tissue distribution.

ADVERSE EFFECTS DUE TO DRUG INTERACTION

The most common drug interactions that are seen in the NICU are shown in Table 62.1. Many of these interactions involve antiepileptic drugs and need to be recognized. Most antiepileptic drugs decrease the effect of commonly used drugs such as corticosteroids and tricyclic antidepressants. Most concerns in the NICU are drugs that decrease the seizure threshold. The carbapenems are one example, and they are contraindicated in patients with acute brain injury at risk of seizures because

---

TABLE 62.1. COMMON DRUG INTERACTIONS IN THE NICU

Warfarin and Valproic Acid
Mode of action: Drug displacement in protein-binding site; a high loading dose reaching a higher serum level may displace warfarin from a valproic acid binding site.

Phenytoin and Fluconazole
Mode of action: Fluconazole inhibits phenytoin metabolism and may increase phenytoin level up to 4 times. Serum concentration monitoring with a reduction in phenytoin dosage is warranted.

Valproic Acid and Carbapenems
Mode of action: The exact mechanism is unknown. Carbapenems, especially meropenem, may inhibit valproic acid absorption. Meropenem may accelerate the renal excretion and may result in low valproic acid serum level and increase risk of seizures. Additionally, carbapenems lower seizure threshold.

Statin and Levofloxacin or Amiodarone
Mode of action: The exact mechanism is unknown, but severe rhabdomyolysis may occur.

Clopidogrel and Omeprazole
Mode of action: Omeprazole inhibits CYP2C19, which is responsible for the conversion of clopidogrel into its active form. The effect of clopidogrel is reduced up to 47%.

---

they intrinsically lower the seizure threshold. The imipenem seizure rates are several-fold higher (up to 30%) than meropenem rates, which are less than 1%, and even the newer carbapenems such as ertapenem may have low risk of seizures. The risk of seizures by imipenem was mostly higher when the dose exceeded 2 g.

DRUG-INDUCED SKIN RASH

Adverse drug reactions manifest themselves in a systemic reaction and many start with skin eruption. Most of these rashes are of no concern and are self-limiting. Recognition requires understanding the defining characteristics of an adverse drug reaction, and also whether there is a likelihood that this explanation is the most valid. Drug reactions usually begin several days following administration of the drug, but drug reactions may occur weeks after the introduction of the drug, and can even produce a toxic epidermal necrolysis to acute generalized exanthematous pustulosis (AGEP). Vancomycin is associated with red man syndrome, which results in significant redness and blanching (Figure 62.1).[8] The typical reactions are shown in Table 62.2. Many of these drug reactions can be treated with topically applied medication, although a more dramatic presentation will have to be treated with a combination of drugs. The treatment of any major emerging drug effect should be the following: epinephrine 1 mg IM, which can be repeated if needed; methylprednisolone 125 mg IV; and diphenhydramine 50 mg IV.[1] A more complicated syndrome is DRESS syndrome (Capsule 62.1).

DRUG-INDUCED ANGIOEDEMA

Angioedema is an uncommon manifestation but can become rapidly problematic, causing difficulty with airway management. The most common drugs used in the NICU that can cause angioedema are angiotensin converting enzyme (ACE) inhibitors. Angioedema is the result of increased plasmakinins and an increase of bradykinin that causes significant leaking vessels, resulting in the rapid development of swelling of lips and posterior pharynx. It may start subtly and then worsen, or there may be a forme fruste of angioedema (Figure 62.2). The rapid development needs to be recognized because when the hypopharynx or larynx becomes involved, intubation might be very difficult or virtually impossible, causing some physicians to proceed with a cricothyrotomy. Most of the time there is a significant time lapse,

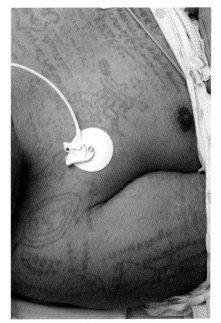

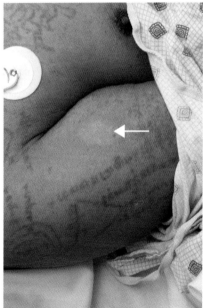

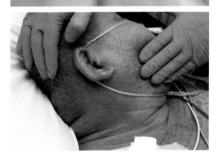

FIGURE 62.1: Marked erythema associated with vancomycin infusion. Note marked blanching (arrow) after pressing with an index finger. Note pustulosis (AGEP).

TABLE 62.2. DRUG-INDUCED DERMATOLOGICAL INJURY

Adverse Drug Reaction			Clinical Pharmacology (DoTS)
Reaction	Paradigm Cause	Associated Features	Time from Drug Exposure to Onset
Acute generalized erythematous pustulosis	Diltiazem	Fever > 38°C, neutrophilia, facial edema	Days to weeks (slow time course with diltiazem)
	Erythromycin	Fever > 38°C, neutrophilia, facial edema	Hours to days (rapid time course with antibiotics)
Angioedema due to Type I hypersensitivity	Penicillin	Anaphylactic shock	Minutes
Drug reaction with eosinophilia and systemic symptoms	Phenytoin	Lymphadenopathy, fever, hepatitis, nephritis, pulmonary infiltrates, eosinophilia	Days to weeks
Exanthems	Ampicillin		Days
Fixed drug eruption	Barbiturates		Hours
Phototoxicity	Amiodarone		Months (reaction appears minutes to hours after sun exposure)
Red person syndrome	Vancomycin	Hypotension	Minutes
Scleromyxedema	Gadolinium contrast media	Systemic fibrosis	Many months
Stevens-Johnson syndrome/ toxic epidermal necrolysis	Carbamazepine	Fever, dysphagia, dysuria, conjunctivitis, leukopenia	Days to weeks

DoTS, *dose*, time-course, susceptibility. Adapted from Ferner RE.[5]

but any patient who develops lip swelling with a recent administration of angiotensin converting enzymes will have to be treated with epinephrine (EpiPen® Auto-Injector), followed by 10 mg IV dexamethasone and 50 mg IV diphenhydramine. Many experts also require the use of fresh frozen plasma to reduce bradykinesis. Elective intubation

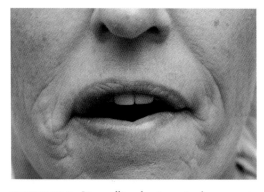

FIGURE 62.2: Lip swelling due to angioedema associated with intravenous tPA. Swelling always starts at the same side of the limb weakness and in this patient on the right.

might be necessary if the swelling progresses.[2,10] The patient needs to be closely monitored, and swelling may subside in several days.

DRUG-INDUCED HYPERPYREXIA

Marked increase in temperature after administration of drugs has been noted with anticholinergics, antidopaminergics, selective serotonin reuptake inhibitors (SSRIs), and tricyclic antidepressants.

Neuroleptic malignant syndrome (NMS) is usually seen after the use of haloperidol and fluphenazine and atypical antipsychotic drugs such as clozapine, risperidone, and olanzapine. Usually the reaction is to the first dose, and results in agitated delirium, mutism and catatonia, and severe muscular rigidity, resulting in marked increase in serum creatine kinase. The patient rapidly becomes dehydrated from fever, and laboratory abnormalities show hypernatremia, hypomagnesemia, and hypocalcemia, which all require correction. SSRIs can cause a serotonin syndrome, but this is a rare condition occurring de novo in the NICU. Many of these patients might be seen in medical ICUs, admitted with confusion and

CAPSULE 62.1   DRESS SYNDROME

The drug reaction with eosinophilia and systemic symptoms (DRESS) syndrome is a poorly understood phenomenon that has been diagnosed using the following diagnostic criteria: (1) macular-papillar rash (see accompanying figure) developing more than 3 weeks after drug initiation; (2) clinical symptoms persisting more than 2 weeks after stopping the drug; (3) fever more than 38°C; (4) transaminase elevation; (5) leucocytosis, atypical lymphocytes, eosinophilia; and (6) lymphadenopathy at multiple sites.[3,4,6] The delayed onset of symptoms 2–6 weeks after initiation for causative drug is a typical feature of DRESS. The pathophysiology is unknown, but there are several susceptible drugs. (Initially DRESS was described as an anticonvulsant, hypersensitivity syndrome.[17]) There is most likely a genetic susceptibility. Some studies have suggested an HHV 6 reactivation as a potential contributor to DRESS development.[9]

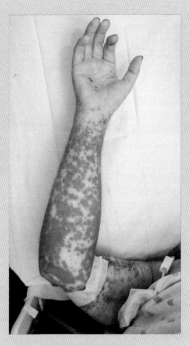

Skin eruption in patient with DRESS.

fever. Serotonin syndrome has characteristic myoclonus, vomiting, and diarrhea. The treatment for NMS is dantrolene 1mg/k IV followed by repeated dose up to 10 mg/k IV. The treatment for severe serotonin syndrome is midazolam infusion to suppress the movements while initiating cyproheptadine (Chapter 8).

ADVERSE EFFECTS DUE TO IVIG AND PLASMA EXCHANGE

Plasma exchange is typically without any significant side effects, and anaphylaxis is uncommon.

Most problems have been seen with patients on ACE inhibitors which should be stopped before plasma exchange. Red blood cell loss is typically small, and hypotension as a result of replacement of plasma responds very well to a single fluid bolus. A transfusion-related acute lung injury is uncommon. Many patients with plasma exchange will have recognizable side effects; these are discussed in chapters on Guillain-Barré syndrome and myasthenia gravis (Chapters 42 and 43). IVIG may have an acute renal failure, but mostly in patients who have IVIG with high sucrose content, and patients

TABLE 62.3. ETIOLOGIES OF EXTRAVASATION BY RISK FACTOR CATEGORY

Category	Risk Factors
Infusion-specific factors	
	Duration of infusion
	Infiltration volume
	Catheter gauge (relative to vein size)
	Inadequately secured catheter
	Catheter type (steel > Teflon > polyurethane)
	Infusion rate
	Catheter location in elbow, ankle, dorsum of hand, or any other point of flexion
	Multiple venous access attempts proximal to site of venous access
	Need for catheter readjustments
Patient-specific factors	
	Patient skin color (darker skin may delay time to detection)
	Hypotension
	Decompensated blood flow
	Peripheral vascular disease
	Raynaud disease
	Prior extravasation injury
	Altered skin and subcutaneous tissue integrity
	Excessive patient movement around venous access site
	Clot formation at cannulation site
	Lymphedema
	Extremes in age
	Altered mental status or inability to verbalize pain
	Peripheral neuropathy or other altered sensory perception
	Variation in venous and arteriolar anatomy
Healthcare-specific factors	
	Lack of knowledge of intravenous access establishment or access skills
	Lack of knowledge of common vesicants
	Distractions or lack of monitoring for infiltration during drug administration of high-risk drugs
	Overnight shift and emergency situations.

Adapted from Reynolds.[11]

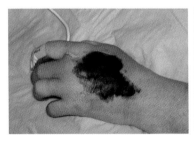 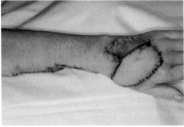

FIGURE 62.3: Blister formation and tissue necrosis after extravasation of vancomycin requiring split thickness skin graft.

with chronic renal failure may be predisposed. Transient fever, chills, urticaria, arthralgias, and hyperglycemia have been described in IVIG but continue to be uncommon side effects and are temporary.

EXTRAVASATION OF DRUGS

Most cannulation sites are in the forearm veins. The medial cubital vein in the antecubital fossa is a site for emergency cannulation. Other peripheral sites are on the dorsum of the palm. Risk factors for extravasation are shown in Table 62.3.[4,13] When extravasation occurs, the cannula should remain in place to administer antidote if applicable.[7] Patients receiving vasopressors require phentolamine (5–10 mg diluted in 10 mL normal saline) within 12 hours of infiltration. The affected extremity should be elevated above the heart, and ice or hot packs should be applied evenly for a 2-hour duration, every 12 hours. A plastic surgeon consult is advised. Infusion of drugs into peripheral catheters may lead to extravasation, and many drugs can lead to sloughing of skin (Figure 62.3). Soft-tissue damage after intravenous administration in a peripheral hand vein (purple glove syndrome) may be associated with marked purple discoloration and edema; however, this complication is rarely seen.[13]

CONCLUSIONS

- Drug side effects are common but are rarely consequential or leading to major comorbidity.
- Drug interactions are complicated and are insufficiently appreciated.
- Polypharmacy changes pharmacodynamics in NICU.
- Major skin lesions may include pustulosis and generalized redness.

REFERENCES

1. Ardern-Jones MR, Friedmann PS. Skin manifestations of drug allergy. *Br J Clin Pharmacol* 2011;71:672–683.
2. Banerji A, Clark S, Blanda M, et al. Multicenter study of patients with angiotensin-converting enzyme inhibitor-induced angioedema who present to the emergency department. *Ann Allergy Asthma Immunol* 2008;100:327–332.
3. Cacoub P, Musette P, Descamps V, et al. The DRESS syndrome: a literature review. *Am J Med* 2011;124:588–597.
4. Descamps V, Ranger-Rogez S. DRESS syndrome. *Joint Bone Spine* 2014;81:15–21.
5. Ferner RE. Adverse drug reactions in dermatology. *Clin Exp Dermatol* 2015;40:105–109.
6. Funck-Brentano E, Duong TA, Bouvresse S, et al. Therapeutic management of DRESS: a retrospective study of 38 cases. *J Am Acad Dermatol* 2015;72:246–252.
7. Heckler FR. Current thoughts on extravasation injuries. *Clin Plast Surg* 1989;16:557–563.
8. Holliman R. "Red man syndrome" associated with rapid vancomycin infusion. *Lancet* 1985;1:1399–1400.
9. Ichiche M, Kiesch N, De Bels D. DRESS syndrome associated with HHV-6 reactivation. *Eur J Intern Med* 2003;14:498–500.
10. Karim MY, Masood A. Fresh-frozen plasma as a treatment for life-threatening ACE-inhibitor angioedema. *J Allergy Clin Immunol* 2002;109:370–371.
11. Reynolds PM, MacLaren R, Mueller SW, Fish DN, Kiser TH. Management of extravasation injuries: a focused evaluation of noncytotoxic medications. *Pharmacotherapy* 2014;34:617–632.
12. Shear NH, Spielberg SP. Anticonvulsant hypersensitivity syndrome: in vitro assessment of risk. *J Clin Invest* 1988;82:1826–1832.
13. Weinstein M. Severe soft-tissue injury following intravenous infusion of phenytoin. *Arch Intern Med* 1989;149:1905.

PART XII

Decisions at the End of Life
and Other Responsibilities

63

The Diagnosis of Brain Death

There are limits beyond which the treatment of catastrophic brain injury cannot go, leaving an irrecoverable condition and persistent coma. A clear dividing line exists between severe brain damage leading to persistent vegetative state, or a minimally conscious state and a neurologic condition associated with complete loss of brain function, also known as brain death.[1,53,128,129]

Brain death in adults is frequently a consequence of severe traumatic brain injury, re-rupture in aneurysmal subarachnoid hemorrhage, and cerebral hemorrhage.[15,16] It is less common in patients with fulminant encephalitis or bacterial meningitis and after anoxic–ischemic encephalopathy from cardiac resuscitation. The prevalence may be declining but has largely to do with recognition and decisions not to do a formal evaluation.[68,71]

Neurologists with experience in critical care neurology and neurosurgeons are commonly involved in the clinical determination of brain death, but staff of any specialty could arrive at the same conclusion. When a neurologist or neurosurgeon is not involved in care or is unavailable for consultation, intensivists or pediatricians typically declare brain death.

Brain death determination, however, is an elaborate task and includes assessment of the proximate cause, interpretation of neuroimaging findings, recognition of conditions that can mimic brain death, full neurologic examination with an apnea test, determination of the indication of confirmatory tests and how to interpret results, management of acute physiologic derangements associated with brain death, and proper documentation.[124,136]

The diagnosis of brain death may lead to organ donation. The early identification of potential organ and tissue donor candidates is important, but the selection of donors can proceed only after the clinical diagnosis of brain death and the consent of family members or a legal representative. The determination of brain death in adults has been reviewed and published as a position paper by the American Academy of Neurology and has been recently revised. The pediatric guidelines were recently updated.[100] Many other works exist, including those specifically directed at brain death determination in neonates and children.[2–4,14–16,27,50,84,91,95,96,115,123,126,128,135] Simulation programs have been developed to teach the complex determination.[55,56,85]

NATIONAL AND INTERNATIONAL CRITERIA

In the United States, legal justification for the determination of death by neurologic criteria is established in the Uniform Determination of Death Act,[5] but US neurologists or neurosurgeons should comply with state law and hospital policies and with any other modifications that may be in place.

In 1995, the Quality Standards Subcommittee of the American Academy of Neurology (AAN) published guidelines for the determination of brain death in adults. The 2010 update was heavily vetted and provided overtly conservative instructions and strict criteria to determine brain death.[135] The AAN guideline was provided as an educational service to practicing neurologists, neurosurgeons, neurointensivists and intensivists. Adherence to the AAN guidelines is voluntary. A survey in leading hospitals in the United States found major differences compared with the AAN guideline.[45] Variations were found in required prerequisites, the lowest acceptable core temperature, the number of required examinations, or the number of physicians required to be involved in the declaration. Differences in expert consensus during the review of the hospital guidelines may have contributed to these variations.[45] A recent survey of 508 unique hospital policies revealed the new AAN guidelines have been incorporated in a substantial number of policies but significant variability remains for brain death

---

CAPSULE 63.1   INTERNATIONAL BRAIN DEATH CRITERIA

There are significant differences in brain death protocols throughout countries in the world. There are striking differences concerning number of physicians, qualifications of physicians, observations time, and need for ancillary tests. Some differences are actually consequential and technically one person could already have been declared brain death in one country but not in another. Apprehensions about errors and physicians' skills may have introduced these "safe guards," but the situation is clearly unwanted. Ancillary tests are skewed toward bedside tests and are mandated in 28 of 70 practice guidelines (40%) in countries of the European Union. It is strange to see test are needed in one European country but not in a neighboring country. Globally, the number of physicians varies from one to four, and in some countries only seasoned physicians with at least associate professor status are allowed to make the determination. Equally troubling is the great variation in time of observation. Many countries, without any justification, require a 24-hour interval in patients who become brain dead after cardiac resuscitation. It is possible that cultural attitudes have modelled these guidelines. Japan has constructed even more complex criteria. (These criteria include a CT scan showing irreparable lesions, the ciliospinal reflex being tested, the apnea test being performed after the loss of seven brainstem reflexes and only after an isoelectric EEG, and exclusion of children less than 6-years-old). In the future, a world-wide consensus on more simplified criteria for brain death may be achieved with the cooperation of multiple professional organizations. This may be utopian and not expected to happen.

---

determination.[46] Determination by one physician is sufficient in most states, but independent confirmation by another physician is required in the states of California, Connecticut, Florida, Iowa, Kentucky, and Louisiana. In Alaska and Georgia, a registered nurse can be the delegated authority to declare death, according to their statutory criteria, but certification by a physician is needed within 24 hours.[127] Other examples of differences in the United States are that only a physician in the neurosciences can make the determination in Virginia, and that the right to have a religious exemption is accepted in New Jersey and New York.[127] The amendments in these states require physicians to honor the request to continue medical care in a brain-dead body.

There is a broad acceptance of the neurologic state of brain death throughout the world. However, brain death guidelines are very different among countries (Capsule 63.1).[50,127] A workable set of (simplified) criteria for brain death should be a priority for professional organizations, but frustratingly there is very little consensus how to get there.[127]

CLINICAL DIAGNOSIS OF BRAIN DEATH

The clinical diagnosis of brain death is equivalent to irreversible loss of all brain and brainstem function.

Loss of consciousness, lack of a coordinated motor response to pain stimuli, absence of brainstem reflexes, and apnea must be documented. In adults, there are no published reports in peer-reviewed medical journals of recovery of neurologic function after a comprehensive determination of brain death using the AAN practice parameter.[135] The procedure of brain death determination is summarized in Figure 63.1, and the principles of neurologic examination are shown in Figure 63.2.

The cause of brain death should be clear from neuroimaging. In most patients, initial cranial computed tomography (CT) reveals diffuse cerebral edema, acute hemispheric mass with profound tissue shift, or multiple hemispheric lesions destroying most of the brain. Obviously, the clinical diagnosis of brain death should be in doubt in patients with normal CT findings. However, this situation occurs in patients with a severe, prolonged anoxic–ischemic insult to the brain. In these patients, the clinical diagnosis of brain death should be made only if there is a high degree of certainty about the mechanism that led to brain death. In addition, a cerebrospinal fluid (CSF) examination is warranted to detect infection in patients with initially normal CT scans. In many patients with such a fulminant meningitis or encephalitis, diffuse edema of the brain will appear on CT scans.

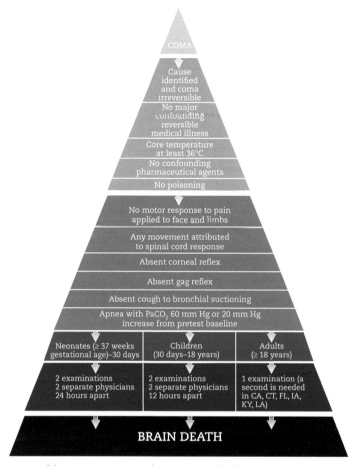

FIGURE 63.1: Summary of the necessary steps to diagnose brain death.

Confounders in Brain Death Determination

Confounding factors that mimic or partly mimic brain death should be excluded.[55,56,131]

Several studies have been published on the recognition of mimics of brain death, including fulminant Guillain-Barré syndrome, organophosphate intoxication, high cervical spinal cord injury, lidocaine toxicity, baclofen overdose, and prolonged vecuronium clearance.[35,66,94,99,106,107,119] In none of the patients described in these articles was a complete brain death examination performed, despite the use of "brain death" in the title or body of the paper.

Hypothermia may blunt brainstem reflexes, but only if core temperatures are below 32°C. With core temperatures below 27°C, brainstem reflexes most likely become absent.[33,37] The influence of any drug effect should be excluded. Routine drug screens may be helpful but mostly when testing is requested for a specific drug or poison. Drug screens may detect alcohol, barbiturates, antiepileptics, benzodiazepines, antihistamines, antidepressants, antipsychotics, amphetamines, narcotics, and analgesics. The diagnosis of brain death most likely can be made when blood levels of barbiturates are subtherapeutic; however, data are lacking in adults. In brain-dead children with therapeutic levels of barbiturates, no change in isoelectric electroencephalograms (EEG) was noted during a decrease of barbiturates in the blood to subtherapeutic or undetectable levels.[73] In extremely high doses, barbiturates also may reduce cerebral blood flow through a mechanism of vasoconstriction, but a more likely explanation for reduced flow is a marked decrease in metabolic demand. The effect of high doses of barbiturates on cerebral blood flow in patients is not known. It is inappropriate to replace a clinical examination confounded by sedative agents such as barbiturates with a test of cerebral blood flow.

The clinical diagnosis of brain death is probably not reliable in patients investigated at the time of an acute severe metabolic or endocrine

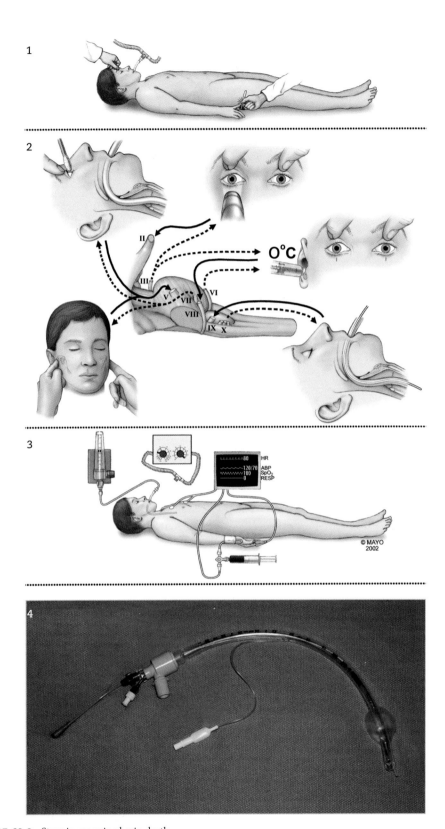

FIGURE 63.2: Steps in assessing brain death.

In part 1, the physician determines that there is no motor response and the eyes do not open when a painful stimulus is applied to the supraorbital nerve or nail bed. In part 2, a clinical assessment of brainstem reflexes is undertaken. The tested cranial nerves are indicated by Roman numerals; the solid arrows represent afferent limbs, and the broken arrows efferent limbs. Depicted are the absence of grimacing or eye opening with deep pressure on both condyles at the level of the temporomandibular joint (afferent nerve V and efferent nerve VII), the absent corneal reflex elicited

derangement, but clear threshold values are not known. In addition, alcohol intoxication and head and spine injury are often closely linked. The condition of patients with apnea and quadriplegia due to traumatic cervical spine distraction and alcohol intoxication may superficially mimic brain death if the brainstem reflexes are not carefully examined.[101] Alcohol has a plasma half-life of 10 mL/hour, and the limit for determination of brain death would be similar to the limit for driving, which in most US states is 0.8, or 800 mg/L.

In summary, to overcome the pitfalls of misdiagnosis, the following prerequisites are needed: (1) definite clinical, neuroimaging, or CSF evidence of an acute central nervous system catastrophe compatible with brain death; (2) lack of complicating medical conditions that may confound clinical assessment (no severe electrolyte, acid–base, or endocrine disturbance); (3) no drug intoxication or poisoning; and (4) core temperature of at least 32°C but preferably normothermia (≥ 36°C). Testing of brain function can proceed only after these requirements have been satisfied.

PRACTICE OF BRAIN DEATH DETERMINATION
The following guidance has been proposed.[126,128,135,136]

Coma or Unresponsiveness
Motor responses of the limbs to painful stimuli should be absent after pressure on the supraorbital nerve, nail-bed pressure stimulus, or simultaneous pressure on both temporomandibular condyles.

One should be aware of several pitfalls. Motor responses may be absent from high cervical cord injury.[101,125] Motor responses (usually brief finger flexion without coordinated responses) of spinal origin may occur spontaneously during apnea testing, often during hypoxic or hypotensive episodes, or during pain stimuli. Sometimes these movements are synchronous with the mechanical ventilator cycle.[07]

Prior use of neuromuscular blocking agents can produce prolonged weakness.[97] If neuromuscular blocking agents have recently been administered, examination with a bedside peripheral nerve stimulator is needed. A train-of-four stimulus should result in four thumb twitches when the neuromuscular blocking agent has been fully washed out.

Absence of Brainstem Reflexes
Pupils
The response to bright light should be absent in both eyes. Round, oval, or irregularly shaped pupils are compatible with brain death. Most pupils in brain death are in mid-position (6–7 mm).[78] Dilated pupils are compatible with brain death because intact sympathetic cervical pathways connected with the radially arranged fibers of the dilator muscle may remain intact. Miosis is very uncommon but can occur with massive pontine destruction.

Many drugs can influence pupil size, but light response remains intact. In conventional doses, atropine given intravenously has no marked influence on pupillary response.[39,43] A report of fixed, dilated pupils after extremely high doses of dopamine has not been confirmed.[92] Because nicotine receptors are absent in the iris, neuromuscular blocking drugs do not noticeably influence pupil size.[42] Topical ocular instillation of drugs and trauma to the cornea or bulbus oculi can cause abnormalities in pupil size and

---

by touching the edge of the cornea (V and VII), the absent light reflex (II and III), the absent oculovestibular response toward the side of the cold stimulus provided by ice water (pen marks at the level of the pupils can be used as reference) (VIII and III and VI), and the absent cough reflex elicited through the introduction of a suction catheter deep in the trachea (IX and X). In part 3, the apnea test is performed; the disconnection of the ventilator and the use of apneic diffusion oxygenation require precautionary measures. The core temperature should be ≥ 36˚C, the systolic blood pressure should be 90 mm Hg or higher, and the fluid balance should be positive for 6 hours. After preoxygenation (the fraction of inspired oxygen should be 1.0 for 10 minutes), the ventilation rate should be decreased. The ventilator should be disconnected if the partial pressure of arterial oxygen reaches 200 mm Hg or higher and if the partial pressure of arterial carbon dioxide reaches 40 mm Hg or higher. In part 4, the oxygen catheter should be at the carina (delivering oxygen at a rate of 6 L/min) shown here is the position of the oxygen catheter in an endotracheal tube. The physician should observe the chest and the abdominal wall for respiration for 8–10 minutes and should monitor the patient for changes in vital functions. If there is a partial pressure of arterial carbon dioxide of 60 mm Hg or higher or an increase of more than 20 mm Hg from the normal baseline value, apnea is confirmed.

ABP, arterial blood pressure; HR, heart rate; RESP, respirations; SpO2, oxygen saturation measured by pulse oximetry.

From Wijdicks EFM. The clinical diagnosis of Brain death. *N Eng J Med* 2001;344:1215–1221. Used with permission.

can produce nonreactive pupils. Preexisting anatomic abnormalities of the iris or effects of previous surgery should be excluded.

Ocular Movements

Ocular movements are absent after head turning and caloric testing with ice water. (Testing is done only when no fractures or instability of the cervical spine are apparent. The cervical spine must be imaged to exclude potential fractures or instability, or both.) The oculocephalic reflex, elicited by fast turning of the head from middle position to 90 degrees on both sides, normally results in eye deviation to the opposite side of the head turning. Vertical eye movements should be tested with brisk neck flexion. Eyelid opening and vertical and horizontal eye movements must be absent in brain death.

Caloric testing should be done with the head elevated to 30 degrees during irrigation of the tympanum on each side with 50 mL of ice water. Tympanum irrigation can be best accomplished by inserting a small suction catheter into the external auditory canal and connecting it to a 50 mL syringe filled with ice water. One may consider marking the lower eyelid at the level of the pupil with a felt-tip pen to make sure the eyes have not moved after caloric testing. Tonic deviation of the eyes directed to the cold caloric stimulus is absent. The investigator should allow up to 1 minute after injection, and the time between stimulation on each side should be several minutes.

Drugs that can diminish or completely abolish the caloric response are sedatives, aminoglycosides, tricyclic antidepressants, anticholinergics, antiepileptic drugs, and chemotherapeutic agents. After traumatic head injury or facial trauma, lid edema and chemosis of the conjunctiva may restrict movement of the globes. Clotted blood or cerumen may diminish the caloric response, and repeat testing is required after otologic inspection and flushing out. Basal fracture of the petrous bone abolishes the caloric response unilaterally only and may be identified by an ecchymotic mastoid process.

Facial Sensation and Facial Motor Response

Corneal reflexes should be absent and can be tested by briefly tapping the cornea with a throat swab. The jaw often has drooped. The jaw reflex should be absent. Grimacing to pain can be tested by using standard pain stimuli.

One should be aware that severe facial trauma may diminish all brainstem reflexes.

Pharyngeal and Tracheal Reflexes

Lack of a cough response to tracheal suctioning should be demonstrated. Usually, a suction catheter is advanced to the level of the carina. Movement of the endotracheal tube up and down may not be sufficient to stimulate cough.

Apnea

An important component of the clinical diagnosis of brain death is the demonstration of apnea. Loss of brainstem function produces loss of breathing and vasomotor control, which results in apnea and hypotension. Hypotension (from many possible causes) is frequently present at the time of the clinical diagnosis of brain death, but blood pressure can depend on intravascular volume reduced by concomitant diabetes insipidus and on the dose of vasopressors.[31] Hypotension is not an absolute criterion for the diagnosis of brain death, but in the vast majority of cases, increasing doses of vasopressors are needed.

Apnea is due to the destruction of ventrolateral medullary structures. The respiratory neurons are controlled by central chemo-receptors that sense changes in pH of the CSF, and these accurately reflect changes in arterial P_{CO_2}.[19] There are many other mechanical and chemical stimuli and inhibitory influences to the respiratory neurons of the brainstem.

It is not known at what arterial P_{CO_2} level the chemoreceptors of the respiratory center are maximally stimulated in hyperoxygenated patients with brainstem destruction. Target arterial P_{CO_2} of 60 mm Hg is derived from findings in a small number of patients who had respiratory efforts after induction of hypercapnia. Lower target levels have been suggested, because one study showed that four patients made effective normal breathing efforts at lower arterial P_{CO_2} values (range, 30–37 mm Hg; mean, 34 mm Hg). At higher arterial P_{CO_2} values (range, 41–51 mm Hg), respiratory-like movements have been observed.[110] These movements are ineffective for ventilation and consist of shoulder elevation and adduction, back arching, and intercostal expansion. These respiratory-like efforts produce negligible tidal volumes and virtually no inspiratory force. In patients we have seen who otherwise fulfilled the clinical criteria for brain death, breathing also began at a much lower arterial P_{CO_2} level (approximately 30–40 mm Hg). In these patients with a preserved breathing trigger but otherwise completely absent brainstem reflexes, breathing starts within minutes after disconnection from the ventilator, assuming the arterial P_{CO_2} has been normalized before testing. Repeat testing often shows apnea. This may take 24 to 48 hours.

Brain death should be differentiated from an unusual clinical entity, recently pathologically confirmed, of isolated preserved medulla function.[132] Traces of cough response after repeated stimuli, no need for vasopressors to support blood pressure, and retained tachycardia after intravenous injection of atropine are salient features of this comatose state ("medulla man"). Technically, the clinical diagnosis of brain death cannot be made, but it is very unlikely that patients survive beyond a vegetative state. In this comatose state, the typical accelerating disintegration of systemic functions leading to cardiac arrest may be absent.[132]

The target arterial P_{CO_2} levels of the apnea tests in brain death determination may be higher in patients with chronic hypercapnia ("CO_2 retainers"). Typically, these patients have severe chronic obstructive pulmonary disease, bronchiectasis, sleep apnea, and morbid obesity. In the absence of a concomitant metabolic acidosis, chronic hypercapnia can be suspected in patients with increased serum concentrations of bicarbonate.[38] If the initial arterial blood gas determination confirms chronic hypercapnia in these patients, the apnea test result could be unreliable, and a confirmatory test may be needed.

Hypocapnia can be expected in patients with acute catastrophic structural damage to the central nervous system. In many instances, hypocapnia is caused by high tidal volumes associated with mechanical ventilation, by hyperventilation instituted to decrease intracranial pressure, or by hypothermia. Hypocapnia can be corrected by decreasing either the rate or the tidal volume for several minutes to change the minute volume.

Three studies on the technique of apnea tests have been published, and they have included apneic oxygenation-diffusion,[134] the use of T-piece with a continuous positive airway pressure (CPAP) valve,[121] and exogenously administered carbon dioxide (CO_2).[76] No comparative studies have been done.

In our study on apnea testing in 212 patients, we used preoxygenation and an apneic oxygenation diffusion technique.[134] In none of the patients did resumption of breathing occur after the initial apnea test documented absent respiratory drive.[134] In 16 patients (7%), apnea testing was not attempted due to inability to maintain a stable blood pressure, the presence of high positive end-expiratory pressure requirements, and refractory hypoxemia despite pretest oxygenation

using 100% oxygen for 10 minutes. The apnea test was aborted in 3% of patients due to acute hypotension or hypoxemia after disconnection from the ventilator. Failure to complete the apnea test occurred more often in patients with increased A–a gradient and pretest acidosis.[139]

One study in 20 adults examined disconnection of the ventilator using a T-piece and continuous positive airway pressure (CPAP valve of 10 cm of water and oxygen administration at 12 L/minute).[81] Apnea testing could be completed in patients with the additional use of a CPAP valve and therefore may be an alternative method in patients who fail an apnea test using a standard method of preoxygenation and an endotracheal catheter placed at the carina. Studies have suggested monitoring of the apnea test with transcutaneous CO_2 partial pressure monitoring. However, comparison with predicting arterial P_{CO_2} rise using an estimated 3 mm Hg increase per minute has not been performed. It is unclear whether this device reduces blood gas testing (and thus cost) during the apnea test, and this device may not be universally present in ICUs.[121]

Apnea testing is greatly facilitated by a starting arterial P_{CO_2} value of 40 mm Hg, because the target level of 60 mm Hg is generally reached 6 to 8 minutes after disconnection from the ventilator. (The estimated arterial P_{CO_2} increase is from 3 to 6 mm Hg per minute.[32]) Failure to reach the arterial P_{CO_2} target (60 mm Hg, or a 20 mm Hg increase above the normal baseline) may be due to relative hypothermia (32°–36°C) and a high flow of oxygen (> 10 L/min) that washes out, rather than provides, oxygen. Use of high-flow oxygen (10–15 L/minute) has also been linked to pneumothorax, but the causality is doubtful.[140] Pneumothorax may be seen more often in patients with progression to brain death who had cardiopulmonary resuscitation or polytrauma.

Cardiac arrhythmias are side effects of severe hypercapnia and respiratory acidosis, occurring mostly in patients with severe hypoxia.[31] Oxygenation may be inadequate, for example, in patients with severe pulmonary disease, acute respiratory distress syndrome, or neurogenic pulmonary edema. The most common abnormalities are premature ventricular contractions, ventricular tachycardia, and hypotension. Severe hypotension (change in mean arterial pressure of > 15%) has been observed in well-oxygenated patients in whom arterial P_{CO_2} values reached very high levels (average, 90 mm Hg).[61,136] Respiratory acidosis can be implicated as a cause of myocardial depression. Administration of 100% oxygen through a catheter placed at the level of the carina secures adequate oxygenation during apnea testing. We found that lack of preoxygenation increased the chance of hypotension.[41]

The literature does not provide evidence to favor one method over another.[10,13,30,86,112] Apnea testing by carbon dioxide augmentation was studied in 34 patients. After preoxygenation, carbon dioxide was insufflated at 1 L/minute; at 1 and 2 minutes later, $PaCO_2$ was checked, followed by disconnection for respiratory movements. The main advantage is that respiratory movements can be observed when $PaCO_2$ is at a target level, rather than after waiting for the $PaCO_2$ value to increase during continuous observation of the patient for 8–10 minutes. The main objections are that the equipment is not readily available in most units and that, most important, there is a danger of overcompensation to hypercapnia and acidosis, potentially leading to hypotension and cardiac arrhythmias. In Lang's studies,[75,76] however, severe hypercapnia and acidosis actually depresses the respiratory drive. PCO_2 values ranged from 60 to 80 mm Hg after 1 minute and from 70 to 95 mm Hg after 2 minutes of insufflation.

Another method of apnea testing is hypoventilation. This method involves a sudden decrease in minute ventilation to 1 L/minute through a decrease in the tidal volume (500 mL) and the ventilator rate (2 breaths/min) with end-tidal PCO_2 monitoring. This method undoubtedly has value, but end-tidal PCO_2 may not reflect $PaCO_2$ in patients with neurogenic pulmonary edema, and the method is more time-consuming (> 15 minutes may be required to reach target PCO_2 values). Determination of apnea by reliance on the ventilator alarm may be misleading, and we and others have noted "breathing efforts" recorded on the ventilator display in apneic patients (ventilator self-cycling).[133,137]

The apnea test using the apneic oxygen diffusion method is usually safe when performed with a strict protocol. The induced moderate respiratory acidosis should have significant effect on left ventricular function.[93] Severe respiratory acidosis (pH < 7.0 mm Hg) and severe hypoxemia (PO_2 < 60 mm Hg), however, can induce significant cardiac arrhythmias, including ventricular fibrillation.

Important changes in vital signs (e.g., marked hypotension, severe cardiac arrhythmias) during the apnea test may be related to inadequate precautions. Therefore, the following prerequisites are suggested: (a) core temperature > 36°C, (b) systolic blood pressure ≥ 90 mm Hg, (c) positive fluid balance in the past 6 hours, (d) arterial PCO_2 ≥ 40 mm Hg, and (e) arterial PO_2 ≥ 200 mm Hg.

One should look closely for respiratory movements. Respiration is defined as abdominal or chest excursions that produce adequate tidal volumes. If present, respiration can be expected early in the apnea test. When respiratory-like movements occur, they can be expected at the end of the apnea test, often when oxygenation may have become marginal. The main components of brain death determination have been summarized in Figure 63.1.

Clinical Observations Compatible with the Diagnosis of Brain Death

Several studies described spontaneous and reflex movements in brain death, and included single

---

TABLE 63.1. PITFALLS OF ANCILLARY TESTS

Cerebral angiogram

- Injection aortic arch or individually catheterizing cerebral arteries may make a difference in result. Force of the injection may determine filling or not.
- No guidelines for interpretation

Transcranial Doppler

- Technical difficulties and skill may make a difference in result
- Normal early in anoxic-ischemic brain injury and in primary infratentorial lesions without extreme hydrocephalus

Electroencephalography

- ICU Artifacts
- Measures mostly cortical activity

Somatosensory evoked potentials

- Absent in patients with catastrophic CNS lesions but who are not brain dead

MR angiogram

- Certain techniques or gadolinium use may make a difference in result

CT angiogram

- Interpretation difficulties due to rapid acquisition time
- Retained blood flow in many arterial territories of uncertain significance

Nuclear brain scan

- Areas of perfusion in thalamus in anoxic ischemic brain injury or in patients with a skull defect

---

reports of facial myokymias, transient eyelid opening, transient bilateral finger tremor, repetitive leg movements, ocular microtremor, and cyclical constriction and dilatation in light-fixed pupils.[7,17,23,59,65,113,116] One study of 144 patients pronounced brain dead found 55% of 144 patients had retained plantar reflexes, either flexion or "stimulation-induced undulating toe flexion." None of the patients had a Babinski sign.[25] One report documented plantar flexion and flexion synergy bilaterally, and these signs remained for 32 hours after the determination of brain death.[141]

Some studies suggested that the ventilator may sense small changes in tubing flow and provide a breath that could suggest breathing effort by the patient where none exists.[133] This phenomenon is more common in current ventilators and in patients who have had chest tubes placed. Changes in transpleural pressure from the heartbeat itself may also trigger the ventilator. These studies emphasize that the determination of apnea can only be assessed reliably with disconnection from the ventilator.

Respiratory acidosis, hypoxia, or quick neck flexion may generate spinal cord responses. Spontaneous movements of the limbs from spinal mechanisms can occur and are more frequent in young adults.[63,64,110] These spinal reflexes include flexion in arms, or fingers, slowly raising of all limbs or one limb off the bed ("Lazarus sign"), grasping movements, spontaneous jerking of one leg, and walking-like movements. Multifocal vigorous myoclonus in the shoulders is occasionally seen in young patients, and its spinal origin is confirmed by an isoelectric EEG. Stepping movements in the legs (an exaggerated alternating triple-flexion response) may occur just before all brainstem function disappears.

Respiratory-like movements are characterized by shoulder elevation and adduction, back arching, and intercostal expansion without any significant measurable tidal volume.

Other, much less common, responses are profuse sweating, blushing, tachycardia, and sudden increases in blood pressure.[23] These hemodynamic responses can sometimes be elicited by neck flexion.[72] Muscle stretch reflexes, superficial abdominal reflexes, and Babinski signs are of spinal origin and thus do not invalidate a diagnosis of brain death. Patients may have initial plantar flexion of the great toe followed by sequential brief plantar flexion of the second, third, fourth, and fifth toes after snapping of one of the toes ("undulating toe flexion sign").[59]

ANCILLARY TESTS

Brain death is a clinical diagnosis. In adults, an ancillary test is not mandated in the United States, the United Kingdom, and the majority of European countries. The AAN decided to recommend one examination only. In six states a second physician is requires to sign off, but it is not clear if this requires a second examination after a certain interval. The statutory language does not indicate exactly how the second physician requirement must be implemented. (It is of interest that two states in the US recently dropped the second physician requirement.) In the United States, an ancillary test could be used for patients in whom some specific components of clinical testing cannot be reliably evaluated, but it should not replace neurologic examination if major confounders are present. Clinical experience with ancillary tests other than EEG, transcranial Doppler ultrasonography, and conventional angiography is limited. Studies reporting the results of ancillary tests did not use blind assessment of the results, did not assess interobserver variation, and generally did not perform tests in control subjects with catastrophic central nervous system lesions who were not brain dead. In addition, many tests require costly equipment and well-trained technicians. Unfortunately, some physicians may supplement a clinical examination with a laboratory test and then agonize over why the results are conflicting. There are false positive results[44] (confirmatory test suggests brain death but patient does not meet criteria) and false negative results (patient is clinically brain dead but laboratory tests suggest otherwise), and some are summarized in Table 63.1.[48] There are also disparities between confirmatory tests.[70] One striking example is a patient with isoelectric EEG, absent somatosensory potentials but normal nuclear scan.[51] At least in adults, when a methodically precise clinical examination has been performed, confirmatory tests should be ordered sparingly, if at all. Ancillary testing showing activity or blood flow proves no survival and no ancillary testing to date has improved (and thereby questioned) prior methods of clinical diagnosis.

EEG has been traditionally used as a confirmatory test, and earlier studies found a good correlation with total brain necrosis,[80,130] but many other ancillary tests have been used. Consensus criteria have been reported for EEG[117] and transcranial Doppler ultrasonography.[28]

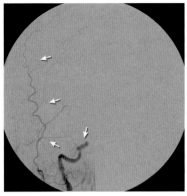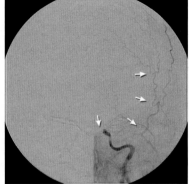

FIGURE 63.3: Cerebral angiogram showing lack of intracranial flow and presence of extracranial flow (*arrows*).

Conventional Cerebral Angiography
Technique
Four-vessel angiography with arch injection is done in the radiology suite. Iodinated contrast medium is injected under high pressure in both the anterior and the posterior circulations. The procedure takes less than an hour.[18,20,47,77]

Result
Intracerebral filling is absent when arteries enter the dura (Figure 63.3). The external carotid circulation is patent and fills rapidly. At times, delayed filling of the superior longitudinal sinus is seen.

Disadvantage
There is a small risk of contrast nephrotoxicity and theoretically this could decrease the acceptance rate in organ recipients.

Electroencephalography
Technique
Usually, a 16- or 18-channel instrument is used with guidelines developed by the American Electroencephalographic Society for recording brain death.[12,26,48,54,57,69,117]

Result
No electrical activity occurs above 2 µV at a sensitivity of 2 µV/mm with filter setting at 0.1 or 0.3 second and 70 Hz. Recording should continue for at least 30 minutes (Chapter 24).

Disadvantage
Considerable artifacts (intravenous pumps, mechanical ventilator) due to high-gain settings in the ICU may limit interpretation.

Nuclear Brain Scan
Technique
The isotope technetium 99m hexamethylpropyleneamine oxime (^{99m}Tc-HMPAO) should be injected within 30 minutes of reconstitution.[36,79,138] A portable gamma camera produces planar views within 5 to 10 minutes. Correct intravenous injection can be checked by taking additional chest and abdominal images.

Result
No uptake occurs in the brain parenchyma ("hollow skull" or "empty light bulb" sign) (Figure 63.4).

Disadvantages
The costs are high, and the technique is not widely available; expertise is variable.

Transcranial Doppler Ultrasonography
Technique
A portable 2-MHz pulsed Doppler instrument can be used at the bedside. Two intracranial arteries should be insulated (middle cerebral artery through the temporal bone above the zygomatic arch and the vertebral or basilar arteries through the suboccipital transcranial window). The transorbital window and the middle cerebral artery may be used and may increase the detection of typical flow patterns.[28,49,52,54,74,100,103,111]

Result
Transcranial Doppler signals that have been reported in brain death are described in Chapter 24. Lack of transcranial Doppler signals cannot be interpreted as confirmatory of brain death,

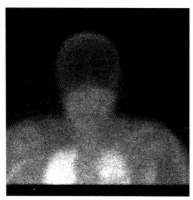
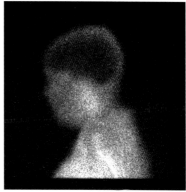

FIGURE 63.4: Single-photon emission computed tomography with no uptake in brain parenchyma, but uptake elsewhere.

because 10% of patients may not have temporal insonation windows. Possibly an exception can be made in patients who had transcranial Doppler signals during admission that disappeared at the time of brain death.

Disadvantages

Transcranial Doppler velocities can be affected by marked changes in arterial Pco_2, hematocrit, and cardiac output. Transcranial Doppler ultrasonography requires considerable practice and skill.

Somatosensory Evoked Potentials
Technique

A portable instrument can be used at the bedside. Median nerve stimulation is performed on both sides.[6,11,21,40,118]

Result

N20–P22 response is bilaterally absent.

Miscellaneous Tests

Some of these tests have been done in only small series of patients and are not widely adopted as confirmatory tests.

Several studies examined both magnetic resonance imaging (MRI) and MR angiography.[58,67,83,89] One study in 15 patients documented loss of flow voids in cavernous portion of the carotid artery with MR angiography. This study compared these results with cerebral angiography in nine patients, and findings matched in eight patients (done 1–2 days later in six patients). Spotty flow voids on MRI were found in one patient with no intracranial flow on cerebral angiogram.[89] One study compared 20 brain dead patients with 10 comatose patients, and found that MR angiography revealed absent arterial flow in the intracerebral circulation only in patients diagnosed as brain dead.[67]

Several studies suggested the use of CT angiography and compared the results with an isoelectric EEG, cerebral angiography, or normal controls.[8,22,29,34,105] One study showed intracranial blood flow in 10 of 21 (50%) patients with isoelectric EEGs. In another study of 43 patients with absent intracranial flow on cerebral angiography, CT angiography demonstrated intracranial blood flow in 13 (30%) patients. Both studies challenged the results of a smaller study showing no blood flow in 15 patients when compared to EEG or cerebral angiography. One study of 105 patients diagnosed clinically as brain dead found residual opacified vessels in both pericallosal arteries in 56%, one pericallosal artery in 41%, both cortical segments of the middle cerebral artery in 18%, one cortical segment of the middle cerebral artery in 20%, one internal cerebral vein in 5%, great cerebral vein in 5%, and basilar artery in 6%.[34] The authors then simplified the reading of a CT angiogram using a 4-point system (1 point for nonpacified vessels; right and left cortical segment of the middle cerebral artery plus right and left internal cerebral vein) and found a sensitivity of 85.7%. A specificity of 100% was found in a comparison with EEG and cerebral angiogram, although only in 12 and 10 patients, respectively. One study found cerebral circulatory arrest on CT angiogram but preserved flow on transcranial Doppler.[44] Computed tomography angiography (Figure 63.5) is widely used in Europe and Canada, but studies remain underpowered, lack

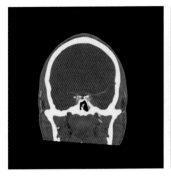 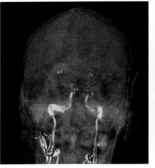 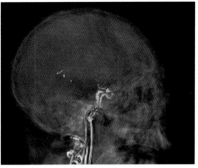

FIGURE 63.5: CTA in a patient fulfilling clinical criteria of brain death. (CTA was performed at the request of the attending general intensivist.) Ambiguous result with largely extracranial circulation uptake (red haze over skull) but some intracranial flow. Note intracranial contrast in middle cerebral arteries.

comparison with other ancillary studies in large number of patients, and residual opacification of vessels remains common.[104]

Two studies suggested the use of nasopharyngeal electrode recording of SSEPs to confirm brain death.[109,122] One study of 181 comatose patients compared nasopharyngeal electrode SSEP recording with the brain death clinical examination, and found that the disappearance of P14—presumably generated in the medial lemniscus and cuneate nucleus—is a reliable sign of brain death.[122] This study suggests that P14 recordings using midfrontal scalp–nasopharyngeal montage could be a valuable confirmatory test. The technique, however, has not been used on a routine basis, interobserver variability studies have not been performed, and absent P14 recordings have been found in 10% of comatose patients using other montages.[109,122]

PRIMARY BRAINSTEM DEATH

Acute catastrophic injury may involve the brainstem only. In most instances, this is a destructive pontine hemorrhage, acute basilar artery embolus, or a head injury that involves primarily the brainstem. The brain hemispheres remain initially unaffected unless acute hydrocephalus—from obstruction at the fourth ventricle or aqueduct—increases the intracranial pressure and stops intracranial flow. A destructive primary brainstem lesion is not common, and many patients will have preserved function of the medulla oblongata (cough reflex and breathing drive). When all is lost, brainstem injury is as irreversible as a lesion that involves the hemispheres and brainstem, and it is therefore unnecessary to perform an ancillary test to demonstrate injury to the hemispheres. In fact,

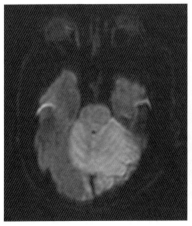 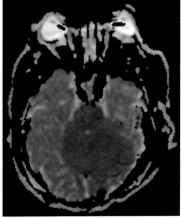

FIGURE 63.6: MRI (DWI and ADC mapping) shows destroyed brainstem and large part of the cerebellum in a patient fullfilling all clinical criteria for brain death.(Kindly provided by Dr Rabinstein.).

these tests often will show preserved blood flow when the intracranial pressure has not increased to extreme values, and electroencephalography may show nonreactive alpha or spindle coma patterns MRI may only show the primary lesion (Figure 63.6).

DETERMINATION OF BRAIN DEATH IN CHILDREN

The current guidelines in children were developed by a task force of the American Academy of Pediatrics.[9,88,136] A study of 93 brain death determinations in children found significant variations in practices.[90] In 25% of patients, the apnea test was not performed, and lack of clear documentation was frequently observed.

MANAGEMENT OF THE BRAIN DEAD DONOR

Support of the potential organ and tissue donor is complex.[24,62,82,108,114] In the United States, the organ procurement officer (OPO) is directing the medical care toward organ retrieval (Chapter 65). Many physiologic changes occur during the development of brain death, and appropriate management guarantees successful procurement. The criteria for becoming a potential organ donor are at the discretion of the organ harvest teams and change frequently. Organ or tissue donation is contraindicated in patients with a possible or demonstrated transmittable disease. This includes patients at high risk for exposure to human immunodeficiency virus (e.g., related to homosexual practice, prostitution, hemophilia, recent skin-piercing treatment) or who recently had treatment with human pituitary extracts.

The most significant initial management problems pertain to hypotension or diabetes insipidus, or both.[102] Hypotension has many potential causes. These include decreased left ventricular function, loss of systemic vascular resistance, and rewarming of a hypothermic patient with resultant vasodilatation, but hypotension can also be related to hypovolemia. Hypovolemia can be a result of insufficient fluid resuscitation in patients with diabetes insipidus or a lingering effect of aggressive osmotic diuresis in an attempt to reverse cerebral edema. Hypovolemia can be reversed with isotonic saline or colloids. Dopamine or phenylephrine is indicated if blood pressure cannot be initially controlled by fluid resuscitation alone. Alternatively, if ventricular

dysfunction is severe by echocardiography, dobutamine can be considered (5–10 μg/kg/min). However, in many patients blood pressure can be well maintained with a vasopressin infusion of 0.5 units per hour alone. Diabetes insipidus can be expected in many patients and can be countered by intravenous desmopressin 2 to 4 μg IV in 2 divided doses daily. Its use can be gauged by urine output (e.g., > 300 mL/hr for 2 successive hours).[98] Altered thyroid function has been found in brain dead patients, but it is unclear whether triiodothyronine replacement therapy improves myocardial function (although some studies have found improved ejection fraction after administration of the hormone).[60] Whether this replacement therapy may decrease inotropic therapy is not known. The organ procurement organization staff will often use this additional therapy in patients with poorly controlled blood pressures, and a bolus of 0.6 μg of T_3 may result in significant improvement.

Cardiac arrhythmias are most troublesome in patients with brain death. Hypocalcemia, hypomagnesemia, hypokalemia, hypothermia, use of vasopressors, and severe hypoxemia all may contribute. Brain death leads to autonomic uncoupling, but also to marked coronary perfusion pressure, possibly due to direct endothelial damage.[120] Terminal rhythms include complete heart block, ventricular tachycardia, and sinus bradycardia progressing to asystole. Pulmonary management is standard with assist control mode and low tidal volumes. Methylprednisolone 15 mg/kg IV could improve oxygenation.

CONCLUSIONS

- Brain death can be determined accurately with a neurologic examination but only after hypothermia, drug effects, and acute metabolic derangements have been excluded.
- Apnea testing requires an apneic oxygenation method aiming at P_{CO_2} of 60 mm Hg, or an increase of 20 mm Hg above baseline. With an estimated increase of 3–6 mm Hg per minute, 8 minutes is required to reach the target.
- Preoxygenation, increasing temperature to normothermia, and adequate fluid status reduce complications during apnea testing.
- Diabetes insipidus and hypotension are best treated with infusions of norepinephrine and vasopressin.

REFERENCES

1. Guidelines for the determination of death. Report of the medical consultants on the diagnosis of death to the President's Commission for the Study of Ethical Problems in Medicine and Biomedical and Behavioral Research. *JAMA* 1981;246:2184–2186.

2. Practice parameters for determining brain death in adults (summary statement). The Quality Standards Subcommittee of the American Academy of Neurology. *Neurology* 1995;45:1012–1014.

3. Report of Special Task Force. Guidelines for the determination of brain death in children. American Academy of Pediatrics Task Force on Brain Death in Children. *Pediatrics* 1987;80:298–300.

4. Report of the Ad Hoc Committee of the Harvard Medical School to Examine the Definition of Brain Death. A definition of irreversible coma. *JAMA* 1968;205:337–340.

5. Uniform Determination of Death Act, 12 Uniform Laws Annotated (U.L.A.) 589 (West 1993 and West Suppl. 1997).

6. Anziska BJ, Cracco RQ. Short latency somatosensory evoked potentials in brain dead patients. *Arch Neurol* 1980;37:222–225.

7. Araullo ML, Frank JI, Goldenberg FD, Rosengart AJ. Transient bilateral finger tremor after brain death. *Neurology* 2007;68:E22.

8. Arnold H, Kuhne D, Rohr W, Heller M. Contrast bolus technique with rapid CT scanning: a reliable diagnostic tool for the determination of brain death. *Neuroradiology* 1981;22:129–132.

9. Ashwal S. Brain death in the newborn: current perspectives. *Clin Perinatol* 1997;24:859–882.

10. Belsh JM, Blatt R, Schiffman PL. Apnea testing in brain death. *Arch Intern Med* 1986;146: 2385–2388.

11. Belsh JM, Chokroverty S. Short-latency somatosensory evoked potentials in brain-dead patients. *Electroencephalogr Clin Neurophysiol* 1987;68:75–78.

12. Bennett DR. The EEG in determination of brain death. *Ann N Y Acad Sci* 1978;315:110–120.

13. Benzel EC, Mashburn JP, Conrad S, Modling D. Apnea testing for the determination of brain death: a modified protocol: technical note. *J Neurosurg* 1992;76:1029–1031.

14. Bernat JL. How much of the brain must die in brain death? *J Clin Ethics* 1992;3:21–26.

15. Black PM. Brain death (first of two parts). *N Engl J Med* 1978;299:338–344.

16. Black PM. Brain death (second of two parts). *N Engl J Med* 1978;299:393–401.

17. Bolger C, Bojanic S, Phillips J, et al. Ocular microtremor in brain stem death. *Neurosurgery* 1999;44:1201–1206.

18. Bradac GB, Simon RS. Angiography in brain death. *Neuroradiology* 1974;7:25–28.

19. Bruce EN, Cherniack NS. Central chemoreceptors. *J Appl Physiol (1985)* 1987;62:389–402.

20. Cantu RC. Brain death as determined by cerebral arteriography. *Lancet* 1973;1:1391–1392.

21. Chancellor AM, Frith RW, Shaw NA. Somatosensory evoked potentials following severe head injury: loss of the thalamic potential with brain death. *J Neurol Sci* 1988;87:255–263.

22. Combes JC, Chomel A, Ricolfi F, d'Athis P, Freysz M. Reliability of computed tomographic angiography in the diagnosis of brain death. *Transplant Proc* 2007;39:16–20.

23. Conci F, Procaccio F, Arosio M, Boselli L. Viscerosomatic and viscero-visceral reflexes in brain death. *J Neurol Neurosurg Psychiatry* 1986;49: 695–698.

24. Darby JM, Stein K, Grenvik A, Stuart SA. Approach to management of the heartbeating 'brain dead' organ donor. *JAMA* 1989;261:2222–2228.

25. de Freitas GR, Andre C. Absence of the Babinski sign in brain death: a prospective study of 144 cases. *J Neurol* 2005;252:106–107.

26. Deliyannakis E, Ioannou F, Davaroukas A. Brainstem death with persistence of bioelectric activity of the cerebral hemispheres. *Clin Electroencephalogr* 1975;6:75–79.

27. Dobb GJ, Weekes JW. Clinical confirmation of brain death. *Anaesth Intensive Care* 1995;23: 37–43.

28. Ducrocq X, Hassler W, Moritake K, et al. Consensus opinion on diagnosis of cerebral circulatory arrest using Doppler-sonography: Task Force Group on cerebral death of the Neurosonology Research Group of the World Federation of Neurology. *J Neurol Sci* 1998;159:145–150.

29. Dupas B, Gayet-Delacroix M, Villers D, et al. Diagnosis of brain death using two-phase spiral CT. *AJNR Am J Neuroradiol* 1998;19:641–647.

30. Earnest MP, Beresford HR, McIntyre HB. Testing for apnea in suspected brain death: methods used by 129 clinicians. *Neurology* 1986;36:542–544.

31. Ebata T, Watanabe Y, Amaha K, Hosaka Y, Takagi S. Hemodynamic changes during the apnoea test for diagnosis of brain death. *Can J Anaesth* 1991;38:436–440.

32. Eger EI, Severinghaus JW. The rate of rise of $PaCO_2$ in the apneic anesthetized patient. *Anesthesiology* 1961;22:419–425.

33. Fischbeck KH, Simon RP. Neurological manifestations of accidental hypothermia. *Ann Neurol* 1981;10:384–387.

34. Frampas E, Videcoq M, de Kerviler E, et al. CT angiography for brain death diagnosis. *AJNR Am J Neuroradiol* 2009;30:1566–1570.

35. Friedman Y, Lee L, Wherrett JR, Ashby P, Carpenter S. Simulation of brain death from fulminant de-efferentation. *Can J Neurol Sci* 2003;30:397–404.

36. George MS. Establishing brain death: the potential role of nuclear medicine in the search for a reliable confirmatory test. *Eur J Nucl Med* 1991;18:75–77.

37. Gilbert M, Busund R, Skagseth A, Nilsen PA, Solbo JP. Resuscitation from accidental hypothermia of 13.7 degrees C with circulatory arrest. *Lancet* 2000;355:375–376.

38. Glauser FL, Fairman RP, Bechard D. The causes and evaluation of chronic hypercapnea. *Chest* 1987;91:755–759.

39. Goetting MG, Contreras E. Systemic atropine administration during cardiac arrest does not cause fixed and dilated pupils. *Ann Emerg Med* 1991;20:55–57.

40. Goldie WD, Chiappa KH, Young RR, Brooks EB. Brainstem auditory and short-latency somatosensory evoked responses in brain death. *Neurology* 1981;31:248–256.

41. Goudreau JL, Wijdicks EFM, Emery SF. Complications during apnea testing in the determination of brain death: predisposing factors. *Neurology* 2000;55:1045–1048.

42. Gray AT, Krejci ST, Larson MD. Neuromuscular blocking drugs do not alter the pupillary light reflex of anesthetized humans. *Arch Neurol* 1997;54:579–584.

43. Greenan J, Prasad J. Comparison of the ocular effects of atropine or glycopyrrolate with two I.V. induction agents. *Br J Anaesth* 1985;57:180–183.

44. Greer DM, Strozyk D, Schwamm LH. False positive CT angiography in brain death. *Neurocrit Care* 2009;11:272–275.

45. Greer DM, Varelas PN, Haque S, Wijdicks EFM. Variability of brain death determination guidelines in leading US neurologic institutions. *Neurology* 2008;70:284–289.

46. Greer DM, Wang HH, Robinson JD, Varelas PN, Henderson GV, Wijdicks EFM. Variability of brain death policies in the United States. *JAMA Neurol* 2016;73:213–218.

47. Greitz T, Gordon E, Kolmodin G, Widen L. Aortocranial and carotid angiography in determination of brain death. *Neuroradiology* 1973;5: 13–19.

48. Grigg MM, Kelly MA, Celesia GG, Ghobrial MW, Ross ER. Electroencephalographic activity after brain death. *Arch Neurol* 1987;44: 948–954.

49. Hadani M, Bruk B, Ram Z, et al. Application of transcranial doppler ultrasonography for the diagnosis of brain death. *Intens Care Med* 1999;25:822–828.

50. Hammer MD, Crippen D. Brain death and withdrawal of support. *Surg Clin N Am* 2006;86:1541–1551.

51. Hansen AV, Lavin PJ, Moody EB, Sandler MP. False-negative cerebral radionuclide flow study, in brain death, caused by a ventricular drain. *Clin Nucl Med* 1993;18:502–505.

52. Hassler W, Steinmetz H, Gawlowski J. Transcranial Doppler ultrasonography in raised intracranial pressure and in intracranial circulatory arrest. *J Neurosurg* 1988;68:745–751.

53. Haupt WF, Rudolf J. European brain death codes: a comparison of national guidelines. *J Neurol* 1999;246:432–437.

54. Heran MK, Heran NS, Shemie SD. A review of ancillary tests in evaluating brain death. *Can J Neurol Sci* 2008;35:409–419.

55. Hocker S, Schumacher D, Mandrekar J, Wijdicks EFM. Testing confounders in brain death determination: a new simulation model. *Neurocrit Care*. 2015;23:401–408.

56. Hocker S, Wijdicks EFM. Simulation training in brain death determination. *Semin Neurol* 2015;35:180–188.

57. Hughes JR. Limitations of the EEG in coma and brain death. *Ann N Y Acad Sci* 1978;315:121–136.

58. Ishii K, Onuma T, Kinoshita T, et al. Brain death: MR and MR angiography. *AJNR Am J Neuroradiol* 1996;17:731–735.

59. Jain S, DeGeorgia M. Brain death-associated reflexes and automatisms. *Neurocrit Care* 2005;3:122–126.

60. Jeevanandam V, Todd B, Regillo T, et al. Reversal of donor myocardial dysfunction by triiodothyronine replacement therapy. *J Heart Lung Transplant* 1994;13:681–687.

61. Jeret JS, Benjamin JL. Risk of hypotension during apnea testing. *Arch Neurol* 1994;51:595–599.

62. Jordan CA, Snyder JV. Intensive care and intraoperative management of the brain-dead organ donor. *Transplant Proc* 1987;19:21–25.

63. Jordan JE, Dyess E, Cliett J. Unusual spontaneous movements in brain-dead patients. *Neurology* 1985;35:1082.

64. Jorgensen EO. Spinal man after brain death: the unilateral extension-pronation reflex of the upper limb as an indication of brain death. *Acta Neurochir (Wien)* 1973;28:259–273.

65. Jung KY, Han SG, Lee KH, Chung CS. Repetitive leg movements mimicking periodic leg movement during sleep in a brain-dead patient. *Eur J Neurol* 2006;13:e3-e4.

66. Kainuma M, Miyake T, Kanno T. Extremely prolonged vecuronium clearance in a brain death case. *Anesthesiology* 2001;95:1023–1024.

67. Karantanas AH, Hadjigeorgiou GM, Paterakis K, Sfiras D, Komnos A. Contribution of MRI and MR angiography in early diagnosis of brain death. *Eur Radiol* 2002;12:2710–2716.

68. Kompanje EJ, de Groot YJ, Bakker J. Is organ donation from brain dead donors reaching an inescapable and desirable nadir? *Transplantation* 2011;91:1177–1180.

69. Korein J, Maccario M. A prospective study on the diagnosis of cerebral death. [Abstract]. *Electroencephalogr Clin Neurophysiol* 1971;31: 103–104.

70. Kramer AH. Ancillary testing in brain death. *Semin Neurol* 2015;35:125–138.

71. Kramer AH, Zygun DA, Doig CJ, Zuege DJ. Incidence of neurologic death among patients with brain injury: a cohort study in a Canadian health region. *CMAJ* 2013;185:E838-E845.

72. Kuwagata Y, Sugimoto H, Yoshioka T, Sugimoto T. Hemodynamic response with passive neck flexion in brain death. *Neurosurgery* 1991;29:239–241.

73. LaMancusa J, Cooper R, Vieth R, Wright F. The effects of the falling therapeutic and subtherapeutic barbiturate blood levels on electrocerebral silence in clinically brain-dead children. *Clin Electroencephalogr* 1991;22:112–117.

74. Lampl Y, Gilad R, Eschel Y, et al. Diagnosing brain death using the transcranial Doppler with a transorbital approach. *Arch Neurol* 2002;59:58–60.

75. Lang CJ. Apnea testing by artificial CO2 augmentation. *Neurology* 1995;45:966–969.

76. Lang CJ, Heckmann JG, Erbguth F, et al. Transcutaneous and intra-arterial blood gas monitoring: a comparison during apnoea testing for the determination of brain death. *Eur J Emerg Med* 2002;9:51–56.

77. Langfitt TW, Kassell NF. Non-filling of cerebral vessels during angiography: correlation with intracranial pressure. *Acta Neurochir (Wien)* 1966;14:96–104.

78. Larson MD, Muhiudeen I. Pupillometric analysis of the 'absent light reflex.' *Arch Neurol* 1995;52:369–372.

79. Laurin NR, Driedger AA, Hurwitz GA, et al. Cerebral perfusion imaging with technetium-99m HM-PAO in brain death and severe central nervous system injury. *J Nucl Med* 1989;30:1627–1635.

80. Leestma JE, Hughes JR, Diamond ER. Temporal correlates in brain death. EEG and clinical relationships to the respirator brain. *Arch Neurol* 1984;41·147–152.

81. Levesque S, Lessard MR, Nicole PC, et al. Efficacy of a T-piece system and a continuous positive airway pressure system for apnea testing in the diagnosis of brain death. *Crit Care Med* 2006;34:2213–2216.

82. Lindop MJ. Basic principles of donor management for multiorgan removal. *Transplant Proc* 1991;23:2463–2464.

83. Lovblad KO, Bassetti C. Diffusion-weighted magnetic resonance imaging in brain death. *Stroke* 2000;31:539–542.

84. Lynch J, Eldadah MK. Brain-death criteria currently used by pediatric intensivists. *Clin Pediatr (Phila)* 1992;31:457–460.

85. MacDougall BJ, Robinson JD, Kappus L, Sudikoff SN, Greer DM. Simulation-based training in brain death determination. *Neurocrit Care* 2014;21:383–391.

86. Marks SJ, Zisfein J. Apneic oxygenation in apnea tests for brain death: a controlled trial. *Arch Neurol* 1990;47:1066–1068.

87. Marti-Fabregas J, Lopez-Navidad A, Caballero F, Otermin P. Decerebrate-like posturing with mechanical ventilation in brain death. *Neurology* 2000;54:224–227.

88. Mathur M, Ashwal S. Pediatric brain death determination. *Semin Neurol* 2015;35:116–124.

89. Matsumura A, Meguro K, Tsurushima H, et al. Magnetic resonance imaging of brain death. *Neurol Med Chir (Tokyo)* 1996;36:166–171.

90. Mejia RE, Pollack MM. Variability in brain death determination practices in children. *JAMA* 1995;274:550–553.

91. Nakagawa TA, Ashwal S, Mathur M, Mysore M. Guidelines for the determination of brain death in infants and children: an update of the 1987 task force recommendations-executive summary. *Ann Neurol* 2012;71:573–585.

92. Ong GL, Bruning HA. Dilated fixed pupils due to administration of high doses of dopamine hydrochloride. *Crit Care Med* 1981;9:658–659.

93. Orliaguet GA, Catoire P, Liu N, Beydon L, Bonnet F. Transesophageal echocardiographic assessment of left ventricular function during apnea testing for brain death. *Transplantation* 1994;58:655–658.

94. Ostermann ME, Young B, Sibbald WJ, Nicolle MW. Coma mimicking brain death following baclofen overdose. *Intens Care Med* 2000;26:1144–1146.

95. Pallis C. ABC of brain stem death: the position in the USA and elsewhere. *Br Med J (Clin Res Ed)* 1983;286:209–210.

96. Pallis C. Brainstem death. In: Vinken PJ, Bruyn GW, Klawans HL, Braakman R, eds. *Handbook*

of Clinical Neurology. Amsterdam: Elsevier Science Publishers; 1990:441–496.

97. Partridge BL, Abrams JH, Bazemore C, Rubin R. Prolonged neuromuscular blockade after long-term infusion of vecuronium bromide in the intensive care unit. *Crit Care Med* 1990;18:1177–1179.

98. Pennefather SH, Bullock RE, Mantle D, Dark JH. Use of low dose arginine vasopressin to support brain-dead organ donors. *Transplantation* 1995;59:58–62.

99. Peter JV, Prabhakar AT, Pichamuthu K. In-laws, insecticide—and a mimic of brain death. *Lancet* 2008;371:622.

100. Petty GW, Mohr JP, Pedley TA, et al. The role of transcranial Doppler in confirming brain death: sensitivity, specificity, and suggestions for performance and interpretation. *Neurology* 1990;40:300–303.

101. Plotkin SR, Ning MM. Traumatic cervical spine disruption. *N Engl J Med* 2001;345:1134–1135.

102. Power BM, Van Heerden PV. The physiological changes associated with brain death: current concepts and implications for treatment of the brain dead organ donor. *Anaesth Intensive Care* 1995;23:26–36.

103. Powers AD, Graeber MC, Smith RR. Transcranial Doppler ultrasonography in the determination of brain death. *Neurosurgery* 1989;24:884–889.

104. Quesnel C, Fulgencio JP, Adrie C, et al. Limitations of computed tomographic angiography in the diagnosis of brain death. *Intens Care Med* 2007;33:2129–2135.

105. Rappaport ZH, Brinker RA, Rovit RL. Evaluation of brain death by contrast-enhanced computerized cranial tomography. *Neurosurgery* 1978;2:230–232.

106. Richard IH, LaPointe M, Wax P, Risher W. Nonbarbiturate, drug-induced reversible loss of brainstem reflexes. *Neurology* 1998;51:639–640.

107. Rivas S, Douds GL, Ostdahl RH, Harbaugh KS. Fulminant Guillain-Barre syndrome after closed head injury: a potentially reversible cause of an ominous examination: case report. *J Neurosurg* 2008;108:595–600.

108. Robertson KM, Cook DR. Perioperative management of the multiorgan donor. *Anesth Analg* 1990;70:546–556.

109. Roncucci P, Lepori P, Mok MS, et al. Nasopharyngeal electrode recording of somatosensory evoked potentials as an indicator in brain death. *Anaesth Intensive Care* 1999;27:20–25.

110. Ropper AH. Unusual spontaneous movements in brain-dead patients. *Neurology* 1984;34:1089–1092.

111. Ropper AH, Kehne SM, Wechsler L. Transcranial Doppler in brain death. *Neurology* 1987;37:1733–1735.

112. Ropper AH, Kennedy SK, Russell L. Apnea testing in the diagnosis of brain death: clinical and physiological observations. *J Neurosurg* 1981;55:942–946.

113. Santamaria J, Orteu N, Iranzo A, Tolosa E. Eye opening in brain death. *J Neurol* 1999;246:720–722.

114. Shah VR. Aggressive management of multiorgan donor. *Transplant Proc* 2008;40: 1087–1090.

115. Shemie SD, Doig C, Dickens B, et al. Severe brain injury to neurological determination of death: Canadian forum recommendations. *CMAJ* 2006;174:S1–S13.

116. Shlugman D, Parulekar M, Elston JS, Farmery A. Abnormal pupillary activity in a brainstem-dead patient. *Br J Anaesth* 2001;86:717–720.

117. Society AE. Guideline three: minimum technical standards for EEG recording in suspected cerebral death. *J Clin Neurophysiol* 1994;11:10–13.

118. Stohr M, Riffel B, Trost E, Ullrich A. Short-latency somatosensory evoked potentials in brain death. *J Neurol* 1987;234:211–214.

119. Stojkovic T, Verdin M, Hurtevent JF, et al. Guillain-Barre syndrome resembling brainstem death in a patient with brain injury. *J Neurol* 2001;248:430–432.

120. Szabo G, Buhmann V, Bahrle S, Vahl CF, Hagl S. Brain death impairs coronary endothelial function. *Transplantation* 2002;73:1846–1848.

121. Vivien B, Marmion F, Roche S, et al. An evaluation of transcutaneous carbon dioxide partial pressure monitoring during apnea testing in brain-dead patients. *Anesthesiology* 2006;104:701–707.

122. Wagner W. Scalp, earlobe and nasopharyngeal recordings of the median nerve somatosensory evoked P14 potential in coma and brain death: detailed latency and amplitude analysis in 181 patients. *Brain* 1996;119: 1507–1521.

123. Walker AE. *Cerebral Death.* 2nd ed. Baltimore, MD: Urban & Schwarzenberg; 1981.

124. Wang MY, Wallace P, Gruen JP. Brain death documentation: analysis and issues. *Neurosurgery* 2002;51:731–735.

125. Waters CE, French G, Burt M. Difficulty in brainstem death testing in the presence of high spinal cord injury. *Br J Anaesth* 2004;92:760–764.

126. Wijdicks EFM. Brain death guidelines explained. *Semin Neurol* 2015;35:105–115.

127. Wijdicks EFM. Brain death worldwide: accepted fact but no global consensus in diagnostic criteria. *Neurology* 2002;58:20–25.

128. Wijdicks EFM. The clinical determination of brain death: rational and reliable. *Semin Neurol* 2015;35:103–104.

129. Wijdicks EFM. The diagnosis of brain death. *N Engl J Med* 2001;344:1215–1221.

130. Wijdicks EFM. The neurologist and Harvard criteria for brain death. *Neurology* 2003;61: 970–976.

131. Wijdicks EFM. Pitfalls and slip-ups in brain death determination. *Neurol Res* 2013;35:169–173.

132. Wijdicks EFM, Atkinson JL, Okazaki H. Isolated medulla oblongata function after severe traumatic brain injury. *J Neurol Neurosurg Psychiatry* 2001;70:127–129.

133. Wijdicks EFM, Manno EM, Holets SR. Ventilator self-cycling may falsely suggest patient effort during brain death determination. *Neurology* 2005;65:774.

134. Wijdicks EFM, Rabinstein AA, Manno EM, Atkinson JD. Pronouncing brain death: contemporary practice and safety of the apnea test. *Neurology* 2008;71:1240–1244.

135. Wijdicks EFM, Varelas PN, Gronseth GS, Greer DM. Evidence-based guideline update: determining brain death in adults: report of the Quality Standards Subcommittee of the American Academy of Neurology. *Neurology* 2010;74: 1911–1918.

136. Wijdicks EFM. *Brain Death*. 2nd ed. New York: Oxford University Press; 2011.

137. Willatts SM, Drummond G. Brainstem death and ventilator trigger settings. *Anaesthesia* 2000;55: 676–677.

138. Yatim A, Mercatello A, Coronel B, et al. 99mTc-HMPAO cerebral scintigraphy in the diagnosis of brain death. *Transplant Proc* 1991;23:2491.

139. Yee AH, Mandrekar J, Rabinstein AA, Wijdicks EFM. Predictors of apnea test failure during brain death determination. *Neurocrit Care* 2010;12:352–355.

140. Zisfein J, Marks SJ. Tension pneumothorax and apnea tests. *Anesthesiology* 1999;91:326.

141. Zubkov AY, Wijdicks EFM. Plantar flexion and flexion synergy in brain death. *Neurology* 2008;70:e74.

64

Donation after Cardiac Death

The United States has a major shortage of organ and tissue donors, as do most other countries. This situation is concerning. The current state of the shortage is monitored through data collected by the United Network of Organ Sharing (UNOS). The UNOS waiting list continues to increase (far over 100,000 potential recipients), and only a third of the patients are eligible for transplantation.

Only a small proportion of the devastatingly injured patients who might become donors fulfill the clinical criteria of brain death (5%–10% of all comatose patients admitted to intensive care units [ICUs]).[7,39] Therefore, in an attempt to reduce this major shortage of organs, protocols have been designed for the timely retrieval of organs from patients who have died of cardiac arrest.[15,23]

As a result of rigorous discussion and careful review, many institutions in the United States have protocols of donation after cardiac death (DCD) in place.[14] The medical decisions made in such cases are difficult: the attending physician must determine the certainty of irreversible, unsurvivable poor outcome, evaluate whether a patient might be eligible for organ donation after circulatory arrest, and finally estimate the likelihood of cardiac arrest after extubation.

This chapter discusses the currently accepted procedures and practices when DCD is considered. In the United States, ICU physicians who consider withdrawal of life support for any patient with a catastrophic neurologic injury are obliged to contact organ procurement agencies that could subsequently initiate discussion on possible organ and tissue donation after circulatory arrest.

DEFINITION AND POLICIES OF DONATION AFTER CARDIAC DEATH

The Uniform Determination of Death Act defines death in two ways: (1) irreversible cessation of circulatory and respiratory functions, and (2) irreversible cessation of the entire brain, or brain death. In brain death, the burden of proof has been with the neurologist or neurosurgeon; in the Act's first definition of death, the burden of proof is with any ICU physician. The definition of cardio-pulmonary arrest has become a matter of debate, echoing the concerns raised during the introduction of proposals to determine death by neurologic criteria. This serious sticking point was best voiced by Lears: "Are we manipulating the death of some person to benefit others?"[21] This is contrary to reality; such a concern can be explained. Beginning as early as 1950, physicians recognized the need for a reliable set of criteria for (brain) death to stop the administration of futile care. In contrast, criteria for non-heart-beating patients are specifically devised to promote organ donation and to resolve the worldwide organ shortage.[3,14,16]

The DCD protocols are operational in many major medical institutions in the United States.[6,41] In some countries (e.g., Canada), national recommendations for DCD and donation after circulatory death have been published.[27,35,36,40,42] DCD protocols vary in countries belonging to the European Union (e.g., objection in Germany, but acceptance in Spain), and the situation is even less clear in Asian countries.[18,20,22] Some countries have laws allowing presumed consent, which could markedly facilitate the execution of these protocols.

A wide range of opinions has emerged, from use of a DCD protocol in the field ("donors from the streets")[1] to use of the protocol in tertiary centers.[2,24,28] Proponents of DCD protocols have argued that a major source of organs is lost, while the disparity between demand and supply is increasing. Transplant surgeons continue to strongly argue that the function of donated organs, including pancreas, lung, and liver, depends on the length of time from retrieval to transplant.[8,25,29,31,36,37,44] Long delay in organ retrieval after donor death produces so-called warm ischemia, which could potentially damage the donor organs.

In 2002, UNOS defined an expanded kidney donor criteria protocol, which included (1) age greater than 60 years, or (2) age 50 to 59 years with any two of three criteria—history of hypertension, death from stroke, or a serum creatinine value greater than 1.5 mg/dL. The outcome of expanded transplant criteria is similar to that of standard criteria, but graft survival was less in some studies using these expanded criteria.[9,10,37]

An argument could be made that the complexity of this protocol should be an incentive to search for other creative solutions to this pressing problem of donor shortage. The real difficulty is in defining irreversible cardiac death: How does the physician make this determination of death,[4,5] and according to what standards? The proposed interval between cardiac stand-still and retrieval of organs varies much and has little support in published data.

There is a considerable variability in DCD donation protocols. Terminology is unclear and observation times are variable.[17] Variability also exists outside the United States, notably in the United Kingdom.[13,30] The Pittsburgh Protocol, introduced in 1992, allows death to be certified on the basis of exclusively cardiopulmonary criteria that require asystole for 2 minutes before procurement proceeds. A conference in Maastricht, the Netherlands, identified four categories of patient status that could provide non-heart-beating donors (Capsule 64.1). This protocol required 10 minutes of cardiopulmonary arrest and was based on the concept that this time was needed for the brain to die. The Institute of Medicine outlined recommendations in 1997 and supported these protocols as a means of providing a possible source of organs ("determination of death in controlled non-heart-beating donors by cessation of cardiopulmonary function for at least 5 minutes by electrocardiographic and arterial pressure monitoring"). It is unclear whether an extension from 2 minutes to 5 minutes is truly

satisfying to skeptics.[26,32,34,43] Most protocols in the United States have concluded that 5 minutes of circulatory arrest are sufficient and are not associated with autoresuscitation (i.e., the spontaneous restarting of the heart with effective pumping after the heart had stopped).

Our study in 12 patients with monitoring electrocardiogram (ECG) tracings for at least 10 minutes after cardiac arrest found two recordings with a salvo of 5 to 20 heartbeats (Figure 64.1a) at 1.5 and 6 minutes after asystole, followed by ECG silence.[45] The arterial catheter in two of these patients did not record measurable tracings during cardiac activity. Four recordings showed broad, undefined complexes at 5, 7, 9, and 10 minutes after initial cardiac arrest but without any recognizable rhythm. Our observations suggest that these ECG recordings are of short duration, often showing bizarre complexes that can neither generate a meaningful contraction nor produce an arterial pulse. A typical pattern is the appearance of an atrial pacemaker, bradycardia, and progressive shifts of ST segments ending in asystole or ventricular tachycardia and asystole (Figure 64.1b). In a neurologic catastrophe, autoresuscitation is an unlikely phenomenon, if present at all.

In our neurosciences intensive care unit (NICU), DCD is considered when patients with a catastrophic brain injury do not seem to progress to brain death and family members have decided, in conjunction with the attending physician, that further care is not warranted. The prediction of respiratory arrest after extubation is not perfectly reliable. A mini apnea test providing oxygen followed by brief disconnection or breathing on a continuous positive airway pressure of 5 cm of water may show the patient developing an irregular respiratory drive and rapid deoxygenation. However, the absence of respiratory distress does not mean that the patient will continue to breathe after extubation. Failure to

---

CAPSULE 64.1   MAASTRICHT CLASSIFICATION OF NON-HEART-BEATING DONORS

Category I	Dead on arrival
Category II	Unsuccessful resuscitation
Category III	Awaiting cardiac arrest
Category IV	Cardiac arrest in a brain-dead donor
Category V	Unexpected cardiac arrest in a critically ill patient

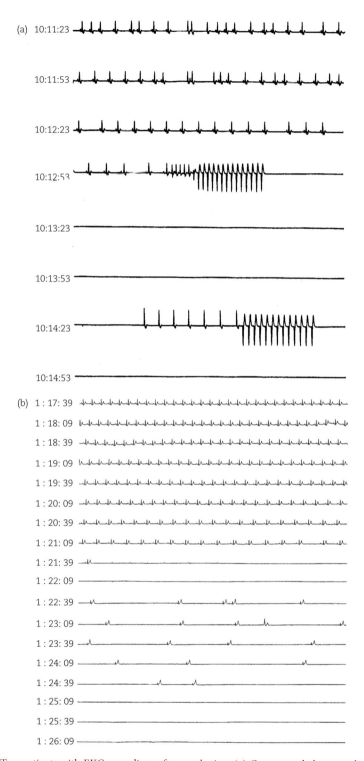

FIGURE 64.1: Two patients with EKG recordings after extubation. (a) Compressed electrocardiogram recordings in an apneic patient with catastrophic neurologic injury and a brief run of heart beats (1.5 minutes) after asystole. (b) Compressed electrocardiogram recordings in an apneic patient with catastrophic neurologic injury and gradual appearance of a "dying heart" pattern and asystole.

From Wijdicks EFM, Diringer MN. Electrocardiographic activity after terminal cardiac arrest in neuro catastrophes. *Neurology* 2004;62:673–674. With permission of *Neurology*.

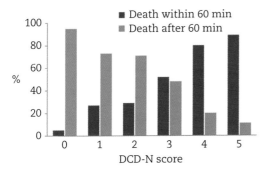

FIGURE 64.2: The DCD-N scale predicts death within 1 hour. Taking into account the presence or absence of corneal reflexes (one point), absent cough reflex (two points), absent motor response or extensor responses (one point), or an increased oxygenation index of > 3 [100 x (FiO$_2$ x mean airway pressure in cm H$_2$0/PaO$_2$ in mm Hg)] (one point). Graph shows probabilities.

protect the airway may be a major component, and that cannot be predicted a priori. A recent study found a large number of abdominal transplants are not possible due to unsuccessful DCD organ donation.[38]

In our preliminary retrospective analysis of 75 patients with a catastrophic neurologic injury who died within 1 hour after extubation, four major predictors for respiratory arrest were found (loss of corneal reflexes, absent cough reflex, motor response extensor or none, and an increased oxygenation index). The probability of respiratory arrest within 60 minutes after extubation in the presence of a single variable ranged from 65% (e.g., abnormal motor response) to 76% (absent cough reflex). The probability increased to 93% in patients with all four variables.[46] We have developed a prediction scale (the DCD-N scale) that accurately predicts death within 1 hour. Taking into account the presence or absence of corneal reflexes (one point), absent cough reflex (two points), absent motor response or extensor responses (one point), or an increased oxygenation index of > 3 (one point) (Figure 64.2). If all of these components are present, less than 10% of the patients will survive beyond 1 hour. This is important information when planning DCD.[33]

PROCEDURE OF DONATION AFTER CARDIAC DEATH

To proceed with DCD, a strict protocol should be followed (Table 64.1 and Figure 64.3) Generally, the protocol can only proceed if the transplantation

TABLE 64.1. PREREQUISITES IN DONATION AFTER CARDIAC DEATH PROTOCOL

Eligibility criteria are satisfied.[a]
All procedures have been explained to the patient's relatives or proxy.
Consent has been given for withdrawal of support (comfort care).
Consent has been given for organ donation.
The appropriateness of the opioids or sedatives for the patients' needs has been determined and discussed with the family.
Family support has been provided.
Death will be determined by a physician with no moral objections to this practice and who is separate from the organ procurement team.

[a] Excluded from the protocol are prior history of intravenous drug use; sepsis or other serious infection; active malignancies; prior infections with human T-cell leukemia-lymphoma virus; systemic viral infection; and prior related disease.

team is not involved with any discussions or management until circulatory arrest occurs.

Adequate explanation to the patient's family and adequate communication about DCD are necessary.[19] After explanation of all the procedures and after consent has been given to proceed, the patient is transferred to the operating room while ventilation and hemodynamic support are maintained. A full surgical team prepares the patient and covers the patient fully with drapes. The family then arrives and the patient is extubated. About 50% of the patients will develop a gasping respiration, rapid deoxygenation, and loss of blood pressure. The family

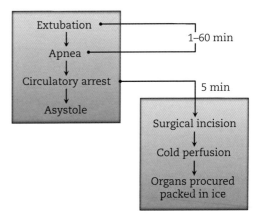

FIGURE 64.3: Timeline for DCD protocol in the operating room.

leaves at the moment of circulatory arrest and the surgical team enters the operating room 5 minutes later.

The experience for the family seeing their loved one in the operating room is a much different one than in the NICU. For family members, it is difficult to be close to the patient while trying not to violate the sterility. The operating room and its uninviting environment—despite all its good intentions and compassion of the staff—may add an additional level of emotion.

In our experience, some families may opt out of a DCD procedure when they realize the long time it takes to come to closure, in particular when the patient does not proceed to circulatory arrest and returns to the ICU. This is in contrast to brain death determination, when family members say their goodbyes before a donation procedure is started.

Circulatory arrest is determined by observing an arterial line showing no reading, followed by confirmation of the absent carotid pulse. A bedside echocardiogram might be used to document absent ventricular contraction if there is uncertainty, but with a draped patient is difficult to do. A 5-minute waiting period starts right at that moment. The transplantation team has determined beforehand which organs to harvest. The harvesting involves the kidneys most of the time and the liver occasionally. Recently, lungs have been harvested, but in adults, per DCD protocols, the heart has not been used.

Finally, there are two important issues. First, the use of opioids and sedatives after withdrawal of the ventilator may be of some concern. The patient is comatose, and therefore, opioids or sedatives are not necessary. However, small doses are allowed if tachypnea occurs after withdrawal of support, potentially suggesting discomfort of the patient. These opioids and sedatives should be administered by the attending physician and should never be directed by the organ procurement team.[26]

Second, the definition of time to abort the organ harvesting procedure in the operating suite is arbitrary. Most protocols have set a time of 60 minutes. This time period is a reflection of the "acceptable" warm ischemia time (time from extubation and withdrawal of support until infusion of cold artificial preservative solutions) and differs with each organ (liver < 30 minutes; kidney and pancreas < 60 minutes; lungs < 45–60 minutes). When a patient does not proceed to circulatory arrest, the patient is transferred to the ICU or ward to receive further palliative care.[11,12]

CONCLUSIONS

- Donation after cardiac death has been accepted as an alternative procedure for organ donation, mostly for patients who have a catastrophic neurologic disease and as part of the implementation of withdrawal of life support.
- The impact on the donor pool is small, but donation using DCD protocols has gradually increased over the years.
- In most recent DCD data sets, 30% of patients do not proceed to cardiac arrest in the operating suite.
- Better prediction is possible using the DCD-N score.

REFERENCES

1. Alvarez J, del Barrio R, Arias J, et al. Non-heart-beating donors from the streets: an increasing donor pool source. *Transplantation* 2000;70:314–317.
2. Alvarez J, del Barrio R, Arias J, et al. Non-heart-beating donors: estimated actual potential. *Transplant Proc* 2001;33:1101–1103.
3. Bell MD. Non-heart beating organ donation: in urgent need of intensive care. *Br J Anaesth* 2008;100:738–741.
4. Bernat JL. Are organ donors after cardiac death really dead? *J Clin Ethics* 2006;17:122–132.
5. Bernat JL. The boundaries of organ donation after circulatory death. *N Engl J Med* 2008;359:669–671.
6. Bernat JL, D'Alessandro AM, Port FK, et al. Report of a National Conference on Donation after cardiac death. *Am J Transplant* 2006;6:281–291.
7. Bustos JL, Surt K, Soratti C. Glasgow coma scale 7 or less surveillance program for brain death identification in Argentina: epidemiology and outcome. *Transplant Proc* 2006;38:3697–3699.
8. Clayton HA, Swift SM, Turner JM, James RF, Bell PR. Non-heart-beating organ donors: a potential source of islets for transplantation? *Transplantation* 2000;69:2094–2098.
9. Cohen B, Smits JM, Haase B, et al. Expanding the donor pool to increase renal transplantation. *Nephrol Dial Transplant* 2005;20:34–41.
10. D'Alessandro AM, Peltier JW, Phelps JE. Increasing organ donations after cardiac death by increasing DCD support among health care professionals: a case report. *Am J Transplant* 2008;8:897–904.
11. DeVita MA. The death watch: certifying death using cardiac criteria. *Prog Transplant* 2001;11:58–66.
12. DeVita MA, Brooks MM, Zawistowski C, et al. Donors after cardiac death: validation of

identification criteria (DVIC) study for predictors of rapid death. *Am J Transplant* 2008;8:432–441.

13. Dominguez-Gil B, Haase-Kromwijk B, Van Leiden H, et al. Current situation of donation after circulatory death in European countries. *Transpl Int* 2011;24:676–686.

14. DuBois JM, DeVita M. Donation after cardiac death in the United States: how to move forward. *Crit Care Med* 2006;34:3045–3047.

15. Elgharably H, Shafii AE, Mason DP. Expanding the donor pool: donation after cardiac death. *Thorac Surg Clin* 2015;25:35–46.

16. Elliott MJ, Mallory G, Jr., Khagani A. Transplantation from non-heart-beating donors. *Lancet* 2001;357:819–820.

17. Fugate JE, Stadtler M, Rabinstein AA, Wijdicks EFM. Variability in donation after cardiac death protocols: a national survey. *Transplantation* 2011;91:386–389.

18. Fung JJ. Use of non-heart-beating donors. *Transplant Proc* 2000;32:1510–1511.

19. Kelso CM, Lyckholm LJ, Coyne PJ, Smith TJ. Palliative care consultation in the process of organ donation after cardiac death. *J Palliat Med* 2007;10:118–126.

20. Kompanje EJ, Bakker J, Slieker FJ, Ijzermans JN, Maas AI. Organ donations and unused potential donations in traumatic brain injury, subarachnoid hemorrhage and intracerebral hemorrhage. *Intensive Care Med* 2006;32:217–222.

21. Lears L. Obtaining organs from non-heart-beating cadavers. *Health Care Ethics USA* 1996;4:6–7.

22. Malaise J, Van Deynse D, Dumont V, et al. Non-heart-beating donor, 10-year experience in a Belgian transplant center. *Transplant Proc* 2007;39:2578–2579.

23. Manara AR, Murphy PG, O'Callaghan G. Donation after circulatory death. *Br J Anaesth* 2012;108 Suppl 1:i108–121.

24. Mandell MS, Zamudio S, Seem D, et al. National evaluation of healthcare provider attitudes toward organ donation after cardiac death. *Crit Care Med* 2006;34:2952–2958.

25. Mason DP, Murthy SC, Gonzalez-Stawinski GV, et al. Early experience with lung transplantation using donors after cardiac death. *J Heart Lung Transplant* 2008;27:561–563.

26. Institute of Medicine. *Organ Donation: Opportunities for Action.* Washington, DC: National Academies Press; 2006.

27. Murphy P, Manara A, Bell D, Smith M. Controlled non-heart beating organ donation: neither the whole solution nor a step too far. *Anaesthesia* 2008;63:526–530.

28. Neyrinck A, Van Raemdonck D, Monbaliu D. Donation after circulatory death: current status. *Curr Opin Anaesthesiol* 2013;26:382–390.

29. Nguyen JH, Bonatti H, Dickson RC, et al. Long-term outcomes of donation after cardiac death liver allografts from a single center. *Clin Transplant* 2009;23:168–173.

30. Patel S, Martin JR, Marino PS. Donation after circulatory death: a national survey of current practice in England in 2012. *Crit Care Med* 2014;42:2219–2224.

31. Petersen SR. Done vida—donate life: a surgeon's perspective of organ donation. *Am J Surg* 2007;194:701–708.

32. Phua J, Lim TK, Zygun DA, Doig CJ. Pro/con debate: in patients who are potential candidates for organ donation after cardiac death, starting medications and/or interventions for the sole purpose of making the organs more viable is an acceptable practice. *Crit Care* 2007;11:211.

33. Rabinstein AA, Yee AH, Mandrekar J, et al. Prediction of potential for organ donation after cardiac death in patients in neurocritical state: a prospective observational study. *Lancet Neurol* 2012;11:414–419.

34. Rady MY, Verheijde JL, McGregor J. Organ procurement after cardiocirculatory death: a critical analysis. *J Intensive Care Med* 2008;23:303–312.

35. Ridley S, Bonner S, Bray K, et al. UK guidance for non-heart-beating donation. *Br J Anaesth* 2005;95:592–595.

36. Roels L, Spaight C, Smits J, Cohen B. Donation patterns in four European countries: data from the donor action database. *Transplantation* 2008;86:1738–1743.

37. Saidi RF, Elias N, Kawai T, et al. Outcome of kidney transplantation using expanded criteria donors and donation after cardiac death kidneys: realities and costs. *Am J Transplant* 2007;7:2769–2774.

38. Scalea JR, Redfield RR, Rizzari MD, et al. When Do DCD Donors Die?: outcomes and implications of DCD at a high-volume, single-center OPO in the United States. *Ann Surg* 2016;263:211–216.

39. Senouci K, Guerrini P, Diene E, et al. A survey on patients admitted in severe coma: implications for brain death identification and organ donation. *Intens Care Med* 2004;30:38–44.

40. Shemie SD, Baker AJ, Knoll G, et al. National recommendations for donation after cardiocirculatory death in Canada: donation after cardiocirculatory death in Canada. *CMAJ* 2006;175:S1.

41. Steinbrook R. Organ donation after cardiac death. *N Engl J Med* 2007;357:209–213.

42. Thomas I, Caborn S, Manara AR. Experiences in the development of non-heart beating organ donation scheme in a regional neurosciences intensive care unit. *Br J Anaesth* 2008;100:820–826.

43. Vincent JL, Brimioulle S. Non-heart-beating donation: ethical aspects. *Transplant Proc* 2009;41:576–578.

44. Wells AC, Rushworth L, Thiru S, et al. Donor kidney disease and transplant outcome for kidneys donated after cardiac death. *Br J Surg* 2009;96:299–304.

45. Wijdicks EFM, Diringer MN. Electrocardiographic activity after terminal cardiac arrest in neurocatastrophes. *Neurology* 2004;62:673–674.

46. Yee AH, Rabinstein AA, Thapa P, Mandrekar J, Wijdicks EFM. Factors influencing time to death after withdrawal of life support in neurocritical patients. *Neurology* 2010;74:1380–1385.

65

Organ Procurement

Depending on the country—comparatively low in Israel, Switzerland, and Brazil—recovery of tissue and vital organs proceeds in 60%–80% of patients who have been declared brain dead. Organ donors in the United States are managed by representatives (organ procurement coordinators) of the organ donation organization UNOS (United Network of Organ Sharing). The UNOS (www. unos.org) administers over 50 federally regulated organ procurement organizations (OPOs). In addition, public and professional education programs and better acknowledgment of true organ donor potential have become more urgent. The involvement of care by the neurointensivist usually stops abruptly when brain death has been determined and consent has been given by family members to proceed with procurement. For the practitioner, it is crucially important to understand the policies surrounding organ donation.[1,2,4,11] This chapter provides some additional insights into the organ donor process in the United States and the explanation of this process to family members.[8,15]

ORGAN PROCUREMENT ORGANIZATIONS

In the United States, the OPOs are independent, private, nonprofit organizations; a specific geographic area has been assigned to each OPO by the Health Care Financing Authority (HCFA). All OPOs are funded by the HCFA and the transplant centers that receive organs recovered by the OPO. OPOs respond to organ donor referrals, organ donor case management, and donor family aftercare. OPO coordinators generally have a background as a nurse, physician assistant, or paramedic. (In some European countries, physicians are involved.)

With transfer of the potential donor to the OPOs, medical suitability for organ donation will be relegated to them, which is to say that this determination is ultimately based on the probability of successfully transplanting at least one organ. The final decision on suitability is left to the discretion of the transplant surgeon.

The process of asking for consent to donate organs is variable throughout the world but typically goes through several steps (Figure 65.1). In the United States it is preferred that neither medical nor nursing staff mentions the topic of donation to families. As public education and experiences with organ donation and transplantation increase, more families, however, approach physicians or nurses about their donation options. When pressed by the family, time should be allowed to answer specific questions, but details should be deferred to the OPOs. Family members decline donation if organ donation is prematurely mentioned, and they may later refuse to speak with the OPO. If a family mentions no interest in donation to nursing staff, OPOs will respectfully request to meet with families to explain the procedure and the benefits to them; in some situations, a better understanding could lead to consent. In any event, all OPOs train individuals not to broach the topic of donation before a determination of brain death has been completed.

ORGAN DONATION REQUESTS

Most organ procurement officers have a presumptive model for consent. That is, families will actively have to state a reason that they would not want to proceed.[12,13]

Many reasons may explain refusal to obtain consent. In a recent experience, it became clear that procrastination with brain death examination reduces the number of conversions to donation and was 10%–20% lower than the usual 50%–60% acceptance rate.[9] The decision to donate organs decreases as the time to declare brain death increases. Families at the bedside of a dying patient in the intensive care unit (ICU) are under tremendous duress. Often the family must spend another night in the ICU, and often they question why further testing is required, and even more, why a second examination is needed if a loved one is, in fact, dead. Although it has been argued that family observation of brain death testing may be

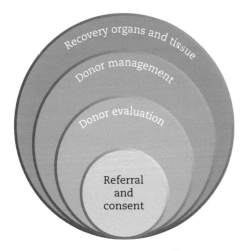

FIGURE 65.1: The multistep process of organ donation.

helpful for those families who are having difficulty understanding the concept of brain death, there are little data that their actual presence will have a convincing effect.[3,5,7,10,14]

Transition from a catastrophic brain injury to brain death usually takes some time, and regular discussions with family members are needed. However, once brain death is diagnosed and communicated, its finality always comes as a shock, and such an experience is difficult to change, even with regular meetings.[6] The OPO usually meets with the family soon after the neurointensivist has met with the family, and often this brief delay provides the family with some time to recuperate. The OPO then systematically discusses the time of death and the benefit of organ donation with high success rates, the time it takes to assess for donor suitability, and the preparatory tests needed. The long, complex preparation may take 36 hours. The family is told that when donation is allowed, the OPO coordinator is going to assume care of the patient, but the nursing staff will remain involved and available. The family says the last goodbyes before the patient goes to the operating room, but they may leave earlier if they wish. The organ donation process should be explained in two parts: the evaluation and placement phase, and organ recovery in the operating room. The family should understand that all of the organs will be tested to determine suitability for transplantation, and testing may include blood tests, chest X-rays, coronary angiography, and possibly liver biopsy. After the organs are evaluated, they are matched with recipients on the waiting list. The OPO then discusses the operation and explains that it is one incision, exactly as it is with heart or abdominal surgery. A single incision is made from below the navel to just above the sternum. After the surgery, the incision is closed the donor is transferred to the medical examiner (if an autopsy is planned) or to the funeral home. The utmost respect and dignity are guaranteed. The family should be reassured that organ donation generally does not interfere with the type of funeral service (such as an open casket funeral). After this explanation, the OPO will have the next of kin sign a consent form with a nurse as

---

CAPSULE 65.1   UNOS BOARD OF DIRECTORS RECOMMENDATIONS ON ORGAN DONATION

The following persons may become donees of anatomical gifts for the purposes stated:

Any hospital, physician, or surgeon, or procurement organization for transplantation therapy, medical or dental education, research, or advancement of medical or dental science.

Any accredited medical or dental school, college or university for education, research, advancement of medical or dental science, or therapy.

(a) Designated individual for transplantation or therapy needed by that individual

(b) The gift may be made to a designated donee or without designating a donee. If the donee is not designated or if the donee is not available or rejects the anatomical gift, the anatomical gift may be accepted by any hospital.

(c) If the donee knows of the decedent's refusal or contrary indications to make an anatomical gift or that an anatomical gift by a member of a class having priority to act is opposed by a member of the same class or a prior class under Section 3 (a), the donee may not accept the anatomical gift.

(d) Donation of organ may not be made in a manner which discriminates against a person or class of persons on the basis of race, national origin, religion, gender or similar characteristic.

Source: UNOS Website: www.unos.org/resources/bioethics.

witness and then will go over the medical history. The consent will apply to all possible organs, and this should be clarified. The family is also asked if there are specific indications of prior intention; a driver's license designation of the potential donor is an important example.

The consent rate for OPO coordinators approaching the family alone for organ donation is higher than a hospital staff member. With a growing number of experienced neurointensivists, the differences may not be that large.

Declining or accepting organ or tissue donation may be a result of personal and cultural values and fear of mutilation of the body. Multiple reasons are listed by families when declining organ donation. Donors of Hispanic descent were four times more likely to decline, and African Americans were seven times more likely to decline. Other than the known objections, there are misconceptions, which may be exacerbated by the way the health care team approaches the family, long delay to discuss organ donation, and a preconceived notion by family members that older age would not qualify. Families who have had more specific conversations about organ donation in the past are more likely to donate. In our experience, failure to consent for donation is often simple—families do not want to deal with it and move on. Utilitarian arguments ("many persons' lives can be saved," "many die on a waiting list") do not carry any weight with families who refuse organ or tissue donation. Closure comes for them when the patient is moved to the funeral home.

There are often questions about the costs of organ procurement. The family should be assured that the entire cost of the organ donation process is paid for by the OPO. Generally, this includes all costs from the time of the brain death declaration and consent until the donor's care is transferred after the organ recovery to the medical examiner or funeral home. (Paying the donor as a compensation for organ or tissue donation, however, is a much more complex ethical problem. Paying the family of the organ donor can be corrosive, particularly if the amount is extraordinary, and many would consider this inappropriate.)

Families who consent to organ donation may request directing of the transplantable organs to family members or to friends. Any person who is in need of an organ transplant and has a relation with family members can receive this as a gift. Most commonly this practice is a donation by living donors, but this can also apply to brain death donors. It is important for physicians

to ensure that the determination of brain death has been fully separated from any discussion on organ donation, removing a possible conflict of interest. Donating a gift to family members in donation after cardiac death (DCD) protocols might be more problematic because withdrawal of care could be seen as a way to facilitate organ donation. If family members could agree, the organ procurement agency would have to contact these family members. Family members, however, are unable to put certain restrictions on organ donation (e.g., refusal to donate organ to a patient who might receive a liver transplant after alcohol abuse). Another very problematic occasionally encountered concern is that some family members do not wish to donate to another race. However, in the overwhelming proportion of cases the gift of life to another person is unbiased and leaves many of us gratified. Families may experience more pain and grief when they hear their loved one cannot donate for whatever reason. Physicians should make every effort and it starts with recognizing this opportunity. UNOS has summarized their recommendations for organ donation (Capsule 65.1).

CONCLUSIONS

- Organ donation agencies become involved before brain death declaration but are operational only after brain death declaration.
- Most families understand the process of organ donation very well and agree to proceed in 60%–80% of cases.
- Discussions about organ donation are detailed and are the responsibility of organ donation agencies.
- The neurointensivist plays an important coordinating role in the process of organ donation.

REFERENCES

1. Al-Khafaji A, Elder M, Lebovitz DJ, et al. Protocolized fluid therapy in brain-dead donors: the multicenter randomized MOnIToR trial. *Intens Care Med* 2015;41:418–426.
2. Al-Khafaji A, Murugan R, Kellum JA. What's new in organ donation: better care of the dead for the living. *Intens Care Med* 2013;39:2031–2033.
3. Berntzen H, Bjork IT. Experiences of donor families after consenting to organ donation: a qualitative study. *Intens Crit Care Nurs* 2014;30:266–274.
4. Dikdan GS, Mora-Esteves C, Koneru B. Review of randomized clinical trials of donor management and organ preservation in deceased

donors: opportunities and issues. *Transplantation* 2012;94:425–441.

5. Doran M. The presence of family during brain stem death testing. *Intens Crit Care Nurs* 2004;20:32–37.

6. Kompanje EJ. Families and brain death. *Semin Neurol* 2015;35:169–173.

7. Kompanje EJ, de Groot YJ, Bakker J, Ijzermans JN. A national multicenter trial on family presence during brain death determination: the FABRA study. *Neurocrit Care* 2012;17:301–308.

8. Lustbader D. Organ donation: practicalities and ethical conundrums. *Am J Crit Care* 2014; 23:81–84.

9. Lustbader D, O'Hara D, Wijdicks EFM, et al. Second brain death examination may negatively affect organ donation. *Neurology* 2011;76:119–124.

10. Pugh J, Clarke L, Gray J, et al. Presence of relatives during testing for brain stem death: questionnaire study. *BMJ* 2000;321:1505–1506.

11. Sally M, Malinoski D. Current research on organ donor management. *Anesthesiol Clin* 2013;31: 737–748.

12. Siminoff L, Mercer MB, Graham G, Burant C. The reasons families donate organs for transplantation: implications for policy and practice. *J Trauma* 2007;62:969–978.

13. Siminoff LA, Agyemang AA, Traino HM. Consent to organ donation: a review. *Prog Transplant* 2013; 23:99–104.

14. Tawil I, Brown LH, Comfort D, et al. Family presence during brain death evaluation: a randomized controlled trial. *Crit Care Med* 2014;42:934–942.

15. Wijdicks EFM. Brain death. *Handb Clin Neurol* 2013;118:191–203.

66

Ethical and Legal Matters

There is little doubt that practicing physicians in any intensive care unit (ICU) will be confronted with ethical quandaries. In critically ill neurologic patients, these disputes mostly pertain to the appropriateness of high-level care provided to the patient. Regular review of the effects of the patient's treatment is one of the universal principles of critical care neurology. Seeing patients improve is most satisfying, but due to the nature of some acute neurologic disorders, many patients remain unchanged or may even deteriorate despite multiple interventions. When advance directives have been written, the family's opinions and interpretations of the patient's wishes may also affect the level of care.[14,44] Decisions that are ethically strained commonly involve the futility of care, and some of the uncertainties and biases surrounding that issue are discussed in this chapter.

Legal vulnerability is inherent in this profession, so this closing chapter also touches briefly on this very difficult subject, particularly focusing on risk avoidance and the neurointensivist as expert witness.

ETHICAL CONTROVERSIES

The most controversial topics within the neurosciences intensive care unit (NICU) are considered here. Not all of these matters are addressed by the law, and some physicians have decided to opt out of (e.g., active euthanasia). A detailed account of bioethics and US law as they pertain to comatose patients can be found elsewhere.[66] The critical care management of devastating brain injury when it pertains to best ethical management has been recently reviewed by the Neurocritical Care Society.[55]

Futility and Its Consequences

Futility is defined as "a useless act or gesture"[38] (from the Latin *futilis*, "leaky"). In classical mythology, futility refers to the punishment of the 50 daughters of Danaus, who killed their husbands on their wedding night and were condemned

to carry water from the river in leaky jars for all eternity.[38]

Futility is value laden.[11,39] Continuous support of a devastatingly injured patient with no hope for recovery or even awakening from coma may seem futile to some but not to others.[63,65,66] Futility is hard to define, and there have been questionable ways of defining it. No success in the last 100 patients under similar circumstances has been proposed as another way to define poor outcome, but recoveries are often vividly remembered by physicians, while failures are less memorable. Attempts to define futility in percentages of treatment success (e.g., less than 1% chance of recovery) arrive at a loose definition, and the thresholds may look arbitrary to family members. Nevertheless, albeit imprecise, the determination of futility remains a pragmatic judgment necessary to daily practice. Without it, the patient, physician, and family remain at a standstill.

Neurologists have no ethical duty to exhaustively provide futile interventions. But some neurologists believe that something about the definition of futility of care is still unconvincing, and certainly not many physicians argue that futility is a simple commonsense notion.[51,52,64] Physicians—particularly the more experienced ones—are more cautious about prognostication, knowing only too well how risky this undertaking can be.

Helft and colleagues[28] noted that "the illusion of futility is the mistaken assumption that it is an objective entity." Dunphy[17] eloquently summarized the problem: "The incoherence of futility stems, no doubt, from different people at the same time, and the same people at different times, using the word to mean many things." In a more pragmatic sense, futility usually is best characterized as a clear appreciation of a hopeless situation, and an obvious disparity between the prediction of fatal outcome and aggressiveness of care in the NICU. The term can be used to denote that a certain goal is not worth pursuing, that intervention has no pathophysiologic rationale, and that prior therapies have already failed.[5]

A unilateral decision on futility of care is complex because it can be construed as polarizing, and a second opinion from a colleague may be warranted.[10] Moreover, a study surveying families 1 year after end-of-life treatment discussions suggested that conflict sometimes arises between family members and medical staff over communication and unprofessional staff behavior.

As physicians, we judge some things incorrectly, and we often unconsciously tack on our own skewed experiences (Capsule 66.1). We continue to make mistakes in prognostication because hard data on long-term outcome are lacking in many disorders. We may also underestimate how much some patients and relatives consider life worth living.[33] These decisions are even more difficult to make in younger patients. In fact, only a few neurologic injuries to the brain or spinal cord exist in which the chance of recovery is infinitesimal. One recent illustration involved a comatose patient with aneurysmal subarachnoid hemorrhage. *New England Journal of Medicine* readers were asked to choose among several options of care. The results showed marked diversity of opinion throughout the world.[31,53] A recent article shows wide variability in opinions of physicians working in intensive care units (Figure 66.1).[40]

Orders Not to Resuscitate

Patients are resuscitated unless it is explicitly directed otherwise. A do-not-resuscitate (DNR) directive is justified when quality of life is very poor or absent, as in a persistent vegetative state; when upper brainstem reflexes are lost after emergency neurosurgical procedure; with persistent locked-in syndrome in basilar artery occlusion; after the clinical diagnosis of brain death; and in other catastrophic conditions when a severely disabled state is anticipated.[13] A DNR statement may have also been noted in an advance directive before admission (Chapter 15), but often the DNR order is written during the hospital stay.[48] Most hospitalized patients would want to discuss DNR orders with their physicians, but data are unknown or difficult to obtain in the NICU.[49] Other surveys suggest that few would want resuscitation in elderly debilitated patients.[35]

The DNR order implies withholding cardiopulmonary resuscitation, but all other treatment continues. Concerns that DNR orders may lead to suboptimal management are real but are difficult to demonstrate or prove. When DNR is discussed, family members and the patient should understand that cardiopulmonary resuscitation implies placement of a mechanical ventilator, is a complicated procedure (unlike jump-starting a car), and is successful in only a third of patients (and possibly even fewer).

Cardiopulmonary resuscitation, despite known questionable long-term outcome, is more successful in the general ICU.[42,50] In our study in the NICU, cardiorespiratory resuscitation was performed in 21 patients, but only 33% had return of pulse and blood pressure. As expected, cardiopulmonary resuscitation in deteriorating neurologic patients is mostly unsuccessful. In addition, some patients had a cardiac arrest soon after transfer out of the NICU, and none survived.[48]

Limited DNR orders (no intubation or defibrillation), or so-called *slow codes*[24,27,41,43] (delay in calling; deliberately ineffective attempt), are troublesome, and are deceiving.

Terminal Extubation and Withdrawal of Support

The main principles of compassionate end-of-life care in the medical ICU have recently been published.[32] The judicial determinations of withholding and withdrawing life-sustaining treatment are discussed in review articles and are not considered further in this chapter.[1,4,25] Withdrawal and withholding of life support are considered ethically equivalent.[4] The practice is prevalent in many ICUs around the world, but not all (e.g., the UK and Japan).[21,30,46,68] The prevailing judicial opinion in court decisions in the United States is that artificial feeding is a medical treatment. A number of court cases and a number of states have accepted nutrition and hydration as medical interventions.[37]

The circumstances of withdrawal of support in the NICU have rarely been reported in detail.[16,36] In one study from New York, terminal extubation was done in 43% of patients with decisions on withdrawal of support; median survival was 7 hours, and almost 70% died within 24 hours. Opioids were used to relieve agonal or labored breathing in this study.[36] Other studies emerged that scrutinized the reasons and justifications for withdrawal of support in patients admitted to the NICU. Withdrawal of mechanical ventilation was less likely in patients of African American ethnicity and more likely in comatose patients or patients with a diagnosis of subarachnoid hemorrhage or ischemic stroke.[16]

A retrospective study on withdrawal of support in patients with cerebral supratentorial hemorrhage found a bias toward elderly patients and

CAPSULE 66.1   SELF-FULFILLING PROPHECY IN NEUROCRITICAL CARE

One could argue that determination of a prognosis is a prophecy in itself. Determination of prognosis in the first weeks of an acute neurologic illness cannot ignore some element of unpredictability. Physicians have the duty to prognosticate, but many are ambivalent—and rightly so. Christakis has identified the "ritualization of pessimism and optimism" as a means of handling uncertainty.

If certain conditions are perceived by a pessimistic neurologist as hopeless (based on clinical experience) and care is withdrawn, thus leading to death, this can be perceived as a self-fulfilling prophecy. In other words, we could cause the outcome to be poor because of our preconceptions. If physicians believe that a self-fulfilling prophecy may influence outcome, it will constrain their decision-making process.

The contrary position is that patients can recover, but only with an aggressive effort. Optimistic physicians may overestimate survival, and this position may add false hope to a certain fate. A common argument is that by giving the patient time to recover, he will recover and often dramatically so. The impact of physician bias and outcome is summarized in the accompanying illustration.

There are four possible scenarios. Aggressive care may result in good outcome, including in patients with poor prognosis. Less aggressive or less attentive care may result in poor outcome. Examples are the following:

1. Early stage of myasthenic crisis; plasma exchange leads to rapid improvement (positive self-fulfilling prophecy; physician is vigilant);

2. Large frontal lobar hematoma with high INR and mass effect, early administration of factor VII, and early evacuation of hematoma (positive self-negating prophecy, physician doubles effort);

3. Ischemic stroke with minimal deficit and diabetes; development of hyperosmolar hyperglycemic coma, cardiac arrest (negative self-negating prophecy, physician fails to order laboratory tests);

4. Comatose patient with a massive ganglionic hemorrhage remains unchanged or even worsens, extubation and death (negative self-fulfilling prophecy, physician withdraws care).

Positive self-fulfilling prophecy	Positive self-negating prophecy
Predict good outcome Aggressive care Good outcome	Predict poor outcome Aggressive care Good outcome
Negative self-negating prophecy	Negative self-fullling prophecy
Predict good outcome Less attentive care Poor outcome	Predict poor outcome Less attentive care Poor outcome

Illustration from Christakis N. *Death Foretold: Prophesy and Prognosis in Medical Care.* Chicago: University of Chicago Press; 2001. With permission of the publisher.

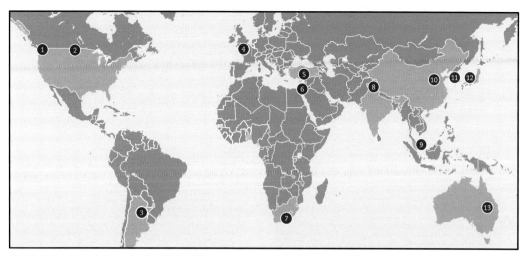

In the **USA**, and in most of the developed world, the majority deaths in the ICU are preceded by a decision to withhold or withdraw life-sustaining treatments. It is often commented that there is tremendous variability between countries. However, there is tremendous variability from ICU to ICU within countries (including the USA and England) and even from physician to physician; variability that is not explained by patient, family, or ICU characteristics. In fact, there is as much variability within countries and ICUs as between countries.

The basis for the decision to withdraw life support should depend on patients' and families' goals and preferences as well as physicians' perspectives. Ideally, we should use the full spectrum of decision-making—from parentalism (doctor decides) through to shared decision-making to autonomy (patient or family decide). Where we are on this spectrum should be determined by the patient's prognosis, by the treatments that are available, and by the patient or family preferences for the role they choose to play in decision-making.

J Randall Curtis, Cambia Palliative Care Center of Excellence, Division of Pulmonary and Critical Care Medicine, University of Washington, Seattle, WA, USA.

As prognosticators and communicators, neurologists are neither unhinged optimists nor paralyzing doomsayers. Acute brain injury is often a major setback in critically ill patients and a tenable reason to de-escalate care. Such a decision is straightforward when catastrophic neurological illness—often a severe diffuse cortical, diencephalic, or brainstem injury—occurs in a patient whose wishes are known.

The expectation that the patient will lack cognition, autonomy, and dignity can determine resuscitative measures. In the USA, decisions are ideally reached after multiple discussions using a shared decision-making model. Disputes about futility of care can often achieve a conciliatory solution after carefully conducted family conferences. Yet, irrational hope or mistrust can result in continuation of care despite very poor prognosis. Legal fear and complacency can drive this decision. Lacking alternatives such as adjudicating hospital tribunals, disputes might have to be litigated in court.

Eelco Wijdicks and Alejandro Rabinstein, Mayo Clinic, Rochester, MN, USA

In **Argentina**, physicians base the clinical decision to withdraw life support on the history of the disease, which means how widespread it is, number of treatments, success of these different approaches, impact of treatment on the quality of life, patient expectation, dignity, and family and patient's feelings and beliefs. This decision would be made following failure of the treatment that had been based on the best clinical evidence, and takes account of the limitations of futile interventions where physicians are faced with the boundaries of overtreatment. Ideally, at this point, the physician who personally followed up the case and spoke to both the patient and relatives should be involved. There are no specific guidelines in our country to instruct us on this matter. I believe that such guidelines would facilitate the approach to the decision; however, when dealing with such a delicate situation, personal decisions must be respected. The philosophy in Argentina is to use all resources available, but this notion must be weighed against the potential harm of overtreatment. The best results are obtained when the decisions are made collaboratively, with the primary physician, intensivists, and the family.

Nestor Wainsztein, FLENI Institute, Buenos Aires, Argentina

With most intensive care unit (ICU) patients now dying as the result of a decision to withhold or withdraw life-sustaining therapies, there is continuing debate and discussion about how this end-of-life process should be managed. In **Belgium**, euthanasia has been legal since 2002, allowing patients in certain carefully defined situations and under strict conditions to request a physician to perform euthanasia.

However, this law does not apply to most ICU patients, who are generally not in a position to request euthanasia, and the legalities of end-of-life practices are less clearly defined, particularly in terms of administering drugs that can hasten death. To acknowledge and support current practice in Belgium, and indeed in other countries, the Belgian Society of Intensive Care has stated that shortening the dying process with use of medication, such as analgesics or sedatives, may sometimes be appropriate, even in the absence of discomfort, and can actually improve the quality of dying. In a recent survey of physicians certifying deaths in Belgium, about one fourth of all deaths were listed as being preceded by intensified alleviation of pain and other symptoms with the use of drugs, with possible shortening of life. Patient and family input is an important aspect of end-of-life decision-making in Belgium, but final decisions remain the responsibility of the doctor in charge, supported by a consensus within the ICU team. The World Federation of Societies of Intensive and Critical Care Medicine has a task force working on these issues. We can only say that the attitudes are extremely variable around the globe, so that it is difficult to find common values—perhaps the only consensus we could reach is around the important principle of proportionality of care, that should be applied everywhere. The concept of futile therapy should be abandoned, because it is inadequate and potentially misleading. We are working on the establishment of patterns for different regions, so that people could recognize themselves in one or another of these patterns.

Jean-Louis Vincent, Erasmus University Hospital, Brussels, Belguim, and President, World Federation of Societies of Intensive and Critical Care Medicine, Brussels, Belguim

In **Turkey**, patients and their families have rights to decide on diagnostic and treatment options offered to them, so they have the right to refuse any treatment. However, there are no medical guidelines or legal regulations about end-of-life care, and do-not-resuscitate or related orders and advanced directives are not legal, although some kind of withholding or withdrawing life support may occur during daily practice when treatment is thought to be futile. In addition, there are huge variations among physicians in terms of understanding and attitudes at the end of life, probably because of religious and cultural differences or differences in resources. Therefore, there are serious conflicts in medical practice, and physicians and other health-care staff face continuous ethical dilemmas and pressures.

Arzu Topeli, Hacettepe University Faculty of Medicine, Ankara, Turkey

In **Israel** as in most other countries, the physician decides when the patient will most likely die and life-sustaining treatments should be limited. What is very different to other countries is that life-sustaining therapies are not withdrawn. This is based on culture, religion, and law. The Israeli Terminally Ill Law 2005 prohibits stopping continuous life-prolonging treatments, but allows stopping intermittent life-prolonging therapies. Discontinuing intermittent life-sustaining therapies is regarded as omitting a therapy rather than withdrawal. The Law is based on Halacha or Jewish law where the value and sanctity of human life is infinite and beyond measure. Although the omission of life-sustaining treatments is allowed, an act that actively and intentionally shortens life is prohibited. The withdrawal of a ventilator, which is considered a continuous form of therapy, shortens life and is forbidden. Halacha considers that not only the ends have to be morally acceptable, but also the means. The Law also regards fluids and food as basic needs and not treatments, requires physicians to care for patients and families, considers palliative care as a citizen's right, and requires that any controversies are taken to ethics committees, not the courts. Decisions are based on the autonomous wishes of the patient, which are based on advance medical directives, the appointment of a surrogate decision maker, and testimony of an incompetent dying patient's wishes by family members or close friends.

Charles Sprung, Department of Anesthesiology and Critical Care Medicine, Hadassah Hebrew University Medical Center, Jerusalem, Israel

FIGURE 66.1: Current views on withdrawal of care from practitioners around the world.

Reproduced from *Lancet Respir Med* 2015;3, with permission.

7 In South Africa, most of the population is served by the primary-care orientated, state-run health system, which has proportionally few ICU beds—mainly in regional or academic hospitals. Decisions to withdraw life support are most often initiated by the intensivist in charge and are usually based on futility. Functional independence is an important outcome as long-term care facilities are minimal. Limited ICU facilities does affect decision making. After ICU team consensus, family assent, but not formal consent, is sought. Families largely trust the doctors and despite the culturally diverse population, religious objection is rare. Challenges include absent families due to distance, language barriers, as well as families in which male-dominated clan elders need to be consulted. There is no formal legal basis for end-of-life decisions, but the courts are guided by what medical peers would regard as reasonable. Euthanasia is illegal. In the health-insurance-funded private sector, most critically ill patients are managed by non-intensivists in open ICUs. Decisions to withdraw life support are made much later in the course of illness and may only be considered when there is medical aid failure.

Lance Michell, Division of Critical Care, University of Cape Town, Cape Town, South Africa

8 Consensus position statements in India favor foregoing of life sustaining treatment when the harm would appear to outweigh the benefit. There appears to be little meaningful debate other than on euthanasia in the public and legal domains. In the context of critical illness, family involvement in day-to-day decision making is the rule. However, economic considerations are usually central to limitation decisions—in most, the expenses are borne by the family, not by the State, and modern medicine is affordable only to some. The national critical and palliative care societies' joint statement has favored the use of the term medically inappropriate over medical futility. Generally it is accepted that the terms are subjective, but the consensus operative principle is "almost certainly will not benefit". The Law Commission of India has directed physicians to respect the wishes of the informed and capable patient. However, for the incapacitated patient, it does not endorse decisions made unilaterally or by proxy. Nor does it recognize instructive directives such as do-not-resuscitate order, advance will, or a durable power of attorney. Likewise, the Supreme Court directs that for the incapacitated patient, passive euthanasia should be validated by a legal process. Not surprisingly, physicians have found these guidelines unworkable. Popular beliefs among the major religions in India have not posed a perceptible barrier to treatment limitations. The composite culture of India glorifies a good death as a fitting culmination of life. Good death is associated with family presence, freedom from distress, preservation of dignity, and a spiritual ambiance.

Pravin Amin, Bombay Hospital Institute of Medical Sciences, Mumbai, India, and Raj Kumar Mani, Nayati Healthcare & Research Pvt. Ltd, Gurgaon, India

9 Attitudes towards end-of-life care in Singaporean intensive care units were explored in the Asian Collaboration for Medical Ethics study. The findings showed that most intensivists would withhold and withdraw life support for patients with no chance of recovering a meaningful life. The likelihood of meaningful survival and the patients' known wishes weigh most heavily in such decisions, and the law in Singapore is aligned with this approach. Nonetheless, as Singapore is a family-centric society, discussions with families are the norm, especially when the prognosis is uncertain. Resources for intensive care are limited, but this does not play a major role in end-of-life care decisions.

Jason Phua, Division of Respiratory and Critical Care Medicine, National University Hospital, Singapore

10 In China, there is neither local nor national legislation governing withdrawal of life-sustaining treatment, and no consensus exists with regards to futile medical treatment. However, the lawsuit against the treating physician in the first reported case of euthanasia in China in 1986 resulted in more cautious and conservative attitudes towards withdrawal of life-sustaining treatment, despite the acquittal of the accused physician.

10 In clinical practice, treatment withdrawal in patients unlikely to make a meaningful recovery, as judged by the treating physician, but often raised by the family, is always a joint decision. Nevertheless, it is not uncommon for the children to override the advanced directives of the patients for do-not resuscitate orders, and insist on aggressive but futile therapy, because filial piety can only be shown when the parent is alive. If this is the case, the physicians usually respect the family decisions and continue life-sustaining treatment. Some families will choose to let the patient die at home, due to religious or cultural values, and sometimes due to financial difficulties.

Bin Du, Peking Union Medical College Hospital, Beijing, China

11 It is very rare to have any advanced directive regarding end-of-life care in critically ill patients. Patients and their families do not like to discuss end-of-life care in the early stages of intensive care. The role of the family is huge. Culturally, South Korean physicians will consult a patients' family at first, and then discuss with the patient only with the agreement of the patient's family. Every measure, especially regarding end-of-life care, is decided after family discussion. In South Korea, it is illegal to quit a life-sustaining measure from a patient, who appears to be terminal, by a physician's unilateral decision. Every South Korean has medical insurance, which is a monopoly managed by our government. However, insurance is on a discounted system, paying around 60-80% of total medical expenses on admission to hospital. Therefore, sometimes issues around medical futility have arisen due to the financial burden on a patient's family. However, resources are a sensitive issue. If we raise this issue of medical expense or resource allocation, we could not make progress on developing guidelines on withholding or withdrawing life-sustaining therapy even in the terminally ill patient in our society. There is increasing consensus regarding proper medical resource allocation between stakeholders for end-of-life care.

Younsuck Koh, Asan Medical Center, University of Ulsan College of Medicine, South Korea

12 The health-insurance system is amazing in Japan, and the economic burden on the family is light. Almost all families request that we take care of patients at any expense. In addition, withdrawal of life support is considered to be illegal. Sometimes a patient's doctor insists on keeping them on life support, even when the intensivist believes it to be of no benefit. It is not unusual for the patient to occupy an ICU bed for a long time. This is ridiculous; however, it is next to impossible to transfer them to a general ward. The family plays a very important role, and rarely accept the option of withdrawing life support. Cultural values occupy an important place in decision-making, but religion is not an issue. The boundaries between definitions concerning medical futility are not clear distinctions.

Masaji Nishimura, University of Tokushima Graduate School, Osaka, Japan

13 Through the College of Intensive Care Medicine, training in intensive care in Australia and New Zealand is strictly controlled via a formal training program and examination process. This results in a relatively homogenous standard of practice in ICUs throughout the region. Most ICUs are closed units run by registered intensivists with the authority and responsibility for all intensive-care decisions. Practicing in Australia, where there are few resource limitations and a western medical training system, we realize modern intensive care can prolong the dying process. While futility cannot be formally defined, we recognize that some severely ill patients have little or no chance of recovery to any meaningful quality of life. This would be stressed in family discussions, often asking the family what the patient would have wanted. With family assent, the intensivist will withdraw therapy for these patients and keep the patient comfortable, often with opiates. In this regard there may be some variety in practice across the region and even within units, but surprisingly little.

Jeffrey Lipman, Royal Brisbane and Women's Hospital, The University of Queensland, Brisbane, QLD, Australia

FIGURE 66.1: (Continued)

dominant hemisphere, and withdrawal was less likely when craniotomy was performed. This study, albeit with very small numbers, suggested that despite intracranial hematomas of large volume, stupor, or coma, functional independence was possible when care was continued. Characteristics in some of these patients were not different from those in whom care was withdrawn.[6] The authors expressed concern about a possible self-fulfilling prophecy by family members or physicians, but retrospective comparisons may not catch important differences.

In our NICU, the suggestion of withdrawal of support is invariably first entertained by family members. Failure to awaken after an emergent neurosurgical procedure, absent upper brainstem reflexes, intercurrent infection or sepsis with prolonged mechanical ventilation, and most important, previously expressed wishes of the patient not to remain in a severely handicapped state are all reasons to withdraw mechanical ventilation and pharmaceutical supportive care.

When a final decision is made that treatment or support is not needed at an aggressive level, the withdrawal of medication, nutrition, and hydration is discussed. Generally, withdrawal of support should be compassionate, with utmost attention to relief of discomfort and symptoms.[7,8,34] Withdrawal of nutrition and hydration does not lead to starvation, because loss of appetite is common in critically ill patients, and some degree of starvation is invariably present. Apart from dryness of the mouth and changes in facial features (decrease in swelling), withdrawal of feeding and hydration leads to a peaceful death in all patients within 2 weeks. Regular swabbing of the mouth provides sufficient comfort.

Sedatives should be administered anticipatorily to achieve a rapid desired effect (arbitrarily defined as a calm, drowsy, non-anxious, or agitated patient).[26] Orders should be p.r.n. rather than automatically escalating. Rapid increase in the dose without a documented reason could potentially cause questioning of intent and in legal proceedings could be challenged by family members. However, a minimally effective dose may not cause a maximal effect.[19,60]

It is not necessary to extubate the patient when further progression will lead to death. However, intubation and maintaining an unobstructed airway should be considered a medical intervention that may prolong dying. Some argue that removal of the tube takes away life, but in fact the brain lesion does. In general, breathing may become slightly more rapid, with associated snoring, and evolves into irregular breathing, inspiratory gasps, and, finally, apnea. (It may be comforting for some family members to know this evolution of the breathing pattern.) In our experience, extubation of a comatose patient results in cardiac arrest, usually without respiratory discomfort or overt stridor.

The time to apnea and cardiac arrest depends on the degree of brainstem involvement, either from direct compression or from direct ischemic or hemorrhagic destruction. Predicting apnea is difficult (Chapter 63). Failure to trigger the ventilator is unreliable, and some patients will breathe after extubation. Thus, a brief disconnection may not provide reliable information about lack of respiratory drive. This information could be important, because some families expect absent breathing after disconnection and become understandably anxious if breathing continues.

Labored breathing remains the most distressing symptom after extubation. It can be managed by elevation of the head and torso, a humidifier, and an intravenous bolus of morphine sulfate, 1–2 mg every 10 minutes until effect. When intravenous access has been removed, opioids (fentanyl, 25 μg with 2 mL of normal saline via nebulizer; morphine sulfate, 5 mg in 2 mL of sterile water) provide relief and comfort.[20] Anticholinergic agents may be used to reduce secretions (e.g., transdermal scopolamine, one patch every 3 days). Vomiting may be reduced with intramuscular administration of promethazine, 25 mg every 4 hours, and intractable hiccups with 5 mg haloperidol intramuscularly. Recurrence of seizures can be treated with fosphenytoin (5 mg PE/kg/day) given intramuscularly.

Active Euthanasia

In active euthanasia, or physician-assisted suicide, a physician commits an act specifically directed to take a patient's life through lethal injection or provides an orally administered drug with specific directions for an overdose. Active euthanasia is rarely performed in the ICU, even in countries where it is legal.[62] A fine line exists between a lethal injection and a large dose of medication given to relieve suffering, with the latter considered appropriate palliative care.[58,59,61] Although legal in some European countries (e.g., Switzerland, Belgium, the Netherlands),[15] assisted suicide remains a controversy with strong opposition in many other countries.[57]

It seems better to avoid altogether the issue of physician-associated suicide in the NICU. Both the American College of Physicians and the American Academy of Neurology have issued position papers against this practice.[2,54]

The US Supreme Court ruled that there is no constitutional right to assisted suicide, but left open the possibility that individual states (e.g., Oregon) can legalize it.[3] The state of Oregon passed the Death with Dignity Act legalizing physician-assisted suicide.[56] In other states, it remains a criminal offense. Some continue to argue that legalizing physician-assisted suicide is an act of compassion, a personal and private decision that harms no one else and respects the patient's choice, particularly when suffering cannot be relieved.

In their monograph, Foley and Hendin[22] argue against euthanasia. In a series of convincing essays, a compelling thesis against this practice is developed. Arguments provided include an abominable lack of knowledge and education on palliative care (including the side effects of palliative drugs) and the danger of casualness. Philosophically, there is the potential for disintegration of trust in the patient–physician relationship when the physician can be allowed to inject lethal doses of medicine. The definition of "terrible suffering" is not a problem-free area, and effective palliation is possible in many, if not most, patients.[22] Other scholars argue that active euthanasia demeans the sacredness of human life. The main argument is that it is a direct violation of a moral prohibition against killing human beings.[18,45] In addition, it has been argued that requests of patients are not truly autonomous and are clouded by underlying, potentially treatable, depression.[7,8,12] Gradually decreasing attention to providing palliative care, which truly can relieve suffering in many patients, is another concern.

In the United States and most other countries, the neurologist must insistently deny euthanasia to any person when requested. One should try not to blur the line between active euthanasia (physician's intent to cause death) and aggressive pharmaceutical treatment to provide comfort (physician's intent to relieve perceived suffering).

LEGAL MATTERS

A general assumption, albeit with little substantive information, is that because ICUs are "high-risk places," they may invite malpractice suits.[23] At the extreme, fear of litigation may hamper entry into intensive care medicine or critical care neurology or may facilitate early departure. This section outlines some of the principles and tangible goals of risk-behavior avoidance.

Liability

Medical errors in the NICU may be technical (e.g., misplacement of catheter, tube, or device; continuation of drug despite adverse drug reaction), judgmental (e.g., misdiagnosis of subarachnoid hemorrhage, spinal cord compression, or brain tumor) or normative (e.g., deception, nondisclosure of risk, breach of confidentiality). Motives for filing malpractice claims in the ICU may involve perceptions of negligence, such as perceived treatment error or delay, missed or delayed diagnosis, equipment misuse, and pharmacologic mishaps. In an NICU, technical-surgical mishaps are prevalent. Clearly, some errors could be considered an associated risk of the surgical procedure. Negligence or error is ultimately a jury determination.

Poor outcome may be due to failure to uphold reasonable standards of practice (e.g., early antibiotics in meningitis, computed tomography [CT] scan in thunderclap headache), but a causal connection between the assumed error and the patient's handicap or death must be established. Injury may be difficult to prove because of the critical illness of the patient and the lack of certain customary standards.

One of the first potential problems is when to admit patients to or transfer them out of the NICU. Potential negligence may be claimed by the plaintiff if other intensivists testify that failure to admit to the NICU or early transfer out of the NICU was a deviation from practice. Examples are failure to admit patients with rapidly worsening Guillain-Barré syndrome or myasthenic crisis for monitoring of respiratory failure, patients with severe traumatic brain injury but minimal initial CT scan abnormalities, and patients with an acute mass in the posterior fossa. More complex sources of legal risk are the type of equipment in the NICU, failure to consult with related specialists, and the skill, experience, and training of other healthcare providers, such as nurses and respiratory care practitioners. Claims have also been filed on the use of physical restraint, disclosing evidence of battery (unconsented, harmful invasion of a patient's bodily integrity).[29]

Disclosure of Mistakes

Serious mistakes can occur in the NICU and may cause permanent morbidity or premature death. Disclosure of mistakes may be deferred because of fear of a negligence suit, punitive responses by colleagues, or a damaged career, failure to accept responsibility ("no proof whatsoever"), or shifting blame to others. Disclosure of overt mistakes to those involved does not appear to increase lawsuits,[69] but failure to do so will cause patients and family to feel betrayed. In fact, concealing mistakes or negligence may increase liability.[9] In addition, some claims are prompted by critical remarks by another physician. Generally self-serving interpretations by physicians are of concern, and uncertainties about a possible cause and effect should be expressed to the patient's family.[67] Often honesty is acknowledged. Explicit acknowledgment of thoughtlessness, its consequences, and therapeutic measures to reduce further harm could be discussed in a separate meeting with the family. Judiciousness and skill are required. If the system is at fault (laboratory errors, pharmacist feedback), more systematic research is needed.

Disclosure may not be warranted or appropriate if failure to respond to a certain problem did no harm (e.g., failure to reverse anticoagulation in a patient already with loss of virtually all brainstem reflexes). In other instances, "mistakes" may be known complications that have been explained to the patient as causing poor outcome, but these cannot truly be considered mistakes (e.g., intracerebral hematoma with thrombolytic agents).

Risk Prevention

There is no prescription for the prevention of a negligence suit. Important measures are knowledge of the scope of practice and adequate documentation. The medical record remains the central focus for determining whether the physician met the standard of care. Entries should be factual and accurate. If the physician is candid, is genuinely good and decent, has a sense of fairness, is open to outside concerns, is willing to listen, and can explain an adverse outcome ("fiduciary relationship"), a persistent desire for malpractice action is reduced. Anyone could argue that open display of pharisaical behavior, unavailability, or egotism and cunning could invite filing a suit.

Expert Witness

The field of neurologic intensive care involves a few, closely knit physicians. Opposition testimony, however, may be obtained from any physician involved in hospital care (so-called hospitalists) that is closely related to the practice.

Proctor[47] summarized the most important questions asked of expert witnesses: "Was it reasonable to have known at such and such a time that a particular substance or procedure was hazardous? And did the people responsible for causing the injury in question act responsibly, given the scientific and ethical standards of the time?"

The court specifically scrutinizes the opinion of the expert for facts, qualifications, and personal experience. Discrediting the qualifications and experience of the expert and pointing out areas of vulnerability are common techniques of cross-examining attorneys. The practices of neurointensivists who see acute neurologic disorders differ substantially. Some may have more expertise in trauma, others in acute stroke and neuromuscular disease. Expert witnesses may remain credible despite selection bias—whether they were chosen because of impressive performance or because of clinical brilliance.

Whether opinions are voiced in depositions or in the courtroom, testimony carries substantial weight and may influence the legal process (settlement or trial) and jury verdict.

CONCLUSION

- Do-not-resuscitate orders should be actively discussed.
- Withdrawal of support is a shared decision.
- Continuous communication may resolve conflicts.
- Adequate documentation, disclosure, and candor should be part of standard care.

REFERENCES

1. Medical futility in end-of-life care: report of the Council on Ethical and Judicial Affairs. *JAMA* 1999;281:937–941.
2. Palliative care in neurology. The American Academy of Neurology Ethics and Humanities Subcommittee. *Neurology* 1996;46:870–872.
3. Washington vs. Glucksberg. *117 S. Ct.* 22581997.
4. Withholding and withdrawing life-sustaining therapy. This Official Statement of the American Thoracic Society was adopted by the ATS Board of Directors, March 1991. *Am Rev Respir Dis* 1991;144:726–731.
5. Abbott KH, Sago JG, Breen CM, Abernethy AP, Tulsky JA. Families looking back: one year after discussion of withdrawal or withholding of life-sustaining support. *Crit Care Med* 2001;29:197–201.
6. Becker KJ, Baxter AB, Cohen WA, et al. Withdrawal of support in intracerebral hemorrhage may lead to self-fulfilling prophecies. *Neurology* 2001;56:766–772.
7. Block SD. Assessing and managing depression in the terminally ill patient. ACP-ASIM End-of-Life Care Consensus Panel. American College of Physicians—American Society of Internal Medicine. *Ann Intern Med* 2000;132:209–218.
8. Block SD. Perspectives on care at the close of life: psychological considerations, growth, and transcendence at the end of life: the art of the possible. *JAMA* 2001;285:2898–2905.
9. Brennan TA, Leape LL, Laird NM, et al. Incidence of adverse events and negligence in hospitalized patients: results of the Harvard Medical Practice Study I. *N Engl J Med* 1991;324:370–376.
10. Burns JP, Truog RD. Futility: a concept in evolution. *Chest* 2007;132:1987–1993.
11. Coggon J. Problems with claims that sanctity leads to 'pro-life' law, and reasons for doubting it to be a convincing 'middle way.' *Med Law* 2008;27:203–213.
12. Conwell Y, Caine ED. Rational suicide and the right to die: reality and myth. *N Engl J Med* 1991;325:1100–1103.
13. Curtis JR, Park DR, Krone MR, Pearlman RA. Use of the medical futility rationale in do-not-attempt-resuscitation orders. *JAMA* 1995;273:124–128.
14. Danis M, Patrick DL, Southerland LI, Green ML. Patients' and families' preferences for medical intensive care. *JAMA* 1988;260:797–802.
15. Deliens L, van der Wal G. The euthanasia law in Belgium and the Netherlands. *Lancet* 2003;362:1239–1240.
16. Diringer MN, Edwards DF, Aiyagari V, Hollingsworth H. Factors associated with

withdrawal of mechanical ventilation in a neurol-ogy/neurosurgery intensive care unit. *Crit Care Med* 2001;29:1792–1797.

17. Dunphy K. Futilitarianism: knowing how much is enough in end-of-life health care. *Palliat Med* 2000;14:313–322.

18. Emanuel EJ. Euthanasia and physician-assisted suicide: a review of the empirical data from the United States. *Arch Intern Med* 2002;162:142–152.

19. Epker JL, Bakker J, Kompanje EJ. The use of opioids and sedatives and time until death after withdrawing mechanical ventilation and vasoac-tive drugs in a dutch intensive care unit. *Anesth Analg* 2011;112:628–634.

20. Farncombe M, Chater S. Clinical application of nebulized opioids for treatment of dyspnoea in patients with malignant disease. *Support Care Cancer* 1994;2:184–187.

21. Ferrand E, Robert R, Ingrand P, Lemaire F. Withholding and withdrawal of life support in intensive-care units in France: a prospective survey. French LATAREA Group. *Lancet* 2001;357:9–14.

22. Foley KM, Hendin H. *The Case Against Assisted Suicide: For the Right to End-of-Life Care.* Baltimore, MD: Johns Hopkins University Press; 2004.

23. Furrow BR, Greaney TL, Johnson SH, Jost TS, Schwartz RL. *Health Law: Cases, Materials and Problems.* 3rd ed. St. Paul, MN: West Publishing; 1997.

24. Gazelle G. The slow code: should anyone rush to its defense? *N Engl J Med* 1998;338:467–469.

25. Gostin LO. Deciding life and death in the court-room: from Quinlan to Cruzan, Glucksberg, and Vacco—a brief history and analysis of con-stitutional protection of the 'right to die.' *Jama* 1997;278:1523–1528.

26. Hawryluck LA, Harvey WR, Lemieux-Charles L, Singer PA. Consensus guidelines on analgesia and sedation in dying intensive care unit patients. *BMC Med Ethics* 2002;3:E3.

27. Heffner JE, Barbieri C. Compliance with do-not-resuscitate orders for hospitalized patients trans-ported to radiology departments. *Ann Intern Med* 1998;129:801–805.

28. Helft PR, Siegler M, Lantos J. The rise and fall of the futility movement. *N Engl J Med* 2000; 343:293–296.

29. Kapp MB. Physical restraint use in critical care: legal issues. *AACN Clin Issues* 1996;7: 579–584.

30. Keenan SP, Busche KD, Chen LM, et al. A ret-rospective review of a large cohort of patients undergoing the process of withholding or with-drawal of life support. *Crit Care Med* 1997;25: 1324–1331.

31. Kritek PA, Slutsky AS, Hudson LD. Clinical decisions. Care of an unresponsive patient with a poor prognosis: polling results. *N Engl J Med* 2009;360:e15.

32. Lanken PN, Terry PB, Delisser HM, et al. An official American Thoracic Society clinical policy statement: palliative care for patients with respi-ratory diseases and critical illnesses. *Am J Respir Crit Care Med* 2008;177:912–927.

33. Larach DR, Larach DB, Larach MG. A life worth living: seven years after craniectomy. *Neurocrit Care* 2009;11:106–111.

34. Levy MM. End-of-life care in the intensive care unit: can we do better? *Crit Care Med* 2001;29: N56–N61.

35. Marco CA, Schears RM. Societal opinions regard-ing CPR. *Am J Emerg Med* 2002;20:207–211.

36. Mayer SA, Kossoff SB. Withdrawal of life support in the neurological intensive care unit. *Neurology* 1999;52:1602–1609.

37. Meisel A. *The Right to Die.* 2nd ed. New York: Wiley Law Publications; 1995.

38. Merriam-Webster. Merriam-Webster's Collegiate Dictionary. 11th ed. Springfield, MA: Merriam-Webster; 2003.

39. Misak CJ, White DB, Truog RD. Medical futil-ity: a new look at an old problem. *Chest* 2014; 146:1667–1672.

40. Morgan J. How do you decide when to withdraw life support? *Lancet Respir Med* 2015;3:430–431.

41. Muller JH. Shades of blue: the negotiation of limited codes by medical residents. *Soc Sci Med* 1992;34:885–898.

42. Murphy DJ, Burrows D, Santilli S, et al. The influ-ence of the probability of survival on patients' preferences regarding cardiopulmonary resusci-tation. *N Engl J Med* 1994;330:545–549.

43. Novack DH, Detering BJ, Arnold R, et al. Physicians' attitudes toward using deception to resolve difficult ethical problems. *JAMA* 1989; 261:2980–2985.

44. Nyman DJ, Sprung CL. End-of-life decision mak-ing in the intensive care unit. *Intens Care Med* 2000;26:1414–1420.

45. Pellegrino ED. Doctors must not kill. *J Clin Ethics* 1992;3:95–102.

46. Prendergast TJ, Luce JM. Increasing incidence of withholding and withdrawal of life support from the critically ill. *Am J Respir Crit Care Med* 1997;155:15–20.

47. Proctor RN. Expert witnesses take the stand. *Nature* 2000;407:15–16.

48. Rabinstein AA, McClelland RL, Wijdicks EFM, Manno EM, Atkinson JL. Cardiopulmonary resus-citation in critically ill neurologic-neurosurgical patients. *Mayo Clinic Proc* 2004;79:1391–1395.

49. Reilly BM, Magnussen CR, Ross J, et al. Can we talk? Inpatient discussions about advance directives in a community hospital: attending

physicians' attitudes, their inpatients' wishes, and reported experience. *Arch Intern Med* 1994;154:2299–2308.

50. Robinson EM. An ethical analysis of cardiopulmonary resuscitation for elders in acute care. *AACN Clin Issues* 2002;13:132–144.

51. Rubin SB. *When Doctors Say No: The Battleground of Medical Futility*. Bloomington: Indiana University Press; 1998.

52. Schneiderman LJ, Jecker NS, Jonsen AR. Medical futility: its meaning and ethical implications. *Ann Intern Med* 1990;112:949–954.

53. Slutsky AS, Hudson LD. Clinical decisions: care of an unresponsive patient with a poor prognosis. *N Engl J Med* 2009;360:527–531.

54. Snyder L, Sulmasy DP. Physician-assisted suicide. *Ann Intern Med* 2001;135:209–216.

55. Souter MJ, Blissitt PA, Blosser S, et al. Recommendations for the critical care management of devastating brain injury: prognostication, psychosocial, and ethical management: a position statement for healthcare professionals from the Neurocritical Care Society. *Neurocrit Care* 2015 Aug;23(1):4–13.

56. Steinbrook R. Physician-assisted suicide in Oregon: an uncertain future. *N Engl J Med* 2002; 346:460–464.

57. Stone K. When a patient chooses death: divided attitudes. *Lancet Neurol* 2009;8:882–883.

58. Truog RD. End-of-life decision-making in the United States. *Eur J Anaesthesiol Suppl* 2008; 42:43–50.

59. Truog RD. Not euthanasia, simply compassionate clinical care. *Crit Care Med* 2008;36:1387–1388; author reply 1389.

60. Truog RD, Brock DW, White DB. Should patients receive general anesthesia prior to

extubation at the end of life? *Crit Care Med* 2012;40:631–633.

61. Truog RD, Campbell ML, Curtis JR, et al. Recommendations for end-of-life care in the intensive care unit: a consensus statement by the American College [corrected] of Critical Care Medicine. *Crit Care Med* 2008;36:953–963.

62. van der Heide A, Onwuteaka-Philipsen BD, Rurup ML, et al. End-of-life practices in the Netherlands under the Euthanasia Act. *N Engl J Med* 2007;356:1957–1965.

63. Wijdicks EFM. Minimally conscious state vs. persistent vegetative state: the case of Terry (Wallis) vs. the case of Terri (Schiavo). *Mayo Clinic Proc* 2006;81:1155–1158.

64. Wijdicks EFM, Rabinstein AA. Absolutely no hope? Some ambiguity of futility of care in devastating acute stroke. *Crit Care Med* 2004;32:2332–2342.

65. Wijdicks EFM, Rabinstein AA. The family conference: end-of-life guidelines at work for comatose patients. *Neurology* 2007;68:1092–1094.

66. Wijdicks EFM. Law and bioethics. In *The Comatose Patient*. New York: Oxford University Press; 2014:278–298.

67. Witman AB, Park DM, Hardin SB. How do patients want physicians to handle mistakes? A survey of internal medicine patients in an academic setting. *Arch Intern Med* 1996;156:2565–2569.

68. Wood GG, Martin E. Withholding and withdrawing life-sustaining therapy in a Canadian intensive care unit. *Can J Anaesth* 1995;42:186–191.

69. Wu AW, Folkman S, McPhee SJ, Lo B. Do house officers learn from their mistakes? *JAMA* 1991;265:2089–2094.

PART XIII

Formulas and Scales

Formulas and Tables for Titrating Therapy

This appendix provides common formulas and nomograms for calculations needed in the daily care of critically ill neurologic patients. The focus is on patients with an acute neurologic disorder. Standard critical care textbooks and pharmaceutical textbooks in critical care can be consulted as well, and ideally should be available in every neurosciences intensive care unit (NICU). Calculations can also be found on the Internet (www.medcalc.com).

GAS EXCHANGE CALCULATION

FIO_2 Fraction of inspired oxygen: 0.21–1.0

PB Barometric pressure at sea level: 760 mm Hg

PH_2O Partial pressure of H_2O: 47 mm Hg (at 37°C)

$$RQ = \frac{VCO_2}{VO_2} = normal = 0.8$$

Calculation for alveolar-arterial (A – a) PO_2 gradient

1. $PAO_2 = FIO_2(PB - PH_2O) - \dfrac{PACO_2}{RQ}$

   $= FIO_2(713) - \dfrac{PAO_2}{0.8}$

2. Measure PO_2 from blood gas

   $PAO_2 - PO_2 = 10 - 20$ mm Hg

WATER DEFICIT

Total body water deficit $= 0.6 \times$ body weight $(kg) \times \left(\dfrac{serum\,Na}{140 - 1} \right)$ (assuming 140 mmol/L is desired serum sodium)

OSMOLAL GAP

Calculated plasma osmolarity $= 2 \times (Na) + \dfrac{(glucose)}{18} + \dfrac{(blood\,urea\,nitrogen\,[BUN])}{2.8}$

   $= mOsm/kg$

Measured plasma osmolarity $= 275–295$ mOsm/kg
Osmolar gap = measured Posm–Pcalc $= \leq 10$ mOsm/kg

ANION GAP

$$\text{Anion gap} = \text{unmeasured anions} - \text{unmeasured cations}$$
$$= Na^+ - (Cl^- + HCO_3^-)$$
$$= 12 \text{ mEq/L}$$

ADULT ENTERAL NUTRITION FORMULARY

Formula (Brand)	kcal/ mL	Protein (g/L)	Osmolality (mOsm/kg)	Volume to Meet US RDA	Indications for Use
Osmolite HN	1.06	44	300	1,320	Standard formula
Promote	1.0	62.5	340	1,000	Stressed patients with higher protein requirements and intact hepatic and renal function
Osmolite	1.06	37	300	1,887	Patients with lower protein requirements or protein restriction
Peptamen	1.0	40	270 (unflavored) 380 (flavored)	1,500	Patients with severe gastrointestinal disease or pancreatic insufficiency
Sustacal Plus	1.52	61	670	1,184	Hypercaloric oral supplement
Nutren 1.5	1.5	60	410 (unflavored)	1,000	Hypercaloric tube-feeding formula

RDA, recommended dietary allowance.
Note: Propofol provides 1.1 kcal/mL.

DOSAGE ADJUSTMENT OF ANTIMICROBIAL AGENTS IN RENAL FAILURE[*]

	Glomerular Filtration Rate (mL/min)		
	> 50	10–50	< 10
Aminoglycosides			
Gentamicin	8–12	12	24
Tobramycin	8–12	12	24
Antifungal agents			
Amphotericin B	24	24	24–36
Flucytosine	6	12–24	24–48
Antiviral agents			
Acyclovir	8	24	48
Amantadine	12–24	48–72	168
Cephalosporins			
Cefamandole	6	6–8	8
Cefazolin	6	12	24–48
Cefotaxime	6–8	8–12	12–24
Cefoxitin	8	8–12	24–48
Cephalothin	6	6	8–12
Antibiotics			
Clindamycin	None	None	None
Erythromycin	None	None	None
Metronidazole	8	8–12	12–24
Penicillins			
Amoxicillin	6	6–12	12–16
Ampicillin	6	6–12	12–16
Carbenicillin	8–12	12–24	24–48
Dicloxacillin	None	None	None
Nafcillin	None	None	None
Penicillin G	6–8	8–12	12–16
Piperacillin	4–6	6–8	8
Ticarcillin	8–12	12–24	24–28
Sulfas/trimethoprim			
Sulfamethoxazole	12	18	24
Trimethoprim	12	18	24
Tetracyclines			
Doxycycline	12	12–18	18–24
Minocycline	None	None	None
Vancomycin	12–24	72–240	240

[*] Interval extension in hours.

Modified from Bennett WM, Arnoff GR, Golper TA, et al. *Drug Prescribing in Renal Failure.*

Philadelphia: American College of Physicians; 1987. With permission of the publisher.

DRUGS THAT ALTER ANTIEPILEPTIC DRUG (AED) CONCENTRATIONS

Mechanism of Drug Interaction	Carbamazepine	Phenobarbital	Phenytoin	Valproic Acid
Changes in AED absorption			Antacids Enteral feedings	
Protein-binding displacement			Salicylates Sulfas Valproic acid	Salicylates
Enzyme inhibition of AED	Cimetidine Danazol Diltiazem Erythromycin Fluoxetine Isoniazid Propoxyphene Valproic acid Verapamil	Chloramphenicol Cimetidine Isoniazid Valproic acid	Amiodarone Chloramphenicol Cimetidine Ciprofloxacin Disulfiram Isoniazid Omeprazole Phenylbutazone Propoxyphene	
Enzyme induction of AED	Phenobarbital Phenytoin Primidone	Carbamazepine Ethanol Phenytoin	Carbamazepine Ethanol Phenobarbital	Carbamazepine Phenobarbital Primidone Phenytoin
Enzyme induction of AED on other drugs	Clonazepam Doxycycline Ethosuximide Theophylline Valproic acid Warfarin	Carbamazepine Chlorpromazine Corticosteroids Doxycycline Oral contraceptives Phenytoin Quinidine Tricyclic antidepressants Warfarin	Carbamazepine Corticosteroids Doxycycline Folic acid Oral contraceptives Primidone Pyridoxine Quinidine Vitamin D Warfarin	
Enzyme inhibition				Ethosuximide Phenobarbital Phenytoin Primidone

MODIFIED NATIONAL INSTITUTES OF HEALTH STROKE SCALE*

Item Number	Item Name	Score
1A	Level of consciousness	0 = alert; responsive 1 = not alert; verbally arousable 2 = not alert; only responsive to repeated stimuli 3 = totally unresponsive
1B	Level of consciousness questions	0 = answers both correctly 1 = answers one correctly 2 = answers neither correctly
1C	Level of consciousness commands	0 = performs both tasks correctly 1 = performs one task correctly 2 = performs neither task
2	Gaze	0 = normal 1 = partial gaze palsy 2 = forced gaze deviation
3	Visual fields	0 = no visual loss 1 = partial hemianopsia 2 = complete hemianopsia
5a	Left arm	0 = no drift 1 = drift before 10 seconds 2 = falls before 10 seconds 3 = no effort against gravity 4 = no movement
5b	Right arm	0 = no drift 1 = drift before 10 seconds 2 = falls before 10 seconds 3 = no effort against gravity 4 = no movement
6a	Left leg	0 = no drift 1 = drift before 5 seconds 2 = falls before 5 seconds 3 = no effort against gravity 4 = no movement
6b	Right leg	0 = no drift 1 = drift before 5 seconds 2 = falls before 5 seconds 3 = no effort against gravity 4 = no movement
8	Sensory	0 = normal 1 = abnormal
9	Language	0 = normal 1 = mild aphasia 2 = severe aphasia 3 = mute or global aphasia
11	Neglect	0 = normal 1 = mild 2 = severe

*The item numbers correspond to the numbering in the original scale to allow easy identification of the changes. From Lyden PD, Lu M, Levine SR, et al. A modified National Institutes of Health Stroke Scale for use in stroke clinical trials: preliminary reliability and validity. *Stroke* 2001;32:1310–1317. With permission of the American Heart Association.

TABLE 8.2 DETERMINING
THE INTRACRANIAL HEMORRHAGE
(ICH) SCORE

Component	ICH Score Points
Glasgow Coma Scale (GCS)	
3–4	2
5–12	1
13–15	0
ICH volume (mL)	
> 30	1
< 30	0
Intraventricular hemorrhage (IVH)	
Yes	1
No	0
Infratentorial origin of ICH	
Yes	1
No	0
Age (years)	
> 80	1
< 80	0
Total ICH score	0-6

ICH, intracerebral hemorrhage; GCS = GCS score on initial presentation (or after resuscitation).
ICH volume on initial CT calculated using ABC12 method.
IVH indicates presence of any intraventricular hemorrhage on initial computed tomography.
From Hemphill JC, 3rd, Bonovich DC, Besmertis L, Manley GT, Johnston SC. The ICH score: a simple, reliable grading scale for intracerebral hemorrhage. *Stroke* 2001;32:891–897.

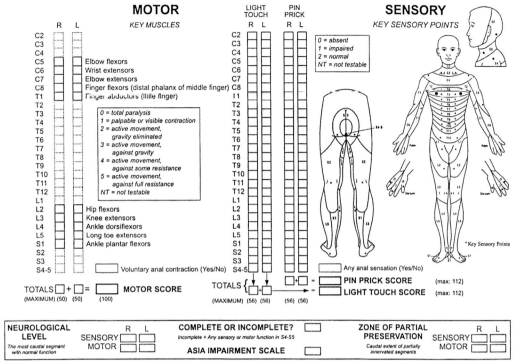

STANDARD NEUROLOGICAL CLASSIFICATION OF SPINAL CORD INJURY

MOTOR
KEY MUSCLES

	R	L	
C2			
C3			
C4			
C5			Elbow flexors
C6			Wrist extensors
C7			Elbow extensors
C8			Finger flexors (distal phalanx of middle finger)
T1			Finger abductors (little finger)
T2			
T3			
T4			
T5			
T6			
T7			
T8			
T9			
T10			
T11			
T12			
L1			
L2			Hip flexors
L3			Knee extensors
L4			Ankle dorsiflexors
L5			Long toe extensors
S1			Ankle plantar flexors
S2			
S3			
S4-5			

0 = total paralysis
1 = palpable or visible contraction
2 = active movement, gravity eliminated
3 = active movement, against gravity
4 = active movement, against some resistance
5 = active movement, against full resistance
NT = not testable

☐ Voluntary anal contraction (Yes/No)

TOTALS ☐ + ☐ = ☐ **MOTOR SCORE**
(MAXIMUM) (50) (50) (100)

LIGHT TOUCH / PIN PRICK

	LIGHT TOUCH R L	PIN PRICK R L
C2		
C3		
C4		
C5		
C6		
C7		
C8		
T1		
T2		
T3		
T4		
T5		
T6		
T7		
T8		
T9		
T10		
T11		
T12		
L1		
L2		
L3		
L4		
L5		
S1		
S2		
S3		
S4-5		

0 = absent
1 = impaired
2 = normal
NT = not testable

☐ Any anal sensation (Yes/No)

TOTALS { ☐ + ☐ = ☐ **PIN PRICK SCORE** (max: 112)
☐ + ☐ = ☐ **LIGHT TOUCH SCORE** (max: 112)
(MAXIMUM) (56) (56) (56) (56)

SENSORY
KEY SENSORY POINTS

* Key Sensory Points

NEUROLOGICAL LEVEL		R	L	COMPLETE OR INCOMPLETE? ☐	ZONE OF PARTIAL PRESERVATION		R	L
The most caudal segment with normal function	SENSORY			*Incomplete = Any sensory or motor function in S4-S5*	Caudal extent of partially innervated segments	SENSORY		
	MOTOR			**ASIA IMPAIRMENT SCALE** ☐		MOTOR		

This form may be copied freely but should not be altered without permission from the American Spinal Injury Association.

2000 Rev.

PART XIV

Guidelines

Guidelines, Consensus Statements, and Evidence-Based Reviews Related to Critical Care Neurology

This section collects the most valuable manuscripts. All pertain to the practice of emergency and critical care neurology. Interpretation of a guideline as an undisputed directive is not justified. Professional organizations provide guidelines as an educational service to practicing physicians and adherence to guidelines remains voluntary. Guidelines and consensus statements do not constitute standard of care. Moreover, there is limited success of clinical practice guidelines in changing decision making— or even changing attitude. These documents however keep us informed and articulate peer opinion.

GENERAL INTENSIVE CARE

2015 American Heart Association Guidelines Update for Cardiopulmonary Resuscitation and Emergency Cardiovascular Care. Part 1: Executive Summary: 2015 American Heart Association Guidelines Update for Cardiopulmonary Resuscitation and Emergency Cardiovascular Care.

Neumar RW, Shuster M, Callaway CW, et al. *Circulation* 2015;132(18 Suppl 2):S315–367.

2014 AHA/ACC guideline for the management of patients with non-ST-elevation acute coronary syndromes: a report of the American College of Cardiology/American Heart Association Task Force on Practice Guidelines.

Amsterdam EA, Wenger NK, Brindis RG, Casey DE Jr, Ganiats, TG, Holmes DR Jr, Jaffe AS, Jneid H, Kelly RF, Kontos MC, Levine GN, Liebson PR, Mukherjee D, Peterson ED, Sabatine MS, Smalling RW, Zieman SJ; ACC/AHA Task Force Members. *Circulation* 2014;130:e344–e426.

Nutrition support in clinical practice: review of published data and recommendations for future research directions. Summary of a conference sponsored by the National Institutes of Health, American Society for Parenteral and Enteral Nutrition, and American Society for Clinical Nutrition.

Klein S, Kinney J, Jeejeebhoy K, et al. *Am J Clin Nutr* 1997;66:683–706.

A.S.P.E.N. Clinical guidelines: nutrition support of hospitalized adult patients with obesity.

Choban P, Dickerson R, Malone A, Worthington P, Compher C; American Society for Parenteral and Enteral Nutrition. *JPEN J Parenter Enteral Nutr* 2013;37:714–744.

ACC/AHA 2007 guidelines on perioperative cardiovascular evaluation and care for noncardiac surgery: executive summary. A report of the American College of Cardiology/American Heart Association Task Force on practice guidelines (writing committee to revise the 2002 guidelines on perioperative cardiovascular evaluation for noncardiac surgery).

Fleisher LA, Beckman JA, Brown KA, Calkins H, Chaikof EL, Fleischmann KE, Freeman WK, et al. *Circulation* 2007;115:1971–1996.

Clinical practice guidelines for the management of pain, agitation, and delirium in adult patients in the intensive care unit.

Barr J, Fraser GL, Puntillo K, Ely EW, Gelinas C, Dasta JF, Davidson JE, Devlin JW, Kress JP, Joffe AM, Coursin DB, Herr DL, Tung A, Robinson BR, Fontaine DK, Ramsay MA, Riker RR, Sessler CN, Pun B, Skrobik Y, Jaeschke R. *Crit Care Med* 2013;41:263–306.

Hyponatremia in neurosurgical patients: clinical guidelines development.

Rahman M, Friedman WA. *Neurosurgery* 2009;65:925–935.

Guideline for Reversal of Antithrombotics in Intracranial Hemorrhage. A Statement for Healthcare Professionals from the Neurocritical Care Society and Society of Critical Care Medicine

Frontera JA, Lewin III JJ, Rabinstein AA, et al. *Neurocrit Care* 2016;24:6–46.

Antithrombotic and thrombolytic therapy.

Geerts WH, Bergqvist D, Pineo GF, Heit JA, Samama CM, Lassen MR, Colwell CW; American College of Chest Physicians. American College of Chest Physicians evidence-based clinical practice guidelines; 8th edition. *Chest* 2008;133:67S–968S.

Guidelines for evaluation of new fever in critically ill adult patients: 2008 update from the American College of Critical Care Medicine and the Infectious Diseases Society of America.

O'Grady NP, Barie PS, Bartlett JG, Bleck T, Carroll K, Kalil AC, Linden P, Maki DG, Nierman D, Pasculle W, Masur H; American College of Critical Care Medicine, Infectious Diseases Society of America. *Crit Care Med* 2008;36:1330–1349.

Recommendations for the diagnosis and management of corticosteroid insufficiency in critically ill adult patients: consensus statements from an international task force by the American College of Critical Care Medicine.

Marik PE, Pastores SM, Annane D, Meduri GU, Sprung CL, Arlt W, Keh D, Briegel J, Beishuizen A, Dimopoulou I, Tsagarakis S, Singer M, Chrousos GP, Zaloga G, Bokhari F, Vogeser M; American College of Critical Care Medicine. *Crit Care Med* 2008;36:1937–1949.

Developing a New Definition and Assessing New Clinical Criteria for Septic Shock For the Third International Consensus Definitions for Sepsis and Septic Shock (Sepsis-3).

Shankar-Hari MD, Phillips GS, Levy ML, et al. for the Sepsis Definition Task Force. *JAMA* 2016;315:775–787.

Infectious Diseases Society of America/ American Thoracic Society consensus guidelines on the management of community-acquired pneumonia in adults.

Mandell LA, Wunderink RG, Anzueto A, Bartlett JG, Campbell GD, Dean NC, Dowell SF, File TM Jr., Musher DM, Niederman MS, Torres A, Whitney CG. *Clin Infect Dis* 2007;44:S27–S72.

Guidelines for the management of adults with hospital-acquired, ventilator-associated, and healthcare-associated pneumonia. Official statement of the American Thoracic Society and the Infectious Diseases Society of America.

Am J Respir Crit Care Med 2005;171:388–416.

Guidelines for the inter- and intrahospital transport of critically ill patients.

Warren J, Fromm RE Jr., Orr RA, Rotello LC, Horst HM. *Crit Care Med* 2004;32:256–262.

American Thoracic Society, the European Respiratory Society, the European Society of Intensive Care Medicine, and the Society de Reanimation de Langue Française: International Consensus Conferences in Intensive Care Medicine: noninvasive positive pressure ventilation in acute respiratory failure.

Am J Respir Crit Care Med 2001;163:283–291.

Evidence-based guidelines for weaning and discontinuing ventilatory support.

MacIntyre NR. *Chest* 2001;120:375S–396S.

American Association for Respiratory Care: consensus statement on the essentials of mechanical ventilators—1992.

Respir Care 1992;37:1000–1008.

Prophylaxis of Venous Thrombosis in Neurocritical Care Patients: An Evidence-Based Guideline: A Statement for Healthcare

Professionals from the NeurocriticalCare Society

Nyquist P, Bautista C, Jichici D, et al. Prophylaxis of Venous Thrombosis in Neurocritical Care Patients: An Evidence-Based Guideline. A Statement for Healthcare Professionals from the Neurocritical Care Society. *Neurocrit Care* 2016;24:46–60.

The Insertion and Management of External Ventricular Drains: An Evidence- Based Consensus Statement. A Statement for Healthcare Professionals from the Neurocritical Care Society.

Fried HI, Nathan B, Rowe SA, et al. The Insertion and Management of External Ventricular Drains: An Evidence-Based Consensus Statement. A Statement for Healthcare Professionals from the Neurocritical Care Society. *Neurocrit Care* 2016;24:61–82.

STROKE

Evidence-based guidelines for the management of large hemispheric infarction: a statement for health care professionals from the Neurocritical Care Society and the German Society for Neuro-intensive Care and Emergency Medicine.

Torbey MT, Bösel J, Rhoney DH, Rincon F, Staykov D, Amar AP, Varelas PN, Jüttler E, Olson D, Huttner HB, Zweckberger K, Sheth KN, Dohmen C, Brambrink AM, Mayer SA, Zaidat OO, Hacke W, Schwab S. *Neurocrit Care* 2015;22:146–164.

Recommendations for the management of cerebral and cerebellar infarction with swelling: a statement for healthcare professionals from the American Heart Association/American Stroke Association.

Wijdicks EFM, Sheth KN, Carter BS, Greer DM, Kasner SE, Kimberly WT, Schwab S, Smith EE, Tamargo RJ, Wintermark M; American Heart Association Stroke Council. *Stroke* 2014;45:1222–1238.

2015 American Heart Association/American Stroke Association Focused Update of the 2013 Guidelines for the Early Management of Patients With Acute Ischemic Stroke Regarding Endovascular Treatment A Guideline for

Healthcare Professionals From the American Heart Association/American Stroke Association

Powers WJ, Derdeyn CP, MD, Biller J, et al. on behalf of the American Heart Association Stroke Council. *Stroke* 2015;46:3024–3039.

Scientific Rationale for the Inclusion and Exclusion Criteria for Intravenous Alteplase in Acute Ischemic Stroke A Statement for Healthcare Professionals From the American Heart Association/American Stroke Association

Demaerschalk BM, Kleindorfer DO, Adeoye OM, et al. *Stroke* 2016 published online.

Society for Neuroscience in Anesthesiology and Critical Care Expert consensus statement: anesthetic management of endovascular treatment for acute ischemic stroke: endorsed by the Society of NeuroInterventional Surgery and the Neurocritical Care Society.

Talke PO, Sharma D, Heyer EJ, Bergese SD, Blackham KA, Stevens RD. *J Neurosurg Anesthesiol* 2014;26:95–108.

Endovascular therapy of acute ischemic stroke: report of the Standards of Practice Committee of the Society of NeuroInterventional Surgery.

Blackham KA, Meyers PM, Abruzzo TA, Albuquerque FC, Fiorella D, Fraser J, Frei D, Gandhi CD, Heck DV, Hirsch JA, Hsu DP, Hussain MS, Jayaraman M, Narayanan S, Prestigiacomo C, Sunshine JL; Society for NeuroInterventional Surgery. *J Neurointerv Surg* 2012;4:87–93.

2011 ASA/ACCF/AHA/AANN/AANS/ACR/ ASNR/CNS/SAIP/SCAI/SIR/SNIS/ SVM/ SVS guideline on the management of patients with extracranial carotid and vertebral artery disease: executive summary.

American College of Cardiology Foundation/ American Heart Association Task Force; American Stroke Association; American Association of Neuroscience Nurses; American Association of Neurological Surgeons; American College of Radiology; American Society of Neuroradiology; Congress of Neurological Surgeons; Society of Atherosclerosis Imaging and Prevention; Society for Cardiovascular Angiography and Interventions; Society of Interventional Radiology; Society of NeuroInterventional Surgery; Society for Vascular Medicine; Society for Vascular Surgery; American Academy of Neurology; Society of Cardiovascular Computed Tomography, Brott TG, Halperin JL, Abbara S, Bacharach JM, Barr JD, Bush RL, Cates CU, Creager MA, Fowler SB, Friday G, Hertzberg VS, McIff EB, Moore WS, Panagos PD, Riles TS, Rosenwasser RH, Taylor AJ. *J Neurointerv Surg* 2011;3:100–130.

Guidelines for the management of aneurysmal subarachnoid hemorrhage: a statement for healthcare professionals from a special writing group of the Stroke Council, American Heart Association.

Bederson JB, Connolly ES, Batjer HH, Dacey RG, Dion JE, Diringer MN, Dildner JE, et al. *Stroke* 2009;40:994–1025.

Guidelines for the early management of patients with ischemic stroke: a guideline for healthcare professionals from the American Heart Association/American Stroke Association Stroke Council.

Jauch EC, Saver JL, Adams HP, et al. *Stroke* 2013;44:870–947.

Guidelines for the management of spontaneous intracerebral hemorrhage: a guideline for healthcare professionals from the American Heart Association/American Stroke Association.

Morgenstern LB, Hemphill JC 3rd, Anderson C, Becker K, Broderick JP, Connolly ES Jr, Greenberg SM, Huang JN, MacDonald RL, Messé SR, Mitchell PH, Selim M, Tamargo RJ; American Heart Association Stroke Council and Council on Cardiovascular Nursing. *Stroke*. 2010;41:2108–2129.

Practice parameter: prediction of outcome in comatose survivors after cardiopulmonary resuscitation (an evidence-based review): report of the Quality Standards Subcommittee of the American Academy of Neurology.

Wijdicks EFM, Hijdra A, Young GB, Bassetti CL, Wiebe S; Quality Standards Subcommittee

of the American Academy of Neurology. *Neurology* 2006;67:203–210.

Evidence-based guideline: Reducing brain injury following cardiopulmonary resuscitation

Geocadin RG, Wijdicks EFM, Armstrong MJ, et al. Neurology 2016 in press

TRAUMATIC HEAD INJURY

Guidelines for the management of severe traumatic brain injury: antiseizure prophylaxis.

Brain Trauma Foundation; American Association of Neurological Surgeons; Congress of Neurological Surgeons. *J Neurotrauma* 2007;24(Suppl 1):S83–S86.

Guidelines for the management of severe traumatic brain injury: deep vein thrombosis prophylaxis.

Brain Trauma Foundation; American Association of Neurological Surgeons; Congress of Neurological Surgeons. *J Neurotrauma* 2007;24:S32–S36.

Guidelines for the management of severe traumatic brain injury: infection prophylaxis.

Brain Trauma Foundation; American Association of Neurological Surgeons; Congress of Neurological Surgeons. *J Neurotrauma* 2007;24(Suppl 1):S26–S31.

Guidelines for the management of severe traumatic brain injury: nutrition.

Brain Trauma Foundation; American Association of Neurological Surgeons; Congress of Neurological Surgeons. *J Neurotrauma* 2007;24(Suppl 1):S77–S82.

Guidelines for the management of severe traumatic brain injury: oxygenation and blood pressure.

Badjatia N, Carney N, Crocco TJ, Fallat ME, Hennes HM, Jagoda AS, Jernigan S, Lerner EB, Letarte PB, Moriarty T, Pons PT, Sasser S, Scalea TM, Schleien C, Wright DW. *Brain Trauma Foundation* 2007;16–25.

Guidelines for the prehospital management of severe traumatic brain injury: airway, ventilation, and oxygenation. 2nd edition. Treatment: airway, ventilation, and oxygenation.

Badjatia N, Carney N, Crocco TJ, Fallat ME, Hennes HM, Jagoda AS, Jernigan S, Lerner EB, Letarte PB, Moriarty T, Pons PT, Sasser S, Scalea TM, Schleien C, Wright DW. *Brain Trauma Foundation* 2007;42–60.

Surgical management of acute epidural hematomas.

Bullock MR, Chesnut R, Ghajar J, Gordon D, Hartl R, Newell DW, Servadei F, Walters BC, Wilberger JE; Surgical Management of Traumatic Brain Injury Author Group. *Neurosurgery* 2006;58(3 Suppl):S2–7, S2–15.

Surgical management of acute subdural hematomas.

Bullock MR, Chesnut R, Ghajar J, Gordon D, Hartl R, Newell DW, Servadei F, Walters BC, Wilberger JE; Surgical Management of Traumatic Brain Injury Author Group. *Neurosurgery* 2006;S2–16, S2–24.

Surgical management of traumatic parenchymal lesions.

Bullock MR, Chesnut R, Ghajar J, Gordon D, Hartl R, Newell DW, Servadei F, Walters BC, Wilberger J; Surgical Management of Traumatic Brain Injury Author Group. *Neurosurgery* 2006;58(3 Suppl):S2–25, S2–46.

SEIZURES

Recommendations on the use of EEG monitoring in critically ill patients: consensus statement from the neurointensive care section of the ESICM.

Claassen J, Taccone FS, Horn P, Holtkamp M, Stocchetti N, Oddo M; Neurointensive Care Section of the European Society of Intensive Care Medicine. *Intensive Care Med* 2013;39:1337–1351.

Guidelines for the evaluation and management of status epilepticus.

Glauser T, Shinnar S, Gloss D, et al. Evidence-Based Guideline: Treatment of Convulsive

Status Epilepticus in Children and Adults: Report of the Guideline Committee of the American Epilepsy Society. *Epilepsy Currents* 2016;16:48–61.

Brophy GM, Bell R, Claassen J, et al; Neurocritical Care Society Status Epilepticus Guideline Writing Committee. *Neurocrit Care* 2012;17:3–23.

Practice parameter: evaluating an apparent unprovoked first seizure in adults (an evidence-based review). Report of the Quality Standards Subcommittee of the American Academy of Neurology and the American Epilepsy Society.

Krumholz A, Wiebe S, Gronseth G, Shinnar S, Levisohn P, Ting T, Hopp J, Shafer P, Morris H, Seiden L, Barkley G, French J; Quality Standards Subcommittee of the American Academy of Neurology, American Epilepsy Society. *Neurology* 2007;69:1996–2007.

Reassessment: neuroimaging in the emergency patient presenting with seizure (an evidence-based review). Report of the Therapeutics and Technology Assessment Subcommittee of the American Academy of Neurology.

Harden CL, Huff JS, Schwartz TH, Dubinsky RM, Zimmerman RD, Weinstein S, Foltin JC, Theodore WH; Therapeutics and Technology Assessment Subcommittee of the American Academy of Neurology. *Neurology* 2007;30;69:1772–1780.

Efficacy and tolerability of the new antiepileptic drugs I: treatment of new onset epilepsy. Report of the Therapeutics and Technology Assessment Subcommittee and Quality Standards Subcommittee of the American Academy of Neurology and the American Epilepsy Society.

French JA, Kanner AM, Bautista J, Abou-Khalil B, Browne T, Harden CL, Theodore WH, Bazil C, Stern J, Schachter SC, Bergen D, Hirtz D, Montouris GD, Nespeca M, Gidal B, Marks WJ, Turk WR, Fischer JH, Bourgeois B, Wilner A, Faught RE Jr, Sachdeo RC, Beydoun A, Glauser TA. *Neurology* 2004;62:1252–1260.

Efficacy and tolerability of the new antiepileptic drugs II: treatment of refractory epilepsy. Report of the Therapeutics and Technology Assessment Subcommittee and Quality Standards

Subcommittee of the American Academy of Neurology and the American Epilepsy Society.

French JA, Kanner AM, Bautista J, Abou-Khalil B, Browne T, Harden CL, Theodore WH, Bazil C, Stern J, Schachter SC, Bergen D, Hirtz D, Montouris GD, Nespeca M, Gidal B, Marks WJ, Turk WR, Fischer JH, Bourgeois B, Wilner A, Faught RE Jr, Sachdeo RC, Beydoun A, Glauser TA. *Neurology* 2004;62:1261–1273.

Practice parameter: antiepileptic drug prophylaxis in severe traumatic brain injury. Report of the Quality Standards Subcommittee of the American Academy of Neurology.

Chang BS, Lowenstein DH. *Neurology* 2003;60:10–16.

NEUROIMMUNOLOGY

Practice parameter: immunotherapy for Guillain-Barré syndrome. Report of the Quality Standards Subcommittee of the American Academy of Neurology.

Hughes RA, Wijdicks EFM, Barohn R, Benson E, Cornblath Dr, Hahn AF, Meythaler JM, Miller RG, Sladky JT, et al. *Neurology* 2003;61:736–740.

CNS INFECTIONS

The management of encephalitis: clinical practice guidelines by the Infectious Diseases Society of America.

Tunkel AR, Glaser CA, Bloch KC, Sejvar JJ, Marra CM, Roos KL, Hartman BJ, Kaplan SL, Scheld WM, Whitley RJ. *Clin Infect Dis* 2008;47:303–327.

Practice guidelines for the management of bacterial and fungal meningitis.

Tunkel AR, Hartman BJ, Kaplan SL, Kaufman BA, Roos KL, Scheld WM, Whitley RJ. *Clin Infect Dis* 2004;39:1267–1284.

Perfect JR, Dismukes WE, Dromer F, et al. Clinical Practice Guidelines for the Management of Cryptococcal Disease: 2010 Update by the Infectious Diseases Society of America. *Clinical Infectious Diseases* 2010;50:291–322.

END-OF-LIFE CARE

International guideline development for the determination of death.

Shemie SD, Hornby L, Baker A, Teitelbaum J, Torrance S, Young K, Capron AM, Bernat JL, Noel L; The International Guidelines for Determination of Death phase 1 participants, in collaboration with the World Health Organization. *Intens Care Med* 2014;40:788–797.

Evidence-based guideline update: determining brain death in adults. Report of the Quality Standards Subcommittee of the American Academy of Neurology.

Wijdicks EFM, Varelas PN, Gronseth GS, Greer DM; American Academy of Neurology. *Neurology* 2010;74:1911–1918.

End-of-Life Care Task Force. An official American Thoracic Society clinical policy statement: palliative care for patients with respiratory diseases and critical illnesses.

Lanken PN, Terry PB, Delisser HM, et al. *Am J Respir Crit Care Med* 2008;178: 912–927.

Recommendations for end-of-life care in the intensive care unit: a consensus statement by the American College of Critical Care Medicine.

Truog RD, Campbell ML, Curtis JR, et al. *Crit Care Med* 2008;36:953–963.

Position statement on laws and regulations concerning life-sustaining treatment, including artificial nutrition and hydration, for patients lacking decision-making capacity.

Bacon D, Williams MA, Gordon J. *Neurology* 2007;68:1097–1100.

Clinical practice guidelines for support of the family in the patient-centered intensive care unit: American College of Critical Care Medicine Task Force 2004–2005.

Davidson JE, Powers K, Hedayat KM, Tieszen M, Kon AA, Shepard E, Spuhler V, Todres ID, Levy M, Barr J, Ghandi R, Hirsch G, Armstrong D; American College of Critical Care Medicine Task Force 2004–2005. *Crit Care Med* 2007;35:605–622.

INDEX

References to tables, figures and capsules are denoted by an italicized *t, f,* and *c.*